Principles of Neurosurgery: A Concise Text

Principles of Neurosurgery: A Concise Text

Editors

Forhad H. Chowdhury
Mainul Haque Sarker
Mohammod Raziul Haque
Khandkar Ali Kawsar
Jalal Uddin Mohammod Rumi

MDPI

Basel • Beijing • Wuhan • Barcelona • Belgrade • Novi Sad • Cluj • Manchester

Editors
Forhad H. Chowdhury
National Institute of Neurosciences and Hospital
Dhaka, Bangladesh

Khandkar Ali Kawsar
Royal Infirmary of Edinburgh
Edinburgh, UK

Mainul Haque Sarker
Dhaka Medical College and Hospital
Dhaka, Bangladesh

Jalal Uddin Mohammod Rumi
National Institute of Neurosciences and Hospital
Dhaka, Bangladesh

Mohammod Raziul Haque
Dhaka Medical College and Hospital
Dhaka, Bangladesh

Editorial Office
MDPI AG
Grosspeteranlage 5
4052 Basel, Switzerland

For citation purposes, cite as indicated below:

Lastname, A.A.; Lastname, B.B.; Lastname, C.C. *Book Title.* Series Title (optional). Year, Page Range.

ISBN 978-3-0365-6923-9 (Hbk)
ISBN 978-3-0365-6922-2 (PDF)
doi.org/10.3390/books978-3-0365-6922-2

Dedication

Dedicated to the readers of the book.

Contents

About the Editiors

Dr. Forhad H. Chowdhury, after having MBBS from Sir Salimullah Medical College, Dhaka in 1998 he accomplished FCPS in surgery in 2005 and MS in Neurosurgery in 2008. He did Fellowship training in micro-neurosurgery in KEM Hospital, Mumbai, India under Professor Atul Goel. Now, he is working as Associate Professor of Neurosurgery in National Institute of Neurosciences and Hospital, Dhaka, Bangladesh. He presented in many international neurosurgical conferences. He has nearly hundred publications in highly impacted international and local journals. He has an extensive work experiences in cadaveric neurosurgical microscopic and endoscopic anatomy including white fiber dissection. He is regarded as pioneer EC-IC bypass surgeon in Bangladesh.

Prof. Mainul Haque Sarker graduated (MBBS) from Dhaka Medical College under University of Dhaka in 1982 and completed Board of Specialist Qualification Examination in Neurosurgery from Postgraduate Medical University, Budapest, Hungary in December 1992. Professor Sarker joinned as Assistant Professor of Neurosurgery in 1992 in Bangladesh and accomplished MS in Neurosurgery under Dhaka University, Bangladesh in 1999. He served as assistant professor, associate professor and professor in different government institute including Dhaka Medical College. Now, he is working as a senior consultant of Neurosurgery in Ibn Sina Specialized Hospital, Dhaka, Bangladesh He has got a number of publications both in national and international journals.

Prof. Mohammod Raziul Haque, after having MBBS from Dhaka Medical College, Dhaka; he accomplished FCPS in surgery in and MS in Neurosurgery. He has extensive training in micro-neurosurgery including Fellowship training in micro-neurosurgery in Sweden. He served as assistant professor, associate professor and professor in different government institute including Dhaka Medical College. Now, he is working as consultant of Neurosurgery in Bangladesh Specialized Hospital, Dhaka, Bangladesh. He presented in many international neurosurgical conferences. He has nearly seventy publications in highly impacted international and local journals.He has an extensive work experiences in cadaveric neurosurgical microscopic and endoscopic anatomy. He is regarded as pioneer endo-skull base surgeon in Bangladesh.

Dr. Khandkar Ali Kawsar is a Consultant in Neurosurgery and Major Trauma at the Royal Infirmary of Edinburgh. He graduated from Dhaka Medical College in Bangladesh, where he also earned his FCPS in Surgery and a Master's in Neurosurgery. Additionally, he obtained his MRCS from the Royal College of Surgeons of England, followed by his FRCS in Neurosurgery.Dr. Kawsar received his neurosurgical training across Dhaka, Dundee, Birmingham, London, and Leeds, and completed fellowships in endoscopic and lateral skull base surgery as well as complex spine surgery in the UK. He has presented at numerous national and international conferences, receiving several awards for his work. His research has been published in prestigious, high-impact neurosurgery journals, and *Nature Scientific Reports*. He has contributed chapters to online medical books and FRCS preparatory courses. In addition to his scholarly contributions, Dr. Kawsar creates original medical illustrations for his written work. He also serves as a tutor for the FRCS (Neurosurgery) course and is in the process of becoming an examiner for the Royal College of Surgeons of England. Currently, he is leading couple of projects aimed at introducing new services at the Royal Infirmary of Edinburgh.

Dr. Jalal Uddin Mohammod Rumi graduated from Sir Salimullah Medical College on 1998, subsequently completed his post Graduation in general surgery and neurosurgery in 2010 and 2015 respectively. He is a pioneering figure in the field of functional neurosurgery in Bangladesh. Renowned for his expertise and innovative approaches, As a leader in his field, he has been instrumental in developing neurosurgical practices in Bangladesh, bringing cutting-edge treatments to patients suffering from debilitating conditions like epilepsy and Parkinson's disease. Dr. Rumi's dedication to improving patient care and advancing medical knowledge has made him a key figure in the country's healthcare landscape. Now, he is working as Associate Professor of Neurosurgery in National Institute of Neurosciences and Hospital, Dhaka, Bangladesh.

Contributors

Abul Khair, FCPS
Retired, Prof., Department of Neurosurgery, Bhongobhondhu Sheikh Mujib Medical University (BSMMU), Dhaka, Bangladesh

Aminul Hasanat, MD
Associate Prof., Department of Neuro-anesthesiology, National Institute of Neurosciences and Hospital, Dhaka, Bangladesh

Atul H. Goel, MCh
Prof., Seth G.S. Medical College and KEM Hospital, Mumbai, India

Bipin Chaurasia, MS
Dr., Department of Neurosurgery, Neurosurgery Clinic, Birgunj, Nepal

Esma Azam Zico, MS
Dr., Department of Neurosurgery, Dhaka Medical College and Hospital, Dhaka, Bangladesh

Kazi Mohibur Rahman, MD
Prof., Department of Neurology, National Institute of Neurosciences and Hospital, Dhaka, Bangladesh

Lutful Anwar Quadery, FRCS
Prof., Department of Neurosurgery, Chittagong Medical College and Hospital, Chittagong, Bangladesh

Md Bayazidur Rahman, MBBS
Dr., Department of Neurosurgery, National Institute of Neurosciences and Hospital, Dhaka, Bangladesh

Md Moshiur Rahman, MS
Asst. Prof., Department of Neurosurgery, Holy Family Red Crescent Medical College and Hospital, Dhaka, Bangladesh

Mohammad Samsul Arifin MS
Dr., Department of Neurosurgery, National Institute of Neurosciences and Hospital, Dhaka, Bangladesh

Mohammod Abdul Hyee, MD
Prof., Department of Neurology, Ibn Sina Specialized Hospital, Dhaka, Bangladesh

Mohammod Bodrul Alam Mondal, MD
Prof., Department of Neurology, National Institute of Neurosciences and Hospital, Dhaka, Bangladesh

Mohammod Habibur Rahman, MD
Asst. Prof., Department of Neurology, National Institute of Neurosciences and Hospital, Dhaka, Bangladesh

Mohammod Hossain, MS
Prof., Department of Neurosurgery, Bhongobhondhu Sheikh Mujib Medical University (BSMMU), Dhaka, Bangladesh

Mohammod Selim Sahi, MD
Associate Prof., Department of Neurology, National Institute of Neurosciences and Hospital, Dhaka, Bangladesh

Mohammod Zahed Hossain, FCPS, MS
Prof., Department of Neurosurgery, National Institute of Neurosciences and Hospital, Dhaka, Bangladesh

M.S. Zahirul Haque Chowdhury, MD
Prof., Department of Neurology, National Institute of Neurosciences and Hospital, Dhaka, Bangladesh

Muhammed Shamsul Arefin, MD
Asst. Prof., Department of Neuro-anesthesiology, National Institute of Neurosciences and Hospital, Dhaka, Bangladesh

Nausher Alam, FCPS
Prof., Department of Neurosurgery, Women Medical College and Hospital, Uttara, Dhaka, Bangladesh

Nazmin Ahmed, MS
Dr., Department of Neurosurgery, Ibrahim cardiac Hospital and Research Institute, Dhaka, Bangladesh

Nur Mohammad, MS
Dr., Department of Neurosurgery, National Institute of Neurosciences and Hospital, Dhaka, Bangladesh

Patwary Mohammod Faruque, FCPS
Dr., Department of Neurosurgery, Bangladesh Specialized Hospital, Shamoly, Dhaka, Bangladesh

Quazi Deen Mohammod, FCPS, MD
Prof., Department of Neurology, National Institute of Neurosciences and Hospital, Dhaka, Bangladesh

Rakibul Haque, MS
Dr., Department of Neurosurgery,
National Institute of Neurosciences and Hospital, Dhaka, Bangladesh

Rakibul Islam, MS
Dr., Department of Neurosurgery,
National Institute of Neurosciences and Hospital, Dhaka, Bangladesh

Rashed Mahmud, MS
Asst. Prof., Department of Neurosurgery Dhaka Medical College and Hospital, Dhaka, Bangladesh

Riad Habib, MS
Dr., Department of Neurosurgery, Enam Medical College and Hospital, Dhaka, Bangladesh

Robert Ahmed Khan, MS
Asst. Prof., Department of Neurosurgery,
Bhongobhondhu Sheikh Mujib Medical University (BSMMU), Dhaka, Bangladesh

Shamsul Alam, MS
Asst. Prof., Department of Neurosurgery,
Bhongobhondhu Sheikh Mujib Medical University (BSMMU), Dhaka, Bangladesh

Sharif Uddin Khan, MD
Prof., Department of Neurology,
National Institute of Neurosciences and Hospital, Dhaka, Bangladesh

Sirajee Shafiqul Islam, MD
Associate Prof., Department of Interventional Neurology
National Institute of Neurosciences and Hospital, Dhaka, Bangladesh

S.I.M. Khairun Nabi Khan, MS
Associate Prof., Department of Neurosurgery
Bhongobhondhu Sheikh Mujib Medical University (BSMMU), Dhaka, Bangladesh

S.M. Monir Hossain, MBBS
Dr., Department of Neurosurgery,
National Institute of Neurosciences and Hospital, Dhaka, Bangladesh

S.M. Noman Khaled Chowdhury, MS
Prof., Department of Neurosurgery, Chittagong Medical College and Hospital, Chittagong, Bangladesh

Syed Ariful Islam, FCPS
Dr., Consultant, Department of Anesthesia,
Sir Salimullah Medical College and Mitford Hospital, Dhaka, Bangladesh

Syeda Neyamot-e-Ferdousi, MS
Dr., Department of Neurosurgery,
National Institute of Neurosciences and Hospital, Dhaka, Bangladesh

Taslim Uddin, FCPS
Prof., Department of Physical Medicine and Rehabilitation, Bhongobhondhu Sheikh Mujib Medical University (BSMMU), Dhaka, Bangladesh

Preface

Students and physicians frequently tend to regard neurosurgery as a difficult subject. Neurosurgery is a vast subject in medical sciences and includes multiple subspecialties, expanding day by day with respect to knowledge, technique, skill, and safety. Before deep diving into the neurosurgical ocean, one should start with the fundamentals of general neurosurgery, covering all of its branches. So, a beginner or neurosurgical student must read through a concise textbook of neurosurgery containing updated basic information on neurosurgical principles and practices. Many students have a hard time obtaining a concise neurosurgical textbook covering all aspects of neurosurgery. Including general neurosurgery, neurosurgery has many branches, such as vascular neurosurgery, stereotactic neurosurgery and functional neurosurgery, epilepsy surgery, oncological neurosurgery, skull-base surgery, spinal neurosurgery, peripheral nerve surgery, pediatric neurosurgery, endoscopic and minimally invasive neurosurgery, endovascular or interventional neurosurgery, neuro-robotics (new and developing), and neuro-stem cell transplantation (also new and developing).

This book will be very useful to those sitting for neurosurgery postgraduate and board examinations or looking for a concise explanation of the concept of neurosurgery. This book is based on recent and established scientific data, covering all parts of neurosurgery that can greatly help such individuals, including practicing neurosurgeons and neuroscientists. Here, more emphasis will be placed on common neurosurgical conditions without ignoring less frequent conditions. More than 400 selective and representative pictures and drawings are included.

Here, neurosurgical conditions are described briefly in regard to epidemiology, pathology and pathogenesis, clinical presentations, investigations, and management principles, including surgery and surgical principles. The descriptions provided are slightly more comprehensive for more frequent neurosurgical conditions. Figures and drawings are used to depict pathologies, pathological anatomy, radiology, and pre- and post-operative demonstrations. Once again, pictures are used frequently for more common conditions. Tables and boxes are used as needed. Operative details and techniques are outside the scope of this book; however, some details of common operations are included. Overlapping is avoided as much as possible, although some overlapping is inevitable.

This book was written by a group of authors who have completed their post-graduate training and have successfully been practicing neurosurgery in Bangladesh and abroad, holding posts ranging from assistant professors/associate specialists to professors/consultants.

We sought to make the difficult topics easier by using simple language without compromising the scientific information. We compiled a number of figures (for which there is no copyright issue) to provide a better understanding of the written text. We cited the current gold-standard practices used across the globe and drew on our local management experience, pertaining to techniques that can be practiced in many countries, including ours.

A summary of the chapters is given below.

In chapter 1, the history of neurosurgery is described, encompassing the global history of neurosurgery starting from the prehistoric period. There are interesting facts that have been cited here as part of the history of neurosurgery. There is also an account of the evolution of modern neurosurgical care in Bangladesh.

In chapter 2, we describe how a patient should be evaluated to reach a neurosurgical diagnosis. The different tests that can be used to differentiate lesions in different parts of the nervous system are mentioned in this chapter. Some important interpretations and pictorial descriptions are given to provide a better understanding.

In chapter 3, the basics of neuroanesthesia are discussed. This discussion revolves around the areas that are important for neurosurgeons to learn about so that they can carry out safe neurosurgical procedures.

In chapter 4, the investigations that must be carried out to reach a neurosurgical diagnosis are discussed. Some imaging pictures are included to provide a better understanding of the chapter. The interpretation of imaging is also mentioned.

In chapter 5, congenital abnormalities in relation to neurosurgery are described. This chapter includes pediatric disorders of both the brain and spine. Signs, symptoms, investigations, and surgical management are described.

In chapter 6, hydrocephalus is elaborated on, starting with pediatric hydrocephalus and then proceeding to describe different types of hydrocephalus. The causes, clinical features, and treatment modalities are described. Emergency and long-term management of hydrocephalus are elaborated on. Different types of shunts and endoscopic approaches to treating hydrocephalus are also discussed. This chapter also includes the rare causes of hydrocephalus and the corresponding treatment modalities.

Chapter 7 elaborates on idiopathic intracranial hypertension. Signs, symptoms, risk factors, and diagnostic criteria from the recent journal articles and recommendations have been compiled. A discussion of the different treatment modalities concludes this chapter.

In Chapter 8, CSF leak is discussed. Both traumatic and non-traumatic cranial CSF leak and spinal CSF leak are discussed. Diagnostic investigations and their interpretations are meticulously described. Treatment modalities are also sufficiently described.

In Chapter 9, brain injury and its clinical presentation, investigation, and management options are described. Some important surgical procedures are also discussed, which will help the reader to acquire the details of some surgical procedures. Long-term sequelae and their management are described as well. Brain injuries caused by gunshots and sharp weapons are included in this chapter, along with some photographs. Cranial vascular injuries and their management are included at the end of this chapter.

In Chapter 10, ischemic stroke, cerebrovascular occlusive diseases and venous Ischemia are discussed. The physiology and anatomy of cerebral blood supply are elaborated on. The clinical picture associated with the occlusion of blood supply to specific areas of the brain is described. History, clinical findings and investigations are all mentioned, along with interpretations and management. Different syndromes resulting from ischemia are included in this chapter. Some treatment options, like arterial bypasses in the management of an MCA stenosis, may be intriguing for the readers. The causes, investigations and management of cerebral venous thrombosis are also part of this chapter.

In Chapter 11, spontaneous cerebral hematoma, its causes, sites of hemorrhages, interpretation of investigations to diagnose the temporal profile and management are described. Surgical procedures to remove hematoma via the burrhole procedure or open procedure, or the instillation of urokinase are discussed. The prediction of mortality and rehabilitation are also included in this chapter.

In Chapter 12, intracranial aneurysm and subarachnoid hemorrhages are discussed. The causes and location of hemorrhages, diagnosis, investigation and treatment of subarachnoid hemorrhages are all mentioned. Clipping and coiling are described, along with some nice illustrations. Aneurysms found in different vessels are discussed separately.

Chapter 13 deals with arteriovenous malformations. Different AVMs are presented. The types are specified using Spetzler–Martin grading and further modifications. In this chapter, microsurgical excision of AVMs is described, along with the postoperative care and outcomes.

In Chapter 14, cerebral AV fistulas are elaborated on. The classification of different AV fistulas, clinical manifestations, risk factors and treatment modalities are described. Rare events like the vein of Galen malformation, pial AV fistula, etc., are included.

In Chapter 15, caroticocavernous fistulas are discussed. A nice demonstration of anatomy and pathology opens the chapter. Classification, pathophysiology, clinical presentation, investigation and treatment are discussed.

In Chapter 16, cerebral cavernous malformations and developmental venous anomalies are discussed. Clinical presentation, investigation and treatment modalities of cavernomas and developmental venous anomalies are included in this chapter.

In Chapter 17, another vascular disorder, moyamoya disease, is discussed. The pathophysiology, presentation, investigation and treatment modalities of moyamoya are discussed.

In Chapter 18, the revolutionary endovascular procedure is discussed. This chapter starts with the history. Then, different types of coiling are described. The current modern methods, e.g., flow diversion, stenting, embolization, etc., are also brought into the discussion. Stenting in different types of vascular neurosurgeries is also illustrated. Cranial AVMs and dural AVFs, and their grading, presentation, investigation and treatment are rediscussed. Both open and endovascular approaches are discussed.

Chapter 19 describes the management of cranial infection. The authors dig into the underlying causes, types of microorganisms (e.g., bacterial, viral, fungal, or parasitic), clinical features and treatment options for both typical and atypical infections. The latest guidelines are also described. Special tests for atypical presentations and atypical infections are all outlined in this chapter. Shunt hardware infection is another concern in neurosurgery, which is also discussed in this chapter.

In Chapter 20, brain tumours are discussed. The latest classification of these tumours and their management is elaborated on. Both supra- and infratentorial benign and malignant lesions are discussed in this chapter.

Imaging investigations and other tumour markers and their interpretation are included in the discussion. Rarer tumours are also discussed. Both surgical and medical management is discussed for tumours where medical management plays a role. Some pictures of large tumours found in our local patients are included.

In Chapter 21, surgical management of all commoner skull base tumours is discussed in short along with short orientation of skull base surgical approaches used for removal of skull base tumors.

In Chapter 22, spinal anatomy and spinal biomechanics are described. The sagittal balance of the spine and important angles which are often missed by neurosurgeons and used by orthopaedic surgeons are discussed in a straightforward manner.

In Chapter 23, spinal injury and its classification and treatment are discussed. The graphical representation of spinal injury illustrated in this chapter helps identify the types of fracture and understand the ideal way of managing them. Some landmark papers regarding spinal injury management are referenced. Complications associated with spinal injury, which can be fatal if left untreated, are also discussed.

In Chapter 24, a very common neurosurgical problem—spinal degenerative diseases—is discussed. Lumbar degenerative disc disease is elaborated on in the first part of the chapter. In the second part, cervical degenerative changes are included. Upper cervical spine degenerative changes, atlantoaxial instability, atlanto-occipital dislocation, etc., are also discussed. Treatment modalities are cited, along with some good illustrations.

In Chapter 25, spinal tumours are the topic of discussion. The epidemiology, classification, clinical features, and treatment strategies for all sorts of tumours, be it intradural, intramedullary, or extradural, are discussed. Rare spinal cord tumours and tumour-like conditions are also discussed.

Chapter 26 is dedicated to spinal infection. Its predisposing factors, aetiopathogenesis, clinical presentation, diagnosis, and both nonsurgical and surgical management are discussed. Due to the prevalence of spinal tuberculosis, different types of presentation, investigation, and treatment modalities of it are described. Some rare parasitic infections are also described, along with interesting perioperative findings.

In Chapter 27, spinal vascular lesions are elaborated on. The chapter opens with a discussion of the spinal vascular anatomy. Different types of vascular lesions are described, along with relevant studies. The treatment options in relation to different types of lesions are listed. Pictures of some rare malformations are included in this chapter.

In Chapter 28, endoscopic neurosurgery is detailed. The chapter opens the discussion with the history of endoscopy. Pictures of endoscopic instruments are provided and their use to treat different types of neurosurgical pathologies is outlined. Some very common procedures are discussed in detail to facilitate the reader to perform the procedures themselves. Some other pathologies, which are not commonly treated using neuroendoscopes, are also included in this chapter due to their potential to be treated as neuroendoscopic procedures. Moreover, some very advanced neuroendoscopic procedures are included in this chapter. Complications that may occur during neuroendoscopy are also discussed.

In Chapter 29, dementia is discussed. The causes of dementia are listed. Different types of memory are described. Medical and surgical causes like NPH are detailed in this chapter along with treatments. Difficulties in the diagnosis and treatment of NPH are discussed.

In Chapter 30, movement disorders and some other areas of functional neurosurgery are discussed. Different methods of surgery for movement disorders like tremor, Parkinson's disease, dystonia, etc., are discussed in this chapter. Spasticity, its types, clinical features, and both non- surgical and surgical treatment are explored in this chapter. Torticollis, trigeminal neuralgia, hemifacial spasms, glossopharyngeal neuralgia, intractable pain surgery, etc., are discussed.

Chapter 31 covers epilepsy and epilepsy surgery. Definitions and classifications of seizures open the discussion. Presurgical evaluation is appropriately emphasized. Neurophysiology assessment, functional MRI, neuropsychological testing, the Wada test, electrical cortical stimulation, etc., are discussed and put into context regarding how these approaches support epilepsy surgery. Different neurosurgical methods to treat epilepsy are elaborated upon in the later part of the chapter.

In Chapter 32, peripheral nerve surgery is discussed. Peripheral nerve anatomy and physiology are described, followed by classifications of peripheral nerve injury. Diagnostic tests like nerve conduction studies, EMG, and MRI are described along with interpretations. Different treatment approaches are provided. Both benign and malignant peripheral nerve tumors and their diagnoses, investigations, and treatments are described. Entrapment neuropathy and its surgery are included at the end.

In Chapter 33, the interesting topic of future directions in neurosurgery is included. Types of neuro-robots and their advantages and applications in neurosurgery are mentioned. Another future direction, neuro stem cell therapy, and its application in neurosurgery will intrigue readers. Gene therapy may be a game-changer in the future, as is described in this topic. Research on different topics like hydrocephalus are discussed.

In Chapter 34, brief descriptions of neurological medical diseases, which are important for neurosurgeons, are listed. Some of these diseases, like encephalitis, multiple sclerosis, motor neuron disease, peripheral neuropathy, myasthenia gravis, inherited myopathies, muscular dystrophy, neurometabolic disorders, etc., overlap in their neurosurgical diagnosis and can be confusing. This chapter was written to briefly shed light on these conditions.

In Chapter 35, neurorehabilitation in neurosurgery is discussed. Rehabilitation is a very important aspect for improving outcomes following neurosurgical management. This chapter discusses these aspects concisely.

Forhad H. Chowdhury, Mohammod Raziul Haque, Mainul Haque Sarker,
Khandkar Ali Kawsar, Jalal Uddin Mohammod Rumi
Editors

Acknowledgements

Special thanks to Mrs. Suborna Forhad Chowdhury and Mohammod Shamim Miah for their support.

Section I: The History of Neurosurgery, Branches of Neurosurgery, and Clinical Evaluation

History of Neurosurgery: Around the World and in Bangladesh

Forhad H. Chowdhury, Lutful Anwar Quadery and S.M. Noman Khaled Chowdhury

Abstract: Thousands of years were needed for neurosurgery to evolve into its present form. The entire history of neurosurgery is vast and beyond the scope of this book. This evolutionary history, spanning from the pre-historic era to the 21st century, is described sequentially in this chapter in brief. Here, the genesis of neurosurgery, including important developmental events, as well as relevant honorable neurosurgeons or neuroscientists are described. In the second part of this chapter, the history of the development of neurosurgery in Bangladesh is described in brief.

Abbreviations

AD	Anno Domini
BC	before Christ
BCE	before common era
CNS	central nervous system
CT	computed tomography
MRI	magnetic resonance imaging

1. History of Neurosurgery—Worldwide

1.1. Introduction

The practice of neurosurgery was started about 8000 to 10,000 years ago in the form of the trephination of skull (Viswanathan 1995). The Incas seem to have used a technique called trepanation starting in the late Stone age (Andrushko and Verano 2008). So, the historical journey of neurosurgical evolution started from the prehistoric stone age and continues to this day. Most of the historic development of modern neurosurgery took place in the last century.

1.2. Historical Ages

1.2.1. Prehistoric Age

The process of making a hole in the skull to expose the underlying brain and meninges has been practiced since the Neolithic era. These crude operations performed with very crude instruments were generally successful. In the late 18th century, anthropologists started to find skulls with intriguing holes in the gross eye that had been created for treatment purposes. Such types of trephined skulls have been found in different parts of the world, including Europe, Africa, South and North America, New Zealand, and New Guinea. It is believed that these holes in the skull were made for the treatment of head injuries via skull fracturing or to bring out a 'confined demon' in the brain (i.e., for superstitious reasons or treating psychiatric disorders!!) (Viswanathan 1995; Goodrich 2005).

1.2.2. Ancient Egyptian Age

The Edwin Smith Surgical Papyrus is the most ancient document pertaining to surgical techniques. Many physicians participated in writing this papyrus at different times from the 30th century BCE to the 17th century BCE in the Nile valley, Egypt. The first writer is unknown, but some believe 'Imhotep' was the first author (30th BCE) and that the last one was the 'Scribe' (1650 BCE). These inscriptions prove that Egyptian medical practitioners could recognize head and spinal injuries as they would elevate a fractured skull if needed (Viswanathan 1995; Goodrich 2005; Ballance 1922; Frey 1985–1986; Helgason 1987; Hughes 1988; Pickett 1992; Sachs 1952).

1.2.3. Ancient Indian Subcontinent Era

The ancient Indian surgeon Sushruta, who is considered the 'father of surgery', lived sometime between the 30th and 26th century BCE. The first written record of trephination was found in a manuscript he wrote called "Sushruta Shamhita". Many of the neurosurgical operations performed by Sushruta (the master surgeon of that time) were recorded in the Sushruta Samhita (Pasztor 1980; Nadkarni et al. 2002). He was born and practiced medicine on the banks of the Gangas river. It was said that he was born in Shologhar, SreeNagar, Munshigonj (Bikrampur), near Dhaka in modern Bangladesh (at that time, Bangladesh was part of Ancient India), and that he later migrated to Vanaras (in modern India).

1.2.4. Ancient Greek Era

The ancient Greeks contributed greatly to the evolution of neurological surgery. One man in particular made extraordinary efforts, not merely in terms of neurosurgical practices but also with respect to general medicine, and that man was Hippocrates (460–370 BCE). Hippocrates used conventional methods and created fresh approaches to the treatment of various illnesses, including spinal and spinal cord injuries. His beliefs and practices serve as the foundation for much of modern medicine. He distinguished medicine from mysticism in religion and classified current medical knowledge as a scientific field. He was also the first to stress the value of a solid moral foundation for those who practice medicine. Young doctors obtaining their licenses still swear the Hippocratic Oath, which is a summary of this ideology. Hippocrates, along with some of his pupils and successors, established a precise and extensive collection of texts that covered examination methods and remedies. A number of surgical volumes were included in the *Corpus Hippocraticum*, all of which are believed to have been written by Hippocrates alone. One of these texts, *Injuries of the Head*, discusses how to treat different kinds of head injuries using various methods. Additionally, but not in extensive detail, anatomy is covered. Hippocrates produced some of the most notable observations in the field of neuroscience. Sutures shaped like the Greek letters "T", "X", or "I" are discussed by him. His diploe and arachnoid granulation descriptions are also quite interesting. Observations and the earliest description of 'subarachnoid hemorrhage' come from this school. Hippocrates stated that the body was made up of four humors, all of which were in balance in a normal individual. These humors were classified by temperature as well as consistency: (i) warm and dry—(blood), (ii) cold and dry—(yellow bile), (iii) warm and wet—(black bile), and (iv) cold and wet—mucus. Each diagnosis pointed to an imbalance in these four humors. Every treatment offered in the Hippocratic tradition aimed to reestablish this equilibrium. Trephining was one method of restoring this balance in the case of a head injury.

Five patterns of head and skull injuries were noted by Hippocrates:

1. Fissures—which are always associated with a cerebral contusion;
2. Contusion of bone—due to crushing or bruising;
3. Depressed fracture—a fracture of the internal table as well as a depression of the external table;
4. Impression (by pointed or sharp weapons)—an injury that does not penetrate the skull;
5. Fractures.

Trephination was advised for all the above types, excluding Type 4 and those associated with widespread comminuted fragments of bones. Trephining was also forbidden if the injury was on a suture. Dural tear was, rightfully so, of great concern to Hippocrates. He described techniques for safe trephination without damaging dura and the brain. Treatment for spine dislocation was also highlighted, in addition to that for head injuries. The discovery of links between spinal injuries as well as a variety of symptoms throughout the body shows some early understanding of the pathways of the nervous system. For instance, sensory problems and urinary incontinence have both been connected to leg paralysis. It was believed that cervical spine dislocations were the cause of paralyzed chewing and swallowing, paresis of the tongue, and paralysis of all four limbs, the bladder, and the rectum. Treatments for these pathological disorders were prescribed to be extended and counter-extended (Viswanathan 1995; Goodrich 2005; Ballance 1922; Sachs 1952; Majno 1975; Margotta 1967; Rutkow 1993; Zimmerman and Ilz 1967).

From the area of the Bosporus to the bustling school of Alexandria came Herophilus of Chalcedon (325–280 BCE), a great, early anatomist. Unlike his predecessors, he dissected both human bodies as well as animal bodies. Besides his many contributions to anatomy, he is also remembered for his error in anatomic physiology regarding the 'rete mirabile'(Goodrich 2005).

Aulus Cornelius Celcus (25BC–50AD) made a number of interesting observations in neurological surgery, including extradural hematomas. Rufus of Ephesus (fl AD 100) and Galen of Pergamus (Claudius Galaneus, AD 129–200) made many contributions to neuroanatomy with neurosurgical implications. Galen provided a more realistic approach to head injury than Hippocrates (Viswanathan 1995; Goodrich 2005; Ballance 1922; Sachs 1952; Majno 1975; Margotta 1967; Rutkow 1993; Zimmerman and Ilz 1967). Paul of Aegina from the sixth century (AD 625–690) was a great surgeon, writer, and teacher. He described some pathophysiological mechanisms in neonatal hydrocephalus, and his antiseptic technique involving the use of wine in the wound management of the head was unique (Goodrich 2005; Paulus 1844–1847).

1.2.5. The Arabic Medicine Era

From approximately 750 to 1200 AD, the main intellectual hub of medicine was in the Arabic and Byzantine cultures. Arabic schools translated and systemized the surviving Greek and Roman texts. Avicenna, Rhazes, Albucasis, Averroes, and many others contributed tremendously to medicine and teaching, including with respect to our understanding of neurology. At that time, physicians rarely performed surgery, and it was considered a menial task. So, the role of surgeon was downgraded. Albucasis (936–1013AD) mainly focused on surgeries such as neurosurgery. The catgut suture with a needle was first introduced by Albucasis (Goodrich 2005; Avicenna 1556; Albuccasis 1519).

1.2.6. The Medieval European Age

Constantinus Africanus (1020–1087) infused Arabic medical science into the school of Salerno and, from there, Europe (Constantinus 1536). Roger of Salerno was a great surgeon and the first Italian surgical writer. He pioneered the techniques of nerve repair for when a nerve was severed. An extraordinary inventive surgeon (Cornor 1937), Theoderic Borgognoni of Cervia (1205–1298) is remembered for his 'clean' aseptic technique and the introduction of the "soporific sponge" (a combination of opium, hemlock mandragora, and other ingredients) to help a patient tolerate surgery (Theodoric Bishop of Cervia 1955–1966). William of Saliceto (1210–1277), Leonard of Bertapalia (1380?–1460), Lanfranchi of Milan (1250–1306), and Guy de Chauliac (1298–1368) were the important medieval surgeons who contributed to varying extents to neurosurgical development (Goodrich 2005).

1.2.7. The Anatomic Exploration Age

In the sixteenth century, there was a great deal of anatomical exploration. Leonardo da Vinci (1452–1519) drew crude diagrams of many neuro-structures (cranial nerves, the optic chiasm, the brachial and lumbar plexus, the ventricular system, etc.) (Goodrich 2005). One individual stands out as a remarkable contributor to the medical and surgical achievements made throughout the Renaissance. Despite the fact that Ambroise Pare (1510–1590) did not specifically contribute to neurosurgery, he had a significant impact on modernizing the entire field of surgery at the time. He represents both the demise of long-standing ties to historic tradition as well as a firm drive toward modernism. Pare was born the son of a modest cabinet manufacturer in a village in Northwest France. He was an apprentice to a number of barber-surgeons. At the age of just 15, Pare left for Paris to continue his formal anatomical and surgical education. Pare was the first to observe the prevalence of brain abscesses due to skull fractures as well as the fact that liver abscesses were generated as a consequence of a pyemic infection after a head injury. The skull, brain, and spine appear to have been subjected to successful procedures by Pare. He suggested trephining in a variety of conditions, the most prevalent of which were cases where matter was stuck between the dura and the brain. He invented a device that applies traction to the spine in the event of a dislocation. Along with some of his own anatomical works, he also wrote a masterwork on Vesalius' Fabrica. The act of making Vesalius' work available to surgeons for the first time had a significant influence on Renaissance surgery. Pare was first regarded with little respect by professional French surgeons due to his modest upbringing and early days as a barber-surgeon. In 1554, he was eventually welcomed into the College of St. Come, a prominent surgeon's society, albeit grudgingly. Beginning in 1536 and lasting until shortly before his death, he worked mostly as a military surgeon. He then served as chief physician to four French kings in succession: Henry II, Francis II, Charles IX, and Henry III (Viswanathan 1995; Goodrich 2005; Sachs 1952; Rutkow 1993; Zimmerman and Ilz 1967; Walker 1951).

Giacomo Berangario da Capri (1460–1530), Johannes Dryander (1500–1560), Volcher Coiter (1534–1576), Giovanni Andrea della Croce (1509?–1580), and Charles Estienne (1504–1564) are other Renaissance individuals who made contributions to surgical and neurosurgical development (Goodrich 2005).

Andreas Vesalius is essential to any understanding of Renaissance surgery in the sixteenth century. De Humani Corporis Fabrica Libri Septem (*On the Fabric of the Human Body*), one of the most important books on human anatomy, was written by Andreas Vesalius (1514–1564), a 16th-century Flemish anatomist and physician. In it, he included a section on brain anatomy with amazing illustrations. Many people consider Vesalius to be the founder of modern anatomy. He was born in the city of Brussels in the Habsburg Netherlands. Before serving as the imperial physician at the court of Emperor Charles V, he was a professor at the University of Padua. He made a fascinating addition to the field of hydrocephalus. He held the belief that the brain and nervous system are the centers of the mind and emotion, in contrast to the widely held Aristotelian idea that the heart is the body's core. Additionally, he believed that the brain rather than the heart is where nerves actually start. Vesalius found that nerves were not empty after researching the optic nerve (Goodrich 2005; O'Malley 1964; Vesalius at 500 2013).

1.2.8. Seventeenth Century

The 17th century, like the Renaissance, was a period of spectacular growth in science and medical science. Thomas Willis (1621–1675) originally investigated the brain and later published the famous 'cerebri Anatome' in London in 1664 (Willis 1664). The arterial circle at the base of the brain was named after him (the 'Circle of Willis'). He also introduced the word 'Neurology'. Humphrey Ridly (1653–1708), Wilhelm Fabricus von Hilden (1560–1634), Johann Schultes of Ulm (1595–1645), and James Yonge (1646–1721) were dedicated physicians and anatomists who contributed to neurosurgical development (Goodrich 2005).

1.2.9. The Venturous Eighteen Century

The 18th century was a time of dazzling activities in the scientific and medical sphere. Attempts to use neurosurgery for diseases other than those related to trauma were a major shift at this time. Percivall Pott (1714–1788) made numerous contributions to this novel surgical method in England. He was the first to demonstrate the pathologies of specific diseases in detail. Despite the fact that choosing a specialty was not yet a common practice, some regard Pott, who made significant contributions to the field of neurosurgery, as a very early neurosurgeon. The "puffy tumor" is one of Pott's most well-known descriptions. He described tuberculous spondylitis, which was named "Pott's disease" after him, though he was unaware of the underlying causative organism, i.e., Mycobacterium Tuberculosis. Certain notions expressed by Pott in relation to the practice of surgery demonstrated his commitment to his work. He highlighted the need for improved surgical techniques over increased speed. Pott also pointed out that a surgeon's success is dependent on more than just manual skills. He emphasized the importance of being able to assess whether to operate and claimed that this capacity can only be gained via experience, not through books (Viswanathan 1995; Goodrich 2005; Sachs 1952; Rutkow 1993; Flamm 1992; Walker 1951).

John Hunter (1728–1793) is evoked for his legacy in describing vascular disorders, in which he figured out the nature of collateral circulation (Hunter 1974). 'Huntarian ligation' was a useful, popular vascular procedure in the past. Benjamin Bell (1749–1806), Lorenz Heister (1683–1758), Francois-Sauveur Morand (1697–1773), Domenico Cotugno (1736–1822), Louis Sebastian Saucerotte (1741–1814), and Daniel Turner (1667–1741) were the 'Torch'-bearing scientists in neurosurgical development in the 18th century (Goodrich 2005).

1.2.10. Great Moments of the 19th and 20th Centuries

Neuropathological Exploration

In the first half of the 19th century, neuropathological understanding, the improvement of surgical techniques, and great advancements in anesthesia set the background for the boom in neurosurgery. John Abernethy (1764–1831), Sir Charles Bell (1774–1842), and Jean Cruveilhier (1791–1874) were key men in describing neuropathological aspects of nervous system diseases (Bright 1827).

Great Advancements in Anesthesia and Infection Control

Due to improvements in the conditions in which surgeons were allowed to work, the nineteenth century saw major advancements in all fields of surgery. However, the real pioneer of anesthesia was Crawford Williamson Long (1815–1878), who introduced anesthesia through the inhalation of ether (Anaya-Prado and Schadegg-Peña 2015). Patients could undergo long hours of surgery painlessly thanks to the inventions of ether (by J.C Warren) and chloroform (by J.Y Simpson) in 1846 and 1847, respectively. This affordance gave surgeons more time to focus on finishing operations successfully rather than operating at breakneck speed to finish surgery without anesthesia. Joseph Lister, an English surgeon, pioneered the utilization of carbolic acid as an antiseptic in 1867. He read Louis Pasteur's papers, which refuted the idea of spontaneous genesis and established bacteria as the source of infections. This had a huge impact on surgical methods, leading to the introduction of antiseptic surgery. He introduced the use of aseptic surgical tools (steam sterilizer, the scrub brush, and Halsted's rubber gloves) in a clean operating room, revolutionizing neurosurgery (Goodrich 2005).

Cerebral Localization

Diagnoses of CNS diseases were not certain until the concept of cerebral localization was devised. Up to 1860, it was thought that the brain acts as a singular entity. Then, GT Fritsch, E Hitzig, and Paul Broca introduced the concept of the localization of cerebral functions. Paul Broca (1824–1880) along with Ernest Auburtin (1825–1893?) discovered a localized speech area in the cerebral hemisphere of a patient with an exposed frontal lobe caused by a failed suicidal gunshot injury. The application of pressure to the third frontal convolution on the left side using a spatula deactivated this patient's speaking capacity (Broca 1861). Later, Karl Wernicke (1848–1904) identified the sensory speech area (Wernicke's area). David Ferrier (1843–1928) localized many brain functions through the use of ablation. The founder of modern neurology, John Hughlings Jackson (1835–1911), identified many functions of localized areas in the cerebrum via electrical stimulation and devised the idea of epilepsy. Robert Barthlow (1831–1904) also worked on cerebral localization. Sir Rickman Godlee (1859–1925) and Sir William Gowers (1845–1915) used cerebral localization techniques for the removal of cerebral tumors (Goodrich 2005).

Advances in Surgical Techniques

Though many important developments led to important paradigm shifts in general surgery and neurological surgery, neurological surgery progressed more slowly, as this branch relied largely on the allied sciences (i.e., neuroanatomy, neurophysiology, neuropathology, neuroradiology, etc.). William MacEwen (1848–1924), a Scottish neurosurgeon, is regarded as a giant in this field. He was a forerunner in establishing this subject as a specialty, and he pioneered numerous methods for diagnosing and treating brain tumors. One of these diagnostic techniques involves tapping the skull as well as listening for the "cracked-pot sound", which denotes hydrocephalus. In addition, MacEwen is renowned for being the first to conduct a craniotomy based only on neurological symptoms and signs rather than any other lesion-related symptoms or signs. On 27 July 1879, MacEwen removed a meningioma, allowing a patient to leave the hospital shortly after. She was able to return to her regular life in a few months. MacEwen noted that numerous symptoms, such as the left pupil contracting; a dull, fixed aching on the left side of the brow; and spasms on the contralateral side of the body, provoked him to perform surgery. One of MacEwen's major gifts was his deductive method of thinking, which revealed the symbiotic relationship between neurologists and neurosurgeons (Viswanathan 1995; Goodrich 2005; Sachs 1952; Rutkow 1993; Zimmerman and Ilz 1967; Bingham 1986; Bucy 1985; Laws 1985; Stone 1985; Walker 1951; Wilkins 1965).

Father of Neurosurgery

Victor Horsley (1857–1916) was one of England's first neurosurgeons, undertaking several neurological studies concerning cerebral function and the electric currents created in the brain, and many consider him the father of neurosurgery. He started his career primarily as a neurologist, and it was not until 1885, when he was 28 years old, that he was recruited as an assistant surgeon at University College Hospital. The following year, he was elevated to the rank of surgeon at the National Hospital for the Paralyzed and Epileptic, which is where nervous diseases are treated most frequently in England. Over his years as a surgeon, Horsley created unique techniques and materials that dramatically increased the success rate of neurosurgery. Bone wax, which was developed to stop bleeding from the bone margins and is still used in cranial surgery today, was one of these significant discoveries. Being the surgeon who carried out the first successful operation to cure an extramedullary spinal tumor in 1888, he is also considered one of the founders of modern spinal surgery. In the cited instance, the patient had experienced considerable agony as well as abdominal and lower-limb partial paralysis. Additional tests carried out by Horsley revealed a tumor in the spinal cord at the fifth vertebra to be the source of the symptoms. He bravely cut into the dura after exposing the chord and opening the spinal column, but he did not discover any signs of a lesion. By increasing the height of the incision, he was able to further open the meninges. He eventually discovered the tumor, which he successfully removed with no difficulties. Horsley received a letter from this patient after a year, in which he represented himself as being in excellent health and capable of working up to 16 h each day. Horsely and Clarke designed the first stereotactic therapy for brain pathologies, inspiring the subsequent designs (Viswanathan 1995; Goodrich 2005; Sachs 1952; Rutkow 1993; Zimmerman and Ilz 1967; Bingham 1986; Bucy 1985; Laws 1985; Stone 1985; Walker 1951; Wilkins 1965). Sir Charles A. Balance (1856–1936) from London, UK; Joseph Pancoast (1805–1882) and William Williams Keen (1837–1932) form Philadelphia, USA; the father of German Neurosurgery, Fedor Krause (1857–1937); and Antony Chipault (1866–1920), the father of

French Neurosurgery, are the individuals who should be mentioned for their extraordinary contribution to 19th century neurological surgery (Goodrich 2005).

American Neuroscientists and Fathers of Modern Neurosurgery

William Williams Keen (1837–1932) from America made remarkable strides in neurosurgery. He wrote the eight-volume series *Surgery* from 1906 to 1921. One of its volumes, *Principles and Practice,* was regarded as the "clinical bible" in the first several decades of the 20th century. "Keen's point", which is used for a ventricular tap during shunt operations, was named after him. He devised the operation techniques for treating spasmodic torticollis.

He brought the Gigli saw to America in 1898, after it was first described in Europe in 1897 (Viswanathan 1995; Goodrich 2005; Stone 1985). The first American monograph on brain surgery was authored by Allan Starr (1854–1932), a distinguished New York neurologist who was not a neurosurgeon. Working very closely with the general surgeon Charles McBurney (1845–1913), he realized cerebral surgery could be accomplished safely. He was very interested in neurosurgical matters. During an operation, he used to stand on the side of the operating table when the surgeon was operating to serve as a coach (Starr 1983). In 1923, Harvey Cushing stated the following about Allen Starr: 'I am confident that if Allen Starr, in view of his position in neurology and his interest in surgical matters, had taken to the scalpel rather than the pen we would now be thirty years ahead in these matters, and I am sure his finger must many times have itched when he stood alongside an operating table and saw the operator he was coaching hopelessly fumble with the brain' (Goodrich 2005).

Many great physicians have contributed to the history of neurological surgery, but one individual almost single-handedly propelled neurosurgery into the modern day. Harvey Cushing, the pioneer of modern neurosurgery, lived from 1869 until 1939. On 8 April 1869, Harvey Williams Cushing was born in Cleveland, Ohio, where the fourth generation of Cushing's family had moved to pursue a profession in medicine. He moved on to Harvard Medical School, where he graduated with honors in 1895. Cushing became interested in neurosurgery after studying under Victor Horsley in England. When he returned to the United States, he was offered a position at The Johns Hopkins Hospital in Baltimore, Maryland, where he could focus entirely on neurological cases. Surgery of the brain was challenging at the time, owing to inadequate hemorrhage control techniques. Cushing made some of his most inventive contributions to neurosurgery in 1904 while attempting to tackle this problem, including the pneumatic cranial tourniquet, the hefty rubber ring, firm digital pressure, and the reflection of hemostats clipped to either side of the cut scalp. Cushing invented the silver hemostatic clips, which were used to reduce meningeal hemorrhage after dural opening, in 1911. Cushing went on to invent astringents, coagulants, and suction mechanisms, all of which had a significant impact on a neurosurgeon's capacity to work for longer periods than ever before. Cushing's other achievements include his research on trigeminal neuralgia and the treatment procedure he developed as a result (Gasserian ganglion excision), as well as his considerable work on the pituitary body. He experimented successfully with infiltration anesthetic and operational intervention in neonatal cerebral hemorrhage and created an "ether chart" for the operating theater on which pulse, breathing, blood pressure, and other vital signs could be monitored. Cushing was also an accomplished novelist and educator. His numerous articles on neurology include *Meningiomas, The Pituitary Body and its Disorders* (1912), *Studies in Intracranial Physiology and Surgery* (1926), *Classification of the tumors of the Glioma Group* (1926), and others (1938) (Goodrich 2005). He also wrote biographies of famous Renaissance anatomist Andreas Vesalius and 18th-century Italian physiologist Luigi Galvanas, the latter of whom made fundamental advances in the understanding of electricity and its uses in medicine. Cushing won the Pulitzer Prize for *The Life of Sir William Osier,* a two-volume book, in 1926. He made significant contributions to the institutions that supported his studies. He gave his vast personal library to his undergraduate alma mater, Yale University, a collection now known as the "Harvey Cushing Collection of Books and Manuscripts". Cushing was also an artist, rumored to be able to draw on a blackboard with both hands at the same time. For his writings and lectures, he frequently created his own pictures. Following surgery, he was commonly seen doodling in the operating theater, often without even taking off his gloves. Cushing was described as austere and frigid by many people, while he was reported to be friendly and gracious to those he knew well. He was regarded with great respect and adoration by prominent surgeons around the world, and the Harvey Cushing Society, a group of American neurosurgeons, was created in America in his honor. Despite the fact that several of his contemporaries also made contributions to this profession, Cushing's combined contributions to medicine, literature, and education set him apart from his contemporaries. He raised neurosurgery to new and famous heights, becoming one of history's most extraordinary people, not merely in the field of medicine (Viswanathan 1995; Goodrich 2005; Sachs 1952; Rutkow 1993; Bucy 1985; Walker 1951; Wilkins 1965).

Walter Edward Dandy was an American neurosurgeon as well as scientist who lived from 1886 until 1946. He is recognized as one of the pioneers of neurosurgery along with Harvey Cushing and Victor Horsley. Dandy is credited with a number of neurosurgical firsts, such as the first explanation of CSF circulation in the brain, surgical intervention for hydrocephalus, the development of air ventriculography and pneumoencephalography, the description of brain endoscopy, the establishment of the first intensive care unit, and the first clipping of an intracranial aneurysm, which launched cerebrovascular neurosurgery. During his 40-year medical career, Dandy wrote five books and produced more than 160 peer-reviewed publications, all the while managing a full-time, groundbreaking neurosurgery practice, where, in his prime years, he performed almost 1000 procedures annually (Goodrich 2005; Fox 1984; Sherman et al. 2006).

Leo Davidoff (1898–1975), emigrant son of a cobbler from Lithuania and disciple of Harvey Cushing, was a great neurosurgeon of the 20th century with over 200 publications who pioneered neuroradiology and its associated tools, including the pneumoencephalogram. In the area of spine surgery, Charles Elsberg (1871–1948) and Charles Frazier (1870–1936), two remarkable American individuals, emerged and made contributions in the first quarter of the 20th century. They contributed many spinal surgical techniques and innovations including myelotomy and the two-stage removal of intramedullary tumors. Jean Athanase Sicard (1872–1929) advanced the myelography technique by introducing radio-opaque dye in CSF through a lumbar puncture. Antonio C. de Egas Moniz (1874–1955) from Lisbon introduced the cerebral angiogram via an arterial puncture. The combination of a pneumo-encephalogram with a cerebral angiogram offered neurosurgeons the first details of intracranial contents. The invention of penicillin in 1929 by Alexander Flamming (1881–1955) heralded the new era of medicine and surgery (Goodrich 2005). Neurosurgery began to be regarded as a specialty distinct from other fields of surgery around this period. Those who opted to concentrate on this field struggled hard for recognition, which did not completely transpire until the early twentieth century.

Microneurosurgery and the Fathers of Microneurosurgery

Mahmut Gazi Yasargil (1925–), a Turkish neurosurgeon, changed the paradigm of neurosurgery by converting it into microneurosurgery (Figure 1). Between 1931 and 1943, he studied medicine at Friedrich Schiller University in Jena, Germany, after attending Ankara Atatürk Lisesi and Ankara University in Ankara, Turkey. His brilliance in creating microsurgical procedures for utilization in cerebrovascular neurosurgery changed the lives of individuals with previously incurable conditions. Microneurosurgery was developed in collaboration with Raymond M. P. Donaghy, M.D., at the University of Vermont. Until his retirement in 1993, he performed laboratory studies and clinical trials of micro methods in Zurich, completing 7500 intracranial procedures. Yaşargil used his own inventions to cure epilepsy and successfully treat brain cancers. From 1953 to 1993, he worked as a resident, chief resident, professor, and chairman of the department. At the Congress of Neurological Surgeons Annual Meeting in 1999, he was named "Neurosurgery's Man of the Century 1950–1999". He is credited as the father of microneurosurgery. He continues to practice microneurosurgery, conduct research, and teach.

Yaşargil is regarded as one of the best neurosurgeons of the 20th century, alongside Harvey Cushing. He has aided three generations of neurosurgeons by outlining what is achievable in neurosurgery and then showing how to get there. He has trained about 3000 colleagues from all continents as well as surgical specialists in the micro-neurosurgical anatomical laboratory in Zurich. As an invited visitor, he has attended hundreds of national and international neurosurgical congresses, symposia, and courses. Yaşargil has written 330 papers and 13 monographs about his surgical experiences. *Microneurosurgery* (1984–1996, Georg Thieme Verlag Stuttgart–New York) is a six-volume compilation of his extensive experience and a significant contribution to the neurosurgery literature (Yasargil 1969; Yasargil 1985; Yasargil 1986; Rogers 2015; Flamm 1999; Tew 1999).

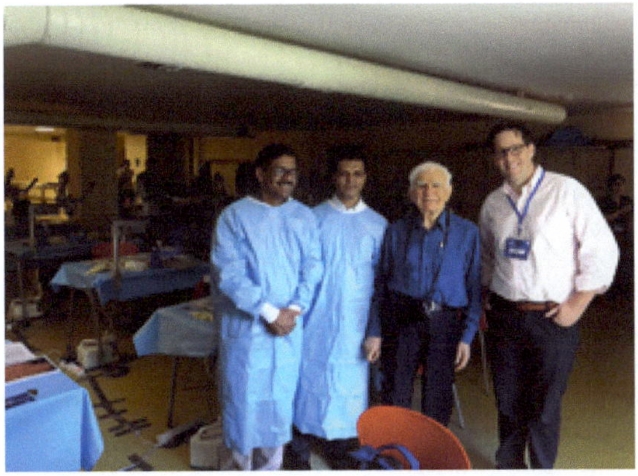

Figure 1. From left to right, Prof. Mohammod Raziul Haque, Dr. Forhad H. Chowdhury, Prof. Gazi Yasargil, and another neurosurgeon. Source: Photo by authors.

Development of Neuro-Imaging

Two inventions revolutionized neuroradiology and neurosurgery: one is the CT scan, and the other is MRI. CT was developed in 1972 by Godfrey Hounsfield of EMI Laboratories in England and Allan Cormack of Tufts University in Massachusetts, both of whom were born in South Africa. For their contributions to medicine and research, Hounsfield and Cormack were later given the Nobel Peace Prize (Richmond 2004). The origins of nuclear MR can be traced back to Isidor Isaac Rabi's groundbreaking research conducted in 1938. For this accomplishment, he received the Nobel Prize in Physics in 1944. Felix Bloch as well as Edward Mills Purcell continued this research into solids and liquids after that, for which they shared the 1952 Nobel Prize in Physics. Future medical applications were hinted at by Raymond Damadian's 1971 proposal that malignant and healthy tissue can be distinguished using MR relaxation lengths. Paul Lauterbur demonstrated in 1973 that an image could be created using nuclear MR. In 2003, Lauterbur and Sir Peter Mansfield received the Nobel Prize in Physiology or Medicine in recognition of their groundbreaking accomplishments. It was not until 1977 that their theory became a reality (Edelman 2014).

Guido Guglielmi's work at UCLA revolutionized the coil embolization of intracranial aneurysms when he realized that electricity could be used as a controlled release mechanism for coils. In 1991, he published two papers on the embolization of brain aneurysms using detachable platinum coils (Guglielmi's coils). Aneurysm treatment has thus become more accessible and safer. This affordance ushered in a new era of neurosurgery known as endovascular neurosurgery (Vaidya et al. 2008).

2. History of Neurosurgery in Bangladesh

2.1. Introduction

Bangladesh is a small South Asian country with a land area of about 147570 square kilometers. It was a part of British India until 14 August 1947, when it was annexed by Pakistan and given the name East Pakistan. The country's health sector was underdeveloped because it was a low-income country. As a result, establishing a highly advanced super-specialized subject of medical science such as neurosurgery in this country was not easy. Professor Omar V. Jooma (also known as Jooma Khan) used to travel from Karachi to Dhaka to provide neurosurgical consultation, particularly for patients with head injuries, during the Pakistan period (Hossain 2016).

2.2. Beginning of Neurosurgery in Bangladesh

In Bangladesh, the year 1970 is seen as a historic moment in neurosurgery. Professor Rashid Uddin Ahmad (1937–2016), after completing his FRCS and five years of Neurosurgery training in Edinburgh under Professor Francis John Gillingham, returned to East Pakistan in 1970 and established the first Neurosurgery unit at the then Institute of Postgraduate Medicine and Research (IPGMR), which housed only six indoor beds. Thus, he is the founder of neurosurgery in Bangladesh. Professor Rashid Uddin Ahmad also served as an honorary colonel in the Combined Military Hospital in Dhaka and as a consultant neurosurgeon. When the IPGMR became the

Bangabandhu Sheikh Mujib Medical University (BSMMU) in 1998, he was the first chairman of the neurosurgery department (Khan et al. 2019).

Professor A. H. M. Ahsanullah (1937–2014) began practicing neurosurgery at the IPGMR in 1972, after finishing his neurosurgical studies in Turkey. Despite the fact that Professor Rashid Uddin Ahmad founded the neurosurgery unit at IPGMR, he was forced to flee the country during Bangladesh's liberation war in 1971. Until 1978, Professor A. H. M. Ahsanullah was the only neurosurgeon at the IPGMR, performing all of the neurosurgical unit's tasks (Khan et al. 2019).

Professor Ata Alahi Khan (1939–2016) returned to Bangladesh in 1975 after completing his FRCS and neurosurgical training in the United Kingdom. In that year, he launched the Neurosurgery unit at Dhaka Medical College and Hospital. He went on to become a professor and the head of the neurosurgery department at Dhaka Medical College and Hospital, where he stayed for a long time. In 1997, he established the MS (neurosurgery) post-graduate course at Dhaka Medical College. Professor Alahi formerly served as the President of the Bangladesh Society of Neurosurgeons. In appreciation of his achievements in the neurosurgical branch of medical science both nationally and globally, the Bangladesh College of Physicians and Surgeons (BCPS) awarded him a fellowship in neurosurgery (Khan et al. 2019).

In 1978, Professor Lutful Anwar Quadery (born 1941) founded the Neurosurgical unit at Chittagong Medical College and Hospital. Professor L. A. Quadery is his moniker. He received neurosurgery training in Bristol, Glasgow, Liverpool, and London after receiving his FRCS in 1971. After returning to Bangladesh from the United Kingdom (UK) in 1978, this passionate man took the initiative and created a neurosurgery department in Chittagong, a city outside of the main city of Dhaka. He began his work with the aid of the General Surgery Department, and at first, he only had 20 beds for neurosurgery patients. Professor M. A. Matin, the then health minister of the Peoples Republic of Bangladesh, launched a dedicated Neurosurgical unit in 1979. Since then, this department has been assisting individuals with various neurosurgical disorders in the south and east of Bangladesh. Professor L. A. Quadery was also the president of the Bangladesh Society of Neurosurgeons and played a key role in the development of neurosurgery in this country (Khan et al. 2019).

2.3. Development of Neurosurgical Centers

At present, neurosurgical services are widely available throughout the country. Now, all neurosurgical services, including cerebrovascular surgery and functional neurosurgery, are available in Bangladesh.

The public neurosurgical centers in Bangladesh are listed below:

- National Institute of Neurosciences and Hospital (NINS&H): This hospital began its journey in September of 2012, employing all of the latest neurosurgical equipment. It is located in Sher-e-Bangla Nagar, Dhaka's health district, and it is Bangladesh's sole government-run tertiary-care neuroscience center. This institute has 175 beds dedicated to neurosurgery patients. This facility offers neurosurgery subspecialties such as clinical neurosurgery, pediatric neurosurgery, traumatic neurosurgery, vascular neurosurgery, and stereotactic radiosurgery. The MS (neurosurgery) program has been available here since 2015.
- Bangabandhu Sheikh Mujib Medical University (BSMMU): Bangabandhu Sheikh Mujib Medical University, founded on 30 April 1998, is the country's main postgraduate medical institution. It is descended from IPGMR, which was the country's first neurosurgical center to offer emergency neurosurgery services in 1970. It now has a neurosurgery department with 95 indoor beds and sophisticated neurosurgery operating rooms. BSMMU is the central institute that oversees the country's post-secondary education.
- Dhaka Medical College and Hospital (DMC&H): This is Bangladesh's largest neurosurgery center. This facility was founded in 1975. It now has 290 beds for patients undergoing neurosurgery. The MS (neurosurgery) program has been available here since 1997.
- Chittagong Medical College and Hospital (CMC&H): Neurosurgery was first practiced here in 1978. Outside of the capital city, Dhaka, this is the first and largest neurosurgery center. It currently contains an 88-bed neurosurgery ward, although this center must handle on average 150 neurosurgical patients in the inpatient department. Since 2002, this center has offered a post-graduate course in MS (neurosurgery).
- Combined Military Hospital (CMH): Neurosurgery was first practiced here in 1987. Colonel (Dr.) Majed Bakht was the first neurosurgeon to work at CMH, having completed his fellowship in Germany. In Dhaka Cantonment, he established an autonomous neurosurgery center equipped with all current neurosurgical equipment.
- Rajshahi Medical College and Hospital: This institute was established as a neurosurgical unit in 1991.

- Sher E Bangla Medical College and Hospital: This institute was established as a neurosurgical unit in 1992.
- Sir Salimullah Medical College and Mitford Hospital: This institute was established as a neurosurgical unit in 1994.
- Sylhet MAG Osmani Medical College and Hospital: This institute was established as a neurosurgical unit in 1996.
- Mymensingh Medical College and Hospital: This institute was established as a neurosurgical unit in 1997.
- Rangpur Medical College and Hospital: This institute was established as a neurosurgical unit in July 2007.
- Shaheed Ziaur Rahman Medical College, Bogra: This institute was established as a neurosurgical unit in 2010.
- Comilla Medical College and Hospital: This institute was established as a neurosurgical unit in 2012
- Dinajpur Medical College and Hospital: This institute was established as a neurosurgical unit in 2012.
- Shaheed Sheikh Abu Naser Specialized Hospital, Khulna: This institute was established as a neurosurgical unit in 2012.
- Faridpur Medical College: This institute was established as a neurosurgical unit in 2012.

Private neurosurgical centers:

- United Hospital, Dhaka
- Evercare Hospital Dhaka (Apollo Hospital)
- Square Hospitals Ltd, Dhaka
- Green Life Hospitals Ltd, Dhaka
- Ibn Sina Specialized Hospital, Dhaka
- Bangladesh Specialized Hospital Limited, Dhaka.
- BIRDEM General Hospital
- Islami Bank central Hospital
- Holy Family Red Crescent Medical College and Hospital
- Metropolitan Medical Center Limited, Dhaka

2.4. Evolution of Neurosurgical Investigations in Bangladesh

In the early days of neurosurgery in Bangladesh, the diagnostic services available were as follows:

- Ordinary X-rays;
- Direct-puncture cerebral angiography;
- Burr hole ventriculography;
- Lumbar air encephalography;
- Isotope brain scans;
- Myelograms.

In Bangladesh, CT scans were available in 1987, while MRI scans were available in 1996. Various sections of the country now have modern CT and MRI devices. MRS, MR tractography, CT and MR Angiography, Digital Subtraction Angiography (DSA), and PET scanning are also available.

2.5. The Making of Neurosurgeons

The year 1997 was a momentous occasion in Bangladeshi neurosurgery. In this year, the first Bangladeshi post-graduate neurosurgery program was developed. The University of Dhaka established the MS (neurosurgery) Course at IPGMR and Dhaka Medical College. It was a five-year academic program divided into three parts (Part 1, 2, and 3). In 2002, the University of Chittagong established the MS (neurosurgery) program at Chittagong Medical College.

In 2010, it was replaced by a five-year residency program at Banghabandhu Sheikh Mujib Medical University (BSMMU) in Dhaka, which was divided into two parts (Phases A and B). In 2015, the National Institute of Neurosciences and Hospital (NINS) began offering an MS course. Over 170 candidates have finished this MS course and are now practicing neurosurgery. Approximately one hundred residents are currently enrolled in various stages of this program.

The Bangladesh College of Physicians and Surgeons (BCPS) also provides a Neurosurgery FCPS degree. These post-graduate courses also attract international students.

2.6. Improving the Skills of Our Neurosurgeons

Well-wishing, friendly countries have provided Bangladesh with several opportunities for fellowship and training in neurosurgery since the outset. Our neurosurgeons were initially trained in the United Kingdom,

Turkey, Germany, and Singapore. As a result, countries such as Japan, Australia, the United States, Russia, India, South Korea, Hungary, and others assist us in improving our neurosurgical skills by providing specific training and fellowships. Of course, Japan has provided significant support for Bangladesh in all aspects of neurosurgery (training, fellowships, scholarships, seminars, workshops, and instrumental support), and new neurosurgeons have benefited, helping to improve the perception of neurosurgery. Pakistani Professor Iftekhar Ali Raja assisted the Bangladesh Society of Neurosurgeons (BSNS) in joining the World Federation of Neurosurgical Societies (WFNS). Following that, the WFNS organized a series of seminars, cadaveric workshops, live surgical workshops, and education courses in Dhaka to help our neurosurgeons improve their skills. Prof. Madjid Samii, Prof. Maurice Choux, Prof. Hirotoshi Sano, Prof. Tetsu Kanno, Prof. Yoko Kato, Prof. P. S. Ramani, Prof. Mehmet Zilelli, Prof. Atul Goel, Prof. Basant kumar Misra, Dr. T. N. Janakiram, Prof. Keki Turel, and Prof. R. P. Sen Gupta are among the world-renowned neurosurgeons who came to Bangladesh as faculty members involved in various workshops and seminars to help young neurosurgeons develop skills and knowledge.

2.7. Neurosurgical Societies

Our prominent society, the Bangladesh Society of Neurosurgeons, was founded in 1998. The society now has 200 members who are actively involved. The Bangladesh Neurospine Society was founded in 2015. Bangladesh is a founding member of the Asian Congress of Neurological Surgeons (founded in 1993), the South Asian Association of Neurosurgeons (founded in 1999), and the World Federation of Neurosurgical Societies (founded in 2000).

2.8. The Bangladesh Journal of Neurosurgery (BJNS)

The Bangladesh Journal of Neurosurgery (BJNS) is the flagship journal of the Bangladesh Society of Neurosurgeons. Its first volume was published in July 2011. It is published twice a year.

3. Conclusions

Neurosurgery is currently one of the biggest subspecialties in medicine, and it has many sub-specialties. It has taken nearly 10,000 years for it to take shape in the 21st century, a time when we can operate with minimum risk of mortality or morbidity, including infections. The performance of surgery in the wrong location is now very rare due to advanced neuro-imaging techniques, i.e., CT scans and MRI. Today's neurosurgery is a far cry and daydream compared to that practiced by our Asclepiad ancestors.

Author Contributions: Conceptualization, methodology, validation, formal analysis, investigation, resources, data curation, F.H.C., L.A.Q. and S.M.N.K.C.; writing—original draft preparation, writing—review and editing, visualization, supervision, F.H.C. and L.A.Q. All authors have read and agreed to the published version of the manuscript.

Funding: This research received no external funding.

Acknowledgments: I (Prof. L. A. Quadery) am grateful to Prof. Md. Kamal Uddin, ex-head of the department of neurosurgery of Chittagong Medical College and Hospital, Dr. Mahfujul Quader, assistant professor of neurosurgery of Chittagong Medical College and Hospital, and other neurosurgeon colleagues for assisting me in preparing this chapter.

Conflicts of Interest: The authors declare no conflicts of interest.

References

Albuccasis, Abu al-Qasim al-Zahrawi. 1519. *Liber Theoricae Necnon Practicae Alsaharavii*. Augsburg: Sigmund Grimm & Marcus Wirsung.

Anaya-Prado, Roberto, and Daniel Schadegg-Peña. 2015. Crawford Williamson Long: The True Pioneer of Surgical Anesthesia. *Journal of Investigative Surgery* 28: 181–87. [CrossRef] [PubMed]

Andrushko, Valerie A., and John W. Verano. 2008. Prehistoric trepanation in the Cuzco region of Peru: A view into an ancient Andean practice. *American Journal of Physical Anthropology* 137: 4–13. [CrossRef] [PubMed]

Avicenna. 1556. *Liber Canonis, de Medicinis Cordialibus, et cantica*. Basel: Joannes Haruagios.

Ballance, Sir Charles A. 1922. *The Thomas Vicary Lecture: A Glimpse into the History of the Surgery of the Brain*. London: MacMillan & Co. Ltd.

Bingham, William F. 1986. W. W. Keen and the Dawn of American Neurosurgery. *Journal of Neurosurgery* 64: 705–12. [CrossRef] [PubMed]

Bright, Richard. 1827. *Report of Medical Cases*. London: Longman, Rees, Orme Brown, and Greene.

Broca, Paul. 1861. Ramerques sur le siege de la faculte du language articule suivie d une observation d'aphemie (perte de la parole). *Bulletins de la Société Anatomique de Paris* 36: 330–57.
Bucy, Paul C. 1985. Scotland: The Birthplace of Surgical Neurologv. *Journal of Neurology, Neurosurgery, and Psychiatry* 48: 965–76. [CrossRef] [PubMed]
Constantinus Africanus. 1536. *Constantini Africani Post Hippocratem et Galenum*. Basel: Hernicus Petrus.
Cornor, George W. 1937. The Bamberg Surgery. *Bulletin of the Institute of the History of Medicine* 5: 1–32.
Edelman, Robert R. 2014. The History of MR Imaging as Seen through the Pages of Radiology. *Radiology* 273: S181–S200. [CrossRef]
Flamm, Eugene S. 1992. Percivall Pott: An 18th century. *Journal of Neurosurgery* 76: 319–26. [CrossRef]
Flamm, Eugene. 1999. Professor M. Gazi Yasargil: An Appreciation by Former Apprentice. *Neurosurgery* 45: 1015–18. [CrossRef]
Fox, William Lloyd. 1984. *Dandy of Johns Hopkins*. Baltimore: Williams and Wilkins.
Frey, Emil F. 1985–1986. The Earliest Medical Texts. *Clio Medica* 20: 79–85.
Goodrich, James Tait. 2005. Landmarks in the history of neurosurgery. In *Principles of Neurosurgery*. Edited by Setty S. Rengachary and Richard G. Ellenbogen. New York: Elsevier Mosby, pp. 1–38.
Helgason, Cathy M. 1987. Commentary on the Significance for Modern Neurology of the 17th Century B.C. Surgical Papyrus. *The Canadian Journal of Neurological Sciences* 14: 560–63. [PubMed]
Hossain, Sheikh S. 2016. Neurosurgery in Bangladesh: Past, Present and Future. *Journal of National Institute of Neurosciences Bangladesh* 2: 46–47. [CrossRef]
Hughes, J. Trevor. 1988. The Edwin Smith Surgical Papyrus: An Analysis of the First Case Reports of Spinal Cord Injuries. *Paraplegia* 26: 71–82. [CrossRef] [PubMed]
Hunter, John. 1974. *A Treatise on the Blood, Inflammation, and Gun-Shot Wounds*. London: J. Richardson.
Khan, Akhlakh, A. T. M. Mosharef, Narendra Shalike, and Kanak K. Barua. 2019. Evolution of Neurosurgery in Bangladesh. *Bangladesh Journal of Neurosurgery* 8: 57–62. [CrossRef]
Laws, Edward R. 1985. Tradition in Neurosurgery: Doing Well What Has Been Done Before. *Neurosurgery* 16: 739–53. [CrossRef]
Majno, Guido. 1975. *The Healing Hand: Man and Wound in the Ancient World*. Cambridge: Harvard University Press.
Margotta, Robert. 1967. *The Story of Medicine*. New York: Golden Press, p. 14.
Nadkarni, T. D., A. Goel, and S. K. Pandya. 2002. Neurosurgery in India. *Journal of Postgraduate Medicine* 48: 332.
O'Malley, Charles Donald. 1964. *Andreas Vesalius of Brussels, 1514–1564*. Berkeley: University of California Press, pp. 21–27.
Pasztor, Emil. 1980. *Concise Neurosurgery*. Basel: S Karger.
Paulus Aeginetes. 1844–1847. *Seven books of Paulus Aegineta*. Translated by F. Adams. London: Sydemhan Society.
Pickett, A. C. 1992. The Oath of Imhotep: In Recognition of African Contributions to Western Medicine. *Journal of the National Medical Association* 84: 636–37.
Richmond, Caroline. 2004. Obituary-Sir Godfrey Hounsfield. *BMJ* 329: 687. [CrossRef]
Rogers, Larry. 2015. *Yasargil: Father of Modern Neurosurgery*. Virginia Beach: Koehler Books. ISBN 978-1-63393-182-4.
Rutkow, Ira M. 1993. *Surgery: An Illustrated History*. St. Louis: Mosby Yearbook Inc.
Sachs, Ernest. 1952. *The History and Development of Neurological Surgery*. New York: Paul B. Hoeber Inc.
Sherman, Irving J., Ryan M. Kretzer, and Rafael J. Tamargo. 2006. Personal recollections of Walter E. Dandy and his brain team. *Journal of Neurosurgery* 105: 487–93. [CrossRef]
Starr, M. Allen. 1983. *Brain Surgery*. New York: William Wood & Co.
Stone, James L. 1985. WW Keen: America's Pioneer Neurological Surgeon. *Neurosurgery* 17: 997–1007. [CrossRef]
Tew, John M. 1999. M. Gazi Yasargil: Neurosurgery's Man of the Century. *Neurosurgery* 45: 1010. [CrossRef] [PubMed]
Theodoric Bishop of Cervia. 1955–1966. *The surgery of Theodoric, Ca.AD 1267*. Translated by E. Campbell, and J. Colton. New York: Appleton-century-Crofts.
Vaidya, Sandeep, Kathleen R. Tozer, and Jarvis Chen. 2008. An Overview of Embolic Agents. *Seminars in Interventional Radiology* 25: 204–15. [CrossRef] [PubMed]
Vesalius at 500. 2013. Available online: https://circulatingnow.nlm.nih.gov/2013/12/31/andreas-vesalius-at-500/ (accessed on 12 October 2024).
Viswanathan, Savitha. 1995. The History of Neurosurgery. Thesis. Rochester Institute of Technology. Available online: http://scholarworks.rit.edu/theses (accessed on 12 December 2020).

Walker, Earl A. 1951. *A History of Neurological Surgery*. Baltimore: The Williams and Wilkins Co.
Wilkins, Robert H. 1965. *Neurosurgical Classics*. New York: Johnson Reprint Corporation.
Willis, Thomas. 1664. *Crebri Anatome: Cui Accessit Nervorum Descriptio et Usus*. London: J. Flesher.
Yasargil, Gazi. 1969. *Microsurgery Applied to Neurosurgery*. New York: Thieme.
Yasargil, Mahmut Gazi. 1985. *Microneurosurgery Tomo I: Microsurgical Anatomy of the Basal Cisterns and Vessels of the Brain, Diagnostic Studies, General Operative Techniques and Pathological Considerations of the Intracranial Aneurysms*. New York: Thieme.
Yasargil, Mahmut Gazi. 1986. *Microneurosurgery Tomo II: Clinical Considerations, Surgery of the Intracranial Aneurysms and Results*. New York: Thieme.
Zimmerman, Leo M., and Veith Ilz. 1967. *Great Ideas in the History of Surgery*. New York: Dover Publications Inc.

Clinical Evaluation of the Nervous System: Neurosurgery and Its Branches

Forhad H. Chowdhury

Abstract: Clinical history taking and examination are the first and fundamental steps of the investigation, diagnosis, and treatment of a patient. Examination of the nervous system is of utmost important for a neurosurgeon. Here, clinical methods for a neurological or neurosurgical patient are briefly mentioned, including history taking for the nervous system; consciousness-level examination; higher-cerebral-function examination; examination of the cranial nerves, limbs, and trunk; examination of posture and gait; and examination for signs of meningeal irritation. Clinical examinations of unconscious and pediatric patients as well as dementia patients are also included in the discussion. In the last part of this chapter, the branches of neurosurgery are listed.

Abbreviations

AVM	arterio-venous malformation
CEA	carotid endarterectomy
ENT	ear, nose, and throat
MMSE	mini mental status examination
A-V	arterio-venous
DBS	deep-brain stimulation
GCS	Glasgow coma scale
MRC	medical research council

1. Clinical History Taking for the Nervous System

Before a patient is clinically examined, their neurological information is obtained. An accurate neurological examination comprises the history of the anatomical site of the pathology, the nature of the pathology, and which physical findings are observed during physical examination. Mastering clinical history taking requires a fundamental understanding of intricate organization and functional localization. It is crucial to recognize and characterize the pattern of a neurological disease over time: the most common symptom patterns are episodic, variable, and progressive. A clear description of the events occurring before, during, and after an episode of neurological symptom presentation is of utmost importance. Different symptom complexes can provide an indication to the neurosurgeon as to whether they are examining a cortical, extrapyramidal, spinal, radicular, peripheral-nerve, or neuromuscular ailment.

The physician begins by asking open-ended questions and concludes by asking specific queries. Depending on the patient's medical history, conditions, and level of competence, a cross history of the patient's attendant is often required. An assiduous examination of previous records is also needed. Data from other systems, past medical history workups, social and family history, and ongoing medication use must all be explored while taking a neurological history.

Loss of consciousness, seizure, dizziness, vertigo, visual impairments, weakness, discomfort, paresthesia, and other recurrent neurologic symptoms are among the most commonly reported major complaints noted in one's clinical history. Cardiac arrhythmias, seizures, migraine episodes, transient ischemia events as a result of a variety of etiologies, vestibular pathology, medication responses, metabolic abnormalities like hypoglycemia, and many others are among the underlying diseases. The most common complaints are sensory problems and pain. Pain, more than any other symptom, helps to pinpoint the location of diseased processes in the body. Pain is frequently coupled with other symptoms that can help with localization and causation. The goal is to pinpoint and focalize the source of the pain. The following data are collected: predisposing factors, quality and the location, radiation, severity, and temporal linkages of pain.

Headache is one of the commonest reasons for visiting a physician across the globe. After careful data gathering and analysis, one of three causal groups will emerge: vascular, myogenic, or traction. Headaches are a common symptom of life-threatening disorders (such as a brain tumor or meningitis, or a subarachnoid hemorrhage). The type and temporal profile of pain, features of pain, prodromes, triggering causes, and related symptoms should all be considered when describing a headache.

A seizure can be a manifestation of many neurological conditions such as cerebral tumors, CNS infections, neurovascular disorders, systemic disorders, neuro-trauma, metabolic disorders, and genetic influences. A thorough history will aid a doctor in ruling out many of these etiologies. The aura, onset, ictus, and postictal phases of a seizure must all be identified.

Neurovascular illness has a long history of being a critical factor in initiating specialized treatments to prevent future events or development. The clinical signs will assist one in determining if the cause of a disease is hemorrhagic or ischemic. When documenting a patient's history in the case of a cerebrovascular illness, start with the presenting symptoms and work your way through each subsequent symptom, just as you would for any other disease. It is essential to compile data on the following: activity at the time of onset (exercise, waking from sleep, and sedentary); symptoms presented; specific neurologic deficiencies; associated symptoms like chest pain, illnesses, and temporal sequences; time course; stroke risk factors; present functional capacity; and so on.

Table 1 lists other neurologic symptoms, which are organized by neurological structure of origin. Open-ended questions asked as part of the Present Illness and System Review will usually reveal these symptoms. When the doctor suspects a condition involving the structure(s) specified, the patient should be questioned about the following information in particular.

Onset, functional status, temporal progression, and detailed indications of the current illness should be obtained via history taking. A review of the neurologic system's processes should be completed. Furthermore, as anomalies are discovered, further questions can be asked, or, when additional complaints are remembered by the patient, their history can be quickly and appropriately supplemented throughout the examination.

Table 1. Symptoms of neurological diseases.

Anatomical Structures	Symptoms
Muscle	Weakness, cramp, hypertrophy, atrophy, myotonia, rhabdomyolysis
Myo-neural junction	Weakness, fluctuation, fasciculation
Peripheral nerve	Paresthesia; pain; hypoesthesia; analgesia; numbness; weakness to paralysis; reduced to absent reflexes; reduced to absent sensitivity to touch, temperature, pain, and vibration
Autonomic nerves	Syncope, orthostatic hypotension, impotence, sweating abnormalities, incontinence, gastrointestinal motility disturbances, cardiovascular reflex abnormalities, secretory disturbances, autonomic hyperreflexia.
Spinal cord	Segmental motor, sensory, and reflex impairments; radicular pain; lower motor findings; upper motor findings; bowel, bladder, and sweating disturbances
Cerebellum	Gait ataxia, dysmetria, incoordination of limbs, hypotonia, titubation, voice abnormalities, eye movement irregularities.
Brainstem	Crossed manifestation (body and face), cranial nerve abnormalities (nuclear and supranuclear), respiratory pattern irregularities, sleep disturbances, impairment of consciousness.
Basal ganglia	Movement disorder, tremors, bradykinesia, disturbances of tone, loss of righting reflex
Cerebral cortex	Mental status irregularities; epilepsy; upper motor symptoms; language, visual, speech, somato-sensory, motor, and hearing abnormalities

Source: Table reprinted from Walker (1990), used with permission.

2. Nervous System—Examination

Systemic disease can cause neurological symptoms, and neurological disease can impact the nervous system. A full general examination must be performed in conjunction with a central nervous system examination. Take note of the following points in particular when conducting examinations of the top of the skull to the bottom and the CNS (Lindsay et al. 2011).

2.1. *Clinical Examination*

2.1.1. Consciousness-Level Evaluation

A wide range of intracranial and systemic diseases result in a shift in consciousness level. To identify whether a patient's condition is deteriorating or improving, accurate examination and recording are required. Teasdale and Jennett established a scale for consciousness-level evaluation in Glasgow in 1974 that is widely accepted for consciousness assessment, discarding the vague terms and scale. EYE opening, VERBAL response, and MOTOR response are used to describe the patient's awareness level (Table 2). The results are repeatable, regardless of the observer's status, and paramedics can assess these metrics just as well as clinicians.

Table 2. Glasgow coma scale (GCS) in brief.

Eye Opening	Best Motor Response	Best Verbal Response
1: spontaneous eye opening 2: eye opening in response to speech 3: eye opening in response to pain 4: none	1: obeys vocal command 2: localizes 3: withdraws 4: flexion 5: extension 6: none	1: oriented 2: confused 3: inappropriate words 4: incomprehensible sounds 5: none

Highest score—15; lowest score—03. Source: Table adapted from Teasdale and Jennett (1974), used with permission.

Glasgow Coma Scale (Teasdale and Jennett 1974, 1976) (Highest total score—15, Lowest total score—03):

(a) Eye opening—Four categories:
- Spontaneously—04
- On speech—03
- On painful stimulation—02
- None—01

(b) Verbal response—Five categories:
- Orientated—05 [The patient knows where they are, including the name of the hospital, and the time, such as the day, month, and year]
- Confused—04 [The patient uses phrases when speaking but is disoriented in terms of time and place]
- Words—03 [The patient utters words occasionally rather than sentences]
- Sounds—02 [The patient utters grunts or groans but no words]
- None—01

(c) Motor response—Five categories:
- Obeys commands—06
- Localizing response to painful stimulation—05 [This consists of the application of a painful stimulus to the supraorbital nerve, such as rubbing of the clinician's thumb in the supraorbital groove, and escalating the pressure until a response is seen. If the individual responds by raising his or her hand above their chin, this is known as 'localizing to pain'. (At this time, applying pressure to the sternum or nail beds may not be enough to distinguish 'localizing' from 'flexing'.)]
- Withdrawal from painful stimulation—04 [If the individual does not exhibit a localized response to supraorbital pressure, turn their head away or apply pressure to the nail bed with a hard object or pen. Take note of the disengagement of the hand in response to pain stimuli.]
- Flexing response to painful stimulation—03 [If the individual does not respond to supraorbital pressure, exert pressure to the nail bed with a pen or a hard instrument. It is worth noting that elbow flexion is also known as 'flexing to pain'. This response may or may not be linked to spastic wrist flexion.]
- Extending response to painful stimulation—02 [Record as the response as 'extending to pain' if elbow extension is provoked as a reaction to the same painful stimulus. This is almost always coupled with spastic wrist flexion.]
- None—01 [Make sure the painful stimuli employed are adequate before placing a patient at this level. The patient's motor reaction may change during the assessment. Supraorbital pain can induce flexion, whereas fingernail pressure can cause extension. Alternatively, one arm may become painful while the other flexes. When this happens, make a note of the strongest response observed during the clinical evaluation session (this finding correlates most with the final result). The arm reaction

should be employed when determining the patient's consciousness level. Leg pain responses are less constant, frequently generating movements that originate in the spinal cord rather than the brain.]

Higher Cognitive Functions

(a) Cognitive skill

- Dominant hemispheric disorders

  Pay attention to the language pattern:
  - hesitant: motor/expressive dysphasia
  - fluent: receptive/sensory dysphasia

Is the individual able to follow basic or complex oral commands? [For example, 'Hold up both arms and place your left fifth finger on your right ear.']

- Dysphasia receptive

Submit a list of things to name to the patient.

- Dysphasia nominale

Is the patient able to comprehend what he or she is reading?

- Dyslexia

Is the patient's handwriting proper?

- Dysgraphia

Solicit a numerical calculation from the patient. [For example, in a serial 7 test, 7 is subtracted sequentially from 100.]

- Dyscalculia

Is it possible for the patient to distinguish objects? [For example, ask the individual to choose an object from a collection of objects.]

- Agnosia
  - Non-dominant hemispheric disorders

Take note of the individual's capacity to navigate the unit or their residence.

- Agnosia in terms of geography

Can the patient dress themself?

- Apraxia Dressing

Notice the individual's ability to duplicate a geometric pattern [for example, have the individual build a star with matchsticks or copy a cube drawing.]

- Apraxia of construction

The Mini Mental Status Examination (MMSE) is utilized in the evaluation of dementia.

(b) Memory test

Testing necessitates alertness, which is impossible to achieve in a patient who is dysphasic or confused.

- Recent memory;
- Short-term memory;
- Long-term memory.

(c) Reasoning and problem solving

To test the patient with regard to two-step calculations, for example, use the following problem: 'I want to buy 12 goods at 7 pence each. How much change will I get from a GBP 1 bill?' The following problems can also be useful:

- Request that the patient reverse three or four random numbers.
- Inquire of the patient about proverbs.
- Ask the patient to sort playing cards into their suits.
- The clinician should compare the patient's current thinking capacity to their expected capabilities based on previous work experience or/and schoolwork.

(d) Emotional state

Note that excitement or anxiety; apathy or depression; uninhibited behavior; emotional behavior; slowness of responses or movement; and personality type or shift are all things to consider.

2.1.2. Cranial Nerve Examination

(i) Olfactory Nerve

Use aromatic non-irritant items that do not stimulate the fifth nerve fibers in the nasal non-olfactory mucosa, such as soap or tobacco, to test both perception and identification. Instruct the patient to close one nostril while sniffing with the opposite.

(ii) Optic Nerve

By measuring reading acuity through a pinhole, refractive error (inadequate focusing on the retina, as in myopia or hypermetropia) can be corrected. A tiny beam of vision is focused on the macula as a result of this.

Visual Fields

Confrontational testing is a form of gross testing. By moving a finger or, more precisely, a 05 mm red pin from the extreme outward end to the point of fixation, you can compare an individual's fields of vision. This diagram depicts 'cone' vision. A 02 mm pin can be used to identify central-field deficiencies, which may only show up as a loss of color vision.

The physiological blind spot can be seen in the temporal section of the visual field. Here, a 02 mm item should vanish.

The individual must focus on the pupil of the examiner.

A Goldmann perimeter is used to examine peripheral vision fields, which are more sensitive to a moving target.

The patient's gaze is drawn to a single location. From the extreme edge, a point of light is moved to the center. On a chart, the patient's position while he or she watches the target is noted. Visual fields are accurately recorded through repeated testing from many directions.

A Goldmann perimeter with a low-intensity light source or a tangent (Bjerrum) screen is used to chart central fields. The Humphrey field analyzer is an alternative method of evaluating central fields that is very sensitive. This is the point at which the individual notices a static light source that is becoming more intense.

Optic Fundus Examination (Ophthalmoscopy)

Request that the individual focus on a faraway object distant from any bright light. Evaluate the individual's right eye using your right eye and the individual's left eye using your left eye. If a fundal examination is impossible due to limited pupil size, dilate the pupil using a fast-acting mydriatic (homatropine). If glaucoma or an acute enlarging lesion is suspected, the aforementioned action is not recommended.

Pupils

Take note of the following:

- Size (large = mydriasis; small = miosis);
- Shape;
- Equality.

Response to light: when light is directed into one of the patient's eyes, observe whether both pupils contract.

Reaction to convergence and accommodation: when the patient's gaze is drawn to a near-point object, observe whether pupil constriction occurs.

(iii) Oculomotor, Trochlear, and Abducens Cranial Nerves

When the third nerve is damaged, it causes problems with regard to eyeball and lid movement, including pupillary response.

Pupil: When exposed to light, the pupil dilates and becomes 'fixed'.

Ptosis: When the eyes are completely open, the eyelid falls over the pupil. Because the levator palpebrae superioris muscle comprises both smooth and skeletal muscle, ptosis can indicate either a sympathetic lesion or third-nerve palsy, with the later being more evident.

Ocular Movement

Ask the patient to keep their head still and follow an item held at arm's length. Keep track of all vertical and horizontal eye movements.

Any misalignment or range restriction should be noted.

Examine eye movements in each of the six gaze directions to determine maximum individual muscle power.

Inquire about double vision (diplopia); the individual is more likely to recognize it before the clinician detects an eye movement limitation. Detect the origin of the external image (from the faulty eye) utilizing a transparent colored lens, if present:

- Note the direction of the greatest displacement of the pictures and locate the pair of muscles implicated.
- Using a clear colored lens, locate the source of the outside picture (from the faulty eye).

Conjugate movement is a term that refers to the movement of both eyes in unison to maintain focus. Take note of the eyes' ability to move conjugately in a vertical or horizontal direction, as well as the propensity for the gaze to be fixed in a single direction.

Nystagmus is a condition in which the usual balance of eye control is disrupted. A slow movement in one direction is followed by a quick movement in the other direction. When the eyes are oriented in the direction of the fast phase, nystagmus is at its peak. The 'direction' of nystagmus is commonly expressed in terms of the rapid phase, which might be vertical or horizontal. Test as you would for other eye movements; however, keep in mind that 'physiological' nystagmus might take place when the eyes stray from the gaze's endpoint. For a left lateral gaze, for example, nystagmus to the left is maximum.

(iv) Trigeminal Nerve

Compare and contrast both sides. Test from the abnormal to the normal areas to map out the sensory deficiency.

Corneal reflex is a reflex of the cornea.

Touch the limbus with a wisp of damp cotton wool to test whether the patient can experience the corresponding sensation. Blinking should be observed on both sides.

Afferent pathway—opthalmic division of V (principal sensory nucleus—light touch).

Efferent pathway—7th nerve.

The most sensitive indication of a fifth-nerve injury is a failure in this test.

Motor Examination

Watch for temporalis muscle thinning and atrophy, which will 'hollow out' the temporalis fossa.

Request that the individual's jaws be clamped together. Feel the masseter and temporalis muscles. Apply pressure on the chin to try to open the patient's jaws. Request that the patient open his or her mouth. If the pterygoid muscles are paretic, the jaw will deviate to the weaker side, where it will be forced over by the properly functioning side's unopposed pterygoid muscles.

Jaw Jerk

Instruct the individual to open their mouth and relax their jaw. Tap their chin with your finger and a hammer:

Slight jerk—this is typical.

Increased jerk-supranuclear damage on both sides.

(v) Facial Nerve

Keep an eye on the individual as they speak and smile, and look for the following:

- Eyelid closure;
- Asymmetrical upward deviation of one angle of the lips;
- Nasolabial fold flattening.

The individual should then be told to execute the following actions:

- Wrinkle their forehead (when looking upwards) (frontalis);
- Keep their eyes closed as the examiner tries to open their eyelids (orbicularis oculi);
- Purse their lips while the examiner presses their cheeks (buccinator);
- Show their teeth (orbicularis oris).

Sugar, sodium chloride, or tartaric acid can all be used to assess taste. In this case, a modest amount of each material is applied anteriorly on the protruded tongue's suitable side.

(vi) Vestibulo-Cochlear Nerve

Cochlear nerve: Test the function of this nerve by speaking numbers into one of the patient's ears while occluding and stroking the external meatus to disguise hearing in the other. If hearing is affected, use an auroscope to analyze the external meatus and tympanic membrane for wax or infection.

1. Weber's test: Hold the base of a tuning fork (vibrating-512 Hz) against the vertex to distinguish conductive deafness (middle ear) from perceptual deafness (nerve-related). Inquire as to whether the sound is louder in one ear than the other.

2. Rinne's test: Place the base of a vibrating tuning fork on the mastoid bone. Ask the patient whether they heard the corresponding note. Hold the tuning fork close to the external ear meatus when the sound fades. Because air conduction via the ear ossicles is higher than bone conduction, the patient should be able to hear again.

Bone conduction is greater than air conduction in conductive deafness.

Both air as well as bone conduction are impeded in nerve deafness.

Specialized investigation is required for additional auditory testing as well as assessment of the vestibular nerve.

(vii) The Glossopharyngeal Nerve and Vagus Nerve

Because they are studied collectively and their actions are rarely hindered singly, these nerves are viewed as a group.

Take note of the patient's voice: if they have vocal cord paresis (vagus nerve palsy), they may have a high-pitched voice. (An ENT specialist should examine the patient's vocal cords.)

Any difficulty swallowing or fluid regurgitation through the nose should be noted.

Instruct the patient to open their mouth and utter 'Ah.' Any imbalance in palatal motions should be noted (X nerve palsy).

Gag reflex: Touch the palate, tonsil, or pharynx on one side of the patient's mouth until the patient 'gags.' Observe palatal contraction symmetry (efferent route—vagus nerve) and compare sensitivity on either side (afferent route—glossopharyngeal nerve). Determine whether the patient exhibits a loss of feeling and/or motor strength due to a lack of gag reflex. (It is impractical to assess taste in the posterior third of the tongue (the ninth nerve).)

(viii) Accessory Nerve

Sternomastoid: Request that the individual rotate their head against applied resistance. Compare the strength and size of each side's muscles. Compare the two sides by having the patient move their head forward against resistance on either side.

Note that the right sternocleidomastoid pulls the head to the left, and the left sternocleidomastoid rotates the head to the right.

Trapezius: Ask the individual to 'shrug' their shoulders and keep them in place against resistance. Compare the strength of each side. Any attempt to depress the shoulders should be resisted by the patient.

(ix) Hypoglossal Nerve

Instruct the individual to open his or her mouth; then, examine their tongue.

Search for atrophy (wasting, increased folds, etc.) as well as fibrillation.

Request that the person expose their tongue. Make a note of any difficulties or deviations. (Note that an apparent deviation can occur in the case of seventh-nerve palsy; if this is the case, evaluate the tongue in relation to the patient's teeth.)

Note whether the patient's protruding tongue deviates toward their weak side.

A tongue that is not protruded cannot travel to the contralateral side.

In this case, the extent of dysphagia and dysarthria is minimal.

2.1.3. Examination—Superior Extremities

(i) Motor System Examination

Appearance (Inspect the Bulk of the Muscle)

Tone of the muscle: Ensure that the individual is calm before assessing their muscle tone by flexing and extending their wrist or elbow alternately.

Muscle Power

Muscle weakness must be evaluated. The grade of weakness is 'scored' utilizing the Medical Research Council (MRC) grading scale.

Grade 0—There are no contractions;
Grade 1—Flickering movement;
Grade 2—Active movement when the effects of gravity are negated;
Grade 3—Active movement is possible against gravity;
Grade 4—Active movement is possible against gravity and resistance;
Grade 5—Normal muscle power.

The following test is simple, rapid, and sensitive if an upper-motor-neuron weakness is suspected (i.e., a weakness resulting from an injury to the descending motor tracts or the motor cortex).

Have the patient hold their arms outstretched and have their hands supinated for up to one minute. The patient's eyes should be shut to negate visual compensation. The weak arm will pronate and slip down with time.

[With the possibility of involvement at the spinal nerve or root level (lower motor neuron), various muscle groups must be tested to assist in identifying the lesion. Consider the nerve and root supply when assessing muscle groups.]

(ii) Sensory System

Pain: A simple approach to checking this essential modality is to prick the patient with a sterilized pin. Ensure that the patient perceives the pin as 'sharp', i.e., painful, before swiftly testing each dermatome.

It is important to note that 'C7' extends down to the middle finger, as this information makes it easier to remember the dermatome distribution. If the pin prick is impeded, map out the extent of the anomaly more carefully, progressing from abnormal to normal locations.

Light touch: A wisp of cotton wool is used to test this response in a similar way.

Temperature: Temperature testing rarely gives you any further information. Utilize a cold object or hot and cold test tubes as necessary.

Joint position sense: Demonstrate 'up and down' movements by gripping the sides of the patient's thumb or finger. With the patient's eyes shut, repeat the procedure. Request that the patient define the movements' direction. With their eyes closed, have the patient touch the tip of their nose with their fingertips or put their forefingers together with their arms outstretched.

Vibration: Place a 128 c/s tuning fork (vibrating) on a bony prominence such as the radius. Request that the patient indicate when the vibrations, if any, have stopped. If you are having trouble, move closer and try again. Vibration testing is useful for detecting demyelinating illness and peripheral neuropathy early on, but it has limited utility elsewhere.

If the aforementioned sensory perceptions are normal but a brain lesion is suspected, tests of the following abilities should be performed:

Two-point discrimination—the ability to distinguish between two blunt points that are applied to a finger at the same time and are 5 mm apart (4 cm for the legs);

Sensory inattention or perceptual rivalry—the inability to notice stimuli (touches or pin pricks) in both limbs at the same time.

Stereognosis—the ability to recognize objects that have been placed in one's hand.

Graphesthesia—the capacity to discern numbers or letters sketched out on one's palm.

(iii) Reflexes

- Biceps jerk;
- Triceps jerk;
- Supinator jerk.

Hoffman's sign: When the examiner flicks the middle finger's fingernail down, the Hoffman reflex induces an involuntary flexion movement of the thumb as well as perhaps the index finger. The thumb flexes and adducts swiftly as a result of the reflexive pathway.

Reflex enhancement: When it is difficult to elicit reflexes, the patient's reflexes can be enhanced by asking them to 'clench their teeth'.

(iv) Co-Ordination

[Ataxia (lack of coordination) is a common symptom of cerebellar illness. Make sure that the patient's proprioception and muscle power are normal before proceeding with this test.]

- Incoordination
- Finger–nose test: Request that the patient touch the tip of their nose with their finger (with their eyes open).

Watch for jerky movements, which could indicate an intention tremor or dysmetria (tremor solely happening on voluntary movements).

Ask the individual to touch the tip of their nose and then your finger as quickly as they can. This can amplify the intention tremor and reveal dysdiadochokinesia, which is the incapability to execute fast alternating motions.

This can also be revealed by having the patient pronate and supinate their forearms quickly or by performing rapid and repetitive tapping movements.

2.1.4. Examination—Trunk

Test light touches and pin pricks in dermatomal distribution as executed for the superior extremities.

Levels to remember:

T5 dermatome—at the nipple level;
T10 dermatome—at the umbilicus level;
T12 dermatome—in the inguinal ligament area.

Abdominal reflexes: Roots T7 to T12 correspond to abdominal reflexes. In each quadrant, lightly scratch or stroke the skin toward the umbilicus. Look for abdominal muscular contractions and record whether they are present or not. (Note that reflexes may not be triggered in cases of obesity, abdominal surgery, or pregnancy.) L1 and L2 are the roots corresponding to the cremasteric reflex. Scratch the inside of the patient's thigh. Observe the testicular elevation caused by the contraction of the cremasteric muscle.

Sphincters: Look for a swollen bladder in the patient's abdomen.

Incontinence, with respect to either urine or feces, should be noted.

During a rectal examination, pay attention to the tone of the anal sphincter.

Roots S4 and S5 correspond to the anal reflexes. A scratch on the skin near the anus causes the anal sphincter to contract reflexively.

2.1.5. Examination—Lower Limbs

(i) Motor System Examination

- Bulk of muscles
- Tone of muscles

Alternate flexing and extending the knee joint while attempting to relax the patient. Take note of the opposition.

Roll the individual's legs from side to side. Then, lift the thigh abruptly and notice the response in the lower leg. The leg kicks will become higher as tone increases.

Clonus: Ensure that the patient is at ease. Ankle flexion should be rapid and sustained. In a typical person, a few oscillatory movements may occur, but if this motion continues, it indicates that tone is increased.

Power of muscle: When examining each muscle group using the MRC scale, nerve and root supply should be kept in mind.

(ii) Sensory System Examination

- Pain
- Light touch
- Joint position sense: To begin, demonstrate the extension and flexion of the big toe. Then, with the patient's eyes closed, ask them to select the direction.

  Test the joint sense of the ankle in the same way if it is lacking.
- Vibration: Place a vibrating tuning fork on the malleolus to test vibration perception. Move upward to the fibular head or the anterior superior iliac spine if the effect is insufficient.

(iii) Reflexes

Knee jerk: Roots L2, L3, and L4. Rest the patient's leg on your arm or hang it over the side of the bed to ensure that it is relaxed. With a hammer, tap the patellar tendon and watch the quadriceps contract. Make a note of any exaggeration or impairment.

Ankle jerk: Roots S1 and S2.Rotate the patient's leg from the outside. Maintain a modest dorsiflexion of the foot. Palpate the tibialis anterior tendon to ensure the foot is relaxed. No ankle jerk will be evoked if this is taut.

Look for contraction of the calf muscle as well as plantarflexion as you tap the Achilles tendon.

Reflex enhancement: Jendrassik's maneuver—when the elicitation of reflexes is difficult, ask the individual to clench his or her teeth or attempt to pull clinched hands apart.

Plantar response: Make sure the patient's big toe is not tense. Stroke the ball of the foot and the lateral aspect of the sole. Take note of the big toe's first movement. Flexibility should be observed.

A pyramidal lesion is characterized by an extension caused by the contraction of the extensor hallucis longus (a 'Babinski' reflex). This is generally accompanied by synchronized knee flexor and tensor fascia lata contractions.

Stimulate the lateral border of the foot to elicit Chaddock's reflex. In the case of upper motor neuron lesions, the big toe expands.

To avoid misinterpretation, avoid touching the sole's interior part or the toes themselves.

2.1.6. Examination of Gait and Posture

Co-Ordination

Request that the individual run his or her heel from the contralateral knee down the shin to their big toe several times. Observe if there is a lack of coordination (ataxia). Request that the patient touch the floor with his or her foot many times. Any dysdiadochokinesia should be noted (difficulty with quickly alternating movements).

Romberg's Test

Request that the individual stand with their heels and feet together and their eyes open and then closed.

Gait

Note the following:

- The width of the patient's stance and the length of their steps;
- Improper leg movements (like unproportionate high steps);
- Instability of gait (gait ataxia);
- Postural motions associated with gait (like pelvic swinging).

Ask the patient to repeat tandem walking, i.e., heel to toe, if their gait is normal. Any instabilities will be amplified as a result.

2.1.7. Signs of Meningeal Irritation

a. Instruct the individual to extend and flex his or her neck.
b. Flex and stretch the individual's neck passively.
c. Kernig's signature.
d. Brudzinski's signature.
e. Check for felt stiffness when moving either actively or passively.

2.2. Examination of an Unconscious Patient

2.2.1. History

Questioning family members, friends, or the ambulance crew is an important component of evaluating an unconscious or uncooperative patient.

Has the patient suffered head trauma recently or in the weeks leading up to admission?

Did the patient pass out unexpectedly?

Was there any limb twitching?

Has the patient had any symptoms in the last several weeks?

Does the patient have a history of systemic sickness?

Is the patient on any kind of medication?

2.2.2. General Examination

General examination is not limited by a lack of patient cooperation, and this may reveal crucial diagnostic signals. Search for signs of needle marks on the arm, a head injury, and proof of tongue biting during a routine medical examination. Take notice of the scent of alcohol as well, but be wary of blaming the patient's clinical condition exclusively on excessive alcohol use.

2.2.3. Neurological Examination

Consciousness Level

This evaluation is extremely important. It provides a baseline against which subsequent tests can be compared, as well as an instant prognostic reference. Examine the patient's consciousness level in terms of spontaneous eye opening, verbal reaction, and motor response, as described previously. It is critical to avoid the temptation of just quoting the patient's overall score, as this information could be deceptive. Avoid any confusion over numbers by assessing the patient's awareness level in terms of real responses, such as 'no eye opening, extension, and no verbal response'.

Eye Movements

Keep an eye out for any unexpected eyeball movements.

The doll's eye (oculocephalic) response should be elicited.

In a comatose patient, flexion/extension or rotation of the head causes transitory eye movements in the contralateral direction of the movement. Observe whether the movements are dysconjugate (i.e., the eyes move in opposite directions) or conjugate (i.e., the eyes move in unison). The midbrain and pontine functions are assessed using these ocular movements.

The oculovestibular reflex should be elicited (caloric testing).

Visual Fields

When 'grimacing' from one side does not cause a 'blink,' the clinician may find a hemianopic field defect in an uncooperative patient.

Facial Weakness

In reaction to bilateral supraorbital pain, the failure to produce a 'grimace' on one side indicates facial weakness.

Limb Weakness

Limb weakness can be identified by comparing the limbs' responses to painful stimuli. A limb weakness is present if pain causes an asymmetric response. (If the person 'localizes' with one upper limb, hold it down and retest to check that the other limb does not have a comparable response.) A pain stimulus delivered to the Achilles tendon or toenails can be used to assess lower-extremity power in a similar way. A localized neuro-deficit is also indicated by differences in tone, plantar responses, or reflexes on each side. In fact, these supplementary features rarely provide persuasive evidence if the clinician is unable to notice a change in response to a painful stimulus.

2.3. Examination of Pediatric Patients

At all ages, including pediatric age, a detailed yet focused history as well as neurological examination are the most crucial first parts of neurological disease diagnosis. Even for a pediatric neurologist and surgeon, neurological examinations of patients in particular pediatric age groups are complex and challenging. Advances in clinical neurophysiology, genetics, neuroimaging, and neuropathological examination have appeared to supplant traditional history taking and physical examination at times in the last two decades; however, no laboratory study can provide the same clues and focus to a diagnosis that clinical findings can. History taking as well as neurological examination procedures are techniques that must be learnt as a student, polished as a resident, and practiced and perfected throughout the carrier of a pediatric neurologist and pediatric neurosurgeon. Furthermore, to localize the value of particular indications that may be applicable to all ages, examinations must be particularly tailored to match age and with the expected developmental skills attained at distinct ages. Extensor plantar responses, hypotonia, and a lack of visual focus may be typical among premature babies, but they are abnormal beyond a few months. "Primitive" reflexes appear to vanish after a certain age, but they are actually inhibited or suppressed and can be re-expressed with disinhibition decades later (Haslam 2013). The details of pediatric neurological examination are outside the scope of this book.

2.4. Examination for Dementia

2.4.1. Mini Mental State Examination (MMSE)

Name:
Date Of Birth:
Hospital Number:

One point is scored for each answer.

	Date:		
ORIENTATION			
Year Season Month Date Time	.../5	.../5	.../5
Country Town District Hospital Ward/Floor	.../5	.../5	.../5
REGISTRATION The examiner names three things (for example, an apple, a table, and a penny) and asks the patient to repeat them (1 point is given for each correct response). Then, the patient repeats the three names until they are correct).	.../3	.../3	.../3
ATTENTION AND CALCULATION Subtract 7 from 100, and then subtract 7 again from the result. Repeat steps 100, 93, 86, 79, and 65 five times more. (Another option is to write "WORLD" backwards: DLROW.)	.../5	.../5	.../5
RECALL Inquire about the three objects you learned about previously.	.../3	.../3	.../3
LANGUAGE			
Ask for the names of two objects (e.g., pen, watch, etc.).	.../2	.../2	.../2
Ask the patient to repeat the phrase "No ifs, ands, or buts".	.../1	.../1	.../1
Give a command that has three stages. Each stage is worth one point. (For example, "Place your right index finger on your nose and then on your left ear").	.../3	.../3	.../3
Request that the patient read and follow a written command written on a piece of paper (e.g., "Close your eyes").	.../1	.../1	.../1
Request that the patient write a sentence. If it is logical and has a subject and a verb, it is given a score of 1.	.../1	.../1	.../1

	Date:		
COPYING: Solicit a pair of intersecting pentagons from the patient. 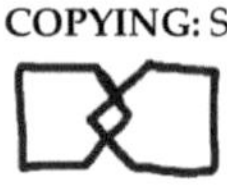	.../1	.../1	.../1
Total:	.../30	.../30	.../30

MMSE scoring:

- 24–30: no cognitive impairment;
- 18–23: mild cognitive impairment;
- 0–17: severe cognitive impairment.

3. Neurosurgery and Its Branches

Neurosurgery, or surgical neurology or neurological surgery, is the branch of medicine that focuses on the prevention, diagnosis, surgical management, and rehabilitation of illnesses of the neurological system, including the brain and skull, spine and spinal cord, peripheral nerves, and neurovascular system.

General neurosurgery is used for treating the majority of neurosurgical issues, encompassing neurotrauma and other neuro-emergencies like cerebral hemorrhages. In the majority of level 1 hospitals, this practice is standard. (American Association of Neurological Surgeons 2012; Esposito et al. 2005).

To handle unusual and difficult situations, specialized departments have been expanded. These specializations coexist with general neurosurgery in more modern hospitals. A neurosurgeon who wishes to practice an advanced specialization in neurosurgery must undergo an additional one to two years of fellowship training.

The branches or divisions of neurosurgery are as follows:

1. Vascular neurosurgery, which includes the surgical clipping of aneurysms, the excision of AVM, the closure of A-V fistula, cerebrovascular bypasses, carotid endarterectomies (CEAs), etc.;
2. Stereotactic neurosurgery and functional neurosurgery, which are used to treat Parkinson's diseases and other movement disorders, spasticity, dystonia, intractable psychiatric disorders, and intractable pain by making lesions in the brain or stimulating it (DBS—deep-brain stimulation);
3. Epilepsy surgery (which includes: 1. a partial or total corpus callosotomy—disconnecting part or all of the corpus callosum to lessen or stop seizure spread and activity and 2. the surgical removal of operable, physiological, and/or anatomical parts or divisions of the brain known to be epileptic foci that cause seizures, as well as the more radical and incredibly rare partial or total lobectomy, or even hemispherectomy—the removal of part or all of one of the brain's lobes or cerebral hemispheres— all of which are ways to stop or lessen seizure spread and activity).
4. Oncological neurosurgery, sometimes known as neurosurgical oncology, is used to treat both benign and malignant central as well as peripheral nervous system cancers in both children and adults, as well as precancerous lesions (including, among others, glioblastoma multiforme and other gliomas; brain stem astrocytoma; brain stem cancer; pontine glioma; tumors of the meninges; medulloblastoma; spinal cancer; secondary metastases of the brain, spine, and nerves; and peripheral nervous system tumors)
5. Skull base surgery
6. Spinal neurosurgery
7. Peripheral nerve surgery
8. Pediatric neurosurgery (for tumors, epilepsy, bleeding, stroke, cognitive functional disorders, or congenital neurosurgical disorders)
9. Endoscopic and minimally invasive neurosurgery
10. Endovascular or interventional neurosurgery
11. Neuro-radiosurgery (stereotactic, gamma knife, and cyber knife)
12. Neuro-robotics (new and developing)
13. Neuro-stem cell transplantation (new and developing)

Funding: This research received no external funding.

Conflicts of Interest: The author declares no conflicts of interest.

References

American Association of Neurological Surgeons. 2012. Ensuring an Adequate Neurosurgical Workforce for the 21st Century. Available online: https://www.aans.org/wp-content/uploads/aans_files/AANS/Advocacy/2012%20News/NeurosurgeryIOMGMEPaper121912.pdf (accessed on 19 December 2012).

Esposito, Thomas J., R. Lawrence II Reed, Richard L. Gamelli, and Fred A. Luchette. 2005. Neurosurgical Coverage: Essential, Desired, or Irrelevant for Good Patient Care and Trauma Center Status. *Transactions of the Meeting of the American Surgical Association* 123: 67–76. [CrossRef] [PubMed]

Haslam, Robert H. A. 2013. Clinical neurological examination of infants and children. *Handbook of Clinical Neurology* 111: 17–25. [CrossRef] [PubMed]

Lindsay, Kenneth W., Ian Bone, and Geraint Fuller. 2011. *Neurology and Neurosurgery Illustrated. General Approach to History and Examination*. London: Elsevier.

Teasdale, Graham, and Bryan Jennett. 1974. Assessment of coma and impaired consciousness. *Lancet* 2: 81–84. [CrossRef] [PubMed]

Teasdale, Graham, and Bryan Jennett. 1976. Assessment and prognosis of coma after head injury. *Acta Neurochirurgica* 34: 45–55. [CrossRef] [PubMed]

Walker, H. Kenneth. 1990. An Overview of the Nervous System. In *Clinical Methods: The History, Physical, and Laboratory Examinations*. Edited by H. Kenneth Walker, W. Dallas Hall and J. Willis Hurst. Boston: Butterworths.

Section II: Neuroanesthesia

Neuroanesthesia and Related Aspects

Syed Ariful Islam, Aminul Hasanat, Muhammad Shamsul Arefin and Forhad H. Chowdhury

Abstract: Neurosurgical procedures are now quite safe due to invaluable advances in neuroanesthesia techniques. During an operation, the maintenance of low ICP is essential both for anesthesiologists and neurosurgeons. So, the basics of ICP and details of the causes of raised ICP as well as its management are described in the first part of this section. The pharmacological drugs utilized for neuroanesthesia are described shortly after, and the steps of practically inducing neuroanesthesia are also mentioned. Inducing neuroanesthesia in special situations (such as aneurysm surgery, sitting-position surgery, post-fossa surgery, etc.) is also discussed in this chapter. Finally, an account of awake craniotomy is also provided in brief.

Abbreviations

ADH	antidiuretic hormone	ICA	internal carotid artery
AVM	arterio-venous malformation	ICP	intracranial pressure
BBB	blood–brain barrier	ICU	intensive care unit
CBF	cerebral blood flow	MAC	minimum alveolar concentration
CBV	cerebral blood volume	MAP	mean arterial pressure
CMRO2	cerebral metabolic rate of O2	NMDA	N-methyl D-aspartate
CNS	central nervous system	NO	nitric oxide
CPR	cardiopulmonary resuscitation	NPPB	normal perfusion pressure breakthrough
CPP	cerebral perfusion pressure	OSA	obstructive sleep apnea
CSF	cerebrospinal fluid	PEEP	positive end-expiratory pressure
CSWS	cerebral salt wasting syndrome	PVC	premature ventricular contraction
CT	computed tomography	SIADH	secretion of inappropriate ADH
CVP	cerebral venous pressure	TBI	traumatic brain injury
DBS	deep-brain stimulation	TIVA	total intravenous anesthesia
DI	diabetes insipidus	VA	ventriculo-atrial
DPH	delayed postoperative hemorrhage	VAE	venous air embolism
EEG	electro-encephalo gram	VT	ventricular tachycardia
HDU	high-dependency unit		

1. Neuro-Anesthesia

1.1. Introduction

The disordered physiology caused by neurosurgical disease and the special demands of neurosurgical techniques pose unique challenges for a neuro-anesthesiologist. The brain is contained in a rigid, closed box, and its function is highly dependent on the (relatively constant) maintenance of the cerebral blood flow within that confined area. Any cerebral injuries and the disease process may jeopardize cerebral circulation in ways that predispose one to cerebral ischemia and ultimately neuronal damage. Anesthetic drugs and techniques have significant effects on both the physiology and pathology of the brain. The alterations they produce in cerebral function can be used to ensure good operating conditions for neurosurgery and to limit the extent of potential perioperative neuronal damage. On the other hand, failure to practice these standard methods in a proper contextual way may lead to disastrous consequences. Modern drugs and monitoring systems grant an anesthesiologist considerable control over cerebral and cardiovascular functions; as a result, many surgical procedures that had been considered very risky even a few decades ago have become routine practices for today's neurosurgeon.

1.2. Disorders of ICP

1.2.1. The Intracranial Pressure

The skull is essentially a closed box containing the brain, which weighs about 1400 g in an adult, and about 150 mL of cerebrospinal fluid (CSF), of which half is in the cranial space and the other half is in the spinal CSF space. The brain (and the spinal cord) also contains a significant amount of both arterial and venous blood in a dynamic state. The cerebral metabolic demand regulates cerebral blood flow (CBF), which is roughly 50 mL per 100 g of brain per minute (on average). Inside the skull vault, a distinct pressure called intracranial pressure (ICP) exists, with a normal value of up to 2 kPa (15 mm Hg). This pressure is the result of many interacting forces, including CSF dynamics, and arterial pressure forcing blood into the skull.

1.2.2. Raised ICP

The four intracranial constituents (brain, CSF, arterial blood, and venous blood), two of which are essentially solid and liquid, are incompressible, but two of them (CSF and venous blood) are connected with low-pressure systems outside the skull. Once intracranial space occupation begins due to any tumor, hematoma, or abscess, the process of a rise in ICP starts (Table 1). The mechanisms that compensate for the presence of a SOL rely on these extracranial connections. As the SOL develops, intracranial CSF is lost to the spinal space of the CSF, and venous blood from the thin-walled cerebral veins is lost to the great veins in the chest. The ICP does not, therefore, rise in the early stages of intracranial space occupation. There is a limit to the amount of space occupation that can be accommodated in this way; once, this limit is reached, the ICP shoots up. The Monroe–Kellie Doctrine addresses this issue, and, according to this theory, the contents of the skull are in a constant-volume state. The total volumes of brain tissues, cerebrospinal fluid (CSF), and intracranial blood are fixed in this way. When the volume of one component is increased, the volume of one or two of the other components is reduced. A decrease in cerebral blood flow or a herniation of the brain is a clinical indication of a component's volume change.

Table 1. Etiologies of intracranial hypertension.

Primary or Intracranial	Secondary or Extracranial (Mostly Related to Faults in the Technique Employed)
Brain neoplasm	Airway obstruction
Trauma (epidural and subdural hematomas, cerebral contusions)	Inadequate muscle relaxation
Nontraumatic brain hemorrhage	Positive end expiratory pressure (PEEP)
Cerebral infarction	Raised Intrathoracic pressure
Hydrocephalus	Hypercarbia or hypoxia
Idiopathic intracranial hypertension	Hypotension (hypovolemia) or hypertension (pain/cough)
Other (example—pneumocephalus, abscesses, cysts)	Volume overload
	Posture (head rotation, Trendelenburg position)
	Hyperpyrexia
	Seizures
	Drug and metabolic (such as, vasodilators)

Source: Table by authors.

If a patient afflicted with such a condition is not treated, the cycle will continue until the patient dies from neurological impairment or a catastrophic herniation. Acute elevations in ICP (plateau waves) lasting 1 to 15 minutes can be linked to periodic rises in arterial blood pressure with a reduction in reflex heart rate (the Cushing response).

The volume of the posterior fossa is much lower than that of the supratentorial space. Any SOL developing in this compartment shows a sharp rise in ICP partly because of its lower volume and partly because it may obstruct CSF flow and hence lead to hydrocephalus at a very early stage.

In patients with a traumatic brain injury (TBI), special aspects should be examined, as lesions might be varied and numerous variables can lead to an increase in ICP (Adelson et al. 2003):

1. Traumatically caused masses—hematomas in the epidural or subdural space, hemorrhagic contusions, foreign bodies, and depressed skull fractures;

2. Cerebral edema;

3. Hyperemia due to vasomotor paralysis or autoregulation loss;

4. Hypoventilation with consequent hypercarbia and cerebral vasodilation;

5. Hydrocephalus caused by a blockage in the route taken by the CSF or its absorption;

6. Mechanical ventilation, posturing, agitation, or Valsalva maneuvers, which result in increased intrathoracic or intra-abdominal pressure.

Vascular engorgement was assumed to be the most important cause of elevated ICP after the evacuation of traumatic mass lesions. According to recent research, cerebral edema is the primary cause in the majority of instances.

Three to ten days after suffering trauma, a secondary increase in ICP is frequently noted, primarily as a result of delayed hematoma formation, such as in the case of epidural hematomas, acute subdural hematomas, and traumatic hemorrhagic contusions with surrounding edema, which may necessitate evacuation (Unterberg et al. 1993). Cerebral vasospasm (Taneda et al. 1996), hypoventilation, and hyponatremia are all possible causes of delayed elevations in ICP.

1.2.3. Symptom and Signs of Raised ICP

A raised ICP (Table 1), either preexisting or developed during anesthesia or surgery, always puts the patient in great danger. In the preoperative assessment of a patient for neuroanesthesia, the issue of raised ICP should always be considered. Although many individuals with high ICP are asymptomatic at first, they eventually develop symptoms and signs such headaches, nausea, vomiting, papilledema, localized neurological impairments, and altered consciousness.

The clinical findings of raised ICP need to be distinguished from those as to the original lesion that produced the raised ICP. Miller suggested that headache, vomiting, papilledema, and drowsiness are the symptoms and signs likely to be due to raised ICP alone, whereas bradycardia, arterial hypertension, and papillary changes, although often occurring together with raised ICP, may arise from brainstem distortion or ischemia (Turner 2003).

1.2.4. Management of Raised ICP

Goals of Therapy

1. Keep the patient's ICP between 20 and 25 mm Hg.
2. Maintain a cerebral perfusion pressure (CPP) of greater than 60 mm Hg by keeping mean arterial pressure (MAP) at a healthy level.
3. Avoid anything that aggravates or causes an increase in ICP.

An outline of the diagnosis and treatment of raised intracranial pressure is shown in Figure 1.

1.3. Pharmacology Related to Neuroanesthesia

1.3.1. Intravenous Anesthetic Agents

Propofol

This drug is the most recent intravenous anesthetic drug in clinical use. It was discovered in 1977 and approved for clinical use in the America in 1989. Over the past few decades, it has replaced thiopental as the leading anesthetic agent mostly because of its excellent kinetic and dynamic profile that is closer to the ideal profile, suitable for short and prolonged use for both anesthesia and sedation (Table 2). Propofol is an alkyl phenol (2,6-isopropylphenol) and highly lipid-soluble; hence, it rapidly crosses the blood–brain barrier (BBB), causing sedation and hypnosis in a dose-dependent manner. However, its amnesic affect is greater in comparison with that of barbiturates and benzodiazepines, and a very high infusion rate may be required to prevent waking if used as the sole anesthetic (Glass 1993).

The electroencephalogram (EEG)-related effects of increasing the propofol concentration include transient beta excitation at low doses followed by a concentration-dependent decrease in median EEG frequency and an increase in EEG amplitude, leading to burst suppression at blood concentrations greater than 8 μg/mL. Propofol also increases the latency and decreases the amplitude of cortical middle-latency auditory evoked potentials in a dose-dependent manner (Thronton et al. 1989).

Although much less frequently than barbiturates and etomidate, propofol has been associated with some excitatory effects, which include occasional involuntary movements, myoclonus, dystonic posturing, and opisthotonos. They are subcortical in origin and do not show any features of epilepsy in an EEG. Propofol has dose-dependent anticonvulsant activity and has been successfully used to control status epilepticus (Rushton and Sneyd 2003).

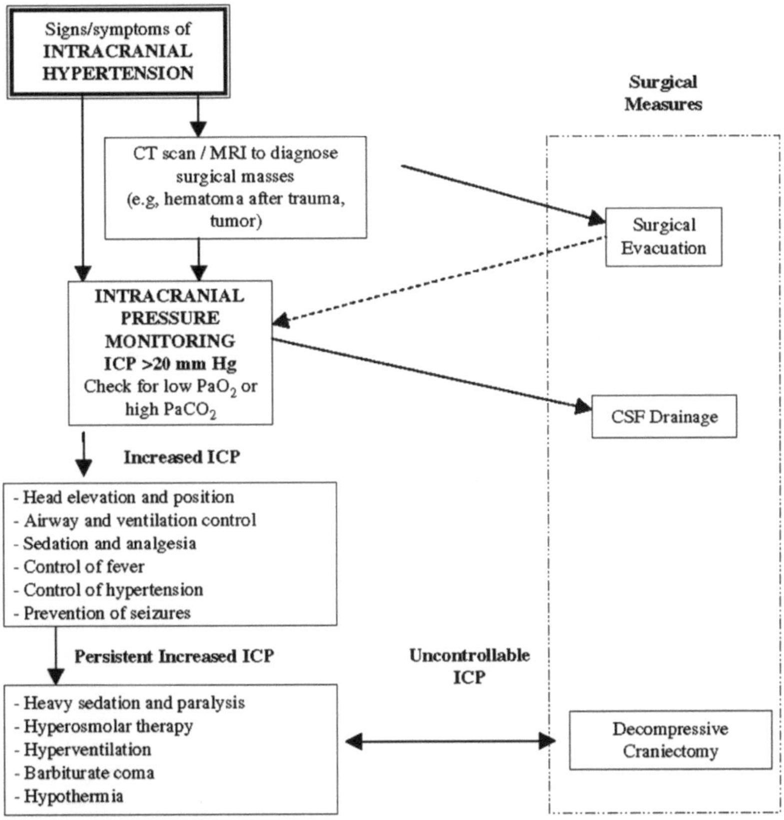

Figure 1. Outline of diagnosis and treatment of raised intracranial pressure. Source: Figure reprinted from Rangel-Castillo et al. (2008), used with permission.

Table 2. Summary of the advantages and disadvantages of this remarkable anesthetic (Propofol).

Advantages	Disadvantages
Pleasant sedation and recovery Rapid onset and easy titration Suitable for both induction as well as maintenance of anesthesia Suppression of airway reflexes Antiemetic effect Safe for patients with porphyria	Pain upon injection It is a lipid emulsion carrier, so it supports bacterial growth Possibility of hypotension, especially with limited cardiovascular reserve. Expensive

Source: Authors' compilation based on data from Rushton and Sneyd (2003).

Propofol reduces cerebral oxygen consumption (cerebral metabolic rate of O2-CMRO2) and cerebral blood flow (CBF), ultimately decreasing ICP in patients with normal or raised ICP. In one study, researchers observed a 32% reduction in CSF pressure following a 1.5 mg/kg bolus injection (Ravussin et al. 1998). Cerebral autoregulation and reactivity to CO_2 are preserved, but MAP and CPP may fall in case of major cardiovascular depression. Propofol can induce a significant drop in CPP (50 mmHg) in patients with high ICP unless measures are taken to sustain mean arterial blood pressure (Butterworth et al. 2013).

Barbiturates

Because of their exceedingly brief duration of action, ultra-short-acting barbiturates are frequently utilized for anesthesia. After their introduction in 1930s, barbiturates, especially thiopental, played a pivotal role in the field of intravenous anesthesia. Although propofol has largely supplanted their role in modern anesthesia, barbiturates (particularly thiopental) still have a prestigious status, especially when neuroprotection is an issue.

Thiopental and methohexital are the only two agents from the barbiturate family that are still being used as intravenous hypnotic agents. Both lead to a decrease in brain electrical activity and metabolism (Box 1). Thiopental depresses CMRO2 in a dose-related manner to a maximum of 55% of the conscious levels when the EEG becomes flat. No further fall in CMRO2 is observed if more thiopental is given. Reduced CMRO2 causes reduced CBF that results in a fall in ICP, and there is evidence that this fall is greater when the ICP is high. CPP is usually maintained or slightly reduced, giving some benefit to the patients with raised ICP.

Both the barbiturates affect EEG results in a dose-dependent manner. The awake α pattern progresses to a higher amplitude and has a slower frequency δ and slower θ waves until burst suppression precedes a flat EEG. Thiopental is a potent anticonvulsant, but methohexital possesses proconvulsant properties (Reddy et al. 1993).

Box 1. Summary of the neuroprotective properties of thiopental.

Decreases CMRO2, CBF and ICP Potent hypnotic with good CVS profile Potent anticonvulsant Antiepileptic Free radical scavenger of CNS (Smith et al. 1980) Facilitates CSF absorption

Etomidate

Etomidate is an imidazole (an organic aromatic heterocyclic compound) derivative. Its ability to quickly induce hypnosis and cause minimal respiratory depression and its high therapeutic index for cardiovascular side-effects make it a good choice during the rapid sequence induction of a compromised patient. A high incidence of myoclonus (50–80%) is observed during the induction of hypnosis in the absence of premedication. It causes increased EEG activity in epileptogenic foci, and this finding has been used during intraoperative mapping prior to surgical ablation. However, in patients receiving etomidate who have no previous history of epilepsy, no clinical or EEG evidence of epileptic seizures has been found; rather, it exhibits potent anticonvulsant characteristics (Modica et al. 1990). Etomidate reduces CBF (36%) and CMRO2 (45%) and thus ICP, but because decreases in CBF occur before decreases in cerebral metabolic activity, there is a risk of cerebral ischemia in areas of critical perfusion.

Increased mortality in a group of patients sedated with etomidate infusions in an ICU was associated with low cortisol levels and attributed to etomidate-induced suppression of adrenal cortisol synthesis. However, the effect of a single bolus is short-lived (6 to 8 h), and the corresponding clinical significance is unclear; hence, etomidate is safe to use for the induction of anesthesia and short-term maintenance (Ledingham and Watt 1993).

Ketamine

Ketamine is the only phencyclidine derivative available for clinical use, and this group of drugs is characterized by an unusual "dissociative" anesthetic state, strong analgesic property, cardiorespiratory stability, and a troublesome emergence phenomenon.

The endpoint of induction is not distinct; in the unique cataleptic state, patients' eyes may remain wide open, and cranial nerve reflexes are more or less preserved, although not necessarily protective. Ketamine bears a complex neuropharmacology. Noncompetitive antagonism of glutamate at N-methyl D-aspartate (NMDA) ligand-gated calcium channels accounts for most of its anesthetic, analgesic, amnestic, and psychomimetic effects. Ketamine also interacts with non-NMDA glutamate receptors, including cholinergic, adrenergic, and opioid receptors. Its ability to inhibit neuronal voltage-dependent sodium channels gives it a local-anesthetic property.

Ketamine increases both CMRO2 and CBF (50–60%) and thereby ICP. This phenomenon is particularly marked in the presence of an intracranial pathology, and it is not coupled with a sympathetically mediated rise in MAP. So, it is conventionally contraindicated for patients with intracranial pathology or if there is a raised ICP.

However, ketamine-induced raised ICP can be attenuated by reducing the P_aCO2 concentration through hyperventilation or using the depressant effects of other intravenous anesthetic drugs. Additionally, according to some investigators, Ketamine may have a neuroprotective effect. Ketamine's blockade of NMDA receptors during periods of increased glutamate concentrations, as commonly found in TBI, may be protective against neuronal cell death.

Emergence reactions include vivid dreams, weird expressions, illusions, and body-image alterations occurring during the first hour of recovery. The incidence of these reactions is higher in adults than in children and in women compared with men, and the psychomimetic side-effects are aggravated by centrally active anticholinergic drugs, including atropine. Premedication with benzodiazepines or a combination of propofol and ketamine are good remedies for these undesirable side effects (Butterworth et al. 2018a).

Benzodiazepines

The primary role of benzodiazepines in anesthesia is sedation and the supplementation of an opioid. Although they have potent sedative, amnestic, and anticonvulsive properties, they provide slow-onset, poor-quality anesthesia when given alone. Their wide range of central effects also includes anxiolysis and centrally mediated muscle relaxation.

Benzodiazepines induce a dose-related decrease in cerebral metabolism as well as cerebral blood circulation and thus should have a beneficial effect on ICP, but hypercarbia and hypoxia from their sedative–depressive effect may cause a dangerous rise in ICP in a patient with compromised intracranial compliance (Butterworth et al. 2018b).

Even though both diazepam and midazolam are excellent anticonvulsants in clinical use, midazolam is the only benzodiazepine suitable for induction during anesthesia and procedural sedation, especially in the case of neuroanesthesia, where an early and clearheaded recovery is highly desirable.

1.3.2. Volatile Anesthetic Agents

Volatile anesthetic agents tend to uncouple the relation between CMRO2 and CBF. This action is well demonstrated by the action of halothane: 1% halothane induces a 26-percent drop in CMRO2 but also a 27-percent increase in CBF and hence a significant increase in ICP (Christensen et al. 1967). Low concentrations of halothane (a mean alveolar concentration (MAC) of 0.6) have little effect on the CBF, but an MAC of 1.1 may triple its effect.

Both isoflurane and sevoflurane are modern ethers and affect the CBF in a less harmful way than halothane (the only hydrocarbon still in use for clinical anesthesia), and both agents significantly reduce CMRO2. However, the cerebral vasodilator effect of sevoflurane is quite a bit weaker than that of isoflurane, and this vapor may be of considerable value in neuroanesthesia because of its low blood gas solubility that allows prompt induction and early recovery.

Sevoflurane and isoflurane cause similar dose-dependent changes in EEG; as the concentration of vapor increases towards an MAC of 1, there is an increase in the voltage amplitude and frequency of the EEG, but above this concentration, both frequency and amplitude start to decrease. Burst suppression occurs at an MAC of 1.5, and at an MAC of 2, the EEG becomes flat.

Nitrous oxide (NO) is the only anesthetic drug that has been used continuously and safely for clinical anesthesia for nearly the last 175 years. It is an inert agent that is not metabolized but induces excellent perioperative analgesia and has a good recovery profile.

However, there are also debates over the use of nitrous oxide to treat the general neurosurgical population; for example, some researchers believe there is a link between nitrous oxide and the development of tension pneumocephalus after surgery, as nitrous oxide may diffuse into air pockets left within the skull following closure of the wound. Moreover, it can further complicate venous air embolism (VAE) if not stopped at the beginning of this event. Like other volatile anesthetics, it induces a significant rise in CBF and ICP, and to add to its odd effects, NO can also induce a slight rise in cerebral metabolism.

1.3.3. Muscle Relaxants

All the neuromuscular blockers are highly charged, and water-soluble molecules hence do not cross the blood–brain barrier (BBB). Therefore, they should not have any direct effects on the CNS. However, the use of suxamethonium (succinylcholine) has been said to cause raised ICP, and a possible explanation for this is that fasciculation causes a rise in intra-abdominal pressure and therefore raised central venous pressure (CVP). But this may not be the entire story. Minton et al. gave succinylcholine to a patient with intracranial space occupation both before and after muscle paralysis had been established with vecuronium. When given before the patient was paralyzed, succinylcholine caused a consistent rise in ICP from a mean of 15 mmHg to 20 mmHg (5 mmHg). After vecuronium had been given, the increase generated by succinylcholine was still present, but it was smaller—with the maximum increase being only 3mmHg. The evidence suggests that increased muscle spindle activity generating afferent neuronal traffic produces an increase in cerebral activity and therefore regional CBF (Minton et al. 1986).

1.4. Practical Conduct Regarding Anesthesia for Neurosurgical Patients

1.4.1. Preanesthetic Evaluation and Preparation

Preanesthetic evaluation is a clinical assessment, risk classification, and optimization process performed before surgery in order to reduce perioperative morbidity and death. The majority of neurosurgery procedures are regarded as moderate to high-risk surgeries and warrant close communication between the surgical and anesthesia teams regarding preoperative findings and possible operative techniques. In this case, the clinical assessment should be carried out in a standard manner, but complications arising from the neurological lesion must be given extra attention; in addition, the patient's position during surgery and the special needs of neuromonitoring are other major issues that require a careful preanesthetic work-up.

1.4.2. Premedication

Heavy premedication, particularly with narcotics and sedatives, should be avoided for neurosurgical patients. Any depression in the level of consciousness or rate of respiration may cause an increase in PaCO2 levels and hence ICP. The administration of anticonvulsant and corticosteroid medication should be continued until surgery. In case of an emergency (and obviously anxiety as well), for adult patients with intracranial tumors, benzodiazepines, especially midazolam, if used in small doses, can induce calmness without affecting ventilation significantly, which will, in turn, help to achieve a sound preanesthetic hemodynamic status. Preanesthetic use of modern antiemetics anticholinergics or H2 blockers does not affect ICP in a noteworthy manner.

1.4.3. Induction of Anesthesia

For patients with a disturbed intracranial-pressure-to-volume relationship, the induction of anesthesia and endotracheal intubation are important periods, especially if a high ICP already exists. Intravenous medications such as propofol, thiopental, or etomidate, which induce a quick, dependable state of unconsciousness without raising ICP, are commonly used to induce hypnosis. Many authorities suggest modest hyperventilation at this point.

1.4.4. Intubation

Once the patient has been rendered unconscious, endotracheal intubation is performed, mostly with the help of a nondepolarizing neuromuscular blocker. The principal author has found rocuronium to be the most convenient in this regard. Succinylcholine administration has been linked to a brief increase in ICP; moreover, it may cause sudden life-threatening hyperkalemia in patients with longstanding paralysis (and many other neurologic conditions) who may have upregulated extra-junctional (premature) nicotinic receptors. However, succinylcholine remains the preferred drug for rapid sequence induction or when a difficult airway is a problem, as hypoxia and hypercarbia are far more dangerous for a patient with intracranial hypertension than the usual side effects of succinylcholine. However, patients' association with malignant hyperthermia, a relatively rare genetic disorder of skeletal muscles, still remains an absolute contraindication for using any depolarizing agent.

A direct laryngoscopy should be performed when profound neuromuscular blockade has been achieved and the patient is in a deep coma. Additional intravenous anesthetic doses, such as IV lidocaine, esmolol, fentanyl, and remifentanyl, have all been successfully utilized to reduce the response to laryngoscopy or other intraoperative stimulations such as pinion placement and skin incision. During induction, arterial hypertension raises CBV and causes cerebral edema. Sustained hypertension can cause considerable increases in ICP, lower CPP, and put one at risk of suffering brain herniation. Excessive blood pressure lowering can be equally harmful, as it impairs CPP.

1.4.5. Positioning

After intubating the trachea and checking that the tube is in the correct position, efforts are focused on establishing a safe and sound connection between the patient and the ventilator. Normally, an armored tube should be used and fixed such that the cerebral venous drainage remains totally unobstructed. Although most craniotomies are accomplished in the supine position, the prone, park bench, and sitting positions are not uncommon, and, in most cases, the skull is kept fixed using a Mayfield head holder. Here, 15–30° head elevation would aid in CSF and venous drainage, and some degree of rotation is needed for comfortable exposure; all the positioning maneuvers can potentially displace or disconnect the breathing unit. Neurosurgical operations may last for several hours, and the airway, venous access, and monitoring equipment must be instituted and secured so that they are completely reliable for the whole operative period. Because the patient's airway cannot be easily evaluated after a surgical drape, and as the operating table is frequently turned 90° or 180° away from the anesthesiologist, the chance of unexpected disconnections occurring may be increased (Butterworth et al. 2018b).

1.4.6. Maintenance of Anesthesia

Throughout the surgery, the anesthesiologist should consider the provision of good intracranial operating conditions when choosing drugs and techniques. The main aims are shown in Box 2 below (Turner 2003).

Box 2. The aims of the maintenance of anesthesia.

1. Maintaining adequate cerebral perfusion pressure
2. Maintaining stable MAP
3. Avoiding factors leading to increased ICP
    a. Hypoxia
    b. Hypercarbia
    c. vasodilating drugs
    d. cerebral venous obstruction
    e. incomplete muscle relaxation
4. Reducing brain bulk
5. Protecting against the sudden development of cerebral ischemia

Inhalation anesthesia, total intravenous techniques (TIVA), or a combination of an opioid, an intravenous hypnotic (most commonly propofol), and a low-dose-inhalation drug can all be used to maintain anesthesia. Rapid emergence and prompt neurological examination are facilitated by TIVA with remifentanil and propofol. Dexmetedomidine, alpha-2 adrenoceptor (a2-AR) agonist, can be used during both awake and unconscious craniotomies, yielding identical results (Butterworth et al. 2018a).

The volatile agents used during the maintenance of anesthesia have been subject to controversy for some time. All these volatile agents increase CBF and thereby have the potential to increase brain bulk and ICP. Some authors have shown that volatile agents may be used quite effectively as long as hyperventilation is employed at the same time. Others have suggested that this is not the case, especially if the compensatory systems for intracranial space occupation are nearing their limits.

The use of nitrous oxide in neuroanesthesia has also been an area of debate and discussion for many years. The main advantage in this regard is that by combining nitrous oxide with other anesthetics and analgesics, the dose of each drug can be minimized to a significant extent so that recovery is likely to occur faster, which may be helpful in postoperative neurological assessment. But the risk is that nitrous oxide can enter a gas-filled cavity and expand it significantly, so in the case of an event of VAE or preexisting pneumocephalus (from trauma or surgery), its effect may be highly detrimental.

Hyperventilation has been an important part of neuroanesthesia for many years because of its ability to reduce ICP by inducing cerebral vasoconstriction. This vasoconstriction also works in favor of fluid reabsorption from the cerebral extracellular space. Consequently, hyperventilation helps to provide improved operative conditions. Intraoperative surgical requirements (a reduction in brain bulk) may call for this technique, but its use in these cases risks increasing cerebral ischemia. Concerns about the fact that hyperventilation "uncoupled" the link between CMRO2 and the CBF, reducing oxygen supply without reducing metabolism, have led to a re-evaluation of this technique. Yet, some authorities suggest a mild hypocapnia (PaCO2 roughly 30–35 mmHg) and others recommend an increased PaO2 for those cases in whom vigorous hyperventilation is planned (Matta et al. 1994).

1.4.7. Intraoperative Muscle Relaxation

Muscle relaxants are typically indicated for most of the neurosurgical procedures that require general anesthesia. Patients' spontaneous movement could lead to an increase in intracranial volume and pressure, greater surgical hemorrhaging, or head and brain injuries from pinions or other surgical devices. It should be remembered that, as resurgence from muscle relaxants begins, abdominal and thoracic muscle tone will recover faster than that of the arm or leg, and a rise in intra-abdominal or intra-thoracic pressures (and therefore in CVP and ICP) may go unobserved. If the brain is found to be tight at any point in surgery, checking that venous drainage from the head is clear and unimpeded is the foremost check that should be carried out, and part of this check is to confirm adequate muscle relaxation.

1.4.8. Reversal of Muscle Relaxation and Extubation

At the end of an operation, the effects of anesthetics and muscle relaxants should have worn off or pharmacologically reversed. This enables real-time monitoring of neurologic function and the early detection of any surgery-related complications. The aim should be to ensure full recovery, but with no coughing, straining, or inadequate breathing events. To avoid the hazards of these potentially dangerous incidences, the reversal of muscle relaxation should not be attempted until the dressing is complete and the patient is off of the head frame.

Delayed awakening may be seen following heavy doses of opioids or sedatives, but metabolic derangement, hypothermia, and perioperative neurological injuries (i.e., ischemia, hematomas, and pneumocephalus) are also common causes. When patients do not respond as expected, they must be taken directly from the operating room to a CT scanner for examination. It is possible that a re-exploration is currently required. If consciousness was depressed prior to surgery or new neurologic deficits are expected as a result of surgery, it may be best to postpone extubation until airway reflexes have returned to a reliable level and the amount of spontaneous ventilation is adequate for avoiding post-anesthesia airway obstruction and hypoventilation. Generally, neurosurgical cases should be cared for in an HDU or ICU after recovery from anesthesia for the close monitoring of vitals and neurologic status.

1.4.9. Fluid Therapy

When the blood–brain barrier is intact, iso-osmolar crystalloid solutions such as lactated Ringer's solution and 0.9% sodium chloride are frequently used since they have no effect on brain water or edema production. Any crystalloid solution provided in significant volumes can increase CBV and ICP in patients with brain tumors, regardless of the crystalloid solution chosen. Glucose-rich fluids are generally avoided as hyperglycemia is common due to corticosteroid therapy; moreover, aqueous glucose solutions leave behind hypo-osmolar free water when the carbohydrate is taken up by the cells, which may adversely affect the water homeostasis of the CNS. Colloid solutions including blood and blood products can be used to restore intravascular volume deficits, while a balanced salt solution is preferred for maintenance.

1.4.10. Postoperative Analgesia

Postoperative pain after neurosurgery has been shown to be less severe than that for other forms of surgery (Dunbar et al. 1999), although some patients experience severe pain, as commonly seen after a frontal craniotomy. Concerns regarding opioids' analgesic side effects such as nausea, vomiting, over-sedation, and increased ICP due to respiratory depression have often resulted in inadequate postoperative pain control measures taken for neurosurgical patients. Due to neurologic impairments, these patients may have trouble articulating their need for analgesics or be entirely unable to do so, adding to the difficulty (Vadivelu et al. 2016).

Risk evaluation, patient education, and, if necessary, the administration of oral drugs begin in the preoperative period. Commonly employed drugs in this regard include opioids (with careful selection, titration, and monitoring), NSAIDs, acetaminophen, gabapentin, and ketamine. While changing surgical procedures may help with pain relief, effective anesthesia administration and the use of various analgesic strategies such as scalp blocks and infiltration or the employment of adjuvants like corticosteroids and alpha-2 adrenergic agonists may be effective components of analgesic strategies applied after neurosurgery.

Multimodal analgesia, nonpharmacological approaches, standardized pain management procedures, and patient empowerment in pain management are all feasible paths to success.

1.5. Special Issues

1.5.1. Anesthesia for Intracranial Aneurysms

The rupture of an intracranial aneurysm is the commonest cause of spontaneous subarachnoid hemorrhage, while patients with unruptured aneurysms usually present with headaches and focal neurological deficits, most commonly third-nerve palsy. Elective clipping or obliteration of the aneurysm via intravascular coiling under angiographic supervision is performed in the operating room or, more commonly, the radiology suite.

During intracranial aneurysm surgery (coiling and clipping), the goals of anesthesia or procedural sedation are to reduce the risk of aneurysm rupture, prevent cerebral ischemia, and facilitate operative exposure. As a result, large changes in systemic blood pressure should be avoided, and CPP should be kept stable. It is reasonable to avoid large drops in ICP before dural opening for patients with cerebral aneurysms without increased ICP and for those with unruptured aneurysms so as not to reduce the tamponading force on the aneurysm's exterior surface. Systemic hypertension may enhance flow in vasospastic arteries, but it may also increase the risk of aneurysm re-bleeding in patients with vasospasms (Pasternak and Lanier 2012).

An exsanguinating hemorrhage can occur as a result of aneurysm surgery due to rupture or re-bleeding. As a result, blood should be made ready before these operations begin. Anesthetic therapy of a ruptured aneurysm includes intensive volume resuscitation to maintain normovolemia, as well as induced hypotension to reduce hemorrhage and allow the neurosurgeon to gain control of the aneurysm. When a burst aneurysm is temporarily clipped to gain control, the systemic blood pressure can be returned to normal or even slightly increased to promote collateral blood flow while the vessel is occluded by the occlusion clip. If prolonged periods of occlusion are required, the injection of suppressing anesthetics, particularly barbiturates, may give protection against regional ischemia or infarction.

Delayed vasospasm is a common complication following both ruptured aneurysms and successful surgical interventions. "Triple H therapy (hypervolemia, hemodilution, and hypertension)" is added to the therapeutic regimen in patients with symptomatic vasospasms who do not respond to nimodipine. Infusions of papaverine, nicardipine, or angioplasty may be used to treat refractory vasospasms. As major fluctuations in both total intravascular volume and systemic blood pressure are very common throughout the perioperative period, hemodynamics monitoring via central venous line and intra-arterial catheters seems appropriate in most cases (Butterworth et al. 2018b).

1.5.2. Vascular Malformations

Low-flow vascular malformations like venous and cavernous angiomas have fewer complications than high-flow vascular lesions like arteriovenous malformations (AVMs) and arteriovenous fistulas. Because AVM resection is usually not an emergency procedure, preexisting medical conditions should be managed as best as possible, and neurological dysfunction caused by hemorrhages, a presumed AVM effect, or preoperative embolic events (infarction, edema, etc.) should be factored into the intraoperative and postoperative management plan.

The possibility of significant, fast, and chronic blood loss is an important consideration during the operation phase. This possibility tempers the choice of intraoperative monitoring, and sufficient blood, as well as access for its administration, must be easily available. Regarding neurosurgical patients, no anesthetic regimen has been rigorously proved to give "cerebral protection". The anesthetic drug chosen must be compatible with safe intracranial surgery, which includes brain relaxation, appropriate blood pressure management, and quick emergence. The following conditions are recommended: euvolemia, normotension, isotonicity, normoglycemia, and mild hypocapnia (Ogilvy et al. 2001).

Cerebral edema and delayed postoperative hemorrhage (DPH) can be troublesome issues during AVM treatment. NPPB (normal perfusion pressure breakthrough) or occlusive hyperemia have been hypothesized to be causes of brain edema and bleeding during or after surgery. According to the NPPB theory, a failure in autoregulation in the region of an ischemic brain around the AVM causes postoperative bleeding and edema. Chronic hypoperfusion in the region of the brain surrounding an AVM may promote maximal chronic vasodilation, resulting in the arteries' incapacity to vasoconstrict in response to the return of normal perfusion pressure after the AVM has been removed. 'Occlusive hyperemia' is an alternative theory for the origin of malignant postoperative edema and bleeding. According to this idea, malignant postoperative hemorrhage and edema are generated by either arterial stagnation and obstruction or venous outflow obstruction, both of which cause malignant postoperative hemorrhages and edema (Mullan et al. 1979).

Hyperventilation, diuretics such as furosemide or mannitol, and induced hypotension may be used as a perioperative solution to rapidly developing cerebral edema. High doses of barbiturates or propofol anesthesia, or a temporary craniectomy with postoperative ventilatory support, may be required in extreme situations (Pasternak and Lanier 2012). However, the etiology of edema and bleeding after brain AVM excision is still unknown, and to reduce the risk of DPH, stringent postoperative blood pressure control and a restrictive IV fluid management regime are required. For combating emergence hypertension, beta blockers are usually employed to pass up vasodilator-induced increases in cerebral blood flow (Niini et al. 2019).

1.5.3. Pituitary Surgery

Pituitary tumor surgery presents unique problems for an anesthesiologist because it combines ideas and techniques from endocrine- and neurosurgery. The anesthesiologist's challenges are multiplied, as the surgical method varies by patient, with some surgeons preferring the transcranial route to others' transsphenoidal approach and some patients undergoing awake craniotomy, functional neurosurgery, and interventional radiology (Venkatraghavan et al. 2006).

The pituitary gland is a master gland, and its tumors present clinically in one of three ways, namely, hormone hyper-secretion syndromes, hormone hypo-secretion, or mass effects, and any of them can ultimately have an extensive effect on human physiology in its entirety. In-depth knowledge of the anatomical as well as pathophysiological effects of the particular tumor in the patient of concern is very crucial for the safe delivery of anesthesia.

Acromegaly, which is caused by an overabundance of growth hormone, can make airway control harder during general anesthesia. Obstructive sleep apnea (OSA) is also common in acromegaly; it can raise the risk of postoperative respiratory obstruction and a compromise. Diabetes mellitus, as well as cardiac abnormalities such as left-ventricular hypertrophy, coronary artery disease, arrhythmias, conduction disturbances, valvular heart diseases, cardiomyopathies, and congestive heart failure, are frequently linked to pituitary hypersecretion, that is, acromegaly and Cushing's disease (Herrmann et al. 2002).

The oral cavity must be secured with throat packs in the trans-sphenoid approach because blood from the dissection of nasal tissues can pool in the oro-pharynx and leak down the endotracheal tube. The position during this approach is also associated with an increased risk of VAE (as a head-up position is required) and postoperative pneumocephalus. Some surgeons request the insertion of a lumbar drain catheter to aid in the dissection of the capsules of suprasellar tumors or to prevent postsurgical CSF rhinorrhea.

Symptomatic syndrome of inappropriate antidiuretic hormone secretion (SIADH), diabetes insipidus (DI), epistaxis, injury to the internal carotid artery (ICA), meningitis, CSF leakage, abdominal wound infection, a new visual deficit, postoperative hemorrhage, and mucocele formation are all postoperative complications of pituitary surgery.

Cortisol replacement is an uncommon routine after pituitary surgery and can be tailored to minimum doses within a few days, but those suffering from Cushing's disease must have heavy suppression of adrenocortical activity and would need to have been given therapeutic steroids for weeks to months.

1.5.4. Diabetes Insipidus (DI)

Diabetes insipidus (DI) is a frequent complication of pituitary and craniopharyngioma surgery and reflects an absence of vasopressin (ADH) as a consequence of the destruction of the posterior pituitary. Moreover, renal tubules may fail to respond to circulating ADH, and another form of DI can ensue, nephrogenic diabetes insipidus, while the first form is called neurogenic DI or vasopressin sensitive DI.

Classic manifestations of DI are polydipsia and a high output of diluted urine despite increased serum osmolarity. Perioperative DI is most likely a result of a reversible assault of the posterior pituitary and usually resolves within days.

After ruling out glycosuria, mannitol administration, and high-output renal failure, the presence of hypotonic (300 mosmol/kg) polyuria (2 mL/kg/h) and an elevated plasma osmolality (>300 mosmol/kg) is required to diagnose acute postoperative cerebral diabetes insipidus. In the acute phase, the plasma sodium concentration may be a more trustworthy guide than osmolality. Adults with a total 24 h production of over 3.5 L of hypotonic urine and a plasma sodium content of more than 143 mmol/L are diagnosed with hypotonic urine.

Antidiuretic medicines should only be administered if a diagnosis of cranial diabetes insipidus has been confirmed, as water overflow can produce cerebral edema and convulsions if not treated properly. Desmopressin (DDAVP) is a hormone produced by the pituitary gland. Antidiuresis is usually achieved by administering 01–0.02 g subcutaneously or intramuscularly (0.4 g for children) and should be accompanied by adequate fluid intake to maintain fluid balance (Seckl and Dunger 1989). There is also an oral preparation and a nasal spray with a metered dose. Until normal water balance is restored, plasma Na+ concentrations and osmolality should be constantly monitored.

1.5.5. Syndrome of Inappropriate Antidiuretic Hormone Secretion (SIADH)

The unsuppressed release of antidiuretic hormone (ADH) from the pituitary gland or nonpituitary sources, as well as its persistent impact on vasopressin receptors, are characteristics of SIADH. This syndrome is characterized by inappropriate (primarily inadequate) water loss via kidneys resulting in hyponatremia as well as hypervolemia (or euvolemia), and it may result from a variety of conditions, including intracranial tumors, brain surgery, meningitis, head injuries, hypothyroidism, porphyria, and carcinoma of the lung.

Hyponatremia is the result of intravascular volume expansion secondary to a hormone-induced increase in the resorption of water by the renal tubules. Serum concentrations of sodium may drop below 110mEq/L, resulting in cerebral edema and convulsions. Schwartz and Bartter developed a clinical profile for SIADH in 1967 that is in use till today and given in the Box 3 below (Bartter and Schwartz 1967).

Box 3. Schwartz and Bartter criteria (of SIADH).

- Serum sodium levels less than 135 mEq/L
- Serum osmolality less than 275 mOsm/kg
- Urine sodium levels greater than 40 mEq/L (due to ADH-mediated free water absorption from renal collecting tubules)
- Urine osmolality more than 100 mOsm/kg
- The absence of clinical evidence of volume depletion (normal skin turgor, blood pressure within the reference range)
- Urine osmolality greater than 100 mOsm/kg
- The lack of other causes of hyponatremia, such as adrenal insufficiency, hypothyroidism, heart failure, pituitary insufficiency, renal illness with salt wastage, hepatic disease, and medicines that affect renal water excretion.
- Fluid restriction is used to treat hyponatremia.

Treatment of SIADH consists of fluid restriction, the antagonism of ADH at renal tubular receptors via demeclocycline, and the intravenous infusion of sodium chloride for correcting hyponatremia. Many of the cases respond well to fluid restrictions alone, but those who manifest acute neurological symptoms may require the administration of hypertonic saline. Conivaptan (intravenous) and tolvaptan (oral) are two more vasopressin receptor antagonists that have been licensed for severe persistent SIADH. By antagonizing V2 receptors, these medicines limit ADH-mediated free water retention and hence correct hyponatremia (Greenberg and Verbalis 2006).

1.5.6. Cerebral Salt-Wasting Syndrome (CSWS)

CSWS is another clinical condition linked with or possibly causing hyponatremia and volume disturbance that at times accompany intracranial problems like head trauma, cranioplasty, brain tumors, intracranial surgery, tubercular meningitis, and, most commonly, aneurysmal subarachnoid hemorrhages. CSWS was first proposed in 1950 by Peters and colleagues and is characterized by hyponatremia, increased urine sodium levels, and hypovolemia. The wastage of salt by the kidneys exhibited in CSWS is not well understood. Disruption of sympathetic neuronal input supplied to the kidneys and natriuresis produced by natriuretic peptides are two proposed mechanisms (Oh and Shin 2014).

Although it is still a matter of debate whether CSWS is a different disorder or a special type of SIADH, it is important to differentiate the two conditions as they are treated with quite converse treatment strategies. Because patients with cerebral salt wasting are hypovolemic while patients with SIADH range from being euvolemic to hypervolemic (Oh and Shin 2014), patients with cerebral salt wasting are given fluids and sodium supplements, while in the case of SIADH, the patients are assigned a course of fluid restriction.

As CSWS is always secondary to aneurysmal subarachnoid hemorrhages or another CNS insult, its treatment should focus primarily on dealing with the underlying disorder. Second, while treating hyponatremia, the patient must be volume-repleted. In cases of mild hyponatremia, this is usually accomplished by infusing isotonic saline, but in cases of moderate to severe hyponatremia, more aggressive sodium replenishment may be required, consisting of using hypertonic saline, such as 3% hypertonic saline, and/or salt tabs (consuming 1–2 g up to three times daily), as well as limiting free water intake. Fludrocortisone has also been recommended by certain professionals for the treatment of cerebral salt wasting (Yee et al. 2010).

1.5.7. Surgery in Posterior Fossa

The posterior cranial fossa (the infratentorial compartment) is a rigid box containing multiple vital structures like the pons and medulla, cerebellum. Small further increases in volume (e.g., for tumors and hematomas) within posterior fossa can result in a considerable rise in pressure and may lead to life-threatening brainstem compression or herniation. Any surgical procedure used for a mass in the posterior fossa can be highly challenging from an anesthetic perspective as it presents an array of potential problems, including possible trauma to the vital centers, obstructive hydrocephalus, pneumocephalus, and, due to an unusual positioning, postural hypotension and air embolism in venous spaces.

1.5.8. Brainstem Injury

In the brainstem, the cardiovascular centers, respiratory control areas, and nuclei of the lower cranial nerves are all close together. Systemic hypertension and bradycardia may result from brainstem manipulation, as well as hypotension and tachycardia. Cardiac dysrhythmias are also common and may range from acute sinus arrhythmia to premature ventricular contraction (PVC) or even life-threatening ventricular tachycardia (VT). These circulatory changes are also features of damage to the respiratory centers. Therefore, continuous monitoring via an ECG is extremely important. Another major complication of surgery in the posterior fossa is postoperative apnea (acquired central hypoventilation syndrome) resulting from brainstem injury or edema, a condition requiring prompt recognition and definitive management.

1.5.9. Sitting Position

Even though surgery for infratentorial tumors can be accomplished in supine, prone, park bench, and lateral positions, the sitting position is sometimes chosen as it improves surgical access by promoting gravity-assisted blood and CSF drainage and thus decreasing ICP. It improves surgical orientations and access to the midline structures and decreases the amount of surgical retraction needed to gain access to deeper structures. These advantages relating to sitting position are sometimes offset by associated cardiovascular instability and the potential hazard of a venous air embolism (VAE).

The depressant effects of anesthetic drugs on myocardial contractility and peripheral vascular tone may add to the troubles of physiologic changes caused by sitting posture. In the event of an abrupt cardiovascular collapse, patients must be quickly returned to the supine position for resuscitative efforts. The complications associated with sitting techniques also include pneumocephalus, macroglossia, quadriplegia, and peripheral nerve injuries. Table 3 summarizes these complications (Porter et al. 1999).

Table 3. Contraindications of sitting position surgery.

Absolute Contraindications	Relative Contraindications
Ventriculo-atrial (VA) shunt	Foramen ovale
Right-to-left cardiac shunt Right-atrial pressure greater than left-atrial pressure Cerebral ischemia when patient is upright and awake	Uncontrolled hypertension
	Extremes of age
	Severe autonomic neuropathy Craniovertebral anomaly or instability

Source: Table adapted from (Porter et al. 1999), used with permission.

Venous Air Embolism (VAE)

While VAE has been described in nearly every field of medicine, seated craniotomy is the quintessential 'at risk' scenario for this potentially fatal occurrence. The other procedures associated with a high incidence of VAE include central venous catheterization, Cesarean delivery, blunt or penetrating trauma, and laparoscopy.

The amount of air entrainment and the pace of buildup are closely associated with VAE morbidity and mortality. The fatal volume for adults has been estimated to be between 200 and 300 mL, or 3 and 5 mL/kg, based on case reports of inadvertent intravascular air delivery. It has been suggested by the cited authors (Toung et al. 2001) that the smaller the required lethal amount, the closer the entrainment vein is to the right heart. A gas air-lock scenario is created quickly if the embolism is significant (about 5 mL/kg). Failure to relieve the tension of the ventricular wall may result in full outflow obstruction from the right ventricle. Right-sided heart failure and cardiovascular collapse occur quickly as a result of this. A venous air embolism may transform into an arterial embolism if a connection between the two systems exists; in that case, the emboli may pass directly to the cerebral or coronary circulation, thereby producing far more serious consequences, even with a smaller volume of air.

Early Detection of VAE: necessitates close clinical monitoring. High-risk instances demand the use of appropriate detection devices as well as a high level of suspicion. The clinical markers in this regard (hypertension, tachycardia, cardiac dysrhythmias, and cyanosis, for example) are usually late manifestations of VAE and are also non-specific. Modern devices and tools such as transesophageal echocardiography, precordial Doppler, contrast-enhanced transcranial Doppler, pulmonary artery catheters, end-tidal carbon dioxide, and end-tidal nitrogen all have a high sensitivity for detecting a VAE, but their use is more expensive and requires more advanced training. At the moment, end-tidal capnography (ETCO2) and precordial Doppler provide the best balance of sensitivity and cost.

Many preventive methods have been suggested, the most essential of which is diligent attention to volume status, as keeping a stable right-atrial pressure reduces the chance of air entrainment. Anti-shock compression garments have also been demonstrated to be useful in raising systemic venous pressure.

Management Highlights for VAE: The prevention of future air entry, a reduction in the entrained volume, and early hemodynamic resuscitation are the main goals of therapy when a VAE is suspected.

- To seal the entrance sites, surgeons should flush the operating site with saline.
- Jugular venous compression lowers head venous return and raises cerebral venous pressure. (1) Repositioning the wound below the level of the right atrium can potentially increase venous pressure at the operating site and (2) volume loading in the intravenous system. (3) The Valsulva maneuver can be used to raise intrathoracic pressure.
- A central venous catheter can be used to aspirate air.
- Using 100-percent oxygen allows nitrogen to be washed out, decreasing the size of air bubbles.
- If nitrous oxide is being used, its use should be stopped immediately because it is 34 times more soluble in blood than nitrogen and can dramatically increase the size of the entrained volume of air.
- The rapid initiation of CPR with defibrillation and chest compressions has been demonstrated to be effective for massive VAEs that result in cardiac stoppage. A closed-chest massage can be used to drive air out of the pulmonary outflow system and into the smaller pulmonary vessels even if cardiac resuscitation is not required (Ericsson et al. 1964).
- Several case reports and case series have been published demonstrating the potential benefits of hyperbaric oxygen therapy (HBO), particularly in the context of a cerebral arterial gas embolism (CAGE) (Burnand and Sebastian 2014).

1.5.10. Awake Craniotomy

Awake craniotomy is increasingly being recognized as the technique of choice for the removal of tumors from eloquent brain areas. It is essentialy useful in epilepsy surgery and deep-brain stimulation (DBS). It has also been employed to treat mycotic aneurysms and arterio-venous malformations in the brain's important sections.

Awake craniotomy is used to maximize tumor removal while maintaining neurological function. A successful awake procedure is built on careful patient selection, precise planning, and well-organized teamwork. All members of the team should interview the patient prior to surgery to establish confidence and engagement. Poor intraoperative patient communication is a common cause of failure. Patient refusal, an altered level of consciousness, a problematic airway, and the possibility of a massive hemorrhage are the major issues that might contraindicate an awake procedure.

Increased lesion excision (through awake procedure) is thought to be beneficial, with emerging evidence of enhanced survival, and it also limits damage to the eloquent cortex and the resultant postoperative neurological impairment. Other benefits include a shorter hospital stay, resulting in lower healthcare costs, and a lower incidence of postoperative problems such as nausea and vomiting (Burnand and Sebastian 2014).

The phrase "awake craniotomy" can be misleading because the patient is not entirely conscious throughout the procedure. Various amounts of sedation, or anesthesia, are required during the more surgically stimulating phases of the process (i.e., during opening and closure). During the mapping operation and the period of lesion resection, the patient is kept completely awake.

Although some patients can be handled with merely sedation, the most typical methods are sedation or an asleep–awake–asleep strategy, with or without airway equipment. For all anesthetic techniques, the patient usually has a scalp block applied (Figure 2) for pain management. The intra-operative challenges are many and include cardiovascular instability, seizures, somnolence, confrontation, airway obstruction, tight brain, oxygen desaturation, and shivering.

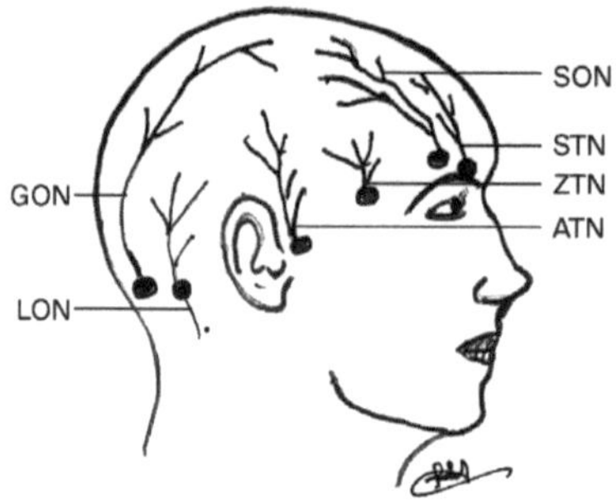

Figure 2. Illustration showing six sensory nerves supplying the scalp that need to be blocked with local anesthetic during a scalp block and an awake craniotomy. SON—supraorbital nerve; STN—supratrochlear nerve; ZTN—zygomatico-temporal nerve; ATN—auriculotemporal nerve; LON—lesser occipital nerve; GON—greater occipital nerve. Source: Figure by authors.

Individual anesthesiologists have different drug preferences. Anesthetics must have a rapid onset and offset, titratability, and minimum drawn-out effects to achieve seamless transitions and ease intraoperative mapping. Propofol, fentanyl, remifentanil, and dexmedetomidine (DEX) are the most regularly utilized anesthetics, while sevoflurane is also used at some facilities. DEX has the distinct advantage of causing minimal respiratory depression while inducing adequate drowsiness and analgesia, and it can be administered alone or in conjunction with other sedatives. It also has the advantage of not enhancing neurologic impairment, unlike propofol or midazolam. Some drugs, such as midazolam, atropine, and scopolamine, should be avoided or taken with caution as a general rule since they can impair neurocognitive function and cause disorientation or delirium. Patients undergoing seizure mapping should avoid taking any medications that reduce epileptiform activity, such as midazolam and anti-convulsant medications (Zhang and Gelb 2018). In case of intra-operative seizure, exposed cerebral cortex should be irrigated with ice-cold normal saline.

Author Contributions: Conceptualization, methodology, S.A.I. and F.H.C.; validation, formal analysis, investigation, resources, data curation, A.H. and M.S.A.; writing—original draft preparation, S.A.I. and F.H.C.; writing—review and editing, visualization, supervision, F.H.C. All authors have read and agreed to the published version of the manuscript.

Funding: This research received no external funding.

Conflicts of Interest: The authors declare no conflicts of interest.

References

Adelson, P. David, Susan L. Bratton, Nancy A. Carney, Randall M. Chesnut, Hugo E. M. du Coudray, Brahm Goldstein, Patrick M. Kochanek, Helen C. Miller, Michael D. Partington, Nathan R. Selden, and et al. 2003. Guidelines for the acute medical management of severe traumatic brain injury in infants, children, and adolescents: Chapter 5. Indications for intracranial pressure monitoring in pediatric patients with severe traumatic brain injury. *Pediatric Critical Care Medicine* 4: S19–S24. [PubMed]

Bartter, Frederic C., and William B. Schwartz. 1967. The syndrome of inappropriate secretion of antidiuretic hormone. *The American Journal of Medicine* 42: 790–806. [CrossRef] [PubMed]

Burnand, Cally, and Joseph Sebastian. 2014. Anaesthesia for awake craniotomy. *Continuing Education in Anaesthesia Critical Care & Pain* 14: 6–11.

Butterworth, John F., IV, David C. Mackey, John D. Wasnick, G. Edward Morgan, and Maged S. Mikhail. 2018a. *Neurophysiology and Anesthesia, Morgan & Mikhail's Clinical Anesthesiology*. New York: McGraw-Hill Education.

Butterworth, John F., IV, David C. Mackey, John D. Wasnick, G. Edward Morgan, and Maged S. Mikhail. 2018b. *Anesthesia for Neurosurgery, Morgan and Mikhail's Clinical Anesthesiology*. New York: McGraw-Hill Education.

Butterworth, John F., IV, David C. Mackey, and John D. Wasnick. 2013. *Intravenous Anesthetics; Morgan& Mikhail's Clinical Anesthesiology*. New York: McGraw-Hill Education.

Christensen, M. Stig, Kai Hoedt-Rasmussen, and Niels Alexander Lassen. 1967. Cerebral vasodilatation by halothane anesthesia in man and its potentiation by hypotension and hypocapnia. *British Journal of Anaesthesia* 39: 927. [CrossRef]

Dunbar, Peter J., Elizabeth Visco, and Arthur M. Lam. 1999. Craniotomy procedures are associated with less analgesic requirements than other surgical procedures. *Anesthesia & Analgesia* 88: 350–40.

Ericsson, J. A., J. D. Gottlieb, and R. B. Sweet. 1964. Closed-chest cardiac massage in the treatment of venous air embolism. *New England Journal of Medicine* 270: 1353–54. [CrossRef]

Glass, Peter S. 1993. Prevention of awareness during total intravenous anesthesia. *Anesthesiology* 78: 399–400. [CrossRef]

Greenberg, Arthur, and Joseph George Verbalis. 2006. Vasopressin receptor antagonists. *Kidney International* 69: 2124–30. [CrossRef]

Herrmann, B. L., C. Bruch, B. Saller, T. Bartel, S. Ferdin, R. Erbel, and K. Mann. 2002. Acromegaly: Evidence for a direct relation between disease activity and cardiac dysfunction in patients without ventricular hypertrophy. *Clinical Endocrinology* 56: 595–602. [CrossRef]

Ledingham, I. McA, and Ian Watt. 1993. Influence of sedation on mortality in critically ill multiple trauma patients. *Lancet* 1: 1270. [CrossRef]

Matta, Basil F., Arthur M. Lam, and Teresa S. Mayberg. 1994. The influence of arterial oxygenation on cerebral venous oxygen saturation during hyperventilation. *Canadian Journal of Anaesthesia* 41: 1041–46. [CrossRef] [PubMed]

Minton, Michael D., Kenneth Grosslight, Joseph A. Stirt, and Robert F. Bedford. 1986. Increases in intracranial pressure from succinylcholine: Prevention by prior non-depolarising blockade. *Anesthesiology* 65: 165. [CrossRef] [PubMed]

Modica, Paul A., Rene Tempelhoff, and Paul F. White. 1990. Pro and anticonvulsant effects of anesthetics. *Anesthesia & Analgesia* 70: 433–44.

Mullan, Sean, Frederick D. Brown, and Nicholas J. Patronas. 1979. Hyperemic and ischemic problems of surgical treatment of arteriovenous malformations. *Journal of Neurosurgery* 51: 757–64. [CrossRef]

Niini, Tarmo, Aki Laakso, Päivi Tanskanen, Mika Niemelä, and Teemu Luostarinen. 2019. Perioperative Treatment of Brain Arteriovenous Malformations Between 2006 and 2014: The Helsinki Protocol. *Neurocritical Care* 31: 346–56. [CrossRef] [PubMed]

Ogilvy, Christopher S., Philip E. Stieg, Issam Awad, Robert D. Brown, Jr., Douglas Kondziolka, Robert Rosenwasser, William L. Young, and George Hademenos. 2001. A Statement for Healthcare Professionals From a Special Writing Group of the Stroke Council, American Stroke Association. *Stroke* 32: 1458–71. [CrossRef] [PubMed]

Oh, Ji Young, and Jae Il Shin. 2014. Syndrome of inappropriate antidiuretic hormone secretion and cerebral/renal salt wasting syndrome: Similarities and differences. *Frontiers in Pediatrics* 2: 146. [CrossRef]

Pasternak, Jeffrey J., and William L. Lanier, Jr. 2012. *Disease Affecting Brain. Stoelting's Anesthesia and Co-Existing Disease*. Philadelphia: Saunders/Elsevier.

Porter, J. M., C. Pidgeon, and A. J. Cunningham. 1999. The sitting position in neurosurgery: A critical appraisal. *British Journal of Anaesthesia* 82: 117–28. [CrossRef]

Rangel-Castillo, Leonardo, Shankar Gopinath, and Claudia S. Robertson. 2008. Management of intracranial hypertension. *Neurologic Clinics* 26: 521–41. [CrossRef]

Ravussin, P., J. P. Guinard, F. Ralley, and D. Thorin. 1998. Effect of Propofol in cerebrospinal fluid pressure and cerebral perfusion pressure in patients undergoing craniotomy. *Anesthesia* 43: 37. [CrossRef]

Reddy, R. V., S. S. Moorthy, Stephen F. Dierdorf, Robert D. Deitch, Jr., and Linda Link. 1993. Excitatory effects and electroencephalographic correlation of etomidate, thiopental, methohexital and propofol. *Anesthesia & Analgesia* 77: 1008–11.

Rushton, Andrew R. A., and J. Robert Sneyd. 2003. Clinical Pharmacology and anesthetic techniques. In *A Practice of Anesthesia by Wylie and Churchill-Davidson*. Edited by Thomas E. J. Healy and Paul R. Knight. Boca Raton: CRC Press.

Seckl, J., and D. Dunger. 1989. Postoperative diabetes insipidus. *BMJ* 298: 2–3. [CrossRef] [PubMed]

Smith, D. S., S. Rehncrona, and B. K. Siesjö. 1980. Barbiturates as protective agents in brain ischemia and as free radical scavengers in vitro. *Acta Physiologica Scandinavica. Supplementum* 492: 129–34. [PubMed]

Taneda, Mamoru, Kazuo Kataoka, Fumiharu Akai, Toshiharu Asai, and Ikuhiro Sakata. 1996. Traumatic subarachnoid hemorrhage as a predictable indicator of delayed ischemic symptoms. *Journal of Neurosurgery* 84: 762–68. [CrossRef] [PubMed]

Thronton, C., M. P. Barrowcliffe, K. M. Konieczko, P. Ventham, C. J. Doré, D. E. Newton, and J. G. Jones. 1989. The auditory evoked response as an indicator of awareness. *BJA: British Journal of Anaesthesia* 63: 113–15. [CrossRef]

Toung, Thomas J., Mark I. Rossberg, and Grover M. Hutchins. 2001. Volume of air in a lethal venous air embolism. *Anesthesiology* 94: 360–61. [CrossRef]

Turner, John M. 2003. *Anesthesia for Neurosurgery, A Practice of Anesthesia by Wylie and Churchill-Davidson*. London: Oxfford University Press.

Unterberg, Andreas, Karl Kiening, Peter Schmiedek, and Wolfgang Lanksch. 1993. Long-term observations of intracranial pressure after severe head injury: The phenomenon of secondary rise of intracranial pressure. *Neurosurgery* 32: 17–23. [CrossRef]

Vadivelu, Nalini, Alice M. Kai, Daniel Tran, Gopal Kodumudi, Aron Legler, and Eugenia Ayrian. 2016. Options for perioperative pain management in neurosurgery. *Journal of Pain Research* 9: 37–47. [CrossRef]

Venkatraghavan, Lakshmi, Pirjo Manninen, Peter Mak, Karolinah Lukitto, Mojgan Hodaie, and Andres Lozano. 2006. Anesthesia for functional neurosurgery: Review of complications. *Journal of Neurosurgical Anesthesiology* 18: 64–67. [CrossRef]

Yee, Alan H., Joseph D. Burns, and Eelco F. M. Wijdicks. 2010. Cerebral salt wasting: Pathophysiology, diagnosis, and treatment. *Neurosurgery Clinics* 21: 339–52. [CrossRef]

Zhang, Kaiyinga, and Adrian W. Gelb. 2018. Awake craniotomy: Indications, benefits, and techniques. *Colombian Journal of Anesthesiology* 46: 46–51. [CrossRef]

Section III: Investigations

Neuro-Imaging, Neuromonitoring, and Other Special Investigations

Forhad H. Chowdhury, Rakibul Islam and Mohammod Zahed Hossain

Abstract: Modern neurosurgery is unimaginable without neuroimaging. Operating neurosurgeons can examine an intracranial pathology virtually (and conceptually) with the help of modern neuroimaging. Neurosurgery has become relatively easy to accomplish due to preoperative and perioperative neuroimaging. Neuroimaging helps in preoperative diagnosis and choosing a per-operative approach, and, perioperatively, it defines pathology precisely and can assess the completeness of resection. Neuromonitoring is very useful in functional preservation during cranial, spinal, and peripheral nerve surgery. In this chapter, X-rays, CT scans, MRI scans, and ultrasonograms are discussed, including with regard to their useful modified (including intraoperative uses) forms. Neuromonitoring (intraoperative neuromonitoring, EEG, ECoG, and neuronavigation) and other special investigations (NCS, EMG, and CSF studies and immunohistochemistry) are discussed briefly in the later part of this chapter.

Abbreviations

AED	anti-epileptic drugs	AFB	acid-fast bacillus
AVM	arteriovenous malformation	AVF	arteriovenous fistula
BAEP	brainstem auditory evoked potential	CBF	cerebral blood flow
CBV	cerebral blood volume.	CNS	central nervous system
CT	computed tomography	CTA	computed tomographic angiogram
CTV	computed tomographic venography	CSF	cerebrospinal fluid
CVST	cerebral vein and dural sinus thrombosis	DSA	digital subtraction angiogram
DTI	diffusion tensor imaging	EC-IC	extracranial–intracranial
ECoG	electrocorticogram	ECS	electrical cortical simulation
EEG	electroencephalogram	EMG	Electromyography
EZ	epileptic zone	fMRI	functional magnetic resonance imaging
GBS	Guillain–Barré syndrome	HF	hemifacial spasm
ICA	internal carotid artery	ICH	intracerebral hemorrhage
ICP	intracranial pressure	IEEG	intracranial EEG
IHC	Immunohistochemistry	IIH	idiopathic intracranial hypertension
MEG	magnetoencephalography	MRI	magnetic resonance imaging
MRA	magnetic resonance angiogram	MEP	motor evoked potential
MRV	magnetic resonance venography	MRS	magnetic resonance spectroscopy
MTP	mean transit time	NAA	N-acetyl aspartate
NSF	nephrogenic systemic fibrosis	PCR	polymerase chain reaction
PET	positron emission tomography	PNS	paranasal sinuses
PW	perfusion weighted	RF	Radiofrequencies
SAH	subarachnoid hemorrhage	SCA	superior cerebellar artery
SPECT	single-photon emission computed tomography	SPGR	spoiled gradient recall
SSEP	somatosensory evoked potential	TBI	traumatic brain injury
TCD	transcranial doppler	TIA	transient ischemic attack
TLE	temporal lobe epilepsy	TM	transverse myelitis
TN	trigeminal neuralgia	TTP	time to peak
USG	ultra sonogram	VEP	visual evoked potential
VA	vertebral artery	VBI	vertebrobasilar insufficiency

1. Neuro-Imaging

1.1. X-Ray

1.1.1. X-Ray—Cranium

A skull X-ray is one of the primary imaging techniques utilized to check the bones of the skull, including the bone structure of the face, the nose, and the paranasal sinuses. It is an easy, quick, and effective method that has been used to view the area that contains the most vital organ of the human body—the brain. It is usually performed after a traumatic head injury. Apart from common AP and lateral views, other special views, such as occipito-mental, Towne's, and oblique views, can be used for different pathologies. An X-ray allows one to inspect any damage resulting from an injury. Other indications include the following:

1. Decalcification and bony tumors as well as osteolytic lesions of the skull and skull base;
2. Skull deformities;
3. Fractures of the skull base or vault or facial bones;
4. Headaches;
5. Osteomyelitis of the skull bones and paranasal sinus (PNS) infections;
6. Infection of the ear and mastoid process and hearing loss;
7. Chronic raised intracranial pressure (ICP) [beaten silver/beaten copper appearances] (Figure 1);
8. Neoplasia of the skull, skull base, brain, meninges, and nose, including the PNSs.

A CT scan of the head is commonly used instead of an X-ray due to its availability and its efficacy in the quick screening of the skull, brain, PNSs, soft tissues, and face.

1.1.2. X-Ray—Spine

X-rays of the spine are used to observe traumatic injuries of the spine, tumors, infections, bone-destructive lesions, and deformities. Besides AP and lateral views, other views such as oblique and open-mouth views can be used. Fractured bones; arthritis; spondylolisthesis; disc degeneration; neoplasms; disorders regarding the curvature of the spine, i.e., kyphosis or scoliosis; and congenital anomalies can all be discovered using neck, back, or lumbar spinal X-rays.

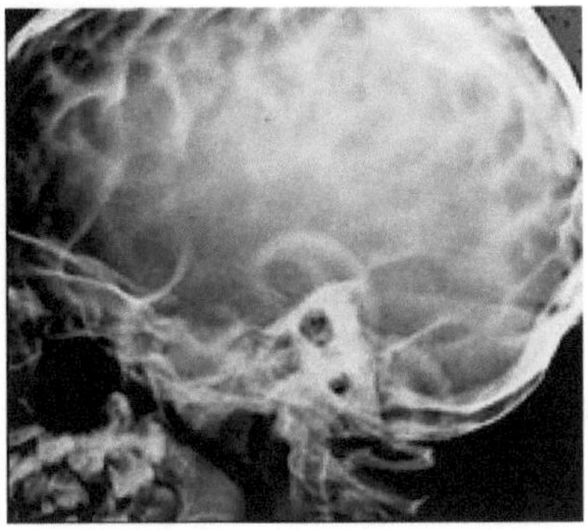

Figure 1. Skull X-ray (lateral view) showing beaten-silver/beaten-copper appearance due to chronic raised ICP. Source: Figure by authors.

1.1.3. Digital Subtraction Angiograms (DSAs) of Brain and Spinal Vessels

DSAs (digital subtraction angiograms) of cerebral and spinal vessels are used to delineate vascular pathologies of the brain and spine (both diagnostic and therapeutic) after injecting radio-opaque dye selectively in cerebral or spinal arteries with an angio-catheter, and X-rays are acquired simultaneously with the digital subtraction of bone.

1.1.4. Peroperative X-Ray/Fluoroscopy/C-Arm and O-Arm X-Rays

A peroperative X-ray is routinely and commonly utilized in spinal surgery for localization and instrumentation.

1.2. CT Scan

1.2.1. Principles of CT Scans

The first computed axial tomographic scanner was designed by Sir Godfrey Hounsfield and Dr. Allan Cormack in 1972, resulting in their receipt of the Nobel Prize in Medicine in 1979. CT scan machines have come a long way since then, with speed and resolution steadily rising (Grossman and Yousem 2003).

The CT scan is a non-invasive technique that has revolutionized research on intracranial diseases since its introduction in the 1970s. In a CT scan, a pencil beam of X-rays passes through the patient's head (spine or other body parts) and is measured by a diametrically oppositely placed detector. Calculation of absorption values for several small blocks of tissue is possible thanks to computer processing and several rotating beams and detectors grouped in a complete circle around the patient's head, spine, or other areas of body (voxels). The traditional CT scan images are created by reconstructing these locations on a two-dimensional screen (pixels). Slices are taken 3–5 mm apart for routine scanning. The most recent "spiral" or "helical" CT scanners utilize a large bank of detectors (multi-slice), and the patient moves through the field during scanning, causing the X-ray beams to follow a helical path. These scanners cut scanning time in half and are especially useful when slices with a length of 1–2 mm are used to provide more anatomical information. These 'high-definition' views enable comprehensive investigation and coronal and sagittal reconstructions. Changing the window level enhances the visibility of tissues with varying X-ray densities. For every scanned level of the spine and head, most centers produce two images: one to reveal bone structures (a bony window) and another to demonstrate soft tissue within and outside the spinal canal or cranium. This allows the creation of 3-D reconstruction images of the head and spine using CT scan data (Figure 2). When a plain CT scan reveals any abnormalities or if definite clinical indications are present, such as a vascular lesions or tumors, an intravenous iodin-containing water-soluble contrast injection is applied (Lindsay et al. 2011).

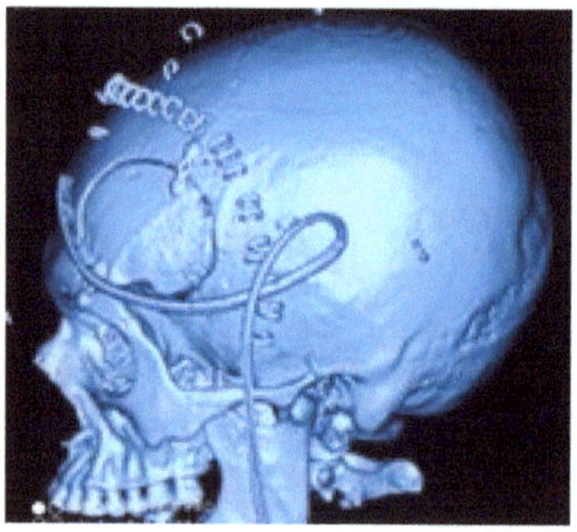

Figure 2. Three-dimensional reconstruction of a head via CT, constituting a lateral view of a post left supraorbital frontolateral craniotomy patient. Source: Figure by authors.

1.2.2. CT Scans of the Brain and Spine

CT scans of the brain and spine are extremely important imaging tools for the screening, diagnosis, and planning of treatment, including surgical intervention. In this modern era of neurosurgery, a neurosurgeon cannot conduct an intracranial operation without CT.

1.2.3. CTA and CTV of the Brain, Neck, and Spine

By using an intravenous contrast medium infusion during scanning, a non-invasive technique for revealing cerebral arteries in 2- and 3-D format can be devised. The capacity to rotate an image 360° allows for a clearer demonstration of vessels and any abnormalities. According to many studies, 3-D CT angiograms are just as good as traditional angiograms at detecting tiny aneurysms. CT arteriograms (Figures 3 and 4) and CT venograms are very useful neuroimaging techniques for the screening and diagnosis of cranial and spinal vascular pathologies including neck vessels (such as cerebral occlusive diseases, Moyamoya disease, carotid stenosis, intracranial aneurysm and AVM, AV fistula, cerebral venous sinus thrombosis, spinal AVM, and AV fistulae). These are essential for the planning of therapeutic options.

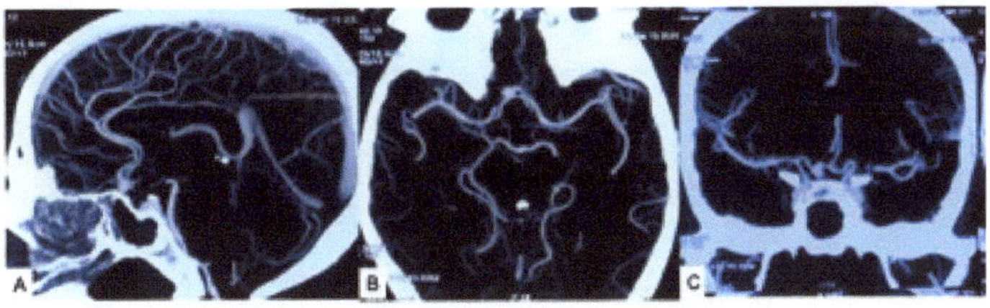

Figure 3. CTA of brain (showing the inside of the brain case); (**A–C**)—sagital, axial, and coronal views, respectively, showing an ACOM aneurysm with otherwise normal vasculature. Source: Figure by authors.

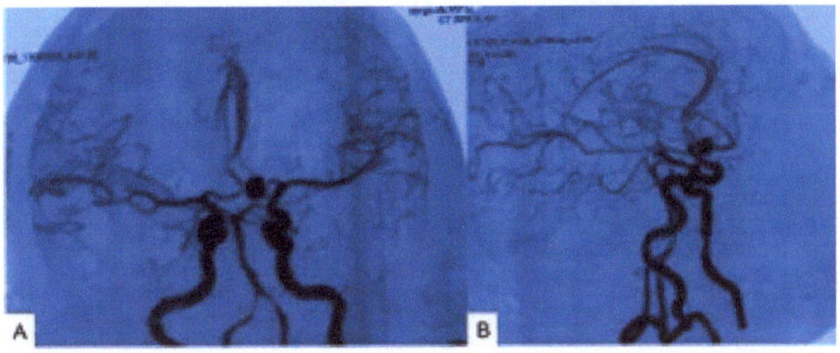

Figure 4. CTA of the brain (**A**—AP view and **B**—lateral view) showing a large ACOM aneurysm. Source: Figure by authors.

1.2.4. Perfusion CT of the Brain

After the intravenous injection of contrast media, it is possible to develop a brain perfusion map, which is very important in assessing acute and chronic ischemic conditions for achieving a diagnosis and selecting therapeutic options. For neurosurgeons, it is very important to create this map alongside conducting a Diamox challenge test in EC-IC bypass in ischemic conditions such as cerebral arterial stenosis/occlusion (Figure 5), Moyamoya disease, etc. Ischemic patches have less contrast and appear to have low density. This method is also useful in predicting the fate of an acute stroke.

1.2.5. SPECT

Single-photon emission computed tomography (SPECT) technology can be used to detect tumor spread in the brain, differentiate between tumor regrowth and radiation-induced necrosis, assess cerebral perfusion in cases of epilepsy and TBI, and diagnose secondary CNS diseases (Golanov et al. 2012).

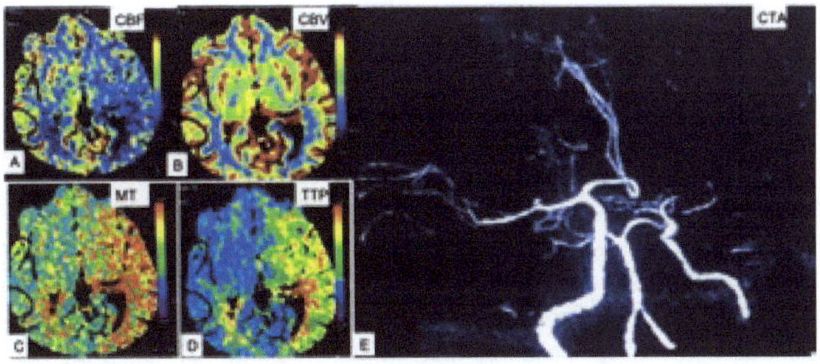

Figure 5. (**A–D**) Perfusion CT scan of the brain in a patient with left MCA occlusion (**E**), showing left MCA territory hypoperfusion. Source: Figure by authors.

1.2.6. PET

PET (positron emission tomography) is a sensitive imaging method that permits one to see real-time brain activity. It provides non-invasive brain measurements of cerebral blood flow (CBF), metabolism, and receptor binding. (Tai and Piccini 2004).

After radioactive "tracers" have been taken into the bloodstream, the FDG-PET/CT 18F-2-fluoro-2-deoxy-D-glucose (FDG) scan records images of cerebral activity. These tracers are "affixed" to a molecule such as glucose (sugar). Glucose is the brain's primary fuel source. The brain's active areas will use glucose at a faster pace than the brain's dormant portions. PET scanning offers a better explanation of how the brain works and aids in the detection of any anomalies. PET is used to detect malignant neoplasms; assess if cancer has spread to the cerebrum; diagnose dementias, e.g., Alzheimer's disease; distinguish between Parkinson's disease and other illnesses; and prepare a patient for epilepsy surgery.

1.2.7. Per Operative CT

A modern well-equipped neurosurgical operation room may have a CT scanner that can be used intra-operatively in cranial and spinal surgery to guide the approach and pathway to pathology or implantation (e.g., a DBS electrode in the brain and screw placement in the pedicle of the spine). It can also be used to check the completeness of the excision of a tumor.

1.2.8. CT Cisternography

In CT cisternography, intrathecal contrast is injected to better locate the source of a CSF leak, increasing the diagnostic yield of conventional CT (Figure 6). Unlike traditional CT imaging, only one investigation is usually required. In most patients with ongoing leaks, CT cisternography demonstrates the exact site of the CSF fistula.

1.3. Magnetic Resonance Imaging (MRI)

MRI is a noninvasive imaging method with superior soft-tissue contrast as well as physiological and functional applications. Since the 1980s, MRI has been a mainstay of non-invasive diagnostic imaging as it does not expose the body to radiation. To obtain comprehensive images, MRI involves the utilization of an intense magnetic field, a quickly altering magnetic field, radio waves, and a computer. However, there are some hazards associated with MRI. As the use of MRI in clinical practice has increased, healthcare workers must learn MRI safety protocols in order to safeguard patients against the hazards associated with this procedure (Feychting 2005).

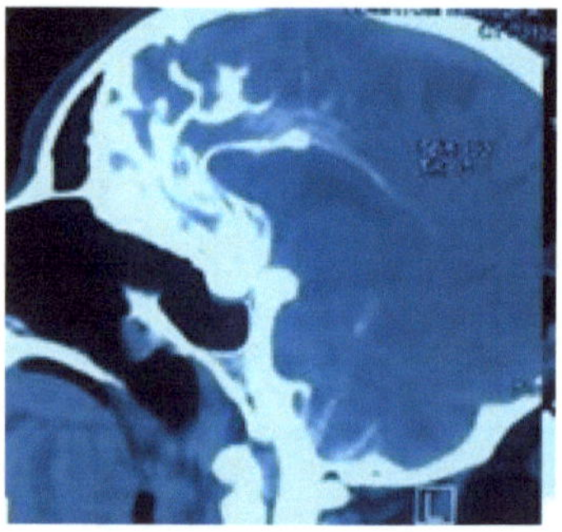

Figure 6. CT cisternogram (sagittal view) showing CSF cisterns at the base of the skull. Source: Figure by authors.

1.3.1. Principles of MRI

An atom's nucleus has angular momentum when it includes unpaired protons, neutrons, or both. Magnetic resonance imaging is based on this feature (MRI). Hydrogen is employed in clinical MRI because it is abundant in the human body. The atoms within the MR magnet are aligned with the magnet's magnetic field. The atoms are exposed to radiofrequency (RF) pulsations to form the MR signal, and the appearance of the image is governed by the pulse sequences utilized. The echo time (TE) is the time between the RF pulse and the signal recording, whereas the repetition time (TR) is the time between RF pulses. T1-weighted scans (short TR/short TE) provide the highest anatomical detail, although T2-weighted images (long TR/long TE) are more commonly used. In MR pictures, there can be a lot of strange artifacts. Unequal distributions in the magnetic field (e.g., those caused by metallic orthopedic devices or past surgical intervention), extraneous RF interference, and movement can all contribute to this. In musculoskeletal MR imaging, surface coils are widely employed to increase the quality of the test by boosting the signal-to-noise proportion over the area of interest (Lindsay et al. 2011; Seeger 1989).

1.3.2. Contraindications of MRI Scanning

Absolute Contraindications of MRI are listed in Box 1.

Box 1. Absolute contraindications of MRI (Seeger 1989).

- Intraocular metallic foreign objects
- Cochlear/ear implants
- Drug/chemical infusion pumps (analgesics, or chemotherapy pumps, insulin delivery)
- Catheters containing metallic parts (Swan–Ganz catheter)
- Residual metallic pieces such as bullets, metal shrapnel, and pellets
- Cerebral aneurysm clips (most of them are now MRI-compatible)
- Cardiac implantable electronic devices (CIEDs) [example: pacemakers]
- Implantable cardioverter defibrillators (ICDs), and cardiac
- Resynchronization therapy (CRT) devices
- Neurostimulator implants
- Piercings
- Dental magnetic implants
- Tissue expanders
- Artificial limbs
- Hearing aids

It is vital to understand that in MRI, some of these things are dangerous, while others are only safe at 1.5 tesla and 3 tesla. All gadgets and implants must be investigated using a certified MRI scanner safety website/the website of the manufacturer. Medical materials, equipment, and implants have been developed from non-ferromagnetic materials for decades and are typically labeled MR-safe or MR-conditional. A device or implant must be considered dangerous for MRI if there is no proof or information about its MRI safety (Seeger 1989).

Relative Contraindications of MRI

There are several relative contraindications (stressing the need for caution before conducting MRI) shown in Box 2.

Box 2. Relative contraindications for MRI (Seeger 1989).

- Peripheral and coronary artery stents
- Intrauterine devices (IUDs)
- Stapes implants
- Penis prostheses
- Inferior vena cava (IVC) filters;
- Medication patches
- Programmable shunts
- (Patients must be informed that they have to ask their providers to readjust their shunts after the scan)
- Tracheostomy/airway stent with metallic part
- Ocular prostheses
- Wire sutures/surgical clips
- Joint replacements/prostheses
- Harrington rods
- Claustrophobia

1.3.3. Gadolinium Contrast MRI

Gadolinium contrast is used to highlight the blood supply in a lesion seen in plain MRI. Gadolinium chelates with various viscosities, stabilities, and types of osmolality are used as MRI contrast agents. Gadolinium is a relatively harmless contrast; but it might induce hypersensitivity reactions in certain people and very rarely nephrogenic systemic fibrosis (NSF) in patients (Seeger 1989).

1.3.4. MRI in Pregnancy

MRI is a useful imaging method for evaluating obstetric and non-obstetric diseases throughout any trimester of pregnancy (Seeger 1989).

1.3.5. MRI Under General Anesthesia

General anesthesia may be needed for pediatric patients, patients with a psychiatric illness, restless patients who have suffered strokes or head injuries, and claustrophobic patients.

1.3.6. MRI of Brain and Spine

MRI of the brain or spine is the minimum requirement for neuro-investigation for a neurosurgeon in the screening, diagnosis, or planning of therapy/surgery of the brain or for spinal disorders including CNS tumors, trauma, stroke, neurovascular diseases, CNS infection, CSF disorders, and skull-base as well as cranial vault pathologies.

1.3.7. MRA and MRV of Brain, Neck, and Spine

MRA and MRV (Figure 7) of brain and neck vessels have almost become a routine investigation for a neurosurgeon. They are utilized in the diagnosis and treatment planning of vascular disorders of the neck and brain as well as in the selection of surgical methods and targets (i.e., cervical and intracranial carotid and vertebral arteries, anterior circulation and posterior circulation aneurysms, AVM, AV fistula, stenosis, occlusion, dissection, and arterial and venous involvement by tumors.) In cases of idiopathic intracranial hypertension (IIH) and cerebral sinus thrombosis, a venogram is recommended.

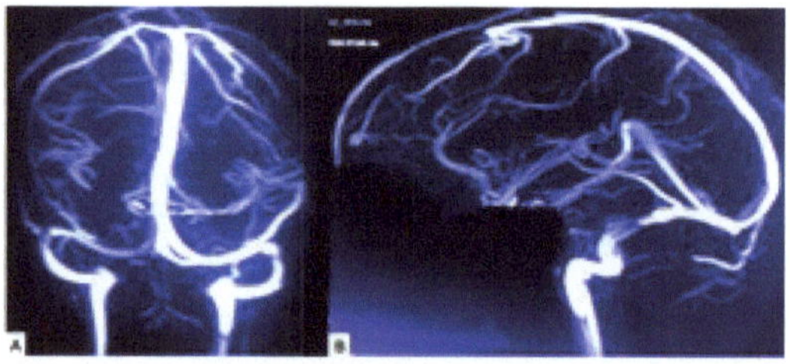

Figure 7. Normal MRV of the brain; (**A**) P/A view and (**B**) lateral view. Source: Figure by authors.

1.3.8. Perfusion MRI of the Brain (Especially for Ischemia)

MR perfusion imaging refers to a group of recently discovered techniques for measuring brain perfusion non-invasively using a variety of hemodynamic parameters. These approaches have become critical diagnostic and therapeutic tools for treating patients with cerebrovascular disease and other brain illnesses. The evaluation of tissues at risk following an acute stroke, the noninvasive histologic examination of cancers, the evaluation of neurodegenerative disorders like Alzheimer's disease, and the evaluation of the effects of medications used to treat these conditions are all possible applications (Petrella and Provenzale 2000).

This technique is very important in assessing acute (penumbra and infarcts) and chronic ischemic conditions (chronic ischemic brain parenchyma) for the diagnosis and selection of therapeutic options. For neurosurgeons, it is very essential to perform it along with a Diamox challenge test in EC-IC bypass in cerebral ischemic pathologies such as cerebral arterial stenosis/occlusion, Moyamoya disease, etc. Like perfusion CT of the brain, perfusion MRI is used to calculate hemodynamic measurements such as cerebral blood volume (CBV), time to peak (TTP), cerebral blood flow (CBF), and mean transit time (MTP).

1.3.9. DTI and Tractography

Diffusion-tensor imaging (DTI) is a noninvasive imaging technique for examining the connections between white matter tracts and connectomes. In DTI, signal contrast is created by variations in the Brownian movement of water molecules in the brain parenchyma. Postprocessed DTI scalars may be used to measure alterations in brain tissue generated by disease, disease progression, and therapeutic responses for a variety of neurological diseases and conditions, including gliomas, multiple sclerosis, Alzheimer's disease, Parkinson's disease, epilepsy, infarction, language or motor disorders, traumatic brain injuries, spinal cord trauma, and depression (Tae et al. 2018). In gliomas or other intra-axial tumors, the white matter tract can be displaced, split, infiltrated, or destroyed by the tumor; in this regard, preoperative DTI and tractography help in surgical planning (Figure 8), neuromonitoring during operation, and postoperative result prediction.

1.3.10. fMRI of Brain

By detecting variations in blood flow, functional MRI (fMRI) determines brain activities. The fact that cerebral blood flow as well as neural activation are chronologically linked is the basis for this approach (Logothetis et al. 2001).

When a part of the brain is working properly, blood circulation to that part of the brain increases. The blood-oxygen-level-dependent (BOLD) contrast (American College of Radiology and Radiological Society of North America 2011) was discovered by Seiji Ogawain in 1990 and is utilized in the primary version of fMRI. The cited researchers used functional magnetic resonance imaging (fMRI) to map the brain and uncover areas involved in critical tasks like moving, speaking, sensing, and planning. This is helpful for planning brain surgery as well as radiation therapy (Figure 9).

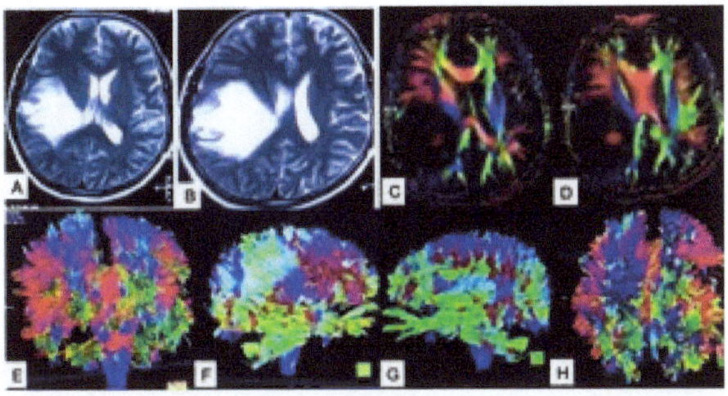

Figure 8. (**A**,**B**) MRI of brain T2W images showing right fronto-parieto-ganglionic glioma. (**C**,**D**) MR diffuse tensor imaging (DTI) of same patient in axial views showing displacement of adjacent white fiber tracts. (**E–H**) Tractography of the same patient in different views. Source: Figure by authors.

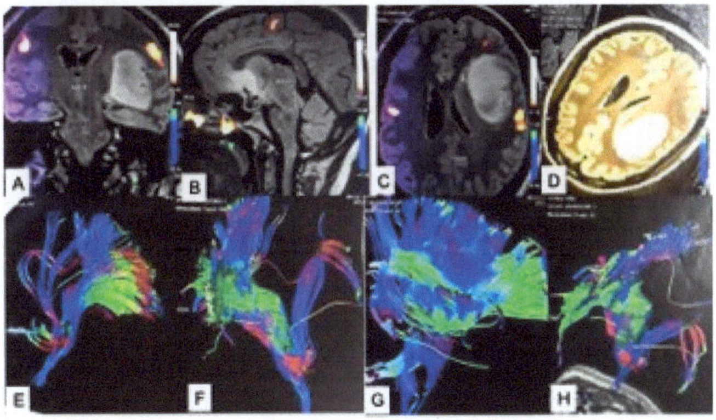

Figure 9. (**A–D**) fMRI of the brain, with coronal, sagittal, and axial views showing cortical functional areas in a patient with insular glioma. (**E–H**) MR tractography of same patient showing reduced and displaced cortico-spinal and cortico-nuclear tracts on the left side. Source: Figure by authors.

Clinicians can use fMRI to map the brain and identify the effects of tumors, strokes, head and brain trauma, diseases like Alzheimer's, and developmental anomalies like autism (Box 3) (American College of Radiology and Radiological Society of North America 2011; Subbaraju et al. 2018).

Box 3. Indications of fMRI.

- Intractable/drug-resistant epilepsy surgery
  Temporal lobe excision
  Epileptic lesion involving eloquent areas
  Cortical dysplasia (CD), involving eloquent areas causing intractable seizure
- Glioma involving eloquent areas
  (For planning surgery)
- Cerebral AVM and other intrinsic lesion involving eloquent areas
- To see the shifting of eloquent areas in diseased eloquent areas
  (i.e., low-grade gliomas, AVM, cavernoma, trauma, infarcts)
- Dementia
- Research in neurosciences

1.3.11. Magnetic Resonance Spectroscopy (MRS)

The predominant source of a signal in MRI is protons that stay within water, as well as molecules of fat, which are nearly a thousand times commoner than the molecules identified with MRS. As the more abundant signal is typically used in MRI to make very clear 2D images, whereas a signal is commonly collected from a single isolated spot known as a "voxel" in MRS, MRS can be utilized to analyze the relative quantities and physical qualities of a number of biochemicals usually referred to as "metabolites" due to their activity in metabolism (Figure 10).

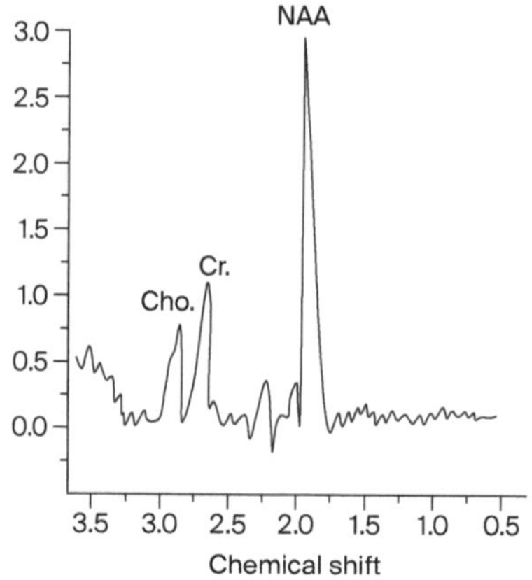

Figure 10. Schematic drawing showing normal MRS of brain. Cho.—choline, Cr.—creatine, and NAA—N-acetyl aspartate. Source: Figure by authors.

The biochemicals (metabolites) that can be studied in this regard include choline-containing molecules (used to construct cell membranes), creatine (an energy-metabolizing chemical), glucose and inositol (both sugars), alanine and lactate (both amino acids), and N-acetylaspartate (Tae et al. 2018).

MRS, also known as nuclear magnetic resonance (NMR) spectroscopy, is a non-invasive technique for studying metabolic changes in cerebral neoplasms, strokes, epilepsy, depression, Alzheimer's disease, and other brain diseases (Preul et al. 1996). MRS findings may be very confusing. MRS findings for different neurosurgical conditions are shown in Table 1.

1.3.12. iMRI (Intraoperative MRI)

Intraoperative MRI is available at only a few neurosurgical centers, where one can check the completeness of the excision of an intracranial tumor.

1.3.13. MR Cisternography

For a CSF fistula, MR cisternography can be performed, as is the case for CT cisternography. T1-weighted imaging is performed routinely in the axial, coronal, and sagittal planes. In the coronal, axial, and sagittal planes, a T2W spinecho sequence is acquired with fat saturation. To see how posture affects the distribution of CSF, MRI is performed in both the supine and prone positions. In one case, a CSF leak was thought to have occurred when CSF was linked to the subarachnoid space outside the skull or herniation of the CSF was noticed (Wang et al. 2011).

Table 1. MRS findings for different neurosurgical conditions.

Conditions	Findings
Glioma (MRS can increase our ability to predict grades.)	NAA and creatine levels drop as the grade rises, whereas choline, lipid, and lactate levels rise. Choline levels are raised beyond the contrast enhancement margins in gliomas, indicating cellular invasion.
Non-glial neoplasms	Generally, non-glial neoplasms will have very few, if any, NAA peaks.
Radiation effects	It can be difficult to tell the difference between radiation alteration and tumor recurrence. Choline levels are elevated in a recurrent tumor, whereas NAA, choline, and creatine levels are all lower in a radiation transformation.
Infarction and ischemia	As the brain transitions to anaerobic metabolism, lactate levels will rise. When there is an infarction, lipids are released, and peaks appear.
Infection	NAA is not present in any of the processes that degrade normal brain tissue. Lactate, alanine, cytosolic acid, and acetate levels are all elevated/present in bacterial abscess cavities. Choline levels are low or nonexistent in toxoplasmosis but high in lymphoma, helping to distinguish between the two diseases.
White matter disorders	Increased myoinositol levels may be seen in progressive multifocal leukoencephalopathy (PML). Raised NAA levels are seen in Canavan illness.
Mitochondrial diseases	Leigh syndrome: high choline, low NAA, and, occasionally, high lactate levels

Source: Authors' compilation based on data from Horská and Barker (2010).

1.3.14. MRI for Cranial Nerves Protocol

Cranial nerve dysfunctions can be caused by disease processes inside the cranial nerves or by neoplasms, inflammation, infections, or traumatic damage to nearby structures. In the investigation of the cranial nerves, MRI is the gold-standard technique. The finest sequences for visualizing the cisternal segments are steady-state free procession (SSFP) images, which show dark cranial nerves on a brilliant cerebrospinal fluid background (CSF) (Romano et al. 2019).

The trigeminal nerve (TN) protocol for trigeminal neuralgia (Figure 11), the facial nerve protocol for hemifacial (HF) spasms, the glossopharyngeal and lower cranial nerve protocol for glossopharyngeal neuralgia and spasmodic torticollis, and the optic nerve (ON) protocol for idiopathic intracranial hypertension (IIH) are some of the most commonly used MRI protocols.

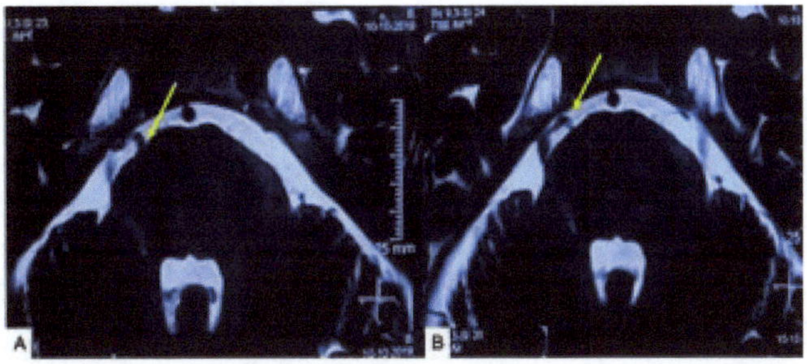

Figure 11. MRI in the TN protocol images (**A**,**B**) showing an artery at the REZ of the right trigeminal nerve causing neuralgia. Source: Figure by authors.

1.3.15. MRI in Epilepsy Protocol

Traditional MRI does not contain spoiled gradient recalled (SPGR) or magnetization prepared rapid gradient echo (MPRAGE) T1-weighted images that improve gray/white matter separation, which is important for understanding cortical architecture. If TLE is suspected, T1-weighted MPRAGE or SPGR pictures of the entire brain from nasion to inion and the epilepsy protocol MRI at 1.5T or 3.0T 1.5 mm slice thickness in the coronal oblique plane with no intervening gap in between are used. Coronal-and-axial-fluid-attenuated inversion recovery (FLAIR) sequences with a 2–3 mm slice thickness and a 0–1 mm interslice gap are also included in an epilepsy MRI protocol. The axial and coronal sequences are T2-weighted thin-slices (3 mm) (Passaro 2020).

1.3.16. MRI Cavernoma Protocol

The most sensitive sequences for cavernomas are gradient echo sequences. As a result, they are the ideal method for detecting cavernomas in patients with numerous lesions.

1.4. USG of the Head

When a probe (i.e., a transducer) with a frequency of 5–10 MHz is attached to the skin's surface, a portion of the ultrasonic waves produced are reflected back and detected by the same probe from structures with varying acoustic resistance. Electrical energy is converted from refracted waves and shown as a two-dimensional image (negative mode).

The reflected waves undergo a frequency shift proportional to the velocity of flowing blood when the probe is pointed towards moving entities, such as RBCs within a blood artery lumen (the Doppler effect). Either continuous wave (CW) or pulsed wave (PW) ultrasound is used Doppler ultrasonography. The former keeps track of frequency shifts over the probe's entire journey. A frequency shift is recorded using pulsed ultrasound at a given depth (Lindsay et al. 2011). Brain ultrasonography (duplex scanning, which includes B-mode and Doppler) can be utilized to assess brain architecture and disease, as well as cerebral circulation via blood flow velocity studies (Robba et al. 2019).

Ultrasound can penetrate the thinner sections of the skull at lower frequencies (2 MHz). When this is combined with a pulsed system, accurate flow velocity measurements in the posterior, middle, and anterior cerebral arteries, as well as the basilar artery, can be obtained. In extracranial stenotic/occlusive vascular disease, this procedure can be utilized to measure intracranial hemodynamics. Vasospasms are detected in subarachnoid hemorrhages (Lindsay et al. 2011). Thus, transcranial color-coded duplex sonography is a generally safe, non-invasive, repeatable bedside technique with a lot of potential for treating neurocritical care patients in a variety of clinical scenarios (Table 2), such as traumatic brain injury, hydrocephalus, aneurysmal subarachnoid hemorrhage, and the diagnosis of cerebral circulatory arrest (Robba et al. 2019).

Table 2. Common uses USG in neurosurgery.

Patients and the Method of USG Employed	Pathologies
In neonates, infants, and children—through an unclosed fontanel/through a burr hole	Congenital brain anomalies, hydrocephalus, cerebral aqueductal stenosis, vein Galan malformation
Older children and adults—through burr holes/bony defects/craniectomy	Congenital brain anomalies, hydrocephalus, cerebral aqueductal stenosis, vein Galan malformation, arachnoid cyst, tumour
Adults—focused ultrasound ablation	Lesioning in movement disorder
Adults—transcranial doppler (through thin bone)	Cerebral vasospasm in a subarachnoid hemorrhage
Children and adults—duplex scan	Carotid, vertebral, and other neck vessels; dissection; atherosclerosis; aneurysms; occlusion; and thrombosis
Children and adults—perioperative (after a burr hole and craniotomy)	For identification of lesions, especially deep, small lesions, and assessing the completeness of the resection of a tumor.
Children and adults—in ICU through TCD	Follow up on a head injury patient.

TCD—Transcranial doppler. Source: Table by authors.

2. Neuromonitoring (Perioperative Neuromonitoring, EEG, ECoG, and Neuronavigation) and Other Special Investigations (NCS, EMG, and CSF Studies and Immunohistochemistry)

2.1. Nerve Conduction Study (NCS)/Nerve Conduction Velocity (NCV) Analysis and Electromyography (EMG)

These methods are jointly used for neurosurgical conditions of peripheral nerves, especially peripheral nerve injuries and entrapments, for which surgery is commonly indicated. It is also indicated for the diagnosis of other peripheral neuropathies and to differentiate them from surgical etiologies.

2.2. Electroencephalography (EEG)

An electroencephalograph records the electrical activity of the brain in real time. Interictal scalp EEG is the first investigation carried out for seizure disorders. Routine EEG very rarely records actual seizures, except generalized absence seizures. However, routine EEG has important limitations. With multiple recordings, epileptiform EEG abnormality is detected in more than 90% of epilepsy patients (Salinsky et al. 1987).

Video-EEG Monitoring (VEM) is considered a cornerstone of the presurgical evaluation in epilepsy. Ictal EEG activity can be analyzed in the context of time-locked signs and symptoms. VEM gives better opportunities for the analysis of seizure semiology. The interpretations are more accurate when ictal events are analyzed in conjunction with simultaneously acquired EEG recordings.

Intracranial electroencephalography (IEEG)/Invasive EEG is an invasive procedure and utilized only when non-invasive tools fail to define EZ adequately (Jayakar et al. 2016).

There are subdural grid and strip electrodes and depth electrodes of multiple configurations for IEEG. Intracranial EEG signals may be recorded intraoperatively or extra-operatively. Craniotomy, the placement of subdural and depth electrodes, and the recording of electrical activity intraoperatively are collectively known as electrocorticography (EcoG) (Figure 12). Strips can be inserted through burr holes. Craniotomy is needed for grid placement. Depth electrodes can be placed through the burr, via craniotomy, or under neuronavigation guidance, but they are more commonly placed using the stereotactic method. Based on noninvasive evaluation, a hypothesis is made regarding a presumptive epileptic zone (EZ). Electrodes are placed to cover the EZ and an irritative zone and adjacent EC. Cortical stimulation mapping can be conducted through IEEG electrodes after EEG recording is completed. AED should be restarted before electrocortical stimulation (ECS).

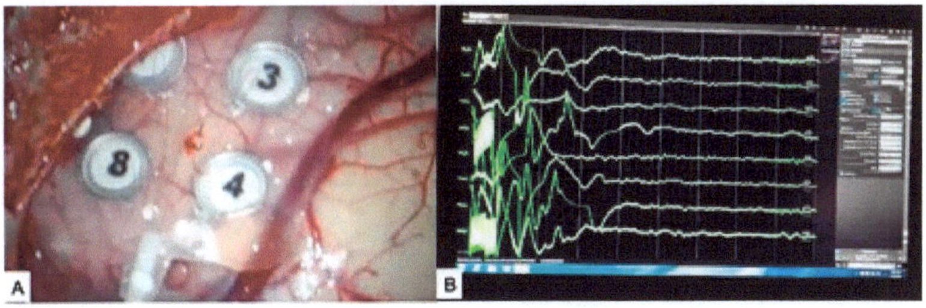

Figure 12. Perioperative electro-corticogram (ECoG). (**A**) Electrode on brain cortical surface after craniotomy and durotomy. (**B**) Tracing of ECoG. Source: Figure by authors.

2.3. Magnetoencephalogram (MEG)

A magnetoencephalogram is a promising noninvasive tool for defining the epileptogenic cortex and delineating the eloquent cortex. The neurophysiological process that generates the MEG signal is exactly the same as that which produces the EEG signal (Barth 1993). Magnetoencephaloghaphy is also useful in the localization of the sensory motor cortex, primary auditory cortex, and the language area. However, it has a huge operational cost.

2.4. Perioperative Neuromonitoring

2.4.1. Motor Nerve Monitoring

This technique is commonly used for the identification and preservation of motor cranial and spinal nerves in surgeries related to them. The levator palpabrae superioris muscle connected to the oculomotor nerve is used for cavernous sinus and superior orbital fissure surgery. Facial nerve monitoring is commonly conducted for vestibular schwannoma (Figure 13) and petrous bone involving surgeries. Vagus, accessory, and hypoglossal nerve monitoring are used in jugular foramen and adjacent area surgery. For vagus monitoring, the cricothyroid muscle can be used. Spinal motor nerve monitoring is used for spinal tumors (especially intramedullary tumors), spinal instrumentations (especially deformity-corrective surgery, e.g., for scoliosis), myelomeningocele, myelocele, lipo-meningocele or tethered cord syndrome, peripheral nerve injury repair, or plexopathy surgery.

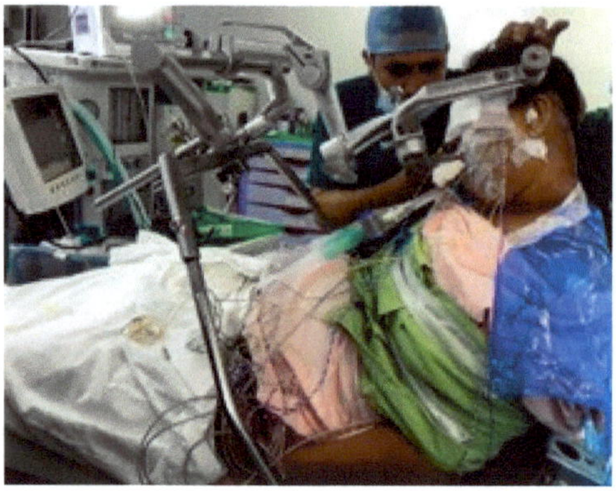

Figure 13. Placement of facial-nerve-monitoring equipment before removal of vestibular schwannoma in sitting posture. Source: Photo by authors.

2.4.2. Motor Evoked Potential (MEP) and Somato-Sensory Evoked Potential (SSEP)

These metrics are used during any surgery that may be related to complete motor (motor cortex to voluntary muscle) or sensory (peripheral sensory receptor to sensory cortex) pathways in order to check the integrity of the pathway.

2.4.3. Electrocorticogram (ECOG)

An ECOG is used during epilepsy surgery after opening a dura to identify the cortex responsible for the seizure (Figure 12) and to check for any residual responsible areas after cortical/lesional excision. It is also utilized for defining the central sulcus (as identified via phase reversal).

2.4.4. Visual Evoked Potential (VEP)

VEP can be used to ensure the safety and integrity of the visual pathway during surgeries related to visual pathways (i.e., visual apparatus tumors, occipital lobe surgery, etc.).

2.4.5. Brainstem Auditory Evoked Potential (BAEP) or Brainstem Auditory Evoked Potential (BAEP)

Brainstem auditory evoked potentials (BAEPs) are the electrical signals generated by the CNS within the first 10 ms after a transient acoustic stimulus. They are utilized for neurodiagnostic testing, intraoperative monitoring (e.g., acoustic schwannoma surgery and other surgeries related to hearing pathways), hearing screening/audiometry, head injuries, comas, brain death, and neurophysiological research.

2.4.6. Awake Craniotomy for Live Neuromonitoring

An awake craniotomy can be safely and expertly applied to psychologically stable patients for surgery involving the eloquent cortex (such as Broca's area, the primary motor area, etc.) or eloquent white mater (such as internal capsules, optic radiation, etc.) where the patient performs specific functions (such as limb movement, speech, etc.) at the time of the pathology's removal (Figures 14 and 15).

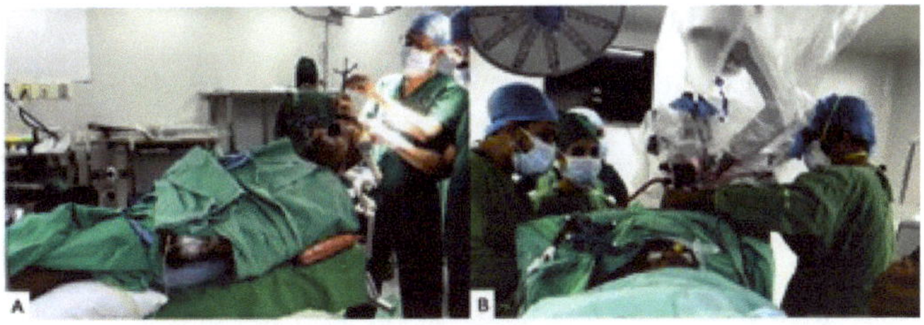

Figure 14. Pictures of awake craniotomy. (**A**) Position of patient and registration of neuronavigation. (**B**) Perioperative picture, showing the performance of an awake craniotomy. Source: Photos by authors.

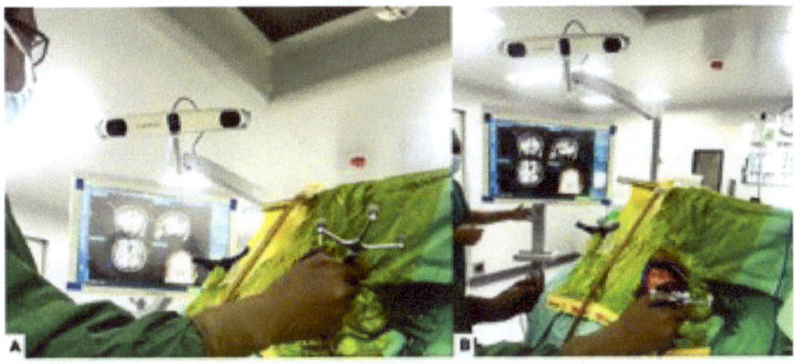

Figure 15. (**A**,**B**) Perioperative use of neuronavigation in awake craniotomy. Source: Photos by authors.

2.4.7. Stereotactic Navigation

The Cartesian coordinate system is based on three mutually perpendicular coordinate axes: the *xx* axis, the *yy* axis, and the *zz* axis. Thus, any point in space may be defined by *x*, *y*, and *z* values. Stereotactic surgery is based on the Cartesian coordinate system. By using computed tomography, magnetic resonance imaging (MRI), and Cartesian-co-ordinate-based stereotactic frames, anywhere deep in the brain can be reached/approached in a minimally invasive, precise, and reproducible manner. Modern stereotactic planning software helps in MRI and CT scan image fusion and trajectory planning, which eventually reduce surgical complications significantly. Biopsies, radiosurgery, deep-brain stimulation, radiofrequency ablation, the insertion of a depth electrode, and the suction of a hematoma or abscess are all indications for intracranial stereotactic surgery.

2.4.8. Neuronavigation

In image-guided neuronavigation, the concept of stereotaxis is applied. The brain is assumed to be a geometric volume that can be divided into three imaginary intersecting spatial planes that are orthogonal to each other using the Cartesian coordinate system (horizontal, frontal, and sagittal). Any site within the brain can be identified by measuring the distance between these three intersecting planes. This process provides precise neurosurgical guidance by transforming medical images into point-to-point maps of the corresponding locations within the brain by referencing this coordinate system of the brain with a parallel coordinate system of the 3-D image data of the patient, which are shown on the console of the computer workstation (Figures 14 and 15). Functional imaging methods such as magnetoencephalography (MEG), fMRI, and PET have been combined with neuronavigation to allow surgery in the vicinity of eloquent cerebral areas with little morbidity. The use of intraoperative MRI, which provides real-time images of residual lesions and allows for the testing of brain displacement during surgery, improves the spatial precision of today's neuronavigation systems (Ganslandt et al. 2002).

In order to relate the surgical techniques employed to images gathered both pre- and intraoperatively, each neuronavigation system follows the same steps: retrieving preoperative pictures; registration; intraoperative localization; intraoperative control; acquiring intraoperative images and fusing them with preoperative images; visualization; and operation (Ivanov and Ciurea 2009).

2.4.9. ICP Monitoring

An increased ICP can occur in cases with intracranial pathological conditions such as severe traumatic brain injuries, intracranial neoplasms, aneurysmal subarachnoid hemorrhage, and cerebral edema. The importance of the early detection and treatment of increased ICP cannot be overstated. ICP management has the ability to influence outcomes, especially when care is targeted, personalized, and supported with data from alternative monitors.

2.4.10. Jugular Venous Oximetry

This technique allows for intraoperative cerebral desaturation detection and anesthetic interventions such as improving hyperventilation therapy and managing perfusion pressure, fluids, and oxygenation to optimize cerebral physiology.

2.4.11. Intra-Operative Utilization of Dyes

Dyes are used in identifying CSF leakage, tumor identification, and intra-operative angiography. Fluorescein has been used intrathecally to identify CSF leaks, but there is risk of seizure associated with its use (Raza et al. 2016).

Fluorescein has also been used IV to help mark areas of the brain parenchyma where there is a breakage of the blood–brain barrier (BBB), e.g., in tumors. It has also been used to perform intraoperative "visible angiograms" during the removal of AVMs or during aneurysm clipping (Greenberg 2010).

Intraoperative angiography is performed using indocyanine green (ICG). This procedure can be performed under regular light; in some cases, near-infrared illumination can be used for a better view. It can only be applied to surface vessels. With big or wide-neck aneurysms or thick-walled atherosclerotic arteries, it may be less reliable (Greenberg 2010).

When tumor cells take up nonfluorescent 5-ALA, this process causes the production and accumulation of fluorescent protoporphyrin IX (PpIX). As a result of a broken BBB, enhanced neovascularization, and overexpression of membrane transporters in malignancy, there is greater ALA absorption in brain tumors. PpIX, which is collected specifically in malignant tissue, emits a red-violet light after being excited with blue light transmitted from a particular filter attachment on an operational microscope, allowing the surgeon to remove the red-violet tumor in a gross total fashion (Belykh et al. 2020).

2.4.12. CSF Study

CSF for research is often obtained via lumbar or ventricular taps, with a cisterna magna tap being used only very infrequently. A lumbar tap is contraindicated for an intracranial-space-occupying lesion (ICSOL), especially in the case of a posterior fossa tumor, wherein it may provoke tonsillar herniation through the foramen magnum, leading to death. A CSF study is commonly indicated for infective conditions (bacterial, viral, and fungal), including tuberculosis, demyelinating conditions (multiple sclerosis (MS), Guillain–Barre syndrome (GBS), and transverse myelitis (TM), wherein protein content is high), subarachnoid hemorrhages, etc. Very high protein content is found in GBS, bilateral acoustic schwannoma, and Froin's syndrome. Bacteria (including tuberculosis), viruses, and fungi can be identified by Gram and acid-fast bacillus (AFB) staining, the culturing of a precipitate of CSF in culture media, or by identifying genomic sequences (via PCR—polymerase chain reaction). CSF can also be used for serological studies, especially in neuro-cystocercosis, neuro-syphilis, hydatid disease, and toxoplasmosis (using ELISA, CFT, RIA, etc.).

2.4.13. Immunohistochemistry (IHC)

The IHC markers for CNS and PNS tumors can be broadly classified into three groups: (1) IHC markers utilized for diagnostic purposes, (2) IHC markers utilized for prognostic purposes, and (3) other IHC markers (Table 3) (Jaiswal 2016).

Table 3. IHC markers for CNS tumors.

Aims	Types	IHC Markers
For diagnosis	For glial cell tumors	S-100, GFAP
	For neuronal neoplasms	Synaptophysin, Beta-tubulin, NSE, Neurofilament, GFAP +/−, MAP-2
	For meningeal neoplasms	EMA, S-100, Vimentin, CK
	For choroid plexus neoplasms	CK, Transthyretin, S-100,
	For lymphomas	LAC, T-cell and B-cell markers
	For Schwann cell neoplasms	Leu 7, S-100,
	For germ cell neoplasms	AFP, PLAP, HCG, HPL
	For melanocytic neoplasms	HMB-45, MART-1(Melan-A), S-100, Microphthalmia transcription factor
	For vascular origin neoplasms	CD34, VEGF, Factor VIII, *Ulex europaeus*
	For pituitary neoplasms	PRL, ACTH, GH, MSH, FSH, LH, TSH
	For neuroendocrine neoplasms	Synaptophysin, Chromogranin
	For ATRT	INI-1/SMARCB-1
For prognosis	Cell cycle/proliferation markers	MIB-1, PNCA, Ki-67, BrdU,
	Tumor suppressor gene/oncogene protein	p53 tumor suppressor gene, C-myc oncogene, Retinoblastoma tumor suppressor gene (Rb)
	Growth factors/receptors	EGER
Other IHC markers		IDH-1and-2, BRAF, ATRX

IHC—Immunohistochemistry, GFAP—glial fibrillary acidic protein, CK—cytokeratin, NSE—neuron-specific enolase, MAP-2—Microtubule-associated protein-2, EMA—epithelial membrane antigen, LCA—leukocyte common antigen, AFP—alpha fetoprotein, HCG—human chorionic gonadotrophin, PLAP—placental alkaline phosphatase, HPL—human placental lactogen, HMB-45—human melanoma black-45, VEGF—vascular endothelial growth factor, PRL—prolactin, GH—growth hormone, ACTH—adrenocorticotrophin hormone, MSH—melanocyte-stimulating hormone, LH—luteinizing hormone, FSH—follicle-stimulating hormone, TSH—thyroid-stimulating hormone, ATRT—atypical teratoid/rhabdoid tumor, MIB-1—molecular immunology borstel-1, Ki-67—Kiel antibody-67, PCNA—proliferating cell nuclear antigen, BrdU—bromodeoxyuridine, EGFR—epidermal growth factor receptor, IDH-1&2—isocitrate dehydrogenase-1&2, ARTX—alpha-thalassemia/mental retardation syndrome X-linked (Jaiswal 2016). Source: Reprinted from Jaiswal (2016), used with permission.

Special molecular traits are part of the definition of a subset of CNS neoplasms in the 4th edition of the WHO Classification of CNS Tumors, which was published in 2016. This integrated 'histo-molecular' classification system provides for a significantly more exact diagnosis of diffuse gliomas and embryonal CNS malignancies, especially diffuse gliomas. IDH1/IDH2 mutations, 1p/19q codeletion, and mutations in histone H3 genes are all defining molecular markers for diffuse gliomas. According to the WHO's 2016 Classification, medulloblastomas, the commonest embryonal CNS neoplasms, are split into four molecularly characterized groups: WNT-signaling-pathway-activated, SHH-signaling-pathway-activated and tumor protein p53 gene (TP53) mutant, SHH-activated and TP53-wildtype, and non-WNT/non-SHH-activated. The diagnosis of various other CNS cancers, such as RELA fusion-positive ependymoma, atypical teratoid rhabdoid tumors (ATs/RTs), embryonal tumors with multilayered rosettes, and solitary fibrous tumors/hemangiopericytoma, is likewise dependent on molecular features. For further molecular characterization of several of these malignancies, immunohistochemistry is a useful alternative. Furthermore, genome-wide methylation profiling is a promising new approach to the diagnosis of CNS tumors (Kristensen et al. 2019).

2.4.14. Sample (Tissue/Granulation Tissue/PUS) for Histology, IHC, PCR, Cultures, and Staining

Sample specimens collected via/during surgical intervention should be collected appropriately. For histopathological examination, PCR, and immunohistochemistry, part(s) of specimens should be preserved in 10% formalin solution in container(s). For cultures, more than one specimen needs to be preserved in a sterile container without any preservative (including normal saline); commonly, three containers are used for 1. pyogenic aerobic bacteria, 2. fungal cultures (Sabouraud dextrose agar media), and 3. tubercular cultures. For anaerobic cultures, collection, transport, and inoculation in Robertson cooked meat medium necessitate special techniques and preparation. For Gram, AFB, or fungal staining, more specimens (without preservative) in different containers are required.

Author Contributions: Conceptualization, methodology, validation, formal analysis, investigation, resources, data curation, F.H.C. and R.I.; writing—original draft preparation, writing—review and editing, visualization, supervision, F.H.C. and M.Z.H. All authors have read and agreed to the published version of the manuscript.

Funding: This research received no external funding.

Conflicts of Interest: The authors declare no conflicts of interest.

References

American College of Radiology and Radiological Society of North America. 2011. Functional MR Imaging (fMRI)-Brain. May 24. Available online: https://www.radiologyinfo.org/en/info/fmribrain (accessed on 30 December 2011).

Barth, Daniel S. 1993. The neurophysiological basis of epileptiform magnetic fields and localization of neocortical sources. *Journal of Clinical Neurophysiology* 10: 99–107. [CrossRef] [PubMed]

Belykh, Evgenii, Kurt V. Shaffer, Chaoqun Lin, Vadim A. Byvaltsev, Mark C. Preul, and Lukui Chen. 2020. Blood-Brain Barrier, Blood-Brain Tumor Barrier, and Fluorescence-Guided Neurosurgical Oncology: Delivering Optical Labels to Brain Tumors. *Frontiers in Oncology* 10: 739. [CrossRef] [PubMed]

Feychting, Maria. 2005. Health effects of static magnetic fields—A review of the epidemiological evidence. *Progress in Biophysics and Molecular Biology* 87: 241–46. [CrossRef] [PubMed]

Ganslandt, O., S. Behari, J. Gralla, R. Fahlbusch, and C. Nimsky. 2002. Neuronavigation: Concept, techniques and applications. *Neuro India* 50: 244.

Golanov, A. V., T. M. Kotel'nikova, A. G. Melikian, M. B. Dolgushin, V. S. Sorokin, O. I. Soboleva, E. V. Khokhlova, G. E. Gorlachev, and S. A. Krasnianskiĭ. 2012. Application of SPECT/CT in neurosurgical practice. *Zhurnal Voprosy Neirokhirurgii Imeni NN Burdenko* 76: 85–91.

Greenberg, Mark S. 2010. *Handbook of Neurosurgery*. New York: Thieme.

Grossman, Robert I., and David. M. Yousem. 2003. *Techniques in Neuroimaging. Neuroradiology: The Requisites*. Philadelphia: Mosby.

Horská, Alena, and Peter B. Barker. 2010. Imaging of brain tumors: MR spectroscopy and metabolic imaging. *Neuroimaging Clinics* 20: 293–310. [CrossRef]

Ivanov, Marcel, and Alexandru Vlad Ciurea. 2009. Neuronavigation. Principles. Surgical technique. *Journal of Medicine and Life* 2: 29–35.

Jaiswal, Sushila. 2016. Role of immunohistochemistry in the diagnosis of central nervous system tumors. *Neurology India* 64: 502–12. [CrossRef]

Jayakar, Prasanna, Jean Gotman, A. Simon Harvey, André Palmini, Laura Tassi, Donald Schomer, Francois Dubeau, Fabrice Bartolomei, Alice Yu, Pavel Kršek, and et al. 2016. Diagnostic utility of invasive EEG for epilepsy surgery: Indications, modalities, and techniques. *Epilepsia* 57: 1735–47. [CrossRef]

Kristensen, Bjarne W., Loudy P. Priesterbach-Ackley, Jeanette K. Petersen, and Pieter Wesseling. 2019. Molecular pathology of tumors of the central nervous system. *Annals of Oncology* 30: 1265–78. [CrossRef]

Lindsay, Kenneth W., Ian Bone, and Geraint Fuller. 2011. *Neurology and Neurosurgery Illustrated. General Approach to History and Examination*. London: Churchill Livingstone Elsevier.

Logothetis, Nikos K., Jon Pauls, Mark Auguth, Torsten Trinath, and Axel Oeltermann. 2001. Neurophysiological investigation of the basis of the fMRI signal. *Nature* 412: 150–57. [CrossRef] [PubMed]

Passaro, Erasmo A. 2020. Neuroimaging in Epilepsy. Available online: https://emedicine.medscape.com/article/1155295-overview?form=fpf (accessed on 25 July 2022).

Petrella, Jeffrey R., and James M. Provenzale. 2000. MR Perfusion Imaging of the Brain: Techniques and Applications. *American Journal of Roentgenology* 175: 207–19. [CrossRef] [PubMed]

Preul, Mark C., Zografos Caramanos, D. Louis Collins, Jean-Guy Villemure, Richard Leblanc, Andre Olivier, Ronald Pokrupa, and Douglas L. Arnold. 1996. Accurate, noninvasive diagnosis of human brain tumors by using proton magnetic resonance spectroscopy. *Nature Medicine* 2: 323–25. [CrossRef] [PubMed]

Raza, Shaan M., Matei A. Banu, Angela Donaldson, Kunal S. Patel, Vijay K. Anand, and Theodore H. Schwartz. 2016. Sensitivity and specificity of intrathecal fluorescein and white light excitation for detecting intraoperative cerebrospinal fluid leak in endoscopic skull base surgery: A prospective study. *Journal of Neurosurgery* 124: 621–26. [CrossRef]

Robba, Chiara, Alberto Goffi, Thomas Geeraerts, Danilo Cardim, Gabriele Via, Marek Czosnyka, Soojin Park, Aarti Sarwal, Llewellyn Padayachy, Frank Rasulo, and et al. 2019. Brain ultrasonography: Methodology, basic and advanced principles and clinical applications. A narrative review. *Intensive Care Medicine* 45: 913–27. [CrossRef]

Romano, Nicola, Margherita Federici, and Antonio Castaldi. 2019. Imaging of cranial nerves: A pictorial overview. *Insights Imaging* 10: 33. [CrossRef]

Salinsky, Martin, Roy Kanter, and Richard M. Dasheiff. 1987. Effectiveness of multiple EEGs in supporting the diagnosis of epilepsy: An operational curve. *Epilepsia* 28: 331–34. [CrossRef]

Seeger, Leanne L. 1989. Physical principles of magnetic resonance imaging. *Clinical Orthopaedics and Related Research* 244: 7–16. [CrossRef]

Subbaraju, Vigneshwaran, Suresh Sundaram, and Sundararajan Narasimhan. 2018. Identification of lateralized compensatory neural activities within the social brain due to autism spectrum disorder in adolescent males. *European Journal of Neuroscience* 47: 631–42. [CrossRef]

Tae, Woo-Suk, Byung-Joo Ham, Sung-Bom Pyun, Shin-Hyuk Kang, and Byung-Jo Kim. 2018. Current Clinical Applications of Diffusion-Tensor Imaging in Neurological Disorders. *Journal of Clinical Neurology* 14: 129–40. [CrossRef]

Tai, Y. F., and Paola Piccini. 2004. Applications of positron emission tomography (PET) in neurology. *Journal of Neurology, Neurosurgery & Psychiatry* 75: 669–76. [CrossRef]

Wang, Xuhui, Minhui Xu, Hong Liang, and Lunshan Xu. 2011. Comparison of CT and MRI in diagnosis of cerebrospinal leak induced by multiple fractures of skull base. *Radiology and Oncology* 45: 91–96. [CrossRef] [PubMed]

Section IV: Congenital Disorders

Congenital Abnormalities of CNS

Mainul Haque Sarker, Rashed Mahmud and Forhad H. Chowdhury

Abstract: Abnormalities in the development of the neural tube result congenital anomalies of the central nervous system, which can range from mild to extensive anomalies and involve any part of nervous system. In this chapter, common neurosurgical congenital anomalies are discussed. In the early part of this chapter, cranial anomalies are summarized, including congenital hydrocephalus, cerebral aqueductal stenosis, craniosynostosis, and encephalocele. Common spinal defects like meningocele, myelomeningocele, lipomyelocele, and tethered cord syndrome are discussed in the middle of this chapter. Craniospinal anomalies, especially Chiari malformation and syringomyelia, are very important in clinical practice. Finally, arachnoid cysts are discussed briefly.

Abbreviations

AqS	aqueductal stenosis	BPC	Blakes pouch cyst
CNS	central nervous system	CSF	cerebrospinal fluid
CSO	Craniosynostosis	CT	computed tomography
CVJ	cranio-vertebral junction	DWC	Dandy–Walker cyst
DWV	Dandy–Walker variant	DWM	Dandy–Walker malformation
ETV	endoscopic third ventriculostomy	HA	Headache
HCP	hydrocephalus.	ICP	intracranial pressure
MM	myelo-meningocele	MRI	magnetic resonance imaging
OFC	occipito-frontal circumference	PICA	posterior inferior cerebellar artery
SCM	split-cord malformation	TC	tethered cord syndrome
VP shunt	ventriculo-peritoneal shunt		

1. Introduction

Disorders of the anatomy of the central nervous system (CNS) that develop in the womb and are present at birth are known as congenital anomalies of the CNS. The symptoms and prognoses for congenital malformations vary depending on their type and severity. Some are diagnosed at birth, while others may remain undetected until adolescence or adulthood.

Causes of congenital anomalies:

- Genetic factors (most common);
- Multifactorial etiology: alcohol, tobacco, smoking, drugs/medications, vitamins, environmental toxins, toxic chemicals, and several viruses that can infect the fetus while in the uterus;
- Idiopathic mechanisms.

Common congenital CNS abnormalities:

A. Primary Cranial Anomalies
   - (i) Cerebral aqueductal stenosis;
   - (ii) Congenital hydrocephalus;
   - (iii) Craniofacial anomalies (a. craniosynostosis; b. encephalocele);
   - (iv) Dandy–Walker malformation;
   - (v) Arachnoid cysts;
   - (vi) Others.

B. Primary Spinal Anomalies
   - (i) Spinal dysraphism;
   - (ii) Tethered cord syndrome;
   - (iii) Klippel–Feil syndrome;
   - (iv) Others.

C. Primary Craniospinal Anomalies
   - (i) Chiari malformation;
   - (ii) Neural tube defects;
   - (iii) Others.

2. Cranial Congenital Anomaly

2.1. Cerebral Aqueductal Stenosis with Hydrocephalus

Aqueductal stenosis (AqS) is the narrowing of the Sylvian aqueduct such that the CSF flow in the ventricular pathway is obstructed (Figures 1–3).

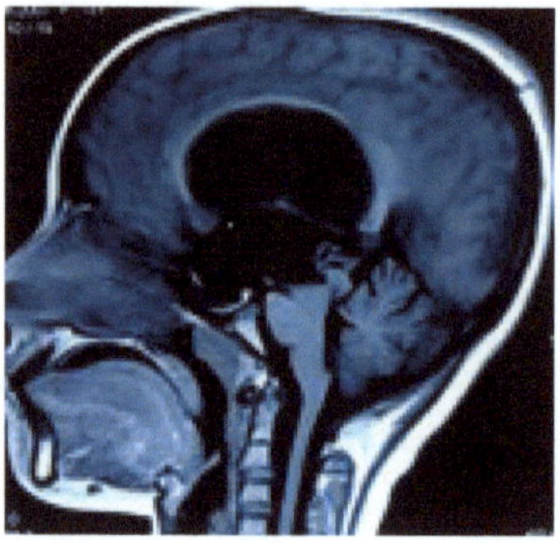

Figure 1. MRI of the brain (sagittal view) showing triventricular HCP due to cerebral aqueductal stenosis (CAS). Source: Figure by authors.

2.1.1. Etiology

1. Congenital: The anomaly may occur alongside neurofibromatosis (NF) or Chiari malformation.
2. Acquired: The anomaly may be due to the causes cited below:
    (a) Inflammation as a sequalae hemorrhage and infections, e.g., tuberculosis (TB), intra-uterine infections, etc.;
    (b) Tumors, particularly brainstem astrocytoma (including tectal plate gliomas) and lipoma;
    (c) Quadrigeminal plate arachnoid cysts.

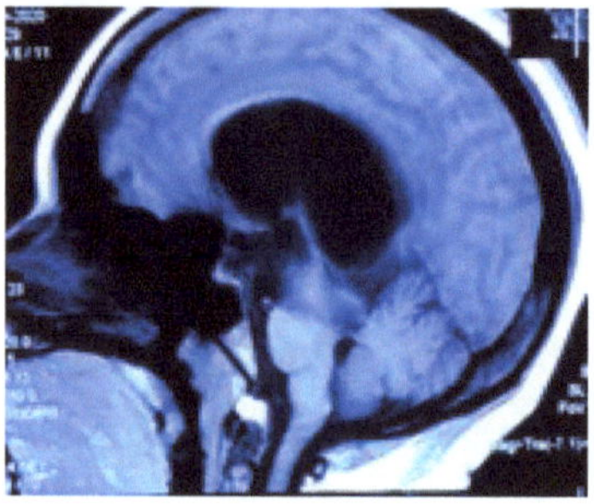

Figure 2. MRI of the brain (sagittal section) showing CAS. Source: Figufre by authors.

2.1.2. Aqueductal Stenosis in Infants

AqS (Chowdhury et al. 2017; Greenberg 2010) is a common etiology of congenital hydrocephalus (HCP) (accounting for up to 70% of cases), and, rarely, it is the outcome of hydrocephalus.

Types of congenital AqS: The four varieties of congenital AqS described by Russell (Nag and Falconer 1966):

1. Forking: As a result of the partial fusion of the median fissure, the aqueduct is split into many independent channels. These channels may re-connect to form a single aqueduct, or they may come to an abrupt halt and form a dead-end. This variety usually occurs in conjunction with other developmental anomalies (spina bifida and lipomyelocele).

2. Periaqueductal gliosis: Here, the aqueduct starts out partially obstructed. To overcome this partial block, the pressure in the third ventricle is increased. This produces more stress on the aqueduct, resulting in greater injury to the epithelial lining of the third ventricle, causing gliosis and glial cell proliferation, which ultimately obstructs the aqueduct.

3. True stenosis: This variety consists of narrowing present since birth. This narrowing results from an unusual folding of the neuro-epithelial plate.

4. Septum formation: Here, a membrane composed of glial cells forms across the aqueduct (Figure 3). The commonest site is at the lower and distal portion of the aqueduct. It obstructs the canal totally.

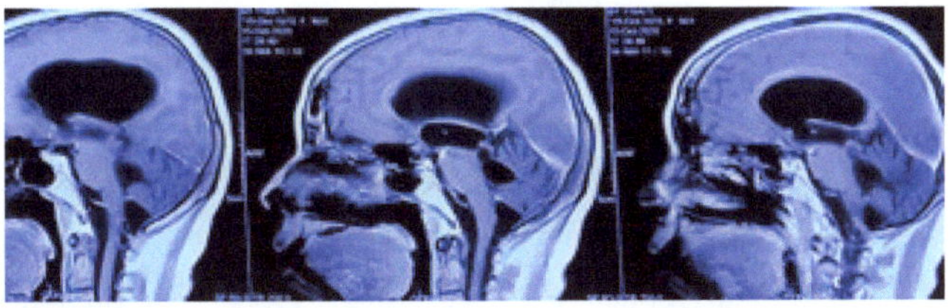

Figure 3. MRI of the brain (sagittal sections) showing CAS with HCP due to septations. Source: Figure by authors.

2.1.3. Aqueductal Stenosis in Adulthood

Most patients present with this anomaly between the ages of 1 and 5, but it may emerge at as late as 47 years of age. The cause of this late presentation is unknown. AqS may be an overlooked cause of "normal pressure hydrocephus" in an adult (Vanneste and Hyman 1986). Although most cases remain benign, there may be elevated ICP and sudden death.

2.1.4. Clinical Features

Most cases occur in childhood, but some may present in adulthood.

Symptoms:

- Headache: This is the most common symptom, and it is caused by raised ICP.
- Visual disturbance: This consists of blurring of vision, loss of acuity, and upward gaze palsy.
- Cognitive difficulty and developmental delay.
- Gait disturbance and frequent falling.
- Endocrine abnormalities, including menstrual irregularity, hypothyroidism, and hirsutism.

Signs:

- Papilledema (the commonest sign);
- Reduced peripheral vision and increased blind spots, while visual fields may be normal;
- Intellectual impairment;
- Others: ataxia, pyramidal tract signs, hemiparesis/paraparesis, spasticity, Babinski sign, anosmia.

2.1.5. Evaluation

MRI is the primary choice for investigation. It will show the disappearance of the usual CSF flow void in the aqueduct. Contrast should be injected to exclude tumors. CT scans can also be used for diagnosis and evaluation. USG can also be used as screening test for younger children.

2.1.6. Treatment

- Endoscopic third ventriculostomy: Possibility of failure of ETV is higher in younger children (age < 06 months);
- Ventriculo-peritoneal shunt.

2.2. Congenital Hydrocephalus

Hydrocephalus (HCP) is an unusual collection of CSF within the ventricular system of the brain. Congenital hydrocephalus is when a child is born with an excessive accumulation of CSF within the brain (Figures 1–6).

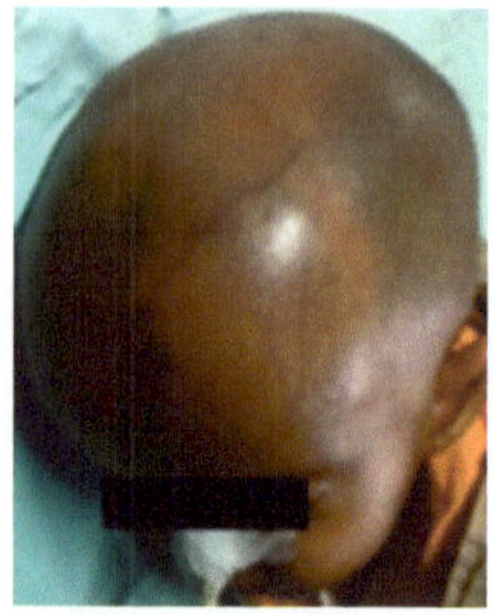

Figure 4. Head of a patient with HCP showing enlarged head, tense fontanels, and a shiny scalp with a sunset eye sign. Source: Photo by authors.

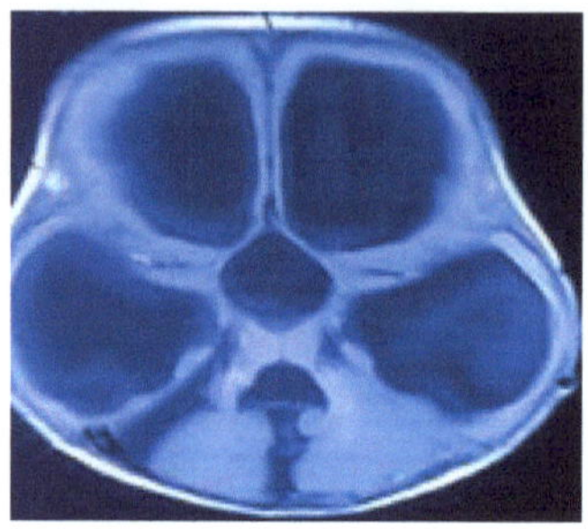

Figure 5. MRI of the brain (axial section) showing HCP with Dandy–Walker Variant (DWV). Source: Figure by authors.

2.2.1. Common Causes of Congenital Hydrocephalus

(i) Aqueductal stenosis;
(ii) Neural tube defects;
(iii) Dandy–Walker syndrome;
(iv) Type 1 and type 2 Chiari malformations;
(v) Genetic mutation.

2.2.2. Symptoms and Signs

(a) In young children:
- Unusually large head;
- Cranial growth > facial growth;
- Thin, transparent scalp;
- Scalp veins show engorgement along with flow reversal from intracranial sinuses due to ↑ICP;
- Fontanelles are full and bulging;
- Irritability, poor head control, nausea, and vomiting;
- Downward gaze;
- Hyperactive reflexes.

(b) In older pediatric patients (with unyielding cranial vault) and adults
- Features of raised ICP: headache, nausea, vomiting, papilledema;
- Gait changes;
- Downward gaze;
- Abducens nerve palsy;
- Initially, slowly increasing ventricles may be asymptomatic.

2.2.3. Treatment

- ETV;
- VP shunt.

2.2.4. Fourth-Ventricular Outflow Obstruction (FVOO)

This is a very rare congenital anomaly where atresia of the foramen Magendie and Luschka cause hydrocephalus with pan-ventriculomegaly (Figure 6). The treatment options are ETV or a VP shunt.

2.2.5. Foramen of Monro Stenosis/Atresia

It is an extremely rare anomaly causing univentricular hydrocephalus.

2.3. Craniosynostosis (Craniostenosis)

Craniosynostosis (CSO) is a condition where one or more sutures close too early, causing impairment of normal brain development and skull growth, increased pressure inside the head, and a change in the skull or facial structures from a normal symmetric appearance. CSO is rarely associated with hydrocephalus (HCP) (Golabi et al. 1987).

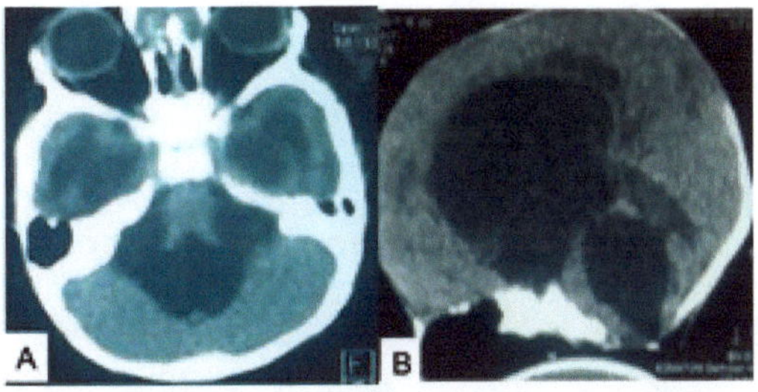

Figure 6. CT scan of the head (**A**) axial and (**B**) sagittal views) showing fourth-ventricular obstruction (FVOO) due to foramen Magendie and Luschka atresia. Source: Figure by authors.

2.3.1. Types

(a) Sagittal synostosis
- This is the commonest form of CSO involving a single suture, and 80% of cases are male.
- It results in dolichocephaly or scaphocephaly (a boat-shaped skull) associated with frontal bossing, a marked occiput, and a palpable, keel-like sagittal ridge.
- In this condition, OFC remains near to normal, but the biparietal diameter is significantly reduced.
- Affected individuals may present with features of elevated ICP.
- Treatment—Surgery: Within the first 36 months of life, a linear strip craniectomy should be performed, removing the sagittal suture from the bregma to the lambda. The strip's width should be at least 3 cm.

(b) Coronal synostosis
- About 18% of CSO cases are coronal synostosis, and they are more common in females.
- In Crouzons syndrome, this condition is associated with abnormalities of sphenoid, orbital, and facial bones.
- In Apert's syndrome, features of Crouzons syndrome plus syndactyly are present (Renier et al. 1996).
  Unilateral coronal CSO is called plagiocephaly, featuring a flattened or concave forehead on the afflicted side above the eye (the normal side appears to protrude unnaturally) and a supra-orbital edge that is higher than that one the normal side (presenting a harlequin eye sign in a skull X-ray). Amblyopia can occur when the orbit spins out on the abnormal side.
- If left untreated, the cheeks flatten, and the nose moves to the usual side (the root of the nose develops a tendency to deviate towards deformity). Bilateral coronal CSO (e.g., Aperts) brachycephaly is characterized by a broad, flattened forehead.
- The corrective surgery in this case is a simple strip craniectomy of the affected suture or a frontal craniotomy (unilateral or bilateral), advancing the lateral canthus by taking off the orbital bar.

(c) Metopic synostosis
- Here, the frontal bone is divided into two similar parts at birth by the frontal/metopic suture, which results in a pointed forehead with a midline ridge (trigonocephaly).

- Many of affected individuals are cognitively handicapped and have a 19p chromosomal issue.

(d) Lambdoid synostosis
- Males are more likely to have this condition than females (with a male/female ratio = 4:1), and the right-sided suture is affected in 70% of instances.
- It commonly appears between the ages of 3 and 18 months; however, it can appear as early as 1–2 months.
- Positional flattening (lazy lambdoid) causes confusion, which might be caused by limited movement in patients who always rest in the supine position with their head on the same side.
- Abnormal postures: congenital torticollis, congenital cervical spine abnormalities

2.3.2. Clinical Findings

- The occiput is flattened. It could be either unilateral or bilateral.
- Unilateral lambdoid synostosis results in a rhomboid skull, with the ipsilateral ear located anterior and inferior to the contralateral ear when severe; bilateral lambdoid synostosis results in brachycephaly with anterio-inferiorly displaced auricles in severe cases (Muakkassa et al. 1984).

2.3.3. Treatment

- Nonsurgical management (McComb 1991).
  Despite the fact that most patients recuperate, permanent deformity is a common occurrence.
- In 85% of situations, repositioning is effective. In this process, patients are placed on the side that is not affected or on their abdomen. Torticollis-related occipital flattening in infants should be treated aggressively with physical therapy, and remission should be seen within 3–6 months.
- Molding helmets (Clarren 1981) may be used to treat more severe involvement. Surgery is required only 20% of the time. The best time to conduct surgery is when an afflicted child is between the ages of 6 and 18.
- Surgical alternatives include a simple unilateral suture removal and repair by a craniofacial team.

2.4. Encephalocele

The term encephalocele (also known as cephalocele or meningoencephalocele) refers to intracranial material protruding through a calvarial or skull-base defect. Until proven differently, a nasal polyp like a mass in a baby should be regarded as an encephalocele.

2.4.1. Some Related Terminologies

Cranium bifidum: congenital fusion failure of cranial bones in the midline.
Encephalocele: when meninges and cerebral tissue protrude through the defect.
Meningocele: when meninges and CSF come through the defect.

2.4.2. Classification

The following classification scheme is based on the work by Suwanwella and Suwanwella (Suwanwela and Suwanwela 1972):

1. Occipital, often affecting vascular structures
2. Cranial vault, constituting about 80% of encephaloceles in the developed world
   (a) Interfrontal;
   (b) Anterior fontanelle;
   (c) Interparietal, often including a vascular component;
   (d) Temporal;
   (e) Posterior fontanelle.
3. Fronto-ethmoidal: (synonym—sincipital) (constituting 15% of encephaloceles), wherein there is an exterior opening on the face in one of the following three areas:
   (a) Nasofrontal: an outer defect in the nasion;
   (b) Naso-ethmoidal: a defect between the nasal bone and nasal cartilage;
   (c) Naso-orbital: a defect in the antero-inferior part of medial orbital wall.
4. Basal: This form constitutes 1.5% of encephaloceles;

(a) Transethmoidal: projection into the nasal cavity through a defect in the cribriform plate;
(b) Spheno-ethmoidal: the defect projects into posterior nasal cavity;
(c) Transsphenoidal: through the patent craniopharyngeal canal (foramen cecum), it projects into the nasopharynx or sphenoid sinus;
(d) Fronto-sphenoidal or spheno-orbital: the pathway is the superior orbital fissure, protruding into the orbit;

5. Posterior fossa: commonly contains cerebellar tissue and a ventricular part.

Basal Encephalocele

This consists of the developmental failure of skull-base ossification. This is the sole group of encephaloceles that does not generate soft tissue swelling that can be seen. CSF leaks or recurrent meningitis are possible symptoms. The majority of babies are stillborn; however, some make it to the age of 17. Basal encephaloceles consist of the following subtypes:

(a) Midline basal encephalocele
   (i) Transsphenoidal: A defect in the foramen cecum that protrudes into the sphenoid sinus or nasopharynx;
   (ii) Transethmoidal: A defect in the Cribriform plate;
   (iii) Sphenoethmoidal: A defect in the Sphenoid and ethmoid bones.
(b) Lateral basal encephalocele
   (i) Sphenomaxillary: A defect in the maxillary sinus and orbital fissure that protrudes into the pterygopalatine fossa;
   (ii) Sphenoorbital or fronto sphenoidal: A defect in the superior orbital fissure that protrudes into the orbit.

Cranial Vault Encephalocele

These encephaloceles may be of the following subtypes:

- Anterior fontanelle;
- Posterior fontanelle;
- Interfrontal;
- Interparietal;
- Temporal.

Frontoethmoidal (Sincipital) Encephalocele

In this type, there is an external opening in the face in one of three areas:

(a) Nasofrontal: an outer gap in the nasion;
(b) Naso-ethmoidal: a defect that stays between nasal bone and cartilage;
(c) Naso-orbital: a gap in the antero-inferior zone of the medial orbital wall.

Occipital Encephalocele

In this type of encephalocele, there is a failure in primary neural tube closure. The defect may be in the occipital bone or foramen magnum. It often involves vascular structures. The surgical removal of the sac and its contents is followed by a watertight dural closure. Hydrocephalus is common in this condition and may require different treatment. If there is a substantial quantity of cerebral tissue in the encephalocele, the ventricles expand into the mass, or there is HCP, the prognosis is usually poor. An occipital encephalocele may be of two subtypes:

Low occipital: A defect that continues into the foramen magnum.

High occipital: A defect that stops at the foramen magnum.

Posterior Fossa Encephalocele

Generally, this type contains cerebellar tissue and a ventricular part.

2.5. Other Cranial Congenital Abnormalities

2.5.1. Dandy–Walker Malformation (DWM)

This malformation is a deformed and wrapped-in-a-neuroglial-vascular-membrane larger posterior cranial fossa with partial (hypoplasia) or total aplasia of the vermis and cystic enlargement of the fourth ventricle. Dandy and Blackfan first characterized this condition in 1914, and Benda called it Dandy–Walker deformity 40 years later (Incesu and Khosla 2008). Hydrocephalus is a common occurrence in this condition.

Differential Diagnoses of DWM

Developmental disorders associated with posterior fossa CSF (or CSF-like) accumulations include (Calabro et al. 2000) the following:

1. Dandy–Walker malformation (DWM);
2. Dandy–Walker variant (DWV), which is defined as a case wherein one or more of the Dandy–Walker requirements are missing. Vermian hypoplasia and cystic distension of the fourth ventricle without expansion of the posterior fossa are examples of this (Figure 5).
3. Persistent Blakes pouch cyst (BPC): This consists of panventriculomegaly with a connected fourth ventricle and a posterior fossa cyst, with or without hypoplasia of both the cerebellar vermis and the medial portions of the cerebellar hemispheres.
4. Retrocerebellar arachnoid cyst: A cyst that pushes the fourth ventricle and the cerebellum anteriorly, a process that has the potential to have a mass effect. Here, the vermis is in good condition (Figure 7).
5. Joubert's syndrome: In this case, the cerebellar vermis is absent or underdeveloped.
6. Enlarged (mega) cisterna magna: Subsequent to an enlarged cisterna magna, an enlarged posterior fossa develops. The vermis and fourth ventricle are normal, and the cerebellum does not have a large impact.

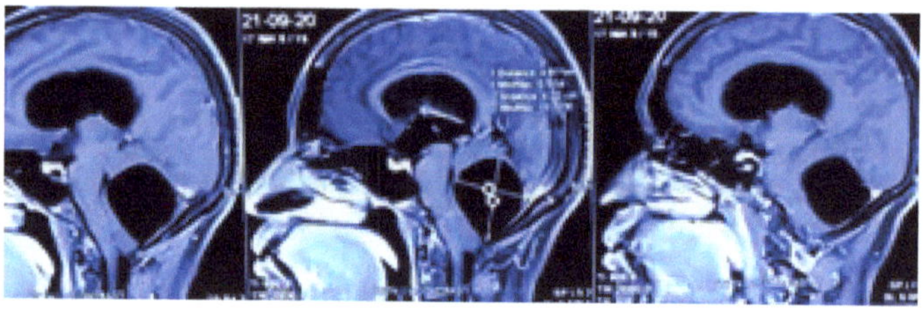

Figure 7. Contrast MRI of the brain showing a retrocerebellar arachnoid cyst causing HCP. Source: Figure by authors.

Differentiating Features

DWC: DWM and DWVs may refer to the Dandy–Walker Complex, a group of developmental disorders (DW) (Forzano et al. 2007).

BPC nor retrocerebellar arachnoid cysts: Although neither BPC nor retrocerebellar arachnoid cysts (Figure 7) undergo vermian agenesis, they may appear to be DWMs. The fourth ventricular choroid plexus is normal in arachnoid cysts, missing in Dandy–Walker malformations, and pushed into the superior cyst wall in BPC.

Arachnoid cyst and mega cisterna magna: An intrathecal enhanced CT scan (wherein iodinated contrast is injected into the CSF through a ventricular catheter, and then CT is performed) will reveal a large cisterna magna that interacts with the ventricular system, but DWM as well as most arachnoid cysts are non-interactive.

Pathophysiology and Risk Factors

The cause of DWM is not known, but it is probably caused by dysembryogenesis of the roof of the fetal rhombencephalon, and not as a result of the failure of the genesis of the fourth ventricular outlets, as previously thought (Forzano et al. 2007). This produces cerebellar vermian aplasia with a large posterior fossa cyst connected to an expanded fourth ventricle (Incesu and Khosla 2008).

Associated abnormalities: Stringed CNS anomalies are aplasia of the corpus callosum in 17% of cases, and 7% have an occipital encephalocele. Extra physical findings include heterotopias, spinal dysraphism, spinal cord syrinx, a small head (microcephaly), dermoid tumors, porencephaly, and Klippel–Feil syndrome. An expanded posterior fossa with superiorly displaced torcular herophili is also common. Atresia of the Magendie as well as Luschka foramen may be present (Raimondi et al. 1969).

Systemic abnormalities may be associated with each other and include (Hirsch et al. 1984) facial anomalies (e.g., hemangiomas, a palatal cleft, macroglossia, and a dysmorphic face), ocular anomalies (e.g., coloboma, dysgenesis of the retina, and small orbits and eyes (microphthalmia)). Cardiovascular abnormalities may include atrial/ventricular septal defects, patent ductus arteriosus, coarctation of the aorta, and dextrocardia. When considering surgery for these patients, the possibility of a cardiac abnormality must be taken into consideration.

Treatment

- If HCP is absent, conduct a follow up.
- If HCP is present, the shunting of the cyst of the posterior fossa is required.
  Solely shunting the lateral ventricles is not recommended as there is a risk of potential trans-tentorial herniation (Mohanty et al. 2006).
  The patency of the aqueduct of Sylvius must be investigated; otherwise, a VP shunt should be inserted simultaneously. When the aqueduct is patent, an endoscopic third ventriculostomy can be attempted.
- Prognosis: Because the severity of the deformity varies, the prognosis varies as well. According to certain pediatric neurosurgery studies, fatality rates range from 12% to 50%, albeit this figure is improving with newer shunting procedures. Only half of affected patients have a normal IQ. Common symptoms include ataxia, spasticity, and impaired fine motor coordination. Seizures affect 15% of afflicted people.

3. Spinal Congenital Anomalies

3.1. Spinal Dysraphism (Spina Bifida)

The word "spinal dysraphism" refers to a group of disorders that affect the spine, spinal cord, or nerve roots and are present at birth. It occurs as a result of the neural tube's incomplete construction or the abnormal development of structures connected to the neural tube and surrounding somites.

3.1.1. Types

A. Spina bifida occulta;
B. Spina bifida aperta, which consists of the following entities:
   a. Meningoceles;
   b. Myelomeningoceles;
   c. Lipomeningoceles;

3.1.2. Spina Bifida Occulta

A lack of a spinal process and a varied amount of lamina are both congenital. There are no apparent meninges or neural tissue. There may be overlaying cutaneous manifestations, and a deficiency may be visible.

3.1.3. Meningocele

- Only meninges herniate through this defect; no neural elements are present. The spinal cord is usually normal. The mass is usually seen in the midline of the lower back. Most meningoceles are well covered with skin (Figure 8).
- Surgery may be delayed or avoided in asymptomatic infants with normal neurologic results and full-thickness skin covering.
- To prevent meningitis, patients with leaking cerebrospinal fluid or a thin skin covering should undergo prompt surgical therapy, which includes sac excision and repair with a watertight dural closure.

3.1.4. Myelomeningocele (MM)

A myelomeningocele is a congenital defect in vertebral arches featuring cystic swelling over the area of the defect encompassing meninges, the spinal nerve root, and the spinal cord itself and that has left the vertebral canal (Figures 9–11).

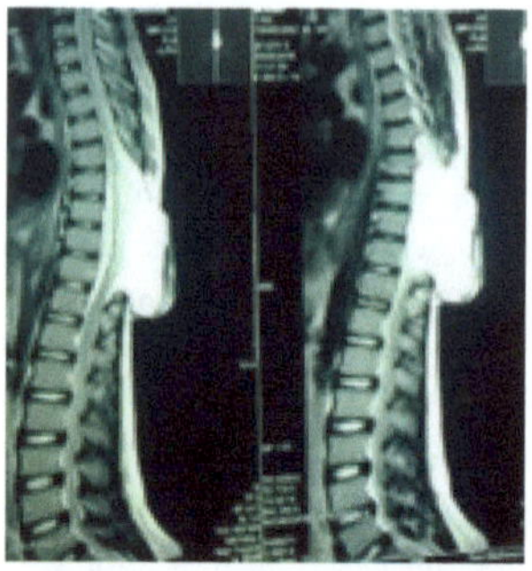

Figure 8. MRI of dorsal spine (sagittal views) showing dorsal meningocele. Source: Figure by authors.

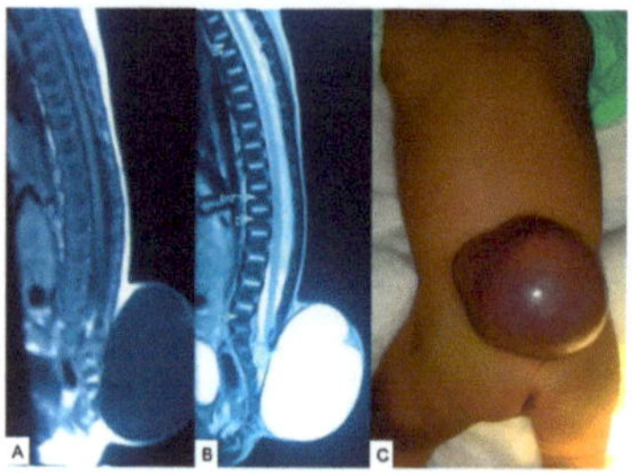

Figure 9. (**A**,**B**) MRI of dorsal spine (sagittal views) showing a lumbo-sacral myelomeningocele (MM). (**C**) Myelomeningocele after positioning a patient for surgical excision. Source: Figure by authors.

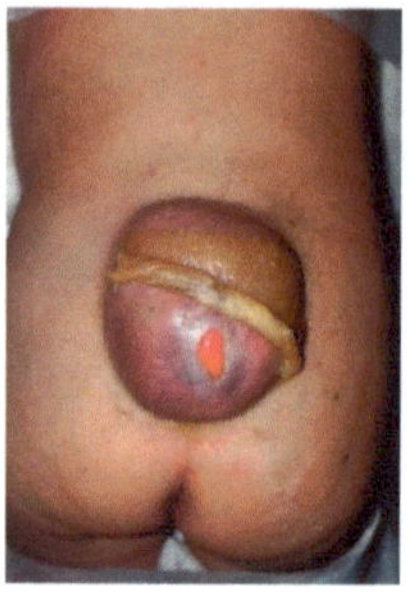

Figure 10. Lumbo-sacral MM seen after positioning of patient for surgical excision. Source: Photo by authors.

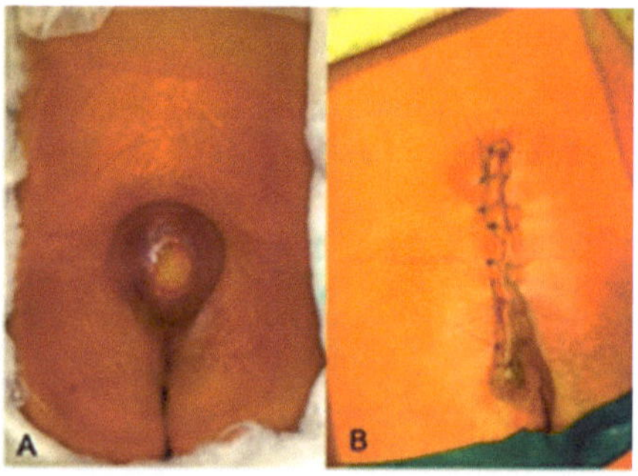

Figure 11. (**A**) Lumbo-sacral MM seen after positioning the patient for surgical excision; (**B**) perioperative view after excision. Source: Photos by authors.

Hydrocephalus in MM

A total of 65–85% of MM patients develop hydrocephalus (HCP), and 5–10% of MM cases may have overt hydrocephalus at delivery (Stein and Schut 1979). HCP affects almost 80% of MM patients before they reach the age of six months. The majority of MM patients have a Chiari type-2 malformation. Closing the MM defect can turn latent hydrocephalus into active hydrocephalus via blocking a CSF outflow route. The lower the abnormality in the neuro-axis (sacrum), the less likely it is that hydrocephalus will occur. However, regardless of the spinal level, the danger of hydrocephalus development should always be recognized.

Clinical Features

- Approximately 75% of MMs are present in the lumbosacral region. MMs induce bowel and bladder incontinence, as well as anesthesia in the perineal area, when it is present in the lower sacral region, but it does not impair motor function.
- MMs in the mid-thoracic region typically feature a growing neurologic deficit and may even present with complete paralysis of all muscles of the lower limbs.
- MMs in the upper thoracic or cervical region are normally accompanied by a minimal neurodeficit and are not associated with hydrocephalus in the majority of instances, but they may occur alongside neurogenic bladder and intestine dysfunction in certain situations.

Surgical Management

Timing of MM Surgical Closure: Although there is no evidence that early closure of an MM defect leads to improved neurologic function, there is evidence that it leads to a lower infection rate. If the membrane is intact, the MM should be closed within 24 h (after 36 h, the lesion will have been colonized, and the chance of postoperative infection is high).

MM Defect Closure and VP Shunting at the Same Time: Most neurosurgeons forestall shunting for at least three days after MM repair in cases without HCP. MM repair and VP shunt insertion can be performed simultaneously in MM cases with obvious HCP at birth without an increased risk of infection and with a shorter hospital stay (Epstein et al. 1985; Hubballah and Hoffman 1987).

These procedures could also lower the likelihood of MM repair failure previously existing at the time preceding shunting. In this combined procedure, the patient is positioned so that they are lying down with their head rotated to the right (to reveal the occiput on the right side) and their right knee and thigh flexed to reveal their right flank (one can consider utilizing the left flank to avoid confusion with an appendicectomy incision scar later in life).

Surgical Technique of MM Repair

General principles (McLone 1980): Keep the exposed neural tissue wet to avoid desiccation. Make use of a latex-free setting (this decreases the chance of stimulating a latex allergy and hypersensitivity due to maternal antibodies that may have transferred across the placenta). Scrubbing chemical or antimicrobial solutions should not come into contact with the neural placode. Monopolar cautery should not be used. Avoid putting tension on the neuronal placode at any time during the closure.

(i) The placode should be sharply separated from the surrounding arachnoid membrane and ectodermal elements. Retained fragments of cutaneous epithelium, which can cause a dermoid cyst, should be removed from the placode.
(ii) Reconstitute the neural tube by gently folding the placode towards the midline and securing the pia with small, nonabsorbable monofilament sutures.
(iii) The thickened filum terminal, if it can be located, should be sectioned.
(iv) Identify the dural–dermis boundary. Circumferentially incise the dura at the boundary, separate it from subcutaneous tissues, and move it towards the midline, where it should be closed.
(v) Ensure water-tight dural closure.
(vi) Move the skin by separating it from the underlying normal fascia.
(vii) Do not apply tension to the neural placode at any point during closure (Figure 11).

Postoperative Care

(i) The patient is kept in prone position to avoid the placement of pressure on the incision.

(ii) A barrier dressing below the incision is used to avoid contamination from urine or stool.
(iii) Daily measurements of OFC and weekly head ultrasounds are obtained to check for progressive ventriculomegaly (especially in children who do not have shunts).
(iv) Routine bladder catheterization is ensured.
(v) Orthopedic and urological consultations for the correction of limb, hip, and bladder function are conducted.

3.2. Other Spinal Anomalies

3.2.1. Klippel–Feil Syndrome

The fusion of two or more cervical vertebrae is a congenital condition. The fusing of merely the bodies of the vertebrae (congenital block vertebrae) to the complete vertebrae is possible (including the neural arch). Flattened vertebral bodies and hypoplastic or missing disc gaps are common in involved vertebral bodies. Hemivertebrae can also be found. The neural foramina are smaller and more oval-shaped than typical foramina. Cervical stenosis is a rather uncommon condition. Iniencephaly is an uncommon condition characterized by a complete lack of the posterior components, a large foramen magnum, and a permanent hyperextension posture.

Presentation

Classical clinical triad (all three are present in <50%):

1. A low posterior hairline;
2. A shortened neck (brevicollis);
3. Limitation of neck motion (may not be evident if <3 vertebrae are fused, if fusion is limited only to the lower cervical levels (Gray et al. 1964), or if hypermobility of non-fused segments compensates for this lack of mobility). Limitation of movement is more common in terms of rotation than flexion–extension or lateral bending.
   Symptoms are not due to the fused vertebrae but result from non-fused segments that possibly become hypermobile, leading to instability or degenerative arthritic changes.
4. Visceral abnormalities:
   (a) Kidneys: ↑albumin excretion in urine, ↑BUN, and ↑ creatinine levels.
   (b) Respiratory: wheezing.
   (c) CVS: irregular heartbeat, complete heart block.

Investigations

(i) Urine: ↑albumin; ↓urinary volume.
(ii) Blood: ↑BUN and ↑creatinine.
(iii) Radiology: vertebral fusion between C2-5, scoliosis, spina bifida, atlanto-axial dislocation.

Treatment

A. Pain killers, muscle relaxant, and physiotherapy. If the condition does not improve, surgery is required.
B. The surgical options are as follows:
   (i) Correction of cranio-vertebral instability and decompression of the spinal cord;
   (ii) Cervical discectomy and fusion;
   (iii) Scoliosis surgery.

3.2.2. Tethered Cord Syndrome (TCS)

Tissue attachments that impede the mobility of the spinal cord within the spinal canal cause this neurological condition. The conus medullaris is unusually low here. TCS is generally accompanied by a short and thickened filum terminale or an intradural lipoma. (Figure 12).

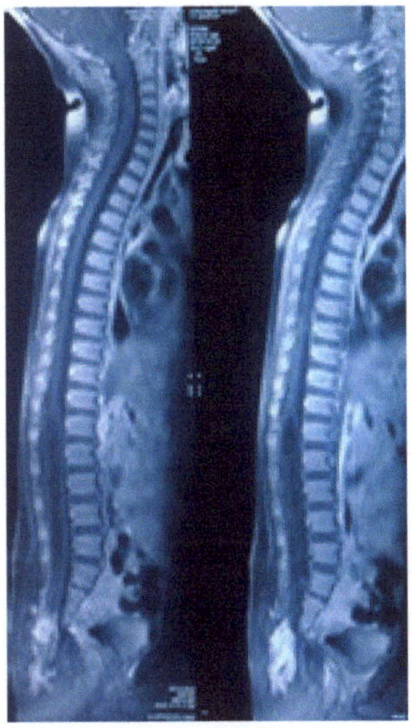

Figure 12. MRI of the spine (sagittal views) showing tethered cord and syringomyelia with sacral lipoma. The patient also had Chiari malformation. Source: Figure by authors.

TCS is most commonly seen in cases of myelomeningoceles (MMs). If an MM patient has deteriorating scoliosis, progressively increasing spasticity, increasing gait disturbances, and worsening urodynamics and the condition is painful, the individual should be considered to have tethered cord syndrome until proof suggests otherwise (Park et al. 1985).

Progressive scoliosis can be observed at the same time as a tethered cord is seen. Early release of the spinal cord may induce an elevation in scoliosis status.

Presentations

TCS is mostly noted in children. Children and adults have different clinical presentations. The symptoms and signs may develop during or after the lengthening of the spine. Comparison of childhood versus adult tethered cord syndrome is shown in Table 1.

Table 1. Comparison of childhood versus adult tethered cord syndrome.

Clinical Presentation	Adult TCS	Pediatric TCS
Pain	Common	Rare
Swelling	Less common	Frequent
Leg weakness	Frequent	Less frequent than adult
Sensory impairment	In 15%	In 18%
Sphincteric dysfunction	In 65% adult TCS	In 18% pediatric TCS
Orthopedic deformity	In 30%	In 16%
Cutaneous stigmata (tufts of hair, dimples, and capillary angioma/naevus flammeus)	In 80–100% cases	In <50% cases
Lipomeningocele	In 40%	In 13%
Meningocele & meningomyelocele	Very rare	Relatively frequent
Dermal sinus	In 10% patient	In 1% patient
Aggravating factor	Trauma	Growth spurts

Source: Authors' compilation based on data from Pang and Wilberger (1982); Shukla et al. (2018).

Evaluation

Radiography: A conus medullaris with a thickened filum terminale (diameter > 2 mm) and a low-lying conus medullaris (below L2) are observed. It can be difficult to tell the difference between a tethered cord and a conus that is naturally low-lying (here, the filum diameter is normal).

Pre-operative cystometrogram: This is especially necessary if the patient is continent

Surgical Treatment

(a) If only a thickened and shortened filum is observed, untethering by sectioning the filum should be performed.
(b) If lipoma is also present, it may be excised along with filum (if it can be easily separated from nervous tissues) or debulking.
(c) Perioperative differentiation of filum terminale from nerve roots:
    (i) Filum has typical squiggly vessels on its surface.
    (ii) Microscopically, filum has a typical whiter appearance than the nerve root.
    (iii) Ligament-like strands can be observed running within it.

Outcome

- It is normally impossible to permanently untether a cord in the case of an MM; but, after 2–4 untetherings, a growing MM-afflicted child's growth may be complete, and tethering may be discontinued.
- Untethered cases from childhood may return later in life, particularly during the adolescent growth spurt.
- Among adults, surgical release is generally effective and good for pain elevation, but bladder function return is poor.

4. Cranio-Spinal and Other Anomalies

4.1. Chiari Malformation

Chiari malformations are a group of four different forms of anomalies of the hindbrain that are unrelated to one another. Types 1 and 2 are the most common Chiari malformations. The remaining types are made up of a small number of examples.

4.1.1. Chiari Type 1 Malformation

- Elongated, peg-shaped cerebellar tonsils, also known as primary cerebellar ectopia (Spillane et al. 1957), and adult Chiari malformation (as it is commonly identified in the 2nd/third decade of life).
- Extends below FM into the upper cervical spinal canal (Figures 13 and 14).
- Unlike Chiari malformation-2, the medulla oblangata is not shifted downward, the brainstem is unaffected, the lower cranial nerves are not lengthened, and the higher cervical spinal nerves do not run upward.
- Syringomyelia affects 30–70% of patients.
- Hydrocephalus has been linked to Chiari type 1 malformation patients.

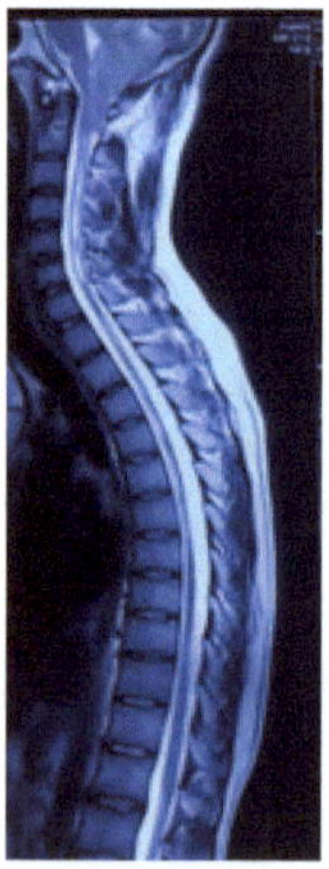

Figure 13. MRI of spine and cranio-vertebral junction (CVJ) showing type 1 Chiari malformation with syringomyelia. Source: Figure by authors.

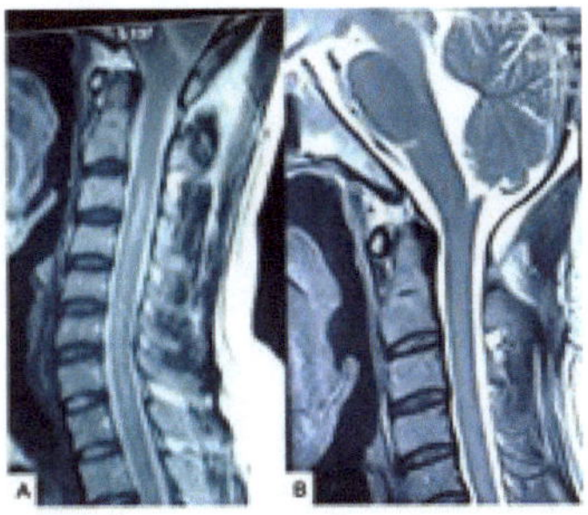

Figure 14. (**A**) preoperative MRI of cranio-vertebral junction (CVJ) and cervical spine (sagittal views) showing type 1 Chiari malformation with syringomyelia. (**B**) Post-operative MRI after three months of operation. Source: Figure by authors.

Associations

Chiari type 1 is usually associated with the following:

1. Base-of-the-skull and CV junction anomalies:
   (i) An underdeveloped occipital bone;
   (ii) Smaller and shallow posterior fossa;
   (iii) Platybasia;
   (iv) Basilar invagination;
   (v) Hypermobility of CVJ.
2. Spine-related abnormality:
   (i) Klippel–Feil syndrome;
   (ii) Occipitalization of atlas;
   (iii) Retroflexion of odontoid process;
   (iv) Scoliosis.
3. Meninges-related abnormalities
   (i) Low-lying tentorium;
   (ii) Thickened arachnoid/scar/fibrosis around brainstem and tonsils near to the foramen magnum;
   (iii) Veils of arachnoid that obstruct fourth-ventricular outflow.
4. Brain-related abnormalities
   (i) Space-occupying lesion in posterior fossa;
   (ii) Intracranial-space-occupying lesion;
   (iii) Craniosynostosis (especially cases involving all sutures).
5. Ventricle- and cistern-related abnormalities
   (i) Hydrocephalus;
   (ii) Elongated fourth ventricle;
   (iii) Retrocerebellar CSF spaces are obliterated or diminished.
6. Following LP shunt or multiple LP (acquired Chiari 1 malformation)

Symptoms

(i) This condition has an adult onset, and the average age at presentation is 41 years. There is a slight female preponderance.
(ii) The most common symptom is headache (sub-occipital HA, often detected via neck extension or valsalva).
(iii) Weakness of limb(s) and/or unsteadiness.
(iv) Loss of temperature sensation.
(v) Painless burns.

Signs

Three prime patterns of clustering of signs:

1. Compression syndrome of the foramen magnum: ataxia, sensory, and corticospinal neuro-deficits; Babinski sign; and lower-cranial-nerve palsies.

2. Central cord syndrome: hand atrophy, upper limb weakness, lower-limb weakness, dissociated sensory loss, and hyperactive deep tendon reflexes.
3. Cerebellar syndrome: ataxia, downbeat nystagmus during vertical movement, and dysarthria.

Evaluation

(i) MRI of the brain and cervical spine is the investigation of choice (Figures 13 and 14).
(ii) Traditionally tonsillar descend >5 mm is defined as pathologic, with 3–5 mm being borderline.
(iii) Most cases are associated with syringomyelia.

Indications for Surgery

Early surgery is advised for clinically symptomatic cases. Asymptomatic cases can be followed up and operated on when the patient becomes symptomatic. Symptomatic patients who are stable for years can be followed up, and surgery is recommended when the patient deteriorates.

Surgical Techniques

Posterior fossa decompression via sub-occipital craniectomy with augmented duroplasty with or without cervical laminectomy of C_1 (sometimes C_2 or C_2). The goal of surgery is to decompress the brainstem as well as reestablish normal CSF flow at the craniospinal junction.

Surgical Complications

Sleep apnea, respiratory depression, CSF leak, cerebellar herniation, vascular injuries (PICA), etc.

4.1.2. Chiari Type 2 Malformation

This condition is also known as Arnold–Chiari malformation

Pathology

Almost all neonatal Chari II patients have a myelomeningocele, which is caused by an in utero CSF leak in turn caused by open spinal dysraphism. Patients with Chiari II who do not have a myelomeningocele are considered to have had a smaller neural tube defect or have had the defect closed in utero.

Major Findings

(i) Caudally dislocated cervico-medullary junction, pons, medulla, and fourth ventricle.
(ii) Cerebellar tonsils are situated at or below the level of the foramen magnum.
(iii) Normal cervicomedullary junction flexure is replaced by a "kink-like" deformity.
(iv) Others: Beaking of tectum, hydrocephalus, bony abnormalities such as abnormalities of cervicomedullary junction, assimilation of C1, platybasia, basilar invagination (BI), Klippel–Feil deformity, etc.

Presentation

Onset is commonly in the neonatal stage and rare in adulthood. Neonates develop rapid neurological deterioration with profound brain stem dysfunction. Patients may present with the following symptoms (Pollack et al. 1992; Park et al. 1983):

1. Swallowing difficulties (neurogenic dysphagia);
2. Apneic spells, which are more common in neonates;
3. Stridor, which occurs as a result of vagus nerve paresis and is commonly transient but may progress to respiratory arrest;
4. Aspiration;
5. Arm weakness, which may result in quadriparesis;
6. Nystagmus, especially downbeat nystagmus.

Evaluation

Cranial and cervical MRI is the investigation of choice. The potential findings are as follows:

A medulla-situated "Z" bend deformity, a cerebellar peg, tectal fusion ("tectal beaking"), increased interthalamic adhesion, extension of the medulla, low levels of attachment of the tentorium, hydrocephalus, syringomyelia, a trapped fourth ventricle, and corpus callosum agenesis/dysgenesis.

Surgical Technique

If hydrocephalus has developed, CSF shunting is performed. Expeditious posterior fossa decompression should be performed if neurogenic dysphagia, stridor, or apneic events occur.

Decompression of the cerebellar tonsils via suboccipital craniectomy with cervical laminectomy with augmented duroplasty is used. In cases with a significant syringomyelic cavity, a syringo-subarachnoid shunt is also placed.

4.1.3. Other Chiari Malformations

Chiari type 0: Patients with syringohydromyelia but no hindbrain herniation who improve after posterior fossa decompression are classified as Chiari type-0 (Iskandar et al. 1998).

Chiari type 1.5: The whole cervicomedullary junction (including the obex) is located below the foramen magnum, and suboccipital decompression with or without duroplasty has little effect.

Chiari type 3: Chiari type 3 is a rare condition. The cerebellum dislocates below the foramen magnum, resulting in an occipital encephalocele. Some individuals have an occipital and high cervical encephalocele combined with herniation of the medulla, fourth ventricle, and entire cerebellum. According to certain sources, occipital encephaloceles are linked to cerebellar and medulla caudal displacement. The majority of cases have a poor prognosis since they are life-threatening.

Chiari type 4: Type 4 Chiari was originally identified as cerebellar hypoplasia without herniation (Chiari 1895).

4.1.4. Syringomyelia

Syringomyelia is a general term referring to a pathology in which a cyst or cavity is formed within the spinal cord (Figures 13–15).

Etiologies

A. Primary syringomyelia: the absence of an identifiable cause

B. Secondary syringomyelia: due to partial obstruction of the spinal subarachnoid space. Etiologies are:

1. Chiari I malformation: the commonest cause of syrinx.
2. Post-inflammatory: (a) postinfectious—meningitis; (b) chemical or other sterile inflammations.
3. Post-traumatic: (a) severe post-traumatic kyphotic deformity, (b) arachnoid scarring, and (c) severe trauma to the spinal cord and/or its coverings.
4. Postsurgical: many years after uneventful intradural tumor resection (e.g., neurofibromas).
5. Basilar arachnoiditis: (a) idiopathic and (b) postinfectious.
6. Basilar invagination with a narrow foramen magnum.
7. Dandy–Walker syndrome.

Presentations

1. Dissociative sensory loss: Pain and temperature sensations are lost, but touch as well as joint position awareness are preserved. Painless ulcerations from unnoticed injuries and/or burns are also exhibited.

2. Cervical and occipital pain are the most common. Dysthetic pain in the sensory loss distribution is also exhibited.

3. Hand and arm weakness due to lower motor neuron weakness.

4. Painless (neurogenic) arthropathies (Charcot's joints) characterized by a loss of pain and temperature sensation, particularly in the shoulder and neck.

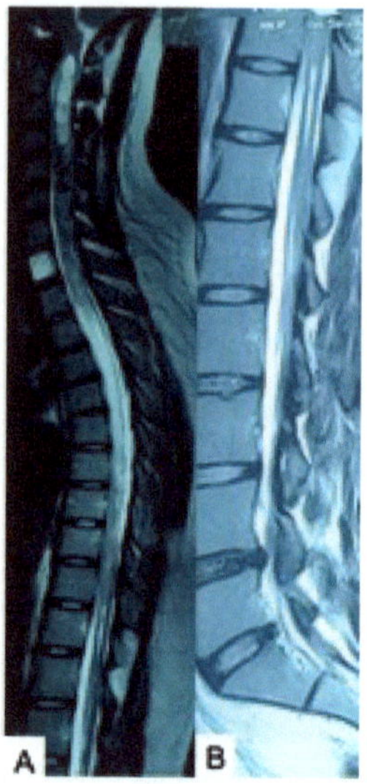

Figure 15. MRI of the spine (sagittal images): (**A**) CVJ and cervico-dorsal spine and (**B**) dorso-lumbar spine showing syringomyelia without an obvious etiology (possibly Chiari-0). Source: Figure by authors.

Evaluation

MRI

Treatment

Treatment of the underlying cause.

4.1.5. Split-Cord Malformation (SCM)

A split-cord malformation (SCM) is a type of concealed spinal dysraphism and tethered spinal cord condition that is rather uncommon. The majority of these instances appear in infancy, with neurocutaneous stigmata being a common early symptom. SCM accounts for almost one-third of all occurrences of spinal dysraphism, in which the spinal cord is separated into two equal or unequal halves across a section of its length (Figure 16). All double spinal cords, which seem to have a common embryological genesis, are classified as SCMs. Two hemicords, each one with its own central canal as well as the surrounding pia, are contained within a distinct dural tube and divided by a dural-sheathed stiff osseocartilaginous/bony median septum in Type I SCMs. Diastematomyelia is a term used to describe this condition, which involves spinal anomalies. Overlying skin abnormalities such as nevi, hypertrichosis, lipomas, dimples, or hemangiomas affect two-thirds of the population. The majority of these patients have an orthopedic foot abnormality. Tethering of the cord is the most prevalent cause of symptoms, which can typically be alleviated by untethering. The dura must be reconstructed as a single tube once the bony septum is removed. A nonrigid fibrous median septum separates two hemicords within a single dural tube in Type II SCM. Diplomyelia is a term that has been used to describe this condition. Nerve roots protrude from each hemicord. At the level of the split, there are usually no abnormalities in the spine, but there is usually spina bifida occulta in the lumbosacral region. One treatment consists of surgically untethering the chord. Surgical removal of the spur and detethering of the filum are also employed (Chowdhury et al. 2016; Hoffman 1992).

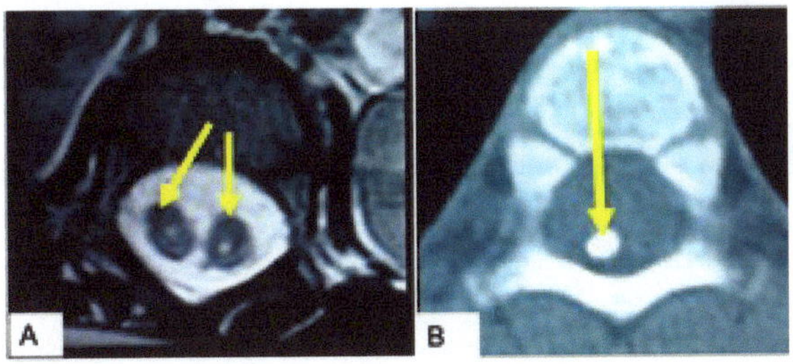

Figure 16. Split cord malformation (SCM). (**A**) MRI of the dorsal spine (axial view) diplomyelia and (**B**) CT scan of dorsal spine (axial view) showing bony septum. Source: Figure by authors.

4.1.6. Arachnoid Cyst (Leptomeningeal Cysts)

Arachnoid cysts (ACs) are congenital anomalies that occur during embryonic development via the duplication of the arachnoid mater (intra-arachnoid cysts), and they contain CSF-like fluid. They do not communicate with the ventricular or subarachnoid CSF. They may have septations and are typically lined with meningothelial cells. ACs can also develop in the spinal canal. Their incidence is 0.5% in autopsy series. ACs constitute 1% of intracranial-space-occupying lesions. The male/female incidence ratio is 4:1. ACs are more common on the left side (Figure 17).

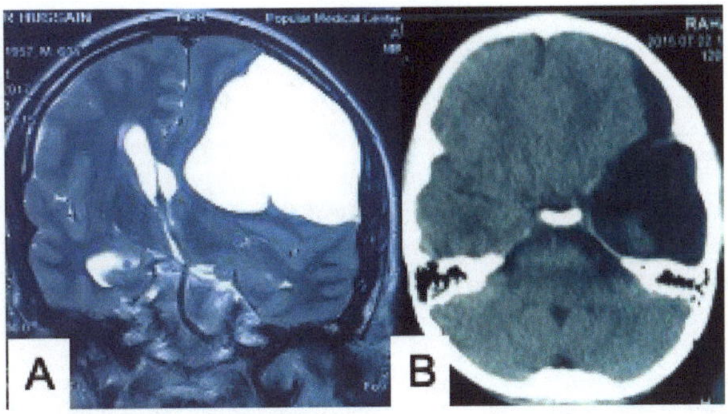

Figure 17. (**A**) MRI of the brain showing left-sided hemispheric symptomatic arachnoid cyst. (**B**) CT scan of the head showing a left temporal AC with hypoplastic temporal lobe. Source: Figure by authors.

There are two varieties of histological ACs:

- Simple arachnoid cysts: In these, the lining cells are capable of active CSF production;
- Complex ACs: Here, the lining may contain neuroglia, ependyma, and other tissue types.

Distributions of AC is (Sinha and Brown 2004):

Sylvian fissure, 49%;
Supracolicular, 10%;
Sellar and supra sellar, 9%;
Cerebral convexity, 4%;
Cerebellopontine angle, 11%;
Vermian, 9%;
Interhemispheric, 5%;
And clival, 3%.

Clinical Presentation

Most ACs are symptomless. Symptomatic ones commonly present in early childhood. The clinical presentation differs with the location of the arachnoid cyst and often appears mild in contrast to the size.

Clinical Features

- Features of intracranial hypertension;
- Sudden deterioration (due to hemorrhage);
- Location related focal signs and symptoms;
- Endocrine symptoms and visual impairment (suprasellar cysts);

- Seizures;
- As a focal swelling of the skull;
- Incidental finding.

Evaluation

- CT scan of the head
- MRI of the brain and spine: This combination is better than CT in distinguishing the CSF contained in ACs from the cystic tumor. It may exhibit cyst walls.
- Cisternograms and/or ventriculograms

Treatment

Incidental ACs: follow up.

Symptomatic ACs:

- Cysto-ventriculostomy (endoscopic/microscopic);
- Cysto-cisternostomy (endoscopic/microscopic);
- Excision/marsupialization;
- Cyst shunting (cysto-peritoneal) and/or CSF shunting.

Even after successful management, a part of the AC may remain because of the re-modeling of the bone and the great shift of the brain (Greenberg 2010; Chowdhury et al. 2018; VanDer Meche and Braakman 1983; Mayr et al. 1982; Pierre-Kahn et al. 1990; Altschuler et al. 1990; Hopf and Perneczky 1998; Sinha and Brown 2004).

Spinal Arachnoid Cysts (SACs)

A SAC nearly always occurs in the thoracic spine. A neurenteric cyst is a differential diagnosis for a ventral SAC. Most are extradural and can be associated with kyphosis, scoliosis, or spina bifida. Intradural spinal arachnoid cysts may be of congenital origin or may be caused by infection or trauma. They are commonly asymptomatic but can cause paraplegia. MRI of the spine is the most useful investigation. Symptomatic SACs need surgical (percutaneous/open) treatment (Greenberg 2010; Chowdhury et al. 2018; VanDer Meche and Braakman 1983; Mayr et al. 1982; Pierre-Kahn et al. 1990; Altschuler et al. 1990; Hopf and Perneczky 1998; Sinha and Brown 2004).

Author Contributions: Conceptualization, methodology, validation, formal analysis, investigation, resources, data curation, M.H.S., R.M. and F.H.C.; writing—original draft preparation, R.M.; writing—review and editing, visualization, supervision, F.H.C. All authors have read and agreed to the published version of the manuscript.

Funding: This research received no external funding.

Conflicts of Interest: The authors declare no conflicts of interest.

References

Altschuler, Eric. M., Charles A. Jungreis, Laligam N. Sekhar, Peter J. Jannetta, and Peter E. Sheptak. 1990. Operative treatment of intracranial epidermoid cysts and cholesterol granulomas: Report of 21 cases. *Neurosurgery* 26: 606–14. [CrossRef] [PubMed]

Calabro, F., T. Arcuri, and J. R. Jinkins. 2000. Blake's pouch cyst: An entity within the Dandy-Walker continuum. *Neuroradiology* 42: 290–95. [CrossRef] [PubMed]

Chiari, H. 1895. Über veränderungen des kleinhirns des pons und der medulla oblongata in folge von congenitaler hydrocephalie des grosshirns. Denkschr der Kais Akad Wiss Wien math. *Naturw* 63: 71–116.

Chowdhury, Forhad H., Mohammod R. Haque, and Nur Mohammod. 2016. Split Cord Malformation-1 (SCM): Characteristic Neuro-imaging. *Journal of National Institute of Neurosciences Bangladesh* 2: 103. [CrossRef]

Chowdhury, Forhad H., Mohammod R. Haque, Khandkar A. Kawsar, Mainul H. Sarker, and Abdul Fazal Mohammod M. Haque. 2017. Result of Endoscopic Third Ventriculostomy for Hydrocephalus Caused by Cerebral Aqueductal Stenosis in Infant Patients. *Indian Journal of Neurosurgery* 6: 189–97. [CrossRef]

Chowdhury, Forhad H., Mohammod R. Haque, Noman K. Chowdhury, Shamsul I. Khan, and Noor Mohammod. 2018. Endoscopic Surgical Management of Intracranial Symptomatic Arachnoid Cyst. *Iranian Journal of Neurosurgery* 4: 61–74. [CrossRef]

Clarren, Sterling K. 1981. Plagiocephaly and torticollis: Etiology, natural history, and helmet treatment. *The Journal of Pediatrics* 98: 92–95. [CrossRef]

Epstein, Nancy E., Alan D. Rosenthal, Joseph Zito, and Michael Osipoff. 1985. Shunt Placement and Myelomeningocele Repair: Simultaneous versus Sequential Shunting. *Child's Nervous System* 1: 145–47. [CrossRef]

Forzano, F., S. Mansour, A. Ierullo, T. Homfray, and B. Thilaganathan. 2007. Posterior fossa malformation in fetuses: A report of 56 further cases and a review of the literature. *Prenatal Diagnosis* 27: 495–501. [CrossRef]

Golabi, Mahin, Michael S. B. Edwards, and Douglas K. Ousterhout. 1987. Craniosynostosis and Hydrocephalus. *Neurosurgery* 21: 63–67. [CrossRef]

Gray, S. W., C. B. Romaine, and J. E. Skandalakis. 1964. Congenital Fusion of the Cervical Vertebrae. *Surgery, Gynecology & Obstetrics* 118: 373–85.

Greenberg, Mark S. 2010. *Handbook of Neurosurgery*. New York: Thieme.

Hirsch, Jean-François, Alain Pierre-Kahn, Dominique Renier, Christian Sainte-Rose, and Elizabeth Hoppe-Hirsch. 1984. The Dandy Walker Malformation: A Review of 40 Cases. *Journal of Neurosurgery* 61: 515–22. [CrossRef] [PubMed]

Hoffman, H. J. 1992. Comment on Pand D. et al. Split cord malformation. Part 1: A unified theory of embryology for double spinal cord malformations. *Neurosurgery* 31: 480.

Hopf, Nikolai J., and Axel Perneczky. 1998. Endoscopic neurosurgery and endoscope-assisted microneurosurgery for the treatment of intracranial cysts. *Neurol Surgery* 43: 1330–37.

Hubballah, Malek Y., and Harold J. Hoffman. 1987. Early Repair of Myelomeningocele and Simultaneous Insertion of VP Shunt: Technique and Results. *Neurosurgery* 20: 21–23. [CrossRef]

Incesu, L., and A. Khosla. 2008. Dandy-Walker Malformation. Available online: http://emedicine.medscape.com/article/408059-overview (accessed on 31 January 2021).

Iskandar, Bermans J., Gary L. Hedlund, Paul A. Grabb, and W. Jerry Oakes. 1998. The resolution of syringohydromyelia without hindbrain herniation after posterior fossa decompression. *Journal of Neurosurgery* 89: 212–16. [CrossRef]

Mayr, U., F. Aichner, G. Bauer, I. Mohsenipour, and A. Pallua. 1982. Supratentorial extracerebral cysts of the middle cranial fossa: A report of 23 consecutive cases of the so-called temporal lobe agenesis syndrome. *Neurochirugia* 25: 51–56. [CrossRef]

McComb, J. Gordon. 1991. Treatment of functional lambdoid synostosis. *Neurosurgery Clinics of North America* 2: 665–72. [CrossRef]

McLone, David G. 1980. Technique for Closure of Myelomeningocele. *Childs Brain* 6: 65–73. [CrossRef]

Mohanty, Aaron, Arundhati Biswas, Satyanarayana Satish, Shanti S. Praharaj, and Kolluri V. R. Sastry. 2006. Treatment options for Dandy-Walker malformation. *Journal of Neurosurgery* 105: 348–56. [CrossRef]

Muakkassa, Kamel F., Harold J. Hoffman, David R. Hinton, E. Bruce Hendrick, Robin P. Humphreys, and Judith Ash. 1984. Lambdoid Synostosis: Part 2: Review of Cases Managed at The Hospital for Sick Children, 1972–1982. *Journal of Neurosurgery* 61: 340–47. [CrossRef] [PubMed]

Nag, T. K., and M. A. Falconer. 1966. Non-Tumoral Stenosis of the Aqueduct in Adults. *British Medical Journal* 2: 1168–70. [CrossRef] [PubMed]

Pang, Dachling, and James E. Wilberger, Jr. 1982. Tethered Cord Syndrome in Adults. *Journal of Neurosurgery* 57: 32–47. [CrossRef] [PubMed]

Park, Tae Sung, Hoffman J. Hoffman, Bruce B. Hendrick, and Robin P. Humphreys. 1983. Experience with Surgical Decompression of the Arnold-Chiari Malformation in Young Infants with Myelomeningocele. *Neurosurgery* 13: 147–52. [CrossRef]

Park, T. S., Wayne S. Cail, William M. Maggio, and Diane C. Mitchell. 1985. Progressive Spasticity and Scoliosis in Children with Myelomeningocele: Radiological Investigation and Surgical Treatment. *Journal of Neurosurgery* 62: 367–75. [CrossRef]

Pierre-Kahn, Alain, Laurent Capelle, Raja Brauner, Christian Sainte-Rose, Dominique Renier, Raphaël Rappaport, and Jean-François Hirsch. 1990. Presentation and management of suprasellar arachnoid 25. cysts: Review of20 cases. *Journal of Neurosurgery* 73: 355–59. [CrossRef]

Pollack, Ian F., Dachling Pang, A. Leland Albright, and Donald Krieger. 1992. Outcome Following Hindbrain Decompression of Symptomatic Chiari Malformations in Children Previously Treated with Myelomeningocele Closure and Shunts. *Journal of Neurosurgery* 77: 881–88. [CrossRef]

Raimondi, Anthony J., Gene Samuelson, Luis Yarzagaray, and Thomas Norton. 1969. Atresia of the Foramina of Luschka and Magendie: The Dandy-Walker Cyst. *Journal of Neurosurgery* 31: 202–16. [CrossRef]

Renier, Dominique, Eric Arnaud, Giuseppe Cinalli, Guy Sebag, Michel Zerah, and Daniel Marchac. 1996. Prognosis for Mental Function in Apert's Sydrome. *Journal of Neurosurgery* 85: 66–72. [CrossRef]

Shukla, Mukesh, Jayesh Sardhara, Rabi Narayan Sahu, Pradeep Sharma, Sanjay Behari, Awadesh KumarJaiswal, Arun Kumar Srivastava, Anant Mehrotra, Kuntal Kanti Das, and Kamlesh Singh Bhaisora. 2018. Adult versus pediatric tethered cord syndrome: Clinicoradiological differences and its management. *Asian Journal of Neurosurgery* 13: 264–70. [CrossRef]

Sinha, Saurabh, and Jennifer I. M. Brown. 2004. Familial posterior fossa arachnoid cyst. *Child's Nervous System* 20: 100–3. [CrossRef] [PubMed]

Spillane, John D., Christopher Pallis, and Arthur M. Jones. 1957. Developmental Abnormalities in the Region of the Foramen Magnum. *Brain* 80: 11–52. [CrossRef] [PubMed]

Stein, Sherman C., and Luis Schut. 1979. Hydrocephalus in Myelomeningocele. *Childs Brain* 5: 413–19. [CrossRef] [PubMed]

Suwanwela, Charas, and Nitaya Suwanwela. 1972. A Morphological Classification of Sincipital Encephalomeningoceles. *Journal of Neurosurgery* 36: 201–11. [CrossRef] [PubMed]

VanDer Meche, F. G., and R. Braakman. 1983. Arachnoid cysts in the middle cranial fossa: Cause and treatment of progressive and non-progressive symptoms. *Journal of Neurology, Neurosurgery & Psychiatry* 46: 1102–7. [CrossRef]

Vanneste, J., and R. Hyman. 1986. Non-Tumoral Aqueduct Stenosis and Normal Pressure Hydrocephalus in the Elderly. *Journal of Neurology, Neurosurgery, and Psychiatry* 49: 529–35. [CrossRef]

Section V: CSF Disorders

Hydrocephalus

Shamsul Alam, Riad Habib, Nur Mohammad and Forhad H. Chowdhury

Abstract: Hydrocephalus is one of the commonest neurosurgical pathologies, and a neurosurgeon has to deal with it daily. It has a number of etiologies at any age. The congenital type of hydrocephalus is more common at pediatric age. The commonly applied surgical treatments for this condition are ventriculo-peritoneal (VP) shunts and endoscopic third ventriculostomy (ETV). Etiology, classification, clinical features, radiological findings, and surgical options are discussed in a focused form. A short description of the surgical procedures for hydrocephalus, including the installment of a ventriculo-peritoneal shunt, endoscopic third-ventriculostomy, and external ventricular drainage (EVD), is provided along with possible complications and strategies for complication management. In the later part of this chapter, normal-pressure (NPH) hydrocephalus is discussed.

Abbreviations

CSF	cerebrospinal fluid	CT	computed tomography
ETV	endoscopic third ventriculostomy	EVD	external ventricular drain
FH	frontal horn	HCP	Hydrocephalus
MRI	magnetic resonance imaging	NPH	normal pressure hydrocephalus
OFC	occipito-frontal circumference	TH	temporal horn

1. Introduction

Excessive collection of cerebrospinal fluid (CSF) within the ventricular system is called hydrocephalus (HCP). We know that the brain has a ventricular system, which contains CSF that supports the brain. Due to CSF, the weight of the brain is significantly reduced in the body in individuals with HCP.

Hydrocephalus can strike anyone at any age, but it is more frequent in infants and people over the age of sixty. Most of these instances are recognized before birth, at the time of parturition, or in early infancy (Figure 1) (Greenberg 2010).

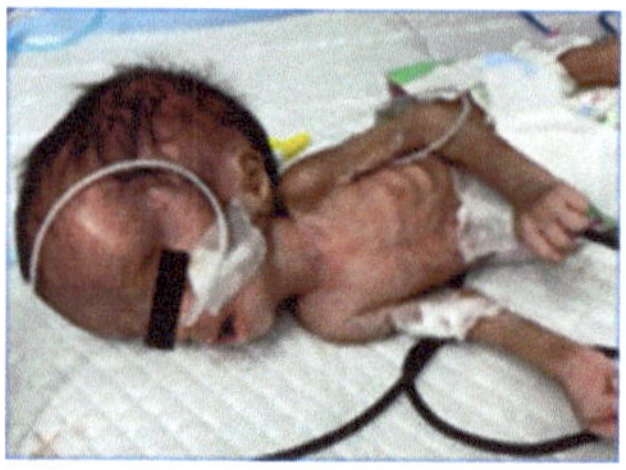

Figure 1. A premature malnourished baby with hydrocephalus. Source: Photo by authors.

2. Etiology

CSF accumulates in the brain either through its excess production, an absorption defect pertaining to it, or its blockage in its pathway. We know CSF is secreted by the lateral ventricular choroid plexus and passes from one ventricle to another lateral ventricle through the foramen of Monro. From the lateral ventricle, CSF passes to the third ventricle and subsequently the fourth ventricle via the aqueduct of Sylvius. Hydrocephalus can be passed down through the offspring, linked to congenital anomalies like spinal dysraphism or encephalocele, or caused by cerebral tumors, head injuries, hematoma, or infections (meningitis). Hydrocephalus is classified into six categories depending on the onset, existence of structural problems, or high vs. normal CSF pressures.

3. Categories of HCP

1. Acquired HCP;
2. Congenital HCP;
3. Communicating HCP;
4. Non communicating HCP (obstructive);

5. Normal-pressure HCP, which is more common in the elderly and marked by enlarged ventricles with normal CSF pressure within the spine.
6. Hydrocephalus ex vacuo, which is common in adults and can occur when the brain is damaged by a degenerative condition, such as Alzheimer's disease, stroke, or head trauma, and in which the brain tissue shrinks.

4. Specific Etiologies of HCP in Pediatric Population

4.1. Congenital

(a) Chiari-2 malformation +/− myelomeningocele;
(b) Chiari-1 malformation;
(c) Primary cerebral aqueductal stenosis;
(d) Secondary cerebral aqueductal gliosis;
(e) Dandy–Walker malformation: Foramina of Luschka and Magendie atresia;
(f) X-linked inherited disorder: rare.

4.2. Acquired

(a) Infectious
- Post-meningitis (Figure 2);
- Cysticercosis.

(b) Post-
- Post-SAH;
- Post-intraventricular hemorrhage (IVH).

(c) Due to mass effect
- Non-neoplastic: such as arteriovenous malformation;
- Neoplastic lesions: e.g., medulloblastoma, colloid cyst of the third ventricle, pituitary tumor, and apoplexy with suprasellar extension (Kalangu et al. 2009).

(d) Postoperative;
(e) Neurosarcoidosis;
(f) Tuberculosis (Figure 3).

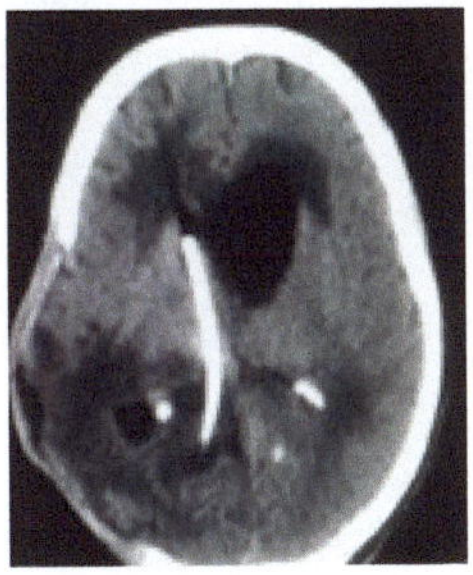

Figure 2. CT scan showing decompressive craniectomy with evidence of a VP shunt. Source: Figure by authors.

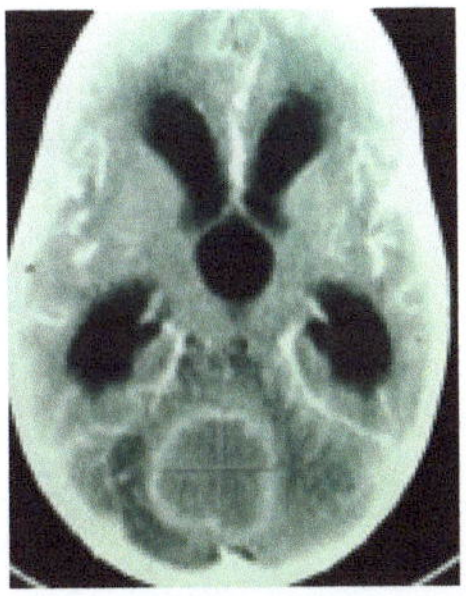

Figure 3. Posterior fossa tuberculoma with triventriculomegally. Source: Figure by authors.

Common etiologies of hydrocephalus are shown in Table 1.

Table 1. Common etiologies of hydrocephalus in pediatric patients.

Etiology
Hemorrhage within ventricle
Myelomeningocele
Neoplasm
Cerebral aqueductal stenosis
Meningitis
Cranial trauma
Others
Idiopathic
Two or more etiologies

Source: Authors' compilation based on data from Kirollos et al. (2019).

5. Classifications of HCP

Hydrocephalus can be classified into various types, which are listed below.

5.1. Noncommunicating Hydrocephalus (Obstructive)

Potential results that can be obtained from lesions that obstruct the CSF pathway from the lateral ventricle to the fourth ventricle and its outlet are noted below:

a. Dilated lateral and third ventricles and a normal-size fourth ventricle;
b. Dilation of the lateral ventricle due to an obstruction at the Forman of Monro, commonly by a colloid cyst;
c. A posterior Fossa mass lesion (tumor, cyst, hematoma), an intraventricular mass lesion (tumor, IVH, cyst), and/or aqueductal stenosis.
d. Lumber puncture is contraindicated in this type of hydrocephalus.

5.2. Communicating Hydrocephalus

This type of hydrocephalus refers to situations in which the intracerebral CSF pathways are active and patent but there is an excessive collection of CSF, commonly from abnormalities in CSF absorption. Here, all four ventricles are dilated. This condition occurs because of meningitis, SAH, adult IVH, and IVH in premature babies. To treat communicating hydrocephalus, a lumber drain can be inserted to decrease intracranial pressure.

6. Clinical Features of HCP

HCP's clinical features vary according to the age limit of the patients. Newborn babies present with enlarge heads and are often born via Caesarean section.

In infancy, the head will grow much larger, with a prominent scalp vein with widened fontanelles. Commonly, the anterior fontanelle closes at 5–15 months' time, and the posterior fontanelle closes at around 2–3 months.

Babies are commonly irritable and cry because of hydrocephalus, and their brains become compressed. Their brain tissue (cortical mantle) becomes thin and varies from a few millimeters to a few centimeters. Normally, the cerebral mantle is 5–6 cm long.

At birth, the head circumference of a baby is 35 cm at 6 months, 39 cm at 1 year, 45 cm at 1.5 years, and 49 cm at 2 years.

Commonly, the head enlarges at a rate of 1–2 cm per month.

6.1. The Various Symptoms of Hydrocephalus

6.1.1. Infants

- Unusually large head size;
- Fastly growing head circumference;
- Bulged and tense fontanelles;
- Prominent and engorged scalp veins;
- Downward deviation of eyes or sunset sign;
- Nausea and vomiting;

- Sleepiness;
- Irritability;
- Seizures.

6.1.2. Children and Adolescents

- Nausea as well as vomiting;
- Papilledema;
- Blurred vision or diplopia;
- Imbalance and gait disturbances;
- Delays in or lack of milestones of development;
- Personality changes;
- Poor concentration;
- Seizures;
- Loss of appetite;
- Urinary incontinence.

6.1.3. Adults

- Headache;
- Nausea as well as vomiting;
- Difficulty walking and gait disturbances;
- Imbalance or incoordination;
- Lethargy;
- Urinary incontinence;
- Visual disturbances;
- Impaired cognitive function skills;
- Loss of memory;
- Mild dementia.

7. Radiological Features

Hydrocephalus is best seen via CT or MRI
Based on experience, a clinician can identify HCP by its characteristics on a CT scan or MRI.

7.1. Specific Imaging Criteria for HCP

1. The width of both temporal horns (THs) of the lateral ventricle is $\geq$2 mm.
2. Both THs are less than 2 mm wide, and the FH/ID ratio is greater than 0:5. (where FH is the greatest width/breath, and ID is the internal diameter from inner-table to inner-table at this level) (Greenberg 2010).

7.2. Other Features Alluding to Hydrocephalus

1. "Mickey Mouse" ventricles (ballooning of the FH of the lateral ventricles) and/or third-ventricular ballooning (the third ventricle is usually slit-like).
2. Periventricular lower density as seen in a CT scan or periventricular higher signal intensity on T2WI as shown via MRI.
3. The FH/ID ratio: <40% is normal, 40–50% is considered borderline, and >50% is hydrocephalus (Omidi-Varmezani 2015).
4. An Evans ratio, i.e., the ratio of FH to BPD (height biparietal diameter calculated in the same CT slice), of >0.3 alludes to hydrocephalus
5. Sagittal view shows thinning and/or superior bending of the corpus callosum (Greenberg 2010).

7.3. Radiological Features in 'Chronic HCP'

1. Beaten copper/silver cranium plain skull X-ray;
2. The third ventricle is herniating into the sellae (as seen via CT scan or MRI);
3. Erosion of sellae turcica;
4. Macrocrania: OFC greater than the 98th percentile;
5. Atrophy of the corpus callosum (Figure 4A);
6. In infantile patients:

(a) Sutural gap (diastasis);
(b) Delay in closure of the fontanelles;
(c) Failure to thrive;
(d) Developmental diverticulum (Figure 4B).

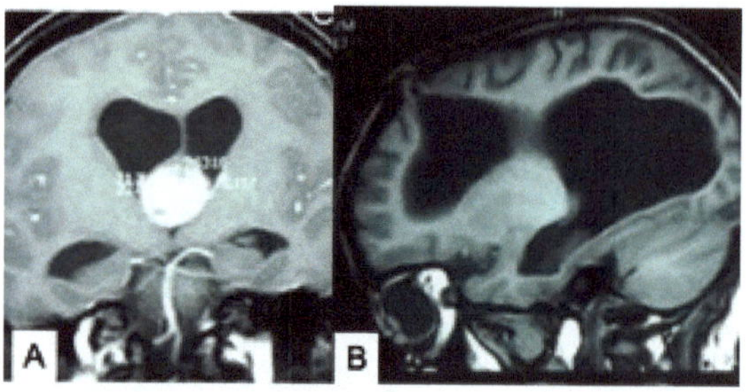

Figure 4. (**A**) MRI shows chronic HCP with diverticulum. (**B**) MRI shows colloid cyst of the 3rd ventricle with biventricular HCP. Source: Figure by authors.

8. Management of HCP

Hydrocephalus needs to be treated to allow normal development of the brain. Otherwise, brain activity such as cognition, motor activity, vision, and urinary control will all gradually decline. HCP strongly affects babies' developmental milestones. Commonly, a baby will raise its head at 3–4 months, crawl at 6–7 months, stand with support at 10–11 months, and be able to walk by year one.

8.1. Endoscopic 3RD Ventriculostomy (ETV)

ETV is an excellent and alternative approach to treating hydrocephalus. For the last 20 years, ETV has worked excellently for most patients. In the case of congenital hydrocephalus occurring when a baby is less than six months old, the surgeons generally do not prefer ETV as it has a more than 50% chance of failure. ETV works better in cases of adult-onset aqueduct stenosis and tumor-related obstructive hydrocephalus. The aim is to create a pathway between the basal cistern and the ventricular system.

8.1.1. Surgical Procedure of ETV

The head is positioned at 30–45-degrees, elevated, and kept straight. There is no need to rotate the head to avoid disorientation. Kocher's point is the commonest point to choose for ETV.

A "U"-shaped skin flap is chosen instead of a linear paramedian wound to allow better closure of the wound.

The optimal burr hole is positioned 3–4 cm laterally from the midline and 1 cm in front of the coronal suture (Oka et al. 1999).

Following the creation of a 10 mm burr hole, the dura is cut in a cruciate fashion. The underlying brain is cauterized, and an incision is made.

After making all preparations, such as employing a camera with a cover, a telescope, a sheath with an obturator, and Fogarty catheters, saline and then the brain canula are introduced through the burr hole.

Clear CSF normally comes out after applying 5–6 cm or less.

At this stage, an ETV telescope is introduced.

The telescope will show the location of the landing, allowing for navigation through the foramen of Monro by revealing the choroid plexus, fornix, and thalamostriate vein so that one can reach the floor of the third ventricle.

The floor of the third ventricle can be identified by the two mammillary bodies in the posterior and infundibular recess in the anterior and the thin or thick membrane (tuberous cinereum) beneath the tuber cinereum Basilar artery pulsation can be observed if the membrane is thin.

The next step is making a puncture in the membrane either with ventriculostomy forceps or by using unipolar or bipolar tips.

Following fenestration, the membrane needs to be dilated at least 4-6 mm, which can be performed either by using a 3F Fogarty catheter or via opening the space using ventriculostomy forceps.

Pulsation of the membrane should now be evident.

Sometimes another membrane is there: it is known as the Liliequist membrane, and it also needs to be punctured to allow the free flow of CSF into the prepontine space.

Hemostasis must be ensured before the withdrawal of the endoscope.

Commonly, hemostasis is achieved via compression using a Fogarty catheter or via direct cauterization.

Profuse irrigation is applied before removing the telescope.

A gel foam is placed in the port, and the wounds in all the layers are closed after the removal of the telescope.

Complications of ETV

The commonest complication of ETV is bleeding; hence, proper hemostasis is mandatory before the closure of an ETV scalp wound. Hemostasis is commonly achieved via continuous irrigation. Another way of achieving hemostasis is the application of either a unipolar or bipolar diathermy. It is recommended to ensure hemostasis in this case and EVD should be employed for safety (Nader et al. 2014).

Success Rate of ETV

ETV success rate is a matter of debate (Quiñones-Hinojosa 2012; Chowdhury et al. 2017) and shown in Table 2.

Favorable clinical as well as radiographic characteristics for ETVare shown in Table 3.

8.2. Choroid Plexus Cauterization

ETV plus choroid plexus cauterization increases the efficacy of ETV. Flexible endoscopic support is required to cauterize the entire length of the choroid plexus on both the right and left sides.

8.3. EVD

EVD is a temporary CSF diversion procedure commonly performed at Kocher's point; however, there are other points at which to perform EVD, such as via Frazier's, Dandy's, and Keene's points. Commonly, EVD is performed using an at least 5 cm subcuticular tunnel; in one study, it was shown that a long subcutaneous tunnel is associated with a reduced chance of brain infection. However, EVD placement after more than two weeks is complicated by meningitis.

Table 2. Third Ventriculostomy success rates according to HCP cause.

Higher Success Rates ($\geq$75%)
Acquired cerebral aqueductal stenosis neoplasms obstructing ventricular CSF outflow Tectal tumour Pineal tumour Thalamic tumour Intraventricular tumour
Intermediate-Level Success Rates (50–70%):
Myelomeningoceles (shunted earlier, in older patients) Congenital cerebral aqueductal stenosis Cystic lesion obstructing CSF flow Arachnoid cysts Dandy–Walker malformation Earlier-shunted patients with difficulties Slit ventricle syndrome Intractable or recurrent shunt infections Intractable or recurrent shunt malfunction
Low Success Rates (<50%)
Myelomeningoceles (not shunted earlier, in neonatal patients) Posthemorrhagic HCP Postinfectious HCP

Source: Authors' compilation based on data from Quiñones-Hinojosa (2012); Chowdhury et al. (2017).

Table 3. Favorable clinical as well as radiographic characteristics for ETV.

Clinical
HCP etiology in a higher or intermediate success group
Age of more than six months at time of HCP diagnosis
Age of more than six months at time of intervention
No history of prior radiation therapies
No history of prior meningitis or hemorrhage
Patient was shunted earlier
Radiographic
Definite proof of ventricular noncommunication
Obstructive type of HCP
Anatomical obstruction of aqueduct
Absence of aqueductal CSF flow void in T2-weighted MRI images
Suitable 3rd ventricular anatomy
Width of foramen of Monro is enough to accommodate endoscope
Rigid endoscope > 7 mm
Flexible endoscope > 4 mm
Third ventricular floor is thin
Downward bulging floor of 3rd ventricle draped over clivus
Basilar artery is posterior to mammillary bodies
Absence of anatomical anomalies related to surgery
AVM or neoplasm obscuring floor of third ventricle
Large massa intermedia
Inadequate space between mammillary bodies, the basilar artery, and the clivus Ectasia of basilar artery

Source: Authors' compilation based on data from Chakraborty et al. (2012); Quiñones-Hinojosa (2012); Chowdhury et al. (2017).

8.3.1. EVD Points

(i) Paine's point: "The junction at 90° angles of the lines measured 2.5 cm above from the floor of the anterior cerebral fossa (lateral orbital roof) and 2.5 cm front to the Sylvian fissure," according to Paine's point definition. The frontal horn base is reached via a ventriculostomy through this site.
(ii) Kocher's point: The entry site is 2–3 cm from the midline, which is roughly the mid-pupillary line from the front of the skull, and 1 cm from the front of the coronal suture, which is nearly 11 cm above from the nasion (this positioning is intended to protect the motor strip).
(iii) Keene's point: The entry point is 2.5–3 cm behind and 2.5–3 cm above the pinna; placement is at the trigone.
(iv) Frazier's point: The entry point is 3–4 cm from the midline laterally and 6–7 cm above the inion.
(v) Dandy's point: The entry point is 2 cm from the midline laterally and 3 cm above the inion (using this point may render the patient more prone to an optic radiation injury than they would be if Frazier's point were used).

EVD is commonly carried out in the case of acute hydrocephalus or obstructive hydrocephalus just before or at the time of primary surgery.

8.3.2. Complications of EVD

1. Bleeding along the tract.
2. EVD migration: The EVD tool can come out through the tract if not secured well.
3. The withdrawal of too much CSF leads to subdural hygroma or hematoma.

8.4. Shunting

Shunting is the most common treatment for hydrocephalus for both the congenital and acquired varieties. Among all shunting procedures, a VP shunt is the commonest, followed by ventriculo-atrial (VA) or ventriculo-pleural shunts.

8.4.1. Ventriculo-Peritoneal Shunt

About 80% of all shunting procedures are VP shunts. This is the only surgery wherein long exposure of the wound can take place, so there is an about 20% chance of shunt infection.

Exposure from the head to the abdomen through the neck is required.

Here, a burr hole is commonly made at Keene's, Frazier's, or Kocher's points and traced up, leading to a subcutaneous Daniel lot. The end of the shunt is introduced into the peritoneal cavity, commonly in the paramedian plane.

Complications of VP Shunt

1. Common complication:
   (i) *Shunt infection:* Shunt infection rates range from 8-15%, with 10% being generally accepted. The greatest risk of shunt infection is within 6 months of its original implementation. Shunt infection is often treated with antibiotics and shunt externalizations.
   (ii) *Shunt obstruction:* Shunt failure occurs when a shunt becomes blocked at either the cranial or caudal ends. Excess protein in the CSF might block the shunt valve at the proximal end. The additional protein will deposit at the drainage point and clog the valve over time. If the shunt is dragged out of the abdominal cavity (as with VP shunts), or if similar protein buildup occurs, the shunt can clog at the end.
   (iii) *Shunt over drainage:* The possible complications of over shunting include the following:
      (a) Slit ventricles;
      (b) Intracranial hypotension;
      (c) Subdural hematoma;
      (d) Craniosynostosis and microcephaly;
      (e) Stenosis or occlusion of sylvian aqueduct;
   (iv) Disconnection or breakage at any point;
   (v) Shunt leaking;
   (vi) Hardware erosion through skin;
   (vii) Seizure;
   (viii) Malposition of catheter tip (Figure 5);
   (ix) Silicon allergy.

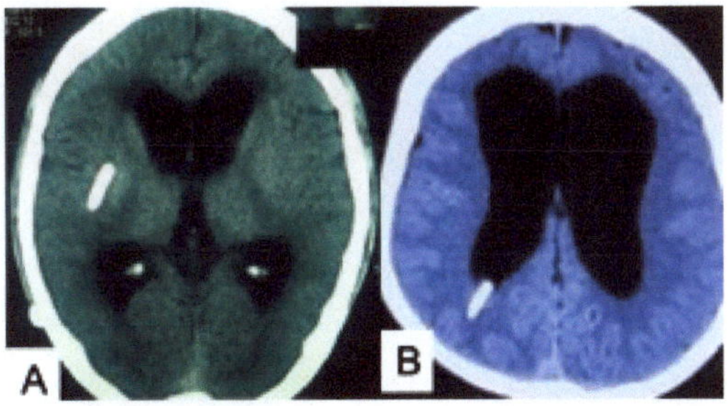

Figure 5. (**A**) CT scan showing that the cranial end of the VP shunt is not in the ventricle; (**B**) CT scan showing that the cranial end of the VP shunt has migrated out of the ventricle. Source: Figure by authors.

2. Others
   (i) Inguinal hernias;
   (ii) The need to lengthen the catheter with growth;
   (iii) Obstructions of peritoneal catheter with growth:
      (a) Omentum;
      (b) Peritoneal cysts;
      (c) Peritoneal adhesion.
3. Complication specific for V-P shunts:
   (i) Peritonitis;
   (ii) Hydrocele;

(iii) CSF ascites;
(iv) The migration of the tip of the shunt or the whole thing into the ventricular system (Figure 6);
(v) Intestinal obstruction;
(vi) Volvulus;
(vii) Intestinal strangulation;
(viii) Over-shunting: Over shunting can cause other complications; such as slit ventricles, intracranial hypotension, subdural hematoma, craniosynostosis, microcephaly, and stenosis or occlusion of sylvian aqueduct.

Shunt Infection

1. Risk factors for shunt infection:
    - Young age of the patient: Waiting until a child is two weeks old before administering antibiotics to treat a myelomeningocele (MM) may reduce the infection rate dramatically.
    - Long operations.
    - Open neural-tube defect.
2. Pathogens:
    - Early infection:
        - Staphylococcus epidermidis
        - Staphylococcus aureus
        - Gram-negative bacilli
        - E. coli and Streptococcus Hemolyticus in neonates.
    - Late infection:
        - Staphylococcus epidermidis
3. Medical treatment/Antibiotics for VP shunt infection:
    - Commonly, the surgeons choose injectable antibiotics, such as Meropenem, Vancomycin, Clindamycin, Linezolid, and Rifampicin.
4. Surgical treatment of shunt infection

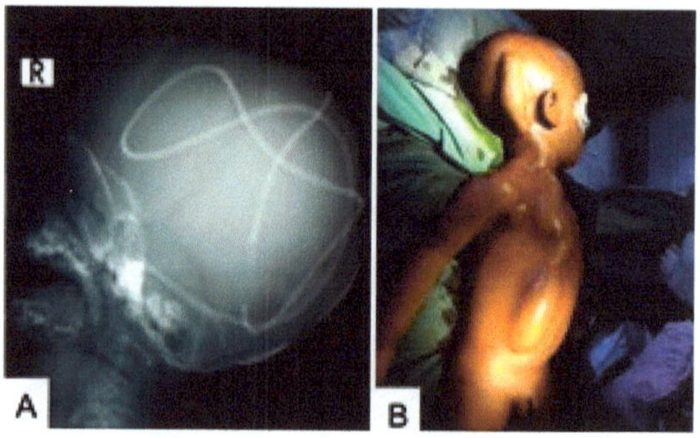

Figure 6. (**A**) X-Ray shows total migration of shunt tube within the brain. (**B**) Picture shows accommodation of CSF within the subcutaneous tunnel because of lower end block. Source: Figure by authors.

Management of a CSF shunt infection usually requires the removal of the shunt as well as the insertion of a temporary ventricular reservoir (Ommaya reservoir) until the infection is over. There are four main methods of managing VP shunt infection:

(i) Appropriate antibiotics;
(ii) Removal of the infected shunt with simultaneous replacement;
(iii) Exteriorization of the shunt with subsequent replacement;
(iv) External ventricular drain (EVD) insertion with removal of the shunt with subsequent shunt re-insertion (this is the best technique, with an over 95% success rate) (Greenberg 2010).

5. VP shunt Replacement
    - VP Shunt externalization:
    Indications:

- VP shunt infection;
- Abdominal pseudocysts;
- Peritonitis.

Contraindications:

- Proximal tube obstruction;
- Valve malfunction;
- Pus in the valve.

- Surgical technique: A small incision is made over the neck along the subcutaneous tube.

Blunt dissection is carried out until the white, shiny VP shunt tube can be seen. Once the tube is observed, the lower end of the VP shunt tube should be gently pulled. All distal tubing removed from the abdomen is connected by a connector system to a closed external drainage system. The wound is closed in layers using an occlusive dressing.

8.4.2. Ventriculo-Atrial (VA) Shunt

The VA shunt is an alternative to the VP shunt. Here, the common facial vein is selected as the area where the lower end of the catheter will be placed. From the common facial vein, the shunt goes to the internal jugular vein and then the right atrium of the heart.

The placement of the lower end by the right atrium can be confirmed via a chest X-ray, where the tip will be located at the D2 level, and at the time of the insertion of the shunt tube, there may be a rhythm change of the heart.

Complications of VA shunt:

- The shunt may be blocked by a blood clot.
- It may be displaced.

8.4.3. Ventriculo-Pleural Shunt

Another alternative shunting technique is the V pleural shunt, where the lower end is placed in the lower chest in the interpleural space, commonly in the fifth or sixth intercostal space and in the mid or posterior axillary line.

Here, the big pleural surface acts as an absorber of CSF (Nader et al. 2014).

8.4.4. Lumbo-Peritoneal Shunt

This is a shunting procedure for the IIH or pseudo-tumor cerebri or communication variety of HCP. It is performed by placing an LP shunt where a lumbar puncture has been made using a 14-bore Touhy needle. The lower end of the shunt is introduced into the peritoneal cavity via a mini laparotomy incision through a subcutaneous tunnel in the flank (Greenberg 2010).

8.4.5. Cysto-Peritoneal Shunt

This is a bypass procedure for encysted cysts such as posterior fossa arachnoid cysts and Sylvia fissure cysts, which compress the loco-regional brain structure.

9. Normal-Pressure Hydrocephalus (NPH)

This condition is typically recognized by noting the following triad of symptoms: dementia, ataxia, and incontinence.

9.1. Epidemiology

According to recent research on probable NPH symptoms, at least 21.2% of nursing home residents have gait impairment, 9.4% have dementia, and 14.7% have incontinence (Shprecher et al. 2008).

9.2. Pathology

NPH is a condition characterized by a decrease in CSF absorption rather than an increase in CSF production. The arachnoid granulations fail to maintain their baseline clearance of CSF, whether due to a known or unknown reason. This is frequently due to fibrosis and scarring, which conceal absorptive surfaces.

Surgical therapy for patients with a severe form of dementia is generally discouraged, even in the presence of gait difficulty and incontinence, independent of radiographic results (Shprecher et al. 2008).

9.3. Radiological Features

The image below show communicating HCP observed via CT (Figure 7A) scan or MRI.

Figure 7B shows that MRI can detect periventricular white matter alterations better than CT scans. These contiguous T2/FLAIR (fluid-attenuated inversion recovery) hyperintensities are assumed to be trans-ependymal edema due to high CSF pressure, but they may seem similar to those seen in small-vessel ischemic illnesses (Shprecher et al. 2008).

9.4. Morphological Changes in MRI

9.4.1. Ventriculomegaly

- Evans' index is increased >0.3;
- The THs of the lateral ventricles are widened by >6 mm;
- Acute callosal angle;
- Superior bowing of the corpus callosum.

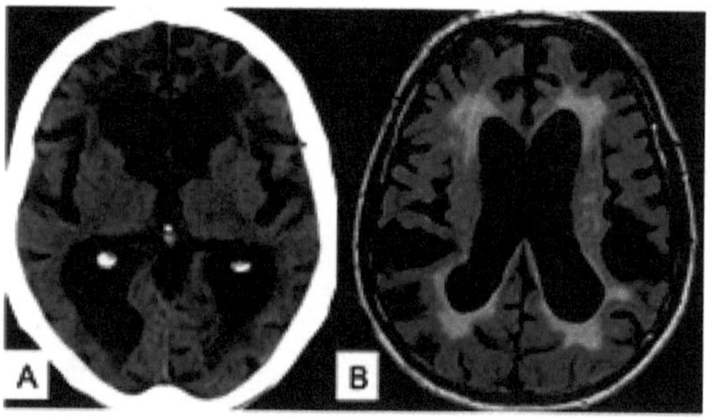

Figure 7. (**A**) CT scan showing ventriculomegaly with periventricular hypodensity suggestive of hydrostatic edema. (**B**) MRI scan shows ventriculomegaly with periventricular high-intensity signal suggestive of hydrostatic edema. Source: Figure by authors.

9.4.2. Disproportionate Alterations in Subarachnoid Spaces

- Expanded Sylvian fissures;
- Compressed high convexity (subarachnoid spaces and sulci are narrow at the vertex and medial/parafalcine region)
- Cingulate sulcus sign: the posterior portion of cingulate sulcus is slenderer than the anterior portion.
- Focal/isolated expansion of sulci on the medial surface or convexity area (sometimes known as transport sulci)

Significantly expanded subarachnoid space hydrocephalus is characterized by ventriculomegaly, Sylvian fissure expansion, and crowding at the vertex.

9.4.3. Cine Phase-Contrast MRI

Phase-contrast CSF flow in films is measured using MRI in terms of stroke volume, which is defined as the average volume of CSF traveling through the cerebral aqueduct in both systole and diastole (Shprecher et al. 2008). A stroke volume of more than 42 micro-liters may indicate that it is probable there will be an improvement after a VP shunt is placed (Scollato et al. 2008).

9.5. Differential Diagnosis of NPH

The possible neuro-imaging differential include the following:

- Normal senile brain;
- Alzheimer's disease with dementia: may demonstrate greater expansion of perihippocampal fissures;
- Obstructive HCP—due to neoplasm (e.g., pineal region, tectal plate, midbrain)

- Lewy body dementia—visual hallucinations as well as delusions are more marked;
- Parkinson's disease—it is important to differentiate one-sided symptoms;
- AIDS–dementia complex—positive HIV immunological test.

Asymmetric rest tremor, lead pipe rigidity, and visual hallucinations may indicate dementia with Lewy bodies (DLB), which induces cognitive abnormalities similar to Alzheimer's disease. Pseudodementia is also a possibility in the differential diagnosis. Aphasia, apraxia, or agnosia might arouse suspicion of dementia with cortical dysfunction, such as Alzheimer's disease (AD), multi-infarct dementia, or frontotemporal dementia, if these symptom appear early (Shprecher et al. 2008). Regardless of ventriculomegaly, a cause other than NPH should be investigated for patients with progressing dementia who do not have gait problems.

9.5.1. Tests for Differentials

Although a high-volume (>40 mL) spinal tap (also known as lumbar tap test) was the first method for diagnosing NPH and predicting shunt response, external lumbar drainage (ELD) is becoming more widely accepted as a more superior predictor for patients who do not respond to a tap test. CSF is drained at a rate of 10–15 cm^3 per hour for 72 h using a lumbar spinal catheter (Shprecher et al. 2008).

9.6. Treatment of NPH

In about 60% of NPH patients, CSF shunting techniques such as ventriculoperitoneal, ventriculopleural, and ventriculoatrial shunting can result in considerable clinical improvement in NPH symptoms (Shprecher et al. 2008).

10. Pineal Cyst and Posterior Fossa Cyst with HCP

Affected patients commonly present with a visual discrepancy and headache (Figure 8).

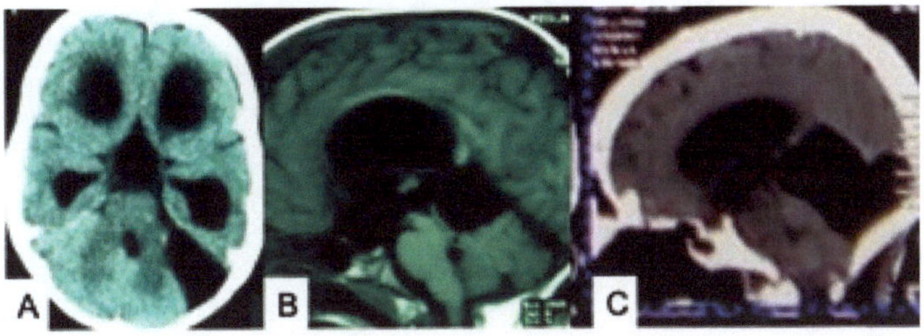

Figure 8. (**A**) CT shows CP angle arachnoid cyst with HCP. (**B**) MRI shows pineal region arachnoid cyst with HCP. (**C**) MRI shows huge pineal region arachnoid cyst with HCP. Source: Figure by authors.

The best treatment is either a endoscopic or microscopic excision of the cyst wall.

11. Trapped Fourth Ventricle

An isolated fourth ventricle can be caused by failure to communicate with either the aqueduct of the Sylvius or the fourth ventricular outlet—the foramen Luschka and Magendie (Figure 9).

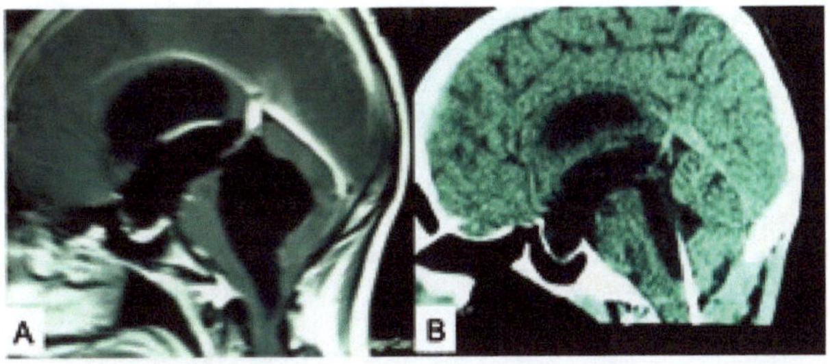

Figure 9. (**A**) MRI shows entrapped and dilated 4th ventricle. (**B**) MRI shows previous entrapped and dilated 4th ventricle treated using a 4th ventricular shunt. Source: Figure by authors.

11.1. *Etiology*

- Post-infective hydrocephalus;
- Chronic shunting of lateral ventricle.

11.2. *Clinical Presentation*

- Headache;
- Recurrent vomiting;
- Decreased consciousness level;
- Ataxia;
- Dysphagia.

11.3. *Surgical Technique*

- A fourth ventricular shunt plus an ETV/VP shunt;
- Opening of fourth ventricular outflow plus an aqueductoplasty +/− stent.

12. Double-Compartment Hydrocephalus

The figure below shows supratentorial and infratentorial hydrocephalus in clinical sequence and separately (Figure 10).

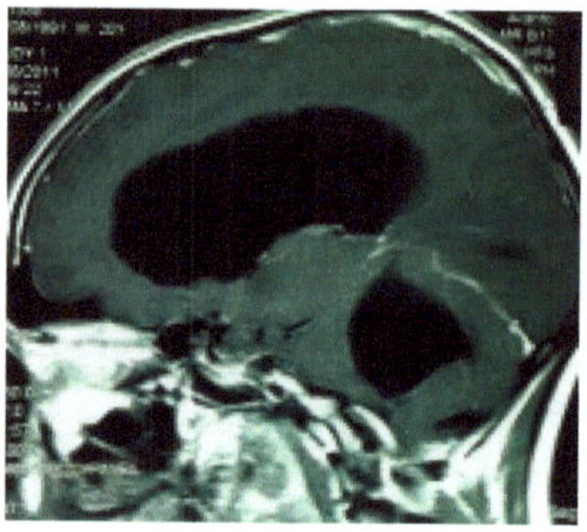

Figure 10. MRI shows double compartmental HCP. Source: Figure by authors.

13. HCP in Dandy–Walker Malformation

Overall, 80% of Dandy–Walker cysts are diagnosed by 1 year of age. The development of hydrocephalus may be explained by a hemorrhage at the time of delivery and subsequent inflammatory blockage of the foramen Luschka. Alternatively, a patient may have congenital aqueductal stenosis. Young children present with delayed motor development and poor head control. Older children present with truncal ataxia and nystagmus.

13.1. *Radiological Diagnosis*

- Cranial ultrasound and a CT scan of head are the initial diagnostic investigations performed. CT has revealed that the cerebellar hemisphere is typically hypoplastic. The tentorium, torcula, and venous sinuses are in higher positions.
- Massively dilated fourth ventricle.
- Concomitant hydrocephalus.

13.2. *Treatment Options*

1. The placement of a proximal bi-compartmental shunt at a single valve using a Y connector and distal tubing.
2. The application of a completely separate VP shunt.
3. Addressing only hydrocephalus using either a VP shunt or via ETV
4. Only ETV of the lateral ventricle, keeping posterior fossa cyst untouched (Nader et al. 2014).

14. Long Standing Overt Ventriculomegaly

LOVA—long-standing overt ventriculomegaly in adults—is a type of chronic hydrocephalus of infantile-onset severe third and lateral ventriculomegaly with a mild clinical presentation in adults. It may be a reactivated form of arrested hydrocephalus wherein compensational factors have failed. Oi et al. described it for the first time in 2000, considering the following criteria: (1) adult-onset hydrocephalus symptoms (headache, cognitive decline, imbalance, gait disturbances, and visual deterioration/diplopia); (2) macrocephaly; (3) overt triventriculomegaly observed via neuroimaging with cortical sulcal effacement and/or destruction of the sella turcica; and (4) no secondary causes of aqueductal stenosis (Oi et al. 2000). It should be differentiated from other types of hydrocephalus without macrocephaly. The clinical features are non-specific low-grade headache, early-morning nausea and occasional vomiting, sometimes insidious visual failure, and normal-pressure-hydrocephalus-like features. Magnetic resonance imaging (MRI) is the gold standard in LOVA diagnostics, combined with clinical and neuropsychological examination.

Treatments includes the following:

1. The conservative approach with regular follow-ups;
2. Endoscopic third ventriculostomy (ETV);
3. The installation of a programmable ventriculo-peritoneal shunt.

Many authors have recommended that endoscopic third ventriculostomy (ETV) is the gold standard for the treatment of LOVA, as it is a triventricular form of hydrocephalus. If ETV fails, a CSF shunt should be used instead (Tuniz et al. 2021).

Author Contributions: Conceptualization, methodology, validation, formal analysis, investigation, resources, data curation, S.A., R.H. and N.M.; writing—original draft preparation, S.A.; writing—review and editing, visualization, supervision, F.H.C. All authors have read and agreed to the published version of the manuscript.

Funding: This research received no external funding.

Conflicts of Interest: The authors declare no conflicts of interest.

References

Chakraborty, Aabir, James M. Drake, and Benjamin C. Warf. 2012. Methods for Cerebrospinal Fluid Diversion in Pediatric Hydrocephalus: From Shunt to Scope. In *Schmidek and Sweet Operative Neurosurgical Techniques*. Edited by Alfredo Quiñones-Hinojosa. Philadelphia: W.B. Saunders, pp. 631–53. [CrossRef]

Chowdhury, Forhad H., Mohammod R. Haque, Khandkar A. Kawsar, Mainul H. Sarker, and Abdul Fazal Mohammod M. Haque. 2017. Result of Endoscopic Third Ventriculostomy for Hydrocephalus Caused by Cerebral Aqueductal Stenosis in Infant Patients. *Indian Journal of Neurosurgery* 6: 189–97. [CrossRef]

Greenberg, Mark S. 2010. *Handbook of Neurosurgery*. New York: Thieme.

Kalangu, Kazadi, Yoko Kato, Gilbert Dechambenoit, and Hirotoshi Sano. 2009. *Essential Practice of Neurosurgery*. Nagoya: Access publishing Co., Ltd.

Kirollos, Ramez W., Adel Helmy, Simon Thomason, and Peter J. A. Hutchinson. 2019. *Oxford Textbook of Neurological Surgery*. Oxford: Oxford University Press.

Nader, Remi, Cristian Gragnaniello, Scott C. Berta, Abdulrahman J. Sabbagh, and Michael L. Levy. 2014. *Neurosurgery Tricks of the Trade: Cranial*. New York: Thieme.

Oi, Shizou, Masami Shimoda, Masayoshi Shibata, Yumie Honda, Kougi Togo, Masaki Shinoda, Ryuichi Tsugane, and Osamu Sato. 2000. Pathophysiology of long-standing overt ventriculomegaly in adults. *Journal of Neurosurgery* 92: 933–40. [CrossRef] [PubMed]

Oka, Kazunari, Yoshiaki Kin, Yoshinori Go, Katsuyuki Hirakawa, Masamichi Tomonaga, Tohru Inoue, and Susumu Yoshioka. 1999. Neuroendoscopic approach to tectal tumors: a consecutive series. *Neurosurgical Focus FOC* 6: E16. Available online: https://thejns.org/focus/view/journals/neurosurg-focus/6/4/article-pE16.xml (accessed on 26 February 2022). [CrossRef]

Omidi-Varmezani, Reza. 2015. Pediatric Hydrocephalus; A Statistical and Historical Approach. *Global Journal of Medical Research* 15: 5–14. Available online: https://medicalresearchjournal.org/index.php/GJMR/article/view/869 (accessed on 30 August 2021).

Quiñones-Hinojosa, Alfredo. 2012. *Schmidek and Sweet: Operative Neurosurgical Techniques E-Book: Indications, Methods and Results*, 6th ed. Philadelphia: Elsevier Saunders.

Scollato, Antanio, R. Tenenbaum, G. Bahl, M. Celerini, B. Salani, and N. Di Lorenzo. 2008. Changes in Aqueductal CSF Stroke Volume and Progression of Symptoms in Patients with Unshunted Idiopathic Normal Pressure 2020. Hydrocephalus. *American Journal of Neuroradiology* 29: 192–7. [CrossRef] [PubMed]

Shprecher, David, Jason Schwalb, and Roger Kurlan. 2008. Normal pressure hydrocephalus: diagnosis and treatment. *Current Neurology and Neuroscience Reports* 8: 371–6. [CrossRef] [PubMed]

Tuniz, Frencesco, Sara Fabbro, Daniele Piccolo, Maria C. Vescovi, Daniele Bagatto, Antanio Cramaro, and Miran Skrap. 2021. Long-Standing Overt Ventriculomegaly in Adults (LOVA): Diagnostic Aspects, CSF Dynamics with Lumbar Infusion Test and Treatment Options in a Consecutive Series with Long-Term Follow-Up. *World Neurosurgery* 156: e30–e40. [CrossRef] [PubMed]

Idiopathic Intracranial Hypertension (IIH)

Syeda Neyamot-e-Ferdousi, Mohammad Samsul Arifin, Mohammod Raziul Haque and Forhad H. Chowdhury

Abstract: Idiopathic intracranial hypertension (IIH) was previously known as pseudotumor cerebri or benign intracranial hypertension. Though rare, it is an important cause of vision loss, especially in women of child-bearing age. It presents clinical features consisting of raised intracranial pressure, including papilledema. Neuroimaging reveals no mass lesions, but a lumbar puncture shows high CSF pressure, while normal findings are revealed by CSF studies. IIH is usually managed using conservative treatment, but surgical intervention is needed for threatened vision and severe resistant headaches. In this chapter, clinical presentation, diagnostic workup, and management principles are summarized. Indications of surgical management along with surgical treatments including optic nerve sheath fenestration, CSF diversion (ventriculoperitoneal shunts and lumboperitoneal shunts), and venous stenting are mentioned in the later part of this chapter.

Abbreviations

BMI	body mass index	CSF	cerebrospinal fluid
CT	computed tomography	ICP	intracranial pressure
IIH	idiopathic intracranial hypertension	LP	lumboperitoneal shunt
MRI	magnetic resonance imaging	OCT	optical coherence tomography
ONSF	optic nerve sheath fenestration	OP	opening pressure
VP	ventriculo-peritoneal		

1. Introduction

Idiopathic intracranial hypertension (IIH) is a seldom-seen illness characterized by increased intracranial pressure (ICP) and papilledema in obese women of childbearing age. Patients with IIH experience chronic disabling headaches as a result of elevated ICP, which is considered to be generated by altered CSF fluid dynamics (Mollan et al. 2016). Considering the modified Dandy criteria (Mollan et al. 2018), IIH is largely a diagnosis of exclusion, in which a rising ICP due to other causes is ruled out. A lumbar puncture (diagnostic) must have an opening pressure (OP) greater than 25cm of CSF, indicating that the cerebrospinal fluid (CSF) is primarily acellular and meets normal biochemical criteria. There must also be papilledema, or swelling of the optic disk. With the exception of empty sellae, neuro-anatomical anomalies in suspected IIH patients are ruled out. With the exception of abducent nerve palsy, patients must also have usual cranial nerve function. Diagnostic criteria of IIH is shown in Table 1.

Table 1. IIH diagnostic criteria.

Diagnostic Criteria of IIH
Papilledema
Normal neurological findings with the exception of sixth nerve palsy
Proof of normal anatomy
Normal CSF constituents
Increased opening pressure (OP) on lumbar puncture (>250 mm CSF)

Source: Table adapted from Mollan et al. (2018), used with permission.

2. Epidemiology

In the Western world, the per annum incidence of IIH is around 0.9/100,000 people, and 3.5/100,000 in females aged 15 to 44. The prevalence of IIH is rising in tandem with the present obesity pandemic. Other demographic studies have found that obese women of reproductive age make up the vast majority of IIH cases. The average age of diagnosis is around 30 years. IIH can affect children, males, and the elderly; however, it is less common in these populations. Males account for less than 10% of IIH sufferers in adulthood. Men with IIH are often overweight, much like women. Males with IIH, on the other hand, may have worse visual acuity than women, according to research. IIH has no obvious racial predisposition. While the bulk of epidemiological studies demonstrate that the incidence of IIH is generally the same across countries, a few studies suggest that IIH is less common among Asians. This is assumed to be due to the lower levels of obesity in various Asian countries (Chen and Wall 2014).

3. Pathogenesis

The pathophysiology of IIH is uncertain; potential theories include aberrant cerebral venous outflow, raised CSF outflow hindrance, obesity-related higher intraabdominal and intracranial venous pressure, abnormal sodium as well as water reabsorption processes, and vitamin A metabolism problems (Bari et al. 2005). The effects of excessive secretion of interstitial fluid as well as extracellular cerebral edema on the blood–brain barrier (BBB) are most likely caused by a pathogenic mechanism: the CSF is generated in a normal way; there are more transactions from the interstitial fluid to the CSF at the trans-ependyma and trans-cerebral pial levels; and there is an increase in resorption of the CSF, and there is a swift venous efflux (Figure 1) (Iencen et al. 2015).

The clinical sign of rapid and possibly turbulent venous flow is tingles in synchronization with an individual's pulse, which are frequent in idiopathic intracranial hypertension. One may consider that an uncertain cause generates impacts on the blood–brain barrier, with the gradual appearance of cerebral edema due to the excess interstitial fluid. The pressure is balanced by the trans-ependymal interchange of edema interstitial fluid from the cerebral parenchyma to the CSF, followed by enhanced resorption of the cerebrospinal fluid, which maintains cerebral blood flow and represents a compensation mechanism (Iencen et al. 2015).

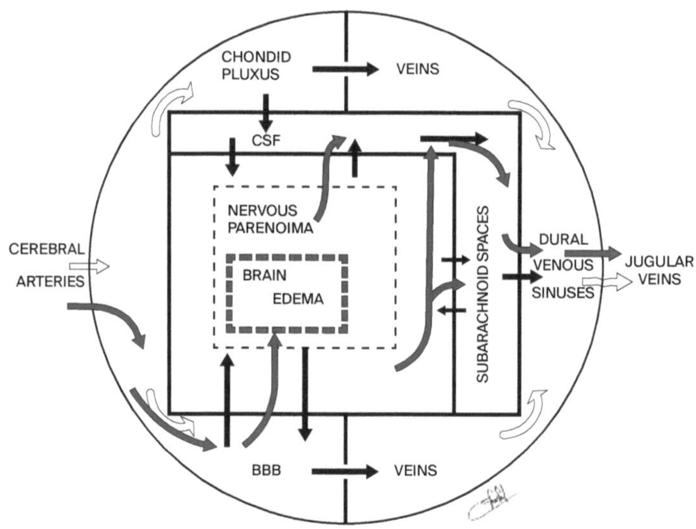

Figure 1. Hydrodynamic model of pathogeny in idiopathic intracranial hypertension. Source: Figure by authors.

When the BBB is gradually damaged, the amount of interstitial fluid grows gradually, and cerebral edema develops (Friedman 2005; Iencean 2003; Iencean 2004; Tabassi et al. 2005; Vorstman et al. 2002; Wraige et al. 2002). The basic ingredient for this balancing mechanism of pressure rise is the interstitial fluid's trans-ependymal and trans-pial route towards the cerebrospinal fluid (Figure 1).

The rise in intracranial pressure is exceedingly slow, and it has a long-term effect (Figure 2). This gradual rise in intracranial pressure permits proper pressure adjustment and near-normal cerebral sanguine flux maintenance. The pathogenic ICP range is extremely high, ranging from 60 to 80 mm Hg, and can remain stable for lengthy periods of time (Figure 2) (Iencen et al. 2015; Wraige et al. 2002).

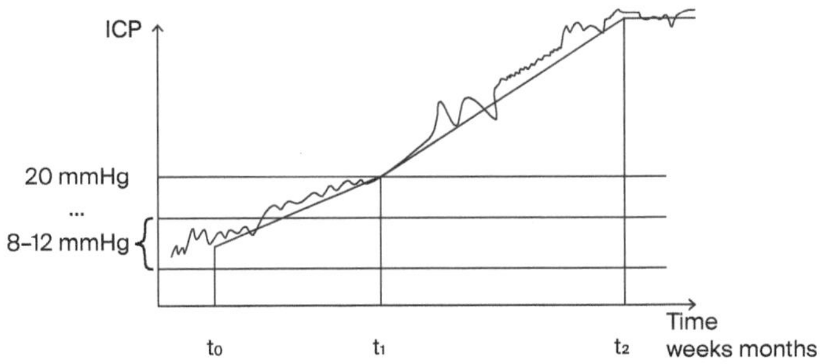

Figure 2. ICP increase in idiopathic intracranial hypertension, with a prolonged infraclinical period and an extremely long duration of pathological pressure value presentation. Source: Figure by authors.

4. Symptoms of IIH

The symptoms of IIH are headache (severe), transient visual obscuration (TVO), blurring of vision, double vision, pulsatile tinnitus, photophobia, retrobulbar pain, and dizziness. According to the International Classification of Headache Disorders, 3rd edition (ICHD-3) (Headache Classification Committee of IHS 2013), most patients with IIH have symptoms such as headaches, which become increasingly worse and more common (Mollan et al. 2018). Headaches caused by increased ICP, like any headaches, can worsen upon waking up and performing the Valsalva maneuver (KesKın et al. 2018).

5. Signs of IIH

Papilledema, visual field loss, and abducent nerve palsy are the most prevalent symptoms of IIH. Papilledema is frequently bilateral and similar; however, it can also be unilateral or asymmetric. Secondary intracranial hypertension caused by cerebral venous thrombosis might have symptoms that are quite similar to those of IIH. It is known that IIH is a long-term disease, which lasts months to years (Whelton et al. 2017). Symptoms of IIH generally worsen slowly; however, a subset has a more fulminant course. The risk factors of IIH are shown in Table 2.

Table 2. Risk factors of IIH.

Major	Others
Gender (>90% of patients afflicted with IIH are female); Obesity.	Addison's disease; Hypoparathyroidism; Steroid discontinuation; Growth hormone utilization in pediatric patients; Malnutrition; Hypervitaminosis A.

Source: Authors' compilation based on data from Chen and Wall (2014).

6. Diagnostic Approach

- The phenotype of headache is extremely variable, and it might be mistaken for various common headache syndromes (Table 1). Investigation and management in this regard are based on symptoms and indicators. For appropriate management, an interdisciplinary approach is essential.
- To exclude malignant hypertension, blood pressure (BP) readings must be as follows: a diastolic blood pressure more than or equivalent to 120 mm Hg and a systolic BP more than or equivalent to 180 mm Hg (Mollan et al. 2018; Whelton et al. 2017).
- Ophthalmological examination: every patient should have confirmed papilledema and a risk evaluation of their visual function. When papilledema is present, the following should be noted:
    - Visual acuity;
    - Pupil evaluation findings;
    - Intraocular pressure;
    - Confrontational visual field test (perimetry) results;
    - Dilated fundoscopy for grading the degree (severity) of the papilledema (Figure 3) and to exclude ocular etiologies for disc edema.

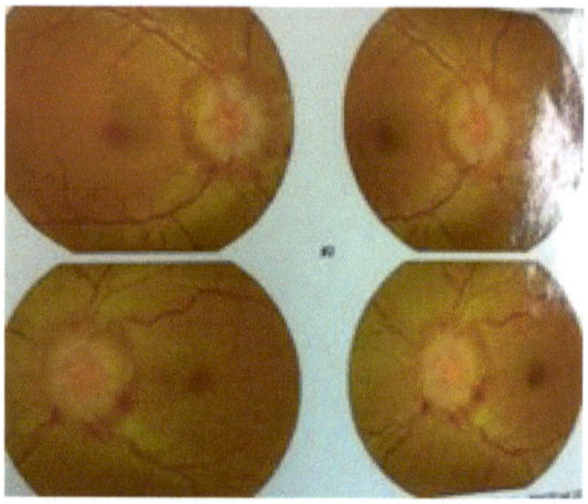

Figure 3. Preoperative fundal photograph of an IIH patient showing advanced papilledema. Source: Figure by authors.

Drawings of the fundus image and significant findings on the optic nerve head should be made and obtained, respectively, whenever possible (hyperemia, hemorrhages, exudate, cotton wool spots, arterio-venous nipping, blurring of the vessels, etc.). The use of photographs and/or optical coherence tomography (OCT) images is beneficial (Mollan et al. 2018). Regular ocular examination is required if visual function is in danger, as this will influence timely management.

- Neurological examination
  - Cranial nerve testing. There must be no cranial nerve dysfunction other than 6th cranial nerve palsy/palsies when IIH is suspected (Mollan et al. 2018).
  - Alternative diagnoses should be considered if other cranial nerves and/or abnormal signs are present.
- Neuroimaging
  - Urgent MRI of the brain and orbit within twenty-four hours; if not possible within twenty four hours, urgent CT scan of brain followed by MRI of the brain if no pathology is found (Mollan et al. 2018).
  - No signs of HCP, a mass, an anatomical or vascular lesion, or aberrant meningeal enhancement should be present.
  - A CT or MR venography must be performed within 24 h to rule out cerebral sinus thrombosis.
  - Features of increased ICP may be found in imaging results, though these are not diagnostic of IIH (Mollan et al. 2018; Degnan and Levy 2011; Hoffmann et al. 2013; Farb et al. 2003; Kelly et al. 2013).

6.1. Neuroimaging Characteristics of Raised ICP

- Empty sellae;
- Partially empty sellae/reduced pituitary height;
- Greater tortuosity and elongation of optic nerve;
- Expanded optic nerve sheath (peri-optic nerve subarachnoid space) (Figure 4);
- Flattened posterior sclera;
- Deflection of the cerebral venous sinuses, involving bilateral transverse sinus narrowing or stenosis of a prime transverse sinus;
- Intraocular projection of the optic nerve head. (Mollan et al. 2018)

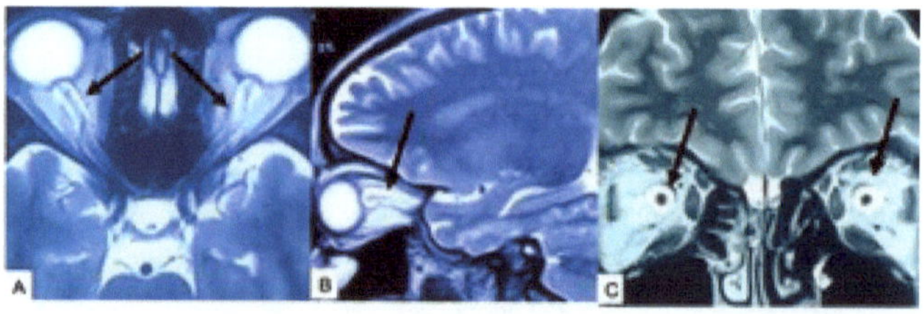

Figure 4. MRI of the brain and orbit: (**A**) axial, (**B**) sagittal, and (**C**) coronal T2W images showing elongated optic nerve with horizontal and vertical kinking, convex optic nerve head invaginating into globe, peri-optic nerve with increased CSF levels, partial empty sella, and normal brain with ventricles. Source: Figure by authors.

6.1.1. Lumbar Puncture

- Patients with papilledema must undergo a lumbar puncture (LP) after normal imaging has been conducted to confirm opening pressure (OP) and normal composition (Mollan et al. 2018).
- In the lateral decubitus posture, measure the LP opening pressure (Friedman et al. 2013). Pressure documentation should take place with the patient in a relaxed state and with their legs extended after the placement of the needle into the CSF space. Allow time for the CSF level to settle before documentation. CSF protein, glucose, and cell count analyses should be conducted.
- To diagnose IIH, a cut-off OP of >250 mm CSF is required per the diagnostic criteria (Friedman et al. 2013).

6.1.2. Exclusion of All Other Possible Causes of Increased ICP

- All patients' should have their medical history thoroughly collected to rule out any secondary reasons for elevated intracranial pressure that have previously been associated with increased ICP.
- To rule out anemia, every patient should be subjected to a complete blood count (Biousse et al. 2003; Mollan et al. 2009).
- If a patient is regarded as abnormal, additional blood testing to rule out secondary reasons may be considered.
- If a patient's condition is regarded as abnormal, further neuroimaging may be considered. More proximal neuroimaging of the neck vessels may be used to rule out internal jugular blockage.

7. Management Principles of IIH

For the optimal management of patients with IIH, there must be seamless interaction between clinician and neurosurgeon to allow smooth joint care between the different specialties. The main goals of treatment of IIH are as follows (Mollan et al. 2018):

1. Mitigate the underlying etiology;
2. Save visual function;
3. Reduce the morbidity due to headache.

IIH management principles: Modify the underlying disease by reducing weight.
Weight loss decreases ICP and is effective in alleviating papilledema and headaches (Sinclair et al. 2010).

- As soon as definitive IIH is established, every patient with a BMI greater than 30 kg/m^2 should be counseled about weight reduction. This should be handled with care.
- It is unknown how much weight reduction is needed to cause a patient to enter remission. It has been noticed that a diagnosis of IIH is related to 5–15% weight gain in the year preceding the diagnosis (Daniels et al. 2007) and that an up to 15% weight reduction is necessary for remission for IIH (Mollan et al. 2018; Sinclair et al. 2010).
- The IIH Treatment Trial (IIHTT) found that combining acetazolamide plus a low-sodium weight-loss diet led to a moderate elevation in visual field function in individuals with mild visual loss when compared to that facilitated by the diet alone. At 6 months, the IIHTT reported better quality-of-life results associated with acetazolamide (Mollan et al. 2014).

The algorithom of managment of IIH is shown in Figure 5.

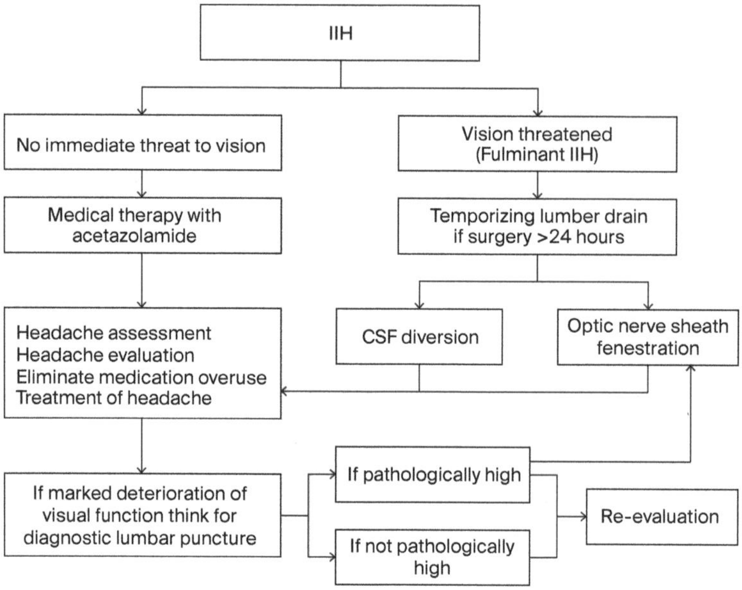

Figure 5. The algorithom of managment of IIH. Source: Authors' compilation based on data from Mollan et al. (2018).

7.1. To Protect Vision

Surgical procedures are indicated for less than 10% of IIH (Friedman et al. 2013) patients who present with a fast progressive reduction in visual function (called fulminant IIH) and require an immediate decrease in ICP to protect their eyesight (Lipton and Michelson 1972; Sodhi et al. 2017). A ventriculoperitoneal (VP) shunt is the most common CSF diversion. A lumboperitoneal (LP) shunt and optic nerve sheath fenestration (ONSF) are two such alternatives. VP shunts are recommended over lumbo-peritoneal shunts (Lipton and Michelson 1972; Sodhi et al. 2017) due to the former's lower reported revision rates (1.8 versus 4.3 revisions per patient, respectively) (Lipton and Michelson 1972; Sinclair et al. 2010).

Many surgical operations, for example, CSF diversion as well as optic nerve sheath fenestration (ONSF), have been shown to be effective in the short term (Mollan et al. 2018; Uretsky 2009). Weight reduction should be used to modify the underlying condition while the procedures are proving effective.

7.2. CSF Diversion

Neurosurgical CSF diversion is the chosen surgical treatment.

- Because of the lower reported number of revisions per patient, a VP shunt should be the recommended CSF diversion method for threatened vision in relation to IIH (Kalyvas et al. 2017).
- An LP shunt could be employed as well.
- When placing VP shunts, it is best to employ neuronavigation.
- To limit the possibility of low-pressure headaches, programable valves containing antigravity or antisiphon systems should be taken into consideration (Mollan et al. 2018).

7.3. Optic Nerve Sheath Fenestration

ONSF is said to have fewer difficulties than CSF diversion (Figure 6), but no cases of fatalities have been found in the literature. Diplopia, ansiocoria, and optic nerve head hemorrhages have all been recorded as transient side effects. More permanent complications, such as branch and central retinal artery occlusions, have been documented on a very infrequent basis. ONSF is sometimes recommended as the first step in the treatment of patients with malignant fulminant IIH as well as those with asymmetrical papilledema causing blindness in one eye (Spitze et al. 2013). If this surgery fails, CSF diversion, which is more intrusive, may be explored (Mollan et al. 2018). Another alternative is ONSF surgery, which is particularly useful for asymmetric papilledema or when visual problems are the most prominent. It has the potential to cause serious consequences such as visual loss, diplopia, and pupillary dysfunction (Chowdhury et al. 2020; Mulla et al. 2015).

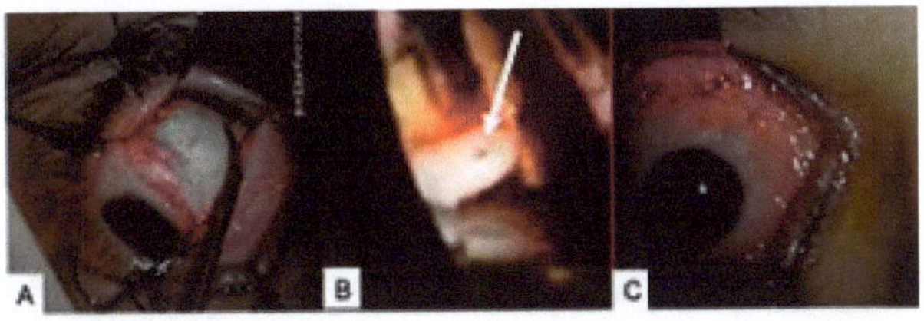

Figure 6. Perioperative pictures of the transconjunctival ONSF approach. (**A**) Right-eye conjunctival incision and approach to optic nerve, (**B**) fenestration on optic nerve sheath, and (**C**) conjunctival repair with sutures. Source: Figure by authors.

7.4. Venous Stenting

Many people with IIH exhibit anatomical anomalies of the cranial venous sinus system observable thanks to advances in venography imaging (Mollan et al. 2018). A narrowing of the prime or both transverse sinuses is one of these anomalies. Stenosis can be caused by the intrinsic dural sinus structure or external compression caused by raised ICP, and lowering ICP might result in the stenosis being resolved.

The degree of narrowing does not appear to be related to ICP or vision loss in a consistent way (Riggeal et al. 2013). In a number of studies, neurovascular stenting has been shown to relieve the symptoms of intracranial hypertension. Many people experience a brief ipsilateral headache after the procedure, especially in the case of stent-adjacent stenosis, which may need retreatment through a third surgery, and artery perforation resulting in acute subdural hematoma, stent migration, and thrombosis in rare cases are possible complications (Mollan et al. 2018).

- Neurovascular stenting's role in IIH has yet to be determined.
- After neurovascular stenting, a long-term antithrombotic drug therapy, is recommended for at least 6 months (Mollan et al. 2018).

7.5. Management of Headache

7.5.1. Lumbar Puncture

Because CSF is released at a rate of 25 mL/hour from the choroid plexus, headache relief after an LP is often short-lived (Wright 1978). As a result, the volume extracted in a so-called therapeutic lumbar tap is quickly replenished. Furthermore, repeated LPs (lumbar punctures) and lumbar–peritoneal shunting have been utilized successfully in the clinical setting. Via lumbar puncture, roughly 30 mL of CSF is drained, or the CSF is drained until the intracranial pressure (as measured via the lumbar technique) is reduced to roughly half of its initial value.

- In spite of the alleviation of headache in nearly 75% of patients, serial LPs are not advised for the treatment of IIH. Many patients experience severe anxiety as a result of LPs, which can lead to acute as well as chronic back pain (Duits et al. 2016).

7.5.2. Acetazolamide

- Acetazolamide, a carbonic anhydrase (CA) inhibitor, is commonly utilized to lower ICP. It is assumed to work by lowering CSF secretion at the choroid plexus.

Two studies showed moderate benefits for acetazolamide for a few outcomes. There is inadequate evidence to advise or reject the efficacy of this drug. Its function and utility are debatable (Biousse et al. 2003; Mollan et al. 2009; Ball et al. 2011).

- It can be used at a maximum dose of 4 g per day (ten Hove et al. 2016); however, Ball et al. (2011) found that 48% of people stopped taking it at 1.5 g because of negative effects.
- A total of 250–500 mg twice a day is a common starting dose of acetazolamide.

7.5.3. Topiramate

Topiramate inhibits hunger by inhibiting carbonic anhydrase. In an uncontrolled open-label study on IIH, it was compared to acetazolamide (Celebisoy et al. 2007). Topiramate has been shown to be effective in the treatment of migraines (Silberstein 2017). With weekly dose increments from 25 mg to 50 mg bd, topiramate may play a role in treating IIH (Mollan et al. 2018; Williams et al. 2017). Topiramate, an anti-epileptic and migraine preventative, was found to be non-inferior to acetazolamide in one trial (Mollan et al. 2014).

7.5.4. Analgesic

In the first few weeks after a diagnosis, short-term painkillers may be beneficial. Nonsteroidal anti-inflammatory medications (NSAIDs) or paracetamol are examples. Indomethacin may provide some benefit due to its ability to lower ICP (Mollan et al. 2018; Liu et al. 2017). Acetazolamide has not been proven to be effective in treating headaches on its own.

8. Definitions

- Idiopathic intracranial: Intracranial hypertension caused by idiopathic factors (IIH). Patients with a high ICP due to an unknown cause meet the criterion.
- Fulminant IIH: Patients with fulminant IIH who meet the criteria for a rapid loss in vision within four weeks of being diagnosed with IIH are said to have fulminant IIH.
- Typical IIH: Females of reproductive age with a body mass index (BMI) more than 30 kg/m^2 are typical IIH patients.
- Atypical IIH: Patients with atypical IIH are not women, are not of reproductive age, or have a BMI of less than 30 kg/m^2. These patients need a more thorough examination to rule out any other potential causes.

Author Contributions: Conceptualization, methodology, validation, formal analysis, investigation, resources, data curation, S.N.-e.-F. and M.S.A.; writing—original draft preparation, S.N.-e.-F., M.S.A. and M.R.H.; writing—review and editing, visualization, supervision, F.H.C. All authors have read and agreed to the published version of the manuscript.

Funding: This research received no external funding.

Conflicts of Interest: The authors declare no conflicts of interest.

References

Bari, Lilla, Rushir Choksi, and E. Steve Roach. 2005. Otitic hydrocephalus revisited. *Archives of Neurology* 62: 824–25. [CrossRef]

Ball, Alexandra K., Andrew Howman, Keith Wheatley, Michael A. Burdon, Timothy Matthews, Andrew S. Jacks, Mark Lawden, Arul Sivaguru, Alexandra Furmston, Steven Howell, and et al. 2011. A randomised controlled trial of treatment for idiopathic intracranial hypertension. *Journal of Neurology* 258: 874–81. [CrossRef] [PubMed]

Biousse, Velerie, Jenet C. Rucker, Catherine Vignal, Isabelle Crassard, Bradley J. Katz, and Nancy J. Newman. 2003. Anemia and papilledema. *American Journal of Ophthalmology* 135: 437–46. [CrossRef] [PubMed]

Celebisoy, Nese, Figen Gökçay, Hadiye Sirin, and O. Akyürekli. 2007. Treatment of idiopathic intracranial hypertension: Topiramate vs acetazolamide, an open-label study. *Acta Neurologica Scandinavica* 116: 322–7. [CrossRef] [PubMed]

Chen, John, and Michael Wall. 2014. Epidemiology and risk factors for idiopathic intracranial hypertension. *International Ophthalmology Clinics* 54: 1–11. [CrossRef]

Chowdhury, Forhad. H., Mohammod R. Haque, Jalal U. M. Rumi, Gurudas Mondal, Mainul H. Sarker, and Qazi D. Mohammod. 2020. Optic Nerve Sheath Fenestration (ONSF). Indications, techniques and results. *Romanian Neurosurgery* XXXIV: 444–51. Available online: www.journals.lapub.co.uk/index.php/roneurosurgery (accessed on 12 July 2021). [CrossRef]

Daniels, Aanthony B., Grant T. Liu, Nicholus J. Volpe, Steven L. Galetta, Mark L. Moster, Nancy J. Newman, Valerie Biousse, Andrew G. Lee, Micheal Wall, Randy Kardon, and et al. 2007. Profiles of obesity, weight gain, and quality of life in idiopathic intracranial hypertension (pseudotumor cerebri). *American Journal of Ophthalmology* 143: 635–41. [CrossRef]

Degnan, Andrew J., and Lucien M. Levy. 2011. Pseudotumor cerebri: Brief review of clinical syndrome and imaging findings. *American Journal of Neuroradiology* 32: 1986–93. [CrossRef]

Duits, Flora H., Pablo Martinez-Lage, Claire Paquet, Sebastiaan Engelborghs, Alberto Lleó, Lucrezia Hausner, José L. Molinuevo, Erik Stomrud, Lucia Farotti, Inez H. G. B. Ramakers, and et al. 2016. Performance and complications of lumbar puncture in memory clinics: Results of the multicenter lumbar puncture feasibility study. *Alzheimer's & Dementia* 12: 154–63.

Farb, Richard I., I. Vanek, J. N. Scott, D. J. Mikulis, R. A. Willinsky, G. Tomlinson, and K. G. terBrugge. 2003. Idiopathic intracranial hypertension: The prevalence and morphology of sinovenous stenosis. *Neurology* 60: 1418–24. [CrossRef]

Friedman, Deborah I., Grant T. Liu, and Kathleen B. Digre. 2013. Revised diagnostic criteria for the pseudotumor cerebri syndrome in adults and children. *Neurology* 81: 1159–65. [CrossRef]

Friedman, Deborah I. 2005. Medication-induced intracranial hypertension in dermatology. *American Journal of Clinical Dermatology* 6: 29–37. [CrossRef] [PubMed]

Headache Classification Committee of the International Headache Society (IHS). 2013. The international classification of headache disorders, 3rd edition (beta version). *Cephalalgia* 33: 629–808.

Hoffmann, Jan, Hans-Jürgen Huppertz, Christoph Schmidt, Hagen Kunte, Lutz Harms, Randolf Klingebiel, and Edzard Wiener. 2013. Morphometric and volumetric MRI changes in idiopathic intracranial hypertension. *Cephalalgia* 33: 1075–84. [CrossRef]

Iencean, S. M. 2003. Idiopathic intracranial hypertension and idiopathic normal pressure hydrocephalus: Diseases with opposite pathogenesis? *Medical Hypotheses* 61: 526–28. [CrossRef]

Iencen, S. M., A. S. Iencean, and A. Tascu. 2015. Pseudotumour cerebri: Idiopathic intracranial hypertension and vascular intracranial hyertension. *Romanian Neurosurgery* 29: 397–409. [CrossRef]

Iencean, Stefan M. 2004. Pattern of increased intracranial pressure and classification of intracranial hypertension. *Journal of Medical Sciences* 4: 52–58. [CrossRef]

Kalyvas, Aristotelis V., Mark Hughes, Cristos Koutsarnakis, Demetrios Moris, Faidon Liakos, Damionos E. Sakas, George Stranjalis, and Ioannis Fouyas. 2017. Efficacy, complications and cost of surgical interventions for idiopathic intracranial hypertension: A systematic review of the literature. *Acta Neurochirurgica* 159: 33–49. [CrossRef]

Kelly, Linda P., Amit M. Saindane, Beau B. Bruce, Maysa A. Ridha, Bryan D. Riggeal, Nancy J. Newman, and Valerie Biousse. 2013. Does bilateral transverse cerebral venous sinus stenosis exist in patients without increased intracranial pressure? *Clinical Neurology and Neurosurgery* 115: 1215–19. [CrossRef] [PubMed]

KesKın, Ahmet O., Fethi İdıman, Derya Kaya, and Behice Bırcan. 2018. Idiopathic Intracranial Hypertension: Etiological factors, Clinical Features, and Prognosis. *Archives of Neuropsychiatry* 57: 23–26. [CrossRef]

Lipton, Howard L., and Paul E. Michelson. 1972. Pseudotumor cerebri syndrome without papilledema. *JAMA* 220: 1591–92. [CrossRef]

Liu, Kenneth C., R. M. Starke, C. Robert Durst, Tony R. Wang, Dale Ding, R. Webster Crowley, and Steven A. Newman. 2017. Venous sinus stenting for reduction of intracranial pressure in IIH: A prospective pilot study. *Journal of Neurosurgery* 127: 1–8. [CrossRef] [PubMed]

Mollan, Susan P., Fizzah Ali, Ghania Hassan-Smith, Hannah F. Botfield, Debohra I. Friedman, and Alexandra J. Sinclair. 2016. Evolving evidence in adult idiopathic intracranial hypertension: Pathophysiology and management. *Journal of Neurology, Neurosurgery & Psychiatry* 87: 982–92. [CrossRef]

Mollan, Susan P., Brenden Davies, Nick C. Silver, Shaw Simon, Conor L. Mallucci, Benjamin R. Wakerley, S. Ramalingam, Anita Krishnan, Swarupsinh V. Chavda, Julie Edwards, and et al. 2018. Idiopathic intracranial hypertension: Consensus guidelines on management. *Journal of Neurology, Neurosurgery & Psychiatry* 89: 1088–100. [CrossRef]

Mollan, Susan P., Alexandra K. Ball, Alexandra J. Sinclair, Carl E. Clarke, Andrew S. Jacks, Michael A. Burdon, and Tim D. Matthews. 2009. Idiopathic intracranial hypertension associated with iron deficiency anaemia: A lesson for management. *European Neurology* 62: 105–85. [CrossRef]

Mollan, Susan P., Keira A. Markey, Jams D. Benzimra, Andrew Jacks, Tim D. Matthews, Michael A. Burdon, and Alex J. Sinclair. 2014. A practical approach to, diagnosis, assessment and management of idiopathic intracranial hypertension. *Practical Neurology* 14: 380–90. [CrossRef]

Mulla, Yasmeen, Keira A. Markey, Rebecca L. Woolley, Smitaa Patel, Susan P. Mollan, and Alexandra J. Sinclair. 2015. Headache determines quality of life in idiopathic intracranial hypertension. *The Journal of Headache and Pain* 16: 45. [CrossRef] [PubMed]

Riggeal, Bryan D., Beau B. Bruce, Amit M. Saindane, Maysa A. Ridha, Linda P. Kelly, Nancy J. Newman, and Valerie Biousse. 2013. Clinical course of idiopathic intracranial hypertension with transverse sinus stenosis. *Neurology* 80: 289–95. [CrossRef]

Silberstein, Stephen D. 2017. Topiramate in migraine prevention: A 2016 perspective. *Headache* 57: 165–78. [CrossRef]

Sinclair, Alexadra J., Michael A. Burdon, Peter G. Nightingale, Alexandra K. Ball, Peter Good, Timothy D. Matthews, Andrew Jacks, Mark Lawden, Carl E. Clarke, Paul M. Stewart, and et al. 2010. Low energy diet and intracranial pressure in women with idiopathic intracranial hypertension: Prospective cohort study. *BMJ* 341: c2701. [CrossRef]

Sodhi, Mohit, Claire A. Sheldon, Bruce Carleton, and Mahyar Etminan. 2017. Oral fluoroquinolones and risk of Sodhi M, Sheldon CA, Carleton B; et al. Oral fluoroquinolones and risk of secondary pseudotumor cerebri syndrome: Nested case-control study. *Neurology* 89: 792–95. [CrossRef]

Spitze, Aarielle, Amina Malik, Nagham Al-Zubidi, Karl Golnik, and Andrew G. Lee. 2013. Optic nerve sheath fenestration vs cerebrospinal diversion procedures: What is the preferred surgical procedure for the treatment of idiopathic intracranial hypertension failing maximum medical therapy? *Journal of Neuro-Ophthalmology* 33: 183–88. [CrossRef] [PubMed]

Tabassi, Abdolreza, Amirali H. Salmasi, and Mahmoud Jalali. 2005. Serum and CSF vitamin A concentrations in idiopathic intracranial hypertension. *Neurology* 64: 1893–96. [CrossRef]

ten Hove, Martin W., Deborah I. Friedman, Anil D. Patel, Isabella Irrcher, Michael Wall, and Michael P. McDermott. 2016. Safety and tolerability of acetazolamide in the idiopathic intracranial hypertension treatment trial. *Journal of Neuro-Ophthalmology* 36: 13–19. [CrossRef]

Uretsky, Scott. 2009. Surgical interventions for idiopathic intracranial hypertension. *Current Opinion in Ophthalmology* 20: 451–55. [CrossRef]

Vorstman, E. B., D. B. Niemann, A. J. Molyneux, and M. G. Pike. 2002. Benign intracranial hypertension associated with arteriovenous malformation. *Developmental Medicine & Child Neurology* 44: 133–35.

Whelton, Paul K., Rrobert M. Carey, Wilbert S. Aronow, Donald E. Casey, Jr., Karen J. Collins, Cheryl Dennison Himmelfarb, Sondra M. DePalma, Samuel Gidding, Kenneth A. Jamerson, Daniel W. Jones, and et al. 2017. ACC/AHA/AAPA/ABC/ACPM/AGS/APhA/ASH/ASPC/NMA/PCNA Guideline for the Prevention, Detection, Evaluation, and Management of High Blood Pressure in Adults: Executive Summary: A Report of the American College of Cardiology/American Heart Association Task Force on Clinical Practice Guidelines. *Hypertension* 71: 1269–324. [PubMed]

Williams, Stefan, Modar Khalil, Asoka Weerasinghe, Anu Sharma, and Richard Davey. 2017. How to do it: Bedside ultrasound to assist lumbar puncture. *Practical Neurology* 17: 47–50. [CrossRef]

Wraige, Elezabeth, Christopher Chandler, and Keith R. Pohl. 2002. Idiopathic intracranial hypertension: Is papilloedema inevitable? *Archives of Disease in Childhood* 87: 223–24. [CrossRef]

Wright, Ernest M. 1978. Transport processes in the formation of the cerebrospinal fluid. *Reviews of Physiology, Biochemistry and Pharmacology* 83: 3–34. [PubMed]

CSF Fistula

Forhad H. Chowdhury, Rakibul Haque, Syeda Neyamot-e-Ferdousi, Rakibul Islam and Md Bayazidur Rahman

Abstract: CSF surrounds the brain and spinal cord, which are contained within the dura mater. Any rift in dura can prompt CSF leakage/fistula. Common sites for CSF fistulas are the nose and ears, known as CSF rhinorrhea and CSF otorrhea, respectively. The etiology of CSF fistula includes neurotrauma, cranial as well as spinal surgery, chronic raised intracranial pressure (ICP), and a spontaneously occurring CSF fistula. Diagnosis and evaluation including 'defect' localization are the main challenge. CT or MR cisternograms assist in the diagnosis and localization of a CSF fistula. An untreated fistula can cause death and morbidity through meningoencephalitis. Treatment options include conservative and surgical treatment. Surgical treatment depends on the site and size of a fistula, associated pathologies, and the surgeon's preferences, which can be endoscopy or microsurgery. In this chapter, the etiology, clinical presentation, evaluation, and treatments of CSF fistulae, especially CSF rhinorrhea, CSF otorrhea, and spinal CSF fistula, are discussed briefly.

Abbreviations

CSF	cerebrospinal fluid	CT	computed tomography
ESS	endoscopic sinus surgery	FESS	functional endoscopic sinus surgery
HCP	hydrocephalus	ICP	intracranial pressure
MRI	magnetic resonance imaging	SSCD	superior semicircular canal dehiscence

1. Introduction

CSF leaks or fistulas happen when CSF escapes via a small rip or crack in the dura mater, which protects the CNS and retains the CSF in place. CSF might leak out through the epidermis, nasal mucosa, or external ear canal due to a rupture or hole. When CSF is lost, the previously cushioned brain sags inside the skull, resulting in a headache, and the intracranial pressure (ICP) within the skull decreases, resulting in intracranial hypotension. CSF fistulas can form anywhere along the spinal column (spinal CSF fistulae) or in the brain (cranial CSF fistulas, i.e., CSF rhinorrhea and CSF otorrhea).

2. CSF Rhinorrhea

The entry of CSF into the nose due to improper connection between the subarachnoid space and the nasal or perinasal sinus mucosa is known as CSF rhinorrhea (Figure 1) (Sumaily 2017).

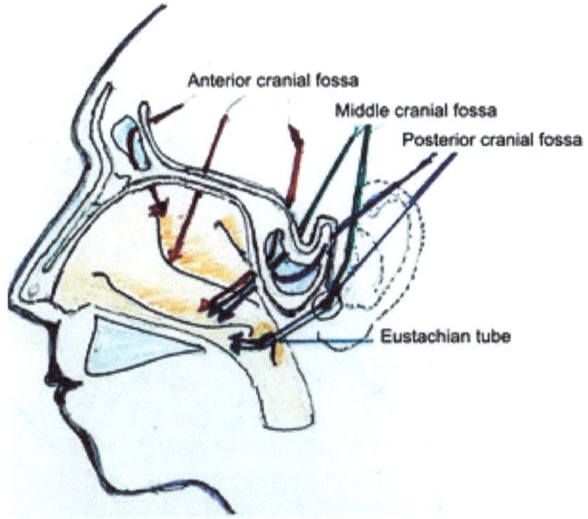

Figure 1. Schematic drawing showing different pathways of CSF rhinorrhea from intracranial fossae to nasal cavity. Source: Figure by authors.

2.1. Etiology

2.1.1. Traumatic

CSF leaks are most commonly caused by trauma (80–90%), caused by either a head injury or iatrogenic factors (Abuabara 2007; Bell et al. 2004; Platt and Parnes 2009; Bumm et al. 2009). Traumatic etiologies (blunt as well as penetrating cranio-facial injuries) account for more than eighty percent of all cases of CSF leaks, with young males being the most commonly affected (Figures 2–6).

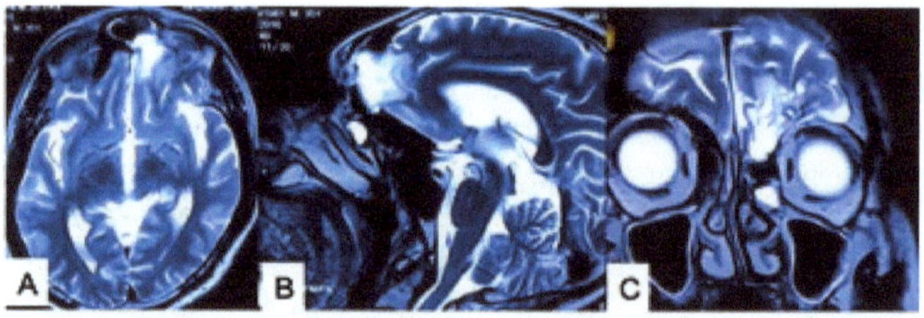

Figure 2. (**A–C**) MRI of the brain T2W images showing post-traumatic CSF rhinorrhea through posterior wall of the left frontal sinus. Source: Figure by authors.

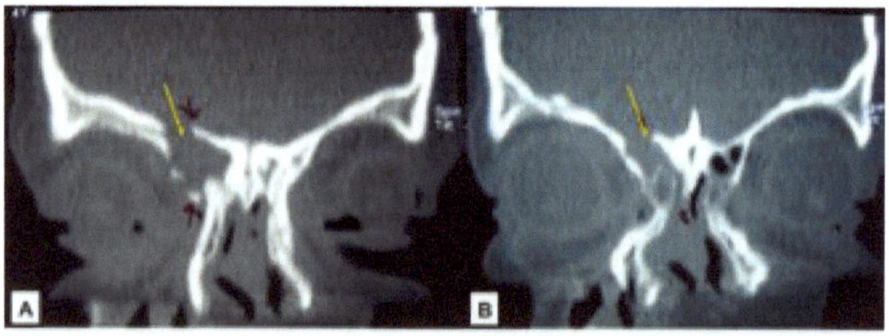

Figure 3. (**A**,**B**) CT scan of anterior skull base (coronal images) in bony window, showing traumatic fractures resulting in a CSF fistula through the ethmoid sinus (arrow marked). Source: Figure by authors.

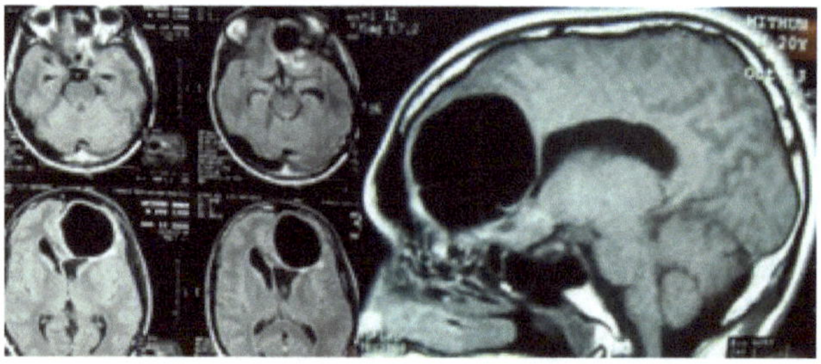

Figure 4. MRI of the brain: axial FLAIR images (left side) and T1W sagittal image (right side) showing post-head injury frontal tension pneumocephalus (with CSF rhinorrhea through ethmoid sinus). Source: Figure by authors.

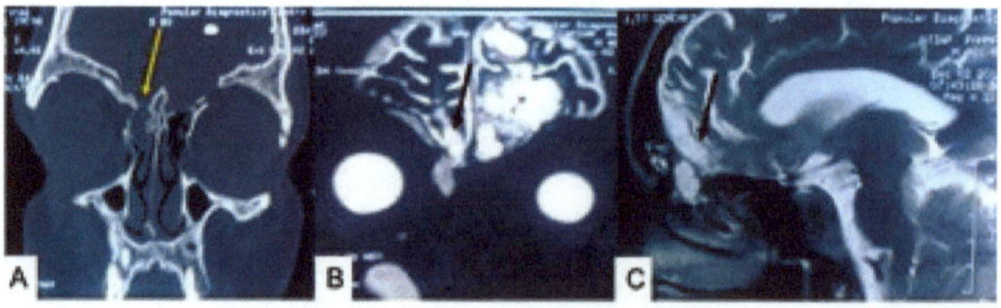

Figure 5. (**A**) CT scan coronal image of bony window showing traumatic fractures (right side) resulting in CSF fistula. (**B**,**C**) MR cisternograms (with a coronal image and a sagittal image, respectively) showing CSF tract through the same defect seen in CT. Source: Figure by auyhors.

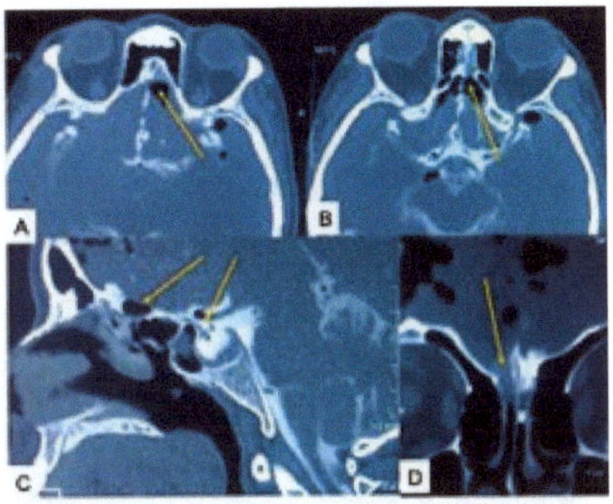

Figure 6. CT cisternogram of a patient with traumatic CSF rhinorrhea: (**A**,**B**) axial images; (**C**) sagittal image; and (**D**) coronal image showing pneumocephalus and a bony defect at the left olfactory fossa and tuberculum sella resulting in a CSF fistula. Source: Figure by authors.

In 12–30% of instances, basilar skull fractures occur, with the anterior cranial fossa being the most prevalently affected area. The dura has greater adhesion to the base of the skull at this level, so traumas can quickly impact it (Patrascu et al. 2017).

CSF leaks are classed as immediate or delayed in terms of occurrence latency: 60% appear in the third or fourth day following the occurrence, 70% appear within the first seven days, and 95% appear within the first three months (Patrascu et al. 2017).

Iatrogenic injury accounts for 16% of traumatic CSF fistula cases. Basically, any surgical procedure conducted around the skull base can cause iatrogenic CSF leaks (Patrascu et al. 2017). The most common causes of iatrogenic CSF leaks in recent decades have been neurosurgical operations (craniotomies and the removal of hypophyseal tumors or suprasellar tumors). FESS (functional endoscopic sinus surgery) has now become the leading etiology of iatrogenic CSF fistulas, accounting for less than 1% of all surgical endoscopic operations. Because of the thickness of the bone of the anterior skull base, the cribriform plate (80%) is the commonest site of lesions observed during endoscopic sinus surgery (ESS) procedures. The frontal sinus (8%), the sphenoid sinus (4%), and the posterior fovea ethmoidalis are other common sites of injury. Iatrogenic CSF fistulas usually occur in just 50% of patients within seven days after surgery, unlike traumatic leakage. The majority of the time, when the leakage occurs, the patients have already been discharged. When there is a possibility of a CSF leak, it is critical to tell patients about the commonest symptoms (Patrascu et al. 2017).

2.1.2. Spontaneous

Spontaneous leaks can occur as a result of elevated intracranial pressure (Figures 7–12) or when intracranial pressure is normal (Schlosser et al. 2006; Schlosser and Bolger 2003; Lopatin et al. 2003; Banks et al. 2009). In forty-five percent of non-traumatic CSF fistulas, leaking at high pressure seems to be implicated (Patrascu et al. 2017). Many causes of raised ICP have been identified in the literature, although the idiopathic mechanism remains the most common. CSF pressure variations affect the anterior cranial base dura, potentially leading to dural deficiency in bone floor defects due to a variety of reasons (respiration and artery pressure fluctuations and Valsalva-like actions during nasal blowing).

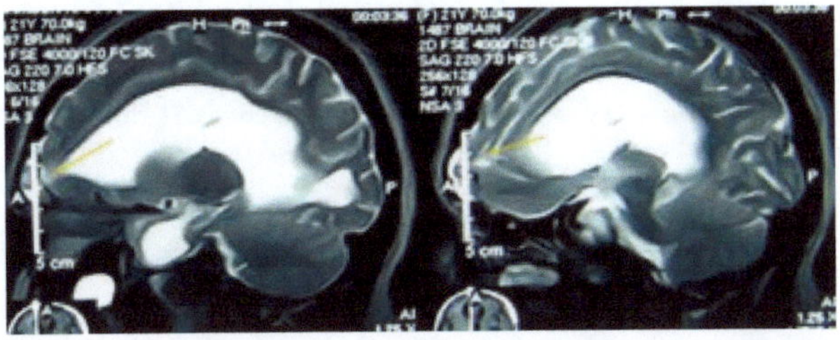

Figure 7. MRI of the brain (T2W sagittal images) showing spontaneous trans-frontal sinus CSF fistula due to chronic increased intracranial pressure (hydrocephalus). Source: Figure by authors.

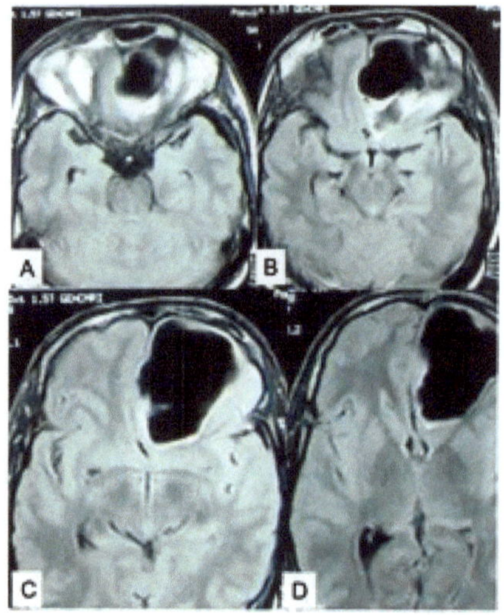

Figure 8. (**A–D**) MRI of the brain (axial FLAIR images) showing frontal tension pneumocephalus in a spontaneous CSF fistula (through left frontal sinus) case. Source: Figure by authors.

The pressure applied to the thin bone areas of the anterior skull base (lateral lamella of the cribriform plate, the sphenoidal sinus lateral recess) determines ischemia via vascular pressure, bony thickening, and bone shaping, along with gap creation, regardless of the reasons for high intracranial pressure. The dura can herniate and create meningoceles through this opening, or the cerebral parenchyma can herniate through it if the breach is large enough (creating an encephalocele) (Woodworth et al. 2008). Patients with spontaneous CSF rhinorrhea showed several contemporaneous bone abnormalities in the skull base according to research by Lieberman et al. (Lieberman et al. 2015). According to the researchers, intracranial hypertension was discovered to be a decisive factor in the formation of these abnormalities. There have also been occurrences of CSF leaks linked to normal ICP, constituting 55% of spontaneous cases of CSF fistulas (Patrascu et al. 2017).

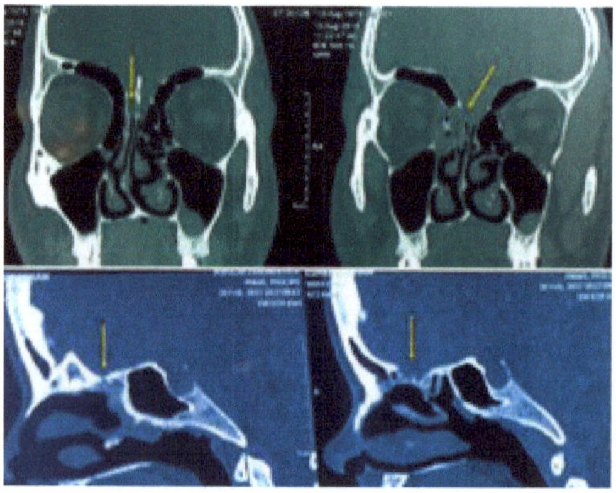

Figure 9. CT scan of head and skull base (bony window) (axial (**upper**) and sagittal (**lower**) images) showing bone gap in right olfactory fossa resulting in spontaneous CSF rhinorrhea through ethmoid sinus. Source: Figure by authors.

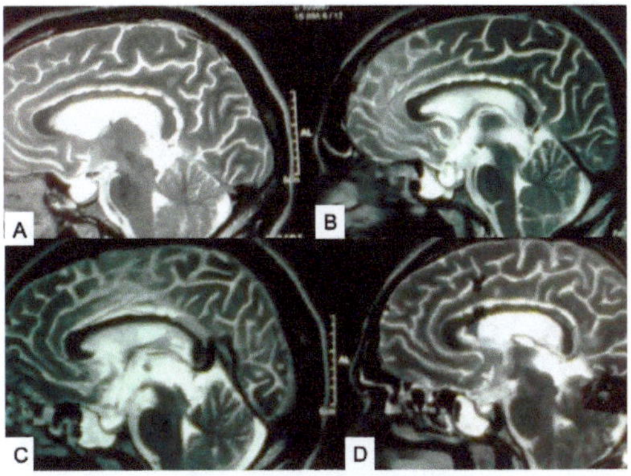

Figure 10. (**A–D**) MRI of the brain (T2W sagittal images) showing spontaneous CSF fistula through sphenoid sinus due to tuberculum sella and sella turcica defects. Source: Figure by auyhors.

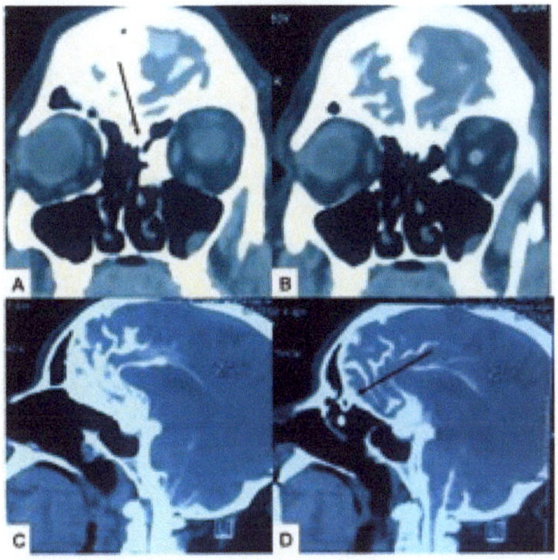

Figure 11. CT cisternogram ((**A,B**) coronal images and (**C,D**) sagittal images) showing spontaneous CSF fistula through left olfactory fossa defect. Source: Figure by authors.

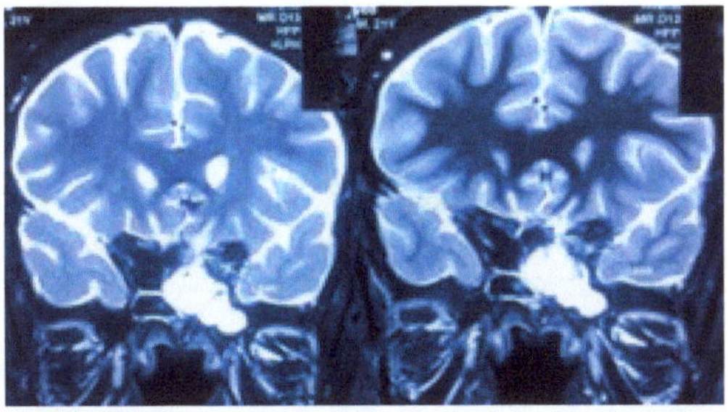

Figure 12. MRI of brain (T2W coronal images) showing spontaneous CSF fistula tract through left plannum sphenoidale and tuberculum sella into the spheno-ethmoidal sinus on left side. Source: Figure by author.

2.1.3. Congenital

Encephaloceles or a persistent craniopharyngeal canal can cause congenital CSF fistulae (Kim et al. 2000) (Figure 13). The capacity for meningeal herniation via the anterior cranial base may be determined by the presence of an anterior neuropore after delivery (meningo-encephaloceles). These are unusually linked to CSF rhinorrhea. Meningo-encephaloceles commonly emerge in the pediatric age group as a transilluminating tumoral mass in the intranasal or extranasal cavity, which increases in size when a child cries (Furstenberg sign). All childhood intranasal tumors, particularly those emerging from the midline, should raise suspicion (Patrascu et al. 2017). Only once the surgeon have carried out imaging studies should he/she proceed with a biopsy (Woodworth et al. 2004). Another congenital lesion that can lead to CSF rhinorrhea is a persistent craniopharyngeal canal. Primary empty sellae syndrome, which is a congenital disease, can result in CSF leakage and is linked to brain tumors, hydrocephalus, and pseudotumor cerebri (Patrascu et al. 2017).

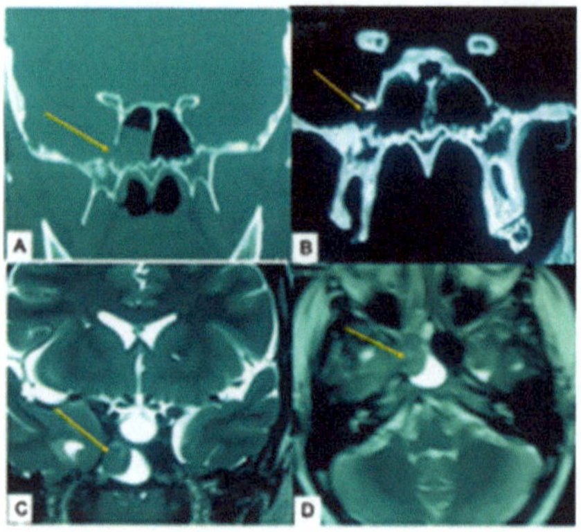

Figure 13. (**A**,**B**) CT scan of skull base (coronal section) showing defect in lateral wall of right sphenoid sinus resulting in a small temporal lobe encephalocele (pushing into the right sphenoid sinus) and CSF rhinorrhea (Sternberg's canal) (**C**,**D**). Source: Figure by authors.

2.1.4. Miscellaneous

Tumors, infection, mucoceles, and radiation can all induce erosion of the base of the skull. CSF rhinorrhea is rarely diagnosed as being caused by these factors. Locally malignant tumors, such as inverted papilloma and other neoplasms (nasopharyngeal carcinoma, osteomas), can also destroy bone in the anterior cranial base. Local inflammation and even dural rupture may result from the mass effect of bone disintegration. Even though tumors may not cause CSF rhinorrhea on their own, resection surgery frequently causes rapid leakage (Sumaily 2017).

2.2. Presentation

Unilateral clear and watery nasal discharge is the commonest indication of CSF rhinorrhea; however, this discharge might be mixed with blood if the trauma occurred recently. The volume of a nasal CSF leak may rise in the supine position. The collection of CSF in one paranasal sinus and its external flow through the nose due to positional changes of the head (the "reservoir sign") can cause intermittent leakage (Meco and Oberascher 2004). Patients may also taste salt. Although most people do not complain of a headache, the presence of a headache raises the risk of excessive ICP and intracranial tumor (Mokri et al. 2000; Mokri et al. 1998). It is crucial to note whether the headache goes away after the CSF leakage has subsided.

Other symptoms may assist one in pinpointing the leak's location in some circumstances. Anosmia (60% of post-traumatic CSF rhinorrhea cases) indicates that the anterior fossa and olfactory region have been injured (Mathias et al. 2016). Lesions of the tuberculum sellae, the posterior ethmoidal sinuses, or the sphenoidal sinus can cause optic nerve dysfunctions (Patrascu et al. 2017). Regardless of whether or not there is a CSF leak, individuals with recurrent meningitis should be investigated for abnormalities that expose the meninges to the upper airways (Bernal-Sprekelsen et al. 2005). Patients may experience nasal bleeding, red eyes, periorbital bruising, visual dysfunction, a loss of smell or cranial nerve palsies (most commonly I–III as well as V–VII), and acute-phase meningitis shortly after the neuro-trauma (Eljamel and Foy 1990; Cassano and Felippu 2009; Scholsem et al. 2008). Patients may develop recurrent nasal watery discharge, intermittent meningitis or cerebral abscesses, headaches, a sweet/salty taste in the nasopharynx, and hyposmia in the chronic phase after the trauma. The probability of the development of recurrent meningitis after trauma ranges from 12.5% to 50%, with a neurological problem incidence of 29.4% (Patrascu et al. 2017; Mokri et al. 1998). The ability to distinguish CSF rhinorrhea from other nasal discharges is still crucial in detecting CSF fistulas.

Patients with obvious CSF rhinorrhea after trauma have a clear diagnosis that just needs to be confirmed. The presence of hemorrhagic clots or nasal bleeding as a result of facial fractures, as well as the interval of CSF rhinorrhea, might also complicate the diagnosis (Yilmazlar et al. 2006).

2.3. *Physical Examination*

Complete rhinologic, otologic, ophthalmologic, and neurologic assessments are included in the physical examination. Encephaloceles or meningoceles can be detected with a physical examination and an intranasal endoscopy. One can detect the existence of a CSF leak by examining a patient when they perform the Valsalva maneuver or when both their internal jugular veins are squeezed simultaneously (Queckenstedt-Stookey test) (Patrascu et al. 2017). Physical examinations may not be definitive in many cases, especially for patients with intermittent CSF leakage (Bolger and Kennedy 1992). The "target sign", which means the ability of CSF to move and generate a bull's-eye stain on filter paper around the central bloody spot, may be seen in some situations. This classic indicator, on the other hand, has poor specificity and can be caused by saliva or tears (Dula and Fales 1993). Physical examination of patients with bilateral CSF rhinorrhea does not reveal anything about the defect's location. Paradoxically, CSF may leak into the contralateral nostril if the midline anatomical structures (crista galli, vomer) are damaged (Patrascu et al. 2017).

2.4. *Laboratory Tests*

The gold-standard beta-2-transferrin test is used to identify the presence of CSF. Beta-2-transferrin is a central nervous system protein generated by neuraminidase activity. Its presence is an indirect indication of CSF rhinorrhea because it is not generally detected in nasal discharge. An amount of 0.5 ml of nasal discharge must be collected for this test. The test is both sensitive (99%) and specific (99%) (Patrascu et al. 2017; Warnecke et al. 2004; Chan et al. 2004). Beta-trace protein, which is detected in the CSF (35-fold higher quantities than serum), cardiac muscle, and plasma, is another test option, but it has poorer specificity than beta-2-transferrin. Renal failure, multiple sclerosis, and intracranial malignancies can all cause its levels to rise (Patrascu et al. 2017).

2.5. *Neuro-Imaging Methods*

After verifying that a patient has CSF rhinorrhea, the next task is to pinpoint the exact location and choose the best treatment.

2.5.1. High-Resolution Computed Tomography (HRCT)

The imaging approach of choice for diagnosing skull base anomalies associated with CSF rhinorrhea is a high-resolution computed tomography examination with axial, coronal, and sagittal reconstructions (Patrascu et al. 2017). The slices should have a thickness of 1 mm (Lund et al. 1994). CT scans can detect skull base deformities caused by iatrogenic or unintentional damage, anatomic disorders such as hydrocephalus (HCP) or pneumocephalus, and tumoral masses (Naidich and Moran 1980). CT scans are advised in all cases of suspected bone abnormalities of the base of the skull.

CT Cisternography

Additionally, a CT scan can be used with an intrathecal contrast material (iophendylate) to perform CT cisternography, a type of imaging. Although this procedure is more intrusive, it is more accurate in pinpointing the specific location of a bone deficiency and a CSF leak. When a patient has an active CSF fistula, CT cisternography has been shown to have a nearly 100% detection rate (Patrascu et al. 2017). This rate of detection is just 60% in the case of intermittent leaks (El Gammal and Brooks 1994). To conduct this research, pledgets must be placed in the anterior plate of the cribriform plate, the middle meatus, or the lateral sphenoethmoidal recess (Patrascu et al. 2017) under endoscopic control. Although this procedure does not offer data, the diagnosis of a fistula is certain when radioactivity is measured through the pledgets.

2.5.2. Magnetic Resonance Imaging (MRI)

Magnetic resonance imaging is another imaging technique employed in this regard, and it has high specificity for soft tissue lesions and CSF. Because of the hyperintense signal available via T2-weighted imaging that is indicative of a CSF leak, MRI can distinguish a CSF leak from other intrasinusal fluid (Jones and Becker 2001). Intrathecal dye injection may be utilized with MRI to improve accuracy. This imaging method has worse sensitivity for detecting abnormalities of the skull base than CT and is significantly more expensive.

MRI Cisternography

Magnetic resonance imaging cisternography with Gadolinium contrast administered intrathecally is a technique whose efficacy has to be proven in more research. In situations of occult CSF fistulas in patients with recurrent meningitis who do not have CSF rhinorrhea, a diagnosis is considerably more challenging, and all neuro-imaging approaches must be balanced to arrive at the best therapeutic decision (Patrascu et al. 2017).

2.6. *Perioperative Intrathecal Fluorescein*

Many surgeons inject fluorescein intrathecally, both preoperatively as well as intraoperatively, to pinpoint the region where a CSF leak is taking place. An endoscope is used to assess the patient 30–60 min later. Fluorescein coloring can usually be seen without any filters in most circumstances. In the case of minor flaws, this fluid can only be detected with filters and black light. This technique has not been approved by the FDA since it has the potential to be neurotoxic in high dosages. This test's accuracy is determined by the area of the dural dehiscence, CSF volume, the time of examination following injection, and fluorescein turnover rate (Patrascu et al. 2017; Liu et al. 2009).

2.7. *Treatment Options for CSF Rhinorrhea*

The management of a CSF fistula can be split into two categories: conservative and surgical. Post-traumatic CSF fistulas are usually resolved with conservative care, although surgical therapy is suggested in the case of spontaneous CSF rhinorrhea. In the case of refractory CSF fistulas, one must use a combination of treatment options, including surveillance, decreasing CSF production, and surgery (intracranial or extracranial procedures) (Patrascu et al. 2017; Albert and Leibrock 2005).

2.7.1. Conservative Treatment

When it comes to post-traumatic leaks, conservative treatment is effective because there is a high chance of spontaneous resolution. In essence, conservative treatment entails bed rest (Gosal et al. 2015). To decrease CSF pressure at the interpeduncular cistern level, the patient has to lie in bed for 7 to 10 days with the head end of the bed raised 15–30 degrees (Patrascu et al. 2017). To reduce the strain and degree of intracranial pressure, stool softeners must be administered. The patient should not strain, blow their nose, or cough, nor should they carry anything heavy. It has been found that 75–80% of all post-traumatic CSF rhinorrhea cases can be resolved spontaneously in 7 days when treated with this method. Acetazolamide, for example, can reduce ICP by inhibiting the Na^+/K^+ ATP-ase activity that produces CSF (Patrascu et al. 2017).

Acetazolamide can thus be used as a supplement in the management of patients who have spontaneous CSF fistulas and high ICP (Carrion et al. 2001; Caballero et al. 2012). A lumbar drain is an additional tool that should be considered when the preceding management has failed for at least 5–7 days. Because it eliminates CSF pressure spikes, continuous draining is favored over intermittent drainage. To avoid side effects of over drainage like nausea, headaches, and vomiting, the suggested CSF drainage rate is around 10–15 cc/hour (Patrascu et al. 2017; Chan et al. 2004).

2.7.2. Surgical Treatment

Surgery is the only effective treatment option in some cases of CSF leakage. Indications of operation are listed in Box 1. The correct surgical treatment of CSF rhinorrhea is determined by the leak's etiology, location, and severity. The following are some general guidelines for dealing with CSF leaks: (1) treat HCP as well as meningitis before undertaking any surgical operations; (2) locate and extend the dural dehiscence; (3) dissect the bone and dural gap; (4) perform direct repair of the dural gap whenever possible; and (5) close the gap with grafts when direct dural repair is not possible (Patrascu et al. 2017).

Box 1. General indications for interventional repair (Patrascu et al. 2017).

1. Repeated meningitis and persistent leaks despite nonsurgical treatment
2. High-CSF-pressure fistulas and HCP
3. Large pneumocephalus (with fluid levels higher than 2 mL) despite conservative treatment
4. Imaging findings indicating a reduced chance of natural dural healing (bone destruction, skull base comminution, soft tissue coverage in the bony edges)
5. Acute post-traumatic/postoperative fistulas that remain or reappear in the 10–13 days after conservative management has been conducted
6. CSF fistulas and congenital cerebral dysplasia, especially after a single episode of meningitis.
7. Intermittent/late fistulae

CT scans should be performed prior to surgery. A stereotactic guided approach is useful in locating the dural gap. For a successful outcome, a multidisciplinary team consisting of an otolaryngologist, an anesthesiologist, and a neurosurgeon is required. The treatment of iatrogenic CSF leaks should take place at the same time as the primary surgery.

Intracranial and extracranial interventions are used to address CSF leaks surgically.

Transcranial Approaches

In cases of comminuted or prolonged skull fractures, as well as hemorrhages in cranial fractures or contusions requiring a craniotomy, intracranial methods are used (Dodson et al. 1994). The fundamental benefit of this approach is that the dural defect may be seen directly.

Endoscopic Endonasal Surgery

Because of its low morbidity (no retraction to the brain or increased risk for anosmia) and wide range of surgical field vision, endoscopic endonasal surgery is now the preferred procedure for treating CSF fistulas. However, in order to insert the graft appropriately in this technique, one must pinpoint the exact location of the fistula (Hegazy et al. 2000; Lee et al. 2004; Lopatin et al. 2003; Marshall et al. 2001). Based on the site of the dural gap, several alternative endoscopic techniques have been devised. The major goal of endoscopic treatment is to expose the dural defect as much as possible, with intrathecal fluorescein being used in low-flow situations (Figure 14). If an encephalocele is discovered, it should be cautiously removed at once. To prevent mucocele formation, the neurosurgeon has to expose 0.2–0.5 cm of the bone around the gap and remove the remaining mucosa inside the defect before fixing it. This also accelerates osteogenesis and enhances graft acceptance (Hegazy et al. 2000; Elmorsy and Khafagy 2014). Various forms of grafts are employed in modern practice; however, their size should not exceed 30% of the defect diameter. Septal cartilage; bone from the septum, mastoid tip, or iliac crest; septal or turbinate mucosa; fascia (fascia lata or the temporal fascia); abdominal/thigh fat; pedicled (septal) flaps; or turbinate flaps are examples of grafting materials (Landeiro et al. 2004). It is worth noting that the pedicled flaps may discolor, fold, or compress. Many factors can impact the choice of graft type, including gap size and site, ICP, personal experience, and material availability (Wetmore et al. 1987). The overlay technique (directly over the gap), the underlay technique (in between the dura and the bone gap), and combination procedures are the three types of grafting techniques. Fibrin glue as well as autologous belly fat are also utilized to strengthen the transplant after it has been placed. As an overlay graft, a mucosal graft from the middle turbinate or septum can be used (Patrascu et al. 2017).

Fasciae (temporalis muscle or fascia lata) provide additional support that aids in sealing the defect.

When all the grafts are put in place, the fistula repair is conducted, using a sponge and non-absorbable nasal packing to put more pressure on the site. Neurosurgeons must carefully avoid obliterating the nearby sinus ostia. The size of the dural gap is an important parameter regarding the number of layers as well as the type of graft material when surgical planning is performed. During dural closure, one must apply the main rule —"watertight closure". When the defect is <2 mm, the graft type is not important for the success of the intervention. For fistula defects of 2–5 mm, it is advised to utilize overlay grafts (mucosal grafts or flaps), without any important dural lesions. If the fractured skull base is of the comminuted type, a composite graft should be used. Composite grafts or mucosa and bone grafts are the preferred treatment for defects larger than 5 mm. For the first 3–5 days after surgery, bed rest with the head end of the bed raised 15–30° is recommended. Antibiotics should be given, and blood pressure (BP) should be managed at a normal level (Patrascu et al. 2017; Jahrsdoerfer et al. 1981).

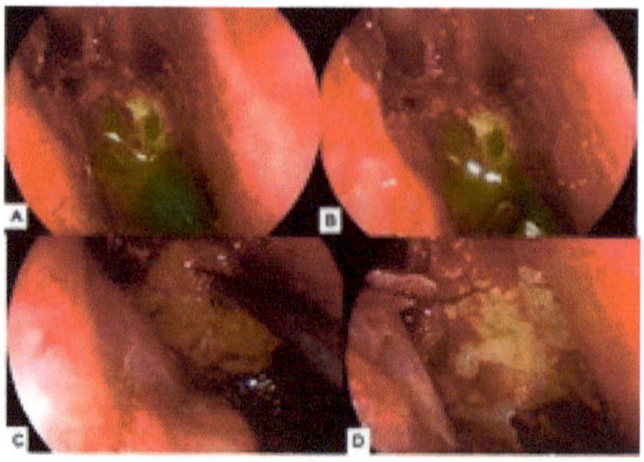

Figure 14. Endoscopic endonasal repair of CSF rhinorrhea (perioperative pictures), (**A**,**B**) showing a dural defect through which fluorescein (injected in the lumbar subarachnoid space)-stained CSF is coming out. (**C**,**D**) Pictures taken after the repair of the fistula with autogenous fat graft. Source: Figure by authors.

3. CSF Otorrhea

Even when CSF leaks through otologic structures, actual ear fluid leakage does not always occur. A rupture in the tympanic membrane or an abnormality in the external ear canal can cause CSF otorrhea; this is frequently the case when the leaking is caused by trauma or previous ear surgery. The CSF flows down the eustachian tube and manifests as a distinct form of CSF rhinorrhea if there is no such abnormality. It must be distinguished from a CSF leak from other parts of the skull base, such as the paranasal sinuses, in this case. It is also vital to realize that the fact that the leak is coming from the nose does not rule out the possibility of an otologic source. The majority of instances involve leaks as a postoperative consequence of base-of-the-skull surgery. According to reports, this problem occurs in 6–12% of such situations (Gacek and Leipzig 1979).

3.1. Congenital Cerebrospinal Fluid Leak

Problems in the otic capsule itself, aberrant patency of routes linked with the otic capsule, and defects far from the otic capsule are all possible congenital causes (Figures 15 and 16). Although congenital causes are more common in youngsters, they can manifest at any age and have even been observed among the elderly (Liao et al. 2016).

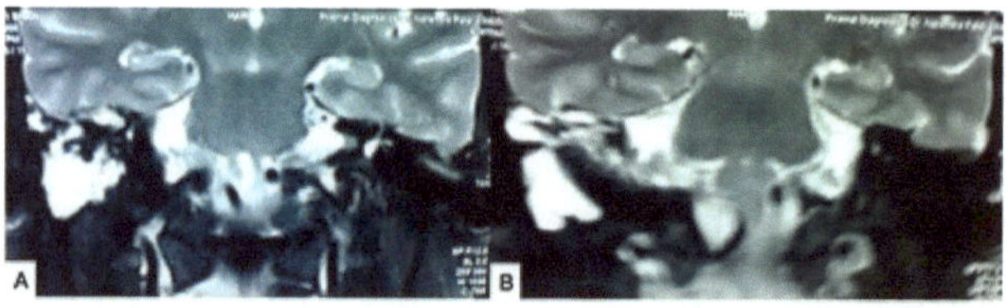

Figure 15. (**A**,**B**) MRI of brain and skull base (coronal T2W images) showing spontaneous CSF fistula (otorrhea) passing through right mastoid air sinus and middle ear cavity (tegmen tympani dehiscence). Source: Figure by authors.

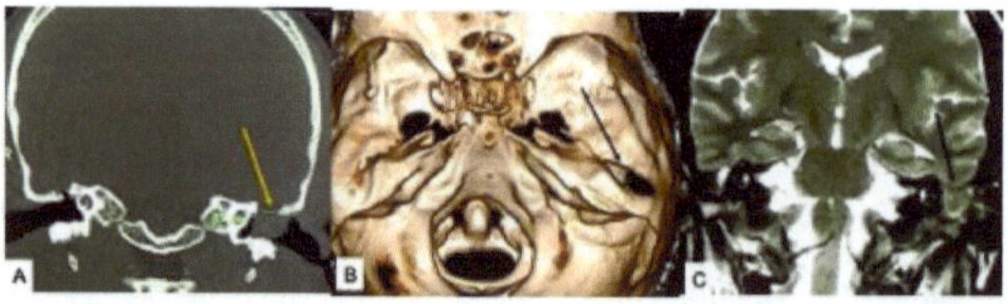

Figure 16. (**A**) CT scan of head coronal image in bony window; (**B**) CT scan 3D reconstruction of skull base showing left middle fossa bony gap on roof of middle ear cavity resulting encephalocele in middle ear cavity with spontaneous CSF otorrhea. (**C**) MRI T2W coronal image showing the encephalocele. Source: Figure by authors.

3.2. *Acquired Cerebrospinal Fluid Leak*

Temporal bone damage, surgery, or viral or neoplastic reasons can all induce acquired leaks (Jackson et al. 1997). Congenital spinal fluid leakage is significantly less prevalent than acquired spinal fluid leakage. The most prevalent etiology of acquired CSF fistulas is postoperative leakage following surgery. It is a well-known side effect of auditory schwannoma removal (Figure 17) and other skull base procedures. These CSF leaks are frequently visible in the first few days after surgery.

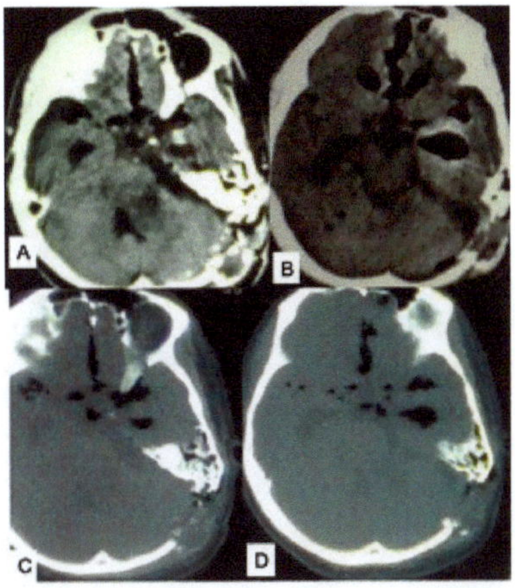

Figure 17. CT scan of head. (**A**,**B**) Axial images and (**C**,**D**) axial images in bony window showing extensive pneumocephalus after retro-sigmoid craniectomy for acoustic schwannoma where CSF rhinorrhea and otorrhea were developed through mastoid air sinus, middle ear cavity, and eustachian tube. Source: Figure by authors.

An acquired CSF leak can also be induced by mastoid surgery for chronic middle ear disease. If the dura is ruptured during surgery, the defect should be corrected as soon as feasible. Commonly, however, the dura is unharmed, but a deficiency in the tegmen's bony plate remains. The constant pulsations of the CSF thin the dura, precipitating the prolapse of the arachnoid and brain through this defect over time. This thin dura may shrink and break spontaneously, ending in a CSF fistula many years after the initial surgery.

Parts of the brain tissue, in addition to the dura, may prolapse through the dural deficiency, producing an encephalocele. Middle ear disorders, particularly cholesteatoma, can cause comparable issues even if surgery is not performed. Cholesteatoma can erode the tegmen plate, allowing dura or brain herniation to develop over time (Leung 2013).

3.3. *Clinical Presentation*

When there is a CSF leakage via the ear, the most common symptom presented is clear watery discharge from the external ear. But this is not always exhibited and only occurs when the eardrum or canal has been damaged in some way. If this is not the case, the CSF leakage could show up as a clear, watery nasal discharge. This discharge can be stationary or intermittent, and it may only be noticeable when the patient strains or leans forward. Some individuals report no discharge at all but instead a weird salty taste in the posterior part of the throat. CSF otorrhea is frequently accompanied by meningitis. It is found in 93% of children and 36% of adults experiencing an isolated CSF leak. Sensorineural hearing loss is another common complication of spontaneous leaks in children, occurring in 82% of cases. Seizures are another possible complication (Jahrsdoerfer et al. 1981; Gacek and Leipzig 1979).

3.4. *Management*

3.4.1. Surgical Treatment

A patient is at high risk of developing meningitis if CSF leaks through their ear structures. In most cases, surgery is required to correct this condition. A pressure dressing with a lumbar drain can often be used to repair leaks that arise as a result of injury or recent skull base surgery. Surgery is advised for patients who have failed to improve following conservative treatment. CSF otorrhea is a broad term that refers to a variety of conditions. The majority of these leaks occur after surgery and are a well-known consequence of acoustic neurinoma surgery (Oh et al. 2019).

Some develop years after being precipitated by tympano-mastoid surgery or erosive pathologies such as cholesteatoma. Some may be caused by congenital anomalies in the inner ear and mastoid development.

Oh et al. discovered a link between CSF otorrhea and superior semicircular canal dehiscence (SSCD) in a retrospective study, showing that 21% of patients with CSF otorrhea had concomitant SSCD, while only 2% of controls had both (Oh et al. 2019; Brodie and Thompson 1997).

A compressive dressing as well as bed rest including head elevation are typically used to address otogenic CSF leaks caused by recent surgery or trauma. Eighty percent of the time, patients with CSF leaks caused by acoustic schwannoma surgery react to this treatment. This is also true for CSF leaks caused by temporal bone fractures, which usually close after 3–4 weeks of conservative treatment (Oliaei et al. 2012).

Surgical correction is the primary treatment for a spontaneous otogenic cerebrospinal fluid leakage. Surgery is reserved for individuals with postsurgical and traumatic leaks who have failed to respond to conservative management. The nature and location of the defect determine the correct surgical approach.

A transcanal technique can often be used to correct spontaneous CSF leaks for children with otic capsule anomalies (such as Mondini deformity). A stapedectomy is frequently performed, and the oval window is erased with soft tissue because patients rarely have the ability to hear.

In some situations of CSF leakage caused by a patent Hyrtl fissure, a transcanal technique can be used. A transmastoid technique is chosen in most situations concerning spontaneous leaking (Assietti et al. 1993).

3.4.2. Medical Therapy

Despite the fact that the presence of a CSF fistula puts a patient at a potential risk for meningitis, the use of preventive antibiotics is controversial. Many people feel that using antibiotics in the absence of an infection selects for resistant bacteria in the normal flora, making it more difficult to treat meningitis when it occurs. Antibiotics should not be applied until signs or symptoms of meningitis appear and a spinal tap confirms the diagnosis. Then, until cultures and sensitivities are returned and determined, respectively, broad-spectrum antibiotics should be used. According to a number of published studies, the risk of meningitis is greatly reduced when preventive antibiotics are administered in cases of post-traumatic CSF leaks, and their administration in this scenario is typically advised (Hanson 2020).

Medication is frequently used to reduce spinal fluid production. Diuretics (e.g., furosemide and hydrochlorothiazide), carbonic anhydrase (CA) inhibitors (e.g., acetazolamide), and steroids are examples of such drugs. These treatments are not utilized as the primary treatment for a CSF leak, but they are helpful supplements. If the output is low throughout the evaluation and diagnosis phase, they may make it difficult to find the fistula (Hanson 2020).

Continuous lumbar CSF drainage may be an effective complement to conservative treatment for a CSF leak caused by surgery or trauma. Uninterrupted CSF outflow reduces the ICP against the leak, allowing natural healing to take place. When the source of the leak is unknown, do not employ a spinal drain as it may obstruct localization and enable air entry into the cranial vault, resulting in pneumocephalus. A lumbar drain may aid healing following surgical repair in cases of spontaneous leakage (Hanson 2020).

Leaks originating in the posterior cerebral fossa anterior to the sigmoid sinus are particularly problematic as there is no arachnoid mesh in this part of the basal cistern. The leakage of CSF from this location is intense and widespread, and fascia alone is ineffective at controlling it. In most cases, a massive fat graft for the obliteration of the mastoid is required (Hanson 2020).

If a CSF leak is caused by a substantial (>1 cm) defect in the middle fossa floor, a combined middle fossa/transmastoid technique is the optimum solution. To determine the source of the leak, a mastoidectomy is performed initially. Attempting to minimize herniated brain tissue is not a good idea. Because these encephaloceles do not include functional brain tissue, they should be removed via bipolar cautery. Use the middle fossa method to fix the defect once it has been found. The middle fossa provides a great view of the defect as well as the possibility of using the lesion's intact bony margins to hold any repair material in place (Hanson 2020).

4. Spinal CSF Leaks

CSF leaks in the spinal axis, like their cranial counterparts, can be classified as traumatic or nontraumatic (or spontaneous).

4.1. *Traumatic Spinal CSF Leaks*

Iatrogenic injuries occurring from surgical, medicinal, or diagnostic operations are examples of traumatic spinal CSF leaks. Patients with a penetrating injury and cutaneous CSF fistula or with headaches after lumbar puncture both have simple diagnoses. Traumatic CSF fistulas have been described from the spinal subarachnoid area to the pleural space (Assietti et al. 1993; Sarwal et al. 1996). The presence of pleural fluid accumulations and symptoms of cerebral hypotension (severe positional headache) should indicate the diagnosis. A CSF leak is diagnosed by the presence of b2-tranferrin in pleural fluid.

4.2. *Spontaneous Spinal CSF Leaks*

The symptoms of spontaneous spinal CSF leaks are similar to those of spinal headache following a lumbar puncture; thus, the corresponding diagnoses should be easy to make. MR imaging of the brain is frequently requested as a result of severe headaches, nausea, and vomiting. Diffuse, significant dural enhancement on contrast-enhanced MR images can be misleading for meningitis or metastatic or inflammatory illnesses (Blank et al. 1997; Bruera et al. 2000; Christoforidis et al. 1998). In 60 to 70% of patients, subdural fluid accumulation suggestive of hygromas is reported. There is usually downward displacement of the cerebellar tonsils and compression of the basal cisterns (Lemole et al. 2001; Blank et al. 1997; Schievink et al. 1998; Thomson 1899).

Other warning signs include cranial neuropathies, such as uni- or bilateral sixth-nerve palsy, temporary visual problems, photophobia, hearing disturbances, facial numbness or paralysis, and stupor due to traction as well as the downward displacement of the brain stem (Berlit et al. 1994; Horton and Fishman 1994; Kosmorsky 1995; Schievink et al. 1998). The literature on spontaneous spinal CSF leaks is a little perplexing. Despite the fact that these symptoms are caused by spontaneous CSF leaks in the spine, patients are diagnosed with "spontaneous intracranial hypotension" (Lemole et al. 2001).

For patients with spontaneous spinal CSF leaks, radionucleotide cisternography is a rather common procedure used for analysis. The escape of CSF from the lumbar subarachnoid space causes rapid uptake of the tracer in the bloodstream, as indicated by the tracer's early presence in the kidneys and bladder in individuals with an active leak (Lemole et al. 2001; Schievink et al. 1998; Kadrie et al. 1976; Molins et al. 1990; Renowden et al. 1995). The location of a spinal CSF leak is occasionally recognized, but the leak is frequently below the study's resolution (Schievink et al. 1998; Kadrie et al. 1976).

If surgery is being considered, CT myelography is needed to locate the leak of CSF and may identify the underlying anatomic deficiency causing the leak, such as a meningeal diverticulum (Schievink et al. 1998). Myelography is frequently used to pinpoint the general location of a leak in preparation for CT scanning. If myelography fails to pinpoint the source of the leak, CT scanning along the complete spinal axis should be performed. Additional axial CSF collections may be visible via MR imaging of the spine, which can help locate the leak's source; however, there is little experience with using spinal MRI for individuals with a spontaneous spinal CSF fistula (Lemole et al. 2001; Matsumura et al. 2000).

4.3. *Treatment of Spinal CSF Leaks*

The treatment of spinal CSF leaks is similar to that used for cranial CSF fistulas. Resting in bed and a brief period of diversionary lumbar CSF drainage are often sufficient in the case of post-traumatic and postoperative CSF leakage. Although simple oversewing of the site can generally resolve postoperative leaks, patients should be monitored for indicators of ongoing leaking, such as positional headaches or the development of a pseudomeningocele. When conservative methods fail to resolve the fistula, surgical exploration should be explored (Lemole et al. 2001).

After surgery, a careful examination typically shows an undiscovered dural rupture that can be repaired using the direct suture method, fibrin glue administration, or both. The correct approach to treating spinal fluid leaks caused by penetrating trauma is determined by the location of the CSF leak, which is best determined via CT myelography. Some success has been found with percutaneous approaches for introducing fibrin glue to the leak location (Lemole et al. 2001; Hughes et al. 1997; Patel et al. 1996).

Fluid replacement and bed rest are the first steps in treating spontaneous spinal CSF fistulas to relive the symptoms of intracranial hypotension. Intravenous caffeine, glucocorticoids, mineralocorticoids, nonsteroidal anti-inflammatory drugs, and salt infusions are some of the medical treatments available. A lumbar epidural blood patch is a more direct and, in some authors opinion, more effective treatment. The findings reported by Szeinfeld et al. (Szeinfeld et al. 1986), revealing that blood injected into the lumbar epidural spaces extended upward and downward to involve eight or more spinal segments, may explain the success of this procedure. Fortunately, these conservative approaches will work for 60 to 70% of patients (Blank et al. 1997; Schievink et al. 1998; Inenaga et al. 2001). Surgical treatment should only be considered if symptoms persist after two sufficient blood patches have been applied.

The cervicothoracic junction or the thoracic spine are the sites of the majority of recorded leaks (Kamada et al. 2000). These leaks were caused by ruptured meningeal diverticula for which surgical confirmation was available. The surgical closure of leaky meningeal diverticula has been linked to positive results (Schievink et al. 1998; Inenaga et al. 2001). Epidural patching combined with fibrin glue has recently been utilized to treat spontaneous spinal CSF fistulas in patients who had previously failed to respond to epidural blood patches (Lemole et al. 2001).

Most meningeal diverticula have no recognized cause, and it is uncertain whether they're congenital or acquired. In some situations, however, an underlying weakening of the spinal meninges is likely to occur, predisposing the development of meningeal diverticula.

5. Conclusions

Anywhere along the craniospinal axis, CSF leaks can occur. Although cranial CSF leaks are most commonly caused by trauma, spontaneous occurrences are becoming more common, especially along the spinal column, where they present as spontaneous intracranial hypotension. Management options vary depending on the cause and degree of the CSF leak, but the general approach is to begin with conservative therapies and progress to more bodily invasive techniques if needed. Patients with substantial volumes of pneumocephalus, extensive base-of-skull fractures, or chronic CSF leakage may require immediate surgical intervention.

Author Contributions: Conceptualization, methodology, validation, formal analysis, investigation, resources, data curation, F.H.C., R.H. and S.N.-e.-F.; writing—original draft preparation, writing—review and editing, visualization, F.H.C., R.I. and M.B.R.; supervision, F.H.C. All authors have read and agreed to the published version of the manuscript.

Funding: This research received no external funding.

Conflicts of Interest: The authors declare no conflicts of interest.

References

Abuabara, Allan. 2007. Cerebrospinal fluidrhinorrhoea: Diagnosis and management. *Medicina Oral, Patología Oral y Cirugía Bucal* 12: E397–E400. [PubMed]

Albert, Bizhan, and L. G. Leibrock. 2005. Neurological approaches to cerebrospinal fluid rhinorrhea. *Ear, Nose, & Throat Journal* 71: 300–5.

Assietti, Roberto, Michael B. Kibble, and Roy A. E. Bakay. 1993. Iatrogenic cerebrospinal fluid fistula to the pleural cavity: Case report and literature review. *Neurosurgery* 33: 1104–8. [CrossRef] [PubMed]

Banks, Caroline A., James N. Palmer, Alexander G. Chiu, Bert W. O'Malley, Jr., Bradford A. Woodworth, and David W. Kennedy. 2009. Endoscopic closure of CSF rhinorrhea: 193 cases over 21 years. *Otolaryngology–Head and Neck Surgery* 140: 826–33. [CrossRef] [PubMed]

Bell, R.Bryan, Eric J. Dierks, Louis Homer, and Bryce E. Potter. 2004. Management of cerebrospinal fluid leak associated with craniomaxillofacial trauma. *Journal of Oral Maxillofacial Surgery* 62: 676–84. [CrossRef]

Bernal-Sprekelsen, Manuel, Isam Alobid, Joaquim Mullol, Francisca Trobat, and Manuel Tomas-Barberan. 2005. Closure of cerebrospinal fluid leaks prevents ascending bacterial meningitis. *Rhinology* 43: 277–81.

Berlit, Peter, Elisabeth Berg-Dammer, and Dietmar Kuehne. 1994. Abducens nerve palsy in spontaneous intracranial hypotension. *Neurology* 44: 1552. [CrossRef]

Blank, S. C., R. A. Shakir, Laurence A. Bindoff, and Nicholas Bradey. 1997. Spontaneous intracranial hypotension: Clinical and magnetic resonance imaging characteristics. *Clinical Neurology Neurosurgery* 99: 199–204. [CrossRef]

Bolger, W. E., and D. W. Kennedy. 1992. Nasal endoscopy in the outpatient clinic. *Otolaryngologic Clinics of North America* 25: 791–802. [CrossRef]

Brodie, Hilary A., and Teresa C. Thompson. 1997. Management of complications from 820 temporal bone fractures. *The American Journal of Otology* 18: 188–97.

Bruera, Osvaldo Carlos, Lucas Bonamico, Jorge Alberto Giglio, Vladimiro Sinay, Jorge Alberto Leston, and Maria de Lourdes Figuerola. 2000. Intracranial hypotension: The nonspecific nature of MRI findings. *Headache* 40: 848–52. [CrossRef] [PubMed]

Bumm, Klaus, Jennifer Heupel, Alessandro Bozzato, Heinrich Iro, and Joachim Hornung. 2009. Localization and infliction pattern of iatrogenic skull base defects following endoscopic sinus surgery at a teaching hospital. *Auris Nasus Larynx* 36: 671–76. [CrossRef] [PubMed]

Caballero, Nadieska, Vidur Bhalla, James A. Stankiewicz, and Kevin C. Welch. 2012. Effect of lumbar drain placement on recurrence of cerebrospinal rhinorrhea after endoscopic repair. *International Forum of Allergy & Rhinology* 2: 222–26. [CrossRef]

Carrion, E., J. H. Hertzog, M. D. Medlock, G. J. Hauser, and H. J. Dalton. 2001. Use of acetazolamide to decrease cerebrospinal fluid production in chronically ventilated patients with ventriculopleural shunts. *Archives in Disease of Childhood* 84: 68–71. [CrossRef] [PubMed]

Cassano, Michele, and Alexandre Felippu. 2009. Endoscopic treatment of cerebrospinal fluid leaks with the use of lower turbinate grafts: A retrospective review of 125 cases. *Rhinology* 47: 362–68. [CrossRef]

Chan, Danny T. M., Wai Sang Poon, Chui Ping Ip, Philip W. Y. Chiu, and Keith Y. C. Goh. 2004. How useful is glucose detection in diagnosing cerebrospinal fluid leak? The rational use of CT and Beta-2 transferrin assay in detection of cerebrospinal fluid fistula. *Asian Journal of Surgery* 27: 39–42. [CrossRef]

Christoforidis, G. A., B. A. Mehta, J. L. Landi, E. J. Czarnecki, and R. A. Piaskowski. 1998. Spontaneous intracranial hypotension: Report of four cases and review of the literature. *Diagnostic Neuroradiology* 40: 636–43. [CrossRef]

Dodson, Edward E., Charles W. Gross, Jason L. Swerdloff, and L. Mark Gustafson. 1994. Transnasal endoscopic repair of cerebrospinal fluid rhinorrhea and skull base defects: A review of twenty-nine cases. *Otolaryngology–Head and Neck Surgery* 111: 600–5. [CrossRef]

Dula, David J., and William Fales. 1993. The 'ring sign': Is it a reliable indicator for cerebral spinal fluid? *Annals of Emergency Medicine* 22: 718–20. [CrossRef]

El Gammal, T., and B. S. Brooks. 1994. MR cisternography: Initial experience in 41 cases. *American Journal of Neuroradiology* 15: 1647–56.

Jones, Nicholas, and Daniel G. Becker. 2001. Advancesin the management of CSF leaks. *BMJ* 322: 122–23. [CrossRef] [PubMed]

Eljamel, M. S. M., and P. M. Foy. 1990. Post-traumatic CSF fistulae, the case for surgical repair. *British Journal of Neurosurgery* 4: 479–83. [CrossRef] [PubMed]

Elmorsy, S. M., and Y. W. Khafagy. 2014. Endoscopic management of spontaneous CSF rhinorrhea with septal graft and middle turbinate rotational flap technique: A review of 31 cases. *Ear, Nose, & Throat Journal* 93: E14–E19.

Gacek, Richard R., and Bruce Leipzig. 1979. Congenital cerebrospinal otorrhea. *Annals of Otology, Rhinology & Laryngology* 88: 358–65.

Gosal, Jaskaran S., Tenzin Gurmey, Gopi K. Kursa, Pravin Salunke, and Sunil K. Gupta. 2015. Is acetazolamide really useful in the management of traumatic cerebrospinal fluid rhinorrhea? *Neurology India* 63: 197–201. [CrossRef]

Hegazy, Hassan M., Ricardo L. Carrau, Carl H. Snyderman, Amin Kassam, and Julie Zweig. 2000. Transnasal endoscopic repair of cerebrospinal fluid rhinorrhea: A metaanalysis. *Laryngoscope* 110: 1166–72. [CrossRef]

Hanson, Matthew B. 2020. CSF Otorrhea Treatment & Management. Available online: https://emedicine.medscape.com/article/883160-treatment?form=fpf (accessed on 22 July 2022).

Horton, Jonathan C., and Robert A. Fishman. 1994. Neurovisual findings in the syndrome of spontaneous intracranial hypotension from dural cerebrospinal fluid leak. *Ophthalmology* 101: 244–51. [CrossRef]

Hughes, R. G., N. S. Jones, and J. J. Robertson. 1997. The endoscopic treatment of cerebrospinal fluid rhinorrhoea: The Nottingham experience. *The Journal of Laryngology & Otology* 111: 125–8. [CrossRef]

Inenaga, Chikanori, Tokutaro Tanaka, Naoki Sakai, and Shigeru Nishizawa. 2001. Diagnostic and surgical strategies for intractable spontaneous intracranial hypotension. *Journal of Neurosurgery* 94: 642–45. [CrossRef]

Jackson, C. Gary, Dennis G. Pappas, Jr., Spiros Manolidis, Michael E. Glasscock, II, Peter G. Von Doersten, Carl R. Hampf, Jack B. Williams, and I. S. Storper. 1997. Brain herniation into the middle ear and mastoid: Concepts in diagnosis and surgical management. *The American Journal of Otology* 18: 198–205.

Jahrsdoerfer, Robert A., William J. Richtsmeier, and Robert W. Cantrell. 1981. Spontaneous CSF Otorrhea. *Archives of Otolaryngology* 107: 257–61. [CrossRef] [PubMed]

Kim, Suzy, Chan H. Park, and Keehyun Park. 2000. Cerebrospinal fluid rhinorrhea caused by a congenital defect of stapes mimicking otorrhea: Radionuclide cisternographic findings. *Clinical Nuclear Medicine* 25: 634–35. [CrossRef] [PubMed]

Kadrie, H., A. A. Driedger, and W. McInnis. 1976. Persistent dural cerebrospinal fluid leak shown by retrograde radionuclide myelography: Case report. *Journal of Nuclear Medicine* 17: 797–99.

Kamada, Masaki, Yoshihisa Fujita, Ryoji Ishii, and Sumiko Endoh. 2000. Spontaneous intracranial hypotension successfully treated by epidural patching with fibrin glue. *Headache* 40: 844–47. [CrossRef]

Kosmorsky, Gregory S. 1995. Spontaneous intracranial hypotension: A review. *Journal of Neuro-Ophthalmology* 15: 79–83. [CrossRef]

Landeiro, José Alberto, Marlo S. Flores, Bruno C. R. Lazaro, and Maria Helena Melo. 2004. Surgical management of cerebrospinal fluid rhinorrhea under endoscopic control. *Neuro-Psychiatric Archives* 62: 827–31. [CrossRef] [PubMed]

Lee, Ta-Jen, Chi-Che Huang, Chi-Cheng Chuang, and Shiang-Fu Huang. 2004. Transnasal Endoscopic Repair of Cerebrospinal Fluid Rhinorrhea and Skull Base Defect: Ten-Year Experience. *Laryngoscope* 114: 1475–81. [CrossRef]

Lemole, G. Michael, Jr., Jeffrey S. Henn, Joseph M. Zabramski, and Volker K. H. Sonntag. 2001. The Management of Cranial and Spinal CSF Leaks. *Barrow Quarterly* 17: 4. Available online: https://www.barrowneuro.org/for-physicians-researchers/education/grand-rounds-publications-media/barrow-quarterly/volume-17-no-4-2001/the-management-of-cranial-and-spinal-csf-leaks/ (accessed on 17 August 2022).

Leung, Randal. 2013. Temporal Bone Encephaloceles, Meningoceles, and CSF Leak, Repair of. In *Encyclopedia of Otolaryngology, Head and Neck Surgery*. Edited by Stilianos E. Kountakis. Berlin/Heidelberg: Springer. [CrossRef]

Liao, Kuo-Hsing, Jia-Yi Wang, Hui-Wen Lin, Tai-Ngar Lui, Kai-Yun Chen, David Hung Tzang Yen, and Mei-Jy Jeng. 2016. Risk of death in patients with post- traumatic cerebrospinal fluid leakage-Analysis of 1773 cases. *Journal of the Chinese Medical Association* 79: 58–64. [CrossRef]

Lieberman, Seth M., Si Chen, Daniel Jethanamest, and Roy R. Casiano. 2015. Spontaneous CSF rhinorrhea: Prevalence of multiple simultaneous skull base defects. *American Journal of Rhinology & Allergy* 29: 77–81. [CrossRef]

Liu, Hai-sheng, Ye-tao Chen, Dong Wang, Hui Liang, Yunpeng Wang, Shi-jie Wang, Yan Wang, Guo-qiang Chen, and Huan-cong Zuo. 2009. The use of topical intranasal fluorescein in endoscopic endonasal repair of cerebrospinal fluid rhinorrhea. *Surgical Neurology* 72: 341–45. [CrossRef] [PubMed]

Lopatin, Andrey S., Dmitry N. Kapitanov, and Alexander A. Potapov. 2003. Endonasal endoscopic repair of spontaneous cerebrospinal fluid leaks. *Archives of Otorhinolaryngology-Head & Neck Surgery* 129: 859–63. [CrossRef]

Lund, V. J., L. Savy, G. Lloyd, and D. Howard. 1994. Optimum imaging and diagcases. *American Journal of Neuroradiology* 15: 1647–56.

Marshall, A. H., N. S. Jones, and I. J. A. Robertson. 2001. CSF rhinorrhoea: The place of endoscopic sinus surgery. *British Journal of Neurosurgery* 15: 8–12. [CrossRef]

Mathias, Tiffany, Joshua Levy, Adil Fatakia, and Edward D. McCoul. 2016. Contemporary approach to the diagnosis and management of cerebrospinal fluid rhinorrhea. *Ochsner Journal* 16: 136–42.

Matsumura, Akira, Izumi Anno, Hiroshi Kimura, Eiichi Ishikawa, and Tadao Nose. 2000. Diagnosis of spontaneous intracranial hypotension by using magnetic resonance myelography. *Journal of Neurosurgery* 92: 873–76. [CrossRef]

Meco, Cem, and Gerhard Oberascher. 2004. Comprehensive algorithm for skull base dural lesion and cerebrospinal fluid fistula diagnosis. *Laryngoscope* 114: 991–99. [CrossRef] [PubMed]

Mokri, B., J. L. Atkinson, and D. G. Piepgras. 2000. Absent headache despite CSF volume depletion (intracranial hypotension). *Neurology* 55: 1722–24. [CrossRef]

Mokri, B., S. F. Hunter, J. L. D Atkinson, and D. G. Piepgras. 1998. Orthostatic headaches caused by CSF leak but with normal CSF pressures. *Neurology* 51: 786–90. [CrossRef]

Molins, A., Alvarez J, J. Sumalla, F. Titus, and A. Codina. 1990. Cisternographic pattern of spontaneous liquoral hypotension. *Cephalalgia* 10: 59–65. [CrossRef]

Naidich, Thomas P., and Christopher J. Moran. 1980. Precise anatomic localization of a traumatic sphenethmoidal cerebrospinal fluid rhinorrhea by metrizamide CT cisterography. *Journal of Neurosurgery* 53: 222–28. [CrossRef] [PubMed]

Oh, Melissa S., Esther X. Vivas, Patricia A. Hudgins, and Douglas E. Mattox. 2019. The Prevalence of Superior Semicircular Canal Dehiscence in Patients with Mastoid Encephalocele or Cerebrospinal Fluid Otorrhea. *Otology & Neurotology* 40: 485–90. [CrossRef]

Oliaei, Sepehr, Hossein Mahboubi, and Hamid R. Djalilian. 2012. Transmastoid approach to temporal bone cerebrospinal fluid leaks. *American Journal of Otolaryngology* 33: 556–61. [CrossRef] [PubMed]

Patel, M. R., W. Louie, and J. Rachlin. 1996. Postoperative cerebrospinal fluid leaks of the lumbosacral spine: Management with percutaneous fibrin glue. *American Journal of Neuroradiology* 17: 495–500. [PubMed]

Patrascu, Elena, Claudiu Manea, and Codrut Sarafoleanu. 2017. Current insights in CSF leaks: A literature review of mechanisms, pathophysiology and treatment options. *Romanian Journal of Rhinolog* 7: 143–51. [CrossRef]

Platt, Michael P., and Steven M. Parnes. 2009. Management of unexpected cerebrospinal fluid leak during endoscopic sinus surgery. *Current Opinion in Otolaryngology & Head and Neck Surgery* 17: 28–32. [CrossRef]

Renowden, S. A., R. Gregory, N. Hyman, and D. Hilton-Jones. 1995. Spontaneous intracranial hypotension. *Journal of Neurology, Neurosurgery and Psychiatry* 59: 511–15. [CrossRef]

Sarwal, Virendar, Rajendar Krishnan Suri, Om Prakash Sharma, Amarjyoti Baruah, Pratibha Singhi, Shivender Gill, and J. Rajiv Bapuraj. 1996. Traumatic subarachnoid-pleural fistula. *The Annals of Thoracic Surgery* 62: 1622–26. [CrossRef]

Schievink, W. I., V. M. Morreale, J. L. Atkinson, F. B. Meyer, D. G. Piepgras, and M. J. Ebersold. 1998. Surgical treatment of spontaneous spinal cerebrospinal fluid leaks. *Journal of Neurosurgery* 88: 243–46. [CrossRef]

Schlosser, Rodney J., Bradford A. Woodworth, Eileen Maloney Wilensky, M. Sean Grady, and William E. Bolger. 2006. Spontaneous cerebrospinal fluid leaks: A variant of benign intracranial hypertension. *Annals of Otology, Rhinology & Laryngology* 115: 495–500. [CrossRef]

Schlosser, Rodney J., and William E. Bolger. 2003. Spontaneous nasal cerebrospinal fluid leaks and empty sella syndrome: A clinical association. *American Journal of Rhinology & Allergy* 17: 91–96. [CrossRef]

Scholsem, Martin, Felix Scholtes, Frèderick Collignon, Pierre Robe, Annie Dubuisson, Bruno Kaschten, Jacques Lenelle, and Didier Martin. 2008. Surgical management of anterior cranial base fractures with cerebrospinal fluid fistulae: A single-institution experience. *Neurosurgery* 62: 463–71. [CrossRef]

Sumaily, Ibrahim. 2017. Current Approach to Cerebrospinal Fluid Rhinorrhea Diagnosis and Management. *Journal of Otolaryngology-ENT Research* 7: 00191.

Szeinfeld, Marcos, Ismael H. Ihmeidan, Mark M. Moser, Rafael Machado, K. John Klose, and Aldo N. Serafini. 1986. Epidural blood patch: Evaluation of the volume and spread of blood injected into the epidural space. *Anesthesiology* 64: 820–22. [CrossRef] [PubMed]

Thomson, St. Clair. 1899. *The Cerebrospinal Fluid: Its Spontaneous Escape from the Nose.* London: Cassel.

Warnecke, Athanasia, Thomas Averbeck, Ulrich Wurster, Meike Harmening, Thomas Lenarz, and Timo Stöver. 2004. Diagnostic relevance of beta2- transferrin for the detection of cerebrospinal fluid fistulas. *Archives of Otorhinolaryngology-Head & Neck Surgery* 130: 1178–84. [CrossRef]

Wetmore, Stephen J., Peter Herrmann, and Ugo Fisch. 1987. Spontaneous cerebrospinal fluid otorrhea. *The American Journal of Otology* 8: 96–102.

Woodworth, Bradford A., Anthony Prince, Alexander G. Chiu, Noam A. Cohen, Rodney J. Schlosser, William E. Bolger, David W. Kennedy, and James N. Palmer. 2008. Spontaneous CSF leaks: A paradigm for definitive repair and management of intracranial hypertension. *Otolaryngology–Head and Neck Surgery* 138: 715–20. [CrossRef] [PubMed]

Woodworth, Bradford A., Rodney J. Schlosser, Russell A. Faust, and William E. Bolger. 2004. Evolutions in the management of congenital intranasal skull base defects. *Arch Otolaryngology–Head and Neck Surgery* 130: 1283–88. [CrossRef]

Yilmazlar, Selcuk, Erhan Arslan, Hasan Kocaeli, Seref Dogan, Kaya Aksoy, Ender Korfali, and Muammer Doygun. 2006. Cerebrospinal fluid leakage complicating skull base fractures: Analysis of 81 cases. *Neurosurgical Review* 29: 64–71. [CrossRef]

Section VI: Head Trauma

Head Injury

Shamsul Alam, Md Moshiur Rahman, Mainul Haque Sarker, Nazmin Ahmed and Forhad H. Chowdhury

Abstract: Head injury/traumatic brain injury (TBI) is the most prevalent etiology of morbidity as well as mortality all round the world, with colossal financial consequences on the healthcare system. The World Health Organization estimated that ten million people experience a head injury per annum. Head injury patients experience long-term cognitive as well as functional problems and medical illnesses like epilepsy, which necessitate long-period or lifelong personal medical and supportive assistance. The common causes of head injury include falls from height, road traffic accidents (RTAs), recreation and sports accidents, physical assault, firearm attacks and accidents, and explosions. TBIs may be mild, moderate, and severe, requiring proper emergency clinical and radiological assessment for appropriate emergency, urgent, or routine management, including ICU management and surgery. This chapter will briefly discuss the principles of the management of TBI patients with regard to issues ranging from emergency management to complication management.

Abbreviations

ABG	arterial blood gas	AEDs	anti epileptic drugs
ABI	ankle–brachial index	ASDH	acute subdural hematoma
APTT	activated partial thromboplastin time	AVF	arterio-venous fistula
ATLS	advanced trauma life support	CBV	cerebral blood volume
CBF	cerebral blood flow	CN	cranial nerve
CCF	carotico-cavernous fistula	CSF	cerebrospinal fluid
CSDH	chronic subdural hematoma	CT	computed tomography
CPP	cerebral perfusion pressure	DC	decompressive craniotomy
CTA	computed tomography angiogram	DVT	deep venous thrombosis
DAI	diffuse axonal injury	EEG	Electroencephalogram
DTI	diffusion tensor imaging	GCS	Glasgow coma scale
EDH	extra-/epidural hematoma	HDU	high-dependency unit
ESS	endoscopic sinus surgery	ICP	intracranial pressure
GRE	gradient echo	INR	international normalized ratio
ICH	intracranial hematoma	MMA	middle meningeal artery
ICU	intensive care unit	PBI	penetrating brain injury
LOC	loss of consciousness	PHIS	post-traumatic head injury syndrome
MRA	magnetic resonance angiogram	PTA	post-traumatic amnesia
MRI	magnetic resonance imaging	SBP	systolic blood pressure
PCA	posterior cerebral artery	SDE	subdural effusion
PPI	proton pump inhibitor	TP	tension pneumocephalus
PT	prothrombin time	TBI	traumatic brain injury
SDH	subdural hematoma	UOP	urinary output
RTA	road traffic accident	AEDs	anti epileptic drugs

1. Introduction

Traumatic brain injury (TBI) is a prevalent etiology of morbidity as well as mortality around the world, with enormous financial consequences for the healthcare system. The World Health Organization believes that ten million people suffer a head injury every year, and the Centers for Disease Control (CDC) and Prevention in the US estimate that 1.7 million people are afflicted by a head injury every year. The expanse of a head injury in the US is estimated to be more than USD 60 billion per year, including medical expenditures and costs due to loss of productivity. Patients with head injuries experience long-term cognitive as well as functional problems and medical illnesses like epilepsy, which necessitate long-period or lifelong personal medical and supportive assistance. The most common causes of head injury differ depending on the affected patient's age. Falls from height are the commonest cause of head injury among those less than 4 years old and elderly people over 75. Road traffic accidents (RTA) are the principal cause of TBI among adolescents. Other major causes of head injuries include recreation-related and sports injuries, physical assault, firearm-related incidents, and blast related injuries among military personnel (Kim and Gean 2011; Greenberg 2010; July and Wahjoepramono 2019).

2. Pathophysiology of Head Injury

The damage to the brain due to TBI is generally classified as primary or secondary. Hematomas and traumatic/diffuse axonal injury (DAI) are primary injuries that arise from direct severe impacts. Secondary brain injuries happen minutes to days following a main injury and consist of a complicated biochemical sequence that is started by the initial primary injury and leads to brain edema and herniation. This classification emphasizes that a brain injury is a continuously progressive trauma that requires appropriate medical as well as surgical treatment consisting of brain oxygenation to relive intracranial pressure (ICP), including cerebral perfusion pressure (CPP), in order to enhance patient healing and stop further trauma. Secondary insults can be triggered by primary head traumas, such as cerebral bleeding, which raises ICP. The gap between mean arterial pressure and ICP is CPP (i.e., the pressure difference pushing oxygen and nutrition supply to the cerebral tissue). CPP is a measure of cerebral blood flow. CPP will decline if the ICP rises owing to a head injury (or the systemic blood pressure lowers), and the cerebral tissue will be ischemic until the normal cerebral autoregulatory mechanism generates compensatory neurovascular vasodilation to provide enough circulation to the parenchyma of the brain. Normal neurovascular autoregulation, on the other hand, is commonly impaired in head injury patients, especially children. Autoregulation appears to be hampered at lower CPP values (under the threshold of 50–60 mm Hg), and, at these levels, the brain is prone to becoming ischemic. Complex cellular as well as biochemical pathways are initiated by ischemia, and the result is reduced glucose and oxygen supply to the cerebral tissue, aggravating brain damage. Extra calcium influx inside the cells leads to mitochondrial malfunction, cellular edema, free-radical generation, and ultimately neuronal death, the last of which is one of the pathophysiologic processes initiated by excitatory neurotransmitters (mainly glutamate) unleashed into the brain parenchyma. (Kim and Gean 2011; Greenberg 2010; July and Wahjoepramono 2019; Kirollos et al. 2019).

3. Incidence and Prevalence of Head Injury

In emerging countries, the overall injury rate is 22.1 per 1000 person years. According to statistics, one person dies from a head injury every 6 to 10 min in India.

Pedestrians, motorbike drivers, and assistants correspond to the highest rates of head injuries in Asia. The majority of people injured in RTAs are pedestrians who are considered vulnerable road users.

Every year, 50 million people are injured around the world.

In total, 1.2 million people are estimated to die due to injuries annually.

The global mortality rate is 97/1,000,000.

Every day, 70% of fatalities (8,500,000) are suffered by people under the age of 45, with 3300 deaths and 6600 catastrophic injuries. In underdeveloped nations, there has been an increase of 80% of TBI (Head Injury Foundation n.d.).

The prevalence of head injuries is high, with men accounting for the majority of cases. The sufferers are mostly illiterate and work as day laborers. The risk factors for a TBI with a difficult course include the following: high-energy injuries, bicycle accidents, RTAs in general, anticoagulant therapy, intoxication with alcohol, age greater than 60 years, and a low GSC score at the time of presentation (Kim and Gean 2011; Gururaj 2002).

4. Etiology of Head Injury

The commonest causes of head injuries are as follows:

- Car accidents, motorcycle accidents, and bicycle accidents;
- Falls from height;
- Child abuse;
- Acts of violence;
- Cycling;
- Football;
- Baseball and softball;
- Explosions and other combat injuries.

5. Risk Factors of Head Injuries

- Children, particularly newborns up to 4 years of age;
- Young adults, particularly between the ages of 15 to 24;
- Adults 60 and older;

- Male sex (any age group);
- Anticoagulant use

(https://www.mayoclinic.org/diseases-conditions/traumatic-brain-injury/symptoms-causes/syc-20378557, accessed on 7 March 2022).

6. NICE Guidelines for Applying CT to Assess Head Injury

- Glasgow Coma Score (GCS) < 13 at any point;
- Focal neurological deficit;
- Suspected open, depressed, or basal skull fracture;
- Seizure;
- Vomiting, >one episode;
- Urgent CT head scan if none of the apply above but the following do:
- Age > 65;
- Coagulopathy (e.g., being on warfarin);
- Dangerous mechanism of injury (CT within 8 h);
- Antegrade amnesia > 30 min (CT within 8 h) (Nader et al. 2014; Habeeb 2017).

7. Principles of Management of Head Injury

In the neuro-intensive care unit, the current head injury management strategy focuses on preventing a cascade of secondary injuries by preserving appropriate brain perfusion. To prevent both hypoxemia and hypotension, which may increase mortality and morbidity, this technique necessitates constant neuromonitoring and blood pressure and oxygenation regulation. Patients with severe autoregulation problems rely solely on blood pressure to continue cerebral circulation to the brain tissue, which is known as "pressure passive" flow.

As a result, enough blood pressure support is essential. Patients with a severe head injury, as defined by a GCS score of 3–8 and a CT scan, have their ICP monitored. External ventricular drainage catheters are commonly used to monitor ICP, but intraparenchymal, subarachnoid, subdural, and extradural devices can also be employed. Raised ICP is linked to a worse prognosis and may indicate cerebral herniation or a potentially weakened CPP. To reduce ICP, strict procedures are utilized. Medical management, such as hyperventilation, hyperosmolar infusion, and proper sedation/analgesia, and surgical treatment, such as external CSF drainage (external ventricular drainage—EVD), cerebral hematoma removal, and, if needed, decompressive craniectomy (DC), are both options. Finally, maintaining an appropriate CPP is critical to minimize ischemic injury; again, the threshold value of CPP is 50–60 mm Hg, and brain ischemia can occur under this value (Brain Trauma Foundation et al. 2008).

7.1. Role of Imaging in Diagnosis and Treatment of Head Injury

Both the diagnosis as well as treatment of a brain injury rely heavily on imaging. Non-contrast CT scanning is the technique of choice for diagnosing head injury in the acute environment because it swiftly and accurately reveals cerebral hemorrhages that necessitate neurosurgical evacuation (Figure 1).

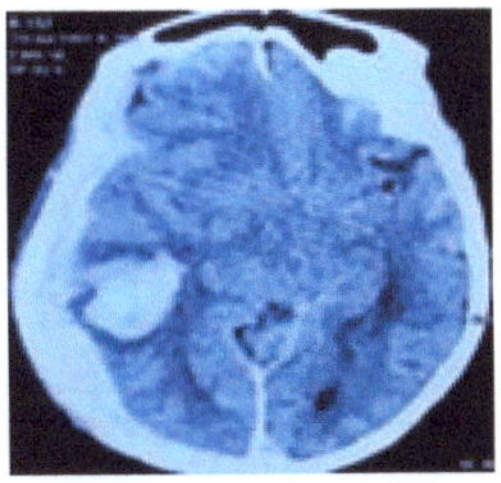

Figure 1. CT scan showing acute SDH and traumatic ICH. Source: Figure by authors.

Extradural, subdural, and subarachnoid/intraventricular hemorrhages and intra-axial brain parenchymal hemorrhages, cortical contusion, DAI, and shear injuries can be easily detected via CT. While CT scans are the gold standard for TBI imaging, magnetic resonance imaging (MRI) provides a higher diagnostic sensitivity for lesions that are not always hemorrhagic, such as cerebral contusions and non-hemorrhagic DAI (Figure 2).

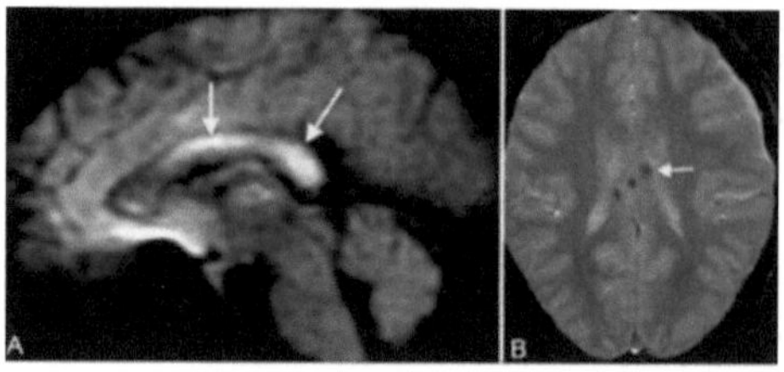

Figure 2. (**A**). MRI in sagittal view in ADC image shows the strong signal along the corpus callosum. (**B**) Axial MRI flair image showing a punctate hemorrhage in the corpus callosum. Source: Figure by authors.

Susceptibility-weighted (SW) and diffusion tensor imaging (DTI) techniques, both of which are based on MRI technology, are better for predicting outcome for brain injury patients. Non-contrast CT scans do not capture physiologic changes in brain perfusion, cerebral blood flow, and parenchymal oxygenation that are linked to the detrimental sequences following TBI that have a major impact on functional outcome. A perfusion CT scan is a neuroimaging technique that uses dynamic scanning images during i.v. contrast injection to show physiologic characteristics such as cerebral blood flow (CBF), cerebral blood volume (CBV), and mean transit time (MTT) (the time required for blood to perfuse a regional brain tissue). Normal cerebral perfusion or hyperemia (high CBF and CBV) observable via perfusion CT for head injury patients has been linked to a better clinical result, while evidence of hypoxia (low CBF and CBV) is linked to a worse clinical outcome (Kim and Gean 2011). DAI disrupts the cytoskeleton as well as axoplasmic flow, resulting in alterations in tissue diffusion that can be seen and measured via DTI. The level of white matter damage in DTI may be related to the severity of cognitive dysfunction as well as the functional result after a head injury. Another very new MRI approach that improves DAI detection sensitivity is SWI. SWI employs a three-dimensional GRE sequence that is high-resolution, velocity-compensated, and founded on both magnitude and phase data. Its sensitivity is higher than that of standard GRE sequences for the identification of hemorrhagic DAI, detecting 4–6 times more microhemorrhages than GRE sequences (Kim and Gean 2011; Qureshi et al. 2016; Badjatia et al. 2008).

7.2. *Management of Head Injury/TBI Including ATLS*

The American College of Surgeons created Advanced Trauma Life Support (ATLS) as a training curriculum for medical doctors in regard to the handling of acute trauma situations. The goal of ATLS is to identify and execute treatment of lethal injuries such as head injuries and polytrauma. The Golden Hour refers to the first hour following a catastrophic injury when emergency treatment is most likely to be effective. The basics of trauma management are as follows:

1. Preparation;
2. Triage;
3. Primary survey with simultaneous resuscitation;
4. Secondary survey;
5. Definitive treatment.

7.2.1. Preparation

The wearing of gloves, a gown, shoe covers, a mask, and head-covering goggles for self-protection is recommended.

7.2.2. Triage

The process of categorizing victims or mass casualties based on their need for treatment and the resources available.

7.2.3. Primary Survey (with Simultaneous Resuscitation)

The primary survey is the first and most important step in assessing patients who have experienced trauma. During this period, life-threatening injuries are detected, and resuscitation must be performed concurrently. ABCDE is a mnemonic for the order in which issues should be dealt with (Maas et al. 1997).

A. Airway Control with Cervical Spine Immobilization

1. Maintenance of airway patency:
   - Lifting of the chin or thrusting of the jaw;
   - Removal of foreign bodies, blood, and vomitus via suction;
   - Nasopharyngeal/oropharyngeal airway clearance.
2. Airway support:
   - Provision of oxygen via a nasal canula/non-breathing mask (high mask) or Ambu bag pumping.
3. Establishment of a definitive airway:
   - Endotracheal tube intubation;
   - Cricothyroidectomy;
   - Tracheostomy.
4. Imobillize the patient;
5. Apply cervical hard collar (Philadelphia collar);
6. Avoid hyperextension of the neck.

B. Breathing and Ventilation

Look for the conditions that impair ventilation, such as the following:

- Tension pneumothorax;
- Massive hemothorax;
- An open pneumothorax;
- A flail chest segment;
- Pulmonary contusion;
- Rib fracture (single or multiple);
- Cardiac tamponade.

If a chest X-ray or HRCT of the chest reveals a hemothorax or tension pneumothorax, then emergency large-caliber tube thoracostomy/water seal drainage of the chest must employed.

Adjuncts to primary survey:

- Hemodynamic monitoring (blood pressure, cardiac rate, and rhythm);
- ECG monitoring;
- Foley catheter placement for urinary output monitoring and to obtain evidence of a possible urethral injury (per-urethral bleeding, perineal hematoma);
- Naso-gastric tube insertion and prevention of gastric dilatation and gastric content regurgitation;
- Respiratory function monitoring with respiratory rate, pulse oximetry, and capnography.
- Analysis of arterial blood gas (ABG);
- CBC, serum electrolytes, blood glucose, serum creatinine, PT, APTT, INR, blood grouping, and cross matching.

Radiographic investigation:

- X-ray of the skull b/v, cervical spine, abdomen, pelvis, and long bones according to the clinical situation;
- CT scan of the head along with the cervical spine;
- HRCT OF CHEST when the chest X-ray presents results that are a cause of concern;
- Ultrasound of the abdomen (Nader et al. 2014; CRASH Trial Collaborators 2004).

C. Circulation Preservation with Bleeding Control

Hemorrhage is the primary etiology of avoidable post-injury mortality. Hypovolemia is induced by significant traumatic hemorrhages. A prolonged shock state leads to multi-organ failure and cell death.

1. Clinical signs of shock:
   - Altered mental status.
   - Pale, cold, and clammy slins. Delayed capillary refill (>3 s).
   - Pulse: rapid (heart rate > 100), thread pulse, or peripherally unpalpable.
   - Arterial hypotension (systolic blood pressure < 120 mm hg).
   - Decreased urinary output (UOP < 0.5 mL/kg/h).
2. Source of bleeding:
   - Scalp, skull, or contused brain tissue;
   - Chest;
   - Abdomen;
   - Pelvis;
   - Long-bone fracture.

3. General management of shock:

Stop bleeding by applying direct pressure, a crepe bandage on the patient's head, and compression or ligation of the superficial temporal artery.

Occult bleeding, either from the pelvis or the long bones, needs to be addressed quickly.

Two large-bore intravenous lines have to be administered, and crystalloid saline must be given.

Urgent blood grouping and cross-matching and rapid blood transfusion are needed to improve the patient's hemodynamic status (Nader et al. 2014; Kalangu et al. 2009).

D. Disability/Neurologic Assessment

The Glasgow Coma Scale (Table 1) is used to conduct a basic neurological examination during the primary survey. The level of consciousness (LOC) of the patient; pupil size, equality, and reaction; lateralizing symptoms; and the level of spinal cord injury are all determined in this way. The Glasgow Coma Scale is a rapid measure for determining state of consciousness and is a predictive factor of patient outcome. A change in LOC necessitates a reassessment of a patient's oxygenation, perfusion, and ventilation. Hypoglycemia and substances such as alcohol might affect one's degree of awareness. If these factors are ruled out, any changes in degree of consciousness are assumed to be the result of traumatic brain damage until proven otherwise.

Table 1. GCS scale (Glasgow coma scale).

	1	2	3	4	5	6
Visual	Eyes closed	Eyes open in response to sharp stimuli	Eyes open in response to sounds	Eyes open without induced stimuli		
Motor	No movement	Movement in response to sharp stimuli	Muscle flexion In response to sharp stimuli	Muscle flexion and bodily movement	Ability to localize touch	Appears to have normal Movement
Verbal	No sounds	Low-intensity sounds	Incoherent words	Understandable words are spoken	Normal conversation	

Highest score—15; lowest score—03. Source: Table adapted from Teasdale and Jennett (1974), used with permission.

E. Exposure (Full) and Environmental Control

The patient should be totally exposed by cutting off their clothes and under garments. Examine them for other signs of injury.

Logroll the patient to examine their back.

Prevent hypothermia by applying a warm blanket and warm IV fluid.

7.2.4. Secondary Survey

The secondary survey is started after the primary survey has been completed and the patient has been adequately resuscitated. It includes the following measures:

- History taking, including the site of the trauma, the nature of the trauma, and its sequelae;
- Complete physical examination (head to-toe) identifying all anatomic injuries;
- Ascertainment of allergy history;
- Medication history, particularly with respect to cardiac anticoagulants such as Ecosprin/clopidogril and diabetic medications
- Determination of medical/pregnancy history;
- Ascertainment of the time when the patient's last meal was eaten.

7.2.5. Definitive Care

According to the clinical and other data, the patient is shifted to the ICU, HDU, or operation theatre for definitive treatment.

All clinical and radiological data are collected for definite surgical treatment or ICU management (Kalangu et al. 2009; Kamel et al. 2011; Cruz 1998).

7.3. Management of Increased ICP

7.3.1. Elevation of Head End of the Bed

- A 30° or reverse Trendelenburg will reduce ICP;
- Set the patient's head as well as neck in a neutral position that improves venous drainage of the brain;
- Avoid compression of internal jugular veins with tight C-collars or fixation of the endotracheal tube.

7.3.2. Osmotic Diuresis

Therapies involving the use of either mannitol or hypertonic saline decrease brain swelling and edema, hence decreasing ICP, which saves some time for preparing the patient for definitive surgery.

Mannitol (Muizelaar et al. 1984):

- Used if the patient's SBP is more than ninety mmHg;
- 20% mannitol, with a bolus dose of 0.25–1 gm/kg, is used as fast infusion over 15–20 min;
- It decreases ICP within thirty minutes, and the duration of this function is 6–8 h;
- Monitor the input/output to continue euvolemia during possible diuresis, and use normal saline to substitute the volume;
- Do not use mannitol as a continuous infusion, as it passes the BBB after long-term infusion and increases cerebral edema.

Hypertonic saline can be more efficacious than mannitol, and it is currently considered a standard agent of care (Kamel et al. 2011).

- Most researchers utilized a 250 mL i.v. bolus of 7.5% saline with dextran;
- A 250 mL initial bolus dose of 3% NaCl solution will decrease ICP and can be administered through a peripheral i.v. channel;
- The expected sodium level is 145–155 mmol/dL;
- Hypertonic saline has a greater osmotic gradient and is less permeable through the BBB than 20% mannitol.

7.4. Seizure Control

Seizures are immediately managed with benzodiazepines and antiepileptic drugs (AEDs), and commonly injections of Phenytoin or Fosphenytoin are administered.

Seizure prophylaxis decreases the severity of seizures, though it does not improve long-term result.

7.4.1. Risk Factors for Post-Traumatic Seizures

- GCS < 10 (initially);
- Contusion of the cerebral cortex;
- Depressed fracture of the skull
- Subdural hematoma (SDH) and/or epidural hematoma (EDH);
- Subarachnoid hemorrhage (SAH) or intra cerebral hematoma;
- Penetrating wound of the head;
- Seizure within first 24 h of TBI;
- Treat any clinically obvious and definite seizures assessed via EEG;
- Consider a prophylactic anti-convulsant for TBI patients with any of the risk factors previously mentioned (Wikem 2019).

7.4.2. Use of Phenytoin or Fosphenytion First-Line Agent According to BTF Guidelines

- The loading dose (Phenytoin equivalent) is 20 mg/kg i.v. and then 100 mg i.v. q8 h for 7 days;
- Assay serum levels to achieve and maintain therapeutic serum levels;
- Levetriacetam may be utilized as an alternative;
- Administer a 20 mg/kg load i.v., followed by 1000 mg i.v. q12 h for 7 days;
- Levetiracetam may have less common but severe adverse effects analogous to those induced by phenytoin (Cruz 1998; Bullock et al. 2006).

7.4.3. Bring Down the Metabolic Rate

- Apply enough sedative and analgesia;
- Prevent hyperthermia and treat fever vigorously.

7.4.4. Barbiturate Coma

- Is used for raised ICP resistance to maximum medical as well as surgical treatment;
- Solely for patients with stable hemodynamics;
- Administer the following:
  - Pentobarbitone (10 mg/kg) over 30 min;
  - Followed by 5 mg/kg/h for 3 h;
  - Then, 1 mg/kg/h.

7.5. Other Critical Care Measures

- Cushing's ulcers (Stress ulcer) prevention with H2 blocker/PPI and sucralfate.
- DVT prevention by using sequential compression devices (SCDs), with no anticoagulation.
- Glycemic control is good, although tight maintenance is not recommended.
- Steroids, particularly methylprednisolone, are contraindicated for head injuries (CRASH Trial Collaborators 2004). Dexamethasone administration is not commonly practiced by any hospitals and institutions in head injury cases. However, some surgeons use it in some severe head injury cases either every 6 or 8 h for a short period of time.
- Routine paralysis is not advised.
- There is a greater risk of pneumonia as well as ICU length of stay (Cruz 1998; Bullock et al. 2006).

7.6. Tetanus Prophylaxis

- Tetanus-prone wound: >6 h after damage, avulsion: >1 cm deep, or crush-type injury: devitalized, polluted, or ischemic tissue;
- If the wound is tetanus-prone, provide 250 units of tetanus immune globulin intramuscularly (Bullock et al. 2006; Kalangu et al. 2009).

8. Skull and Skull Base Fractures

8.1. Classification of Skull and Skull Base Fractures

A. There are different types of skull fractures:
   - Linear skull fractures;
   - Diastatic fractured or sutural fractures:—separation of sutures due to a blunt blow on head with a blunt weapon;
   - Ping-pong fractures;
   - Growing fractures;
   - Compound/comminuted fractures:—fractures with two or more fracture lines that meet, dividing the bone into three or more fragments. When the fragment is not displaced, it resembles a spider's web or a mosaic design;
   - Depressed fractures (Figures 3 and 4):
     - A simple depressed fracture or closed fracture, that is, a fracture in which the inside of the skull is not exposed.
     - A compound depressed fracture or open fracture, in which the inside of the skull is exposed to the exterior environment. This type is commonly associated with a dural tear, which may cause meningitis and or brain abscesses.
     - A technical compound fracture, that is, a type of fracture of the air sinuses that exposes them to the environment outside the skull (Kalangu et al. 2009; Haddad and Arabi 2012).

B. Classification of fractures according to site:
   - Frontal bone fracture;
   - Temporal bone fracture;
   - Parietal bone fracture;
   - Posterior fossa fracture;
   - Orbital bone fracture;
   - Fracture of the basilar skull.

C. Findings of fracture of temporal bone:
   - Boggy temporalis muscle due to extravasation of blood;
   - A bruise posterior to the pinnae, i.e., in the mastoid area (Battle's sign), and otorrhea.

D. Findings of fracture of patrous temporal bone

- Hearing loss, CSF otorrhea, and bulging of the ear drum due to blood or CSF.
- Ipsilateral facial palsy.

E. Findings of mastoid temporal bone fracture

- Otorrhea, rhinorrhea, bulging of ear drum, Battle's sign, tinnitus, and vertigo.

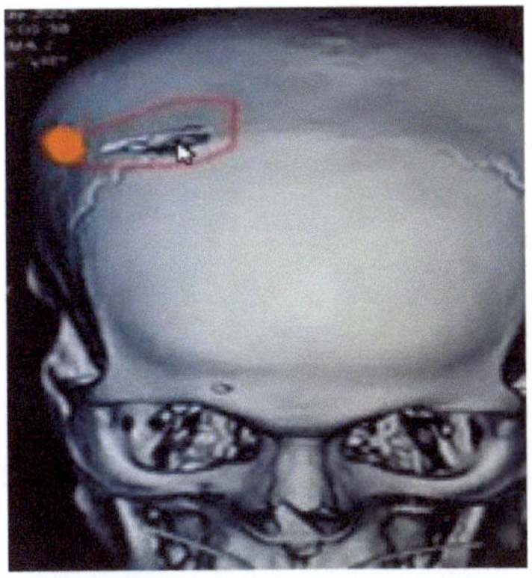

Figure 3. Three-dimensional CT image showing a depressed fracture close to the coronal suture. Source: Figure by authors.

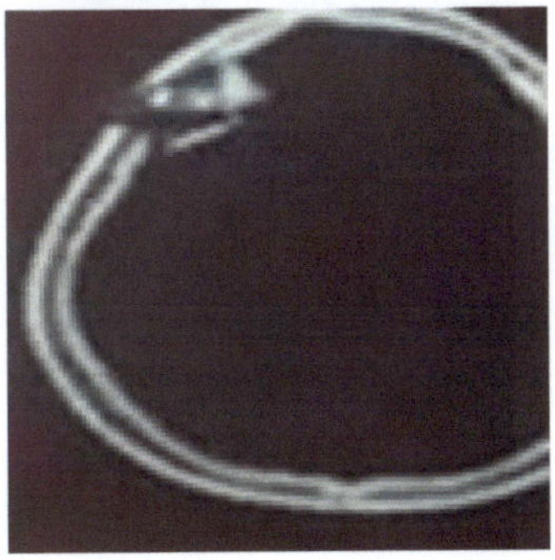

Figure 4. A frontal depressed fracture. Source: Figure by authors.

8.2. Surgical Treatment

Surgical toileting and elevation of the depressed fracture are employed for treatment.

Generous washing with normal saline, povidone iodine, and hydrogen peroxide is required to avoid infection of the depressed fragments and underlying brain. Bone fragments are either removed or repositioned after being washed with antiseptic.

Dural tears need to repair via a direct stitch or augmented via the pericranium.

8.3. Complications of Depressed Fracture

1. Infection leads to meningitis and subsequently brain abscess formation;
2. Epilepsy—early- or late-seizure disorder;
3. CSF leak: A nasal fracture may form a connection between the subarachnoid spaces and paranasal air sinus or middle ear cavity. Rhinorrhea or otorrhea may result. Infection may lead to meningitis and its consequences.

8.4. Pond Fracture/Ping Pong Fracture

Ping pong fractures occur in newborns and young infants when their skulls are relatively flexible and robust, allowing the bone to indent without breaking. This type of fracture gets its name from its resemblance to the depression left by a ping pong ball (Figure 5). Ping pong fractures have been reported in both accidental and non-accidental circumstances, including birth traumas. They are rarely linked to intracranial damage. Depending on the severity of the depression, it can be treated conservatively or surgically (Haddad and Arabi 2012; Khan and Banerjee 2010).

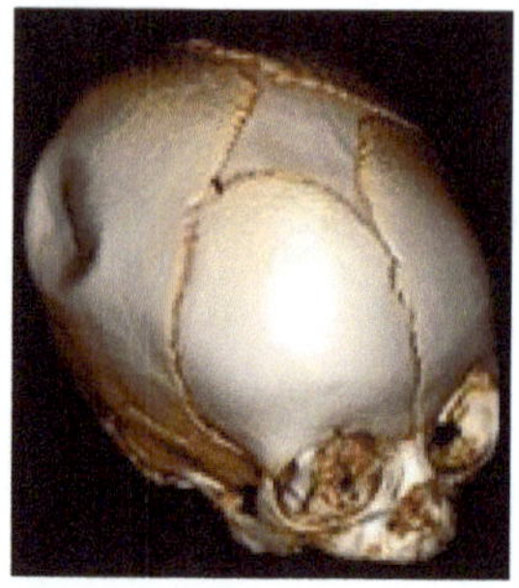

Figure 5. CT scan showing a ping-pong fracture. Source: Figure by authors.

8.5. Growing Fracture

A post-traumatic leptomeningeal cyst or growing fracture is a very rare pediatric head injury. Its formation requires a rapidly growing brain (Figure 6).

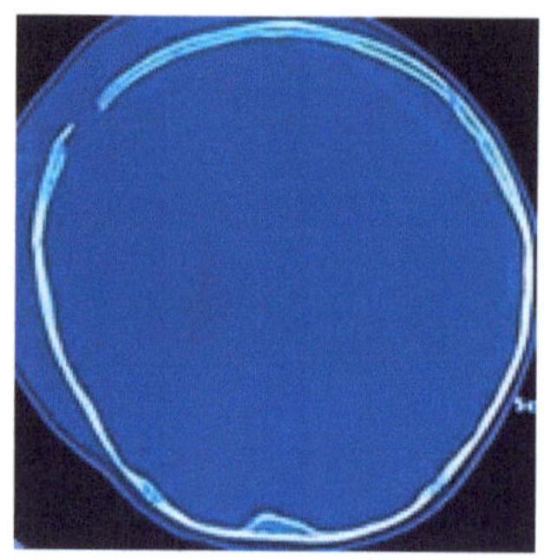

Figure 6. CT scan showing a growing skull fracture. Source: Figure by authors.

Surgical treatment: Craniotomy and closure of the dural defect. Dural augmentation from the pericranium or fascia lata is commonly required to close the defect.

8.6. Skull Base Fracture

Skull base fractures are estimated to constitute 4% of all head trauma cases.

8.6.1. Types

There are three types of skull base fractures:

1. Longitudinal fractures (the causes of these fractures are given below):
   (a) Blunt impact on the face as well as forehead or back of head;
   (b) Compression from front to back or back to front.
2. Transverse fracture—This type of fracture is caused by an impact either on the side of head or by side-to-side compression.
3. Ring fracture.

8.6.2. Clinical Manifestations

A. The frontal, ethmoidal, and sphenoidal sinuses may be involved in a fracture of the anterior skull base (because of direct contact with the chin), resulting in blood loss from the nose or mouth. CSF and even brain matter can seep into the nose (CSF rhinorrhea) in a cribriform fracture. Bilateral preorbital ecchymosis is also known as Raccoon's eyes (black eyes) (Figure 7A).

B. A middle fossa fracture of the basi-occipital or sphenoid bone and sellae turcica may result in bleeding from the mouth.

C. Fracture of the petrous temporal bone (as a result of a direct impact posterior to the ear) may result in blood as well as CSF coming out from the ear (CSF otorrhea), and blood may pass to the oropharynx via the auditory tube or hemorrhage from the ear as a result of the rupture of the posterior branch of the middle meningeal artery.

D. A posterior fossa fracture (resulting from a direct impact to the back of the head) causes bleeding behind the mastoid process and can result in a large hematoma at the back of the neck and ecchymosis of the mastoid process (known as Battle's sign).

E. Fracture of the foramen magnum, cerebellar contusion, and edema can cause fatal cerebellar tonsillar herniation and cranial never injury (stretched or bruised) (Khan and Banerjee 2010; Joswig et al. 2016).

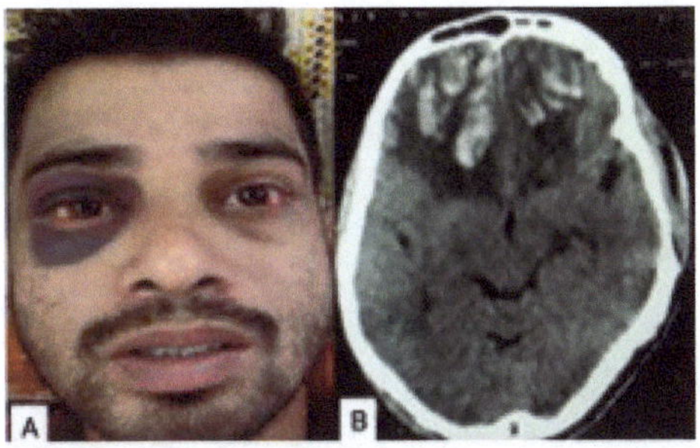

Figure 7. (**A**) Patient with black eye due tofront-basal fracture. (**B**) CT findings showing a bifrontal basal hemorrhagic contusion caused by a road traffic injury. Source: Figure by authors, used with patient's consent.

CT scanning is the most valuable diagnostic process that usually shows fractures of bone, CSF in air sinuses, and pressure in the subdural space or different parts of the intracranial cavities.

8.6.3. Treatment

Conservative treatment consisting of antibiotic administration and bed rest is the usual method of treatment for a skull base fracture.

In the case of optic nerve compression due to depressed bone fragments, surgery is required to decompress the optic nerve.

In most cases, CSF leakage ceases spontaneously in a few days. In this case, when CSF rhinorrhea persists, a lumbar drain and bed rest are options to contemplate before considering surgery to repair the dural defect either via endonasal an endoscopic approach or a bifrontal basal craniotomy. The risk of meningitis is high, and therefore it is essential to treat the patients with broad-spectrum antibiotics for at least two weeks (Khan and Banerjee 2010; Joswig et al. 2016).

9. Cerebral Injury/Brain Injury

TBI is one of the main causes of mortality and morbidity for children and young adults all over the world. Males are two times more likely to suffer a TBI than girls. Falls, automobile collisions, and violence are among the causes. A quick acceleration or deceleration within the brain box, or a complicated mix of movement and sudden impact, causes brain trauma. A multitude of events after the injury may result in a subsequent injury, in addition to the damage suffered at the time of injury.

9.1. Classification of Head (Brain) Injuries

9.1.1. According to Severity

Head injuries may be mild, moderate, or severe depending upon the affected individual's level of consciousness (Table 2).

Table 2. Severit y and level of consciousness.

Severity	GCS	PTA (Post-Traumatic Amnesia)	LOC (Loss Of Consciousness)
Mild	13–15	<1 day	0–30 min
Moderate	9–12	1 to <7 days	>30 min to <24 h
Severe	3–8	>7 days	>24 h

For children under the age of five, a somewhat different version of the GCS is employed. TBIs are classified as mild, moderate, or severe, based on patient's GCS score: Source: Authors' compilation based on data from Greenberg 2010.

Mild/Minor head injury—GCS of 13 or higher: The majority of head injuries are minor. The patient may be conscious or lose consciousness for anywhere from a few seconds to minutes at a time. Confusion, memory problems, headaches, and behavioral issues are all common symptoms. The majority of persons who present with modest head injuries will not experience any further complications. Mild head injuries can be classified into two groups: low-risk and moderate-risk. Low-risk injuries are defined as those causing mild to moderate headaches, dizziness, and nausea. After a thorough assessment, many so-affected individuals require just modest surveillance, and many do not require radiographic evaluation (CT scans). These patients may be discharged if they can be monitored by a trustworthy individual.

Moderate-risk-group patients on anticoagulant treatment, even if they have suffered minor head trauma, should be subjected to radiographic imaging (CT scan) since a slight head injury can escalate into a catastrophic injury.

Moderate head injury—GCS of 9 to 12: These patients may be released if they can be monitored by someone they can trust. Patients on anticoagulant therapy should undergo radiographic imaging (CT scan), even if they have had minimal head trauma, because even a modest head injury can lead to a catastrophic injury.

Severe head injury—GCS of 8 or lower: In this type of injury, for more than six hours, the patient will remain unconscious and in a comatose condition. Because there is a possibility of catastrophic brain damage, severe head injuries require prompt medical attention. An urgent CT scan is required to estimate the severity of the injury.

9.1.2. Types of Head (Brain) Injury According to Brain Parenchymal Injury

Concussion

The most prevalent sort of head injury is concussion. In this case, for a brief amount of time, the patient loses consciousness. A concussion occurs when the brain is jostled or shaken forcefully enough to cause it to bounce against the skull. It varies in severity from minor to severe.

Contusion

A contusion is a bruise on the brain itself. It could be a bleed or an edematous swelling of the brain (Figure 7B).

Cerebral Laceration and Intracranial Hematoma (ICH)

These terms refer to a clot in the brain that forms under the skull. The severity of brain hematomas varies from minor to severe, and they are classified according to their origin. In injury, there is a lack of brain tissue continuity. Pia matter ruptures and subarachnoid hemorrhages are common side effects of surface lacerations. Bone shards tear the brain surface in depressed fractures.

Laceration of brain tissue is caused by any penetrating injury.

In traumatic intracerebral hematoma (ICH), there are four CT findings considered to be significant:

(1) A shift of 5 mm or more in the septum pellucidum, third ventricle, or pineal gland;
(2) Pentagonal cisterna ambient (compressed or collapsed);
(3) Effacement of peripheral sulci (ipsilaterally or diffusely);
(4) Decreased lateral ventricles (uni- or bilateral).

9.1.3. Classification of Head Injuries Depending on Site of Impact

Focal

This type occurs due to a direct overhead impact resulting in a skull fracture, contusion, EDH (extradural hematoma), acute SDH (subdural hematoma), or cerebral laceration, and an intracerebral hematoma may form.

Contusions are multiple small hemorrhages in the surface layers of the brain. They can form at the impact site and/or on the side of the head contralateral to the impact site. A 'coup' injury occurs when a lesion develops at the site of impact, while a 'contrecoup' injury occurs when a lesion occurs on the side of the brain contralateral to the site of impact. The movement of the brain within the skull cavity causes contrecoup contusions (Figures 8 and 9).

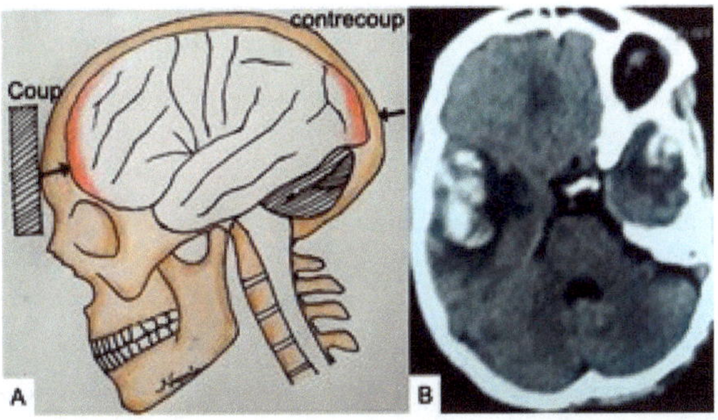

Figure 8. (**A**) Diagrammatic presentation of coup and contrecoup effect. (**B**) CT scan showing a hemorrhagic contusion in both temporal lobes as a result of coup and contrecoup effects. Source: Figure by authors.

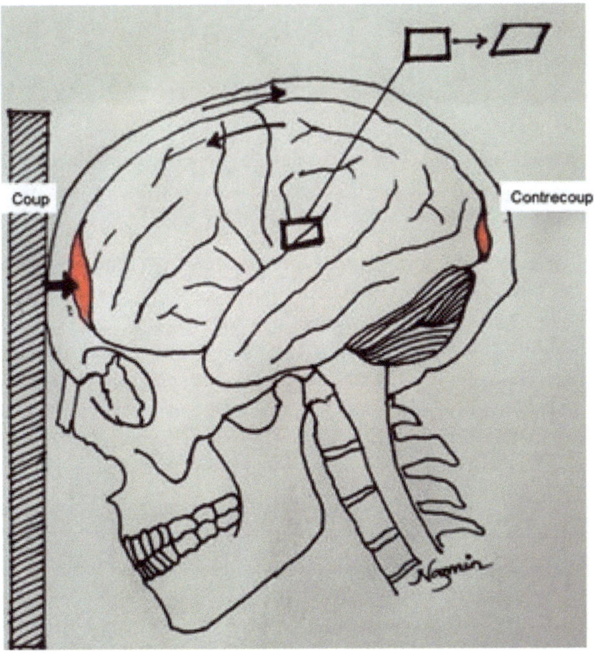

Figure 9. Diagrammatic structure of brain showing coup and contrecoup effects. Source: Figure by authors.

Diffuse Axonal Injury (DAI)

A DAI is a primary brain injury resulting from an accelerating–decelerating impact. The sudden deceleration produces a shearing force that disrupts axons as well as small vessels (Figure 9). Axonal damage results in localized transport failures in the corresponding axon, resulting in swelling and, in some cases, axonal lysis with Wallerian degeneration.

A. Grading of DAI

- Mild DAI: Coma of >6 to 24 h. Mild to severe memory loss as well as mild to moderate impairments follow.
- Moderate DAI: Coma > 24 h. Confusion and long-term amnesia are followed by mild to severe behavioral, memory, and cognitive impairments.
- Severe DAI: With flexor and extensor posturing, the coma can last months. Deficits in cognition, memory, speech, sensorimotor control, and personality are induced.

The effect of a DAI on reticular formation (without a space-occupying lesion observable via CT) induces loss of consciousness (although a DAI can be present alongside subdural or epidural hematomas).

B. Radiological features of DAI

A focal hemorrhagic or edematous lesion in the corpus callosum, parasagittal white matter, septum pellucidum, third-ventricle wall, and/or dorsolateral brainstem can be seen. These lesions are identified as hyperintense lesions in T2W MRI. Because it can identify both hemorrhagic and non-hemorrhagic lesions, MRI is markedly more sensitive than CT (Figure 10).

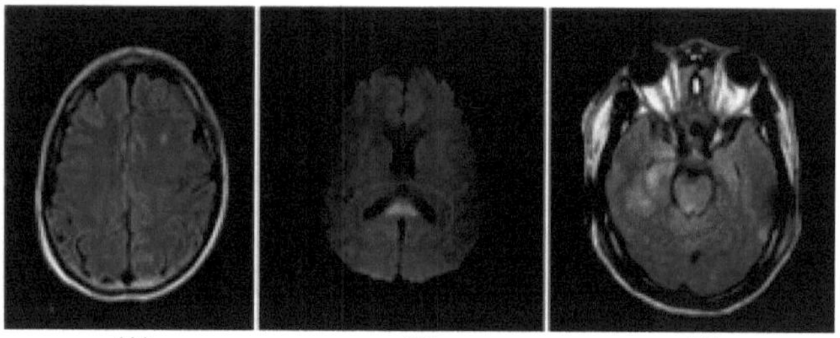

(A) (B) (C)

Figure 10. (**A**) MRI (axial image) shows small hemorrhage in frontal white matter and (**B**) hemorrhage in splenium of corpus callosum. (**C**) MRI image (axial view) showing hemorrhage in the rostral midbrain and medial temporal lobe. Source: Figure by authors.

In gradient recalled echo (GRE) and susceptibility-weighted (SW) images, acute hemorrhagic lesions show localized susceptibility and signal loss due to the paramagnetic effects of deoxyhemoglobin (SWI). When comparing 1.5 Tesla (3T) to 3 Tesla (3T), these susceptibility effects are amplified, with about two times as many hemorrhagic lesions visible at 3T. Non-hemorrhagic lesions are best seen via fluid attenuation inversion recovery (FLAIR) imaging, which makes subcortical as well as periventricular lesions stand out (in comparison to T2W images). Diffusion-weighted imaging (DWI) is also sensitive to DAI and able to detect lesions that are not visible in GRE or FLAIR images. In the acute context, DAI lesions are often hyperintense, with low apparent diffusion coefficient (ADC) values, indicating cytotoxic edema (Kim and Gean 2011; Joswig et al. 2016; Timofeev et al. 2012). Classification of DAI is shown in Table 3.

C. MRI grading of DAIs

MRI can sequentially detect punctuate micro hemorrhages in the white matter, corpus callosum, and midbrain.

Grade I: The hemorrhage is restricted to the cerebral cortex.

Grade II: The hemorrhage is restricted to the corpus callosum.

Grade III: The hemorrhage extends into the midbrain.

D. Outcome of DAI

The average amount of time it takes to regain consciousness is 20–33 days. The median time to regain awake status differs significantly for different groups. If a grade I patient takes 5 days to regain consciousness, grade

II and III patients will take 2 and 4 weeks, respectively. As the MRI grading improves, so does the length of time spent in the ICU and hospital. Finally, depending on the patient, the duration of mechanical ventilation can increase. A hemorrhage in a DAI-type lesion, especially when associated with traumatic space-occupying lesions (such as EDH, SDH, and ICH), is a poor prognosticator. Isolated DAI-type lesions that are not hemorrhagic are not linked to a poor clinical outcomes.

Table 3. Classification of diffuse axonal injuries.

Grade MRI Findings	**Neuropathologic Findings**	**Stage**
1: White matter	Microscopic axonal injury in the white matter of the hemispheres, corpus callosum, brain stem, and/or cerebellum, without hemorrhagic or necrotic lesions in the corpus callosum or superior cerebellar peduncles.	01. Traumatic lesion limited to lobar white matter or the cerebellum only.
2: Brain Stem	Microscopic or macroscopic hemorrhagic or necrotic lesion in the brain stem and corpus callosum	02. Traumatic lesion in the corpus callosum with or without lobar white matter lesion.
3: Cerebellar peduncle	Microscopic or macroscopic injury in the lobar callosum. Hemorrhagic or necrotic lesions in the dorsolateral quadrants of the rostral brain stem.	03. Traumatic lesion in the brain (dorsolateral quadrant of the brain stem and superior cerebellar peduncles) with or without lesions in white matter or the corpus.

Source: Authors' compilation based on data from Pascual and Prieto (2012).

9.1.4. Another Classification of Head Injury (Based on Mode)

Closed head injury—This type of is usually caused by a car accident, a fall, or shaking (for babies). A closed head injury is the result of rapid forward and backward movement as well as shaking of the brain parenchyma inside the brain box.

Penetrating head injury—When the head is penetrated by a sharp cutting instrument, bullet, or pellet.

9.1.5. Another Classification of Head Injury (Based on Timing)

Primary head injury—This type of injury happens at the time of the impact. It can be a focal or diffuse type of injury. EDH, SDH, and traumatic ICH are types of primary head injury.

Secondary head injury—This type refers to changes that occur over time (from hours to days) after a primary brain injury. It involves a series of neuronal, metabolic, and vascular alterations in the brain, all of which contribute to further brain tissue death. Cerebral swelling, cerebral edema, cerebral ischemia and infarct, and brain herniation occur after a primary head injury.

Cerebral Swelling

The literature is divided on whether cerebral edema (Figure 11) or hyperemia with an increased volume of blood is the root etiology of brain swelling. It is possible that both mechanisms are at work. The main mechanism of cerebral swelling, according to popular belief, is cerebral hyperemia caused by dysautoregulation with engorgement of vessels and increased CBF. Vasogenic edema occurs when the BBB is compromised, allowing extracellular water to accumulate, and cytotoxic edema occurs when cell membrane pumps fail, enabling intracellular water to leak. As evidenced by the higher water content observed in this condition, cytotoxic edema may be the primary cause of cerebral swelling among these two forms of edema. Sulcal effacement, basilar cistern compression, and flattening of the ventricular borders are all signs of cerebral edema caused by hyperemia. The attenuation and differentiation of gray and white matter are preserved. Cerebral swelling caused by vasogenic edema, on the other hand, will show up as low-attenuation patches, whereas cytotoxic edema will show up as an absence of a gray–white distinction. Diffuse cerebral swelling is more common in pediatric patients than adults after a head injury, with the prevalence of diffuse swelling being two times greater in children than in adults. Post-traumatic dysautoregulation, which causes vasodilation, hyperemia, and cerebral edema, is more common in children and young adults. When the swelling is significant, the ICP rises and the CPP drops, resulting in cerebral infarction and brain damage. Head raising, controlled moderate hyperventilation, mannitol administration with hyperosmolar therapy, and the careful use of sedatives and analgesics to avoid pain or agitation from raised ICP are all therapeutic strategies used to fight the detrimental effects of cerebral swelling. Decompressive craniectomy (DC) can be performed to try to reduce ICP when it is unresponsive to maximal medical therapy. DC has been shown to reduce ICP and enhance functional outcomes in a number of studies. DC also improves radiologic outcomes by allowing for better viewing of basilar cisterns and a reduction in midline shift, both of which are linked to a better outcome.

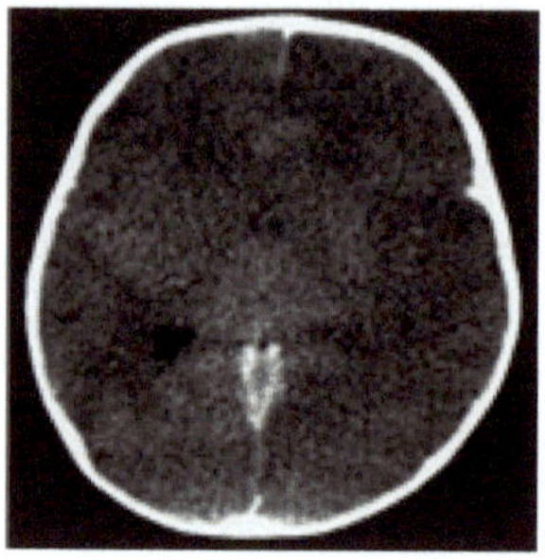

Figure 11. CT scan revealing generalized cerebral edema. Source: Figure by authors.

Cerebral Herniation

Cerebral herniations (Figure 12) are the result of an unmitigated increase in ICP. The process of the cingulate gyrus herniating below the falx cerebri is known as subfalcine herniation or midline shift. When the medial part of the temporal lobe/uncas herniates through the tentorial incisura and compresses the suprasellar cistern, this is known as uncal herniation (Kim and Gean 2011). Caudal herniation of both temporal lobes through the tentorial incisura causes descending transtentorial herniation, compressing the basilar cisterns. The cerebellum extends through the tentorial incisura and effaces the quadrigeminal cistern in upward transtentorial herniation, which happens in the opposite way. The cerebellar tonsillar protrusion into the foramen magnum is known as tonsillar herniation (Kim and Gean 2011). A dilated pupil is a clinical indication of cerebral herniation in the absence of CT imaging results. The herniated medial temporal lobe puts pressure on the same side of the third nerve, resulting in the lack of normal light reflexes exhibited by those with uncal herniation. Cerebral infarction and the Duret hemorrhage, which often occur in the anterior and paramedian midbrain/pons following fast caudal herniation, are two more serious consequences of cerebral herniation. The pathophysiology of the deleterious effects of the Duret hemorrhage is assumed to be either the rupture of the pontine perforator from the basilar artery or venous thrombosis with an infarct (Kim and Gean 2011; Quiñones-Hinojosa 2012; Gooch et al. 2009).

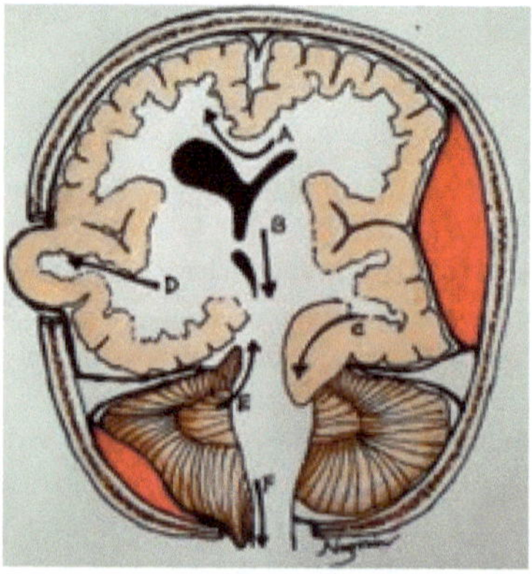

Figure 12. Schematic presentation of different types of brain herniation; A—subfalcine, B—central, C—Uncal, D—transcalvarial, E—upward cerebellar, and F—tonsillar herniation. Source: Figure by authors.

Cerebral Ischemia and Infarction

Cerebral ischemia as well as infarction affect 2% of patients who undergo a CT scan of the head for a head injury and can be caused by multiple factors. Ischemia is usually caused by a blood vessel being mechanically compressed by a brain herniation through the falx cerebri and/or tentorium. In acute subfalcine or uncal herniation, infarctions are due to a mechanical shift of the anterior cerebral artery (ACA) or posterior cerebral artery (PCA) distribution, respectively. In subfalcine herniation, the calloso-marginal branch of the ACA might be squeezed against the free border of the falx, causing infarction. The herniated medial temporal lobe may press the PCA and cause an infarction, or it can compress the anterior choroidal artery and cause an infarction of the internal capsule (the posterior limb) in uncal herniation. Vasospasm is another possible etiology of ischemia and infarction in TBIs. Extra-axial hematomas, which apply a great deal of pressure on the neighboring cortex, can also squeeze cortical veins, resulting in a venous infarction. Lastly, ischemia can occur as a result of direct arterial injury, such as blockage, dissection, or pseudoaneurysm caused by a fracture of the base of the skull.

10. EDH (Extradural Hematoma)

EDHs account for 1% of head trauma. They commonly occur in young adults, commonly following a temporo-parietal skull fracture that disrupts the MMA (middle meningeal artery), causing arterial bleeding between the dura mater and bone.

The main source of bleeding (85%) in the middle meningeal artery and the rest is either the middle meningeal vein or the dural sinus. Fracture of the temporal or frontal bone via trauma or a head fixation pin leads to an injury to the dura and dural blood vessels (main trunk, frontal branch, or parietal branch).

The main site for EDH is the pterion; the other sites are the frontal, occipital, and posterior fossa.

10.1. Presentation

Typical presentations are as follows:

1. Transient (post-traumatic) loss of consciousness (LOC) due to concussion;
2. Followed by a lucid interval for several hours (in 30–40% cases);
3. Followed by obtundation, contralateral hemiparesis, and ipsilateral pupillary dilation.

Other presentations are headache, vomiting, bradycardia, seizure, hyper reflexes, and being Babinski-sign-positive.

Contralateral hemiparesis is the most typical presentation of EDH; however, ipsilateral hemiparesis may occur due to compression of the contralateral cerebral peduncle against the tentorial free margin—the so-called Kernohan's notch phenomenon. It is a false localizing sign.

4. If both pupils are dilated, then the patient may also develop decorticated or decerebrated rigidity.

10.2. CT Appearances of EDH

Classical EDH (Figures 13 and 14) looks like a hyperdense lenticular shape adjacent to the skull. It is limited by sutures as the external dural layer is tightly attached to the sutural line.

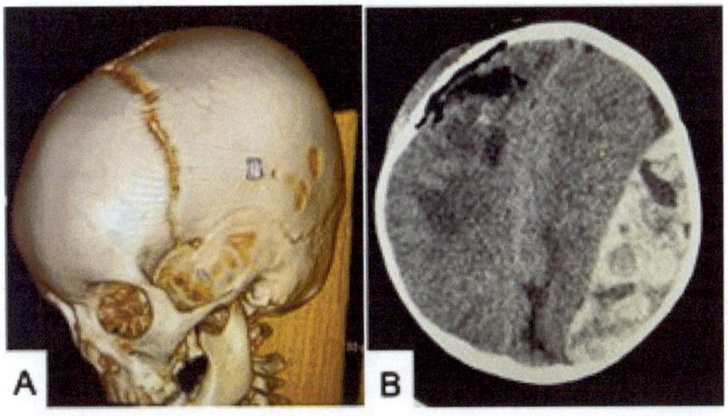

Figure 13. (**A**) A 3D CT scan showing a depressed fragment in temporal bone. (**B**) A huge EDH found in the tempero-parietal region of the same patient. Source: Figure by authors.

A total of 5–20% of EDHs are bilateral. EDHs may extend in the cranial and caudal directions with respect to the tentorium cerebelli. The hematoma volume can be calculated using the formula ABC/2 (for which the CT slice containing the greatest hemorrhage is chosen), where A represents the diameter of the hematoma on that slice, B represents the measurement taken 90° to A, and C represents the approximate number of 10 mm slices containing the hematoma (Kim and Gean 2011).

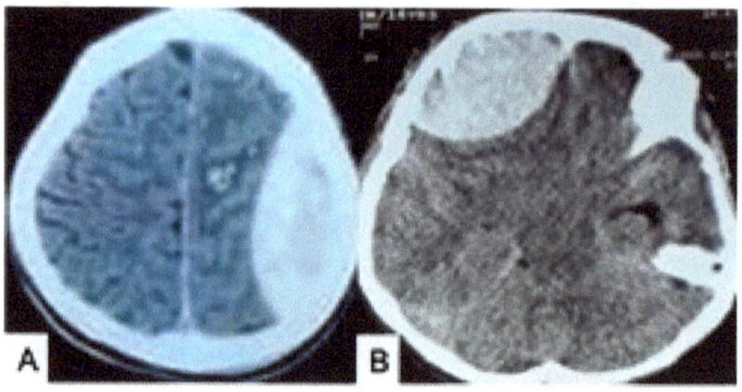

Figure 14. CT scan showing a typical extradural hematoma: (**A**) parietal convexity EDH; (**B**) frontal EDH. Source: Figure by authors.

10.3. Indications for EDH Surgery

1. Surgical evacuation is recommended for epidural hematomas (EDHs) > 30 cm^3 regardless of GCS, according to recent guidelines (Vella et al. 2017).
2. Surgery is also recommended for patients who have EDH and GCS scores less than 9, a clot thickness greater than 15 mm, a midline displacement greater than 5 mm, or localized neurologic impairments.

10.3.1. Conservative Treatment of EDH

Epidural hematomas measuring < 30 cm^3 and that are <15 mm thick and have a <5 mm shift in patients with a GCS > 8 and no focal deficits can be followed up carefully and subjected to serial imaging (with repeat scans every 6–8 h).

Controversy appears to surround the nonsurgical management of acute epidural hematomas that are asymptomatic or nearly so. Regardless of whether this conservative approach may be contemplated for supratentorial hematomas far from the perimesencephalic cistern, many surgeons strongly recommend that all acute epidural hematomas in the temporal fossa or the posterior fossa be immediately removed, even if they are small. This is because these patients may initially appear relatively asymptomatic while harboring a "small" clot. The latter, however, may rapidly enlarge, leading to dramatic, life-threatening changes.

10.3.2. Operative Technique

An extensive fronto-tempro-parietal craniotomy is commonly carried out by keeping the patient's head on a horseshoe head rest or a three pins' head fixator (Figure 15). A wide question-mark- or c-shaped incision is made on the front or back of the external acoustic meatus. Skin along with temporalis muscle are removed as a single flap. Bone fractures (if any), either linear or depressed, are evident following exposure. Multiple burr holes are made. Small blood clots commonly come out through the burr hole. A wide craniotomy is carried out using a high-speed craniotome. Extradural blood clots are removed via suction, irrigation, and a coup scoop or spatula. A common source of bleeding is the middle meningeal artery, in which the blood coagulates, and the vein along with it, in which the blood also coagulates. Sometimes the surgeons need to coagulate and ligate the origin of the MMA at the origin foramen spinosum level.

Following the cauterization and ligation of MMA, the waxing of the foramen spinosum must be conducted.

The application of dural tack-up sutures is always recommended, both centrally and peripherally. This maneuver prevents epidural hematoma re-accumulation, which is particularly relevant for patients with acute hypo-coagulopathic disorders or those in whom a bleeding source was missed intraoperatively because of temporary spontaneous hemostasis (Quiñones-Hinojosa 2012).

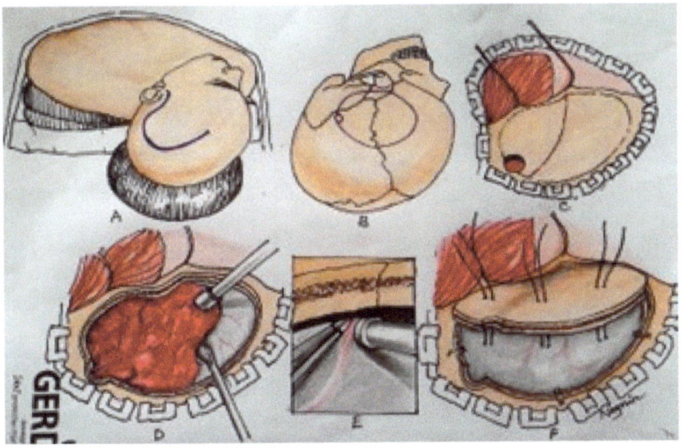

Figure 15. EDH surgical technique via the standard craniotomy. (**A**) The patient is put in the supine position, with a roll placed under their ipsilateral shoulder and their head turned to the opposite side. A large question-mark-shaped skin flap is marked out. If the patient suffers rapid neurologic deterioration due to mass effect, rapid decompression through a large temporal bur hole is initially carried out. (**B**) A large frontotemporal craniotomy is performed, with further exposure of the middle fossa being achieved by removing parts of the lateral sphenoid wing. (**C**) When the bone flap is turned, the hematoma is rapidly removed with suction, irrigation, and cup forceps. (**D**) In most cases, the principal bleeding source is the middle meningeal artery or the bone of its main branches lying in the dura mater, and this blood easily coagulates. (**E**) In other cases, the bleeding may originate either from the foramen spinosum or from a fracture running across the temporal bone, and the hemorrhage can be arrested by plugging it with bone wax. (**F**) After meticulous hemostasis in the epidural space is achieved with bipolar diathermy and hemostatic agents, "tack-up" sutures are placed at the periphery and in the middle of the bone flap, which is then reapplied. Source: Figure by authors.

10.3.3. Causes of Death from EDH

- Respiratory failure;
- Cerebral edema;
- Secondary pontine hemorrhage;
- Herniation of the uncas.

11. Acute Subdural Hematoma (ASDH)

ASDHs is more common than EDH. It occurs due to the rupture of surface or bridging vessels via the acceleration or deceleration types of violent head trauma. Here, blood accumulates between the dura mater and pale brain surface. Another cause of ASDH is associated with a burst temporal or frontal lobe. A rare cause is a rupture of the small cortical artery due to an overlying fracture of the bone.

In descending order of frequency, ASDHs usually occur over the cerebral hemisphere convexities, along the tentorium cerebelli, and along the falx cerebri. ASDHs look crescent-shaped on imaging and do not cross the midline (Figures 16 and 17) (Kim and Gean 2011).

Here, the lucid interval is not typical like that for EDH. In total, 10–40% of individuals with ASDH may experience a lucid interval. Patients commonly deteriorate rapidly.

The poor outcome of ASDHs largely results from simultaneous cerebral cortical injuries such as contusion, brain swellings, and DAI. Overall, 60–80% of patients are in a state of coma during diagnosis. The accumulation of 100–150 mL of blood may be fatal in acute ASDH.

CT scanning is the ideal tool for investigation. CT findings according to time frame are summarized in Table 4.

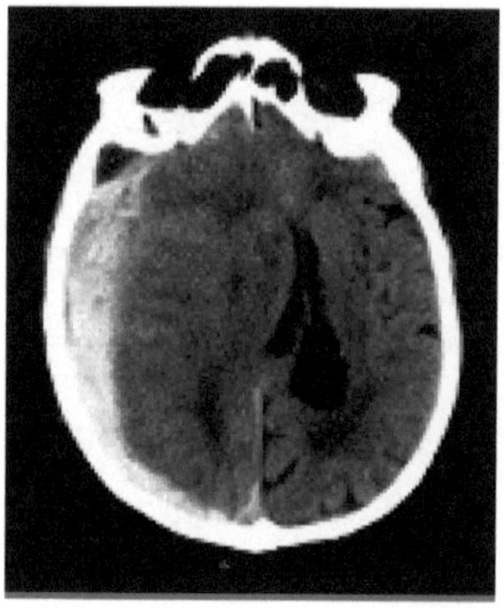

Figure 16. CT scan showing the typical crescentic shape of acute SDH in temporal convexity area with midline shift and biventricular effacement. Source: Figure by authors.

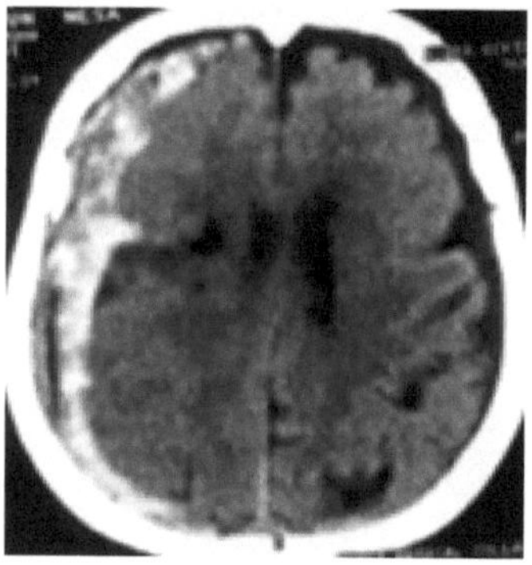

Figure 17. CT scan of the crescentic shapes of an acute subdural hematoma with no midline shift. Source: Figure by authors.

Table 4. ASDH density changes visible on CT scans over time (Figures 16 and 17).

Category	Time Frame	Density on CT
Acute	1–3 days	Hyperdense
Subacute	4 days–2/3 weeks	Isodense
Chronic	Usually, more than 3 weeks and less than 3–4 months	Hypodense (trending toward CSF density)
	After nearly 30–60 days	May take lenticular shape (akin to EDH) with density greater than CSF and less than fresh blood

Source: Authors' compilation based on data from Greenberg (2010); Vella et al. (2017).

11.1. Etiologies

1. Rupture of connecting bridging or veins.
2. Tear of inferior cerebral vein entering the venous sinuses at the skull base.
3. Rift or tear in dural venous sinuses.
4. Damage to cortical veins.
5. Contusion and/or laceration of the brain and dura.
6. Damage to earlier adhesions between the dura and brain.
7. Secondary to pathology, e.g., cerebral tumor, aneurysm, or hematological disorder.
8. Drugs (such as dicoumarol, heparin, and warfarin).

11.2. Management

11.2.1. Indications of Surgery

1. ASDH with a thickness of more than 10 mm, regardless of GCS;
2. ASDH with a midline shift of more than 5 mm, regardless of GCS;
3. GCS < 8 and ICP > 20 mmHg—thickness or midline shift is of less concern;
4. GCS < 8 and asymmetric or fixed and dilated pupils;
5. GCS < 8 and decrease of 2 or more points on GCS after hospital admission;
6. Secondary injury to the brain that is frequently associated with ASDH (Bishokarma 2018).

11.2.2. Surgical Treatment

Treatment consist of a wide craniotomy with a durotomy and removal of the subdural hematoma (Figures 18 and 19).

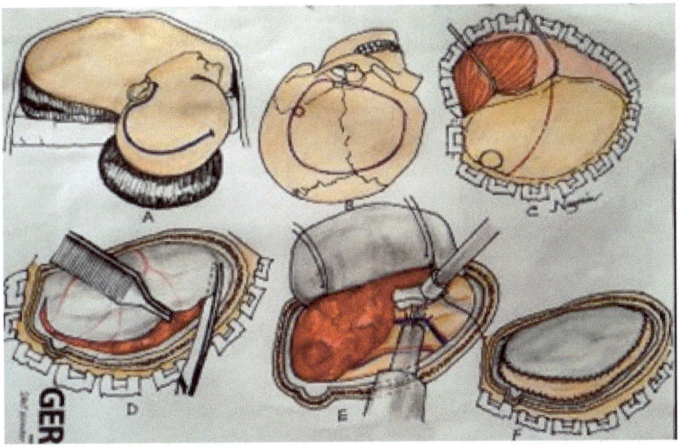

Figure 18. Schematic presentation of surgical evacuation of ASDH: (**A**) patient's position and incision; (**B**) marking indicating the site at which large fronto-parieto-temporal craniotomy will be performed; (**C**) subperiosteal dissection and removal of craniotomy bone flap; (**D**) durotomy; (**E**) evacuation of hematoma via gentle irrigation and suction; (**F**) expansile duroplasty through the pericranium. Source: Figure by authors.

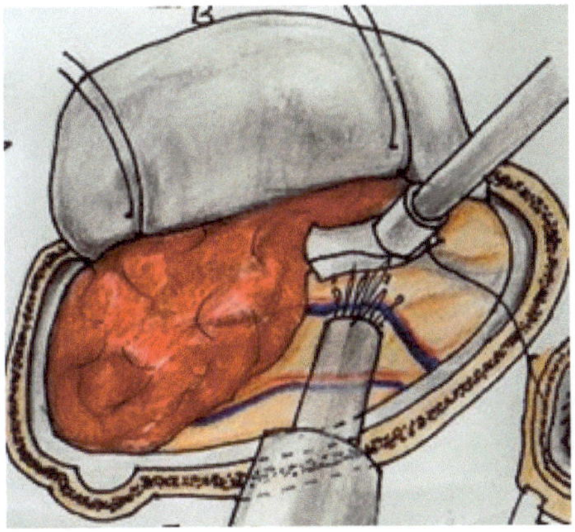

Figure 19. Diagrammatic perioperative picture of acute SDH showing clotted blood being sucked out using a suction device and gentle irrigation. Source: Figure by authors.

In some cases, a duroplasty is needed.

Some cases require a decompressive hemicraniectomy and a duroplasty depending upon the state of brain swelling.

11.2.3. SDH Removal Technique

A standard fronto-temporo parietal trauma craniotomy is performed. Once the bone flap is taken away, inverse U-shaped or Y-shaped or X-shaped (cruciform) dural openings can be adopted depending on the neurosurgeon's experience. A wide cruciate dural incision is carried out. Starting from the area of maximum clot thickness, the clot is evacuated with copious irrigation and suction. A bleeding point on the surface of the brain could be a connecting vein or an artery that can be coagulated via bipolar diathermry, or a hemorrhage could be caused by ragged dural borders or decaying brain tissue. The connecting vein is occasionally visibly avulsed, and it can be effortlessly coagulated with diathermy. Areas of a cortical contusion larger than 1 to 2 cm in diameter, with irreversibly injured brain that appears mottled, should be aspirated gently.

If a tear formed across a venous sinus, the neurosurgeon should be ready to deal with profuse sinus bleeding, and the sinus tear needs to be completely observable. The edge of the craniotomy may have to be expanded toward the sinus; at the same time, profuse bleeding may make this a difficult maneuver. In addition, it may be important to repair the sinus rip properly without interfering with sinus blood flow. In some circumstances, massive red cell transfusions may be required. Sinus ligation may be performed, but neurosutgeons choose to ligate solely the anterior quarter of the superior sagittal sinus while avoiding ligation involving more posterior segments of superior sagittal sinus.

After homeostasis has been ensured, the dura is sealed with a water-tight closure. Depending on the status of the brain, the bone flap is either replaced or preserved in situations where significant brain edema/brain swelling is observed. The reciprocal of intraoperative brain swelling in acute subdural hematomas is found when the hematoma is essentially non-pulsatile. Under these circumstances, visual confirmation of a poorly perfused brain indicates rapid attempts at tissue reperfusion. Because the status of cerebral pressure autoregulation is not usually assessable intraoperatively, caution should be exercised when iatrogenically raising the patient's blood pressure with dopamine, noradrenaline, or both in an attempt to induce re-expansion of the retracted brain.

If rebound brain swelling develops, fast intravenous administration of 25% mannitol (0.75–1 g/kg) should follow along with rapid intravenous fluid replacement. This therapeutic combination is justified because mannitol simultaneously increases CBF and decreases brain volume. Acute subdural hematomas are more frequently associated with contusions than EDH. Brain swelling is also more frequent in acute subdural than epidural hematomas. Therefore, decompressive surgery may be necessary under the following circumstances:

(1) The clot itself is not very thick, but the hemorrhagic contusion is sizable, leading to a mass effect (frequently compressing basilar cisterns);
(2) The clot itself is not very thick, but hemispheric swelling may be pronounced in proportion to the size of the hematoma;
(3) The clot is large and associated with contusions, and acute "rebound" brain swelling is found after clot removal (Quiñones-Hinojosa 2012).

ASDHs do not provide the rewarding outcome that is usually seen for EDH patients after surgical intervention. SDHs are the worst form of traumatic injury affecting the brain.

This is because of associated parenchymal brain injury and the subsequent secondary brain injury that is commonly present with ASDH. Mortality rates range from 40–60%.

11.3. Risk Factors for Worse Outcome

1. Age: younger patients generally have more favorable outcomes than patients older than 65;
2. The period of loss of consciousness and poor GCS;
3. Signs of brain herniation and brain stem injury;
4. Surgery within 2 h of injury has a more favorable outcome and lower mortality rate compared to that for patients who undergo surgery after 2 h.

11.4. Comparison Between EDH and ASDH

Comparison between EDH and ASDH is shown in Table 5.

Table 5. Epidural vs. subdural hematomas.

Hematoma Type	Extradural	Subdural
Site	Between the skull bone and the dura	Between the arachnoid matter and the dura
Involved vessel	Tempero-parietal (most likely vessel)—Middle meningeal artery Frontal—anterior ethmoidal artery Occipital—sigmoid or transverse sinuses Vertex—superior sagittal sinus	Bridging or connecting veins
Symptoms	Lucid interval after period of initial unconsciousness	Slowly incrementing headache and confusion
CT appearance	Biconvex lenticular shape—restricted by suture lines	Crescent-shaped—transcends suture lines

Source: Authors' compilation based on data from Habeeb (2017).

12. Chronic Subdural Hematoma (CSDH)

A CSDH is an encapsulated accumulation of old blood frequently liquefied and situated in between the dura mater and the pial brain surface. The cortical vein may be ruptured with minimum head trauma, particularly for elder individuals with cortical atrophy of the brain.

12.1. Sign and Symptoms of CSDH

The onset of the symptoms of CSDHs is generally delayed by 4–7 weeks.

Clinical features:

- Dementia
- Unconsciousness
- Seizures
- Numbness
- Dizziness
- Amnesia
- Nausea and vomiting
- Changes in personality
- Ataxia and/difficulty walking
- Altered respiratory patterns
- Gaze palsy or abnormal eye movement
- Fluctuating LOC
- Irritability
- Pain
- Headache (either constant or fluctuating)
- loss of orientation
- Weakness
- Anorexia
- Aphasia or slurred speech
- Lake of muscle control
- Deafness or tinnitus
- Blurring of vision

12.2. Neuroimaging

12.2.1. CT Findings of CSDH

CSDHs are crescent-shaped when viewed in a CT scan, having a concave surface away from the skull. A fresh subdural hemorrhage is hyperdense at first, but as cellular materials dissolve, it becomes hypodense. The hemorrhage becomes isodense with brain tissue after 3–14 days and may thus be ignored (Figure 20). It will eventually become more hypodense than brain parenchyma (Figure 21).

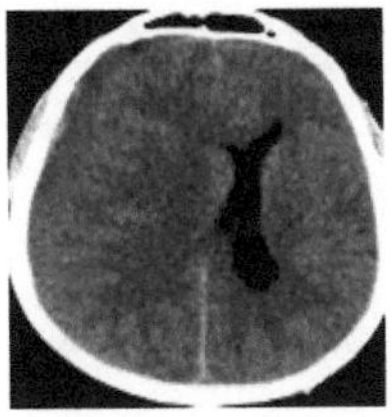

Figure 20. CT scan showing isointense right-sided mass with a midline shift—suggestive of chronic SDH. Source: Figure by authors.

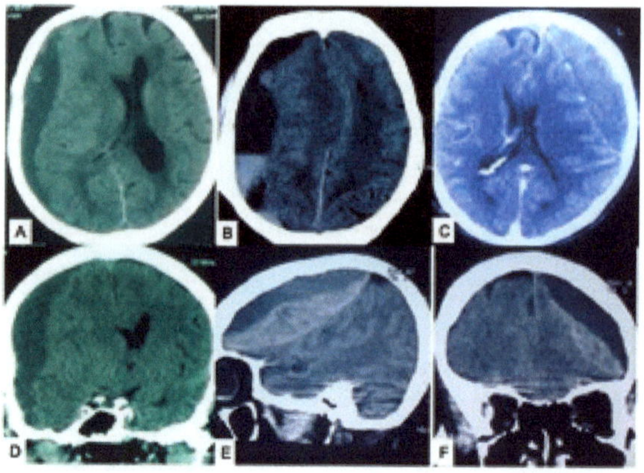

Figure 21. CT head shows fluid levels in chronic SDH (**A–F**). Source: Figure by authors.

12.2.2. MRI Findings

The diagnosis of a CSDH and numerous loculations, intra-hematoma membranes, fresh bleeding, hemolysis, and capsule size is more sensitive when using magnetic resonance imaging (MRI). Primary or metastatic dural illnesses can be detected using contrast-enhanced MRI.

T1: If the hemorrhage is stable, it looks isointense with respect to CSF; nevertheless, if there is a further hemorrhage or infection, it can seem hyperintense with respect to CSF.

T2: The hematoma looks isointense with respect to CSF if it is stable. If the hematoma bleeds again, it will seem hypointense.

12.3. Etiology

Although trauma is the commonest cause of a CSDH, intracranial hypotension and coagulation problems may also be to blame.

12.3.1. Post-Traumatic

In the vast majority of instances, a definitive trauma history can be acquired. Most of these cases involve mild brain damage, while in some situations, moderate to severe injury may be the cause. It is possible for this injury to be minor and go unreported. Some cases may arise as a result of neurosurgical procedures. Bridging/connecting veins in the subdural portion are weaker than those in the subarachnoid portion due to their thin walls, circumferential distribution of collagen fibers, and absence of outside support by arachnoid trabeculae.

Acute SDH or subdural effusion can lead to a CSDH (SDE) (Simmons and Luks 2013). It is suspected that matrix metalloproteinase is involved in the formation of CSDH. Approximately 50% of asymptomatic post-traumatic SDEs develop into CSDHs. Bridging vein rupture, hemorrhage from the wall of hygroma owing to neocapillaries, increased vascular permeability, accelerated fibrinolysis as well as increased protein component in the hygroma are some of the ideas for the etiology of traumatic SDE progressing into CSDH. Inflammatory cytokines are greater in SDE as well as CSDH than in peripheral venous blood. SDE and CSDH are hypothesized to be different stages of the same inflammatory reaction with different signs and symptoms (Kim and Gean 2011; Feng et al. 2008).

12.3.2. Intracranial Hypotension

CSF leaking could result in intracranial hypotension, which could contribute to the development of a CSDH.

12.3.3. Spontaneous Intracranial Hypotension

Without prior trauma or hematological abnormalities, spontaneous intracranial hypotension can be the etiology of CSDH, particularly in young and middle-aged people. Intracranial hypotension can be diagnosed via spinal MRI as well as radionuclide cisternography. Even among elderly patients taking anticoagulants, the existence of a spontaneous spinal CSF fistula should be explored in relation to CSDH (Kim and Gean 2011).

12.4. Pathology

An exterior membrane, a hematoma cavity, and an internal membrane make up a CSDH. Hematoma fluid is usually a non-clotting liquid. Hematomas are usually liquid, but mixed lesions with solid components sometimes occur. The growth of CSDHs has been linked to recurrent hemorrhaging, more exudates from the outer membrane, and CSF entrapment.

Older CSDHs (after 40 days of trauma) generally show numerous capillaries and thin-walled sinusoids along with patent, larger blood vessels. Vessels are commonly occluded by a thrombus in the fibrotic external membrane of a sixty-or-more-day-old hematoma. The external capsule may ossify or calcify in some cases.

Recurrent bleeding, more exudates from the external membrane, osmotic mechanisms, and fast enlargement due to CSF entrapment are probable causes of the expansion of CSDH (Kim and Gean 2011; Quiñones-Hinojosa 2012; Gooch et al. 2009).

12.5. Management

Symptomatic and mass effects generating a CSDH need surgical evacuation.

12.5.1. Burr-Hole Craniostomy

A burr-hole craniostomy is a common procedure for treating a primary, uncomplicated CSDH with a low recurrence risk and low morbidity.

Technique

The patient is put in supine position on a horseshoe headrest in the operation room. To allow for safe tilting of the operating table, the patient is fastened to the table. Based on the patient's comorbidities and the neurosurgeon's preference, general or local anesthesia may be used. At the time of anesthetic induction, a single dosage of prophylactic broad-spectrum antibiotics is administered.

Over the hematoma's maximal width, a pair of 14 mm burr holes are bored around 7 cm apart (commonly one frontal as well as one parietal, with the proper location calculated based on a CT scan). A cruciate incision is used to open the dura mater, which is then coagulated by bipolar diathermy. Using a 50 mL syringe, the subdural collection is flushed away with warmed Ringer solution until the subdural collection becomes clear. A soft catheter can be utilized to irrigate the hematoma cavity across long distances. Through the burr hole, a soft silicon drain with three smooth side holes along with a blunt tip is placed into the subdural space (Figure 22). Gel foam is applied in the burr hole. The skin is closed in multilayers.

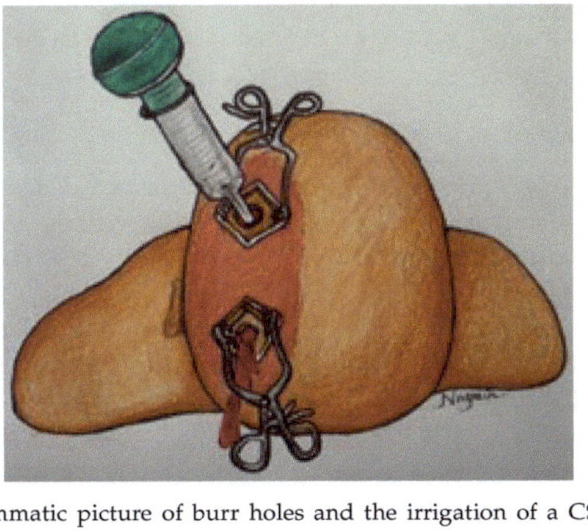

Figure 22. A diagrammatic picture of burr holes and the irrigation of a CSDH. Source: Figure by aurhors.

12.5.2. Mini Craniotomy and Partial Membranectomy

Mini craniotomy and partial membranectomy with irrigation, followed by closed-system drainage, are regarded as a potential management method for CSDHs when there are multiple septations present.

12.5.3. Large Craniotomy with Extended Membranectomy

In non-liquefied and solid hematomas, multilayer intrahematomal loculations, and calcified or organized CSDHs, a larger craniotomy using the 'extended membranectomy' technique may be required, as opposed to a micro craniotomy via the partial membranectomy technique (Kim and Gean 2011; Gooch et al. 2009).

13. Subdural Hygroma

When the arachnoid mater is disrupted, CSF may enter the subdural space, and heavy accumulation of CSF leads to compression of the cerebral parenchyma. A subduro-peritoneal shunt may be required in some cases to treat this hygroma.

14. Traumatic Intracerebral Hematoma (ICH)

This is an acute intracerebral hematoma defined as follows:

- Small ICH—when the size of the hematoma is between 1 and 3 cm;
- Average ICH—when the size of the hematoma size is between 3 and 5 cm;
- Large ICH—when the hematoma is over 5 cm in diameter.
- ICH is conservatively managed in a variety of circumstances:
  (1) In the event of an intracapsular location;
  (2) When there is little or no mass effect (except, perhaps, for the contribution of peri-hematoma edema);
  (3) When there is severe acute hypo-coagulopathy.

Repeat CT 6–8 h after admission or the development of new neurologic localizing signs indicates that it is necessary to re-evaluate these initially small hematomas.

If the intraparenchymal hematoma exhibits a relevant pressure effect upon conducting the first CT scan and is extracapsular, one should consider emergency removal via standard craniotomy and corticectomy while attempting to preserve a layer of clotted blood against the walls of the hematoma cavity. The latter maneuver is conducted to minimize the risk of clot re-accumulation. Proper hemostasias must be ensured before closure of the dura to avoid hemorrhage.

14.1. Surgical Management of Traumatic ICH

14.1.1. Surgical Indication of Evacuation

Yamaki et al. thought that only ICHs greater than 3 cm in diameter were of clinical importance. Surgery should be advised for every patient with an intracerebellar hematoma larger than 3 cm (Yamaki et al. 1990).

McLaurin and McBride treated surgically an ICH that was between 10 and 75 mL in volume. For an ICH in the temporoparietal region (McLaurin and McBride 1956), Andrews et al. suggested that such a procedure should be considered for lesions greater than 30 mL in volume (Andrews et al. 2012).

15. Decompressive Craniotomy (DC) in Head Injury

This term refers to surgical decompressive measures other than cerebral decompression due to hematoma removal alone. In the management of acute traumatic intracranial hypertension associated with brain swelling, decompressive surgery is required for approximately 20% of patients. The main factor governing the acquisition of successful results in decompressive surgery appears to be its timing. Little or no benefit can be found when decompressive procedures are carried out after irreversible bilateral pupillary dilatation has developed. Bifronto-temperoparietal decompressive craniectomy in cases with diffuse traumatic head injury and resistant ICH results in decreased ICP and short ICU stay, according to the DECRA (decompressive craniectomy in diffuse traumatic brain injury) randomized clinical trial. However, when compared to individuals receiving normal care, DC may be linked to poor long-term neurological prognosis and equivalent mortality at 6 months.

15.1. DC Techniques

Large fronto-temperoparietal DC (at least either 12 × 15 cm or 15 cm in diameter) is advised over a mini fronto-temporoparietal DC to allow decreased mortality and better neurological results in cases with severe head injuries (Figure 23).

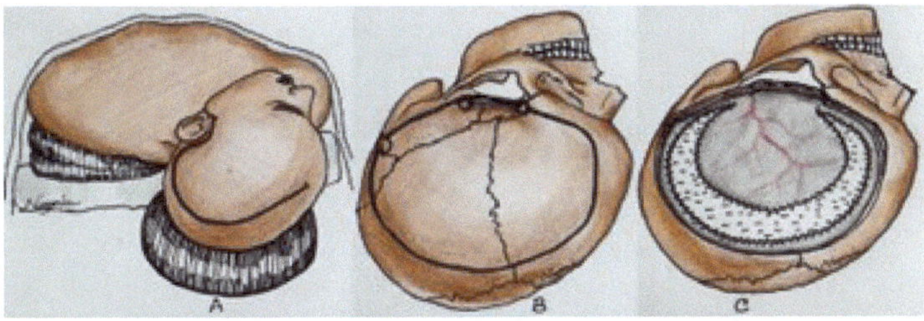

Figure 23. Unilateral decompressive craniectomy. (**A**) The dotted line represents the usual skin incision made during a unilateral decompressive craniectomy. To preserve adequate vascular supply. The length of the incision (distance B) should not exceed its width (distance A). (**B**) A myo-cutaneous flap is depicted. The dotted line represents the usual extent of the craniectomy. (**C**) The dotted line on the dura mater represents our preferred method for opening the dura. Source: Figure by authors.

The dura opens in a C shape, its base running along the sphenoidal ridge. To reduce the risk of harming the protruding brain, the dural incision is made 5–10 mm away from the craniectomy margin. A hemi-craniectomy can be helpful when there is a midline shift and (possible) swelling (e.g., for a SDH with tissue damage). To achieve a sufficient decrease in ICP and reduce the risk of trans-calvarial herniation, the latter of which is linked to brain tissue injuries and cortical venous occlusion at the bone margin, adequate hemi-craniectomies should be performed, and the bone flap should be big enough, with a diameter of at least 11–12 cm antero-posteriorly.

For diffuse (bi-hemispheric) cerebral injuries with intractable intracranial hypertension, bifrontal DC (Figures 24 and 25) is a therapeutic option. A bifrontal DC runs from the anterior cranial fossa floor, posteriorly to the coronal suture and bilaterally to the temporal floor. To permit the brain to expand sufficiently, the dura mater must be opened considerably. The dura is left open with a layer of hemostatic agent, pericranium, or temporalis fascia or closed with dural grafts as well as superior sagittal sinus sectioning or sparing, using various procedures (Bohman and Schuster 2013). The DC must be extended to the floor of the middle cranial fossa in individuals with a temporal lobe contusion or edema producing midbrain compression.

The superior sagittal sinus is divided anteriorly along its attachment to the skull base, and the dura is cut in a C-shaped pattern on each side of the midline (Gooch et al. 2009; Hall 2014; Carney and Ghajar 2007).

Many problems can develop after a decompressive craniotomy, including infection, CSF leaking, and sinking skin flap syndrome (Figure 26).

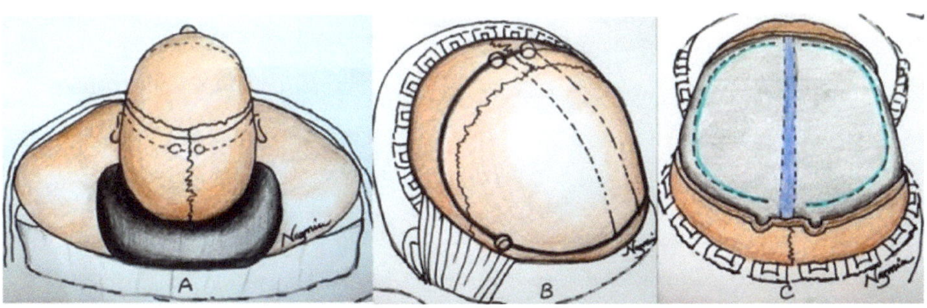

Figure 24. Bifrontal decompressive craniectomy. (**A**) The dotted line represents the usual skin incision made for bifrontal decompressive craniectomy, which should be kept behind the hairline. (**B**) Bi-coronal myo-cutaneous flap is depicted anteriorly. The dotted line on the skull represents the usual extent of a craniectomy. Subtemporal decompression can be seen. (**C**) The bone flap has been removed. The dotted line on the dura mater represents our preferred method for opening the dura. Source: Figure by authors.

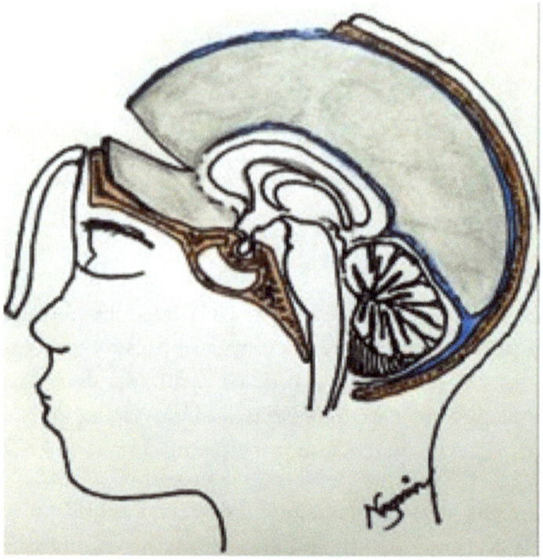

Figure 25. Diagrammatic figure depicting bifrontal decompressive surgery and cutting of falx. Source: Figure by authors.

15.2. Cranioplasty

After a previous DC for TBI or ischemic or hemorrhagic disease or even the excision of cranial tumors, cranialoplasty is a surgical treatment used to reconstruct a cranial vault defect.

Timing of surgery: 1–6 months after decompressive surgery.

Materials used in Cranioplasty:

- Autologous bone graft;
- Titanium (mesh or plate);
- Synthetic substitute of bone (in liquid form);
- Solid biomaterial (customized prefabricated implant matching the appropriate contours as well as shape of the skull) (Gooch et al. 2009; Carney and Ghajar 2007).

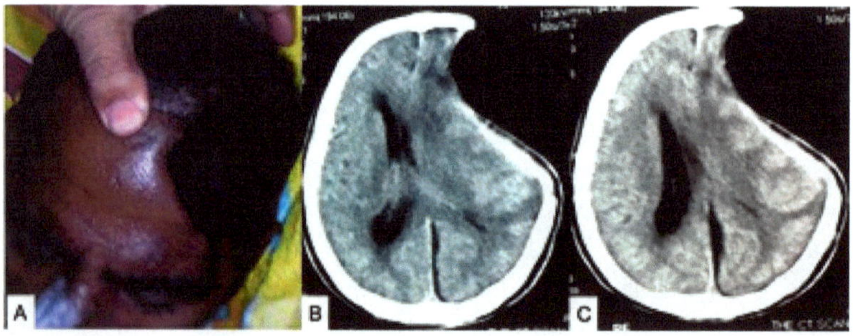

Figure 26. Post-DC sinking skin flap syndrome (SSFS): (**A**) the head of a patient with SSFS; (**B**,**C**) CT scan of the head (axial views) of the patient. Source: Figure by authors.

15.2.1. Procedure

Autologous bone harvested from the abdomen or from a bone bank is laid on the pericranium and fixed using a miniplate and screws or via a custom plate made of titanium or porous plastic (Figures 27 and 28).

First, a CT scan is conducted to measure the defect, and a virtual composite model is created. According to the model, a custom implant that identically matches the shape of the defect of the patient is created. This custom-made implant inserted over the defect through the previous incision or a new incision according to the situation. Implants are secured with the bone adjusted via miniplates or screws. The wound is closed in either single or multiple layers after setting up a subgaleal drain.

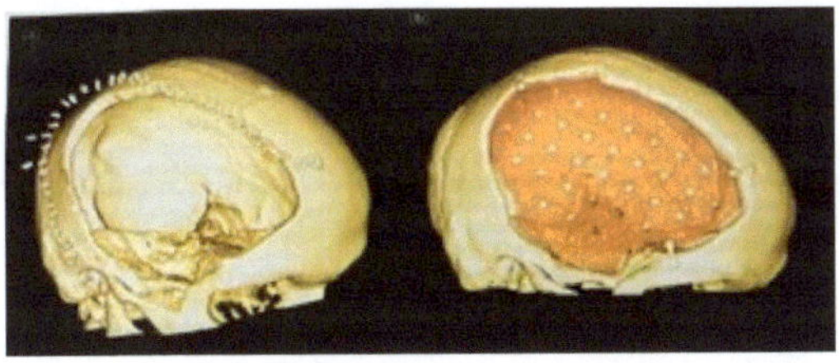

Figure 27. 3-D CT before and after cranioplasty. Source: Figure by authors.

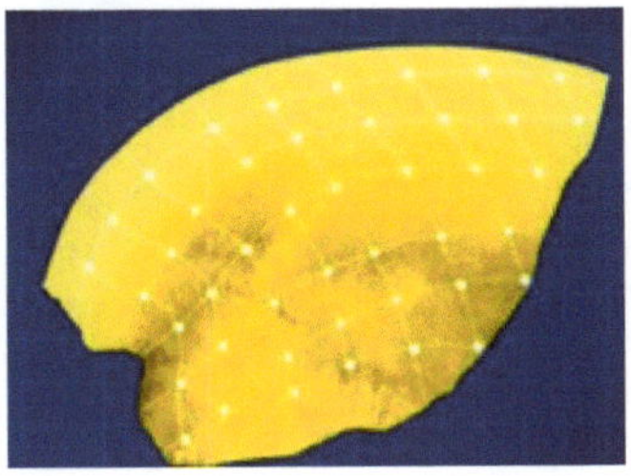

Figure 28. Computer-generated virtual composite. Source: Figure by authors.

15.2.2. Complications of Cranioplasty

- Infection (which may be treated with appropriate antibiotics);
- Postoperative clots needing drainage;
- Wound dehiscence;
- Stroke;
- Seizure;
- DVT and thromboembolism;
- Pneumonia;
- Heart attack;
- Urinary infection.

16. Cerebellar Injury

Cerebellar damage causes sluggish and disorganized motions. When walking, people with cerebellar abnormalities tend to stagger and sway.

Injury to the cerebellum may cause the following symptoms: (1) lack of motor coordination (asynergia), (2) an inability to asses distance and when to stop after indicating a given point to travel towards (dysmetria), (3) an inability to execute fast alternating movements (adiadochokinesia), (4) intention tremors, (5) an ataxic gait, (6) a tendency to fall, (7) hypotonia, and (8) scanning speech and nystagmus.

The fastest recovery happens in the first three months after a moderate TBI, and most people return normal by six months. If an affected individual still has symptoms after 6 months, these symptoms will most likely go away or improve significantly within a year of the incident.

17. Brain Stem Injury

An injury to the brain stem can be catastrophic and deadly.

A brain stem injury can result in dizziness or motor weakness, and more severe forms can cause paralysis, coma, or death.

A brain stem injury can be caused by the following:

1. Stretching of the peduncles;
2. Deceleration against the basi-sphenoid as well as dorsum sellae;
3. Lateral movement of the peduncles against the tentorial margin;
4. Force avulsion of the cranial nerves;
5. Stretching of the brain stem's vascular pedicles.

Brain stem damage can be difficult to recover from, and therapy differs based on the degree of the injury. The initial phase of recuperation is usually started in a hospital or a specialized facility. Physiotherapy can be used to assist a person.

18. Death

According to the Uniform Determination of Death Act proposed in 1981, death is defined as follows:

1. A condition in which circulatory and pulmonary functions are irreversibly lost.
2. Brain death is the irreversible loss of all functioning of the brain. In 1968, the Harvard Medical School Ad Hoc Committee published a definition of brain death or permanent coma as "loss of brain functioning."

18.1. Causes of Death via Head Injury

Head injuries can cause death in the following ways: injury to vital brain centers, such as the posterior hypothalamus, mesencephalon, or medulla oblongata; respiratory failure/paralysis via an uncal or other form of brain herniation caused by a traumatic expanding mass lesion or brain swelling; and other causes, including infection, hypostatic pneumonia, pulmonary embolism, or renal failure.

18.2. Brain Death

The diagnosis of brain death requires three conditions to be met: a persistent coma, no brainstem reflexes, the inability to breath independently.

When a painful stimulus is applied, coma is confirmed. A patient is confirmed to have a coma when he or she does not open their eyes, respond verbally, or move their limbs in reaction to a painful stimulation. During the twentieth century, mechanical breathing and life support technologies allowed patients with serious brain damage to be kept alive in intensive care units (ICUs) for longer periods of time.

It is critical to distinguish brain death from various types of serious brain damage that might result in a vegetative state in which few brain functions are preserved and recovery may take time.

There is no way to reverse the brain stem's permanent loss of function, and even if a ventilator is employed, the heart will eventually stop beating.

18.2.1. Clinical Significance

Before brain death can be determined, certain conditions must be met:

1. There should be evidence of a coma etiology. Confounding disorders, such as severe metabolic, endocrine, and acid–base imbalance, should be ruled out. If a drug overdose is suspected, 5 half-lives of drug clearance should be allowed to pass while adjusting renal and hepatic functioning.
2. The patient's core body temperature should be at least 36 °C.
3. A systolic blood pressure (SBP) of >100 mm of mercury (mmHg) should be observed. Using vasopressors like noradrenaline or dopamine, as well as vasopressin, is a common way to achieve this.

Brain death can be evaluated via clinical tests, the apnea test, and ancillary tests.

I. Physical examination: Physical examination in this case covers the examination of brain stem reflexes and a patient's response to pain.

The administration of painful stimuli to particular locations such as the supraorbital notch, the sternum, and the anterior axillary fold causes a lack of responsiveness to central pain. In brain death, neither eye response nor motor reflexes are detected. It is vital to note that patients with brain death may still have some spinal reflexes.

Reflexes, especially gag reflexes, are lost when the brain dies.

- CN II: Loss of light reflex: pupils should be mid-dilated (4–9 mm) as well as light-insensitive.
- CN III, IV, and VI: Eye motion in response to head movement is lost (doll's eyes).
- CN V and VII: Corneal reflex loss.
- CN VIII: Absence of oculovestibular reflex (Caloric test): The eyes will not migrate toward the irrigated ear when each are irrigated with 60 mL of ice water.
- CN IX: Absence of the gag reflex.
- CN X: Cough reflex loss.

II. Apnea test: This test is positive in case of brain death. When respiratory effort ceases and artificial ventilatory support is temporarily turned off, then $PaCO_2$ levels will rise. The $PaCO_2$ level will be >60 mmHg.

III. Ancillary tests: Ancillary diagnostics for detecting cerebral blood flow stoppage include angiography of the brain; the gold standard for the evaluation of CBF is four-vessel angiography. When there is no blood flow to the brain, this can indicate brain death.

18.2.2. Considerations for and Consequences of Brain Death

Once brain death is diagnosed, the brain is no longer working.

An examination that includes an apnea test is required to diagnose brain death in adults. Recent guidelines, however, advocate two distinct brain death investigations as the minimum norm in youngsters.

If the patient is a probable candidate for organ donation or is pregnant and the decision is made to prolong assistance for the unborn, organ support, with artificial ventilation and drugs to keep normal blood pressure, may be initiated following an announcement of brain dead (Carney and Ghajar 2007).

18.2.3. Vegetative State

In a state of wakefulness, a patient will open their eyes but not react to the external environment. A vegetative patient with a functioning brain stem has the following capacities:

1. Some state of consciousness (awake but not aware);
2. Unassisted normal respiration.

19. Burst Lobe Syndrome

This condition is an intracranial hemorrhage affecting the temporal or frontal lobe, commonly associated with subdural and subarachnoid hemorrhages and contusion (Figure 29). It occurs due to high-energy trauma and results in a high mortality rate.

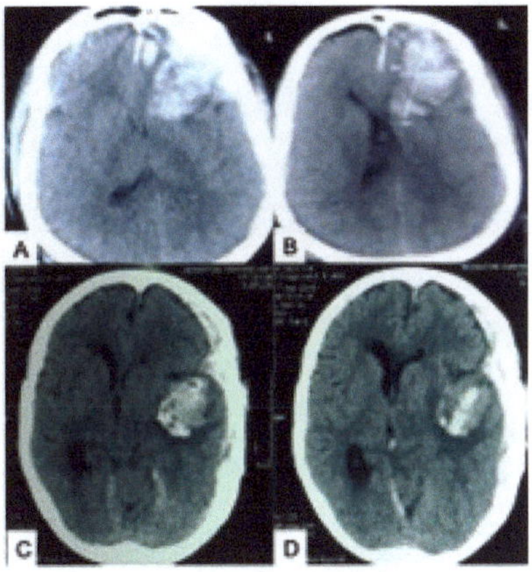

Figure 29. CT scans showing (**A**,**B**) burst frontal lobe; (**C**,**D**) the burst temporal lobe on left side. Source: Figure by authors.

19.1. Kluver–Bucy Syndrome

Kluver–Bucy syndrome is an uncommon behavioral disorder characterized by a bilateral anterior temporal lobe injury. It drives people to put things in their oral cavities and participate in sexual activities that are not appropriate. Visual agnosia (an inability to distinguish objects visually), a lack of typical fear and rage, memory impairment, distractibility, seizures, and dementia are all possible symptoms. Herpes encephalitis may also be linked to this condition (Das and Siddiqui 2021).

19.2. Amnesia Following Head Injury

Post-traumatic amnesia is commonly associated with concussion. Some patients may experience permanent retrograde amnesia. Such patients may make false accusations (Cantu 2001).

20. Penetrating Injury of the Brain

The dura mater is pierced in a penetrating head injury, also known as an open head injury (Mckee and Daneshvar 2015). Penetrating trauma can be produced by high-velocity projectiles (Figures 30 and 31) or low-velocity (Figure 32) items like rods, knives, or bone pieces from a vault bone fracture that penetrates the brain. Penetrating trauma to the head is a medical emergency that can result in permanent impairment or death.

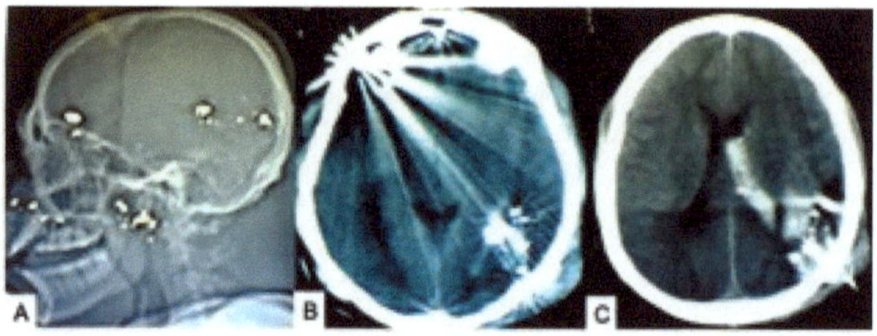

Figure 30. (**A**) X-ray of the skull (lateral view) showing multiple retained bullet fragments in different sites of the head. (**B,C**) CT scan (axial views) showing multiple retained bullet fragments with artifacts and parenchymal and lateral ventricular hemorrhages, respectively. Source: Figure by authors.

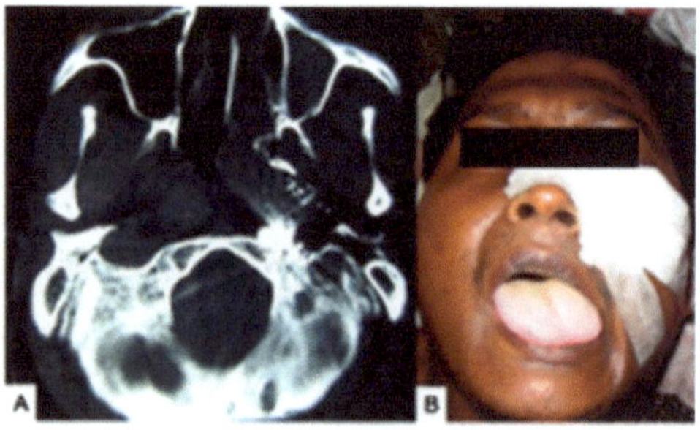

Figure 31. (**A**) CT scan of the head (axial view) (bony window) showing bullet fragments near the left hypoglossal canal that entered through the face. (**B**) Picture of a patient with left hypoglossal palsy. Source: Figure by authors.

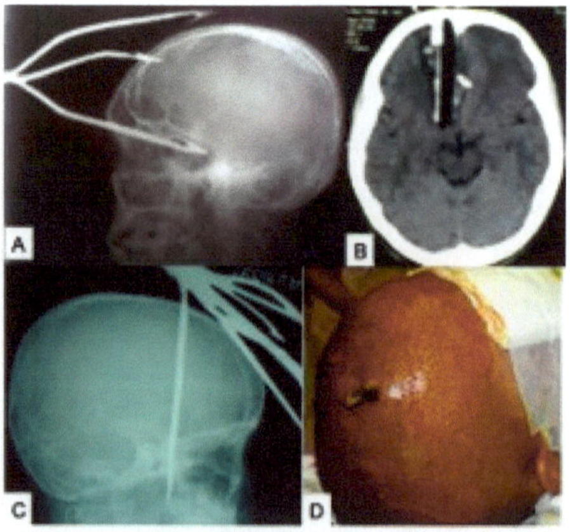

Figure 32. (**A**) X-ray of the head (lateral view) showing penetrating orbitocranial injury caused by a polyspike animal-hunting weapon locally called a 'Teta'. (**B**) CT scan (axial view) of the head showing a penetrating injury caused by a long fragment of wood file. (**C**) Head X-ray (lateral view) showing a penetrating head injury caused by a 'Teta'. (**D**) Painted head of a patient during operation showing a metallic peg nailed into the head by a political rival. Source: Figure by authors.

A penetrating head injury is defined as follows: "A wound where an object passes through the cranium but does not come out." A perforating head injury, on the other hand, occurs when an object moves through the head and comes out through an exit wound (Vinas and Pilitsis 2006). A penetrating brain injury (PBI) is a type of TBI that is a leading cause of death among young people. PBI is the most serious traumatic brain injury and usually counts as all TBIs excluding blunt head injuries (Kim and Gean 2011; van Rein et al. 2019; Kommaraju et al. 2019; Vlček et al. 2018; Cengiz et al. 2019). Penetrating trauma takes place when a foreign instrument pierces the skin, affecting the underlying tissues and leading to an open wound. Such injuries are most commonly caused by gunshots, explosive devices, and stab wounds.

Penetrating injuries can be classified into two categories depending on penetration speed:

- Bullet or shell fragment injuries, direct injury, or shockwave injury to adjacent brain tissue owing to a stretching brain injury are all examples of high-velocity penetration (Figures 30 and 31).
- Low-velocity penetrating injury: Injuries caused by sharp instruments like knives, with direct harm to brain parenchyma, are examples (Figure 32) (Das et al. 2015).
- The following factors influence the outcomes of a penetrating head injury.
- Path and location of intracranial fluid: Injuries wherein intracranial path crosses the midline, moves through the ventricles, or lands in the posterior cranial fossa have a significant mortality rate.
- Energy and velocity of entry: These factors are determined by a weapon or missile's characteristics. This type of injury occurs when energy from an instrument or object is transferred to the skull and the brain parenchyma beneath it. High-velocity projectiles are connected with a high death rate. The square of the velocity determines the kinetic energy involved. Three types of injury mechanisms have been identified.
- Primary injuries happen right away. Secondary brain trauma occurs after an initial injury. The breadth and severity of secondary brain injury have an impact on the final neurologic outcome. As a result, the primary priority in the emergency room is to deter or ameliorate disorders like hypotension, hypoxia, anemia, and hyperpyrexia, which can all exacerbate outcomes.

Certain elements play a role in making vital decisions and have prognostic significance. The following are some examples:

- Wounds at the entry and exit points;
- Intracranial fragments;
- The link between a missile's trajectory and cerebral vessel and air-filled skull base structures;
- The presence of air inside the cranial cavity.

20.1. Management of Penetrating Injuries

Medical and surgical treatment are required for patients who have suffered a penetrating head injury (Maragkos et al. 2018; McGrew et al. 2018; Milton et al. 2017; Elias et al. 2007).

20.1.1. Emergency Medical Management

In cases of penetrating head trauma, neurosurgical consultation is warranted, as many patients with a significant head injury will almost certainly need surgery.

Patient management should be conducted in accordance with ATLS guidelines. In the emergency department, one should not remove any piercing weapons from the skull until a trauma and neurosurgery examination has been conducted. In order to avoid further harm, the external part of the weapon should be stabilized and rendered immobile throughout the patient's transportation.

Conditions where endotracheal intubation is necessary:

- Inability to maintain proper ventilation;
- An insecure airway due to a low level of consciousness;
- Injury to the neck or pharynx.

20.1.2. Surgical Management

The presence of a hematoma is a common reason for conducting a neurosurgical procedure. Large hematomas should be evacuated without delay. Early decompression and cautious brain debridement may be required. In most circumstances, removing a deeply lodged bullet is not necessary. However, there are certain indications that it should be removed. These are the following:

- When there is an injury to the pterion, orbit, or posterior fossa that penetrates the skin;

- When an intracranial hematoma is present;
- When a pseudoaneurysm is present during the initial examination.

For low-velocity missile injuries in which the weapon is still inside the skull in situ, a craniotomy is required. For those who survive the initial damage, some crucial elements can influence the result; these patients rely on rapid as well as early neurosurgical operation, including the capacity to provide a standard level of care in the neurocritical care unit.

20.2. Gunshot Injury to the Head

Due to an increase in gang violence and general homicide rates, in many urban locations across the United States, gunshot injuries to the head are a prominent cause of TBI. Suicide and unintended accidents are two other examples. Suicide-related gunshot injuries to the head have a high death rate and are associated with substantial morbidity among survivors. Individuals who suffer TBIs as a result of self-inflicted gunshot injuries have a higher risk of death as well as a poorer prognosis than those who suffer TBIs as a result of accidental or intentional gunshot wounds (Vlček et al. 2018; UCLA Health 2021; Chotai and Than 2021).

A penetrating wound is defined as one in which the bullet penetrates but does not exit the cranium. A perforating wound occurs when a bullet enters and exits the cranium at the same time. When a projectile passes through the brain, it causes harm due to both direct penetration and the spread of a pressure wave from a high-velocity bullet going through brain tissue (greater than 2000 feet per second) (Chotai and Than 2021). Brain swelling is caused by both bleeding and damage caused by this pressure wave, and it can lead to death.

The severity of damage dealt by a gunshot wound depends on certain factors, such as the gun's caliber, the bullet's size and speed, and the trajectory and location of the injury. As it passes through the brain tissue or vascular structures, a bullet from a gunshot wound to the right frontal pole, located well above the skull base, seems to result in only modest clinical damage. A bullet traveling in a caudal direction from the left frontal pole into the temporal lobe and brainstem, on the other hand, would be fatal because it would pierce the eloquent cerebral parenchyma and injure key vascular structures within the cranial cavity. A bullet directed into vital intracranial vessels can cause a quickly developing blood clot in the brain, compressing crucial brain tissue and leading to immediate death. If the sufferer survives the initial phase, the main confounding situation is increased intracranial pressure (Chotai and Than 2021).

20.2.1. Surgical Treatment

Patients with a gunshot injury to the head should promptly and vigorously be resuscitated when they arrive at the hospital. An immediate CT scan should be conducted if blood pressure and oxygenation are satisfactory. The following considerations guide decisions regarding the surgical treatment of a gunshot wound:

- The spectrum of brainstem function;
- The CT scan findings of head;
- The LOC: According to the Glasgow Coma Scale (GCS), scored from 1 to 15, a patient with a score < 7 or 8 is deemed to be in coma (Chotai and Than 2021).

A fatal end-result is almost inevitable if individuals are in a severe coma with minimal indications of brainstem function as well as no signs of an intracranial hemorrhage. If a CT scan confirms a hematoma, an emergency craniotomy may be performed to remove the clot, debris, and devitalized tissue. Because pressure inside the skull is widespread, a decompressive craniectomy is often performed (Chotai and Than 2021).

20.2.2. Outcomes

Patients with long bullet tracks crossing the deep midline tissues of the cerebrum or brain stem have a poor prognosis. A gunshot that hits the brain's right cerebrum may produce motor and sensory deficiencies on the left side, and vice versa. The control of several tasks such as cognitive functions, speech, memory, and vision are carried out by both cerebral hemispheres. As a result, depending on which lobes of the brain are affected, a person's ability to execute specific activities may be limited (Chotai and Than 2021).

Because each hemisphere is separated into four lobes, a more superficial injury restricted to one hemisphere and one lobe is the "best-case scenario", minimizing the functional losses caused by the trauma. The acute and critical-care stages correspond to the first 1–14 days. The amount of tissue damage, the degree of edema, the pressure inside the brain during the early stage, and the functional extension of the lesion all influence the extent and speed of recovery after an injury. To assist a survivor's functional restoration or adaptation to persistent disabilities, intensive neurorehabilitation may be employed. Recovery from a neurological condition might take anywhere from months to years (Chotai and Than 2021) (Box 1).

Box 1. Factors influencing initial gunshot injuries and outcomes (Chotai and Than 2021; Aarabi et al. 2014).

- The location of the entry and/or exit wound
- The site of the brain injury
- The bullet's fragmentation level
- Bullet caliber and weapon type—high velocity or low velocity
- The shooting range (distance between the gun and the victim)
- The time gap between the infliction of the gunshot wound and beginning of treatment
- The age and overall health status of the patient
- The initial GCS score
- Pupil status (dilation and reactivity)
- The state of the brainstem function and reflexes
- High blood pressure
- The state of oxygenation immediately after the trauma.

21. Pneumocephalus and Tension Pneumocephalus

21.1. Pneumocephalus

Pneumocephalus (Figure 33) is most commonly related to skull disruption, such as incidents following facial and head injury, skull base tumors, otorhinolaryngological surgery, or neurosurgery and, on rare occasions, incidents occurring spontaneously. It can also occur while scuba diving, though this is quite uncommon. Pneumocephalus has also been linked to neurosurgery techniques like deep-brain stimulation, which, while ostensibly safe for the patient, might result in brain displacement and consequent stereotactic inaccuracy (Elias et al. 2007; Sharim et al. 2015). Neurosurgeons strive to limit pneumocephalus volume and, as a result, brain shift during an operation.

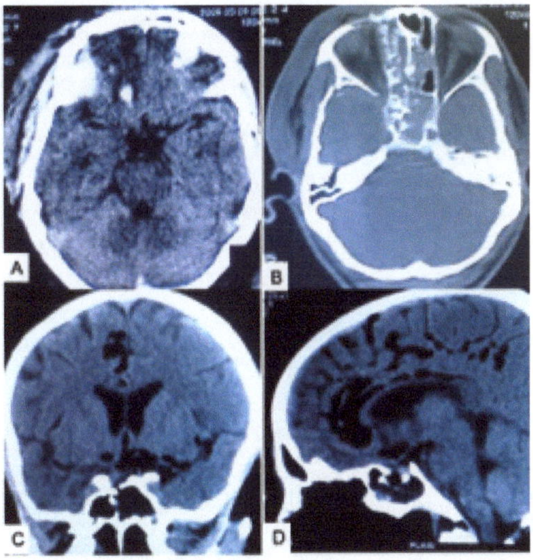

Figure 33. (**A**,**B**) CT scan of the head (axial views) following RTA showing right-side skull base fractures with right frontal contusion. (**C**,**D**) CT scans on the 24th day following RTA (at which point the patient developed CSF rhinorrhea), with coronal and sagittal views, respectively, showing sellar bony gap with pneumocephalus. Source: Figure by authors.

21.2. Tension Pneumocephalus (TP)

Tension pneumocephalus (Figure 34) is a neurosurgical emergency that happens when subdural air creates a pressure effect on the surrounding brain parenchyma, usually as a result of a ball valve system failure that permits air to enter the subdural region only one way. During the early postoperative phase, clinical imaging of neurosurgical patients frequently reveals postsurgical pneumocephalus. The distinction between uncomplicated and tension pneumocephalus is critical in clinical practice since the latter is a neurological emergency. To confidently arrive at an accurate diagnosis, an understanding of the imaging findings regarding tension pneumocephalus and a strong index of suspicion are essential. It is a rare but life-threatening neurosurgical emergency that can happen after head trauma (especially if there are skull base or air sinus fractures), extradural injections, or complicated neurosurgical, spinal, air sinus, or craniofacial surgeries (Simmons and Luks 2013; Sweni et al. 2013; Ishiwata et al. 1988; Monas and Peak 2010). Because the symptoms and signs of TP are not specific, its detection should be carried out by recognizing the characteristic imaging signals of TP as soon as possible, allowing for life-saving emergency decompression (Simmons and Luks 2013; Monas and Peak 2010).

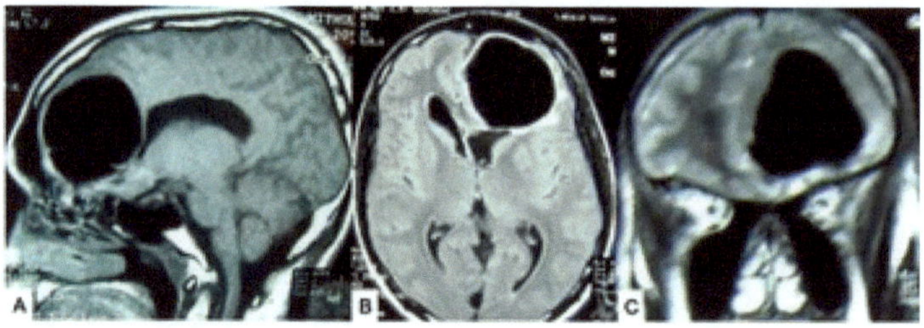

Figure 34. MRI of the brain (**A–C**) (sagittal, axial, and coronal views, respectively) showing tension pneumocephalus with mass effect that requires surgical decompression (through burr hole). Source: Figure by authors.

21.2.1. Clinical Presentation of TP

Tension pneumocephalus manifests itself in a variety of ways:

- Agitation;
- Deterioration of consciousness;
- Specific neurological impairments;
- Cardiac arrest.

There are several etiologies of this condition:

- Recent neurosurgery;
- Trauma with cerebrospinal fluid leaks;
- Infections of the paranasal air sinuses;
- Tumors in the paranasal air sinuses;
- The use of NO (nitrous oxide) as a local anesthetic.

21.2.2. Investigations

A plain X-ray can identify pneumocephalus, but a CT scan or MRI of the brain can identify pneumocephalus along with possible causes and sites of air entry (Figures 33 and 34).

21.2.3. Treatment

Post-traumatic or post-surgery pneumocephalus resolves spontaneously. Tension pneumocephalus requires urgent surgical decompression with treatment of the cause (Figure 34). Pneumocephalus with a spontaneous CSF fistula requires urgent fistula closure.

22. Vascular Injury to the Cranium

Blunt as well as penetrating wounds to the base of the skull might cause vascular damage. In 8.5% of instances, blunt base-of-skull fractures were shown to be linked to neurovascular damage (Feiz-Erfan et al. 2007). A clival fracture and fracture of 'the sellae turcica-sphenoid air sinus complex', in particular, have been linked to vascular damage.

The following are the most common vascular injuries related to head trauma:

- Aneurysms caused by trauma;
- Carotid-cavernous fistulas (CCF) (Figure 35);

- Post-traumatic (arteriovenous) AV fistulas, which are rarely arterial and generally relate to the venous sinuses such as the SSS (the superior sagittal sinus) or lateral sinuses.

Neurovascular injuries can be caused by blunt trauma to the neck, chest, or head that can injure the vessels perfusing the brain; these injuries can be caused by the following:

- Pressure or forceful compression from a seat belt during an MVA;
- Sudden violent movements (such as flexion and extension of the neck) that may occur during an MVA when a vehicle decelerates/accelerates (whiplash injury).

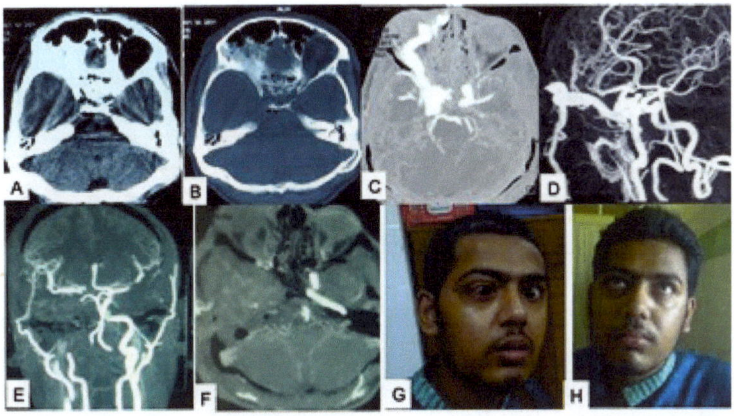

Figure 35. (**A**,**B**) CT scan of head (axial views) showing skull base fractures in sellar and parasellar zones after RTA. (**C**,**D**) CTA of head 3 months after RTA showing rightside high flow CCF. (**E**,**F**) Early postoperative CTA following right STA-MCA bypass occlusion of right ICA in Glasscock triangle (where CCF and right ICA are not seen). (**G**) Photograph of the patient three months after RTA showing ocular clinical features of right CCF. (**H**) Patient three months after microsurgical treatment of CCF. Source: Figure by authors, used with patient's consent.

22.1. Diagnosis

A CT scan and CTA are generally utilized for diagnosing traumatic vascular damage. Catheter angiography is conducted if a vascular injury is suspected but not conclusively seen via CTA. Cerebral DSA is carried out in an angiography suite in a hospital. An arterial catheter is introduced into the artery through the groin, and contrast is injected into the arteries directly, allowing the abnormality to be seen more clearly in the images taken. An MRI of the brain or spine of a patient who has suffered a stroke may be performed in some conditions to assess the patient's spine or brain, and this may also reveal blood vessel injuries.

High-energy injuries have a higher risk of vascular damage, and high-energy blunt trauma is associated with a higher chance of amputation. Damage to nearby tissues and structures may necessitate a one-time intervention or, in the case of severe polytrauma, a multidisciplinary treatment incorporating advanced life support techniques. Irreversible alterations of the neurological and musculoskeletal systems are generally observed after 6 h of limb ischemia, albeit the exact start time must be determined. If the ischemia process is iatrogenic, the time can be calculated from the time when blood flow was interrupted (e.g., pressure dressing, tourniquet).

22.2. Medical Examination

Due to a significant mortality risk in the case of a misdiagnosis, the decision to perform early surgery, particularly when a substantial hemorrhage is obvious, is critical within the first minutes of assessment. With a sensitivity of over 90%, most patients with "hard signals" of vascular injury need prompt surgery; on the contrary, if no "hard sign" is observed, the risk of vascular injury is low (Cheaito et al. 2016).

An algorithm for managing patients with vascular injury to the cranium (like a vascular injury of any other part of the body) is shown below (Figure 36).

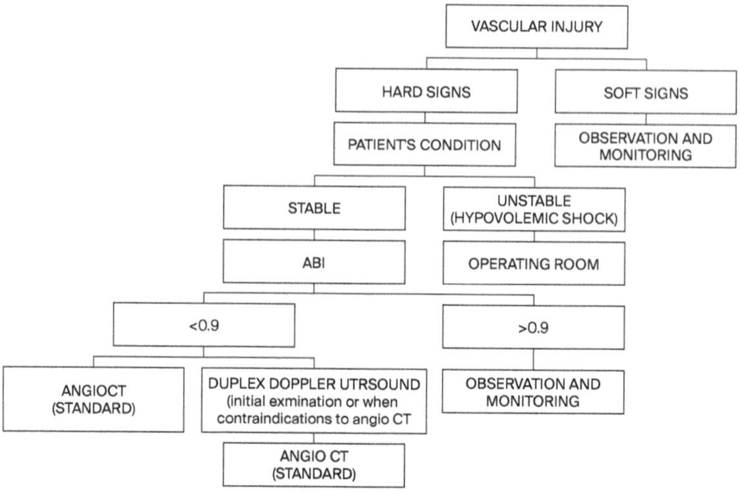

Figure 36. An algorithm for managing patients with vascular injury to the cranium. ABI—ankle–brachial pressure index. Source: Authors' compilation based on data from Krzysztof et al. (2019).

Vascular injuries are uncommon, yet they are among the most serious and complex situations for medical experts to correctly evaluate and treat. The fast development of minimally invasive procedures in numerous neurology departments has increased the extent of iatrogenic vascular damage that can be accounted for. Iatrogenic injuries are common, despite their rarity, as a result of the larger number of minimally invasive operations that require the assistance of a vascular surgeon.

22.3. Treatment

The type of treatment to be applied is determined by the degree of damage. Minor injuries are carefully monitored, and a patient may be prescribed blood thinners to prevent a thrombus from developing as well as detaching and spreading to the cerebrum. A stent can be put endovascularly into an injured artery in more severe cases to keep it open and prevent it from becoming obstructed. The artery may need to be repaired surgically in some cases.

22.4. Dissection of Arteries and Pseudoaneurysm

Dissection of the carotid as well as vertebral arteries is a major cause of stroke in young people, causing up to 25% of strokes in this population (Schievink 2001). Intracranial and extracranial dissections are both possible, with the latter being the more prevalent. These can happen on their own, be linked to certain medical illnesses such as connective tissue diseases (Ehlers–Danlos syndrome, fibromuscular dysplasia, and Marfan syndromes), or happen as a result of a traumatic incident. Carotid and vertebral artery dissections can cause aneurysmal expansions at the dissection site, particularly in the event of subadventitial dissections (Boström and Liliequist 1967). Dissecting pseudoaneurysms are the most common type of pseudoaneurysm. The percentage of dissections that result in pseudoaneurysm development has been observed to range between 5% and 40% (Guillon et al. 1999). They may be fusiform or saccular, and their appearance varies depending on where they are found (Touzé et al. 2001). They can be seen as a sudden occurrence or as a result of a follow-up angiography (MRA/CTA/DSA) (Levy et al. 1994; Nguyen Bui et al. 1993; Provenzale 1995). Because pseudoaneurysms have the potential to develop and become symptomatic.

Management techniques for dissections with associated pseudoaneurysms are not well defined, with some authors claiming that these aneurysmal structures are benign and thus only require medical management with antiplatelet or anticoagulation agents, while others advocate using endovascular or surgical interventions to avoid aneurysm rupture or thrombus formation (Provenzale 1995 Dennis et al. 2012; Holle et al. 2009). Stenting is the most frequently utilized endovascular intervention, with data in the literature progressively supporting its safety and efficacy.

The majority of dissecting pseudoaneurysms will not develop clinical features or exhibit expansion in a follow-up. For dissecting pseudoaneurysms, medical/conservative treatment may be adequate as an initial management strategy. Stenting or other endovascular techniques can safely treat the a few cases of pseudoaneurysms that grow and produce symptoms. Aneurysm site and size, smoking history, and hyperlipidemia are all important influencers of the progression as well as treatment of these conditions.

22.5. *Carotid-Cavernous Fistula (CCF) and AV Fistula*

A CCF is aberrant communication between the carotid artery and/or its branches as well as the cavernous sinus, a major vein. The cavernous sinus (CS) receives blood from the brain, orbit, and pituitary gland and is located behind the eye. A CCF can be either direct (high-flow) (Figure 35) or spontaneous (indirect/low-flow). A CCF can occur due to trauma or spontaneously. A traumatic CCF can arise when the intracavernous carotid artery is ruptured due to a head injury. Injuries ranging from minor falls to severe piercing wounds can cause head trauma. Endovascular treatment can also cause traumatic CCFs. A ruptured cavernous carotid aneurysm is the commonest etiology of spontaneous CCFs; these fistulas, on the other hand, can be congenital arteriovenous connections that occur spontaneously in the presence of collagen vascular disease, atherosclerosis, or hypertension.

22.5.1. Clinical Features

In the days and weeks after a close head trauma, the development of a direct CCF is common. Chemosis, pulsatile proptosis, and ocular bruit are the traditional trifecta that patients exhibit (including blood flow sounds coming from the eye). These fistulas can cause proptosis, diplopia, and vision loss (Figure 35).

The onset of an indirect CCF is usually gradual, with a milder appearance. They do not always exhibit the usual triad of symptoms. Because of the convoluted arterialization of the conjunctiva, patients with a CCF frequently have chronic red eyes. Often, an ocular bruit goes unnoticed.

22.5.2. Treatment

Microvascular neurosurgery or endovascular methods can be used to treat CCFs. Because of the decreased morbidity and mortality, an endovascular method is preferable. However, all CCFs are not susceptible to both types of management.

Endovascular Treatment

Traditional treatment for direct CCFs has involved occlusion of the fistula with deployment of detachable balloons transarterially while preserving the ICA (internal carotid artery). Due to the lack of disposable balloons, further treatment options include a covered stent and transarterial fistula coiling with stent support to keep the ICA open. A transvenous method utilizing platinum coils may be indicated if a transarterial route is impractical or ineffective. This can be carried out either surgically through the superior ophthalmic vein or through the femoral route through the inferior petrosal sinus.

Indirect CCFs can sometimes spontaneously resolve. In low-risk CCFs, manual carotid compression may be undertaken, as it can cure about 30% of fistulas. Compression is not recommended for patients with retrograde cortical venous system filling because of the danger of a cerebral hemorrhage. Either a transarterial or transvenous technique should be used to treat these patients.

Surgical Treatment

CCFs are surgically treated using a craniotomy and surgical clips occluding the ICA distal as well as proximal to the CCF site. The venous outflow is subsequently stopped by packing the cavernous sinus with acrylate glue, fascia, or Surgicel. To prevent a stroke, based up on the cerebral blood flow, a branch of the external carotid artery (ECA) may need to be connected to the MCA (middle cerebral artery), i.e., EC-IC bypass (Figure 35).

22.6. *Traumatic Scalp AV Fistula*

AVFs of the scalp are quite uncommon and mainly occur due to severe injuries to the superficial scalp veins. Car accidents, penetrating trauma from sharp weapon attacks, diving accidents, and iatrogenic causes such as punch-graft hair transplantation and temporomandibular joint arthroscopic surgery are all examples of insults that might cause this. Single case reports (Davis and Nelson 1997; Dogan et al. 2008; Fukuta et al. 1994; Lanzieri et al. 1985; Mathis et al. 1994) constitute the majority of the literature on scalp AVF after hair transplantation. Surgical ligation and excision, selective angiography, and embolization and direct-puncture embolization have all been effective in treating these lesions, with full recuperation in 100% of cases and no documented complications as of yet. Polyvinyl alcohol microparticles, absolute alcohol, coils, acrylic glue, and Onyx material all have been used to successfully embolize scalp AVF (Mathis et al. 1994). Traumatic scalp AVF (Figure 37) is a rare vascular disease in which the high-flow arterial as well as low-flow venous systems communicate (Badejo and Rockwood 1987; Li et al. 2007). There is no capillary bed between the scalp's arterial feeding vessels and the draining veins; therefore, there is a direct connection (Badejo and Rockwood 1987). It manifests as a disfiguring pulsatile swelling with a wide range of clinical symptoms, including local discomfort, headaches, bruits, tinnitus, hemorrhage, epilepsy, and scalp necrosis (Mohanty and Rao 1976).

Open surgical excision (Figure 37), obstruction of the feeding arteries, trans-arterial or trans-venous embolization, and intralesional sclerosant injection all have been used to treat these patients (Badejo and Rockwood 1987).

Hair transplantation treatments, while generally low-risk, can occasionally result in arteriovenous fistulas in the scalp. In the ultimate treatment of these lesions, both open surgical as well as endovascular treatments are often safe and effective. When deciding on the best treatment technique, pay close attention to the anatomy of the fistula. Its appearance after the intervention should also be taken into account.

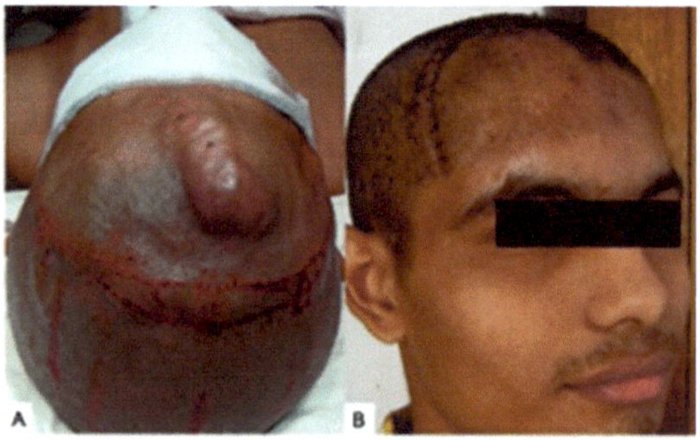

Figure 37. (**A**) Perioperative picture of patient with frontal scalp AV fistula that developed after blunt scalp injury. (**B**) The patient without an AV fistula following an operation. Source: Photos by authors.

22.6.1. Prognosis and Treatment

If left untreated, patients may develop cosmetic flaws. Endovascular occlusion, surgical resection, or direct injection of sclerosing agents are all alternative treatments.

23. Cranial Nerves Injury

Injuries to the cranial nerve (CN) can range from minor annoyances to life-threatening complications. Practitioners in a variety of specialties, including neurosurgery, otolaryngological surgery, head–neck surgery, ophthalmological surgery, oral and maxillofacial surgery, neurology, and general surgery, may encounter patients who may be at risk for these injuries. As a result, anatomic principles, proper history taking, clinical examination, and diagnostic evaluation are all significant components of their professions.

23.1. Facial Nerve Injury

Facial nerve damage has a wide range of consequences that have a substantial influence on one's quality of life. The facial nerve is one of the most frequently injured CNs, and a damaged nerve has a critical impact on various physiologic functions such as tear secretion, saliva secretion, and shutting of the eyelids. Furthermore, the spectacular disfigurement resulting from damage may have social and psychological consequences, making the prevention of iatrogenic nerve injury critical. Therapeutic improvements in recent years have boosted both medicinal and surgical therapeutic options for treating disfigurements, though the surgical option may play an essentially increasing role in the management of iatrogenic nerve injuries.

23.1.1. Traumatic Facial Nerve Injuries

Clinically, the major etiology of seventh-nerve damage is traumatic temporal bone fractures. There are numerous approaches for arranging temporal bone fractures when looking at relevant clinical circumstances. The classification of temporal bone fractures as transverse or longitudinal is one useful paradigm for determining the possibility of seventh-nerve damage. This classification is based on whether the temporal fracture is parallel to the petrous pyramid's long axis. Longitudinal fractures are significantly more common, accounting for 75–95% of all fractures. Only about one-fourth of these injuries result in seventh-nerve impairments. When the nerve is affected, the cause is usually local inflammation, edema, and compression. Transverse fractures, on the other hand, though being significantly less common, have a greater frequency of related seventh-nerve injury, which occurs in almost 50% of cases (Hasso and Ledington 1988). These types of facial nerve damage seem to result in nerve transection and frequently involve occipital damage. Aside from temporal bone fractures, additional common etiologies of traumatic seventh-nerve injury include direct intratemporal fossa injury from penetrating/gunshot wounds as well as extratemporal wounds from a variety of sources.

23.1.2. Surgical Facial Nerve Injury

The occurrence of iatrogenic seventh-nerve injury, especially during tympanic cavity surgery, is quite rare. When it comes to extratemporal injury, parotidectomy is the most common cause. If negative margins cannot be established, malignant tumors, especially those encasing the facial nerve, necessitate the deliberate sacrifice of the seventh nerve. Nerve transection discovered during surgery, whether deliberate or unintentional, should be corrected immediately. Local edema, trauma, nerve manipulation, or still-active local anesthetics are the most common causes of postprocedural facial palsy, even when a surgeon is confident that the nerve is safe.

23.2. Olfactory Nerve Injury

The olfactory nerve is a special sensory nerve that is responsible for olfaction. People who have olfactory nerve dysfunction live a life with lower quality (Svider et al. 2014). Dysgeusia is caused by a distorted or nonexistent sense of olfaction, which makes it difficult to enjoy a meal. The diminished ability to perceive toxic smoke or an adjacent fire is a potentially life-threatening matter for persons with olfactory impairment. In such circumstances, a lack of early diagnosis may result in injuries or fatalities that may have been otherwise avoided.

23.3. Other Cranial Nerves Injuries

Though rare, any cranial nerve can be affected by a traumatic brain injury, especially penetrating injuries (Figure 31). But postsurgical paralysis of cranial (any) nerves is quite common and is conducted according to the approach, the site, and the nature of the pathology.

23.4. Medicolegal Aspects of Cranial Nerve Injury

Iatrogenic cranial nerve injuries may be a possible issue for malpractice since the aforementioned ailments have severe consequences for basic activities connected with sustaining a positive and good quality of life. Malpractice litigation has increased exponentially in the last 30 years, resulting in higher malpractice insurance costs and the exercise of defensive medicine (Brenner and Smith 2004). These developments, in combination with other variables, have attributed to increased healthcare expenses in the US. As a result, practicing surgeons may find it beneficial to learn the fundamental principles and rules of CN injury litigation, particularly for application in preoperative counselling as well as the informed consent process.

24. Traumatic CSF Rhinorrhea and Otorrhea

CSF rhinorrhea or otorrhea indicates that the subarachnoid space is open to the nasal cavity or tympanomastoid cavities. Because such a conection poses a serious risk of intracranial infection, the disease must be appropriately recognized, and the link must be closed. The identification and localization of a CSF leak can be difficult at times. There are also some widespread misconceptions about the utility and precise role of positive contrast computed tomographic cisternography. When there is direct discussion about the exact task being asked of the diagnostic procedure, the interdisciplinary team performs well. The best therapy options for patients will come from effective communication and focused imaging.

CSF leaks can be classified as either acquired or congenital. Trauma, frequently with fractures that result in a dural defect; surgical leaks; infections; and benign or malignant neoplasms are all acquired causes. The most common causes of congenital CSF leaks include developmental bone communication channels and accompanying dural deficits, as well as more serious developmental anomalies such as meningoencephaloceles and inner-ear dysplasia. CSF rhinorrhea is caused by the breach of the partitions that separate the subarachnoid space from the nasal cavity and/or paranasal sinuses. The most prevalent cause of CSF rhinorrhea from the anterior cranial fossa is head trauma, followed by endoscopic sinus surgery (ESS) or more extensive sinonasal operational procedures. A CSF fistula after ESS is thought to occur in less than 1% of cases. Conditions that raise ventricular pressure may have a role in the development of CSF fistulas. Congenital conditions such as developmental meningoencephaloceles, arachnoid granulations, or simply developmental areas of larger-than-normal bone abnormalities can cause CSF fistula. CSF rhinorrhea is a term used to describe an unusually fluid, unilateral nasal discharge caused by CSF leaks. It may also be detected during a search for a cause of meningitis, particularly recurring meningitis caused by bacteria with a nasal origin.

CSF leaks are caused by an osteodural defect that creates an improper connection between the CSF space and the neighboring paranasal air sinus or tympano-mastoid cavity, causing CSF rhinorrhea or otorrhea (Lloyd et al. 2008). The extension of infection from the sinonasal cavity puts affected individuals at risk of meningitis, the prevalence of which can be as high as 19–50% in individuals with persistent leakage (Daudia et al. 2007; Aarabi and Leibrock 1992). In spite of advances in drug treatment, the increasing risk of life-threatening consequences underlines the importance of early diagnosis, the correct dentification of the leak's location, and the execution of quick action to prevent morbidity. Endonasal endoscopic surgery for CSF rhinorrheas has become the standard of therapy due to its higher success rate as well as lower morbidity analogous to transcranial procedures (Zweig et al. 2002). Neuroimaging is important in the preoperative workup because it helps to pinpoint the location of the leak and determine the exact size of the osteodural gap. It also assists in endoscopic repair by promoting real-time anatomical neuro-navigation utilizing multiplanar imaging as well as endoscopic views, allowing the operating neurosurgeon to avoid critical structures (Kacker et al. 2005). CSF leaks are easier to diagnose when imaging is used.

25. Post-Head-Injury Syndromes

Post-traumatic brain injury syndrome (PHIS) is a symptom complex that consists of dizziness, headache, cognitive impairment, and neuropsychiatric symptoms and is a common complication of TBI. Mild TBI can happen when the head is struck, when the head hits an item, or when the brain accelerates or decelerates without any external trauma to the head.

It is divisive, particularly in its extended form. The clinical features are hazy, subjective, and widespread among different people. The patient population is diverse, with varying degrees of head as well as brain trauma.

The features of individual patients may influence how the injury manifests. The pathology that underpins this condition is unknown. Test abnormalities may or may not be present, and when they are, they are not consistent with a clear pattern.

- A loss of consciousness lasting <30 min is considered a mild head injury/concussion.
- PTA (post-traumatic amnesia) is a type of amnesia that lasts less than 24 h after a distressing event has taken place (this is a period wherein people are confused, act strangely, and are unable to remember what has just happened)

It is important that only around 10% of reported minor head injuries/concussions result in loss of consciousness, so do not rely on this as a sole indicator (Dean et al. 2012).

25.1. Symptoms of Concussion

In people who have suffered a moderate head injury, the symptoms of concussion include headache, irritability, difficulty concentrating, dizziness, confusion, nausea, a difficulty processing or memorizing information, light sensitivity, and vision distortion.

Following a minor head injury, there is a small possibility for the development of problems that may demand emergency care in the early stages.

Concussion symptoms usually go away after a few days or a few weeks, but some people may suffer from these symptoms for a much longer period. A symptom group known as "post-concussion syndrome" persists after a mild head injury or concussion (Dean et al. 2012).

25.2. Management of Concussion

While there is no one-size-fits-all treatment for concussion, most people recover effectively with good medical care, plenty of rest, and professional assistance, as needed.

Family members and employers must be notified of the potential implications of a mild head injury/concussion, and suitable measures must be established. These could include not rushing returning to work, limiting short-term stress, and avoiding alcohol (Dean et al. 2012).

Author Contributions: Conceptualization, methodology, validation, formal analysis, investigation, resources, data curation, S.A., M.M.R. and M.H.S.; writing—original draft preparation, S.A. and M.M.R.; writing—review and editing, F.H.C.; visualization, supervision, N.A. and F.H.C. All authors have read and agreed to the published version of the manuscript.

Funding: This research received no external funding.

Conflicts of Interest: The authors declare no conflicts of interest.

References

Aarabi, Bizhan, Babak Tofighi, Joseph A. Kufera, Jeffery Hadley, Edward S. Ahn, Camell Cooper, Jacek M. Malik, Neal J. Naff, Louis Chang, Michael Radley, and et al. 2014. Predictors of outcome in civilian gunshot wounds to the head. *Journal of Neurosurgery* 120: 1138–46. [CrossRef] [PubMed]

Aarabi, Bizhan, and L. G. Leibrock. 1992. Neurosurgical approaches to cerebrospinal fluid rhinorrhea. *Ear, Nose & Throat Journal* 71: 300–305.

Andrews, Charles M., Edward C. Jauch, J. Claude Hemphill, III, Wade S. Smith, and Scott D. Weingart. 2012. Emergency neurological life support: Intracerebral hemorrhage. *Neurocrit Care* 17: S37–S46. [CrossRef] [PubMed]

Badejo, Leke, and Peter Rockwood. 1987. Traumatic arteriovenous fistula of the scalp: Case report. *Journal of Neurosurgery* 66: 773–74. [CrossRef]

Badjatia, Neeraj, Nancy Carney, Todd J. Crocco, Mary E. Fallat, Halim M. A. Hennes, Andrew S. Jagoda, Sarah Jernigan, Peter B. Letarte, E. Brooke Lerner, Thomas M. Moriarty, and et al. 2008. Guidelines for Prehospital Management of Traumatic Brain Injury 2nd Edition. *Prehospital Emergency Care* 12: S1–S52. [CrossRef]

Bishokarma, Suresh. 2018. Head Injury AKA Traumatic Brain Injury. Available online: https://www.slideshare.net/slideshow/head-injury-aka-traumatic-brain-injury/91707862 (accessed on 15 March 2022).

Bohman, Leif-Erik, and James M. Schuster. 2013. Decompressive Craniectomy for Management of Traumatic Brain Injury: An Update. *Current Neurology and Neuroscience Reports* 13: 1–8. [CrossRef] [PubMed]

Boström, Kerstin, and Bengt Liliequist. 1967. Primary dissecting aneurysm of the extracranial part of the internal carotid and vertebral arteries. A report of three cases. *Neurology* 17: 179–86. [CrossRef]

Brain Trauma Foundation, American Association of Neurological Surgeons, and Congress of Neurological Surgeons. 2008. Erratum: Guidelines for the management of severe traumatic brain injury. *Journal of Neurotrauma* 24: S1–106. [CrossRef]

Brenner, R. James, and John J. Smith. 2004. The malpractice liability crisis. *Journal of the American College of Radiology* 1: 18–22. [CrossRef]

Bullock, M. Ross, Randall Chesnut, Jamshid Ghajar, David Gordon, Roger Hartl, David W. Newell, Franco Servadei, Beverly C. Walters, and Jack E. Wilberger. 2006. Surgical Management of Traumatic Brain Injury Author Group: Surgical management of acute epidural hematomas. *Neurosurgery* 58: S7–S15. [CrossRef]

Cantu, Robert C. 2001. Posttraumatic Retrograde and Anterograde Amnesia: Pathophysiology and Implications in Grading and Safe Return to Play. *Journal of Athletic Training* 36: 244–48. [PubMed]

Carney, Nancy A., and Jamshid Ghajar. 2007. Introduction. In *Guidelines for the Management of Severe Traumatic Brain Injury*, 3rd ed. New York: Brain Trauma Foundation, Inc., pp. S1–S2. [CrossRef]

Cengiz, Ozan, Arife Çimen Atalar, Betül Tekin, Nerses Bebek, Betül Baykana, and Candan Gürses. 2019. Impact of seizure-related injuries on quality of life. *Neurological Sciences* 40: 577–83. [CrossRef] [PubMed]

Cheaito, Ali, Areti Tillou, Catherine Lewis, and Henry Cryer. 2016. Management of traumatic blunt IVC injury. *International Journal of Surgery Case Reports* 28: 26–30. [CrossRef] [PubMed]

Chotai, Silky, and Khoi D. Than. 2021. Gunshot Wound Head Trauma. Available online: https://www.aans.org/en/Patients/Neurosurgical-Conditions-and-Treatments/Gunshot-Wound-Head-Trauma (accessed on 23 July 2021).

CRASH Trial Collaborators. 2004. Effect of intravenous corticosteroids on death within 14 days in 10,008 adults with clinically significant head injury (MRC CRASH trial): Randomised placebo-controlled trial. *The Lancet* 364: 1321–28. [CrossRef]

Cruz, Julio. 1998. *Neurologic and Neurosurgical Emergencies*. Philadelphia: WB Saunders.

Das, Joe M., and Waquar Siddiqui. 2021. Kluver-Bucy Syndrome. In *StatPearls*. Treasure Island: StatPearls Publishing. Available online: https://www.ncbi.nlm.nih.gov/books/NBK544221/ (accessed on 10 April 2021).

Das, Joe M., Satheesh Chandra, and Rajmohan B. Prabhakar. 2015. Penetrating brain injury with a bike key: A case report. *Ulusal Travma ve Acil Cerrahi Dergisi* 21: 524–26. [CrossRef]

Daudia, Anu, Debabrata Biswas, and Nick S. Jones. 2007. Risk of meningitis with cerebrospinal fluid rhinorrhea. *Annals of Otology, Rhinology & Laryngology* 116: 902–5. [CrossRef]

Davis, Adam J., and Peter Kim Nelson. 1997. Arteriovenous fistula of the scalp secondary to punch autograft hair transplantation: Angioarchitecture, histopathology, and endovascular and surgical therapy. *Plastic and Reconstructive Surgery* 100: 242–49. [CrossRef]

Dean, Philip J. A., Darragh O'Neill, and Annette Sterr. 2012. Post-concussion syndrome: Prevalence after mild traumatic brain injury in comparison with a sample without head injury. *Brain Injury* 26: 14–26. [CrossRef]

Dennis, Mark, William Talbot Bowen, and Lucy Cho. 2012. *Mechanisms of Clinical Signs*. Chatswood: Elsevier, p. 396e400.

Dogan, Sozen, Celal Cinar, Gulen Demirpolat, and Ahmet Memis. 2008. Endovascular treatment of AVF after hair transplantation. *CardioVascular and Interventional Radiology* 31: S128–S130. [CrossRef]

Hasso, A. N., and J. A. Ledington. 1988. Traumatic injuries of the temporal bone. *Otolaryngologic Clinics of North America* 21: 295–316. [CrossRef]

Elias, W. Jeffrey, Kai-Ming Fu, and Robert C. Frysinger. 2007. Cortical and subcortical brain shift during stereotactic procedures. *Journal of Neurosurgery* 107: 983–88. [CrossRef] [PubMed]

Feiz-Erfan, Iman, Eric M. Horn, Nichola Theodore, Joseph M. Zabramski, Jeffrey D. Klopfenstein, Gregory P. Lekovic, Felipe C. Albuquerque, Shahram Partovi, Pamela W. Goslar, and Scott R. Petersen. 2007. Incidence and pattern of direct blunt neurovascular injury associated with trauma to the skull base. *Journal of Neurosurgery* 107: 364–69. [CrossRef] [PubMed]

Feng, Jun-Feng, Ji-Yao Jiang, Ying-Hui Bao, Yu-Min Liang, and Yao-Hua Pan. 2008. Traumatic subdural effusion evolves into chronic subdural hematoma: Two stages of the same inflammatory reaction? *Medical Hypotheses* 70: 1147–49. [CrossRef]

Fukuta, Keizo, Rick J. Smith, and Ian T. Jackson. 1994. Arteriovenous fistula formation after punch graft hair transplantation in the frontal region. *Plastic and Reconstructive Surgery* 93: 587–89. [CrossRef]

Gooch, M. Reid, Greg E. Gin, Tyler J. Kenning, and John W. German. 2009. Complications of cranioplasty following decompressive craniectomy: Analysis of 62 cases. *Neurosurgical Focus* 26: E9. [CrossRef]

Greenberg, Mark S. 2010. *Handbook of Neurosurgery*. New York: Thieme.

Guillon, B., L. Brunereau, V. Biousse, H. Djouhri, C. Lévy, and M.-G. Bousser. 1999. Long-term follow-up of aneurysms developed during extracranial internal carotid artery dissection. *Neurology* 53: 117–22. [CrossRef] [PubMed]

Gururaj, G. 2002. Epidemiology of traumatic brain injuries: Indian scenario. *Neurological Research* 24: 24–28. [CrossRef]

Habeeb, Salman. 2017. Head injury.ppt. Available online: https://www.slideshare.net/salmanhabeebek/head-injuryppt-75238809 (accessed on 7 March 2022).

Haddad, Samir H., and Yaseen M. Arabi. 2012. Critical care management of severe traumatic brain injury in adults. *Scandinavian Journal of Trauma, Resuscitation and Emergency Medicine* 20: 12. [CrossRef]

Hall, W. A. 2014. Cranioplasty Infection—Adding Insult to injury. *World Neurosurgery* 82: E435–E437. [CrossRef]

Head Injury Foundation. n.d. Traumatic brain injury. Available online: https://indianheadinjuryfoundation.org/traumatic-brain-injury/ (accessed on 6 March 2022).

Holle, D., O. Kastrup, S.-Y. Sheu, and M. Obermann. 2009. Tongue pseudohypertrophy in idiopathic hypoglossal nerve palsy. *Journal of Neurology, Neurosurgery & Psychiatry* 80: 1393. [CrossRef]

Ishiwata, Yusuke, Kazuhiko Fujitsu, Tsunemi Sekino, Hideyo Fujino, Takamichi Kubokura, Kyoji Tsubone, and Takeo Kuwabara. 1988. Subdural tension pneumocephalus following surgery for chronic subdural hematoma. *Journal of Neurosurgery* 68: 58–61. [CrossRef] [PubMed]

Joswig, Holger, Oliver P. Gautschi, Amir El Rahal, Lukas Sveikata, Andrea Bartoli, Gerhard Hildebrandt, Karl Schaller, and Martin N. Stienen. 2016. Cranioplasty: Is Surgical Education Safe? *World Neurosurgery* 91: 81–88. [CrossRef] [PubMed]

July, Julius, and Eka J. Wahjoepramono. 2019. *Neurovascular Surgery: Surgical Approaches for Neurovascular Diseases*. London: Springer Open.

Kacker, Ashutosh, Abtin Tabaee, and Vijay Anand. 2005. Computer-assisted surgical navigation in revision endoscopic sinus surgery. *Otolaryngologic Clinics of North America* 38: 473–82. [CrossRef]

Kalangu, K., Y. Kato, G. Dechamberoit, and H. Sano. 2009. *Essential Practice of Neurosurgery*. Nagoya: Access Publishing Co., Ltd.

Kamel, Hooman, Babak B. Navi, Kazuma Nakagawa, J. Claude Hemphill, III, and Nerissa U. Ko. 2011. Hypertonic saline versus mannitol for the treatment of elevated intracranial pressure: A meta-analysis of randomized clinical trials. *Critical Care Medicine* 39: 554–59. [CrossRef]

Khan, Arshad Ali, and Ashis Banerjee. 2010. The role of prophylactic anticonvulsants in moderate to severe head injury. *International Journal of Emergency Medicine* 3: 187–91. [CrossRef]

Kim, Jane J., and Alisa D. Gean. 2011. Imaging for the diagnosis and management of traumatic brain injury. *Neurotherapeutics* 8: 39–53. [CrossRef]

Kirollos, Ramez W., Adel Helmy, Simon Thomason, and Peter J. A. Hutchinson. 2019. *Oxford Textbook of Neurological Surgery*. Oxford: Oxford University press.

Kommaraju, Kavya, Jeffrey H. Haynes, and Ann M. Ritter. 2019. Evaluating the Role of a Neurosurgery Consultation in Management of Pediatric Isolated Linear Skull Fractures. *Pediatric Neurosurgery* 54: 21–27. [CrossRef]

Krzysztof, Szaniewski, Byrcezk Tomasz, and Sikora Tomasz. 2019. Vascular Trauma. In *Emergency Medicine and Trauma*. Edited by Ozgur Karcioglu and Müge Günalp Eneyli. London: IntechOpen. [CrossRef]

Lanzieri, Charles F., Michael Sacher, Peter M. Som, and Moshe Haimov. 1985. Arteriovenous fistula after hair transplantation. *British Medical Journal* 6: 111–12.

Levy, Claude, Jean Pierre Laissy, Vincent Raveau, Pierre Amarenco, Vincent Servois, Marie Germaine Bousser, and Jean Michel Tubiana. 1994. Carotid and vertebral artery dissections: Three-dimensional time-of-flight MR angiography and MR imaging versus conventional angiography. *Radiology* 190: 97–103. [CrossRef]

Li, Feng, Shugan Zhu, Yuguang Liu, Yu Chen, Lingyi Chi, Gang Chen, Jian Zhang, and Fujun Qu. 2007. Traumatic arteriovenous fistula of the superficial temporal artery. *Journal of Clinical Neuroscience* 14: 95–600. [CrossRef]

Lloyd, Kristen M., John M. DelGaudio, and Patricia A. Hudgins. 2008. Hudgins. Imaging of skull base cerebrospinal fluid leaks in adults. *Radiology* 248: 725–36. [CrossRef] [PubMed]

Maas, A. I., M. Dearden, G. M. Teasdale, R. Braakman, F. Cohadon, F. Iannotti, A. Karimi, F. Lapierre, G. Murray, J. Ohman, and et al. 1997. EBIC-guidelines for management of severe head injury in adults. European Brain Injury Consortium. *Acta Neurochirurgica* 139: 286–94. [CrossRef]

Maragkos, Georgios A., Efstathios Papavassiliou, Martina Stippler, and Aristotelis S. Filippidis. 2018. Civilian Gunshot Wounds to the Head: Prognostic Factors Affecting Mortality: Meta-Analysis of 1774 Patients. *Journal of Neurotrauma* 35: 2605–14. [CrossRef] [PubMed]

Mathis, John M., Andrew J. DeNardo, Mary E. Jensen, Kant Y. Lin, and Jacques E. Dion. 1994. Arteriovenous fistula of the scalp after hair transplantation treated by endovascular embolization. *Annals of Plastic Surgery* 33: 633–37. [CrossRef]

McGrew, Patrick R., Paul J. Chestovich, Jay D. Fisher, Deborah A. Kuhls, Douglas R. Fraser, Purvi P. Patel, Chad W. Katona, Syed Saquib, and John J. Fildes. 2018. Implementation of a CT scan practice guideline for pediatric trauma patients reduces unnecessary scans without impacting outcomes. *Journal of Trauma and Acute Care Surgery* 85: 451–58. [CrossRef]

Mckee, Ann C., and Daniel H. Daneshvar. 2015. The neuropathology of traumatic brain injury. *Handbook of Clinical Neurology* 127: 45–66. [CrossRef] [PubMed]

McLaurin, Robert L., and Bert H. McBride. 1956. Traumatic intracerebral hematoma; review of 16 surgically treated cases. *Annals of Surgery* 143: 294–305. [CrossRef]

Milton, Jason, Alex Rugino, Kailash Narayan, Chris Karas, and Victor Awuor. 2017. A Case-Based Review of the Management of Penetrating Brain Trauma. *Cureus* 9: e1342. [CrossRef]

Mohanty, S., and C. J. Rao. 1976. A large cirsoid aneurysm of the scalp associated with epilepsy. *Journal of Neurology, Neurosurgery and Psychiatry* 39: 835–36. [CrossRef]

Monas, Jessica, and David A. Peak. 2010. Spontaneous tension pneumocephalus resulting from a scalp fistula in a patient with a remotely placed ventriculoperitoneal shunt. *Annals of Emergency Medicine* 56: 378–81. [CrossRef]

Muizelaar, J. Paul, Harry A. Lutz, and Donald P. Becker. 1984. Effect of mannitol on ICP and CBF and correlation with pressure autoregulation in severely head-injured patients. *Journal of Neurosurguery* 61: 700–706. [CrossRef] [PubMed]

Nader, Remi, Cristian Gragnaniello, Scott C. Berta, Abdulrahman J. Sabbagh, and Michael L. Levy. 2014. *Neurosurgery Tricks of the Trade – Cranial.* New York: Thieme.

Nguyen Bui, L., M. Brant-Zawadzki, P. Verghese, and G. Gillan. 1993. Magnetic resonance angiography of cervicocranial dissection. *Stroke* 24: 126–31. [CrossRef]

Pascual, José María, and Ruth Prieto. 2012. Surgical Management of Severe Closed Head Injury in Adults. In *Schmidek and Sweet Operative Neurosurgical Techniques*. Edited by Alfredo Quiñones-Hinojosa. Philadelphia: W.B. Saunders.

Provenzale, James M. 1995. Dissection of the internal carotid and vertebral arteries: Imaging features. *American Journal of Roentgenology* 165: 1099–104. [CrossRef]

Quiñones-Hinojosa, Alfredo. 2012. *Schmidek and Sweet: Operative Neurosurgical Techniques E-Book: Indications, Methods and Results*, 6th ed. Philadelphia: Elsevier Saunders.

Qureshi, Adnan I., Yuko Y. Palesch, William G. Barsan, Daniel F. Hanley, Chung Y. Hsu, Renee L. Martin, Claudia S. Moy, Robert Silbergleit, Thorsten Steiner, Jose I. Suarez, and et al. 2016. ATACH-2 Trial Investigators and the Neurological Emergency Treatment Trials Network. Intensive Blood-Pressure Lowering in Patients with Acute Cerebral Hemorrhage. *New England Journal of Medicine* 375: 1033–43. [CrossRef] [PubMed]

Schievink, Wouter I. 2001. Spontaneous dissection of the carotid and vertebral arteries. *New England Journal of Medicine* 344: 898–906. [CrossRef] [PubMed]

Sharim, Justin, Patrick Pezeshkian, Antonio DeSalles, and Nader Pouratian. 2015. Effect of Cranial Window Diameter During Deep Brain Stimulation Surgery on Volume of Pneumocephalus. *Neuromodulation: Technology at the Neural Interface* 18: 574–79. [CrossRef]

Simmons, Joshua, and Andrew M. Luks. 2013. Tension pneumocephalus: An uncommon cause of altered mental status. *The Journal of Emergency Medicine* 44: 340–43. [CrossRef]

Sweni, Shah, Subramanian Senthilkumaran, Namasivayam Balamurugan, and Ponniah Thirumalaikolundusubramanian. 2013. Tension pneumocephalus: A case report with review of literature. *Emergency Radiology* 20: 573–78. [CrossRef]

Svider, Peter F., Andrew C. Mauro, Jean Anderson Eloy, Michael Setzen, Michael A. Carron, and Adam J. Folbe. 2014. Malodorous consequences: What comprises negligence in anosmia litigation? *International Forum of Allergy & Rhinology* 4: 216–22. [CrossRef]

Timofeev, I., T. Santarius, A. G. Kolias, and P. J. A. Hutchinson. 2012. Decompressive craniectomy—Operative technique and perioperative care. *Advances and Technical Standards in Neurosurgery* 38: 115–36. [CrossRef]

Teasdale, Graham, and Bryan Jennett. 1974. Assessment of coma and impaired consciousness. *Lancet* 2: 81–84. [CrossRef] [PubMed]

Touzé, Emmanuel, Bruno Randoux, Eric Méary, Caroline Arquizan, Jean-François Meder, and Jean-Louis Mas. 2001. Aneurysmal forms of cervical artery dissection: Associated factors and outcome. *Stroke* 32: 418–23. [CrossRef]

UCLA Health. 2021. Neurosurgery—Cranial GunShot Wounds. Available online: https://www.uclahealth.org/neurosurgery/cranial-gunshot-wounds (accessed on 26 May 2021).

van Rein, Eveline A. J., Rogier van der Sluijs, Frank J. Voskens, Koen W. W. Lansink, R. Marijn Houwert, Rob A. Lichtveld, Mariska A. de Jongh, Marcel G. W. Dijkgraaf, Howard R. Champion, Frank J. P. Beeres, and et al. 2019. Development and Validation of a Prediction Model for Prehospital Triage of Trauma Patients. *JAMA Surgery* 154: 421–29. [CrossRef] [PubMed]

Vinas, F. C., and J. Pilitsis. 2006. Penetrating Head Trauma. Available online: http://www.Emedicine.com (accessed on 6 February 2007).

Vlček, M., E. Jaganjac, M. Niedoba, I. Landor, and J. Neumann. 2018. Current treatment procedures for civilian gunshot wounds. *Rozhledy v Chirurgii: Mesicnik Ceskoslovenske Chirurgicke Spolecnosti* 97: 558–62.

Vella, Michael A., Marie L. Crandall, and Mayur B. Patel. 2017. Acute Management of Traumatic Brain Injury. *Surgical Clinics of North America* 97: 1015–30. [CrossRef] [PubMed]

Wikem. 2019. Moderate-to-Severe Traumatic Brain Injury. Available online: https://www.wikem.org/wiki/Moderate-to-severe_traumatic_brain_injury (accessed on 7 March 2022).

Yamaki, T., K. Hirakawa, T. Ueguchi, H. Tenjin, T. Kuboyama, and Y. Nakagawa. 1990. Chronological evaluation of acute traumatic intracerebral haematoma. *Acta Neurochirurgica* 103: 112–15. [CrossRef]

Zweig, Julie L., Ricardo L. Carrau, Scott E. Celin, Carl H. Snyderman, Amin Kassam, and Hassan Hegazy. 2002. Endoscopic repair of acquired encephaloceles, meningoceles, and meningoencephaloceles: Predictors of success. *Skull Base* 12: 133–9. [CrossRef]

Section VII: Neurovascular Diseases and Stroke

Ischemic Stroke, Arterio-Occlusive Diseases and Cerebral Venous Sinus Thrombosis (CVST)

Forhad H. Chowdhury, Quazi Deen Mohammod and M. S. Zahirul Haque Chowdhury

Abstract: There is an excess of 13.7 million strokes per year globally. Globally, there are more than eighty million people currently alive who have had a stroke. Its management, cost and morbidity have a huge social and economic impact on families, societies and countries. Stroke has important predisposing factors that need to be addressed for stroke prevention. Time is a very important factor in the management of acute stroke to avoid mortality and morbidity. An early diagnosis and initiation of appropriate management, including IV thrombolysis, mechanical thrombectomy and emergency surgical interventions (decompression or revascularization), are utterly precious for reasonable outcomes. This chapter will discuss the pathophysiology, presentation, imaging, principles of medical and surgical management, and prevention of ischemic stroke. This chapter will also outline a short discussion of atherosclerotic cerebrovascular disease, cerebral arterial dissection and cerebral venous sinus thrombosis (CVST).

Abbreviations

AAD	atlanto-axial dislocation	ABG	arterial blood gas
ACZ	acetazolamide	ACA	anterior cerebral artery
ADC	apparent deficient co-efficient	AICA	anterior inferior cerebellar artery
ATA	anterior temporal artery	AVM	arterio-venous malformation
BA	basilar artery	BHS	bow hunter's stroke
BP	blood pressure	CAD	cerebral arterial dissection
CBC	complete blood count	CBF	Cerebral blood flow
CBV	cerebral blood volume	CCA	common carotid artery
CCU	coronary care unit	CEA	carotid endarterectomy
CHF	chronic heart failure	CRV	cerebrovascular reserve
CT	computed tomography	CTA	computed tomographic angiogram
CTV	computed tomographic venography	CSF	cerebrospinal fluid
CXR	chest X-ray	CVA	cerebrovascular accident
CVST	cerebral vein and dural sinus thrombosis	DSA	digital subtraction angiogram
DTI	diffusion tensor imaging	DW	diffusion weighted
ECA	external carotid artery	ECG	Electrocardiogram
EC-IC	extracranial–intracranial	EEG	electro encephalogram
ER	emergency room	EVD	external ventricular drainage
FMD	fibro muscular dysplasia	FND	focal neurological deficit
fMRI	functional magnetic resonance imaging	GI	Gastrointestinal
HTN	hypertension	IA	Intraarterial
ICA	internal carotid artery	ICH	intracerebral hemorrhage
ICP	intra cranial pressure	IIH	idiopathic intracranial hypertension
IV	intra venous	LP	lumbar puncture
MCA	middle cerebral artery	MI	myocardial infarction
MRI	magnetic resonance imaging	MRA	magnetic resonance angiogram
MRV	magnetic resonance venography	OA	occipital artery
OEF	oxygen extraction fraction	ONSF	optic nerve sheath fenestration
OP	opening pressure	PAN	polyarteritis nodosa
PCA	posterior cerebral artery	PET	positron emission tomography
PICA	posterior inferior cerebellar artery	PT	prothrombin time
PTT	partial thromboplastin time	PW	perfusion weighted
RIND	reversible ischemic neurological deficit	rtPA	recombinant tissue plasminogen activator
SAH	subarachnoid hemorrhage	SCA	superior cerebellar artery
SPECT	single-photon emission computed tomography	SSS	superior sagittal sinus
TCD	transcranial Doppler	TIA	transient ischemic attack
tPA	tissue plasminogen activator	TS	transverse sinus

U/A	urine analysis	VA	vertebral artery
VBI	vertebrobasilar insufficiency		

1. Ischemic Stroke

There is an excess of 13.7 million strokes per annum globally. The yearly incidence rate is 185/100,000 population. The global prevalence rate is 1083/100,000. Globally, there is an excess of eighty million people currently alive who have had a stroke (GBD 2016 Stroke Collaborators 2019).

1.1. Cerebral Blood Flow and Its Relation to Ischemia

Cerebral blood flow (CBF) at rest is 45–60 mL blood/minute/100 mL of brain tissue.

CBF < 20 mL/min/100 gm of brain tissue results in cerebral ischemia.
CBF < 16–18 mL/min/100 gm of brain tissue causes a flat EEG.
CBF < 15 mL/min/100 gm of brain tissue causes physiologic paralysis.
CBF < 10 mL/min/100 gm of brain tissue leads to infarction (Greenberg 2010).

1.2. Suddenly Developed Focal Neurological Deficit

Patients presenting to the hospital emergency department with sudden development of a new focal neuro-deficit (Greenberg 2010; Lindsay et al. 2011):

- Neoplasm, epilepsy or psychogenic—5%;
- Neurovascular (stroke)—95%;

Ischemic infarct—85%;

- Unknown cause—41%;
- Lacunar infarct—21%;
- Cardiogenic embolus—16%;
- Large artery lesion—11%;
- Tandem arterial pathology—10%;

Hemorrhagic stroke—15%;

- Intracerebral hemorrhage (ICH)—11%. "Hypertensive" hemorrhage, amyloid angiopathy;
- SAH (aneurysmal, AVM)—5%;

Venous infarction—a small proportion of strokes.

1.3. Risk Factors for Stroke

Risk factors are shown in Table 1.

Table 1. Major and other risk factors.

Major Factors	Other Factors
Hypertension	Age
Hypertension—Major risk factor for brain infarction and hemorrhage.	Sex (male > female)
	Race
Cardiac disease	Hereditary
Cardiac failure and cardiomegaly, and arrhythmias, valvular diseases and patent foramen ovale.	Sedentary lifestyle
	Diet and environment
Diabetes mellitus	Polycythemia
Smoking	Oral contraceptives
Hyperlipidemia	Heavy alcohol consumption

Source: Authors' compilation based on data from Greenberg (2010).

1.4. Pathophysiology of TIA and Infarction

When the CBV is compromised (by arterial diseases), i.e., below the 20 mL/min/100 gm brain tissue and a drop-in blood pressure or perfusion pressure (such as arrhythmia, thrombus or embolus) leading the CBV below 15 mL/min/100 gm of brain tissue, it can lead to a TIA. If the CBV improves, the TIA recovers, and if the CBV does not improve and instead decreases under the 10 mL/min/100 gm of brain tissue, a cerebral infarction ensues.

1.5. *Cerebrovascular Reserve (CRV) and Reactivity*

The CRV may be evaluated with a xenon-enhanced CT, perfusion CT, TCD, SPECT or an MRI with perfusion images. The reaction of the CBF to a vasodilator challenge with 1 gm of IV acetazolamide (ACZ) is classified in Table 2.

Table 2. Types of CRVs and reactivity.

Type	Description
Type I	Normal, baseline CBF with 30–60% rise after ACZ challenge
Type II	Reduced baseline CBF with a response (blunted) of <10% rise or <10 mL/100 g/min absolute rise following ACZ challenge
Type III	Reduced baseline CBF with a paradoxical fall in regional CBF after ACZ challenge, alluding a steal phenomenon in areas with the most dilated vessels at the baseline

Source: Authors' compilation based on data from Greenberg (2010).

1.6. *Penumbra and Treatment Rationale of Cerebral Infarction*

With the total lack of blood flow to cerebral neurons, neuronal death occurs within 2 to 3 min. However, in most infarctions, there is a recoverable penumbra (tissue at risk) that survives for a period of time due to poor collateral flow perfusion. If a local cerebral edema from the lesion progresses, these collaterals are compromised and the ischemic penumbra progresses to infarction if flow is not restored. The prevention of this secondary damage drives the management of stroke and has prompted the evolution of dedicated primary stroke centers that offer proper and timely triage and treatment for all potential stroke patients. The current standard of care requires the administration of IV tPA (tissue plasminogen activator) to all eligible patients. In centers with advanced capabilities (comprehensive stroke centers), other management options are also offered (Greenberg 2010; Lindsay et al. 2011).

1.7. *Transient Ischemic Attacks (TIA)*

TIAs are episodes of focal neuro-deficit due to poor blood circulation to the brain. The attacks come on suddenly, last for 24 h or less, and leave no lingering neuro-deficiency. These assaults could be a sign of an impending cerebral infarction. Migraine, partial seizures, hypoglycemia, syncope and hyperventilation are all examples of transient neurological malfunction. After a TIA, 5% of patients suffer cerebral infarction within one week and 12% within three months. A TIA warning occurs in about 10% of people who have a stroke (Greenberg 2010; Lindsay et al. 2011).

1.8. *Clinical Presentation of an Ischemic Stroke*

Patients may present with (TIAs) or features of infarctions. Clinical features depend on the artery that is affected by the disease process (Lindsay et al. 2011).

1.8.1. Clinical Pictures of a TIA

Ninety percent (90%) of TIAs are anterior-circulation (ICA territory) TIAs that include hemiplegia, hemisensory disturbance, dysphasia and mono-ocular blindness (amaurosis fugax). Seven percent (7%) are posterior-circulation (vertebrobasilar territory) TIAs that include unconsciousness, bilateral sensory and motor disturbances, binocular blindness, diplopia, vertigo, tinnitus and dysarthria. Three percent (3%) are indifferentiable between anterior- and posterior-circulation TIAs.

1.8.2. Clinical Pictures of an Infarction

Large Vessel Occlusion—Internal Carotid Artery (ICA) Occlusion

Increasing lumen constriction and thrombosis, or a repeated emboli may manifest in a 'stuttering' manner. The severity of the deficiency varies. An asymptomatic ICA occlusion is possible, or a catastrophic infarction may occur. The initial prodromal symptoms include amaurosis fugax, and a transient hemi-motor or hemisensory disturbance. In the worst-case scenario, the symptoms may be a dwindling of level of consciousness; contralateral homonymous hemianopia, hemiplegia, hemisensory disturbances and gaze palsy; or global aphasia (in the case of the dominant hemisphere). There is an absence of ICA pulsation at the angle of the jaw.

Large Vessel Occlusion—Anterior Cerebral Artery (ACA) Occlusion

A thrombus or embolus can obstruct the ACA. The clinical symptoms vary depending on the location of the blockage (most commonly in relation to the anterior communicating artery) and anatomical variance; for example, an enlargement of the anterior communicating artery might cause both anterior cerebral arteries to emerge from one side. A pre-communicating ACA blockage is well tolerated and may be asymptomatic. In most cases, a distal ACA blockage causes paralysis and cortical sensory loss in the contralateral lower limb, as well as incontinence. Cerebral paraplegia with the paralysis of both lower limbs, cortical sensory loss and incontinence can result from a proximal ACA occlusion when both ACAs originate from one side or an azygos ACA occlusion. The grasping reflex, snout and palmo-mental reflex may be present. An altered level of consciousness and akinetic mutism may be present in the case of an infarction of both sides of the frontal lobe.

Large Vessel Occlusion—Middle Cerebral Artery (MCA) Occlusion

The MCA produces deep branches (lenticulostriate perforating arteries) that supply the anterior limb of the internal capsule and a portion of the basal nuclei. It then travels to the insula of the Sylvian fissure on the lateral surface of the cerebral hemisphere. It produces cortical branches here such as the temporal, frontal and parietal cortical branches.

Clinical features: An embolus or thrombus can obstruct the MCA. The clinical signs and symptoms vary depending on the blockage site and whether the dominant or nondominant hemisphere is affected. When specific cortical branches are occluded, the clinical symptoms are less severe. For example, the involvement of the parietal branches alone can cause Wernicke's dysphasia without limb paresis or sensory problems. Tiny infarcts may be caused by the MCA's deep branches (perforating arteries) (lacunar infarct).

Occlusion at the insula: Again, the symptoms depend on which branch or branches are impacted. If all branches are compromised, there will be contralateral hemiplegia (leg largely spared), contralateral hemianesthesia and hemianopia, aphasia (in the case of the dominant hemisphere), neglect of the contralateral side and clothing difficulties (in the case of the non-dominant hemisphere).

Large Vessel Occlusion—Vertebral Artery (VA) Occlusion

The VA arises from the subclavian artery bilaterally and passes through the foramina transversarium of the cervical vertebrae. It enters the cerebral cavity through the foramen magnum after piercing the dura and arachnoid tissue. It joins with its companion at the pons' lower border to produce the basilar artery. Before creating the basilar artery, the VA and its branches are distributed on the medulla and inferior surface of the cerebellum.

Clinical features: When the VA is blocked down in the neck, anastomotic channels compensate well. When one of the vertebral arteries is hypoplastic, the blockage of the other is analogous to the occlusion of the basilar artery. The flow of the vertebral artery is solely responsible for the posterior inferior cerebellar artery (PICA). As a result, the blockage of the vertebral artery can cause PICA syndrome. The vertebral artery's close proximity to the cervical spine is crucial.

Injury to the intervertebral foramina or the atlanto-axial joints as a result of subluxation can cause intimal damage, thrombus development and embolization in rare cases. Intermittent vertebrobasilar insufficiency can be caused by the compression of the vertebral artery during neck extension.

Posterior Inferior Cerebellar Artery Syndrome (PICA/Lateral Medullary Syndrome)

Cerebellar features include dysarthria, ipsilateral limbs, vertigo, ataxia and nystagmus; and lateral medullary features include ipsilateral Horner's syndrome, and ipsilateral pain and temperature sensation loss in face, ipsilateral laryngeal and pharyngeal paralysis, and contralateral pain and temperature sensation loss in the trunk and limbs.

Large Vessel Occlusion—Basilar Artery (BA) Occlusion

From the medulla to above, the BA nourishes the brain stem, finally dividing into posterior cerebral arteries. Posterior cerebral arteries, long circumflex branches and paramedian branches are the three types of branches of BA.

Clinical features: Diplopia, visual field loss, occasional memory disturbance and a slew of other brain stem symptoms such as vertigo, ataxia, paresis and paresthesia are all frequent prodromal symptoms. Following BA occlusion, complete basilar syndrome develops, which includes the loss of awareness or coma, bilateral motor and sensory deficits, cerebellar symptoms and cranial nerve indications that indicate the amount of blockage. The clinical picture, on the other hand, is diverse and may be asymptomatic. Occlusion of the top of the basilar artery causes infarction of the lateral midbrain, and thalamic, occipital and medial temporal lobes. Visual loss, pupillary abnormalities, gaze palsies, reduced conscious level and behavioral disorders are all symptoms of hemiballismus.

'Locked-in' syndrome and lacunar infarction are caused by obstruction of the paramedian perforating artery.

Large Vessel Occlusion—Posterior Cerebral Artery (PCA) Occlusion

PCAs are the basilar artery's terminal branches. Midbrain structures, the choroid plexus and the posterior thalamus are all served by small perforating branches. The posterior temporal artery supplies the undersurface of the temporal lobe, while the parieto-occipital and calcarine arteries nourish the occipital and visual cortices.

Clinical features: Perforating branches and structures are affected by the proximal blockage of PCA by a thrombus or embolism.

The midbrain syndrome includes third nerve palsy with contralateral hemiplegia (Weber's syndrome), thalamic syndromes such as chorea or hemiballismus with hemisensory impairment, and obstruction of cortical vasculature, which result in visual field loss (homonymous hemianopia) but macular vision sparing. Color and object naming may be affected by posterior cerebral infarction in the dominant hemisphere.

BA Branch Occlusion Syndrome

Superior cerebellar artery (SCA) syndrome: cerebellar features, including gait disturbances and limb ataxia; and lateral midbrain features, including ipsilateral Horner's syndrome and hemisensory loss (pain and temperature sensation loss, including in the face).

Anterior inferior cerebellar artery (AICA) syndrome: cerebellar feature, including limb ataxia; and lateral pontine features, including ipsilateral Horner's syndrome and ipsilateral pain and temperature sensation loss in the face; ipsilateral facial weakness; ipsilateral lateral gaze palsy; and contralateral pain and temperature sensation loss in the trunk and limbs.

Lacunar Infarcts

Different perforators from anterior and posterior circulation can produce different lacunar stroke syndromes.

Anterior circulation lacunar stroke—pure sensory syndrome, pure motor syndrome, etc.

Posterior circulation lacunar stroke—dysarthria/clumsy hand syndrome, ataxic hemiparesis, etc.

1.9. Evaluation and Investigations

1.9.1. History—Key Components to Consider

- Time when the patient was last observed to be normal;
- Current deficit/s and clinical presentation;
- Stroke scale (such as the NIH) score should be assessed and recorded;
- Causes for not starting IV tPA (if any) must be written (Greenberg 2010; Lindsay et al. 2011; Awad 2005).

1.9.2. Investigations

1. CT scan of brain, perfusion CT with a CTA of the brain and neck vessels from the arch of aorta;
2. MRI of the brain as per the ischemic stroke protocol (routine images with DW, ADC, PW images, DTI and tractography, MRA and MRV of the head and neck vessels and fMRI of the brain);
3. Carotid Doppler;
4. Cerebral DSA;
5. CXR P/A view, ECG and echocardiogram;
6. Routine hematological tests (Greenberg 2010; Lindsay et al. 2011; Awad 2005).

1.9.3. Computed Tomography (CT) Scan, CT Angiogram and Perfusion CT

CT Scan

On presentation with the signs and symptoms of a potential stroke, a brain CT scan without contrast should be carried out urgently to exclude hemorrhage (intra- parenchymal or SAH), early signs of ischemia, hematoma, old infarcts or injuries, and other pathologies (e.g., tumor).

Hyperacute (<6 h after stroke): Early signs of an infarction involving large areas of the MCA territory correlate with poor outcomes. Early findings may include the following:

1. Hyperdense artery sign (Figure 1): low sensitivity, but helpful if present;
2. Focal low attenuation within the gray matter;
3. Loss of the gray–white matter interface;
4. Attenuation of the lentiform nucleus;
5. Mass effect
    A. Early: effacement (obscuration) of the cerebral sulci (often subtle);
    B. Late: midline shift in large territory infarction;
6. Absence of the insular ribbon (hypodensity involving the insular area);
7. Enhancement: occurs in only 33%, where stroke becomes isodense (called the "masking" effect) or hyperdense with the normal brain, and, rarely, may be the only sign of an infarction.

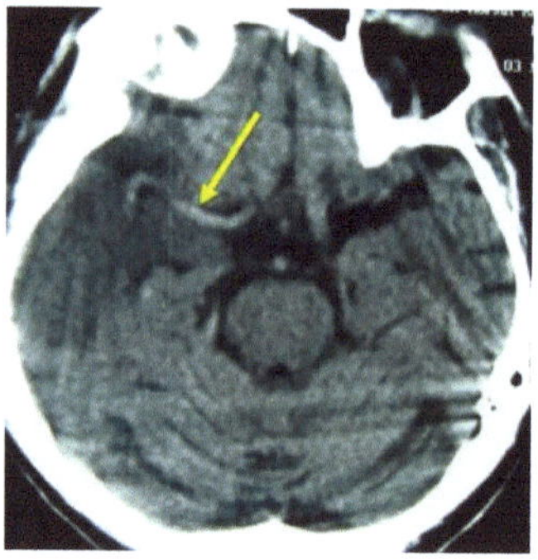

Figure 1. Axial CT scan of the brain showing a right MCA infarct with the 'hyperdense MCA' sign (arrow marked). Source: Figure by authors.

24 h: Most strokes can be identified as a low density by this time.
1–2 weeks: Strokes are starkly demarcated.
3 weeks: Stroke area approaches CSF density.

In 5–10%, there may be a short window (approximately day 7–10) where the stroke turns isodense, known as the "fogging effect". A IV contrast will generally visualize these.

Mass effect: common between days 1 and 25. Then, atrophy is usually seen by week 5 (2 weeks at the earliest). Serial CT scans of the brain have demonstrated that the midline shift increases following ischemic stroke and reaches its highest 2 to 4 days after the event.

Calcifications: Only 1–2% of strokes calcify. Thus, in an adult person, calcifications almost rule out a stroke.

Hyperdense artery sign (Figure 1): The cerebral vessel (usually the MCA) appears as a high density on an unenhanced CT, pointing out an intra-arterial thrombus or embolus. It is found in 12–34% of patients within 24 h of stroke. Sensitivity for an MCA occlusion is low, but specificity is high (although it may also be seen with a carotid dissection).

Contrast enhancement:

1. Many infarcts take up contrast by day 6, most by day 10, and some will contrast enhance up to 5 weeks;
2. Rule of the 2s: 2% contrast enhance at 2 days, 2% contrast enhance at 2 months;
3. Gyral contrast enhancement ("ribbon" enhancement) is frequent, commonly seen by 1 week, and a differential includes inflammatory infiltrating lesions such as lymphoma, neuro-sarcoidosis, etc.;
4. There should not be contrast enhancement at the same time when there is a mass effect (Greenberg 2010; Marks et al. 1999; Tomandl et al. 2003; Lyden et al. 1994; Sims et al. 2005).

CTA

CTA is useful for assessing the location and extent of vascular occlusion in acute ischemic stroke. The findings can direct treatment toward endovascular or microsurgical options when a proximal or significant large vessel occlusion is seen.

Perfusion CT

A perfusion CT identifies salvageable penumbra as a region of mismatch between the CBF and CBV. An infarcted core has a decreased CBF within a region of a decreased CBV (CBF/CBV match). A decreased CBV without a decrease in the CBF (CBF/CBV mismatch) represents a potentially salvageable penumbra.

1.9.4. Magnetic Resonance Imaging (MRI), MR Angiogram (MRA) and MR Perfusion

MRI

With newer, faster acquisition times, MRIs (Figures 2 and 3A,B) are increasingly being utilized in the hyper-acute setting, at times replacing CTs for an initial evaluation. They are more sensitive than CTs (especially DWI–MRIs, particularly within the first 24 h after stroke), especially for imaging the brainstem or a cerebellar infarction.

Contrast MRI: (not used often) several enhancement patterns can be seen:

1. Intravascular contrast enhancement occurs in 75% of 1–3-day-old cortical infarcts, and is thought to be caused by a slow flow and vasodilation (thus, it is not seen with a complete occlusion). It is possible that certain parts of the brain are at a risk of an infarction.
2. Dural enhancement is found in 35% of 1–3-day-old cortical strokes.
3. Parenchymal enhancement has shown as a cortical or subcortical gyral ribbon enhancement in the past. It may not be noticeable for the first 1–2 days, but by the end of the week, it reaches 100% (Greenberg 2010; Lindsay et al. 2011; Awad 2005; Barber et al. 1998).

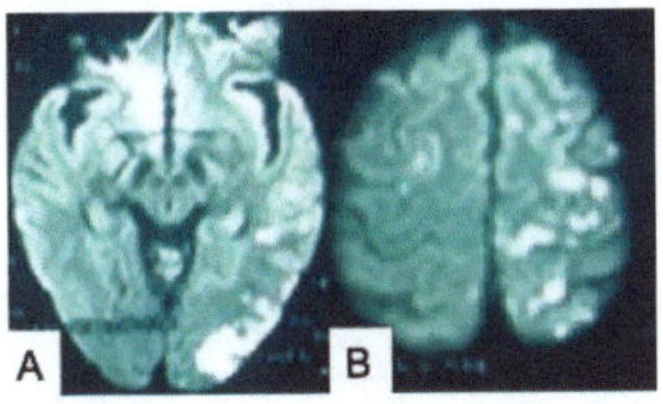

Figure 2. (**A**,**B**) MRI of brain axial DW images showing "strings of beads" as watershed infarcts under ischemic conditions. Source: Figure by authors.

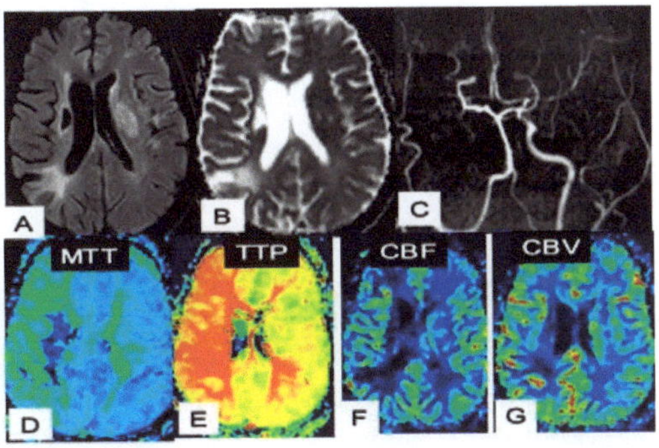

Figure 3. MRI of the brain. (**A**) Axial FLAIR and (**B**) axial T2W image showing multiple infarcts and ischemic zones in both hemispheres. (**C**) MRA of the brain showing an occlusion of the right ICA and scarcity of the right MCA vessels. (**D**–**G**) Perfusion MRI showing ischemic "penumbra". Source: Figure by authors.

MRA

An MRI (Figure 3C) is useful for assessing the site, as well as the extent of a vascular occlusion in acute ischemic stroke, like CTA.

The findings can direct treatment toward endovascular or microsurgical options when a proximal or significant large vessel occlusion is seen.

MRI Perfusion

An MRI perfusion (Figure 3D–G) is akin to a CT perfusion, where areas of a matched DWI and PWI abnormality are thought to represent the infarcted tissue. PWI abnormalities that do not have a DWI correlation are thought to represent a potentially salvageable penumbra.

1.9.5. Emergency Cerebral Digital Subtraction Angiography (DSA)

Digital subtraction angiography is rarely needed and is usually carried out with therapeutic intervention. A DSA should be avoided in unstable patients with a severe disabling neuro-deficit. Indications include the following:

1. An early stroke in the carotid circulation combined with a history of amaurosis fugax, bruit or retinal emboli, etc., could indicate a growing carotid stenosis, thrombogenic ulcerated plaque or carotid dissection;
2. If the diagnosis is still up in the air (e.g., aneurysm, vasculitis);
3. In the face of a growing stenosis, the quick recovery of neuro-deficits suggests a carotid TIA.

The findings include the following:

1. Cut off sign: the vessel abruptly ends at the point of impediment;
2. String sign (Figure 4): a narrow strand of contrast in an artery with a stenosis of high severity;
3. "Luxury perfusion": reactive hyperemia is a well-known brain tissue reaction to damage (Greenberg 2010; Lindsay et al. 2011; Awad 2005).

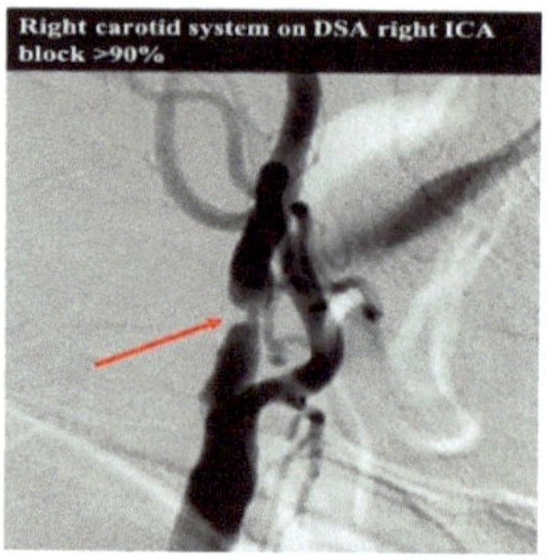

Figure 4. Cerebral DSA right carotid injection showing a high-grade ICA stenosis (string sign is arrow-marked). Source: Figure by authors.

1.10. Management

1.10.1. Aims of Treatment and General Management

Aims of general management and treatment are shown in Table 3.

Table 3. The aims of treatment and general management are shown in the boxes.

Aim of Treatment	General Management
• Reopening of blocked vessels • Preclusion of progression of the present event • Avoidance of immediate complication • Prevention of the development of subsequent events and complication/s • Rehabilitation of the patient	1. Management of airways and oxygenation 2. Maintenance of hydration 3. Maintenance of blood sugar 4. Treatment of hypertension if BP > 185/110 mm of Hg

Source: Authors' compilation based on data from Greenberg (2010), Lindsay et al. (2011) and Awad (2005).

1.10.2. Specific Management

Within 4.5 h of initiation of the event:

- IV thrombolysis (with tPA);
- Failures to respond to IV thrombolysis;

  (i) intraarterial tPA or
  (ii) mechanical embolectomy/clot disruption.

4.5–6 h after onset:

- Intra-arterial tPA/rtPA or
- Mechanical embolectomy/clot disruption.

6–9 h after onset:

- Check perfusion with CT perfusion or MRI-DWI and PWI
- Mechanical embolectomy;
- Balloon angioplasty and stenting likely works by buttresses the clot.

A higher efficacy is noticed in the failure of other available options.

(These times are more applicable to anterior circulation strokes. Posterior circulation occlusions may be treated more aggressively, e.g., IA tPA has been used up to 12 h).

Contra-Indication of Thrombolysis

The contra-indications of thrombolysis include an uncertain onset, spontaneous improvement, brain injury or previous stroke in the previous 3 months, GI surgery in the preceding 21 days, BP > 180/110, on anticoagulant, seizure and hypodensity on CT.

Complications of Thrombolysis

The complications of thrombolysis include intracranial hemorrhage (ICH) following IV tPA.

There is a chance of an increased risk of symptomatic intracerebral hemorrhage with the thrombolysis (6.4–8.8%).

Except in the rare case of a big hematoma, ICH has no bearing on the outcome.

Management of Post-Thrombolysis ICH

1. Discontinuation of tPA infusion and obtaining STAT head CT;
2. Lab investigations: PT, APTT, fibrinogen and platelet count, as well as type and cross;
3. Preparation to inject 6–8 units of cryoprecipitate-containing factor VIII;
4. Preparation to administer 6–8 units of platelets.

Emergency external ventricular drain (EVD) placement or an ICH evacuation, which is needed rarely (Greenberg 2010; Lindsay et al. 2011; Awad 2005; Paciaroni et al. 2008).

1.10.3. Management of Patients Not Undergoing Antithrombotic Therapy

The following recommendations for initial treatment should be continued 48 h following the last neuro deterioration:

1. Frequent vitals and neuro-status checks.
2. Bed rest and nothing except oral and IV fluids.
3. Laboratory investigations:

   (i) Routine: CBC + platelet count, electrolytes, PT/PTT, U/A, ECG, CXR, ABG;
   (ii) At 24 h: CBC, platelet count, cardiac profile, lipid profile, ECG.

4. Oxygen (O2) inhalations as needed.
5. Nursing care:

   (i) Indwelling urinary Foley catheter if consciousness is impaired or indicated;
   (ii) Accurate input–output chart maintenance;
   (iii) Control of blood sugar and maintenance of normoglycemia;
   (iv) Adequate hydration and avoidance of overhydration.

6. Treatment of CHF and arrhythmias. Patients with myocardial ischemia and neurological deficit should be admitted to the CCU.
7. Blood pressure (BP) containment:

    (i) For patients presenting with an HTN: baseline BP must be taken into account. If the patient has a known case of hypertension, the treatment endpoints for the HTN have lower limits at a systolic BP of 180–185 mmHg and diastolic BP of 105–110 mmHg. If the patient has no prior history of an HTN, the treatment endpoints for an HTN have lower limits at a systolic BP of 160–170 mmHg and diastolic BP of 95–105 mmHg.
    (ii) For patients presenting with hypotension (DBP < 70 or SBP < 110):

        a. Administration of IV fluids;
        b. Vasopressors if fluid ineffective or contraindicated.

8. Medications:
   Aspirin 300 mg daily for 14 days or Clopidogrel where aspirin is intolerant.
9. Transfer-to-stroke unit:
   Multidisciplinary care in a stroke unit has been shown to enhance the outcome of stroke patients.
10. Assessment of swallowing capacity:
    After a stroke, aspiration pneumonia is a common consequence. Swallowing should be assessed and a nasogastric tube for fluids and food used if necessary to reduce this risk.

    (i) Swallowing is dangerous;
    (ii) Early mobilization as soon as feasible and patients should be assisted in sitting up and mobilizing.

11. Special situations

    (i) Decompressive hemicraniectomy
    A limited number of young individuals (under 70 years old) with big middle cerebral artery strokes develop significant cytotoxic cerebral edemas that are resistant to medical treatment after 24–72 h. Surgical decompression can save a patient's life and allow them to recuperate within a reasonable amount of time.
    (ii) Other neurosurgical procedures
    When an edema causes compression of the posterior fossa and concomitant hydrocephalus, patients with massive cerebellar infarcts can decline 24–48 h following their stroke. Decompression of the posterior fossa can save a patient's life, and many patients recover fully.

1.10.4. Preclusion of Further Stroke

The identification of risk factors (Table 4), as well as their amendment to minimize the risk of further stroke forms an essential and standard step in long-term treatment.

Table 4. The strategies for prevention (utilized for the treatment of a TIA).

	Prevention of Further Stroke
(i)	Controlling of hypertension.
(ii)	Stopping of tobacco smoking.
(iii)	Correction of hyper-lipidaemia.
(iv)	Give antiplatelet drugs (Clopidogrel or aspirin) to decrease the rate of reinfarction.
(v)	Removal or treatment of embolic source (long-term use of anticoagulation in atrial fibrillation). Stop anticoagulation in disabling a stroke for 14 days as a risk of hemorrhage more than the benefits.
(vi)	Treatment of vascular inflammatory or inflammatory diseases.
(vii)	Avoidance of prothrombogenic drugs (i.e., oral contraceptives).

Source: Authors' compilation based on data from Greenberg (2010) and Lindsay et al. (2011).

1.11. *Cerebellar Infarction*

Cerebellar infarction is seldom seen. Cerebellar infarcts may be categorized as involving the PICA distribution (cerebellar tonsil and/or inferior vermis), superior cerebellar artery distribution (superior hemisphere or superior vermis) or other indeterminate patterns. After developing the signs of brainstem compression, 80% of patients die usually within hours to days. In the majority of cases, the onset is abrupt. The first 12 h following onset are marked by a lack of improvement. Dizziness or vertigo, nausea/vomiting, loss of balance (frequently accompanied by a fall and inability to get up), headache, truncal and appendicular ataxia, nystagmus and dysarthria are common early symptoms. Later findings include features of a raised ICP for the development of triventriculomegaly and brainstem compression. Clinical findings generally increase between 12 and 96 h following the onset (Greenberg 2010; Lindsay et al. 2011; Chen et al. 1992; Vahedi et al. 2007).

1.11.1. Surgical Indications

If any of the following indications appear and medicinal treatment is ineffective, surgical decompression should be performed as soon as possible. If no intervention is made, the findings proceed in the following order: 1. abducent nerve palsy; 2. ipsilateral gaze loss (compression of VI nucleus and lateral gaze center); 3. peripheral facial nerve paresis (compression of facial colliculus); 4. disorientation and somnolence (perhaps owing to developing hydrocephalus); 5. Babinski sign; 6. hemiparesis; 7. lethargy; 8. tiny but responsive pupils; 9. coma; 10. posturing flaccidity; and 11. ataxic respirations.

The results of a CT scan may be normal in the early stages. Compression or obliteration of the basal cisterns or the fourth ventricle may be modest signs of a tight posterior fossa. MRIs (including DWI) are more sensitive for ischemia, especially in the posterior fossa (Greenberg 2010; Lindsay et al. 2011; Chen et al. 1992; Vahedi et al. 2007).

Suboccipital Craniectomy for a Cerebellar Infarction

Unlike the situation with supratentorial masses causing herniation, patients with a deep unconsciousness from direct brainstem compression who are operated upon without delay can make a good recovery. The operation of choice is a suboccipital decompression to include an enlargement of the foramen magnum with removal of an infarcted cerebellum. *(It is very important to identify a lateral medullary syndrome (LMS) that is not accompanied by a change in the sensorium. There is no place for surgical decompression in the LMS since it indicates primary brainstem ischemia and not compression.)*

1.12. Malignant Middle Cerebral Artery (MCA) Territory Infarction

A very different syndrome happens in up to 10% of stroke patients which can cause mortality of up to 80%. Patients often present with findings of severe hemispheric stroke (hemiplegia and deviated eye, as well as head deviation). Most develop drowsiness shortly after admission. There is a continuation of deterioration during the first 2 days; transtentorial herniation usually occurs within 2–4 days of stroke. Mortalities are often accompanied by severe drowsiness, dense hemiplegia, age > 45–50 years, early parenchymal hypodensity involving> 50% of the MCA distribution on CT scan, midline shift > 8–10 mm, early sulcus effacement, as well as a hyperdense artery sign in the MCA. Aggressive surgical therapies in these patients may reduce morbidity and mortality. Treatment options include the following: 1. usual conventional measures to control ICP (mortality is very high); and 2. hemicraniectomy (decompressive craniectomy) with or without the removal of an infarcted brain, especially temporal brain (Greenberg 2010; Lindsay et al. 2011; Vahedi et al. 2007; Gage et al. 2001).

1.12.1. Hemicraniectomy for Malignant MCA Territory Infarction

A hemicraniectomy may decrease mortality to as low as 32–37%, with a surprising decrease in hemiplegia and dominant-side strokes, with only mild-to-moderate aphasia (better outcomes occur with early intervention, especially if surgery is accomplished before any changes linked to herniation occur). The indication guidelines are as follows: 1. age < 70 years; 2. more seriously considered on the nondominant side (commonly right); and 3. clinical and CT evidence of acute, complete ICA/MCA infarcts and direct signs of inevitable or complete severe hemispheric brain swelling (Greenberg 2010).

1.13. TIA and Minor Infarction—Management

The goal of management to avoid later cerebral infarction includes the establishment of a diagnosis, as well as exclusion of other pathologies causing transient neurological symptoms such as migraine and the correction of predisposing factors. Examination of patients is vital for extracranial and neck vascular disease. Hence, the palpation of carotids and upper limb pulses, along with auscultation of the neck for bruits should be routine. The measuring of blood pressure in both arms and examination of the heart are invaluable (Greenberg 2010; Lindsay et al. 2011; Awad 2005; Brott et al. 2016; Sardar et al. 2017; Naylor 2018; Xu et al. 2017; White et al. 2019; Cai and Peng 2017; Pirau and Lui 2020).

1.13.1. Medical Treatment

(i) Controlling hypertension;
(ii) Stopping smoking;
(iii) Correction of lipid abnormality;
(iv) Prescription of antiplatelets (aspirin or Clopidogrel) to decrease the reinfarction;
(v) Removal or treatment of the embolic source.

1.13.2. Surgical and Other Interventional Treatments

Carotid stenosis (Figures 4–6)—High-quality surgical studies have shown that individuals with a carotid stenosis greater than 70% (but not occlusion) and a TIA or minor stroke in carotid territory have a lower risk of a second stroke if they have a carotid endarterectomy. This advantage is contingent on the procedure being performed by a skilled surgeon with a low risk of complications. With higher grades of stenosis and in patients with a hemispheric TIA, the risk of stroke, and consequently, the benefit of surgery is the greatest (as opposed to amaurosis fugax). For patients with lower degrees of stenosis, the risk of consequences outweighs the benefit. In individuals with a stenosis of more than 70%, carotid angioplasty with stenting is an option instead of carotid endarterectomy; however, recent studies have indicated a greater risk of stroke, and perioperative mortality and morbidity are a little higher than CEA, though this was not statistically significant. Other surgical techniques such as the superficial temporal-to-middle cerebral artery (STA–MCA) bypass have no benefit in carotid stenosis.

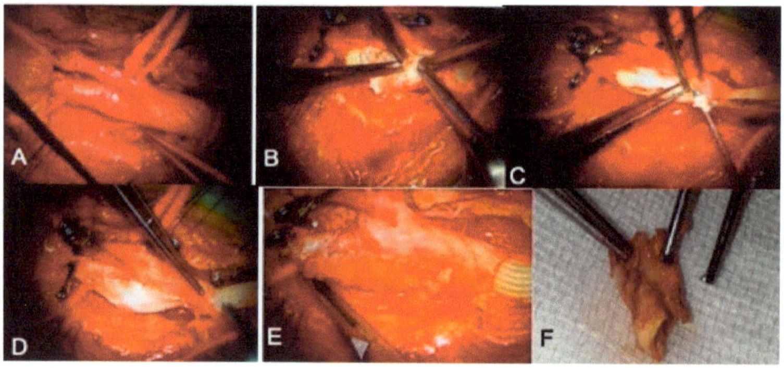

Figure 5. (**A–E**) Preoperative sequential pictures of the right ICA CEA of the patient from Figure 4. (**F**) Atherosclerotic plaque after a CEA. Source: Figure by authors.

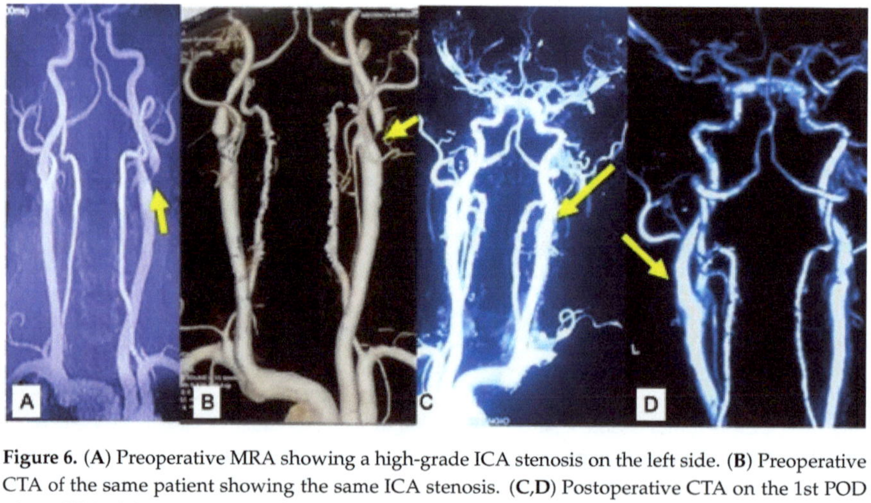

Figure 6. (**A**) Preoperative MRA showing a high-grade ICA stenosis on the left side. (**B**) Preoperative CTA of the same patient showing the same ICA stenosis. (**C,D**) Postoperative CTA on the 1st POD after a CEA of the same patient showing relief of left ICA stenosis. Source: Figure by authors.

1.13.3. Carotid Occlusion

For a carotid occlusion, the surgical options are an EC–IC bypass, CEA with an opening of the ICA and endovascular carotid stenting with a wire-guided catheter-assisted reopening of the ICA. All have definite indications with pros and cons.

1.13.4. MCA or ACA Stenosis

For an MCA or ACA stenosis, an EC–IC bypass is employed in selective cases.

1.13.5. Vertebrobasilar Stenosis

For a vertebrobasilar stenosis, a vertebral artery endarterectomy, VA reimplantation in CCA/ICA/ECA or OA–VA or OA–PICA bypass are employed. The role of these interventions in vertebrobasilar stenosis is not yet established.

2. Atherosclerotic Cerebrovascular Disease

2.1. Carotid Artery

2.1.1. Presentation

The majority (80%) of carotid atherothrombotic strokes occur without warning symptoms. The prevalence of an asymptomatic bruit increases with age (2.3–8.2% in ages 45–75 years). The accuracy of a bruit in predicting an ICA stenosis is 50–83% and sensitivity is as low as 24%. Symptomatic carotid disease may present as a TIA, RIND (reversible ischemic neurological deficit) or CVA, with findings such as amaurosis fugux or monocular blindness (retinal insufficiency or infarction), contralateral motor or sensory TIA (arm and face worse than legs) or language deficits if the dominant hemisphere is involved (MCA symptoms) (Greenberg 2010; Kistler and Furie 2000; Sonecha et al. 2006; Nighoghossian et al. 2005).

2.1.2. Assessment Options

Cerebral DSA

The "gold standard" test for a cerebral DSA is a catheter angiogram (Figures 4 and 6). It cannot be justified as a screening test because it is invasive, costly and risky. Also, unlike duplex Doppler and MRA, it does not provide any information about the thickness of the plaque. It is usually carried out when a simultaneous endovascular intervention is planned if needed.

Duplex Doppler Ultrasound

B-mode image evaluates the artery in a cross-sectional plane, and it is noninvasive. It performs poorly with a "string sign". Its sensitivity is 88% and specificity 76% (Greenberg 2010; Lindsay et al. 2011; Awad 2005; Kaufmann et al. 2007; Heiserman et al. 1996; Koelemay et al. 2004).

Magnetic Resonance Angiography (MRA)

It is noninvasive and can be carried out at the time as an MRI with ischemic stroke protocol in TIA/stroke cases (Figure 6A). It obviates the need for a DSA in some risky symptomatic cases of a carotid stenosis. Sometimes, it overestimates the degree of a stenosis. An MRA has 91% sensitivity and 88% specificity for extracranial carotid disease. It can detect a thrombus or dissection. An MRA is less operator-dependent than Doppler, but is costlier as well as more time-consuming. An MRA is more difficult to perform if the patient is critical and in contraindicated cases. A high-resolution MRI may also detect vulnerable plaques.

Computed Tomography Angiography (CTA)

The results of a CTA (Figure 6B–D) are comparable to that of an MRA. A CTA can be performed within minutes and can display high-resolution images of all vessels from the arch of the aorta through the intracranial/extracranial vessels, including the surrounding soft tissues. In a meta-analysis, the sensitivity and specificity for the identification of a 70–99% stenosis were 85% and 93%, respectively. A CTA may help detect vulnerable plaques. Another potential advantage is the ability to get CT–perfusion images at the same time.

Choice of Imaging Test/Management Decisions

Doppler, CTA or MRA are usually acceptable initial screening tests. In patients having an abnormal screening test, a common protocol is to go for a second confirmatory noninvasive investigation to reassess the carotid bifurcation before the intervention. If noninvasive investigations are not concordant, a DSA should be carried out before the intervention (Greenberg 2010; Lindsay et al. 2011; Awad 2005; Kaufmann et al. 2007; Heiserman et al. 1996; Koelemay et al. 2004).

2.1.3. Treatment

The treatment alternatives are primarily the following:

1. Medical management with antiplatelet therapy and a lipid-lowering agent;
2. Carotid endarterectomy is a time-tested and gold standard treatment;
3. Endovascular carotid angioplasty and stenting, where perioperative mortality and morbidity are little more than the CEA and the long-term results are yet to be established (Greenberg 2010; Lindsay et al. 2011; Awad 2005; Brott et al. 2016; Sardar et al. 2017; Naylor 2018; Cremonesi et al. 2006).

Asymptomatic Carotid Artery Stenosis

Due to the increased frequency of carotid screening, more asymptomatic cases are being diagnosed. In these cases, the chance of a stroke is 2%/year. Large, randomized trials have revealed that moderate surgical benefits are significantly superior than medical management for asymptomatic stenosis >60%. The patient's age, gender and comorbidities (and therefore life expectancy), as well as perioperative complication rate are the factors to consider in the selection of treatment options.

Practice Guideline 33·1: Asymptomatic Carotid Stenosis

For patients with a neurosurgical risk < 3% and life expectancy > 6 years:

In asymptomatic stenosis >60%, carotid endarterectomy (CEA) should be carried out, and a unilateral CEA is also indicated for asymptomatic stenosis> 50% when an atherosclerotic plaque is large, deep, complex or a cavitated ulcer.

An ipsilateral CEA is recommended for a stenosis> 75% with a contralateral ICA stenosis 75–100%, even in patients with a 3–5% surgical risk.

Once again, endovascular angioplasty with stenting is an option (popular option) in these cases with less favorable (minutely) results than a CEA.

Carotid stenting should be carried out with enough procedural quality levels and should be considered instead of a CEA in the presence of the following:

1. Severe cardiovascular comorbidities (such as heart failure) and severe pulmonary disease.
2. Specific situations:

   (i) Laryngeal nerve palsy on the contralateral side;
   (ii) Radio-therapy to the neck;
   (iii) Previously performed CEA with recurrent restenosis;
   (iv) High cervical internal carotid/below the level of a clavicle common carotid stenosis;
   (v) Severe tandem stenosis (Greenberg 2010; Lindsay et al. 2011; Awad 2005; Brott et al. 2016; Sardar et al. 2017; Naylor 2018; Cremonesi et al. 2006).

2.1.4. Totally Occluded Internal Carotid Artery

Introduction

About 10–15% of patients presenting with an ICA territory infarct or TIAs are seen to have a total internal carotid artery occlusion (Figures 7–9). The prevention of a second stroke in symptomatic individuals with a complete carotid blockage is still a difficult task. Following a stroke, the overall rate of a subsequent stroke is 7% per year for all strokes, and 5.9% for ischemic stroke ipsilateral to the blocked carotid artery. These risks persist in spite of treatment with antiplatelets and anticoagulants. The prevalence of an asymptomatic carotid occlusion is unknown, and the incidence of an ipsilateral stroke in never-symptomatic carotid stenosis is negligible.

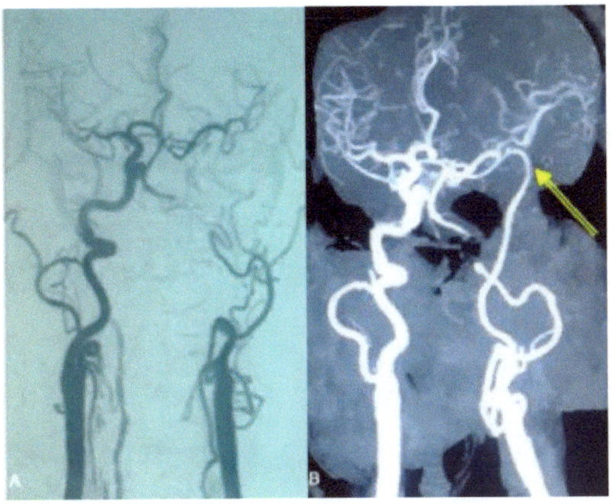

Figure 7. (**A**) CTA showing a chronic occlusion of the left ICA and both VA with presented with a "Crescendo TIA". (**B**) CTA after an urgent left-sided intermediate flow EC–IC bypass (CCA–RAG–MCA) in the same patient. Source: Figure by authors.

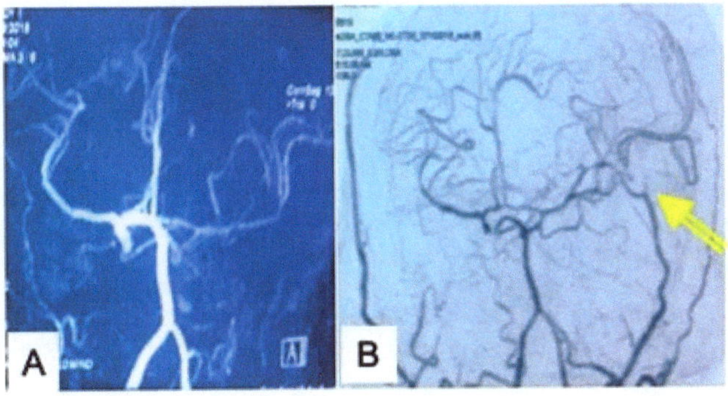

Figure 8. (**A**) Preoperative MRA of the brain showing a bilateral ICA occlusion presented with a recurrent TIA and recurrent strokes. (**B**) Postoperative CTA after a left STA–MCA bypass (arrow-marked). Source: Figure by authors.

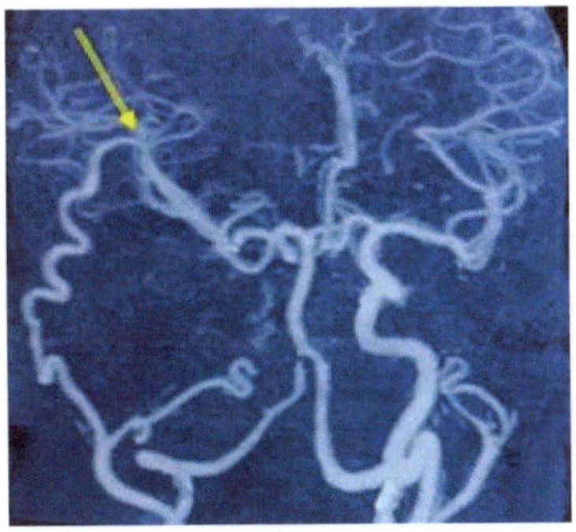

Figure 9. Post-STA–MCA bypass CTA in the case of a right ICA occlusion showing a "robust STA–MCA bypass". Source: Figure by authors.

Presentation

Three types of CVA can occur with an acute carotid artery occlusion:

1. Stump emboli can produce cortical infarcts. Emboli usually go up the external carotid, then through an ECA–ICA anastomosis into the ICA to the embolic infarct.
2. Whole-hemisphere infarction.
3. A watershed infarct hemiparetic TIA (53%), dysphasic TIA (34%), furred neuro-deficit (21%), crescendo TIAs (21%), amaurosis fugax (17%) and an acute hemiplegia (6%) can occur in symptomatic patients. Patients may have the so called "slow carotid stroke" of a carotid occlusion, which is a stuttering progressive stroke. An MRI may show the so called "string of pearls" sign (small areas of intra-parenchymal increased density on DWI) of watershed-type infarcts. Of patients with an acute ICA occlusion with profound neurological deficit, 2–12% make reasonably good recovery, 40–69% have severe neuro-deficit and 16–55% die by the time of follow-up.

Treatment and Surgery

Options include the following:

- Endarterectomy;
- Fogarty balloon catheter embolectomy (utilizing a no. 2 French catheter with a 0.2 mL balloon gently passed 10–12 cm up the ICA from a small arteriotomy made distal to the atheromatous plaque);
- Extracranial–intracranial (EC–IC) bypass (Figures 7–9);
- Endovascular thrombolysis and stenting (although the results of case reports appear promising, randomized controlled trials on cervical carotid thrombolysis and/or stenting are lacking);
- Hybrid techniques for the re-opening of the ICA.

The patency restoration rate is inversely related to the duration of the occlusion. A chronically occluded ICA has a poor patency rate and little gain from re-opening. The retrograde filling of the ICA to petrous or cavernous segment from an ECA anastomosis or contralateral ICA is a good sign of operability.

Operating pearls:

- Emergency operations for an acute neuro-deficit associated with the total occlusion should not be performed after about 2 hrs;
- Extremely poor neuro status (lethargy/coma) is a contraindication to surgery;
- Patients without a persistent neuro-deficit should be operated on as soon as possible;
- If the patient has recurrent TIAs (despite maximal medical therapy) following a recent carotid occlusion and no definite infarct on MRI, an EC–IC bypass surgery should be considered (Greenberg 2010; Xu et al. 2017; White et al. 2019; Powers et al. 2000; Sugg et al. 2005; Powers et al. 1987; Hafner and Tew 1981).

2.2. *Vertebrobasilar Insufficiency (VBI)*

2.2.1. Introduction

VBI may be suspected in a patient with transient episodes of "dizziness" (vertigo without apparent cause) that is initiated by positional changes. The estimated stroke rates are 22–35% over 5 years, or 4.5–7% per year. The risk of infarction after the first VBI–TIA has been estimated to be 22% for the first year.

Depending on the severity of the disorder, VBI can cause a variety of symptoms. Some symptoms may just last a few minutes, while others may last a lifetime. Loss of vision in one or both eyes, diplopia, nausea and vomiting, dizziness or vertigo, slurred speech, numbness or tingling in the hands or feet, changes in mental status (including confusion or loss of consciousness), sudden and severe weakness throughout the body also known as a drop attack, loss of balance and coordination, difficulty swallowing and weakness in a part of the body are all common symptoms of VBI. As with a TIA, the symptoms may come and go.

2.2.2. Clinical Presentation

The diagnostic criteria for VBI are shown in Table 5.

For the clinical diagnosis of VBI, two or more of the following criteria are needed:

- Sensory or motor symptoms or both, happening bilaterally at the same time;
- Diplopia: due to ischemia of the upper brainstem (midbrain) near the ocular nuclei;
- Dysarthria: due to ischemia of the lower brainstem;
- Homonymous hemianopsia: as a result of ischemia of the occipital cortex (this is binocular, where amaurosis fugax which is monocular).

Table 5. Diagnostic criteria for VBI.

"The 5 Ds of VBI" Diagnostic Criteria
Drop attack
Diplopia
Dysarthria
Defect (visual)
Dizziness

Source: Authors' compilation based on data from Greenberg (2010).

2.2.3. Etiology

Atheromatous and stenotic lesions occur most frequently at the VA origin which usually causes VBI. Other atheromatous lesions on the BA or PCA can cause symptoms related to VBI. VBI symptoms may be due to hemodynamic insufficiency (perhaps the most common etiology), including subclavian steal syndrome where reversed flow in the VA due to a proximal stenosis of the subclavian artery and sometime stenosis of both VAs or one VA where the other is hypofunctional.

VBI may sometimes be due to squeezing of the VA at the level of C1–C2 with head turning (bow hunter's syndrome) or anterior atlantoaxial subluxation (e.g., in rheumatoid arthritis) with rotatory atlantoaxial subluxation. Embolism from the ulceration of a plaque or cardiac origin can also cause a vertebrobasilar infarction.

2.2.4. Investigations

An MRI (MRA) is part of the ischemic stroke protocol, CT (with perfusion CT) and CTA, or a six-vessel cranial-selective DSA.

2.2.5. Treatment

Surgical treatments are the main way of management. The options are as follows:

- Vertebral endarterectomy should be carried out in
    - (i) Bilaterally substantial VA stenosis, defined as a stenosis of more than 60% in both arteries;
    - (ii) If the contralateral is hypoplastic, the dominant vertebral artery (VA) has a greater-than-60% stenosis, terminating in the posterior inferior cerebellar artery (PICA), or is obstructed;
    - (iii) Symptomatic embolism thought to be caused by a spinal lesion;
- Transposition of the VA to the ICA, CCA or ECA (with or without a saphenous vein patch graft), or to the thyrocervical trunk or subclavian artery;
- Bypass grafting (for example, occipital artery to the PICA);
- For a Cl-2 posterior reduction, arthrodesis with stabilization may prevent a potentially life-threatening CVA in the cases of os odontoideum, AAD or bow hunter's syndrome.

Anticoagulation is the mainstay of medical treatment. Alternatives to anticoagulants include antiplatelet drugs. The efficacy of either drugs remains unproven. Secondary prevention, like all types of ischemia events, necessitates a multimodal approach that includes blood pressure control, quitting smoking, stringent blood sugar control, statin use and lifestyle changes such as diet and exercise (Greenberg 2010; Lindsay et al. 2011; Awad 2005; Schaller 2008; Kuether et al. 1997; Pirau and Lui 2020; Caplan 2003).

2.2.6. Bow Hunter's Stroke (BHS)

BHS Hemodynamic

Here, VBI (TIA to infarct) is induced by an intermittent VA occlusion resulting from head rotation. It may also occur with forced (e.g., chiropractic neck manipulation) or voluntary head rotation. An occlusion usually involves the VA contralateral to the direction of rotation, and usually occurs at the Cl–C2 junction (due to the immobility of the VA at this location). However, other sites can also be involved. A VA occlusion does not produce clinical symptoms in most individuals due to collateral supply through the contralateral VA and/or the circle of Willis. A symptomatic occlusion usually involves the dominant VA, however, may also occur with a non-dominant VA. Most cases of a BHS occur in patients with an isolated posterior circulation (incompetent posterior communicating arteries).

Contributing Factors to a BHS

1. External VA compression
   - (i) Spondylotic bone spurs: particularly in the foramen transversarium;
   - (ii) Tumors;
   - (iii) Fibrous bands (e.g., proximal to entrance of the VA into the C6 foramen transversarium);
   - (iv) Infectious processes;
   - (v) Trauma.
2. Tethering of the VA
   - (i) At the transverse foramina of Cl and C2;
   - (ii) Along the sulcus arteriosus proximal to where the VA enters the dura;
   - (iii) Defect in the odontoid process;
   - (iv) Atherosclerotic vascular disease.

Diagnosis

A dynamic cerebral DSA is the investigation of choice, but significant consequences can be precipitated during a DSA in patients with a BHS. The involved VA shows loss of flow as the head is rotated from the neutral position to the contralateral side. Carotid injections demonstrate patency of the posterior communicating artery, as well as the presence of any persistent fetal anastomoses.

CT angiogram (CTA): The same precautions are needed as with a dynamic DSA. A CTA is not the initial diagnostic study of choice. If the dynamic DSA is negative, a CTA is not needed. If the dynamic DSA is positive, a CTA with a CT scan of the cervical spine with the craniovertebral junction may be helpful to demonstrate the arterial relationship to the bony anatomy.

Treatment

Conservative: conservative treatment includes anticoagulation with the cervical collar to remind the patient not to turn their head. Surgical treatment is the definitive treatment.

For VA compression at Cl–2:

(i) Cl–2 fusion and fixation after reduction;
(ii) VA decompression: Cl "hemilaminectomy" via a posterior approach.

For compression at other sites: elimination of the source of compression where possible (e.g., sectioning of an offending fibrous band, removal of osteophytic spurs) (Greenberg 2010; Schaller 2008; Pirau and Lui 2020; Lemole et al. 2002).

3. Cerebral Arterial Dissections (CADs)

3.1. Introduction

When intraluminal blood penetrates the layers of the vessel wall, a cerebral arterial dissection occurs. In the young population, a cranial–cervical dissection is responsible for 15–20% of strokes (Rajpal and Naik 2018; Anson and Crowell 1991). In CAD, hemorrhage occurs in the medial layer of an artery which may be spontaneous or post-traumatic, and may be intracranial or extracranial. It usually presents with ipsilateral pain, as well as features of an infarction or subarachnoid hemorrhage (SAH).

3.2. Pathophysiology

A pathological trans-intimal extravasation of blood from the true lumen into the vessel wall either dissects the internal elastic membrane from the intima, causing a narrowing of the true lumen leading to ischemia or infarction, or it may dissect into the sub-adventitial plane, producing an adventitial outpouching from the vessel wall (pseudoaneurysm). Rupture through the vessel wall producing an SAH occurs occasionally.

Subintimal dissections are more common with intracranial dissections, whereas extracranial vessels usually dissect either at the media or between media and adventitia.

CADs primarily affect middle-aged patients with an average age of 45 years (average age of traumatic dissections is slightly lower). CADs are more frequent in men; however, the incidence is unknown, as it often causes mild and transient symptoms. Some internal carotid artery cases (though considered spontaneous) may actually be due to trivial trauma, including violent coughing, nose blowing and simple neck turning. This usually occurs in young women.

The VA was the commonest intracranial site for dissection. VA dissections are less frequent than carotid dissections. Extracranial lesions outnumber intracranial ones. Traumatic dissections frequently occur where the VA crosses bony prominences, e.g., at the Cl–2 junction or where it enters the foramen transversarium (usually at C6). Spontaneous dissections tend to be intracranial and commonly occur on the dominant VA.

Dissecting aneurysms of the VA tends to be fusiform and may be amenable to clipping. Basilar artery dissections tend to present with a brainstem infarction and the prognosis is generally regarded as poor (Greenberg 2010; Lindsay et al. 2011; Rajpal and Naik 2018; Yamaura 1994; CA VAT AS Investigators 2001).

3.3. Etiology of "Spontaneous" Dissections

Etiologies of spontaneous dissection are shown in Table 6.

Table 6. Etiologies of a spontaneous dissection.

Common	Others
Fibromuscular dysplasia (FMD): found in 15% cases	Ehlers–Danlos syndrome
Cystic medial necrosis (or degeneration)	Takayasu's disease
Saccular aneurysm	Medial degeneration
Marfan syndrome	Syphilitic arteritis
Atherosclerosis	Polyarteritis nodosa (PAN)
Strenuous physical exercise	Moyamoya disease
Autosomal dominant polycystic kidney disease	Allergic arteritis
Homocystinuria	Migraine

Source: Authors' compilation based on data from Greenberg (2010), Lindsay et al. (2011), Anson and Crowell (1991) and Halbach et al. (1993).

3.4. Clinical Presentation

The most frequent presentation in patients under 30 years is usually due to an internal carotid (anterior circulation) dissection without an SAH but can present with an SAH (Figure 10). In patients > 30 years, a vertebrobasilar artery (VBA) dissection with an SAH is the most common. Headaches are commonly severe and usually predate neurologic deficits by days or weeks.

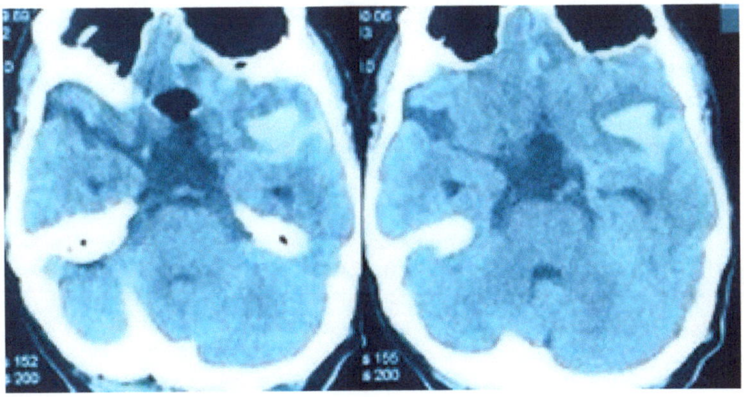

Figure 10. Axial CT scan showing a left Sylvian SAH (the patient presented with features of an SAH with left hemiparesis and aphasia). Source: Figure by authors.

3.4.1. Internal Carotid Dissection

In a spontaneous dissection, the most common initial symptom is an ipsilateral headache. It may also produce a sudden onset of severe pain over the carotid artery (carotidynia). For incomplete Homer's syndrome (oculosympathetic palsy), ptosis and miosis without anhidrosis may occur. A bruit may be heard either by the examiner or by the patient. It may be a cause of infantile and childhood hemiplegia and hemiparesis. Post-traumatic ICA dissections are much more common than spontaneous ones, and are managed like of arterial dissections with the management of other injuries.

3.4.2. Vertebrobasilar System Artery Dissection

In spontaneous extradural dissections, neck pain and severe headache are common, along with TIAs or stroke (usually lateral medullary syndrome or cerebellar infarction, especially in patients with an occlusion of the third or fourth portion of the VA. A VA dissection may be bilateral). Dissecting aneurysms may present with an altered level of consciousness, and may cause an SAH. Rebleeding occurs in 24–30% of these cases presenting with an SAH, making these lesions risky with a very high mortality. Traumatic extradural dissections or pseudoaneurysms may have a similar presentation but can also produce massive external hemorrhage or neck hematomas (Greenberg 2010; Yamaura 1994; Halbach et al. 1993; Welling et al. 1983; Pozzati et al. 1994).

3.5. Evaluation

A CT is very useful for evaluating the brain for an infarction (perfusion CT). Dissections can sometimes be visualized directly. A CTA identifies the CAD with 99% accuracy (Figures 10–12).

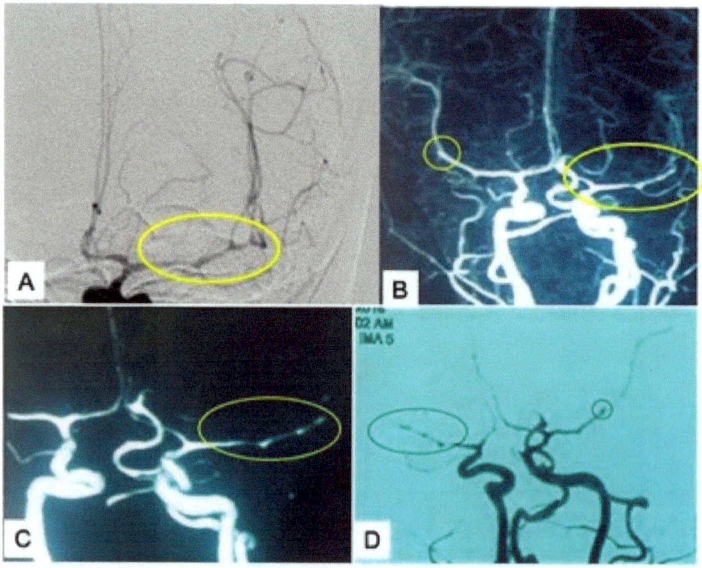

Figure 11. DSA and CTA of the patient from Figure 10. (**A**) Cerebral DSA of the left CCA injection showing a beaded appearance of the left MCA. (**B–D**) CTA of the brain showing beaded appearance of the left MCA, suggesting an MCA dissection. The patient (27-year-old female) also had a right MCA aneurysm (incidental) and dorsal scoliosis. Source: Figure by authors.

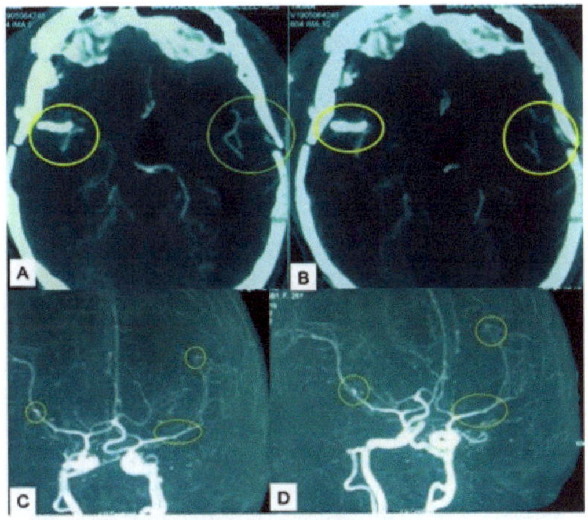

Figure 12. The patient from Figure 10 underwent a left STA–MCA bypass and microsurgical clipping of the right MCA aneurysm in the same sitting. (**A–D**) Postoperative CTA on the first POD. Source: Figure by authors.

The definitive diagnostic study is a cerebral DSA. However, diagnosis is challenging and may be delayed or misinterpreted as a saccular aneurysm or vasospasm. Angiographic findings in CAD are shown in Table 7.

Table 7. Angiography (DSA, CTA, MRA) findings.

(i)	Luminal stenosis ("string sign")		
(ii)	Fusiform dilation with distal or proximal slandering (string and pearl sign)	(vi)	"Double lumen sign": true vessel lumen and an intramural pseudo lumen is the only pathognomonic sign
(iii)	Occlusion of artery		
(iv)	Intimal flap	(vii)	Wavy "ripple" appearance
(v)	Proximal beading ("string of beads" configuration, indicative of an FMD) (Figures 10–12)	(viii)	Severe kinking (frequently bilateral); VBA may show dolichoectasia
A finding of arterial dissections is that they often alter configuration on repeat angiography due to resolve or worsen.			

Source: Authors' compilation based on data from Greenberg (2010), Lindsay et al. (2011), Rajpal and Naik (2018), Eastman et al. (2006) and Kitanaka et al. (1994).

MRI: On T1 weighted magnetic resonance imaging (MRI), an intramural hematoma appears as a region of elevated signal intensity, whereas contrast MRI shows a thick ring-like or railroad-like enhancement corresponding to the twofold lumen (Crescent sign). MRA can also show the details of CAD (Greenberg 2010; Rajpal and Naik 2018; Eastman et al. 2006; Kitanaka et al. 1994).

3.6. *Treatment*

- Extracranial dissections are usually treated medically (anticoagulation).
- Whereas intracranial dissections with SAH are treated surgically (Figures 10–12).
- But treatment should be individualized as case by case.

The clinical presentation, collateral circulation, access-related problems for both surgical and endovascular techniques, the presence of any leptomeningeal anastomoses, and contralateral flow all influence the treatment. After a rebleed, there is a substantial risk of morbidity and mortality, especially in dissecting aneurysms, hence this condition necessitates intensive surgical or endovascular therapy. Heparin, followed by warfarin or antiplatelet medicine, can be used to treat patients with ischemic intracranial dissection. Stenting and balloon dilatation or surgical bypass followed by occlusion or trapping of the affected section are options for patients with acute or recurrent strokes who do not respond to pharmacological treatment. The role of surgical treatment in patients with fusiform dilated aneurysms is clip reconstruction of the vessel, wrapping of the aneurysm, and clipping or trapping of the parent artery and revascularization, especially if there are insufficient leptomeningeal anastomoses or collaterals. Endovascular therapy options include proximal blockage of the parent artery with materials, coils or detachable balloons, proximal and distal trapping of the diseased arterial, or a surgical distal bypass followed by a parental vessel occlusion. The parent vasculature can be preserved using stent-assisted coiling, or the vessel can be remodeled utilizing flow diverters with or without coiling (but with a lack of long-term results, with periprocedural complications) (Greenberg 2010; Rajpal and Naik 2018; Zhang et al. 2016; Uhl et al. 2003; Grigoryan et al. 2016; Gory et al. 2017; Sugita et al. 1981; Anxionnat et al. 2003; Aymard et al. 1991; Kurata et al. 2001; Peluso et al. 2008; Lylyk et al. 2009; Ogata et al. 2017; Ramgren et al. 2005; Kühn et al. 2015).

3.7. Outcome

Based on an evaluation of 260 cases, a mortality of 26% was found. Of the cases, 70% had a favorable outcome (based on the Glasgow Outcome scale) and 5% were poor. Mortality was higher for ICA lesions (49%) than VBA lesions (22%). Mortality was 24% in the SAH group and 29% in non-SAH cases (Yamaura 1994).

4. Cerebrovascular Bypasses

4.1. Introduction

Cerebrovascular bypasses are highly specialized, skill-requiring and assiduous armamentariums for the correction/treatment of many cerebrovascular lesions and some cases of skull base lesions. An extracranial–intracranial (EC–IC) bypass was first introduced and pioneered by Donaghy and Yasargil in 1967.

4.2. Classification

Cerebrovascular bypass can be classified in many ways.

Types of cerebrovascular bypasses:

- EC–IC bypass (Figures 7–9):
  Low flow (blood flow 20–40 mL/min)
  - STA–MCA (superficial temporal artery and middle temporal artery) (Figures 8 and 9);
  - STA–PCA (superficial temporal artery–posterior cerebral artery);
  - STA–SCA (superficial temporal artery–superior cerebellar artery);
  - OC–PICA (occipital artery–posterior inferior cerebellar artery);
  - OC–PCA (occipital artery–posterior cerebral artery);
  - OC–VA bypass.

  Intermediate flow (blood flow 50–80 mL/min) (Figure 7)
  - CCA/ICA/ECA–RA (radial artery) graft–MCA/PCA/SCA bypass;
  - IMA (internal maxillary artery)–MCA bypass.

  High flow
  - CCA/ICA/ECA–GSV (great saphenous vein) graft–MCA/PCA/SCA
- IC–IC (intracranial–intracranial) bypass.
  Side-to-side bypass
  - MCA–MCA (upper trunk and lower trunk) bypass;
  - ACA–ACA (anterior cerebral artery–anterior cerebral artery) bypass;
  - PICA–PICA bypass;
  - PCA–SCA bypass.

  End-to-side bypass
  - ATA (anterior temporal artery)–PCA bypass;
  - ATA–ACA bypass;
  - ATA–MCA(M2) bypass.

  Reimplantation
  - M2 to M2.

  End-to-end re-anastomosis
  - A3–A3;

- M2–M2.

4.3. Indications

- Symptomatic cerebral ischemic conditions (CBV and CBF mismatch on perfusion images or increase O_2 extraction fraction on PET):

  ICA occlusion;
  ICA stenosis;
  MCA/ACA stenosis or occlusion;
  Vertebrobasilar insufficiency (VBI).

- For management of a complex giant or fusiform aneurysm.
- ICA/VA dissection.
- Moyamoya disease and moyamoya syndrome.
- Traumatic arterial injury.
- Skull base tumor where a radical excision is performed (cavernous sinus malignant tumor/fungal mass excision with ICA).

4.4. EC–IC Bypass for Cerebrovascular Ischemia

After the introduction of an EC–IC bypass (Figures 7–9), it became popular rapidly, but after the failure of an EV–IC trial in 1985, it plummeted suddenly. In spite of a graft patency rate of 96%, surgical patients failed to show any superiority over the medical management group. An extensive evaluation showed the failure of the study's inclusion criteria to distinguish between hemodynamic vs. thromboembolic causes of stroke.

4.4.1. Present Recommendation for EC–IC Bypass in Ischemia

Currently, imaging can identify flow-dependent ischemia. Xenon-CT, TCD, SPECT and MRI may be utilized in combination with an acetazolamide challenge test to investigate the cerebrovascular reserve and reactivity. As cerebral perfusion pressure decreases in severe atherosclerotic occlusive disease, cerebral vascular autoregulation fails to maintain an adequate CBF to keep up with metabolic demands. In this situation of "misery perfusion", the oxygen extraction fraction (OEF) of available blood flow will increase. An increased OEF, as quantified by a PET, is an independent predicator of subsequent stroke. Patients with an abnormal response to acetazolamide challenge and/or with an elevated OEF are therefore potential candidates for cerebral revascularization (Greenberg 2010; Crowley et al. 2008; Garrett et al. 2008; Garrett et al. 2009; Kuroda et al. 2001; Lawton 2018).

5. Cerebral Vein and Dural Sinus Thrombosis (CVST)

5.1. Introduction

A CVST is a less frequent cause of stroke, with a yearly incidence of approximately 5/million, most commonly afflicting those in younger age groups and females. Its clinical presentation varies, and thus may delay the diagnosis (Al-Sulaiman 2019; Ferro et al. 2004; Bousser and Ferro 2007; Ferro and Canhão 2014).

Three types of CVST may produce cerebral venous infarctions:

(i) Dural sinus thrombosis;
(ii) Cortical venous thrombosis;
(iii) Deep venous thrombosis.

5.2. Etiologies

Etiological condition are listed in Table 8.

Table 8. Many conditions have been associated with a CVST.

Common	**Others**
Infection, i.e., otitis media, sinusitis, meningitis	Cardiac disease (including CHF)
	Ulcerative colitis
Pregnancy and puerperium	Periarteritis nodosa Sickle cell trait
Oral contraceptives, dehydration, burn and cachexia (malignancy)	Trauma, including closed head injury
	Malignancy, including myeloproliferative disorders
Hypercoagulable state or thrombophilia (protein C, S, antithrombin III and plasminogen deficiency; anti-phospholipid antibodies; systemic lupus erythematosus)	Diabetes mellitus, especially with ketoacidosis
	Homocystinuria

Source: Authors' compilation based on data from Greenberg (2010), Al-Sulaiman (2019) and Dolan and Chowdry (1995).

5.3. Frequency of Involvement of Dural Sinuses and Other Veins

The superior sagittal sinus (SSS), left transverse sinus (TS) and superficial cortical veins are the most commonly involved. Multiple sinuses/veins involvement occur in 71% of cases. The cavernous sinus, straight sinus and deep venous system are rarely involved (Greenberg 2010).

5.4. Pathophysiology

A CVST reduces venous return from the brain tissue and reduces essential circulation to the brain.

This venous engorgement results in cerebral edema. The elevated venous pressure may also result in an infarction and/or hemorrhage. All these sequences may lead to a raised ICP. Hence, the clinical features may be due to a raised ICP, and the focal deficit/s may be due to edema and/or hemorrhage. A brain infarction in this situation is known as a venous infarction (Greenberg 2010; Al-Sulaiman 2019).

5.5. Clinical Features

There are no pathognomonic findings. Many signs and symptoms are due to an elevated ICP. They may present as a syndrome clinically indistinguishable from idiopathic intracranial hypertension (IIH). The anterior 1/3 of the SSS may have a blockage often without symptoms. In the posterior 2/3 occlusion, a venous infarction is more likely to evolve. The middle portion of the SSS occlusion usually causes hypertonia ranging from spastic hemi- or quadri-paresis. A posterior SSS occlusion can cause visual field cuts or cortical blindness, or a massive venous infarct with edema and death. Thrombosis of the TS may occur without symptoms, unless the opposite TS is hypoplastic or aplastic where the clinical presentation is akin to posterior SSS thrombosis. An isolated SSS blockage will not result in a cranial nerve deficit, except visual impairment and sixth nerve palsy from an elevated ICP. An occlusion of the jugular bulb may press the nerves in the jugular foramen, resulting in hoarseness, dysphonia, dysphagia and dyspnea.

A CVST should be diagnosed based on clinical evidence and supported imaging investigations, and should always be investigated in patients who have the following symptoms:

- Symptoms of FNDs in the absence of recognized vascular risk factors;
- New onset of an atypical headache;
- Intracranial hypertension;
- Neuroimaging evidence of hemorrhagic infarctions, particularly if the infarctions are many and do not follow arterial vascular regions (Greenberg 2010; Al-Sulaiman 2019; Kalbag 1984; Stam 2005).

5.6. Diagnosis

5.6.1. CT and CT Venogram (CTV)

May be normal in 10–20% of cases of CVST. The findings include the following:

(i) Hyperdense sinuses and veins (the cord sign which is pathognomonic);
(ii) Intraparenchymal petechial "flame" hemorrhages, seen in 20% of cases;
(iii) Small/slit ventricles are seen in 50% of cases;

(iv) Thrombosis of the SSS may produce a triangular-shaped high density within the sinus;
(v) White matter edema;
(vi) All of the above changes occurring bilaterally;
(vii) Enhancement of the dura around the sinus, intense tentorial enhancement and gyral enhancement on contrast CT;
(viii) CTV shows occluded sinus/veins with evidence of redirected venous flow (Greenberg 2010; Al-Sulaiman 2019; Stam 2005; Perkin 1995).

5.6.2. MRI and MR Venogram (MRV)

An MRI (Figures 13 and 14) is excellent for a diagnosis and follow-up. It demonstrates the absence of venous flow and thrombus; it also demonstrates cerebral parenchymal changes. It can differentiate an occluded sinus from congenital aplasia. An MRI shows cerebral edema and non-acute hemorrhagic changes brilliantly at different stages. An MRV shows occluded sinus/veins, with evidence of redirected venous flow, but tends to overestimate the degree of the occlusion (Greenberg 2010; Al-Sulaiman 2019; Stam 2005; Perkin 1995).

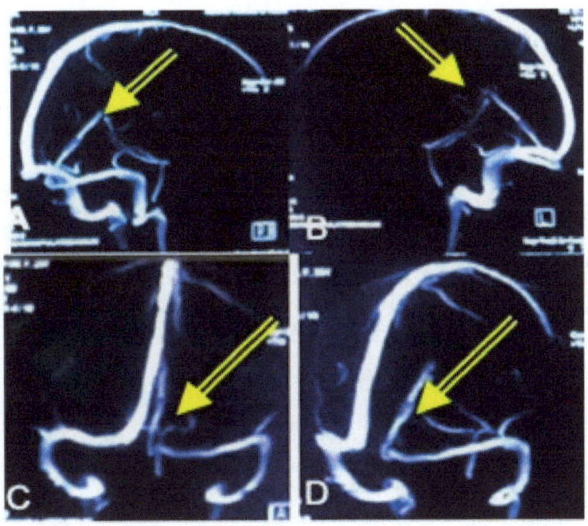

Figure 13. (**A–D**) Normal MRV of the brain where the deep venous system (through the straight sinus) is drained into the right transverse sinus (TS), and the SSS into the left TS. Source: Figure by authors.

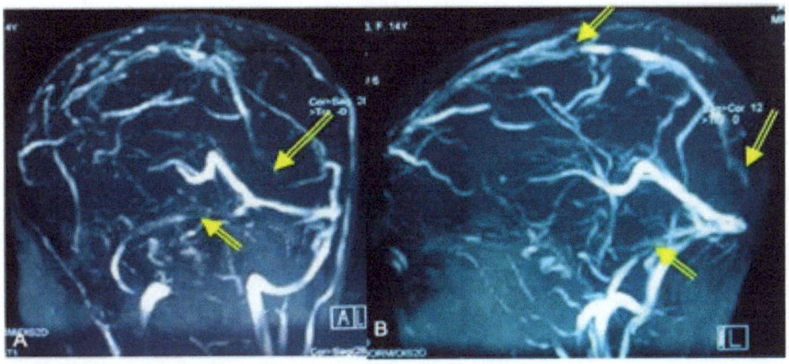

Figure 14. MRV of the brain (**A**,**B**) showing a CVST, especially the SSS and left TS (arrow-marked), where the deep venous drainage system is intact. Source: Figure by authors.

5.6.3. Cerebral DSA

A DSA is better to demonstrate the non-filling of segments of sinuses/veins or filling defects, residual flow and long circulation time, and can find out the areas of reversal of venous flow. Sometimes, a DSA can show a thrombus.

A DSA is often used as a complementary or therapeutic intervention.

5.6.4. Lumbar Puncture (LP)

An OP is usually increased. The CSF may be bloody or xanthochromic.

5.6.5. Hematological Tests

Hematological tests are used to find out predisposing factors when the cause is not known.
An evaluation for thrombophilia and hypercoagulability includes the following:

- Proteins C and S, as well as antithrombin III levels, antiphospholipid antibodies and lupus anticoagulants;
- CBC, factor II level, paroxysmal nocturnal hemoglobinuria panel, serum homocysteine level and leukocyte alkaline phosphatase (Greenberg 2010; Al-Sulaiman 2019; Stam 2005; Perkin 1995).

5.6.6. Ultrasound of the Head in Neonates

An ultrasound can be used in diagnosis of SSS thrombosis in neonates.

5.6.7. Detection of Underlying Disorders

During presentation, laboratory work-up is difficult, as the acute and active process will cause a lot of abnormalities in the coagulation system. The best time to work with these patients up is 3 months after the patient recovers from the acute stage of the disease.

5.7. Prognosis

Prognostic factors are listed in Table 9. Mortality: approximately 30% (range: 5–70%).

Table 9. Poor prognostic factors in CVST.

Poor Prognosticator
Coma
Rapid neurologic deterioration/focal signs
Extremes of age
Male sex
Large hemorrhage
Venous infarct
Deep venous system thrombosis

Source: Authors' compilation based on data from Greenberg (2010).

5.8. Treatment

- Treatment approach should be aggressive as the recovery rate is better than arterial stroke, and mortality and morbidity are very high without appropriate treatment;
- Again, management is intricated as anticoagulation increases the risk of an already increased hemorrhagic infarct, and available measures that lower the ICP may increase blood viscosity and coagulability.

Specific treatment:

(i) Treatment of underlying cause/s when identified (e.g., antibiotics for infection).
(ii) Early systemic heparin therapy—it reduces mortality and morbidity even with the evidence of intracerebral hemorrhage where there is a risk of increasing the size of the hemorrhage.
(iii) Avoidance of steroids and control of blood pressure.
(iv) Control seizures via anticonvulsants.
(v) Maintenance of hydration.
(vi) Monitoring the ICP—if the patient continues to deteriorate, then ventriculostomy or lumbar CSF drainage (continuous or intermittent).
Measures to lower the ICP:

a. Ease of venous drainage by elevation of the head;
b. Hyperventilation;
c. Drain CSF (LP or ventriculostomy);
d. Pentobarbital;
e. Use hyperosmotic and/or loop diuretics last, as they can cause dehydration, hyperosmolarity and hypercoagulability.

(vii) Thrombolytic treatment—systemically or directly into the thrombosed sinus, usually followed with heparin.
(viii) When the patient is deteriorating in spite of the above measures:

- Decompressive craniectomy (± decompressive lobectomy) decreases the ICP, but may not allure the outcome;
- Direct "attack" on thrombosed sinus—sinutomy and sinuplasty with removal of the thrombus.

(ix) Endovascular neurosurgery—success rate is much less with a chronic occlusion.
(x) Visual loss with papilledema may be managed with optic nerve sheath fenestration (ONSF).
(xi) Long-term anticoagulants after resolution of the acute stage with heparin and/or warfarin (3–6 months).

Author Contributions: Conceptualization, methodology, validation, formal analysis, investigation, resources, data curation, F.H.C., Q.D.M. and M.S.Z.H.C.; writing—original draft preparation, writing—review and editing, visualization, supervision, F.H.C. All authors have read and agreed to the published version of the manuscript.

Funding: This research received no external funding.

Conflicts of Interest: The authors declare no conflicts of interest.

References

Al-Sulaiman, Abdulla. 2019. Clinical aspects, diagnosis and management of cerebral vein and dural sinus thrombosis: A literature review. *Saudi Journal of Medicine & Medical Sciences* 7: 137–45.

Anson, Jhon, and Robert M. Crowell. 1991. Cervicocranial arterial dissection. *Neurosurgery* 29: 89–86. [CrossRef]

Anxionnat, René, João Ferreira de Melo Neto, Serge Bracard, Jean Christophe Lacour, Catherine Pinelli, Thierry Civit, and Luc Picard. 2003. Treatment of Hemorrhagic Intracranial Dissections. *Neurosurgery* 53: 289–300; discussion 300–1. [CrossRef] [PubMed]

Awad, Issam A. 2005. Cerebrovascular occlusive disease. In *Principles of Neurosurgery*. Edited by Setti S. Rengachary and Richard G. Ellenbogen. New York: Elsevier Mosby, pp. 197–213.

Aymard, Armand, Y. Pierre Gobin, Jonathan E. Hodes, Siegfried Bien, Daniel Rüfenacht, Daniel Reizine, Bernard George, and Jean J. Merland. 1991. Endovascular occlusion of vertebral arteries in the treatment of unclippable vertebrobasilar aneurysms. *Journal of Neurosurgery* 74: 393–98. [CrossRef] [PubMed]

Barber, P. Alan, D. G. Darby, P. M. Desmond, Q. Yang, R. P. Gerraty, D. Jolley, G. A. Donnan, B. M. Tress, and Stephen M. Davis. 1998. Prediction of stroke outcome with echoplanar perfusion- and diffusion-weighted MRI. *Neurology* 51: 418–26. [CrossRef]

Bousser, Marie-Germaine, and Jose M. Ferro. 2007. Cerebral venous thrombosis: An update. *Lancet Neurology* 6: 162–70. [CrossRef]

Brott, Thomas G., George Howard, Gary S. Roubin, James F. Meschia, Ariane Mackey, William Brooks, Wesley S. Moore, Michael D. Hill, Vito A. Mantese, Wayne M. Clark, and et al. 2016. Long-Term Results of Stenting versus Endarterectomy for Carotid-Artery Stenosis. *The New England Journal of Medicine* 374: 1021–31. [CrossRef] [PubMed]

CA VAT AS Investigators. 2001. Endovascular versus surgical treatment in patients with carotid stenosis in the carotid and vertebral artery transluminal angioplasty study (CA VATAS): A randomized trial. *The Lancet* 357: 1729–37. [CrossRef]

Cai, Bin, and Bin Peng. 2017. Intracranial artery stenosis: Current status of evaluation and treatment in China. *Chronic Diseases and Translational Medicine* 3: 197–206. [CrossRef]

Caplan, Louis R. 2003. Atherosclerotic vertebral artery disease in the neck. *Current Treatment Options in Cardiovascular Medicine* 5: 251–56. [CrossRef]

Chen, Han-Jung, Tao-Chen Lee, and Chi-Peng Wei. 1992. Treatment of cerebellar infarction by decompressive suboccipital. *Stroke* 23: 957–61. [CrossRef] [PubMed]

Cremonesi, Alberto, Carlo Setacci, Angelo Bignamini, Leonardo Bolognese, Francesco Briganti, Germano Di Sciascio, Domenico Inzitari, Gaetano Lanza, Luciano Lupattelli, Salvatore Mangiafico, and et al. 2006. Carotid Artery Stenting. *Stroke* 37: 2400–9. [CrossRef] [PubMed]

Crowley, R. Webster, Ricky Medel, and Aaron S. Dumont. 2008. Evolution of cerebral revascularization techniques. *Neurosurgical Focus* 24: E3. [CrossRef] [PubMed]

Dolan, Robert W., and Khalid Chowdry. 1995. Diagnosis and treatment of intracranial complications of paranasal sinus infections. *Journal of Oral and Maxillofacial Surgery* 53: 1080–87. [CrossRef]

Eastman, Alexander L., David P. Chason, Carlos L. Perez, Amy L. McAnulty, and Joseph P. Minei. 2006. Computed Tomographic Angiography for the Diagnosis of Blunt Cervical Vascular Injury: Is It Ready for Primetime? *The Journal of Trauma and Acute Care Surgery* 60: 925–29. [CrossRef] [PubMed]

Ferro, José M., and Patrícia Canhão. 2014. Cerebral venous sinus thrombosis: Update on diagnosis and management. *Current Cardiology Reports* 16: 523. [CrossRef]

Ferro, José M., Patrícia Canhão, Jan Stam, Marie-Germaine Bousser, and Fernando Barinagarrementeria. 2004. Prognosis of cerebral vein and dural sinus thrombosis: Results of the international study on cerebral vein and dural sinus thrombosis (ISCVT). *Stroke* 35: 664–70. [CrossRef]

Gage, Brian F., Amy D. Waterman, William Shannon, Michael Boechler, Michael W. Rich, and Martha J. Radford. 2001. Validation of Clinical Classification Schemes for Predicting Stroke. *Jama-Journal of The American Medical Association* 285: 2864–70. [CrossRef]

Garrett, Matthew C., Ricardo J. Komotar, Maxwell B. Merkow, Robert M. Starke, Marc L. Otten, and E. Sander Connolly. 2008. The Extracranial–Intracranial Bypass Trial: Implications for future investigations. *Neurosurgical Focus* 24: E4. [CrossRef]

Garrett, Matthew C., Ricardo J. Komotar, Robert M. Starke, Maxwell B. Merkow, Marc L. Otten, Robert R. Sciacca, and E. Sander Connolly. 2009. The efficacy of direct extracranial–intracranial bypass in the treatment of symptomatic hemodynamic failure secondary to athero-occlusive disease: A systematic review. *Clinical Neurology and Neurosurgery* 111: 319–26. [CrossRef]

GBD 2016 Stroke Collaborators. 2019. Global, regional, and national burden of stroke, 1990–2016: A systematic analysis for the Global Burden of Disease Study 2016. *The Lancet Neurology* 18: 439–58. [CrossRef] [PubMed]

Gory, Benjamin, Michel Piotin, Diogo C. Haussen, Henrik Steglich-Arnholm, Markus Holtmannspötter, Julien Labreuche, Christian Taschner, Sebastian Eiden, Raul G. Nogueira, Papanagiotou Panagiotis, and et al. 2017. Thrombectomy in Acute Stroke with Tandem Occlusions from Dissection Versus Atherosclerotic Cause. *Stroke* 48: 3145–48. [CrossRef] [PubMed]

Greenberg, Mark S. 2010. *Handbook of Neurosurgery*. New York: Thieme.

Grigoryan, Mikayel, Diogo C. Haussen, Ameer E. Hassan, Andrey Lima, Jonathan Grossberg, Leticia C. Rebello, Wondwossen Tekle, Michael Frankel, and Raul G. Nogueira. 2016. Endovascular Treatment of Acute Ischemic Stroke Due to Tandem Occlusions: Large Multicenter Series and Systematic Review. *Cerebrovascular Diseases* 41: 306–12. [CrossRef]

Hafner, Charles D., and J. M. Tew. 1981. Surgical management of the totally occluded internal carotid artery. *Surgery* 89: 710–17. [PubMed]

Halbach, Van V., Randall T. Higashida, Christopher F. Dowd, Kenneth W. Fraser, Tony P. Smith, George P. Teitelbaum, Charles B. Wilson, and Grant B. Hieshima. 1993. Endovascular treatment of vertebral artery dissections and pseudoaneurysms. *Journal of Neurosurgery* 79: 183–91. [CrossRef]

Heiserman, Joseph E., Joseph M. Zabramski, Burton P. Drayer, and Paul J. Keller. 1996. Clinical significance of the flow gap in carotid magnetic resonance angiography. *Journal of Neurosurgery* 85: 384–87. [CrossRef]

Kalbag, Ramanand M. 1984. Cerebral Venous thrombosis. In *The Cerebral Venous System and Its Disorders*. Edited by Jhon P. Kapp and Henry H. Schmidek. Orlando: Grune and Stratton, pp. 505–36.

Kaufmann, Timothy J., John Huston III, Jay N. Mandrekar, Cathy D. Schleck, Kent R. Thielen, and David F. Kallmes. 2007. Complications of Diagnostic Cerebral Angiography: Evaluation of 19826 Consecutive Patients. *Radiology* 243: 812–19. [CrossRef]

Kistler, J. Philip, and Karen L. Furie. 2000. Carotid endarterectomy revisited. *The New England Journal of Medicine* 342: 1743–45. [CrossRef]

Kitanaka, Chifumi, Jun-Ichi Tanaki, Masanori Kuwahara, Akira Teraoka, Tomio Sasaki, and Kintomo Takakura. 1994. Nonsurgical treatment of unruptured intracranial vertebral artery dissection with serial follow-up angiography. *Journal of Neurosurgery* 80: 667–74, Erratum in: *Journal of Neurosurgery* 1994, 80: 1132. [CrossRef]

Koelemay, Mark J. W., Paul J. Nederkoorn, Johannes B. Reitsma, and Charles B. Majoie. 2004. Systematic Review of Computed Tomographic Angiography for Assessment of Carotid Artery Disease. *Stroke* 35: 2306–12. [CrossRef]

Kuether, Todd A., Gary M. Nesbit, Wayne M. Clark, and Stanley L. Barnwell. 1997. Rotational Vertebral Artery Occlusion: A Mechanism of Vertebrobasilar Insufficiency. *Neurosurgery* 41: 427–33. [CrossRef] [PubMed]

Kühn, Anna Luisa, Peter Kan, Francesco Massari, J. Diego Lozano, Samuel Y. Hou, Mary Howk, Matthew J. Gounis, Ajay K. Wakhloo, and Ajit S. Puri. 2015. Endovascular reconstruction of unruptured intradural vertebral artery dissecting aneurysms with the Pipeline embolization device. *Journal of NeuroInterventional Surgery* 8: 1048–51. [CrossRef] [PubMed]

Kurata, Akira, Taketomo Ohmomo, Yoshio Miyasaka, Kiyotaka Fujii, Shinichi Kan, and Takao Kitahara. 2001. Coil Embolization for the Treatment of Ruptured Dissecting Vertebral Aneurysms. *American Journal of Neuroradiology* 22: 11–18. [PubMed]

Kuroda, Satoshi, Kiyohiro Houkin, Hiroyasu Kamiyama, Kenji Mitsumori, Yoshinobu Iwasaki, and Hiroshi Abe. 2001. Long-Term Prognosis of Medically Treated Patients with Internal Carotid or Middle Cerebral Artery Occlusion. *Stroke* 32: 2110–16. [CrossRef]

Lawton, Michael T. 2018. *Seven Bypasses-Tenets and Techniques for Revascularization*. New York and Stuttgart: Thieme Publishers.

Lemole, G. Michael, Jeffrey S. Henn, Robert F. Spetzler, and Joseph M. Zabramski. 2002. Bow hunter's stroke. *BNI Quarterly* 17: 4–10.

Lindsay, Kenneth W., Ian Bone, and Geraint Fuller. 2011. *Neurology and Neurosurgery Illustrated. General Approach to History and Examination*. London: C L Elsevier.

Lyden, Patrick, T. Brott, B. Tilley, K. M. Welch, E. J. Mascha, S. Levine, E. C. Haley, J. Grotta, and J. Marler. 1994. Improved reliability of the NIH. Stroke Scale using video training. NINDS. TPA. Stroke Study Group. *Stroke* 25: 2220–26. [CrossRef]

Lylyk, Pedro, Carlos Miranda, Rosana Ceratto, Angel Ferrario, Esteban Scrivano, Hugh Ramirez Luna, Aaron L. Berez, Quang Tran, Peter K. Nelson, and David Fiorella. 2009. Curative endovascular reconstruction of cerebral aneurysms with the pipeline embolization device: The Buenos Aires experience. *Neurosurgery* 64: 632–43. [CrossRef]

Marks, Michael P., Eric B. Holmgren, Allan J. Fox, Suresh Patel, Rudiger von Kummer, and Juergen Froehlich. 1999. Evaluation of Early Computed Tomographic Findings in Acute Ischemic Stroke. *Stroke* 30: 389–92. [CrossRef]

Naylor, A. Ross. 2018. Endarterectomy versus stenting for stroke prevention. *Stroke and Vascular Neurology* 3: e000146. [CrossRef]

Nighoghossian, Norbert, Laurent Derex, and Philippe Douek. 2005. The vulnerable carotid artery plaque: Current imaging method and new perspectives. *Stroke* 36: 2764–72. [CrossRef]

Ogata, Atsushi, Shuji Sakata, Hiroaki Okamoto, and Tatsuya Abe. 2017. Ruptured dissecting aneurysm of the recurrent artery of Heubner: Consideration of pathological findings. *Neurology India* 65: 623–25. [CrossRef] [PubMed]

Paciaroni, Maurizio, Giancarlo Agnelli, Francesco Corea, Walter Ageno, Andrea Alberti, Alessia Lanari, Valeria Caso, Sara Micheli, Luca Bertolani, Michele Venti, and et al. 2008. Early hemorrhagic transformation of brain infarction: Rate, predictive factors, and influence on clinical outcome: Results of a prospective multicenter study. *Stroke* 39: 2249–56. [CrossRef] [PubMed]

Peluso, J. P. P., W. J. van Rooij, M. Sluzewski, G. N. Beute, and C. B. Majoie. 2008. Endovascular Treatment of Symptomatic Intradural Vertebral Dissecting Aneurysms. *American Journal of Neuroradiology* 29: 102–6. [CrossRef] [PubMed]

Perkin, G. D. 1995. Cerebral venous thrombosis: Developments in imaging and treatment. *Journal of Neurology, Neurosurgery and Psychiatry* 59: 1–3. [CrossRef]

Pirau, Letitia, and Forshing Lui. 2020. Vertebrobasilar Insufficiency. [Updated 5 February 2020]. In *StatPearls [Internet]*. Treasure Island: StatPearls Publishing. Available online: https://www.ncbi.nlm.nih.gov/books/NBK482259/ (accessed on 31 July 2021).

Powers, William J., C. P. Derdeyn, S. M. Fritsch, D. A. Carpenter, K. D. Yundt, T. O. Videen, and R. L. Grubb, Jr. 2000. Benign prognosis of never-symptomatic carotid occlusion. *Neurology* 54: 878–82. [CrossRef]

Powers, William J., Gary A. Press, Robert L. Grubb, Jr., Mokhtar Gado, and Marcus E. Raichle. 1987. The effect of hemodynamically significant carotid artery disease on the hemodynamic status of the cerebral circulation. *Annals of Internal Medicine* 106: 27–34. [CrossRef]

Pozzati, Eugenio, Alvaro Andreoli, Paolo Limoni, and Mario Casmiro. 1994. Dissecting aneurysms of the vertebrobasilar system: Study of 16 cases. *Surgical Neurology* 41: 119–24. [CrossRef]

Rajpal, Girish, and Vikas Naik. 2018. Management of intracranial arterial dissection. *Neurology India* 66: 40–42.

Ramgren, B., Mats Cronqvist, Bertil Romner, Lennart Brandt, Stig Holtås, and Elna-Marie Larsson. 2005. Vertebrobasilar dissection with subarachnoid hemorrhage: A retrospective study of 29 patients. *Neuroradiology* 47: 97–104. [CrossRef]

Sardar, Partha, Saurav Chatterjee, Herbert D. Aronow, Amartya Kundu, Preethi Ramchand, Debabrata Mukherjee, Ramez Nairooz, William A. Gray, Christopher J. White, Michael R. Jaff, and et al. 2017. Carotid Artery Stenting Versus Endarterectomy for Stroke Prevention. *Journal of the American College of Cardiology* 69: 2266–75. [CrossRef]

Schaller, Bernhard. 2008. Extracranial-intracranial bypass to reduce the risk of ischemic stroke in intracranial aneurysms of the anterior cerebral circulation: A systematic review. *Journal of Stroke and Cerebrovascular Diseases* 17: 287–98. [CrossRef] [PubMed]

Sims, John R., Guy Rordorf, Eric E. Smith, Walter J. Koroshetz, Michael H. Lev, Ferdinando Buonanno, and Lee H. Schwamm. 2005. Arterial Occlusion Revealed by CT Angiography Predicts NIH Stroke Score and Acute Outcomes after IV tPA Treatment. *American Journal of Neuroradiology* 26: 246–51.

Sonecha, T. N., K. T. Delis, and M. Y. Henein. 2006. Predictive value of asymptomatic cervical bruit for carotid artery disease in coronary artery surgery revisited. *International Journal of Cardiology* 107: 225–29. [CrossRef] [PubMed]

Stam, Jan. 2005. Thrombosis of the Cerebral Veins and Sinuses. *New England Journal of Medicine* 352: 1791–98. [CrossRef]

Sugg, Rebecca M., Marc D. Malkoff, Elizabeth A. Noser, Hashem M. Shaltoni, Raymond Weir, Edwin D. Cacayorin, and James C. Grotta. 2005. Endovascular Recanalization of Internal Carotid Artery Occlusion in Acute Ischemic Stroke. *American Journal of Neuroradiology* 26: 2591–94. [PubMed]

Sugita, Kenichiro, Shigeaki Kobayashi, Toshiki Inoue, and Tatsuo Banno. 1981. New angled fenestrated clips for fusiform vertebral artery aneurysms. *Journal of Neurosurgery* 54: 346–50. [CrossRef]

Tomandl, Bernd F., Ernst Klotz, Rene Handschu, Brigitte Stemper, Frank Reinhardt, Walter J. Huk, K.E. Eberhardt, and Suzanne Fateh-Moghadam. 2003. Comprehensive Imaging of Ischemic Stroke with Multisection CT. *RadioGraphics* 23: 565–92. [CrossRef]

Uhl, E., R. Schmid-Elsaesser, and H. J. Steiger. 2003. Ruptured intracranial dissecting aneurysms: Management considerations with a focus on surgical and endovascular techniques to preserve arterial continuity. *Acta Neurochirurgica* 145: 1073–84. [CrossRef]

Vahedi, Katayoun, Jeannette Hofmeijer, Eric Juettler, Eric Vicaut, Bernard George, Ale Algra, G. Johan Amelink, Peter Schmiedeck, Stefan Schwab, Peter M. Rothwell, and et al. 2007. Early decompressive surgery in malignant infarction of the middle cerebral artery: A pooled analysis of three randomised controlled trials. *The Lancet Neurology* 6: 215–22. [CrossRef]

Welling, Richard E., Assad Taha, Tarun Goel, John Cranley, Raymond Krause, Charles Hafner, and John Tew. 1983. Extracranial carotid artery aneurysms. *Surgery* 93: 319–23.

White, Timothy G., Hussam Abou-Al-Shaar, Jung Park, Jeffrey Katz, David J. Langer, and Amir R. Dehdashti. 2019. Cerebral revascularization after the Carotid Occlusion Surgery Study: What candidates remain, and can we do better? *Neurosurgical Focus* 46: E3. [CrossRef] [PubMed]

Xu, Baofeng, Chao Li, Yunbao Guo, Kan Xu, Yi Yang, and Jinlu Yu. 2017. Current understanding of chronic total occlusion of the internal carotid artery (Review). *Biomedical Reports* 8: 117–25. [CrossRef] [PubMed]

Yamaura, Akira. 1994. Nontraumatic intracranial arterial dissection: Natural history, diagnosis, and treatment. *Contemporary Neurosurgery* 16: 1. [CrossRef]

Zhang, Yisen, Ming Lv, Conghai Zhao, Ying Zhang, Xinjian Yang, and Zhongxue Wu. 2016. Endovascular treatment of ruptured vertebrobasilar dissecting aneurysms: Review of 40 consecutive cases. *Neurology India* 64: 52–61. [CrossRef]

Spontaneous Intracerebral Hematoma

Shamsul Alam and Forhad H. Chowdhury

Abstract: An intracerebral hematoma (ICH) is a stroke which constitutes about 10–15% of all strokes. An ICH is considered an acute deadly event. Patients are characterized by the peak age between 55 and 75 years and male predominance. In 50% of cases, an ICH occurs in deep grey and white matter such as basal ganglia, thalamus and internal capsule; 35% are lobar/hemispheric, and occur due to a rupture of the Charcot–Bouchard micro-aneurysm. Even if the presenting symptoms appear mild at onset, a hematoma progression may lead to rapid neurological deterioration. Here, the etiopathological aspects of an ICH, clinical presentation and progression, imaging and interpretation, as well as principles of management with special attention to surgical management are discussed.

Abbreviations

AVM	arteriovenous malformation	BP	blood pressure
CBF	cerebral blood flow	CNS	central nervous system
CSF	cerebrospinal fluid	CT	computed tomography
EV	external ventricular drain	FFP	fresh frozen plasma
HTN	Hypertension	MRI	magnetic resonance imaging
MRA	magnetic resonance angiogram	MRV	magnetic resonance venogram
ICH	intracerebral hematoma	ICP	intracranial pressure
INR	international normalized ratio	IVH	intraventricular hemorrhage
OTC	over the counter	tPA	tissue plasminogen activator
VTE	venous thromboembolism		

1. Introduction

An intracerebral hematoma (ICH) is another variety of stroke which constitutes about 10–15% of all strokes. An ICH is considered an acute life-threatening event. It generally affects a younger age group rather than older patients, with the peak age of patients between 55 and 75 years. It is characterized by a male predominance. In 50% of cases, an ICH occurs in deep grey and white matter such as basal ganglia, thalamus and internal capsule; 35% are lobar/hemispheric, with 10% being cerebellar and 5% in the brainstem location (Figure 1). The rupture of the Charcot–Bouchard micro-aneurysm developed in small vessels (lenticulostriate, thalamostriate) is a result of longstanding chronic hypertension. Other causes of an ICH are coagulopathy (anticoagulant or chronic liver disease) and underlying vascular abnormalities such as AVM, aneurysm or a hemorrhagic tumor (glioblastoma multiforme, metastasis), drug abuse (such as cocaine, amphetamine) and cortical venous sinus thrombosis. Even if the presenting symptoms appear mild at onset, hematoma progression may lead to rapid neurological deterioration (Kirollos et al. 2019; Fewel et al. 2003; An et al. 2017).

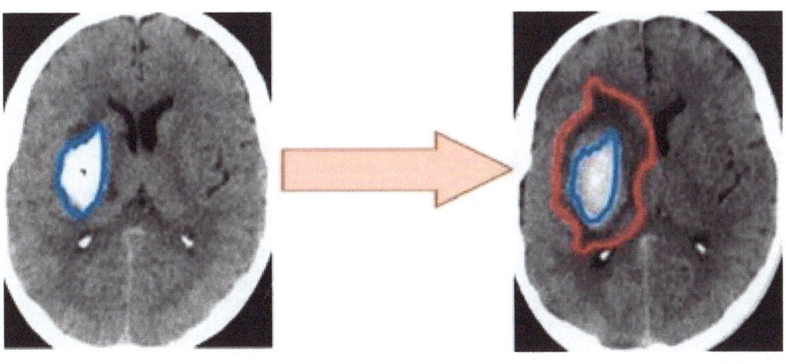

Figure 1. Putaminal hemorrhage with a mild space-occupying effect (**left side**); subsequent edema development around the primary lesion leads to compression of the midline structure (**right side**). Source: Figure by authors.

A hematoma produces ischemic penumbra, resulting in ischemia to the regional brain. Early neurological impairment, poor prognosis and death are all linked to hematoma enlargement. Between baseline and 1-h CT scans, Brott et al. discovered that 26% of ICH patients exhibited a significant bleeding expansion (defined as a 33% rise from the baseline hematoma volume) (i.e., within 4 h of symptom onset). In addition, between the 1-h and 20-h CT scans, 12% of the patients exhibited a hematoma expansion. The progression of a hemorrhage was linked to early neurological impairment. Regardless of how hematoma enlargement is defined, it is an independent predictor of poor outcomes and mortality. The necessity of frequent neurological examinations and early repeat CT scanning, which might alter medical patient care or prompt surgical procedures, is highlighted by the early incidence of hematoma expansion and subsequent neurological deterioration (Qureshi et al. 2009; Fallenius et al. 2019; Cruz and Hopkins 1999; Greenberg 2010). Patients receiving warfarin (or with an international normalized ratio (INR) > 1.5) have an increased tendency of a hematoma expansion compared with patients not receiving warfarin.

2. Intracerebral Hemorrhage in Adults

An intracerebral hemorrhage is the second most common form of a stroke (15–30% of strokes). It has a progressive onset over minutes to hours. The volume of the hematoma correlates highly with morbidity and mortality. Generally, it starts during an activity (seldom during sleep) that may be connected to the elevation in blood pressure (BP) or increased CBF (Fewel et al. 2003; Fallenius et al. 2019; Greenberg 2010).

3. Risk Factors

- Age: risk rises markedly after the age of 55 years and twice with every additional ten years;
- Gender: more common in men;
- Race: higher prevalence in Asians and African Americans;
- Previous stroke: (any type) increases risk to 23:1;
- Alcohol consumption;
- Cigarette smoking;
- Street drugs: cocaine, amphetamines;
- Liver disfunction: coagulopathy (An et al. 2017; Fallenius et al. 2019; Greenberg 2010).

3.1. *Major Risk Factors*

1. Age;
2. Male sex;
3. Hypertension;
4. High alcohol intake;
5. Race—incidence of ICH among the Black population is twice as high as in the White population;

Low serum cholesterol—Japanese population diet has a low cholesterol level (Kirollos et al. 2019; Qureshi et al. 2009; Cruz and Hopkins 1999; Greenberg 2010).

3.2. *Weak Risk Factor*

1. Smoking;
2. Diabetes mellitus (Kirollos et al. 2019).

Frequent sites of ICH are listed in Table 1.

Table 1. Common sites of an ICH.

Percentage (%)	Location
50	Corpus striatum (basal ganglia); putamen is the commonest; along with lenticular nucleus, globus pallidus, internal capsule.
15	Thalamus
10–15	Pons
10	Cerebellum
10–20	Cerebral white matter
1–6	Brain stem

Source: Authors' compilation based on data from Cruz and Hopkins (1999) and Greenberg (2010).

3.3. *Ganglio-Thalamic ICH: Etiologies*

1. Hypertension

(a) Acute hypertension (HTN);
(b) Chronic HTN: degenerative changes within blood vessels.

2. Acutely increased CBF (globally or focally) especially to areas previously rendered ischemic:

(a) Carotid endarterectomy;
(b) Repair of congenital heart defects in children.

3. Previous stroke (embolic or otherwise): hemorrhagic transformation.
4. Vascular anomalies:

(a) AVM rupture;
(b) Aneurysm rupture.

5. Venous angioma rupture.
6. Arteriopathies: amyloid angiopathy, fibrinoid, lipohyalinosis, cerebral.
7. Brain tumor (primary or met).
8. Coagulation or clotting disorders: leukemia, thrombocytopenia, thrombotic thrombocytopenic purpura, aplastic anemia.
9. Patients receiving anticoagulation, thrombolytic, aspirin therapy.
10. CNS infection:

(a) Especially fungal, which attack blood vessels;
(b) Granuloma;
(c) Herpes simplex encephalitis.

11. Venous or dural sinus thrombosis.
12. Drugs:

(a) Substance abuse (alcohol, cocaine, amphetamine);
(b) Drugs that raise BP, alpha-adrenergic agonists (sympathomimetics): phenylpropanolamine, OTC alpha agonists (phenylephrine, ephedrine, pseudoephedrine).

13. Posttraumatic.
14. Pregnancy and puerperium (up to 6 weeks post-partum) most commonly associated with eclampsia or preeclampsia.
15. Postoperative: following carotid endarterectomy, craniotomy.
16. Idiopathic (Fewel et al. 2003; An et al. 2017; Greenberg 2010).

3.4. Lobar Hemorrhage

Lobar hemorrhages have a more benign outcome than ganglionic–thalamic hemorrhages.

Etiologies are (Greenberg 2010):

1. Extension of a deep hemorrhage;
2. Amyloid angiopathy of the brain (the commonest etiology of a lobar ICH in older normotensive sufferers);
3. Trauma;
4. Hemorrhagic changing of an infarct (ischemic);
5. Hemorrhagic;
6. Cerebrovascular malformation (especially AVM);
7. Rupture aneurysm;
8. Idiopathic.

4. Clinical Presentation of an ICH

Classical presentation is sudden the onset and rapid progression of a focal neurological deficit, along with headache, vomiting and an impaired level of consciousness. The severity of presentation depends upon the volume of a hematoma. When a hematoma is significant in volume (>60 mm^3), it causes brain herniation. When the volume of hematomas is more than 85 mL, brain herniation is more prominent and patients may die even after carrying out a proper decompression.

The symptoms and signs of a spontaneous ICH vary according to the site and size. Most cases of an ICH occur during daily routine activity. The neurological signs and symptoms generally increase progressively over minutes to a few hours, in contrast to a cerebral embolism, as well as subarachnoid hemorrhage, where the neurological signs and symptoms are often the highest at onset. However, a few patients with an ICH are comatose or obtunded upon arrival to the emergency department or when first discovered. Headache and vomiting, as well as a reduced level of consciousness develop following an adequately large ICH. Headache and vomiting occur in nearly 50% of patients with an ICH. Headaches may be due to traction on meninges, blood in the cerebrospinal fluid (CSF) or increased intracranial pressure (ICP); they are the most common with lobar and cerebellar hemorrhages. These clinical features are absent with a small ICH; the clinical features in this situation are that of a slowly progressing stroke. Neck stiffness and meningism are seen in ICH with ventricular extension. Coma or stupor in ICH is a perilous sign. The sole exception is a thalamic ICH, where involvement of the reticular activating system is the etiology of stupor or coma rather than diffuse cerebral injury; these sufferers may recover once the ICH is reabsorbed. In putaminal hemorrhage, the spread of an ICH into the putamen commonly takes place along white fiber tracts, resulting in hemiplegia, homonymous hemianopsia, stupor, hemisensory loss, gaze palsy and coma. In the small internal capsule, hemorrhage restricted to the internal capsule may result in mild dysarthria and contralateral hemiparesis, as well as a sensory deficit. Cerebellar hemorrhage generally starts in the dentate nucleus, and spreads into the hemisphere and fourth ventricle. These ICHs result in imbalance, headache, vomiting, gaze palsy, neck stiffness and facial weakness without hemiparesis. Thalamic hemorrhage may extend transversely to the posterior limb of the internal capsule, inferiorly to put pressure on the tectum of the mesencephalon or may rupture into the 3rd ventricle. Symptoms are hemisensory loss, hemiparesis and rarely transient homonymous hemianopsia. Aphasia may result if the ICH affects the dominant cerebral hemisphere, while neglect may result if the ICH affects the nondominant cerebral hemisphere. Lobar hemorrhages vary in their neurologic signs based on the location. Often, the affected lobes are the parietal and occipital lobes. These are linked with a higher frequency of seizures. An occipital ICH commonly presents with a dense contralateral homonymous hemianopsia. The frontal ICH brings about a contralateral paresis or plague of the leg with relative sparing of the arm. A pontine hemorrhage is characterized by a medial ICH that extends into the basal pons. These often lead to deep coma over the first few minutes, probably as a result of the disruption of the reticular activating system. The motor examination may reveal total paralysis. The pupils are pinpointed but react to a strong light. Horizontal gaze palsy, ocular bobbing, facial palsy, deafness and dysarthria can be found when the patient is awake (Ahangar et al. 2019).

5. Diagnostic Imaging

5.1. CT Scan

A CT scan can give the diagnosis of an ICH rapidly. It is quick and can even preform in restless patients without aggressive sedation (Figure 2A–C).

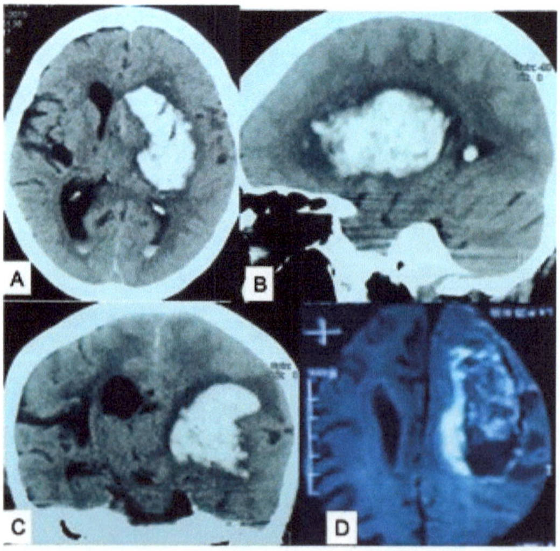

Figure 2. (**A**) CT scan of the brain: axial view showing intraventricular hemorrhage; (**B**) CT scan of the brain: sagittal view showing blood in the ventricle; (**C**) CT scan showing uncal herniation due to an ICH; (**D**) MRI showing an ICH in the frontoparietal lobe. Source: Figure by authors.

5.2. CTA

A CTA is needed in suspicious cases of an AVM and aneurysm ruptures.

5.3. MRI Scan

An MRI scan of the brain (Figure 2D) can clearly rule out bleeding from a cavernous angioma or intratumoral bleed. MRI appearance of an ICH are shown in Table 2.

Table 2. MRI appearance of an ICH in different stages.

Stage	Age	Condition of Hemoglobin	T1WI	T2WI
Hyperacute	<24 h	Oxy-Hgb	Iso	sl ↑
Acute	1–3 d	Deoxy-Hgb	sl ↓	Very ↓
Subacute				
Early > 3d		Met-Hgb	Very ↑	Very ↓
Late > 7d		Met-Hgb	Very ↑	very ↑
Centre > 14 d		Hemichromes	Iso	sl ↑
Chronic Rim		Hemosiderin	sl ↓	Very ↓

Source: Authors' compilation based on data from Greenberg (2010).

5.4. MRV

An MRV depicts the cortical and dural venous sinus and is needed in case of suspected dural venous sinus thrombosis.

Clinical symptoms of an ICH in relation to anatomical localization are shown in Table 3.

Table 3. Typical symptoms of an ICH in relation to the localization.

Typical symptoms of an ICH in Relation to the Localization
Putamen
• Contralateral hemiparesis
• Conjugate gaze deviation to the lesion side
• Homonymous hemianopia
• Aphasia if an ICH is on the dominant side
Thalamus
• Contralateral sensory symptoms
• Initial reduced conscious state progressing to coma
• Hemiparesis
• Hemiataxia (up to 20%)
• Oculomotor symptoms caused by pressure to the midbrain (i.e., Parinaud's syndrome)
• Neuropsychological deficit
Caudate nucleus
• Hemiparesis
• Often intraventricular involvement with meningism
• Pons
• Initial reduced conscious state progressing to coma
• Teraparesis
• Abnormal flexion or extension
• Bilateral cranial nerve deficits in medial lesions
• Tegmental localization: internuclear ophthalmoplegia, dilated pupil and contralateral hemiparesis
Midbrain
• Initial reduced conscious state progressing to coma
• Parinaud's syndrome cerebellum
Initial reduced conscious state progressing to coma
• Ataxia
• Dizziness
• Gaze palsies
• Signs of an elevated ICP

Source: Authors' compilation based on data from An et al. (2017), Qureshi et al. (2009) and Quiñones-Hinojosa (2012).

6. Herniation Syndrome

Uncal herniation (Figure 2C) is the most common herniation which is caused by a temporal lobe hematoma that shift the uncus medically and downward until it is herniated over the tentorium and compress the midbrain.

The earliest sign of an impending uncalled herniation is the unilateral dilated pupil secondary to the compression of the parasympathetic fiber which lies on the periphery of the 3rd nerve. When the uncalled herniation progresses, it is then associated with a rapid decline in the level of consciousness and sign of an ipsilateral or contralateral hemiplegia with an extensor planter response (due to ipsilateral or contralateral compression of cerebral peduncle, respectively). Eventually, a bilateral pupil disloyalty dilatation develops (Greenberg 2010).

There are various separate types of brain herniation that assert the type of herniation taking place:

- Subfalcine herniation;
- Transellar herniation: descending and ascending;
- Transtentorial herniation;
  - Caudal: central herniation as well as uncal herniation;
  - Cranial: ascending transtentorial herniation;
- Tonsillar (cerebellar) herniation;
- Extracranial herniation.

7. Management

7.1. Medical Management

7.1.1. Hypertension Management

Antihypertensive therapy is usually not indicated if the systemic BP is <180 mm Hg. If the systolic BP is 180 to 230 mm of Hg or more and/or the diastolic is 105 to 120 mm of Hg, then oral nifedipine or injectable labetalol is required.

An intracerebral hematoma varies in amount.

Calcium channel blockers (nicardipine or nimodipine, 16.2%), combination alpha- and beta-blockers (labetalol, 14.4%), venodilators (nitroglycerin, 14.9%), a diuretic (furosemide, 12.4%) and arterial vasodilators (furosemide, 12.4%) are among the most commonly prescribed medications (nitroprusside, 12.1%; hydralazine 5.9%). The ATACH 2 experiment used an intravenous infusion of nicardipine, starting at a dose of 5 mg/h and increasing by 2.5 mg every 15 min until the target SBP is reached (maximum dose of 15 mg/h). If the SBP target is not met despite the maximum dose of nicardipine, intravenous labetalol is administered as a second-line drug. The most commonly prescribed medicines in North America are nicardipine and labetalol; both appear to be safe, but nicardipine may be more effective in achieving and maintaining the target blood pressure (Kirollos et al. 2019; Fewel et al. 2003; An et al. 2017; Qureshi et al. 2009; Fallenius et al. 2019; Cruz and Hopkins 1999; Greenberg 2010; Quiñones-Hinojosa 2012; de Oliveira Manoel et al. 2016).

7.1.2. Anticoagulant-Associated ICH

Patients having an ICH on antithrombotic drugs carry a higher threat for an ICH expansion, as well as greater risk for mortality and poor results.

A. Warfarin-Induced ICH

Warfarin is to blame for 9–11% of all ICH cases. When compared to people who do not use anticoagulants, patients on long-term warfarin had an 11-fold increased risk of an ICH. Urgent coagulopathy reversal is required for patients with warfarin-related ICH and an elevated INR (>1.4). Vitamin K can entirely reverse the warfarin effect when administered as a slow intravenous infusion (5–10 mg over 30 min) (de Oliveira Manoel et al. 2016).

The transfusion of fresh frozen plasma (FFP):

- FFP is required when the INR is more than 5.
- Recombinant activated factor VII (rFVIIa) can be utilized for the reversal of warfarin-related coagulopathy.

B. Low-Molecular-Weight Heparin (LMWH)-Induced ICH

Heparin-related ICH affects about 0.1–0.2% of patients receiving continuous infusions. The heparin infusion should be stopped promptly, and 1 mg of protamine sulfate should be given for every 100 units of heparin given in the previous 2–3 h (maximum single dose of 50 mg) (de Oliveira Manoel et al. 2016).

C. Antiplatelet Agent (Ecosprin, Clopidogril)-Related ICH

In ICH, for patients on antiplatelets (APTs), the drug should be stopped instantly and there is an advantage from platelet transfusion.

Desmopressin (DDAVP) was tested in a recent pilot research to see if it could increase platelet function in individuals with an ICH and low platelet activity who were also taking aspirin. Platelet activity was raised by desmopressin (0.4 g/kg IV over 30 min) (de Oliveira Manoel et al. 2016).

7.1.3. Management of Diabetes Mellitus

Uncontrolled diabetes mellitus is one of the prime risk factors and most often associated with an ICH. The control of diabetes is of utmost importance for treatment and also prevention.

7.1.4. Fever

Besides infection, intraventricular hemorrhage may cause a prolonged fever. To return the temperature to normal, a cold saline infusion (4 °C, 2 L at 4 L/h) vs. nasopharyngeal cooling (60 L/min for 1 h) may be needed (de Oliveira Manoel et al. 2016).

7.1.5. Preventing Venous Thromboembolism (VTE)

Patients with an ICH are at an increased risk of a VTE, which has been shown to be up to four times higher than in patients with an ischemic stroke. Intermittent pneumatic compression devices, positioned at the time of hospital admission (strong recommendation and high-quality evidence) are used as an initial prophylaxis, followed by pharmaceutical prophylaxis with LMWH (de Oliveira Manoel et al. 2016).

7.1.6. Dysphagia

After a stroke, dysphagia is widespread, with a reported incidence ranging from 37 to 78%, depending on the method employed to identify it. Dysphagia is linked to a higher risk of pneumonia/pneumonitis (RR 3.17, 95% CI 2.07–4.87). Aspiration pneumonia can be prevented with NG tube feeding (de Oliveira Manoel et al. 2016).

7.1.7. Seizure Prophylaxis

In patients with an ICH, seizure frequency has been found to range between 8.1 and 10.6%, with status epilepticus occurring in 1–2% of cases. Phenytoin has been linked to a higher risk of adverse effects and poorer outcomes. Anticonvulsant prophylaxis is not recommended by the current AHA ICH recommendations (de Oliveira Manoel et al. 2016).

7.1.8. ICP Management

ICP management techniques include the head of the bed elevation of 30 to 45 degrees, CSF draining by an EVD, analgesia and sedation, normocapnic breathing and hypertonic solution administration (e.g., hypertonic saline or mannitol). Barbiturates therapy is indicated in resistant cases of hypothermia (de Oliveira Manoel et al. 2016).

7.2. Surgical Management

Commonly, we need surgical removal +/− decompressive surgery of the brain for hematoma removal (Box 1).

Box 1. Hematoma volume measurement.

The result of the ABC/2 formula is as below: The volume of an ellipsoid is **4/3π(A/2)(B/2)(C/2)**, where A, B and C are the three diameters. If π is estimated to be 3, then the volume of an ellipsoid becomes ABC/2, where A is the greatest diameter on the largest ICH section, B is the diameter right angle to A, and C is the number of axial cuts with ICH multiplied by the section thickness. Frequently, we categorize them according to the volume: Mild—>10 mL Moderate—30 to 60 mL Severe—more than 60 mL of ICH

7.2.1. Surgical Indication of an ICH

(a) Lesions with a marked mass effect, edema or midline shift on imaging;
(b) Symptoms (e.g., hemiparesis/plegia, aphasia, or sometimes just confusion or agitation) due to an increased ICP or mass effect;
(c) Volume: surgery for a moderate and large volume of hematomas;
(d) Continued raised ICP despite therapy;
(e) Quick deterioration (signs of brainstem compression), regardless of the location in a patient considered to be salvageable;
(f) Favorable location (lobar, cerebellar, external capsule, non-dominant hemisphere);
(g) Young patient (especially age $\leq$ 50 years) with a moderate-to-large lobar hematoma who is clinically worsening;
(h) Early intervention: surgery after 24 h from onset of symptoms or deterioration may be of less benefit;
(i) Patients having cerebellar hemorrhages larger than 3 cm in diameter, hydrocephalus or neurological deterioration;
(j) ICH linked with a surgically accessible structural lesion, such as an AVM or tumor (Greenberg 2010).

7.2.2. ICH Score

ICH score can be used for assessment of outcome (Table 4).

Table 4. ICH score.

Component	Points	Total ICH Score	30-Day Mortality (%)
		Glasgow Coma Scale	
3–4 5–12 13–15	2 1 0	0	0–10
		Age (years)	
≥80 <80	1 0	1	7–13
		ICH volume (mL)	
≥30 <30	1 0	2	30–44
		Presence of intraventricular hemorrhage	
Yes No	1 0	3	56–78
		Infra-tentorial origin of ICH	
Yes No	1 0	4	70–100
Total ICH score	0–6	5–6	100

Source: Authors' compilation based on data from de Oliveira Manoel et al. (2016) and Hemphill et al. (2001).

The first column shows the five independent predictors of 30-day mortality based on the original ICH score (Glasgow Coma Scale, age, ICH volume, intraventricular hemorrhage, and infra-tentorial location of ICH). The total score, which ranges from 0 to 6, is the sum of the five components (column 3). The expected 30-day mortality increases as the total score (column 3) rises (column 4). The key factors in selecting the appropriate surgical candidate is the size of the hematoma, age of the patient, comorbidity, location of hematoma (lobar vs. deep) and clinical course of the patient (Greenberg 2010; Hemphill et al. 2001). In our experience, young patients need surgical decompression more than older patients. Some neurosurgeons prefer only bony and dural decompression, keeping the deep-seated hematoma intact. Some prefer hematoma removal, as well as bony and dural decompression.

7.2.3. Surgical Approaches

1. *Trans-Sylvian approach:* Commonly, we use the trans-Sylvian approach (Figures 3 and 4) to remove a basal ganglionic hematoma. It is the shortest and most manageable trajectory for hematoma removal. The cortical opening is very minimal and the insular incision is given depending on the maximum location of the hematoma. Following insular incision and by gentle sucker manipulation, the hematoma commonly comes out spontaneously. The surgeons need controlled suction for gentle decompression. Often, the brain also becomes slack when a hematoma comes out. Interestingly, blood pressure also declines rapidly at this time. Therefore, the surgeons

often do not keep the patient antihypertensive before surgery. The surgeons also try not to administer mannitol if early surgery can be done. Following hematoma evacuation, it is needed to visualize the floor of the hematoma cavity to see the bleeding or oozing point. It needs proper coagulation if there is a bleeding point. Blood pressure needs to be raised at this level for proper hemostasis. Following hemostasis, a dural closure and bone placement are carried out, and the wound is closed in multiple layers.

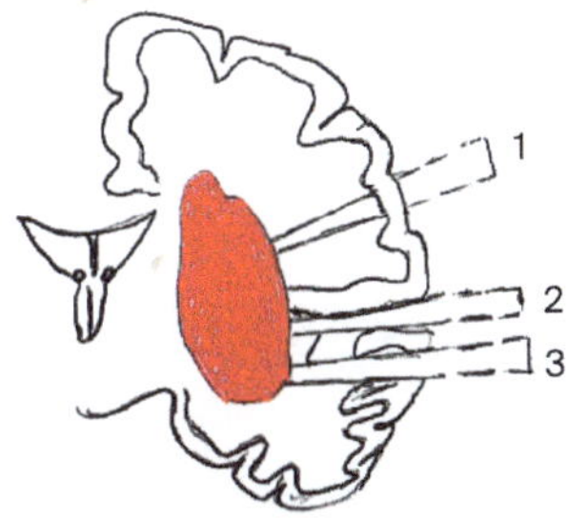

Figure 3. Surgical approaches to an ICH in basal ganglia. Source: Figure by authors.

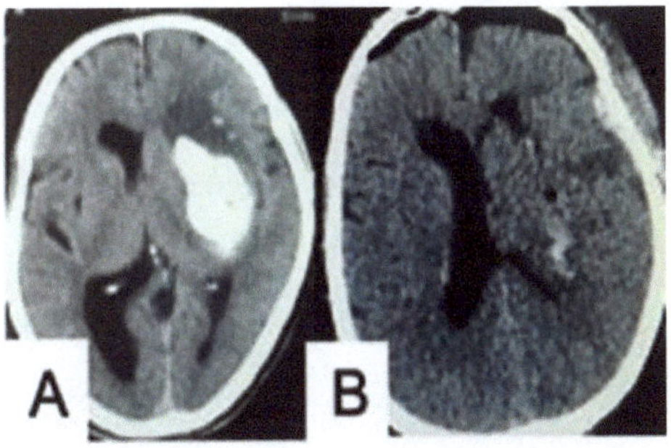

Figure 4. (**A**) CT scan showing a left-sided huge basal ganglionic hematoma. (**B**) Postoperative CT scan showing good removal of the hematoma, with no midline shift. Source: Figure by authors.

Sometimes, in young patients, if the surgeon suspects the patient may have developed brain swelling, he may offer some more bone removal in the temporal area and keep the dura open, with placement of an artificial dura to cover the exposed brain. Following decompression, commonly the bone is harvested in the subcutaneous plane of the abdomen just below the umbilicus. In some cases, the surgeons also offer a resection of the temporalis muscle and keep the bone over the temporal fascia just beneath the scalp to accommodate brain swelling. Figure 4 shows an ICH evacuation through trans-Sylvian approach.

2. *Keyhole endoscopic removal:* In this approach, a 0-degree endoscope and a sheath measuring about 10–17 mm in diameter and 5–10 cm long are needed. An endoscope can be held by an assistant or by an endoscope holder, and the surgeon removes the hematoma by direct endoscopic vision. This approach is carried out along the long trajectory of the hematoma cavity to get the parallel vision of the hematoma cavity by a 0-degree telescope.

It is a minimal, invasive procedure. It also needs proper hemostasis before the removal of the sheath. A hematoma cavity is properly irrigated and any bleeding point needs to be cautery by either monopolar or bipolar cautery. A hematoma cavity can be packed by surgical or gel foam following proper hemostasis to avoid recurrent hemorrhage. Wound is closed in layers keeping dura open and placement of bone commonly not needed as small opening. A hematoma evacuation can be successfully performed by direct endoscopic vision using a 0-degree endoscope. The trajectory of hematoma removal is considered along the longitudinal direction of the hematoma volume. A sheath with an obturator is mandatory to protect the brain as the trajectory is a little long. There are various types and lengths of the plastic sheath with an obturator available. The suction tube must have a teardrop for controlled suction. Fine unipolar or bipolar cautery is required for a proper hemostasis of the hematoma cavity (Kalangu et al. 2009).

3. *Burr hole drainage and irrigation with urokinase* (Macdonald 2018).

4. *EVD for an intraventricular hemorrhage:* External ventricular drains (EVDs) are used to treat ICH patients with an IVH, who have developed an obstructive hydrocephalus. Unfortunately, when there is a lot of IVH

present, the EVD fills up with blood, which clots and obstructs the EVD regularly. The surgeon can provide 5 mg of intraventricular tissue plasminogen activator (tPA) twice a day for 5 days in these instances. If the intracranial pressure (ICP) transduced by the EVD does not rise after each dosage, the EVD is clamped for 30 min to prevent the tPA from leaking out of the ventricle (Quiñones-Hinojosa 2012).

7.2.4. Complication of Surgical Management

1. Rebleed: There may be rebleed in a keyhole hematoma removal approach. Some patients may also develop brain swelling, especially those who are young and hence need to go for decompressive surgery.
2. Residual hematoma (Figure 5A).
3. Brain swelling (Figure 5B).

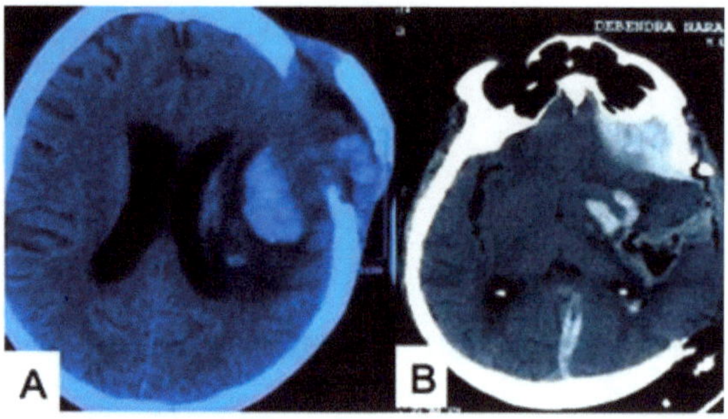

Figure 5. (**A**) CT scan showing brain swelling following surgery. (**B**) CT scan showing a residual hematoma with a perilesional edema, causing a raised ICP and extracalvarial herniation. Source: Figure by authors.

The earliest sign of an impending brain herniation from massive brain swelling is a depressed level of consciousness and a contralateral hemiparesis or ipsilateral hemiparesis (Kernohan's notch phenomenon) with a fixed and dilated ipsilateral pupil. Medical therapy by hyperosmolar therapy, hyperventilation, diuretic therapy, CSF drainage and barbiturate therapy is recommended. Surgical decompressive craniectomy is often required when the medical theory is failed or cannot be initiated.

4. Infection—meningitis and post-meningitis hydrocephalus.

7.2.5. Contraindications of ICH Surgery

1. Elderly patient (age more than 80 years);
2. Poor neurological status (GCS 5 or below);
3. Poor general condition (unable to tolerate general anesthesia);
4. Asymptotic patient with a small blood clot (<3 cm in cerebellar hematoma and <4 cm in lobar location).

7.2.6. 30-Day Mortality

An ICH has a 30-day mortality rate for 44%. Half of the deaths occur within first 2 days.

For pontine and other brainstem ICH, the mortality rate is 75% within 24 h.

For all ICH locations, the volume of an ICH is the highest predictor of 30-day mortality. Patients with a parenchymal bleeding volume of 60 cm^3 or more on their initial CT scan and a GCS of 8 or less had a predicted 30-day mortality of 91% in one research involving 188 cases. Patients with a GCS of 9 or above and a volume less than 30 cm^3 had a predicted 30-day death rate of 19% (Der-Yang Cho et al. 2008).

In individuals with spontaneous intracerebral hemorrhage, the volume of an ICH combined with the initial GCS score is a powerful and simple predictor of 30-day death and morbidity. The basal ganglia are the most prevalent site of a hypertensive ICH, accounting for 60% of all cases, and a basal ganglion ICH is linked with a 50% death risk (Quiñones-Hinojosa 2012). When there is a third ventricular outlet obstruction, a thalamic ICH is nearly invariably treated medically, with the installation of an external ventricular drain. The only study that examined surgical and medicinal treatment for a thalamic ICH found that an endoscopic evacuation had no advantage over medical treatment.

Because of the difficulties in gaining safe surgical access to the brainstem and the morbidity associated with brainstem manipulation required for a hematoma evacuation, most patients with a pontine hematoma are handled conservatively. A pontine ICH is expected to have an 18% death rate during hospitalization and a 69% mortality rate after a year (Quiñones-Hinojosa 2012).

A cerebellar ICH, when large in volume, causes brainstem compression and rapid fatal worsening. A second cause of mortality as well as morbidity for these patients is an ICH causing compression of the 4th ventricle and a subsequent hydrocephalus (Greenberg 2010).

7.3. *Rehabilitation*

It is likely that patients will need specialist rehabilitation. The extent of this will be dependent on their symptoms and how poorly they have been. This is specific to what is available at their local hospital or what the specialist team thinks will benefit the patients the most. This includes medical input from a specialist in rehabilitation, occupational therapy, physiotherapy, language and speech therapy, and dietetic evaluation of nutrition and psychology. It may include the following:

- Specialist inpatient rehabilitation;
- Referral back to the hospital the patient came from for the specialist stroke rehabilitation.

Author Contributions: Conceptualization, methodology, validation, formal analysis, investigation, resources, data curation, writing—original draft preparation, S.A. and F.H.C.; writing—review and editing, visualization, supervision, F.H.C. All authors have read and agreed to the published version of the manuscript.

Funding: This research received no external funding.

Conflicts of Interest: The authors declare no conflicts of interest.

References

Ahangar, Alijan Ahmadi, Shayan Alijanpour, and Mostafa Mostafazdeh Bora. 2019. Clinical Features and Diagnosis of Spontaneous Intracerebral Hemorrhage. *Online Journal of Cardiovascular Research* 1: 513. [CrossRef]

An, Sang Joon, Tae Jung Kim, and Byung-Woo Yoon. 2017. Epidemiology, Risk Factors, and Clinical Features of Intracerebral Hemorrhage: An Update. *Journal of Stroke* 19: 3–10. [CrossRef] [PubMed]

Cho, Der-Yang, Chun-Chung Chen, Han-Chung Lee, Wen-Yuan Lee, and Hong-Lin Lin. 2008. Glasgow Coma Scale and hematoma volume as criteria for treatment of putaminal and thalamic intracerebral hemorrhage. *Surgical Neurology* 70: 628–33. [CrossRef] [PubMed]

Cruz, Julio, and Robert Hopkins. 1999. Neurologic and Neurosurgical Emergencies. *Pediatric Emergency Care* 15: 368. [CrossRef]

de Oliveira Manoel, Airton Leonardo, Alberto Goffi, Fernando Godinho Zampieri, David Turkel-Parrella, Abhijit Duggal, Thomas R. Marotta, R. Loch Macdonald, and Simon Abrahamson. 2016. The critical care management of spontaneous intracranial hemorrhage: A contemporary review. *Critical Care* 20: 272. [CrossRef] [PubMed]

Fallenius, Marika, Markus B. Skrifvars, Matti Reinikainen, Stepani Bendel, Sami Curtze, Gerli Sibolt, Nicolas Martinez-Majander, and Rahul Raj. 2019. Spontaneous Intracerebral Hemorrhage. *Stroke* 50: 2336–43, Erratum in: *Stroke* 2022, 53: e64. [CrossRef] [PubMed]

Fewel, Matthew E., B. Gregory Thompson, and Julian T. Hoff. 2003. Spontaneous intracerebral hemorrhage: A review. *Neurosurgical Focus* 15: 1–16. [CrossRef]

Greenberg, Mark S. 2010. *Handbook of Neurosurgery*. New York: Thieme.

Hemphill, J. Claude, 3rd, David C. Bonovich, Lavrentios Besmertis, Geoffrey T. Manley, and S. Claiborne Johnston. 2001. The ICH Score. *Stroke* 32: 891–97. [CrossRef] [PubMed]

Kalangu, Kazadi, Yoko Kato, Gilbert Dechambenoit, and Hirotoshi Sano. 2009. *Essential Practice of Neurosurgery*. Nagoya: Access publishing Co., Ltd.

Kirollos, Ramez, Adel Helmy, Simon Thomson, and Peter Hutchinson. 2019. *Oxford Textbook of Neurological Surgery*. Oxford: Oxford University Press.

Macdonald, R. Loch. 2018. *Neurosurgical Operative Atlas: Vascular Neurosurgery*. Teningen: Thieme.

Quiñones-Hinojosa, Alfredo. 2012. *Schmidek and Sweet: Operative Neurosurgical Techniques E-Book: Indications, Methods and Results*, 6th ed. Philadelphia: Elsevier Saunders.

Qureshi, Adnan I., A. David Mendelow, and Daniel F. Hanley. 2009. Intracerebral haemorrhage. *The Lancet* 373: 1632–44. [CrossRef] [PubMed]

Subarachnoid Hemorrhage and Intracranial Aneurysm

Shamshul Alam, Forhad H. Chowdhury, Nazmin Ahmed, Mohammod Abdul Hyee and Mohammod Raziul Haque

Abstract: A subarachnoid hemorrhage (SAH) constitutes about 5% of total strokes and occurs due to a ruptured intracranial aneurysm or an AVM. Of aneurysms, 85% are constituent from anterior circulations and the remaining 15% from posterior circulation. Saccular (berry) aneurysms comprise 90% of all intracranial aneurysm morphologies. About 2% of the general population has an intracranial aneurysm, about 1% will have a rupture during their lifetime and 0.5% will die because of an SAH. A ruptured aneurysm usually presents with a sudden, severe thunderclap headache. A CT scan followed by a CTA/MRA/DSA will confirm the diagnosis. Patients are managed in the ICU and need urgent or delayed microsurgical clipping or endovascular coiling to prevent further rupture of the aneurysm. This chapter will include discussion of SAHs and the microsurgical management of different types of intracranial aneurysms in brief. The endovascular management of aneurysms will be discussed in Chapter 18.

Abbreviations

AChA	anterior choroidal artery	ACOM	anterior communicating artery
AVM	arteriovenous malformation	ACA	anterior cerebral artery
AICA	anterior inferior cerebellar artery	BTO	balloon test occlusion
CCF	caroticocavernous fistula	CSF	cerebrospinal fluid
CT	computed tomography	CTA	CT angiogram
DACA	distal anterior cerebral artery	DIND	delayed ischemic neurological deficit
DSA	digital subtraction angiogram	DVT	deep vein thrombosis
EI-IC	Intracranial–extracranial	GCS	Glasgow Coma Scale
ICA	internal carotid artery	IC-IC	intracranial-intracranial
ICMA	intracranial mycotic aneurysm	ICP	intracranial pressure
ICU	intensive care unit	IE	infective endocarditis
IMAX	internal maxillary artery	LOC	loss of consciousness
MCA	middle cerebral artery	MRA	magnetic resonance angiogram
MRI	magnetic resonance imaging	OA	occipital artery
OFZ	orbito-froto-zygomatic	OZ	orbito-zygomatic
PCA	posterior cerebral artery	PCOM	posterior communicating artery
PDR	proximal dural ring	PICA	posterior inferior cerebellar artery
PMF	pterigo-maxillary fissure	PWoM	posterior wall of maxilla
SAH	subarachnoid hemorrhage	SCA	superior cerebellar artery
STA	MCA-superficial temporal artery–middle cerebral artery	TM	temporalis muscle
VA	vertebral artery	WFNS	world federation of neurosurgical society

1. Introduction

A subarachnoid hemorrhage constitutes about 5% of total strokes, which occurs commonly from a ruptured aneurysm of either anterior or posterior circulation. Of aneurysms, 85% are constituent from anterior circulations and the remaining 15% from posterior circulation. Saccular (berry) aneurysms comprise 90% of all aneurysm morphologies, and their rupture is the leading etiology of SAHs. Fusiform aneurysms are responsible for roughly 10%, with posterior circulation being the most prevalent area. An epidemiological study shows that about 2% of the general population has an intracranial aneurysm, about 1% will have rupture during their lifetime and 0.5% will die because of an SAH (Williams and Brown 2013; Greenberg 2010).

2. Etiologies, Types and Frequencies of SAHs

Etiologies:

(a) Aneurysms (70–75%);
(b) Arteriovenous malformation (AVM) (4–5%);
(c) Vasculitides;
(d) Tumor (rarely);
(e) Cerebral artery dissection;
(f) Coagulation disorders;
(g) Dural sinus thrombosis;
(h) Pituitary apoplexy (Greenberg 2010).

Types of aneurysms causing SAH are listed in Table 1.

Table 1. Types of aneurysms causing an SAH.

Types
Saccular
Fusiform (atherosclerotic)
Traumatic
Dissecting
Mycotic
Miliary

Source: Authors' compilation based on data from Cruz and Hopkins (1999).

Intracranial arteries lie in the subarachnoid space and lack an external elastic laminate and have a very thin tunica adventitia. The histological section at the neck of an aneurysm shows a lack of muscle coat and internal elastic lamina (Yamazoe et al. 1990). Frequency distribution of intracranial aneurysms are shown in Table 2.

Table 2. Frequency of aneurysms.

Type of Aneurysm	**Frequency (%)**
ACOM	35
PCOM	25
MCA	20
Basilar top	10
Vertebral artery	5
Others	5
Very few are from an ophthalmic segment aneurysm and ICA bifurcation aneurysm	

Source: Authors' compilation based on data from Greenberg (2010).

When an SAH occurs, blood spreads all over the brain surface and to the cistern; hence, the brain becomes red and swollen (Figure 1). A fresh blood clot found in the basal cistern, interhemispheric fissure and Sylvian fissure. Chemical inflammation from clotting blood surrounding the brain can lead cerebral arteries to spasm in the days after the hemorrhage. An arterial spasm can result in further brain injury.

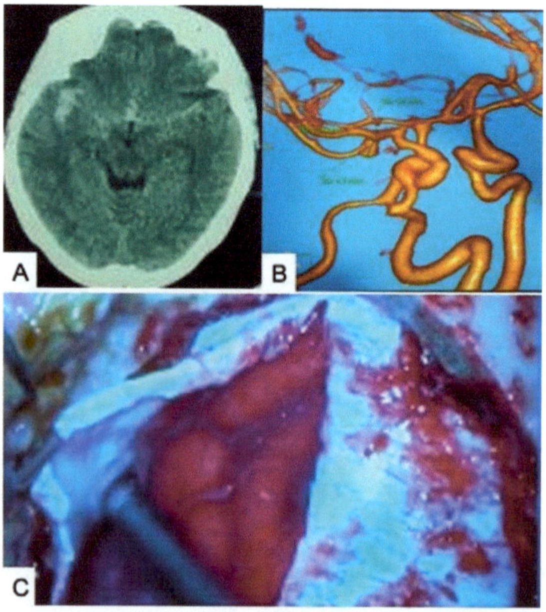

Figure 1. (**A**) CT scan showing an SAH likely from a ruptured right MCA aneurysm. (**B**) CTA showing a small right MCA aneurysm. (**C**) Blood in the subarachnoid space following an opening of the dura in an acute subarachnoid hemorrhage patient. Source: Figure by authors.

It is difficult to finalize which aneurysm has ruptured by only identifying it by seeing a plain CT scan. In the case of an anterior communicating artery aneurysm, there will be bleeding in the anterior circle of Willis, and in the case of a posterior communicating artery aneurysm, there will be bleeding along the tentorial edge. In the case of a middle cerebral artery aneurysm, there will be bleeding in the Sylvian fissure, even in the temporal lobe. A CT angiogram, MR angiogram, digital subtraction angiogram or direct puncture angiogram is the key to diagnose the cause of a subarachnoid hemorrhage. We can only carry out a CT angiogram, and in some cases, we go for a DSA when the aneurysm is giant or complex. An MR angiogram is a good tool for the diagnosis of a ruptured and unruptured aneurysm in the outpatient department (Greenberg 2010).

3. Natural History of Disease

An SAH represents just 5% of all strokes; however, it is associated with significant fatalities, as well as long-term impairments. Between 1984 and 2007, a retrograde cohort study in two large Norwegian populations found a 36% 30-day case fatality rate. Female sex, Japanese or Finnish ancestry, aneurysm size, shape and sites, hypertension, smoking, elderly patients and cocaine misuse are all major risk factors for an aneurysm rupture. The annual rupture rate is 1–1.5% per year and the re-rupture rate is 40–60% within 3 days and gradually decreases over a period of time. The highest risk of a re-rupture is within 24 h (often within 6–12 h) (Williams and Brown 2013; Greenberg 2010).

Neurological injury from the original hemorrhage and re-hemorrhage, and delayed cerebral ischemia (DCI) are the most common causes of death.

4. Morphology of a Saccular Aneurysm

Larger aneurysms are most likely to bleed, whereas individual aneurysm anatomy reveled with a daughter lobe a blend of or dome irregularities that implicate the aneurysm as a culprit of an SAH (Kirollos et al. 2019).

5. Risk Factors for an SAH

Systemic hypertension;
Smoking;
Contraceptive pill;
Substance abuser (cocaine, alcohol);
Pregnancy and parturition;
Advancing age;
Cerebral aneurysm;
Procedure like cerebral angiography or lumbar puncture in patients with an aneurysm (Cruz and Hopkins 1999).

6. Clinical Features

6.1. Symptoms and Signs

The symptoms and signs of an SAH include a sudden, severe, thunder-clap headache; nausea; vomiting; syncopal attack (apoplexy); and neck ache (meningismus); as well as light apprehension. If there is a loss of consciousness (LOC), patients may regain consciousness later. Cranial nerve palsy may occur (for example, oculomotor nerve palsy caused by aneurysm-induced pressure of the oculomotor nerve, resulting in double vision and/or ptosis). Dependent blood can irritate the lumbar nerve roots, causing lower back pain. A sentinel hemorrhage may cause a warning headache (Greenberg 2010; Kirollos et al. 2019).

6.2. Meningismus

Nuchal rigidity;
Kernig sign;
Brudzinski sign;
Ocular hemorrhage (Greenberg 2010).

6.3. Coma Following an SAH

May occur due to the following:

1. Raised intra cranial pressure (ICP);

2. Injury to the brain from intracerebral hemorrhage;
3. Hydrocephalus;
4. Diffuse ischemia;
5. Seizure;
6. Low blood flow (Greenberg 2010).

6.4. Mortality in Aneurysmal SAH

10–15% patients succumb before reaching the hospital;
10% mortality within the subsequent few days;
In general, the mortality is 45% (32–67%);
25% die due to medical complications of an SAH;
8% die from progressive deterioration from the initial hemorrhage;
55–60 years is the common age for an SAH (aneurysmal);
30% of aneurysmal SAHs happen during sleep (Greenberg 2010).

7. Intracranial Aneurysm

Though it is not possible to guess whether an aneurysm will rupture or not, an aneurysm is more possible to rupture when its diameter is 7 mm or over.

7.1. Presentation of a Ruptured Aneurysm

- Sudden, excruciating, severe headache;
- Nausea, as well as vomiting;
- Neck stiffness;
- Blurring of vision or diplopia;
- Photophobia;
- Convulsion;
- Ptosis;
- LOC;
- Subhyaloid (preretinal) hemorrhage;
- Retinal hemorrhage (Williams and Brown 2013; Greenberg 2010; Cruz and Hopkins 1999; Yamazoe et al. 1990; Kirollos et al. 2019).

7.2. Presentation of an Unruptured Aneurysm

Mass effect leads to hemiparesis and compromise vision.

7.3. Diagnosis

CT scan: It is the most common investigation in an acute SAH, as patients are either restless or unconscious, and it takes much less time to get the image.

CT angiogram (CTA): It is a more popular investigation method for an SAH for the defect of an aneurysm of any location. Here, an intravenous contrast agent is pushed by a syringe pump to get the vascular image.

MR angiogram (MRA): It is the best chosen when patients are having a headache without an impaired consciousness level. Here, the contrast agent is not required to get vascular images.

Digital subtraction angiogram (DSA): it is performed for a complex aneurysm.

Direct puncture angiogram

A lumbar puncture can confirm the presence of an SAH even when the hemorrhage is small to declare its presence on a CT scan. Blood mixed CSF comes in SAH in spinal tap (Williams and Brown 2013; Greenberg 2010; Cruz and Hopkins 1999; Yamazoe et al. 1990; Kirollos et al. 2019).

7.4. Gradings

7.4.1. Hunt and Hess Grading

The Hunt and Hess (Hunt and Hess 1968) grading is a predictor of survival that defines the degree of an SAH caused by the burst of an intracranial aneurysm.

(1) Grade 1

(a) Without symptoms or a mild headache, as well as slight stiffness of the neck;
(b) 70% survival.

(2) Grade 2

(a) Moderate-to-severe headache plus neck stiffness, but no neuro-deficit other than cranial nerve palsy;
(b) 60% survival.

(3) Grade 3

(a) Drowsy and minimal neurological deficit;
(b) 50% survival.

(4) Grade 4

(a) Stuporous and moderate-to-severe hemiparesis, with possible early decerebrate rigidity, as well as vegetative disturbances;
(b) 20% survival.

(5) Grade 5

(a) Deep coma and decerebrate rigidity, moribund;
(b) 10% survival.

7.4.2. Fisher Grading

SAH severity and location are important prognostic variables. An SAH is classified utilizing the Fisher grading scale, as follows:

- Grade 1—No SAH found on CT of the head;
- Grade 2—Diffuse or vertically seen SAH < 1 mm thick;
- Grade 3—Diffuse and/or vertical layer of SAH > 1 mm thickness;
- Grade 4—Intraventricular or intracerebral blood with diffuse or no SAH (July and Wahjoepramono 2019).

Comparison between Barrrow Neurological Institute and Fisher grading is shown in Table 3.

Table 3. Analogy between the Barrow Neurological Institute (BNI) and Fisher grading.

Scale	Grade 1	Grade 2	Grade 3	Grade 4	Grade 5
Fisher	No blood	Clot < 1 mm thick	Clot > 1 mm thick	Grade 1 or 2 plus intracerebral or intraventricular hematoma	-
BNI	No blood	Clot < 5 mm thick	Clot 5 to 10 mm thick	Clot 10 to 15 mm thick	Clot > 15 mm thick

Source: Authors' compilation based on data from July and Wahjoepramono (2019) and Greenberg (2010).

7.4.3. WFNS Grading

The World Federation of Neurosurgical Societies (WFNS) grading system utilizes the Glasgow Coma Scale (GCS) and existence of focal neurological deficits for grading the severity of an SAH.

WFNS Classification:

- Grade 1: GCS 15, no neuro-deficits;
- Grade 2: GCS 13–14 without neuro-deficits;
- Grade 3: GCS 13–14 with focal neuro-deficits;
- Grade 4: GCS 7–12, with or without deficits;
- Grade 5: GCS < 7, with or without neuro-deficits (July and Wahjoepramono 2019).

The predisposing factors for the rupture of an aneurysm are shown in Table 4.

Table 4. Risk factors for the rupture of an aneurysm.

PHASES significant risk factors	P—Population–Japanese or Finnish H—Hypertension A—Age > 70 years E—Earlier subarachnoid hemorrhage from another aneurysm S—Site anatomical location of aneurysm
Other postulated risk factors	Female gender Tobacco smoking Familial aneurysm Growth on serial imaging Symptomatic aneurysm

Source: Authors' compilation based on data from Kirollos et al. (2019).

7.5. Treatments of an Intracranial Aneurysm

Various treatments have been proposed for an intracranial aneurysm. The prime objective of treatment is the separation of an aneurysm from the parent artery with its preservation, which can be performed either by clipping or coiling. We prefer clipping rather than coiling because it has both an aneurysm occlusion under direct vision and irrigation of the brain surface and cistern by normal saline and urokinase with an aim to reduce the incidence of vasospasm.

Endovascular coiling is a treatment that is less invasive. A slender catheter with a metal coil at the end is inserted into a blood vessel by a particularly trained neuro-interventionist. The catheter or micro-catheter is inserted into the aneurysm location in the brain. The metal coil is abandoned. It prevents blood from flowing to the aneurysm.

7.5.1. Initial Management Concerns

1. Rebleeding;
2. Hydrocephalus;
3. Delayed ischemic neurologic deficit (DIND);
4. Hyponatremia;
5. DVT, as well as pulmonary embolism;
6. Detecting the source of the SAH.

7.5.2. Targets of Medical Management Related to Secondary Cerebral Injury

Early medical management constitutes the following:

Augmentation of CBF: To carry this out, the prime device is hyperdynamic therapy.

The goals are as follows:

(a) To increase cerebral perfusion pressure (CPP);
(b) To improve blood rheology: RBC aggregability increases after an SAH;
(c) Continuing euvolemia;
(d) Maintenance of a normal ICP (Williams and Brown 2013; Greenberg 2010; Cruz and Hopkins 1999; Hunt and Hess 1968; July and Wahjoepramono 2019; Guo et al. 2011).

7.5.3. Rebleeding

Rebleeding is the most common in the first hour (between 4 and 13.6%), with >33% of patient re-rupture within 3 h and 50% within 6 h of commencement of symptoms. After the day 1, the risk is 1.5% per day for the following 13 days. Overall, 15–20% of patients will bleed again within fourteen days, and 50% will bleed again within 6 months. Furthermore, greater Hunt and Hess grades have been linked to a higher risk of rebleeding. The chance of rebleeding is higher by preoperative ventriculostomy and perhaps lumbar CSF drainage (Greenberg 2010; Kirollos et al. 2019; Guo et al. 2011).

7.5.4. Prevention of Re-Hemorrhage

An optimal way of a reclusion of re-hemorrhage is early microsurgical clipping or coiling.

7.5.5. Hydrocephalus After an SAH

Acute Hydrocephalus

Blood obstructs the CSF passage through the cerebral aqueduct, the 4th ventricular output or the CSF (subarachnoid) space, as well as reabsorption at the level of arachnoid granulations. Aneurysmal rebleeding is more likely in patients who get a ventriculostomy soon after an SAH. It is recommended that an ICP be kept between 15 and 25 mm Hg and that a fast pressure drop be avoided.

Chronic Hydrocephalus

Chronic hydrocephalus is due to either permanent malfunctioning of the arachnoid granulations or adhesion of the pia and arachnoid.

7.5.6. Cerebral Vasospasm

A cerebral vasospasm is most commonly observed following an aneurysmal SAH, but it can also occur after other intracranial hemorrhages (e.g., AVM-induced intraventricular hemorrhage, idiopathic SAH), head injury (with or without SAH), cranial surgery, lumbar tap, meningitis and might even be linked to preeclampsia.

A cerebral vasospasm almost never occurs before the third day after an SAH, with a peak incidence 6–8 days following an SAH and rarely after the 17th day.

Prime time of risk: from 3 to 14 days after an SAH.

Risk factors: higher grade of SAH, more SAH on CT.

No treatment is curative. The prime way of treatment includes euvolemia, as well as hemodynamic augmentation (formerly "triple-H" therapy: hypertension, hypervolemia and hemodilution).

Avoidance of a vasospasm: This can often be accomplished by avoiding hypovolemia and anemia after an SAH CVS is not prevented by early aneurysm therapy (clipping or coiling) (i.e., before the vasospasm). Nowadays, triple-H therapy is not recommended for hyperdynamic therapy (it may invite complications without benefits).

Treatment options for a vasospasm:

1. Pharmacological:
   (a) Smooth muscle relaxants: calcium channel blockers (usually advised for standard utilization); nimodipine (60 mg every 4 hrs continued for 21 days or if the patient is in good neurological condition) does not counteract cerebral vasospasm, but improves neurological outcomes. Endothelin receptor antagonists (still experimental): ETA antagonists (clazosentan); Ryanodine receptor blocker: Dantrolene.
   (b) Intra-arterial papaverine.
2. Intervention:

   Balloon angioplasty;
   Cervical sympathectomy;
   Removal of blood clot.
3. Monitoring all patients of SAH:
   (a) Serial neuro exam;
   (b) Daily CBC;
   (c) Transcranial Doppler monitoring.
4. Specific measures:
   Manage the patient in ICU and place on triple-H therapy.

   Triple-H therapy:
   a. Hypertension: start dopamine at 2.5 μgm/kg/min (renal dose) and titrate up to 15–20 μgm/kg/min. Alternate drugs—levophed, dobutamine.
   b. Hepervolemia: normal saline ± plamanate (200–250 mL/h).
   c. Hemodilution: target hematocrit (Hct): ≤33%. Transfuse for Hct < 25% (Greenberg 2010).

7.5.7. Timing of Aneurysm Surgery

A. **"Early surgery"** (usually, but not accurately defined as ≤48–96 h after an SAH)

Benefits:

1. Virtually eliminates the chance of rebleeding if effective;
2. Makes it easier to treat vasospasm;
3. Allows for the removal of possibly vaso-spasmogenic substances from vascular contact through lavage.

Risks:

1. Inflammation and cerebral edema are at their worst right after an SAH. (a) More cerebral retraction is required. (b) Simultaneously, the brain softens and thus brain retraction is more difficult and injurious.
2. Surgery is hampered by the existence of a firm hematoma which has not had time to disintegrate.
3. Early surgery increases the chance of intraoperative rupture.
4. An increased risk of vasospasm after early surgery for mechano-trauma to the vasculature.
5. Operative mortality is higher.

Factors that favor choosing early surgery:

1. Physical condition is well;
2. Neurological status is well (Hunt and Hess (H and H) grade 1, 2 and 3);
3. Huge volumes of blood in the subarachnoid space, which increases the risk and severity of a future vasospasm;
4. Situations that make management of an unclipped/coiled aneurysm more difficult (for example, uncontrollable blood pressure, frequent and/or uncontrollable convulsions);
5. SAH is associated with a big clot with a mass effect;
6. Rebleeding in the early stages, especially numerous rebleeds;
7. Signs of impending rebleeding.

B. **"Late surgery"** (generally ≥10–14 days after an SAH)

Factors that favor choosing delayed surgery:

1. The patient's poor health and/or elderly age;
2. Patient's poor neurologic condition (H and H grade 4): debatable;
3. Aneurysms that are difficult to clip due to their size or placement, requiring a loose brain intraoperatively (e.g., mid-basilar artery aneurysms or difficult basilar bifurcation, giant aneurysm);
4. CT scan reveals severe cerebral edema;
5. Active vasospasm is present.

7.5.8. Specific Treatment of Intracranial Aneurysm

Various treatments have been proposed for an intracerebral aneurysm. The main aim of the treatment is the exclusion of an aneurysm with an intact parent artery, which can be done either by clipping or coiling.

Endovascular Coiling

Endovascular coiling is a process that is less intrusive. A slender catheter with a metal coil at the end is inserted into a blood vessel by a particularly trained neuro interventionist. The catheter or micro-catheter is inserted into the aneurysm location in the brain. The metal coil is abandoned. It prevents blood from flowing to the aneurysm. Coiling will be discussed in the endovascular chapter (Chapter 18) of this book.

Microsurgical Clipping

We prefer clipping rather than coiling because it has both the aneurysm occlusion under direct vision and irrigation of the brain surface and cistern by normal saline and urokinase with an aim to decrease the incidence of a cerebral vasospasm. We will discuss the clipping of an aneurysm in this chapter. Various patterns and types of clippings are shown in Figures 2–6.

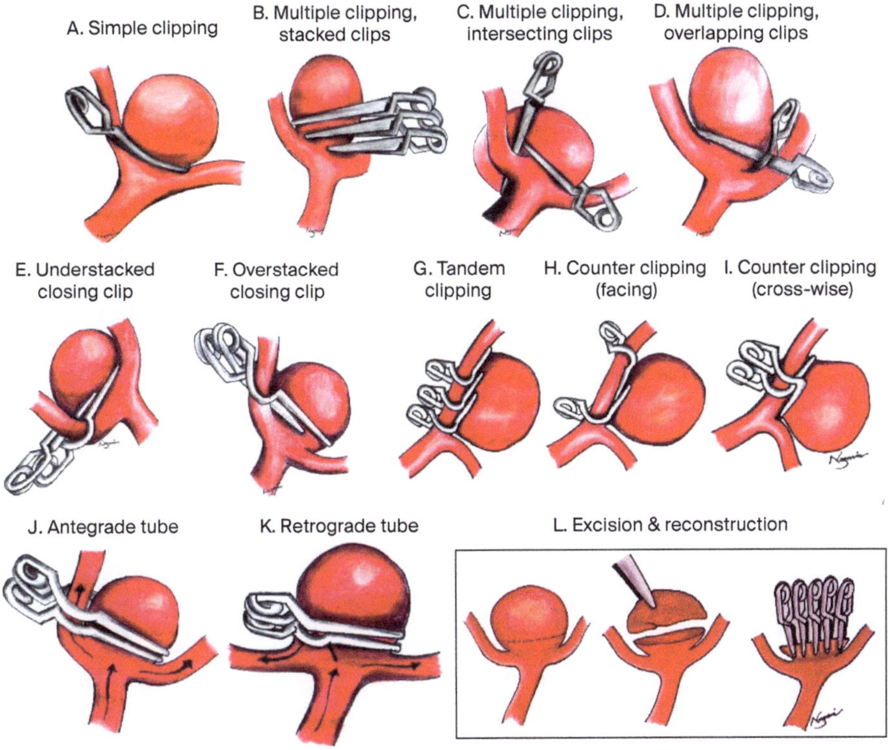

Figure 2. Diagram of various patterns of the clipping of different types of aneurysms. Source: Figure by authors.

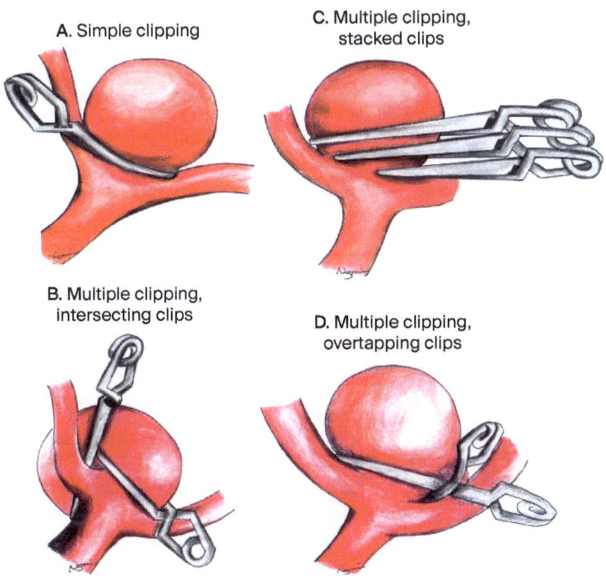

Figure 3. Diagram of various patterns of the clipping of different types of aneurysms. Source: Figure by authors.

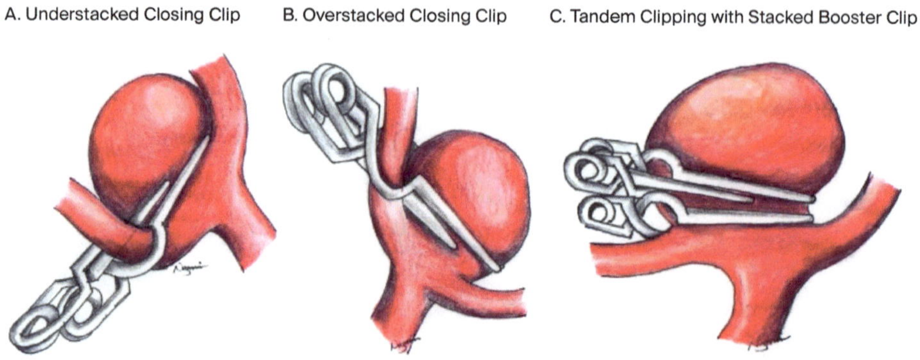

Figure 4. Diagram of various patterns of the clipping of different types of aneurysms (tandem clipping). Source: Figure by authors.

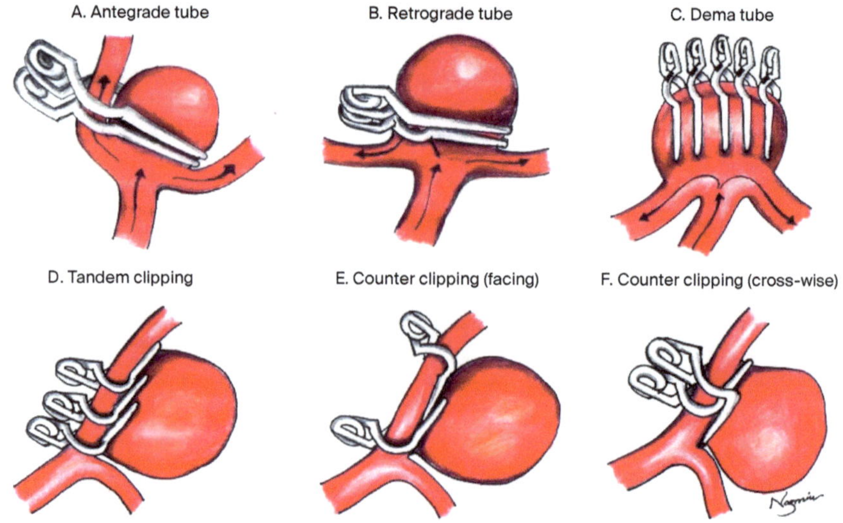

Figure 5. Diagram of various patterns of the clipping of different types of aneurysms (fenestration tubes, tandem angle-fenestrated clipping). Source: Figure by authors.

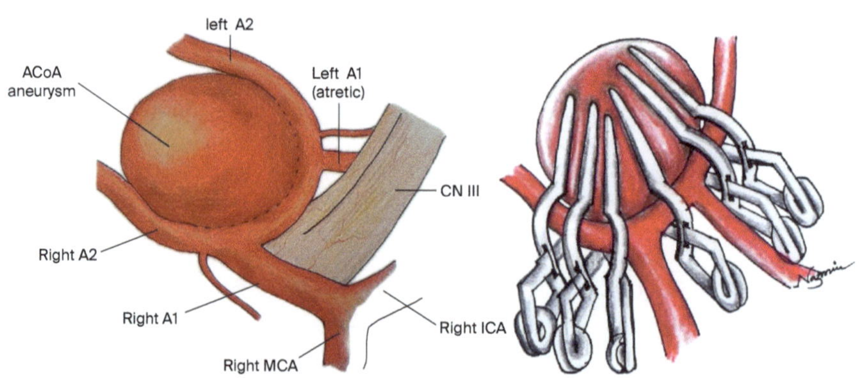

Figure 6. Reverse picket-fence-type clipping in the case of a giant ACOM or MCA aneurysm. Source: Figure by authors.

Comparison between coiling and clipping is shown in Table 5.

Table 5. Coiling vs. clipping with respect to the results.

Coiling	Clipping
Equal risk	Equal risk
22% obliteration/10 years	93% obliteration/10 years
19% retreatment/10 years	<1% retreatment/10 years
2.5 to 6 times higher rebleed rate	2.5 to 6 times lower rebleed rate
Can treat 64% of patients	Can teat >99% of patients
More expensive	Less expensive

Source: Authors' compilation based on data from Spetzler (2018).

Giant Aneurysms

Giant aneurysms are >2.5 cm (about 1 inch) in diameter (Figure 7). Saccular (possibly an inflated "berry" aneurysm) and fusiform aneurysms are the two forms. Of all aneurysms, 3–5% are cerebral aneurysms, the common age of prevalence is 30 to 60 years, the female: male ratio = 3:1 and 35% present as a hemorrhage, with 10% displaying some signs of distant bleeding. About a third of them have a clippable neck (Greenberg 2010; Kalangu et al. 2009).

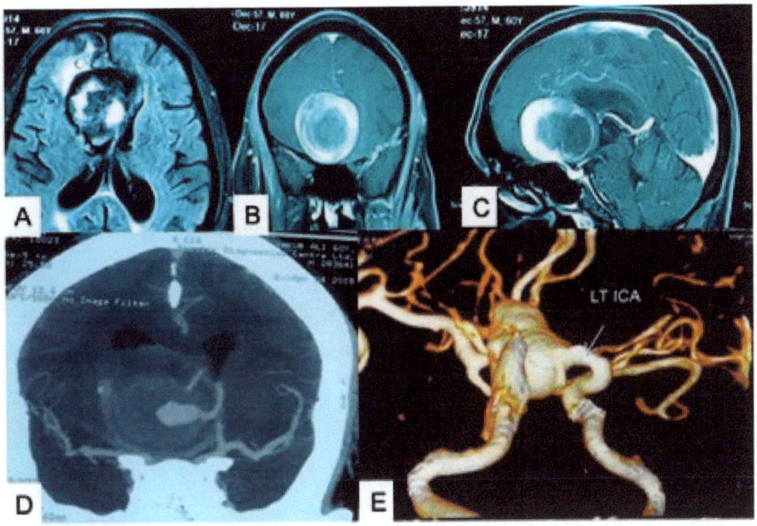

Figure 7. (**A–C**) MRI axial, coronal and sagital view showing a thrombosed ACOM aneurysm. (**D**) CT angiogram in coronal view showing a partially thrombosed ACOM aneurysm. (**E**) CT angiogram showing a giant ACOM aneurysm. Source: Figure by authors.

Tips and tricks for aneurysm surgery:

1. Adequate exposure under the microscope;
2. Meticulous sharp subarachnoid dissection;
3. Gentle brain retraction of brain support for proper vision;
4. Resection of some of the brain portion (gurus rictus);
5. Proximal control of patent artery by temporary clipping;
6. Occlusion of the neck or trapping of an aneurysm by permanent clipping;
7. Never panic during an intraoperative rupture, keep calm, get speedy help from an assistant, double and wide bore sucker, application of cottonoid, use of bipolar and proper clipping or in some cases cotton assistant clipping for a safe outcome;
8. Proper selection of clip length, breath and closing force, where length is commonly 1 $\frac{1}{2}$ of the aneurysm neck diameter. (Lawton 2011)

Tenets of the aneurysm clipping:

- Under the microscope;

- Meticulous sharp subarachnoid dissection;
- Gentle brain retraction;
- Vascular control: proximal control by temporary clipping;
- Temporary clipping;
- Proper selection of clip length (1 $\frac{1}{2}$ of aneurysm neck diameter), breath and closing force;
- Permanent clipping;
- Inspection;
- Brain transgression;
- Intraoperative rupture. (Lawton 2011)

8. Anterior Communicating Artery (ACOM) Aneurysm

ACOM aneurysms are the most common cranial aneurysms and the most complex aneurysms to clip in the anterior circulation (Kirollos et al. 2019; July and Wahjoepramono 2019; Yasargil 1987; Jiménez-Sosa et al. 2017).

8.1. Types of ACOM Arteries

1. Adult-type ACOM arteries comprise 1/3 of A1 thickness; here, the aneurysm location is usually in the A1–A2 junction.
2. Fetal-type ACOM arteries are the same size as A1, and here, the aneurysm location is usually the ACOM itself.
3. There are about 3 to 13 perforators from the ACOM artery with a mean diameter of 250–300 µm (Greenberg 2010). The hypothalamic artery is a perforator, feeding the hypothalamus which is present in only in 10% of all cases. A1 perforators pass through the anterior perforated substance.

Important perforators:

- Recurrent artery of Heubner;
- Hypothalamic perforators.

There are variations in A1. Often, A1 runs over the optic nerve but it may be infraoptic (Figure 8).

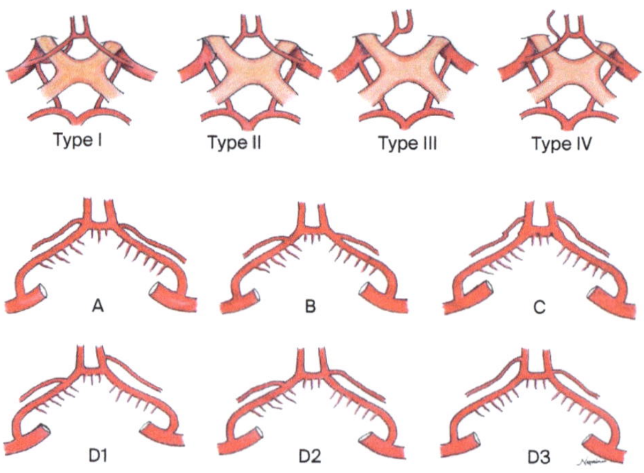

Figure 8. Four different types of an infraoptic A1, as modified after Wong et al. Type 1: infraoptic anastomotic branch between the ICA and ACA in the presence of normal anatomy around the ICA. Type 2: infraoptic A1 with the bifurcation at the level of the ophthalmic origin but no supraoptic A1. Type 3: similar to type 2, except for the absence of contralateral A1. Type 4: an accessory ACA variant. Variations in the origin of Heubner's artery are shown in (**A**–**D**). Recurrent artery of Heubner: The ACOM artery complex is located in the basal frontal lobes, near the hypothalamus, optic apparatus and cognitive/emotional centers, and its arteries supply the motor/sensory cortex, the basal ganglia and internal capsule. Source: Figure by authors.

A recurrent artery of Heubner is an important perforator originating from the initial portion of A2 (Figure 8).

- *Hypothalamic perforators:* originates from the ACOM and present in 10% of the cases.
- *Variation in A1 and A2* (Jiménez-Sosa et al. 2017) is shown in Table 6.

Table 6. Anatomic variants associated with an anterior communicating artery aneurysm.

Dominant A1: fills both A2s
Unilateral hypoplasia of one A1 (25%)
Exclusive filling of the anterior communicating artery by one A1

Source: Authors' compilation based on data from Jiménez-Sosa et al. (2017).

When an ACOM aneurysm ruptures, it presents with an impaired consciousness, and in the case of an unruptured and giant aneurysm, it may present with a bitemporal field defect.

A fenestrated ACOM is shown in Figure 9A. The types of ACOM aneurysms are shown (July and Wahjoepramono 2019) in Figure 9B and a fenestrated A1 is depicted in Figure 9C.

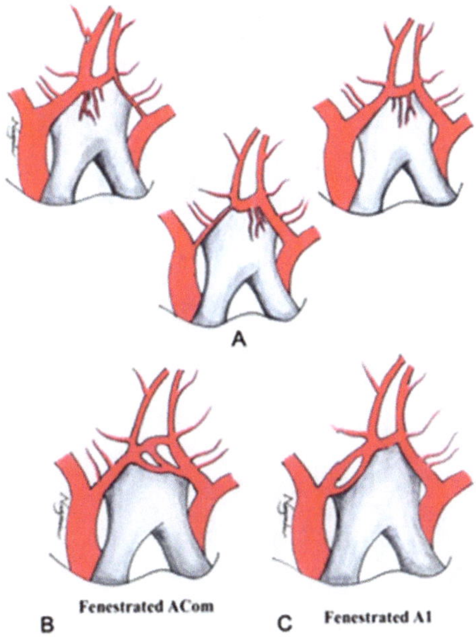

Figure 9. (**A**) Variation in the origin of the hypothalamic arteries; (**B**) Fenestrated ACOM; (**C**) Fenestrated A1. Source: Figure by authors.

In Figure 10, a CT scan of the head shows an SAH of a ruptured ACOM aneurysm and a CTA of the brain shows an ACOM aneurysm.

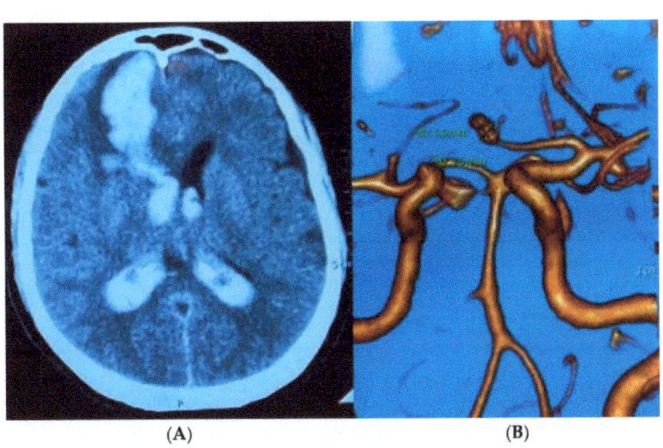

Figure 10. (**A**) CT scan showing basal frontal blood along with intraventricular bleed and no SAH; (**B**) CT angiogram showing an ACOM aneurysm. Various origin-types of ACOM aneurysms are illustrated in Figure 11. Source: Figure by authors.

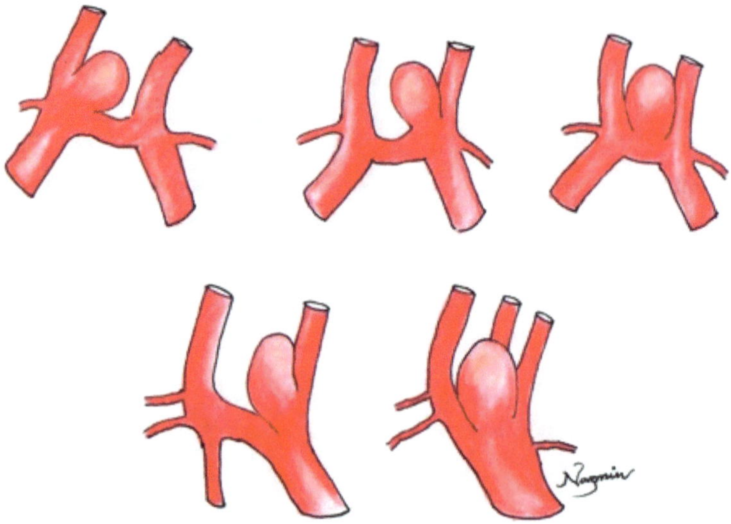

Figure 11. Various sites of origins of an ACOM aneurysm. Source: Figure by authors.

Schematic diagram of different dome directions of an ACOM aneurysm are seen in Figure 12.

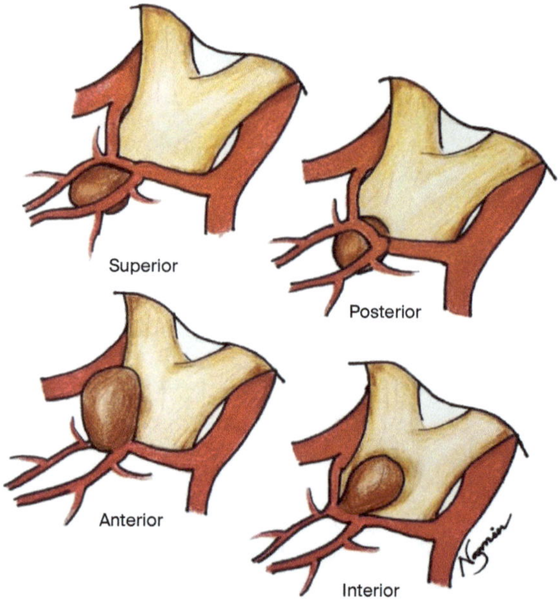

Figure 12. Schematic diagram showing an ACOM aneurysm with different directions, such as the anterior, superior, posterior and inferior directions (July and Wahjoepramono 2019). Source: Figure by authors.

8.2. Surgical Technique

- *Pterional craniotomy*—most ACOM aneurysms are carried out by pterional craniotomy;
- *Bifrontal basal approach* for superiorly directing ACOM aneurysms;
- *Supraorbital keyhole approach* for a small size, both for ruptured and unruptured aneurysms;
- *Orbitozygomatic approach* for giant ACOM aneurysms.

The types of clippings of an ACOM aneurysm are diagrammed in Figure 13.

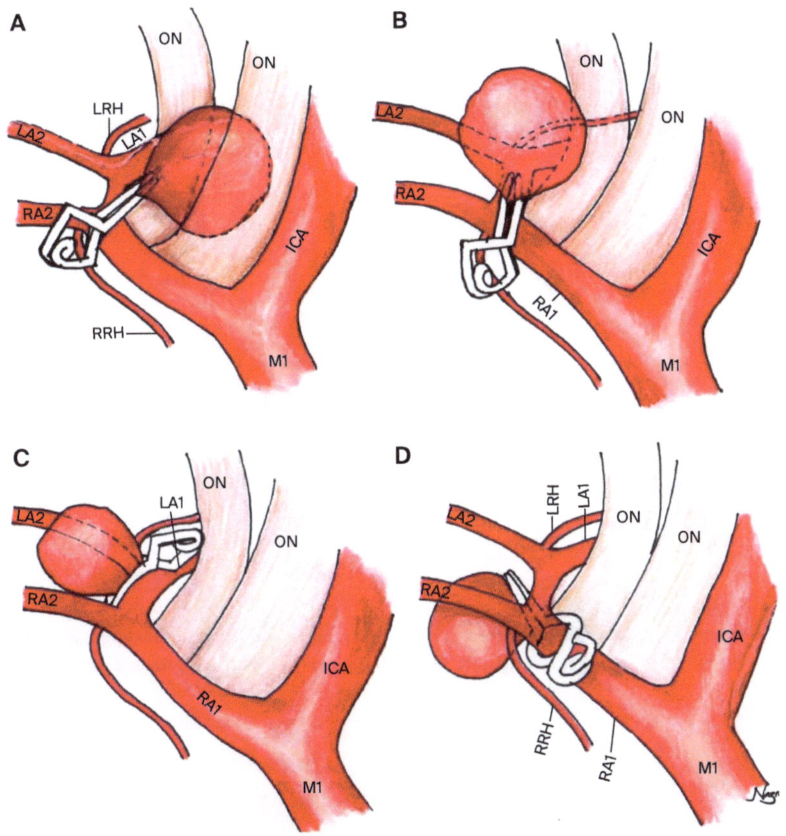

Figure 13. (**A**,**B**) Various types of clippings of an ACOM aneurysm (**C**,**D**). Anteriorly projecting aneurysm. Schematic demonstration of the clip placement. Source: Figure by authors.

8.3. Complications of ACOM Aneurysms

(1) Vasospasm—leads to ischemia in anterior circulation areas and produces leg weakness with incontinence of the bowel and bladder;
(2) Rebleeding;
(3) Hydrocephalus—needs a VP shunt.

9. Posterior Communicating (PCOM) Artery Aneurysm

Posterior communicating artery (PCOM) aneurysms (Kirollos et al. 2019; Lawton 2011; Yasargil 1987) are one of the most common aneurysms following ACOM aneurysms, which constitute about 25% of all aneurysms. The PCOM artery runs parallel and above the 3rd nerve, so an aneurysm of the PCOM produces a pupil involving 3rd nerve palsy (Figure 14), along with headaches.

There are three types of PCOM artery patterns:

1. Adult pattern

   Flow from basilar to posterior cerebral artery (PCA).

2. Fetal pattern

   Flow from the internal carotid artery (ICA) to PCA;
   Hypoplastic P1.

3. Hypoplastic

   Flow from basilar to PCA;
   PCOM gives perforators which supply the internal capsule.

Surgical technique for PCOM aneurysms:

Pterional craniotomy and clipping of an intact PCOM, as well as an anterior choroidal artery are the aim of treatment.

The clipping patterns of a PCOM are illustrated in Figure 15.

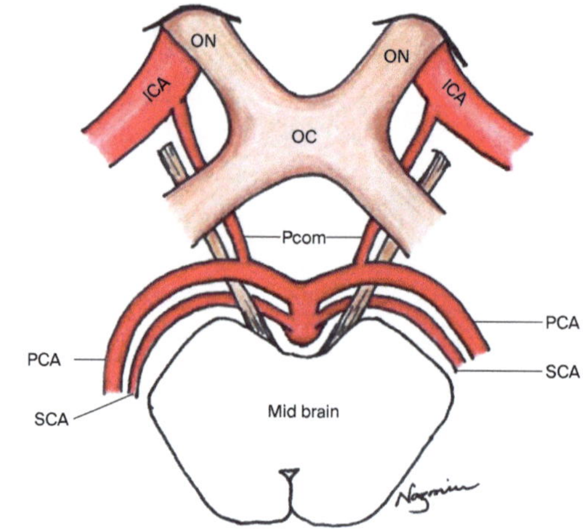

Figure 14. Anterior relationships between the 3rd cranial nerve and the posterior circulation. PCOMA; posterior communicating artery; roman numeral cranial nerves. Source: Figure by authors.

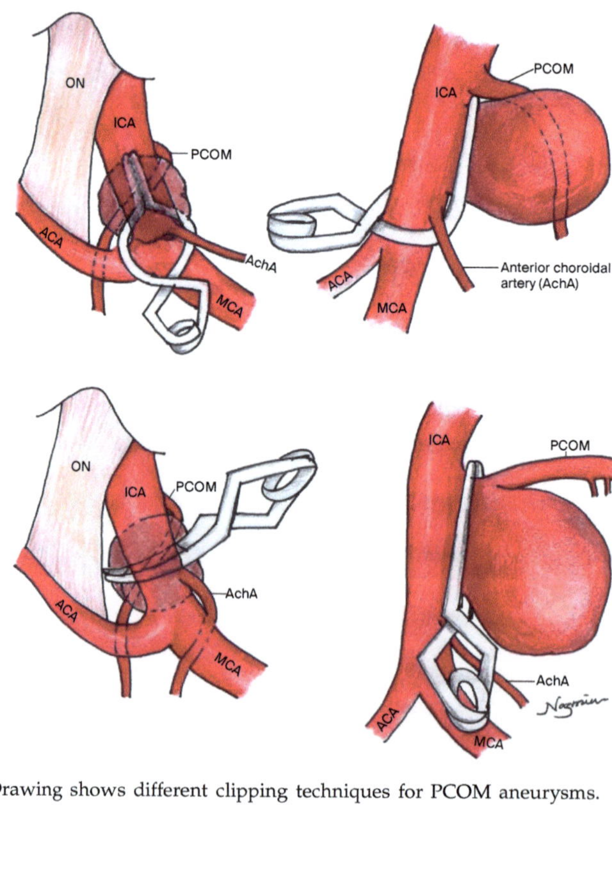

Figure 15. Drawing shows different clipping techniques for PCOM aneurysms. Source: Figure by authors.

10. Middle Cerebral Artery (MCA) Aneurysm

An MCA aneurysm (Lawton 2011; Paulo et al. 2010) constitutes about 20% of intracranial aneurysms, classically arising in the second division of a lateral sulcus (Sylvian fissure). When it ruptures, it commonly presents with aphasia, hemisensory loss, hemiparesis, visual field defects or anosognosia along with a headache and decreasing mentation.

A Sylvia fissure SAH, along with a temporal lobe hematoma, is the common radiological findings (Figure 16).

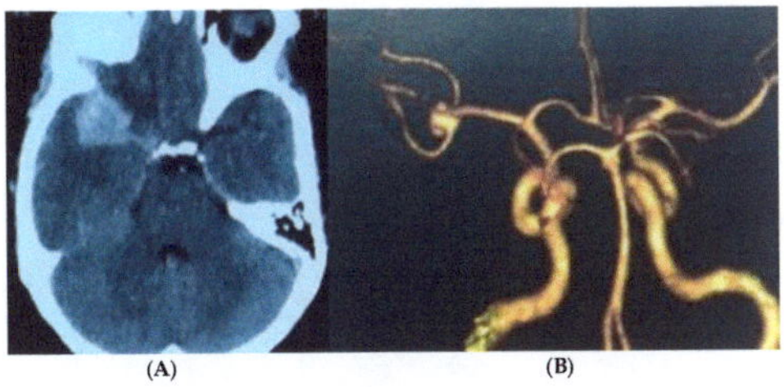

Figure 16. CT scan showing blood in the right Sylvian fissure (**A**) and CT angiogram showing a right MCA aneurysm (**B**). Source: Figure by authors.

10.1. MCA Aneurysm Dome Projection

Dome projection of MCA aneurysm is shown in Figure 17.

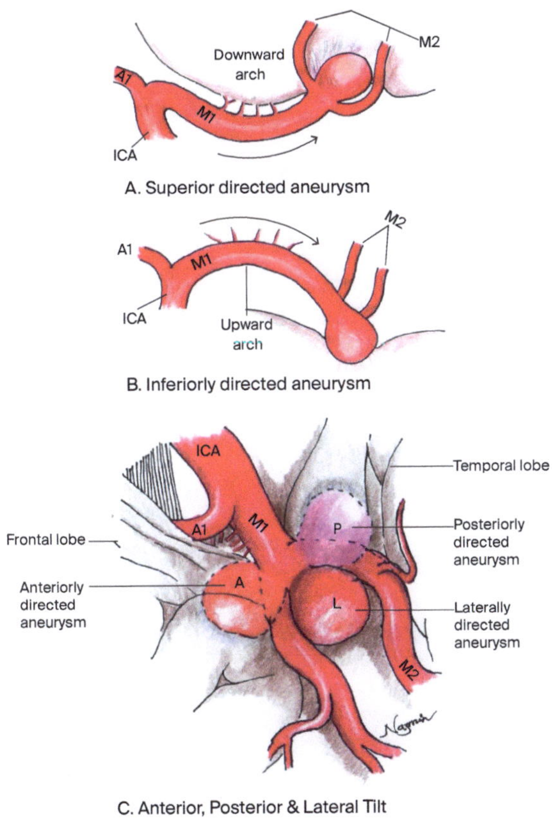

Figure 17. Image shows different directions of an MCA aneurysm; (**A**) superior projection, (**B**) inferior projection, (**C**) L—lateral projection, P—Posterior projection and A—anterior projection. Source: Figure by authors.

10.2. Surgical Technique

Pterional craniotomy with a trans- Sylvian approach is the choice of surgery.

A hematoma needs to be evacuated through the wash of the Sylvian fissure with urokinase-mixed normal saline.

The Sylvian fissure can be exposed either distally to proximally, or proximally to distally.

Proximal control in the M1 artery is needed to make the aneurysm soft, and dissecting the neck is needed for proper clipping and keeping the superior and inferior trunks intact (Figure 18).

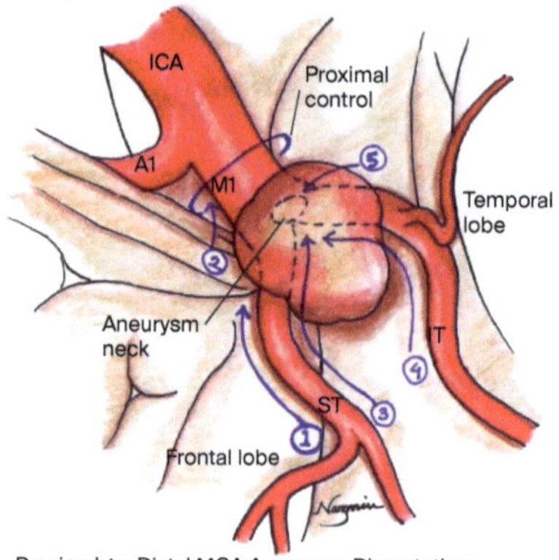

Figure 18. MCA aneurysm dissection strategy: distal-to-proximal dissection. Step 1: following the superior trunk (outer surface); step 2: preparing the M1 segment for proximal control; step 3: following the superior trunk (inner surface); step 4: following the inferior trunk (inner surface); step 5: dissecting the distal neck (blind spot). Source: Figure by authors.

Pterional craniotomy is the approach for an MCA aneurysm. In the case of an acutely ruptured MCA aneurysm with a significant hematoma, we need wide exposure with the aim to evacuate and decompress the hematoma if needed. Those having a hematoma with evidence of a vasospasm need to undergo wide temporal decompression to avoid tentorial herniation.

A trans-Sylvian trajectory is chosen in most of the cases; however, a transcortical trajectory is sometimes chosen when the temporal lobe is swollen and has an underlying hematoma.

The Sylvian vein is commonly dissected from the frontal side and kept to the temporal lobe, but it can also be dissected from the temporal side and kept with the frontal lobe when necessary. Figure 19 shows different types of clip occlusions of an MCA aneurysm.

A keyhole or mini pterional craniotomy is commonly chosen for chronic or unruptured cases of MCA aneurysms.

10.3. Complications

1. Vasospasm of the MCA leading to a massive MCA territory infarction, which may lead to uncal herniation and death of the patient if unnoticed;
2. Rebleed;
3. Hydrocephalus.

10.4. Giant MCA Aneurysm

The MCA is the most common site for the development of a giant aneurysm. About 6% of all MCAs are giant (>25 mm).

A combination of 3D DSA, 3D CTA and MRI data is needed for a complete idea of the vascular anatomy, intraluminal thrombus, calcification and thickness of the wall.

10.4.1. Surgical Technique

The EC–IC and IC–IC bypass are now popular to manage a giant MCA aneurysm.

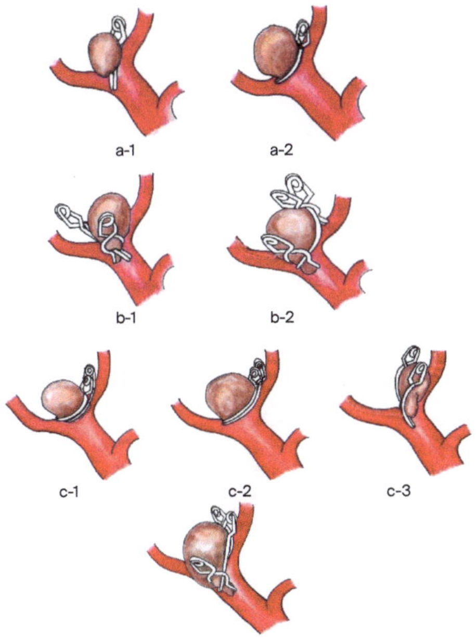

Figure 19. Images showing different clipping techniques for MCA aneurysms. Source: Figure by authors.

11. Basilar Top Aneurysm

Basilar top aneurysms (Kirollos et al. 2019; Lawton 2011; July and Wahjoepramono 2019) are the most common in posterior circulation and constitute about 5–10% of all intracranial aneurysms.

- Basilar artery aneurysms may be either fusiform or saccular;
- Rupture of a basilar artery aneurysm is classically localized to the interpeduncular cistern, though it may extend into the suprasellar cistern.

11.1. Types of Basilar Top Aneurysms

Three types of aneurysms according to the level of aneurysm and dorsum sellae (Figure 20): 1. High riding; 2. normal; 3. low riding.

The carotid is normally fixed at two points: distal dural ring and by the PCOM artery. Thus, for better exposure, we need to mobilize the ICA by cutting the distal dural ring following anterior clinoidectomy and coagulation, and scarify the posterior communicating artery close to the PCA junction. The corridor is often used to reach is carotid oculomotor corridor which can be expanded by mobilizing the 3rd and or 4th nerve (Figure 21), as well as retraction of the tentorium cerebelli by a stitch. Unroofing of the cavernous sinus is carried out by clipping of the aneurysm (Figure 22). Often, long clips are applied, preserving the contralateral posterior cerebral artery and thalamo-perforators.

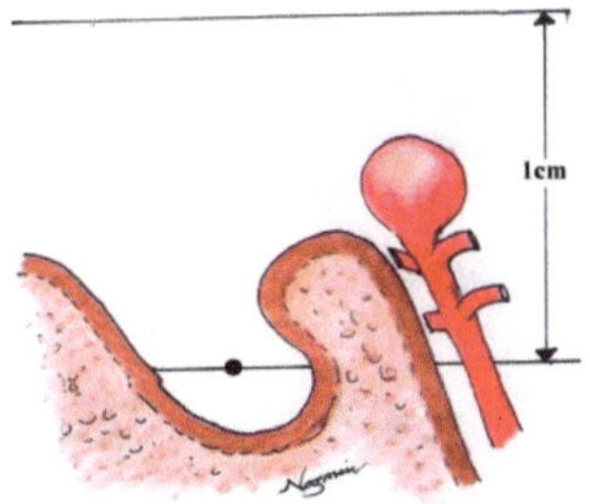

Figure 20. Schematic image showing relation of the basilar top aneurysm and dorsum sella. Source: Figure by authors.

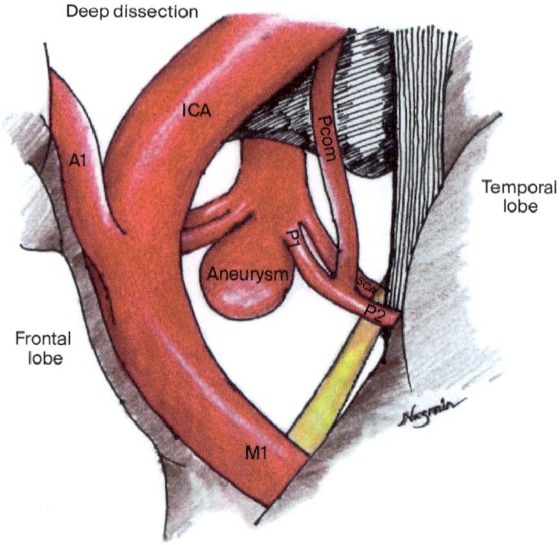

Figure 21. Image showing the PCOM and 3rd nerve reaching the basilar top location. Source: Figure by authors.

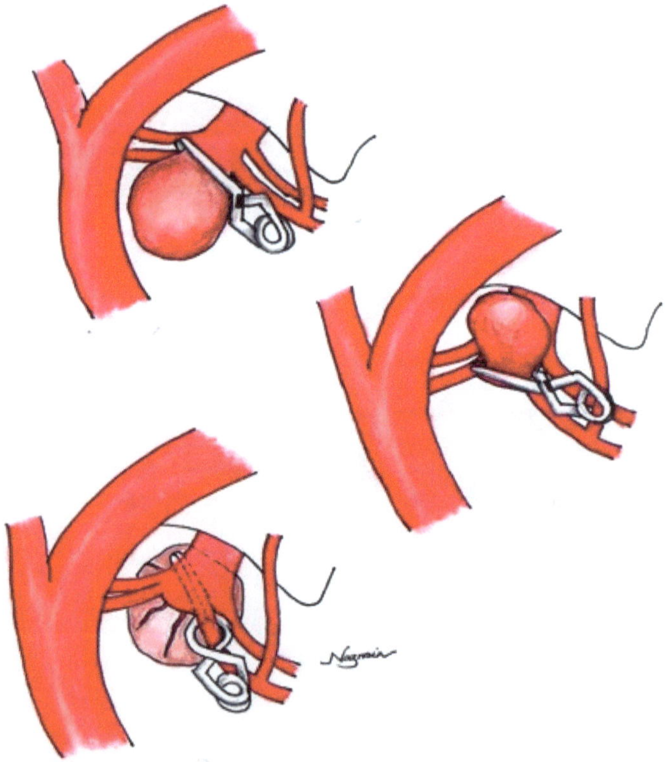

Figure 22. Types of clippings of a basilar top aneurysm. Source: Figure by authors.

In Figure 23, a cerebral DSA shows a basilar top aneurysm.

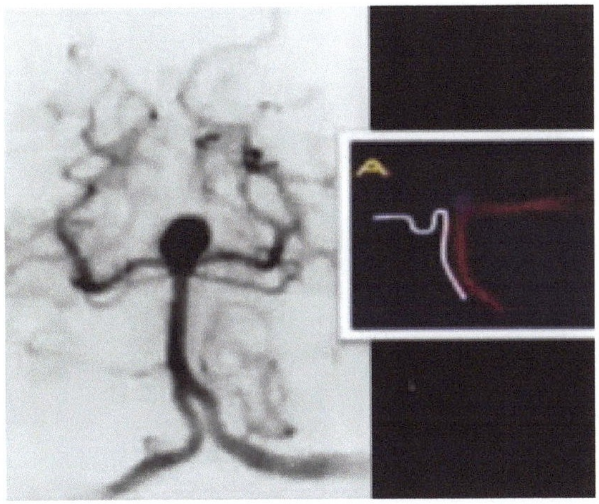

Figure 23. DSA showing a basilar top aneurysm. Source: Figure by authors.

11.2. Microsurgical Approaches

Different surgical approaches to reach the basilar top area are employed as follows:

1. **Extradural temporal approach/trans-cavernous approach/temporopolar extradural approach/trans-Sylvian trans-clinoidal trans-cavernous approach:** for normal or low-riding basilar top aneurysms;
2. **Orbito-zygomatic craniotomy:** for high-riding basilar top aneyrysms; this approach is a versatile approach in neurosurgery and can be carried out in one piece, two pieces or even three pieces;
3. **Pretemporal craniotomy/half-and-half approach:** for normal or low-riding basilar top aneurysms;
4. **Sub-temporal approach for normal-position basilar top aneurysms.**

Details of a craniotomy of frequently used approaches for posterior circulation aneurysm are shown in Table 7.

Table 7. Positioning, skin incision and details of a craniotomy of frequently used approaches for posterior circulation aneurysms at or about the basilar apex level.

Approach	Pterional	Lateral Supraorbital	Orbito-Zygomatic	Anterior Temporal or Temporopolar
Position	Supine position, head rotated 15–20° toward the opposite side, head extension 20°	Supine position, head rotated 15–30° toward the opposite side, head flexion or extension according to the lesion	Supine position, head rotated 30–90° toward the opposite side, neck extension (top point is at the ipsilateral malar eminence)	Supine position, head rotated 30° to the opposite side and slightly elevated above the heart level
Skin incision	Posterior the hairline, beginning at the root of the zygoma and crossing the midline	Posterior the hairline, starting 3 cm cranial to the zygoma to the same-sided midpapillary line	Posterior the hairline, beginning at the root of the zygoma and crossing the midline toward the opposite midpapillary line	Posterior the hairline, beginning at the root of the zygoma, extending backward to the retro-ocular area and crossing the midline
Temporalis muscle (TM) dissection	Interfascial dissection, TM is totally dissected	Myocutaneous flap (only the upper and anterior aspect of the TM is dissected)	Subfascial or interfascial dissection, the TM is totally dissected	Subfascial or interfascial dissection, the TM totally dissected and retracted downward

Table 7. *Cont.*

Approach	Pterional	Lateral Supraorbital	Orbito-Zygomatic	Anterior Temporal or Temporopolar
Site of craniotomy	Frontal bone, squamous temporal bone, pterion	Frontal bone, between zygomatic process of the frontal bone, greater sphenoid wing, as well as superior temporal line	Frontal bone, pterion, squamous temporal bone and orbito-zygomatic osteotomy (orbital roof, orbital rim, lateral orbital wall, as well as zygomatic arch)	Frontal bine, squamous temporal bone pterion and orbito-zygomatic osteotomy can be performed
Size of craniotomy	6 × 6 cm	4 × 4 cm	Nearly 8 × 8 cm (varies based on the necessary temporal or frontal exposure)	Nearly 6–8 cm in diameter
Sphenoid ridge drilling	Up to the superior orbital fissure (SOF)	Not essential	To SOF	To SOF

Source: Authors' compilation based on data from July and Wahjoepramono (2019).

12. ICA Bifurcation Aneurysm

The incidence of ICA bifurcation aneurysms (July and Wahjoepramono 2019; Lawton 2011; van Rooij et al. 2008) is about 2.4% to 4% among all intracranial aneurysms.

An aneurysm fundus projection may be superior (56%), posterior (18%), anterior (20%) or lateral (6%).

12.1. Surgical Technique

- Pterional craniotomy is the approach of choice for this aneurysm, with or without anterior clinoidectomy.
- A single clip or multiple clips are commonly required to secure the neck of the aneurysm.

Figure 24 shows a DSA and CTA with different types of ICA aneurysms.

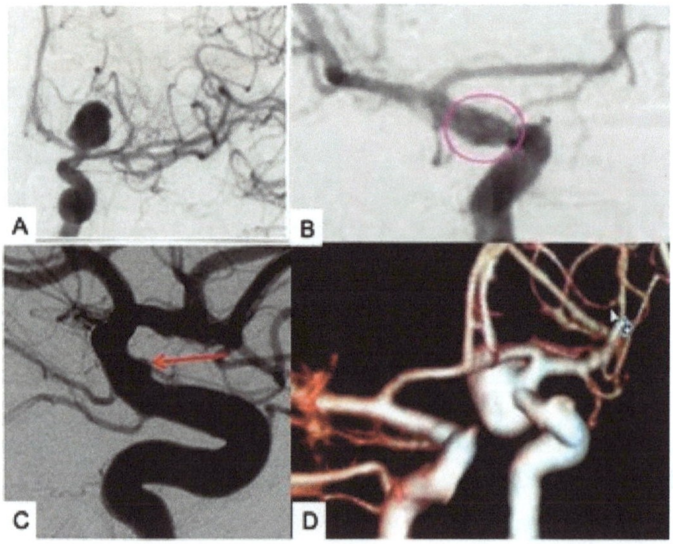

Figure 24. (**A**) DSA showing an ICA bifurcation aneurysm. (**B**) DSA showing the focal dilatation of an ICA. (**C**) DSA showing the focal bulging of an ICA, suggestive of a blood blister aneurysm. (**D**) Huge ICA of a dorsal wall aneurysm. Source: Figure by authors.

13. Blood Blister Aneurysm

A blood-blister-like aneurysm (Gopaul et al. 2015) is a wide-based bulge at the non-branching point of an artery that is unsimilar to saccular (or 'berry') aneurysms that generally occur at the branching points.

It accounts for 0.5–2.0% of ruptured intracranial aneurysms that cause unexpectedly higher mortality, as well as morbidity.

It is small dilatation or focal bulging in the non-branch portion of the supraclinoid ICA opposite to the origin of the PCOM or anterior choroidal artery.

It is frequently tiny (<6 mm), with an average of 3 mm.

- CTA: often negative
- DSA: is the most effective diagnostic imaging

13.1. Surgical Technique

Microsurgical clipping carries a higher danger of tearing the aneurysm or ICA laceration during surgery:

A. Clipping with wrapping;
B. EC-IC arterial bypass plus surgical or endovascular trapping (can be used as the last resort);
C. Endovascular management by a stent assistant coiling or flow-diverting device may be used, but the value is yet to be proven.

14. IC Dorsal Wall Aneurysm

Aneurysms originating from the anterior (dorsal) wall of the ICA (Figure 24D) comprise 0.3 to 1% of all intracranial aneurysms (Gopaul et al. 2015). It is assumed that a blood blister aneurysm may turn to a dorsal wall aneurysm rapidly.

14.1. Surgical Technique

A. Trapping surgery, both with and without an EC–IC bypass has been described; however, due to the delicate nature of the ICA, re-rupture may happen during operation (Figures 25 and 26).
B. Coiling, stent-assisted coiling, flow-diverter and coated stents in endovascular surgery.

Application of a distal ICA temporary clip and suction decompression technique from the neck allows for the collapse of the aneurysm and helps in clipping. In Figure 24B, the fenestrated clipping technique in an ICA dorsal wall aneurysm is shown.

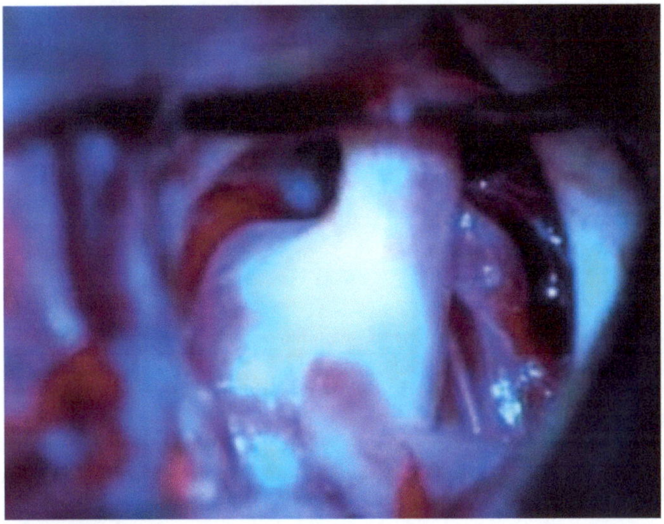

Figure 25. Preoperative picture of an ICA dorsal wall aneurysm. Source: Figure by authors.

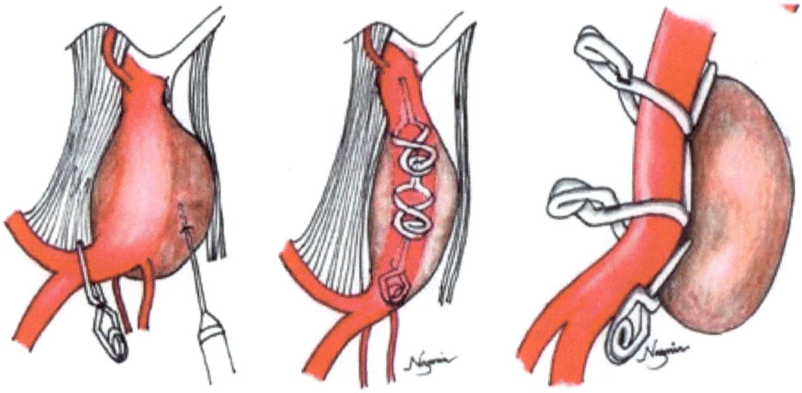

Figure 26. Schematic showing the fenestrated clipping technique for an ICA dorsal wall aneurysm. Source: Figure by authors.

15. Ophthalmic Segment Aneurysm

A supraclinoid ICA, particularly the ophthalmic part of the supraclinoid ICA, is the site of origin of ophthalmic artery aneurysms (Day 1990). An ICA from the distal dural ring to the PCOM artery is included in this segment.

Ophthalmic aneurysms are intradural. Ophthalmic artery aneurysms, superior hypophyseal aneurysms and unusual varieties such as those on the ventral and dorsal surfaces of this ICA segment are among them.

Ophthalmic segment aneurysms, as well as transitional or distal cavernous ICA aneurysms, are all classified as paraclinoid aneurysms (Figure 27).

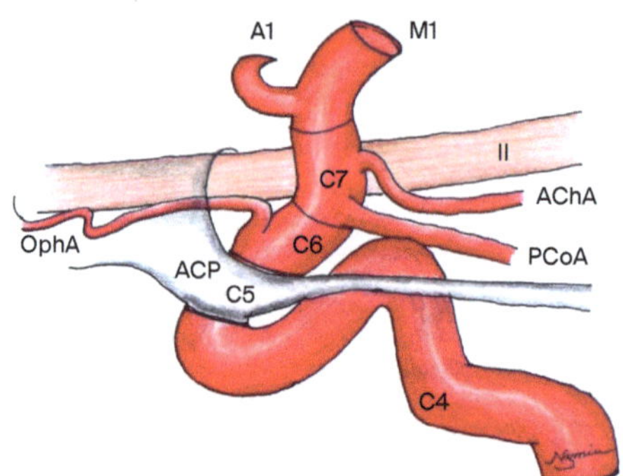

Figure 27. Anterior clinoid process and optic strut, along with an optic foramen and superior orbital fissure. Source: Figure by authors.

15.1. Surgical Technique

- An ophthalmic segment aneurysm, when small, can be managed by pterional craniotomy with anterior clinoidectomy and clipping of the aneurysm neck.
- Clinoidectomy can be performed either by an intradural or extradural route, depending on surgeons' choice and patient status.
- Release of the distal dural ring and getting proximal control, but when the aneurysm is big, it needs exposure of the neck to get vascular proximal control and for suction decompression technique.
- Contralateral pterional approach for an ophthalmic segment aneurysm—when the neck and dome of an aneurysm are redirected toward the contralateral site, then a contralateral pterional craniotomy can be carried out to secure the aneurysm.

16. Paraclinoid Aneurysm

Aneurysms that start at the ICA distal to the proximal dural ring (PDR) and proximal to the PCOM artery, which includes both the ophthalmic and clinoidal segments of the ICA, are known as paraclinoid aneurysms (Otani et al. 2018).

Ocular indications could be the first signs of a gradually expanding paraclinoid ICA aneurysm, which can cause blindness and death if left untreated. A patient with a rapidly increasing paraclinoid aneurysm, on the other hand, may exhibit acute symptoms such as episodic visual loss and headache. The different sites of origin of a paraclinoid aneurysm are shown Figure 28.

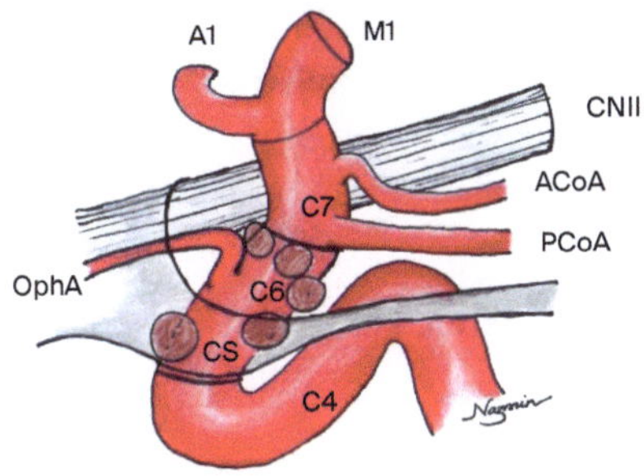

Figure 28. Different sites of the origin of a paraclinoid aneurysm. Source: Figure by authors.

16.1. Surgical Treatment

Obtaining proximal control of the artery, proper dissection of the aneurysm neck and effective clipping of the aneurysm with less handling of the optic nerve are all critical characteristics of the successful surgical therapy of these diseases.

The extracranial cervical carotid and intracranial carotid arteries distal to the aneurysm are temporarily clipped and the aneurysm is aspirated through a catheter insertion into the extracranial carotid (a needle decompression technique similar to suction decompression can be achieved by first trapping the intracranial arterial segment and then puncturing the aneurysm dome with a "butterfly" needle connected to the suction).

Pterional craniotomy:

- Intradural or extradural clinoidectomy;
- Release of the distal dural ring and falciform ligament and mobilization of the optic nerve;
- It needs exposure of the neck for proximal vascular control and the suction decompression technique (Figure 29) of clipping;
- In some case, it needs a high-flow STA–MCA brain bypass and entrapment of the aneurysm.

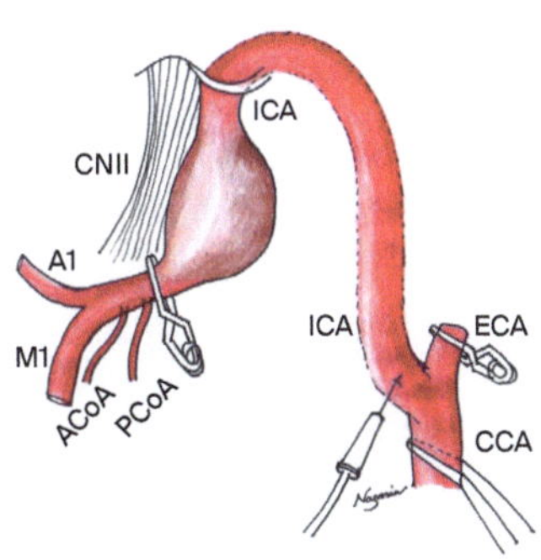

Figure 29. Suction decompression technique. "Dallas" technique for proximal internal carotid aneurysms. Source: Figure by authors.

17. Cavernous Carotid Aneurysm

Cavernous ICA aneurysms (Eddleman et al. 2009) comprise 2–9% of all intracranial aneurysms. The risk assessment of a cavernous ICA aneurysm rupture is limited (Figure 30).

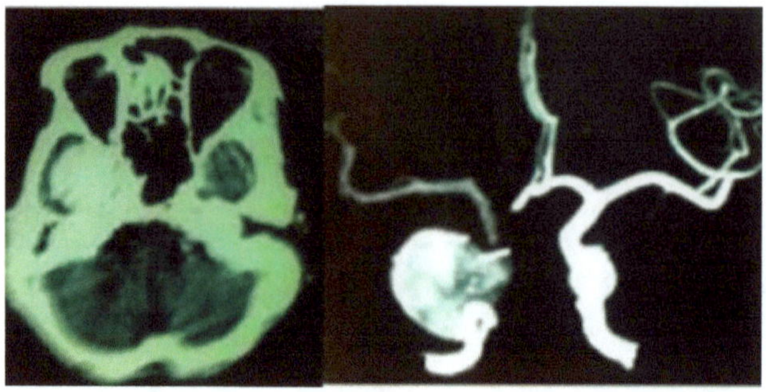

Figure 30. CT scan showing a giant cavernous carotid aneurysm on the left. CT angiogram showing a giant cavernous carotid aneurysm on the right side. Source: Figure by authors.

17.1. Surgical Technique

A carotid cavernous aneurysm seldom needs treatment in the form of carotid ligation at the neck, plus/minus an STA–MCA/high-flow bypass (Figure 31).

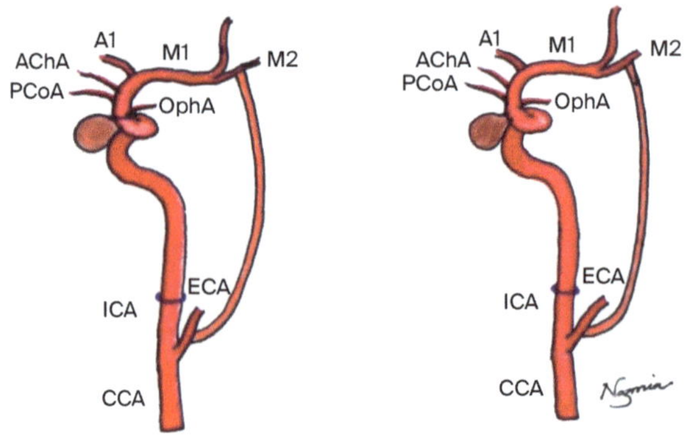

Figure 31. Pictures showing an EC–IC bypass with trapping and without trapping but only neck ligation of an ICA. Source: Figure by authors.

18. DACA (Distal Anterior Cerebral Artery) Aneurysm

Aneurysms of the distal anterior cerebral artery (DACA) (also called pericallosal artery aneurysms) account for around 6% of all intracranial aneurysms (Figure 32). They are found on the anterior cerebral artery's A2–A5 segments, as well as its distant branches (Lehecka et al. 2010).

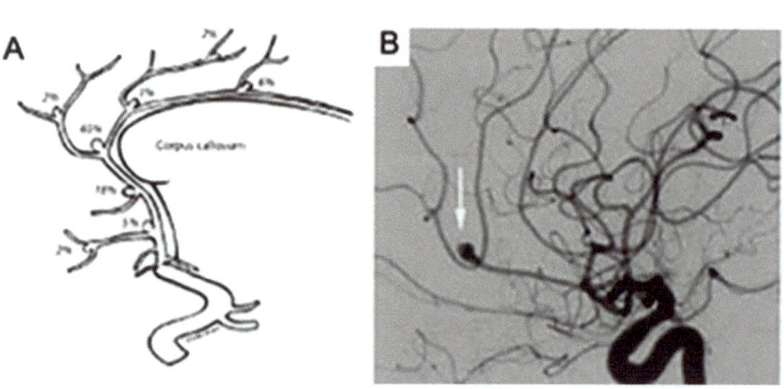

Figure 32. (**A**) Distribution of a DACA aneurysm based on the microneurosurgical division. (**B**) DSA showing a DACA aneurysm. Source: Figure by authors.

18.1. Surgical Technique

The surgical clipping of these aneurysms also presents a unique challenge due to a narrow operative field, dense interhemispheric adhesions, difficulty in locating the aneurysm, associated vascular anomalies, a small pericallosal cistern and occasional problems in attaining proximal control.

The surgical approaches used are a unilateral parasagittal craniotomy or bifrontal craniotomy.

19. PICA Aneurysm

Aneurysms of the vertebral artery–posterior inferior cerebellar artery (VA–PICA) constitute 0.5–3% of all intracranial aneurysms (Figures 33 and 34). Subarachnoid hemorrhage, neck pain, disorientation and coma are the common symptoms and indicators (Singh et al. 2012).

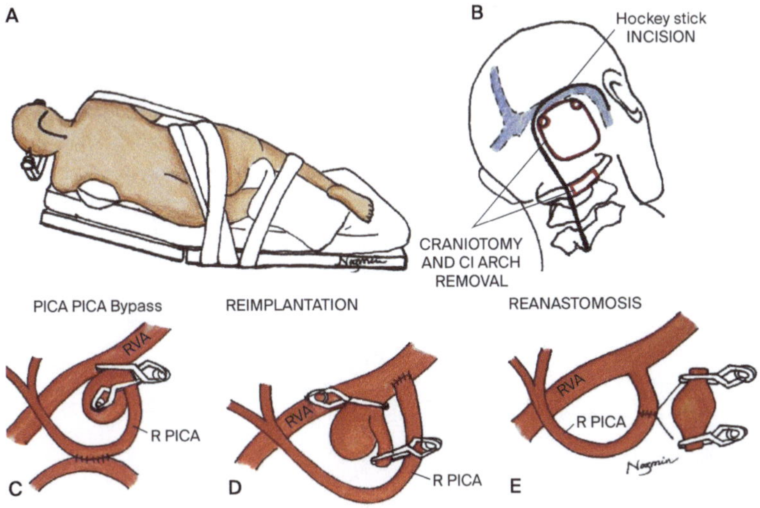

Figure 33. (**A**,**B**) Picture showing the far lateral transcondylar approach for a PICA aneurysm; (**C**) drawing of a PICA–PICA bypass; (**D**) reimplantation of the PICA to VA; (**E**) reanastomosis of the PICA. Figure by authors.

The PICA is divided into five parts along its course; these are anterior medullary (p1), lateral medullary (p2), tonsillomedullary (p3), telovelotonsillar (p4) and cortical (p5) segments.

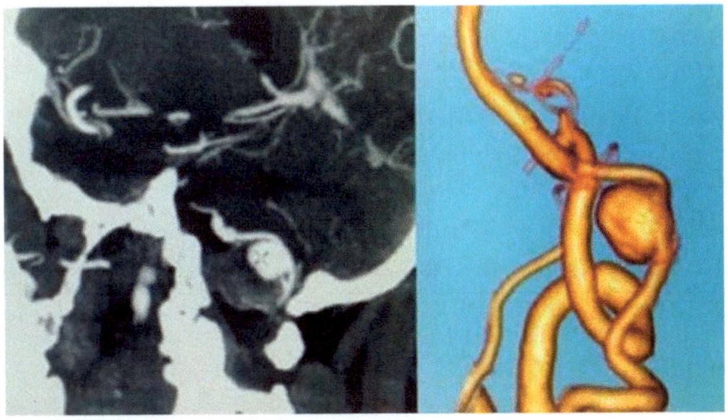

Figure 34. On the left-CT angiogram of a partially thrombosed aneurysm. On the right- CT angiogram of a PICA aneurysm. Source: Figure by authors.

19.1. Surgical Technique

The far-lateral transcondylar approach is the preferred surgical route in the park bench or lateral position (Figure 33).

When direct surgical clipping is not feasible, then a bypass is an alternative way of treatment of PICA aneurysms (Figure 33). A bypass can be:

1. Bypass from a PICA to a PICA;
2. Reimplantation of a PICA in the VA;
3. Reanastomosis after excision of a PICA aneurysm;
4. Using radial an artery graft high-flow bypass from the VA to the PICA;
5. Occipital artery (OA) to a PICA bypass.

20. Dissecting Aneurysm

Dissecting aneurysm (Keedy 2006): The wall of an artery tears (dissects) longitudinally in an aneurysm. This happens because hemorrhage into a vulnerable wall causes the wall to split. This is common in the aorta. Intracranially, it is common in posterior circulation. Often, it is connected to a genetic disorder (Table 8) such as Down's syndrome or Ehlers–Danlos syndrome.

Table 8. Vascular diseases associated with cerebral arterial dissection.

1. Fibromuscular dysplasia
2. Syphilitic arteritis
3. Polyarteritis nodosa
4. Mucoid degeneration of the media
5. Marfan's disease/cystic medial necrosis
6. Atherosclerosis
7. Takayasu's disease
8. Allergic arteritis

Source: Authors' compilation based on data from Yasargil (1987).

20.1. Surgical Technique

It is commonly managed by a high-flow bypass.

21. Mycotic Aneurysm

Mycotic aneurysms (Kirollos et al. 2019) are aneurysms that develop due to a bacterial infection of the artery wall. They are a typical consequence of a bacterial or fungal infection that spreads through the bloodstream. Intracranial mycotic aneurysms (ICMAs) complicate roughly 2 to 3% of infective endocarditis (IE) cases, despite the fact that up to 15 to 29% of IE patients experience neurologic symptoms:

- ICMAs are thought to account for 0.7% to 6.5% of all intracranial aneurysms and complicate 2% to 10% of infective endocarditis cases.
- Endocarditis caused by native or prosthetic valves is frequently associated with an ICMA.
    - Most cases occur with left-sided bacterial endocarditis.
    - Locations of an endocarditis-associated ICMA:

      55%–77% reported in the middle cerebral artery;

      18% reported in the posterior cerebral artery.
- Indirect spread of intracranial bacterial infections, such as meningitis, septic cavernous sinus thrombophlebitis and orbital cellulitis, is a less common cause of an ICMA.

21.1. Surgical Management

Perioperative rupture and clip erosion of the parent artery are the most serious consequences of surgery. In an unruptured aneurysm, the alternative is to postpone surgery and allow for enough time for the aneurysm to turn fibrotic, reducing the risk of perioperative rupture and allowing for direct cutting. It needs systemic antibiotic therapy for 4–6 weeks according to the culture and sensitivity.

22. Anterior Choroidal Artery (AChA) Aneurysm

Aneurysms at the intersection of the AChA and the ICA (Yu et al. 2018) constitute from 2% to 4% of all intracranial aneurysms.

The AChA is a tiny, thin artery that branches off from the posterior communicating artery, 2–5 mm away. The posterior limb of the internal capsule, the optical tract, the lateral geniculate body, the medial temporal lobe and the medial part of the pallidum are all supplied by the AChA.

22.1. Surgical Technique

Pterional craniotomy and clipping of the aneurysm to secure its neck are a feasible approach for this type of aneurysm.

23. Multiple Aneurysms

Approximately 20% of patients who have had an SAH have multiple aneurysms (Diringer 2009). These are common in women and hypertensive patients. They may be in the following combinations:

- Bilateral PCOM aneurysm (Figure 35);
- PCOM and ICA bifurcation aneurysm;
- Bilateral ophthalmic segment aneurysm;
- DACA plus MCA aneurysm;
- ACOM plus MCA aneurysm;
- ACOM plus PCOM aneurysm.

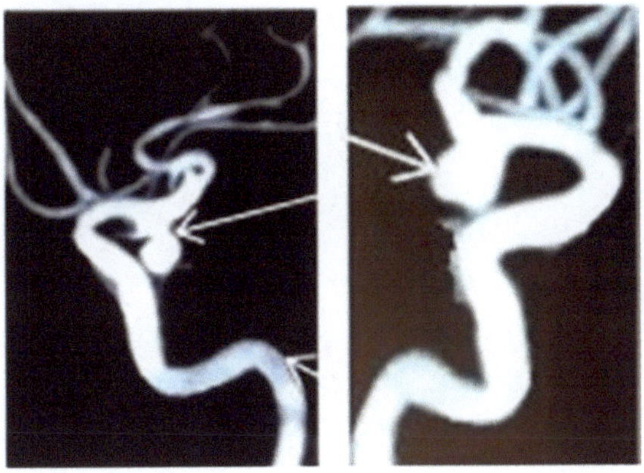

Figure 35. CT angiogram showing a bilateral PCCOM aneurysm. Source: Figure by authors.

24. Management of Giant Aneurysms

24.1. BTO (Balloon Test Occlusion) of the Carotid and Vertebral Artery

Sacrifice of the carotid or vertebral artery, or entrapment of the carotid may be required when treating giant carotid aneurysms or an advanced CCF (carotico- cavernous fistula). A sudden occlusion of the ICA can result in 50% cases of neurological deficits. Therefore, the safety of the carotid artery sacrificed should be assessed by BTO by local anesthesia and keeping the patient awake. The vertebral artery balloon test occlusion is also carried out to evaluate the feasibility of the vertebral artery occlusion in the case of fusiform or dissection posterior circulation aneurysms (Linskey et al. 1994).

24.2. Bypasses for Giant Aneurysms

An STA–MCA bypass is employed for complex aneurysms.

It may be as follows (Figure 36):

- High flow;
- Low flow;
- Protective/insurance bypass;
- Double-barrel bypass (both frontal and parietal branch of STA);

- Bonnet bypass (graft harbor beneath the bone);
- Fourth-generation bypass (endoluminal stitch and exoluminal stitch).

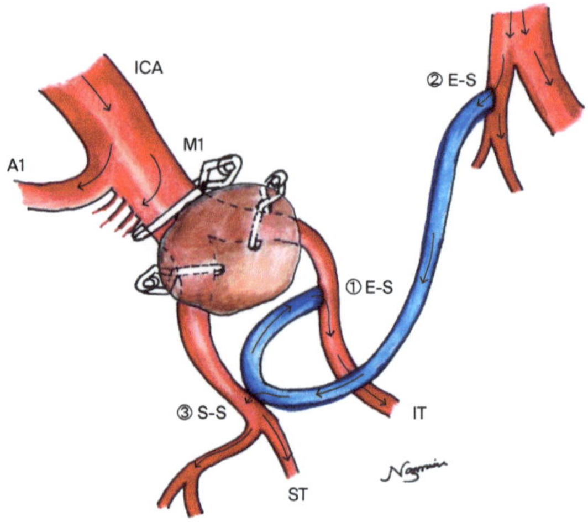

Figure 36. Picture showing the long saphenous graft EC–MCA bypass. End-to-side bypass with an inferior trunk of the MCA and side-to-side bypass with a superior trunk of the MCA. Source: Figure by authors.

Geometry of bypasses:

- End-to-side;
- Side-to-side;
- In situ bypass.

Types of bypasses:

1. End-to-side
    - STA–MCA;
    - STA–PCA;
    - OA–SCA.
2. Side-to-side
    - A3–A3;
    - PICA–PICA;
    - AICA–PICA;
    - M2–M2.

Donor vessels:

1. STA;
2. OA;
3. Radial Artery

[Modified Allen test:

- *Tell the patient to clench his or her fist; if the patient is unable to do so, tighten the person's hand.*
- *Apply occlusive pressure to both the ulnar and radial arteries with your fingers to stop blood flow to the hand.*
- *Relax the patient's hand while continuing occlusive pressure to both arteries, and check to see if the palm and fingers have blanched. If this is not the case, your fingers have not totally obstructed the arteries.*
- *Only assess whether the modified Allen test is positive or negative by releasing the occlusive pressure on the ulnar artery.*
    - *A positive modified Allen test reveals that the ulnar artery has good blood flow if the hand flushes within 5 to 15 s; this normal flushing of the hand is regarded as a positive test.*

- *A negative modified Allen test occurs if the hand does not flush within 5 to 15 s, ulnar circulation is either inadequate or absent; in this case, the radial artery is providing arterial blood to that hand (Benit et al. 1996).]*

4. Saphenous vein
5. IMAX (Nossek et al. 2014)

[In an EC–IC bypass surgery, the internal maxillary artery (IMAX) is a relatively novel donor artery.
There is a necessity for a large skull base drilling while still allowing for appropriate proximal anastomosis space.
The temporalis muscle is separated from the zygomatic process of the frontal bone and the frontal process of the zygomatic bone, and is reflected caudally into the bony gap produced by the zygomatic osteotomy. A palpation of the posterior wall of the maxilla (PWoM) is performed. Following PWoM caudally, the IMAX passes via *the pterygo-maxillary fissure (PMF), which is a constant point.*
The calibers of the IMAX, RAG and MCA are closely matched, making anastomosis assembly easier.
When a long graft is under it, there is a need for a submandibular submuscular tunnel to transfer from the neck to the brain by using chest drain no. 24 or long artery forceps.]

24.3. How to Manage Giant MCA Aneurysms

The most prevalent location for large aneurysms of the anterior circulation is the middle cerebral artery (MCA). The treatment approaches are as follows:

- Aneurysm clipping;
- Clipping or trapping with an EC–IC bypass surgery;
- Endovascular treatment.

However, an acute cerebral infarction is the most common consequence (16%). When M1 is sacrificed or M2 is obstructed, we choose a high-flow bypass (Figure 36) using the saphenous vein or radial artery graft. A low-flow superficial temporal artery distal bypass is usually sufficient for an M3 or M4 blockage (Lee et al. 2018).

24.4. How to Manage Giant ACOM Aneurysms

The treatment of massive intracranial aneurysms, including giant ACOM aneurysms, is debatable, and the final decision should be made by a multidisciplinary team that considers a variety of criteria.

24.4.1. Surgical Technique

The surgical techniques include the cranio-orbito-zygomatic approach and multi-clip reconstruction of an ACOM aneurysm, OZ plus additional interhemispheric craniotomy and side-to-side bypass of A2–A2 or A3–A3 and ligation of preserving one A2, and sacrifice of feeding A1 of the contralateral side (Nakase et al. 2006).

24.5. How to Manage Giant Basilar Top Aneurysms

Ruptured basilar top aneurysms (Ge et al. 2016) can cause a fatal SAH, with a fatality rate of up to 23%. Surgical clipping for basilar tip giant aneurysms remains difficult due to the brainstem's closeness and difficulties providing appropriate exposure, as well as crowding of the arteries in this location. The procedure-related mortality and morbidity can be as high as 9% and 19.4%, respectively.

Endovascular treatment can be feasible but may produce a mass effect and brainstem compression. Hence, a PCA bypass and micro-surgical excisions of the giant aneurysm are the choice by an OZ approach or trans-cavernous approach, or half-and-half approach.

25. Angio Negative SAH

A perimesencephalic SAH is commonly associated with a venous bleed, and angiograms reveal no evidence of aneurysms or other forms of vascular abnormality (Greenberg 2010). A hydrocephalus in the PMH is related to blockage of the tentorial hiatus due to the presence of blood in the perimesencephalic cistern. Angiography is the next line of investigation. If the first angiogram is negative, then a repeat angiogram is obtained after 2 weeks in the form of a 3D DSA.

Genetic disorders linked to the higher risk of aneurysm development are listed in Table 9. Factors influencing the treatment of incidental (unruptured) intracranial aneurysms are listed in Table 10.

Table 9. Genetic disorders linked to the higher risk of aneurysm development.

Disorders
Type IV Ehlers–Danlos syndrome Klinefelter's syndrome Autosomal dominant polycystic kidney disease Tuberous sclerosis Hereditary hemorrhagic telangiectasia Alpha1-antitrypsis deficiency Neurofibromatosis type 1 Alpha-1,4-glucosidase deficiency Noonan's syndrome

Source: Authors' compilation based on data from Yasargil (1987).

Table 10. Factors influencing the treatment of incidental (unruptured) intracranial aneurysms.

Favoring Surgical/Endovascular Treatment	Favoring Follow-Up
Patient factors	
Age less than 70 years Previous SAH form another-site aneurysm	Age > 70 years Significant medical comorbidities
Family incidence of intracranial aneurysms Symptoms due to aneurysm	Patient preference
Size	
Size approaching ≥ mm	Size <7 mm
Location	
Within the CSF space, posterior circulation aneurysm	Clinoidal or intracavernous ICA segment aneurysm Tiny superior hypophyseal artery aneurysm
Shape	
Irregular shape with bleb multilobular (with daughter dome), aspect ratio is high	Regular unilobed Aspect ratio is low

Source: Authors' compilation based on data from Yasargil (1987).

26. SCA Aneurysm

The superior cerebellar artery (SCA) is responsible for roughly 1.7% of all aneurysms. The surgical management of these aneurysms, on the other hand, has its own set of complexities and necessitates meticulous planning, particularly in determining the approach trajectory. Endovascular treatment for all aneurysms has become more common in the last decade, particularly for aneurysms of the posterior circulation, where it has surpassed microsurgical clipping. But, in the Indian subcontinent, endovascular experience is either unavailable or too expensive. For these patients, microsurgical clipping is the primary therapy option (Nair et al. 2015). An SCA aneurysm tends to rupture despite the small aneurysm size (<7 mm). They usually present with an SAH.

An OFZ with a trans-Sylvian approach and temporal craniotomy with a subtemporal approach are commonly used (Nair et al. 2015).

27. Posterior Cerebral Artery (PCA) Aneurysm

Aneurysms of the PCA (van Rooij et al. 2006) are less common, accounting for only 1.2% of all aneurysms. An SAH, oculomotor palsy, visual field deficiency or a combination of these symptoms can be seen clinically. Aneurysms in the PCA can be saccular, fusiform or dissecting, and they can occur in any region of the PCA. If collateral circulation is insufficient, dissecting aneurysms might obstruct the PCA, resulting in homonymous hemianopsia. The aneurysm is selectively occluded or the parent artery is occluded in endovascular or surgical treatment. PCA aneurysm surgery is technically difficult, and the commonly used approach is temporal craniotomy with a subtemporal approach.

28. Vertebral Artery (VA) Aneurysm

Intracranial spontaneous VA dissecting aneurysms are common in people in their third to fifth decades of life, and they are usually linked to high blood pressure. They are present in patients with bleeding or ischemia events.

Patients who have had an intracranial hemorrhage have a 70% chance of having another one. Patients with basilar artery involvement have had poorer clinical outcomes. Surgical and endovascular therapy options are available for a ruptured dissecting VA aneurysm. Surgical or endovascular trapping is a straightforward procedure with positive results. Where the parent artery cannot be sacrificed (in patients with a posterior–inferior cerebellar artery (PICA) or ipsilateral dominant vertebral artery), revascularization may be the best technique to eradicate aneurysms by trapping the dissecting vessel. Flow-diverting and coiling embolization is treated with the help of a stent. The surgical approach used for a VA aneurysm is a far-lateral approach in combination with retromastoid lateral suboccipital craniotomy (Urasyanandana et al. 2017).

Author Contributions: Conceptualization, methodology, validation, formal analysis, investigation, resources, data curation, S.A., F.H.C., N.A. and M.A.H.; writing—original draft preparation, S.A. and F.H.C.; writing—review and editing, F.H.C.; visualization, supervision, F.H.C. and M.R.H. All authors have read and agreed to the published version of the manuscript.

Funding: This research received no external funding.

Conflicts of Interest: The authors declare no conflicts of interest.

References

Benit, Edouard, Pascal Vranckx, Luc Jaspers, Rudi Jackmaert, Chris Poelmans, and Ria Coninx. 1996. Frequency of a positive modified Allen's test in 1,000 consecutive patients undergoing cardiac catheterization. *Catheterization and Cardiovascular Diagnosis* 38: 352–54. [CrossRef]

Cruz, Julio, and Robert Hopkins. 1999. Neurologic and Neurosurgical Emergencies. *Pediatric Emergency Care* 15: 368. [CrossRef]

Day, Arthur L. 1990. Aneurysms of the ophthalmic segment. *Journal of Neurosurgery* 72: 677–91. [CrossRef] [PubMed]

Diringer, Michael N. 2009. Management of aneurysmal subarachnoid hemorrhage. *Critical Care Medicine* 37: 432–40. [CrossRef] [PubMed]

Eddleman, Christopher S., Michael C. Hurley, Bernard R. Bendok, and H. Hunt Batjer. 2009. Cavernous carotid aneurysms: To treat or not to treat? *Neurosurgical Focus* 26: E4. [CrossRef]

Ge, Huijian, Xianli Lv, Hengwei Jin, Zhihua Tian, Youxiang Li, and Hongwei He. 2016. The role of endovascular treatment in unruptured basilar tip aneurysms. *Interventional Neuroradiology* 23: 8–13. [CrossRef]

Gopaul, Roodrajeetsing, Wen Shao Xiao, Jun Yan, and Dang Zong Wei. 2015. Intraoperative rupture of blood blister-like aneurysm: A case report and review of literature. *Chinese Neurosurgical Journal* 1: 14. [CrossRef]

Greenberg, Mark S. 2010. *Handbook of Neurosurgery*. New York: Thieme.

Guo, Lie-Mei, Hong-Yu Zhou, Ji-Wen Xu, Yong Wang, Yong-Ming Qiu, and Ji-Yao Jiang. 2011. Risk Factors Related to Aneurysmal Rebleeding. *World Neurosurgery* 76: 292–98. [CrossRef]

Hunt, William E., and Robert M. Hess. 1968. Surgical Risk as Related to Time of Intervention in the Repair of Intracranial Aneurysms. *Journal of Neurosurgery* 28: 14–20. [CrossRef]

Jiménez-Sosa, Michelle Stephanie, Juan Ramón Cantu-Gonzalez, Rodolfo Morales-Avalos, Oscar de la Garza-Castro, Alejan-dro Quiroga-Garza, Ricardo Pinales-Razo, Guillermo Elizondo-Riojas, Rodrigo E. Elizondo-Omaña, and Santos Guzmán-López. 2017. Anatomical variants of anterior cerebral arterial circle. A study by multidetector computerized 3d tomographic angiography. *International Journal of Morphology* 35: 1121–28. [CrossRef]

July, Julius, and Eka J. Wahjoepramono. 2019. *Neurovascular Surgery*. Singapore: Springer Open.

Kalangu, Kazadi, Yoko Kato, Gilbert Dechambenoit, and Hirotoshi Sano. 2009. *Essential Practice of Neurosurgery*. Nagoya: Access Publishing Co., Ltd.

Keedy, Alexander. 2006. An overview of intracranial aneurysms. *MJM* 9: 141–6. [CrossRef] [PubMed]

Kirollos, Ramez, Adel Helmy, Simon Thomson, and Peter Hutchinson. 2019. *Oxford Textbook of Neurological Surgery*. Oxford: Oxford University Press.

Lawton, Michael T. 2011. *Seven Aneurysms: Tenets and Techniques for Clipping*. New York: Thieme.

Lee, Chien-Hui, Sheng-Tzung Tsai, and Tsung-Lang Chiu. 2018. Superficial temporal artery-middle cerebral artery bypass for the treatment of complex middle cerebral artery aneurysms. *Tzu Chi Medical Journal* 30: 110–15. [CrossRef] [PubMed]

Lehecka, Martin, Reza Dashti, Hanna Lehto, Riku Kivisaari, Mika Niemelä, and Juha Hernesniemi. 2010. Distal anterior cerebral artery aneurysms. *Acta Neurochirurgica Supplement* 107: 15–26. [CrossRef] [PubMed]

Linskey, Mark E., Charles A. Jungreis, Howard Yonas, W. L. Hirsch, Laligam N. Sekhar, Joseph A. Horton, and J. E. Janosky. 1994. Stroke Risk after Abrupt Internal Carotid Artery Sacrifice: Accuracy of Preoperative Assessment with Balloon Test Occlusion and Stable Xenon-Enhanced CT. *American Journal of Neuroradiology* 15: 829–43. [PubMed]

Nair, Prakash, Dilip Panikar, Anup Nair, Shyam Sundar, Parasuraman Ayiramuthu, and Anoop Thomas. 2015. Microsurgical management of aneurysms of the superior cerebellar artery—Lessons learnt: An experience of 14 consecutive cases and review of the literature. *Asian Journal of Neurosurgery* 10: 47. [CrossRef]

Nakase, Hiroyuki, Yasushi Shin, Yukihide Kanemoto, Hideyuki Ohnishi, Tetsuya Morimoto, and Toshisuke Sakaki. 2006. Long-term outcome ofunruptured giant cerebral aneurysms. *Neurologia Medico-Chirurgica* 46: 379–84. [CrossRef]

Nossek, Erez, Peter D. Costantino, Mark Eisenberg, Amir R. Dehdashti, Avi Setton, David J. Chalif, Rafael A. Ortiz, and David J. Langer. 2014. Internal Maxillary Artery-Middle Cerebral Artery Bypass. *Neurosurgery* 75: 87–95. [CrossRef]

Otani, Naoki, Terushige Toyooka, and Kentaro Mori. 2018. *Surgery of Paraclinoid Aneurysm*. Edited by J. July and E. Wahjoepramono. Singapore: Springer, pp. 105–15. [CrossRef]

Paulo, Marques-Sanches, Spagnuolo Edgardo, Martínez Fernando, Pereda Pablo, Tarigo Alejandro, and Verdier Verónica. 2010. Aneurysms of The Middle Cerebral Artery Proximal Segment (M1) Anatomical and Therapeutic Considerations Revision of A Series. Analysis of a series of the pre bifurcation segment aneurysms. *Asian Journal of Neurosurgery* 5: 57–63.

Singh, Rohit K, Sanjay Behari, Vijendra Kumar, Awadhesh K. Jaiswal, and Vijendra K. Jain. 2012. Posterior inferior cerebellar artery aneurysms: Anatomical variations and surgical strategies. *Asian Journal of Neurosurgery* 7: 2–11. [CrossRef]

Spetzler, Robert. 2018. *Aneurysm*. Chengdu: WFNS, China.

Urasyanandana, K., P. Withayasuk, D. Songsaeng, T. Aurboonyawat, E. Chankaew, and A. Churojana. 2017. Ruptured intracranial vertebral artery dissecting aneurysms: An evaluation of prognostic factors of treatment outcome. *Interventional Neuroradiology* 23: 240–48. [CrossRef]

van Rooij, Willem Jan, Menno Sluzewski, and Guus N. Beute. 2006. Endovascular Treatment of Posterior Cerebral Artery Aneurysms. *American Journal of Neuroradiology* 27: 300–5. [PubMed]

van Rooij, Willem Jan, Menno Sluzewski, and Guus N. Beute. 2008. Internal carotid bifurcation aneurysms: Frequency, angiographic anatomy and results of coiling in 50 aneurysms. *Neuroradiology* 50: 583–87. [CrossRef] [PubMed]

Williams, Lindsy N., and Robert D. Brown, Jr. 2013. Management of unruptured intracranial aneurysms. *Neurology Clinical Practice* 3: 99–108. [CrossRef] [PubMed]

Yamazoe, Naohiro, Nobuo Hashimoto, Haruhiko Kikuchi, Yoo Kang, Hideyuki Nakatani, and F. Hazama. 1990. Study of the elastic skeleton of intracranial arteries in animal and human vessels by scanning electron microscopy. *Stroke* 21: 765–70. [CrossRef]

Yasargil, Mahmut Gazi. 1987. *Microneurosurgery: AVM of the Brain—History, Embryology, Pathological Considerations, Hemodynamics, Diagnostic Studies, Microsurgical Anatomy*. Stuttgart: Georg Thieme.

Yu, Jing, Ning Xu, Ying Zhao, and Jinlu Yu. 2018. Clinical importance of the anterior choroidal artery: A review of the literature. *International Journal of Medical Sciences* 15: 368–75. [CrossRef]

Cerebral Arteriovenous Malformation (AVM)

Shamshul Alam, Forhad H. Chowdhury, Nazmin Ahmed and Mainul Haque Sarker

Abstract: An arteriovenous malformation (AVM) is another cause of brain hemorrhage and it comprises about 15% of intracerebral hematomas. It often occurs at a young age. Bleeding from an AVM most often occurs between the ages of 10 and 30 years. It often causes a cerebral hematoma in the frontal lobe, temporal lobe, occipital lobe or parietal lobe, and in some cases, even within the ventricle. Cerebellar AVMs are less frequent. Besides an ICH, another type of presentation of an AVM is seizure disorders, and it is commonly partial seizure. Investigations of a cerebral AVM include a CT scan, MRI of the brain, CTA, MRA and DSA, and sometimes tractography and fMRI are necessary for a diagnosis, as well as a complete and compact understanding of an AVM and the planning of management. The management options for a brain AVM are microsurgical excision, endovascular embolization, radiosurgery or any possible combination of the above three options. Microsurgery is the main option for curative treatment. In this chapter, the pathology, clinical presentation, investigation, grading of AVM, options for treatment, choosing option/s and a brief introduction of microsurgical excisions are mentioned.

Abbreviations

AOVM	angiographically occult vascular malformation	AV	Fistula–arteriovenous fistula
AVM	arteriovenous malformation	CCF	caroticocavernous fistula
CNS	central nervous system	CT	computed tomography
CT	angiogram-computed tomographic angiogram	DSA	digital subtraction angiogram
DVA	developmental venous anomaly	fMRI	functional magnetic resonance imaging
MR	angiogram–magnetic resonance angiogram	MR	scan–magnetic resonance scan
MR	tractography–magnetic resonance tractography		

1. Introduction

An AVM is a nonneoplastic vascular malformation of the CNS. An arteriovenous malformation is another cause of brain hemorrhage and it constitutes about 15% of intracerebral hematomas. It often affects the younger generation. Bleeding from an AVM most often occurs between the ages of 10 and 30 years, which is a little different from an SAH which is common in older or middle-age groups of people. It often causes a cerebral hematoma in the frontal lobe, temporal lobe, occipital lobe or parietal lobe, and in some cases, even within the ventricle. Cerebellar AVMs are less encountered now-a-days. Besides an ICH, another type of presentation of an AVM is seizure disorders, and it commonly partial seizure (Greenberg 2010).

2. Types Vascular Malformations

McCormick described vascular malformation in 1966 (McCormick 1966):

a. Arterio-venous malformation (AVM);
b. Cavernous malformation;
c. Developmental venous anomaly (DVA), formerly venous angioma;
d. Capillary telangiectasia.

Possible additional categories:

1. A direct fistula is also known as an arteriovenous fistula (AV fistula). One or numerous dilated arteriolar direct connections to a draining vein sans an intervening nidus is the pathology of an AV fistula. These have high pressure, as well as high flow with a low frequency of hemorrhage. They are generally amenable to endovascular techniques. Examples include the following:

   (i) Carotid–cavernous fistula (CCF);
   (ii) Vein of Galen malformation (aneurysm);
   (iii) Dural AVM.

2. For a mixed or unclassified angioma, 11% are angiographically occult vascular malformations (AOVMs) (July and Wahjoepramono 2019).

3. Components of an AVM

An AVM consists of the following (Figure 1):

- Feeding artery;
- Nidus;
- Draining vein/veins.

AVM-related arteries:

- Feeding artery—terminal artery of either the anterior, middle or posterior cerebral arteries.
- Transit artery (en passage)—branches to the AVM nidus but does not end into the nidus.

  The choroidal feeding artery and perforating artery are examples of such a type.
- Bystander artery—normal artery that does not send supply to the AVM nidus but travels alongside or near to the nidus (Spetzler et al. 2015).

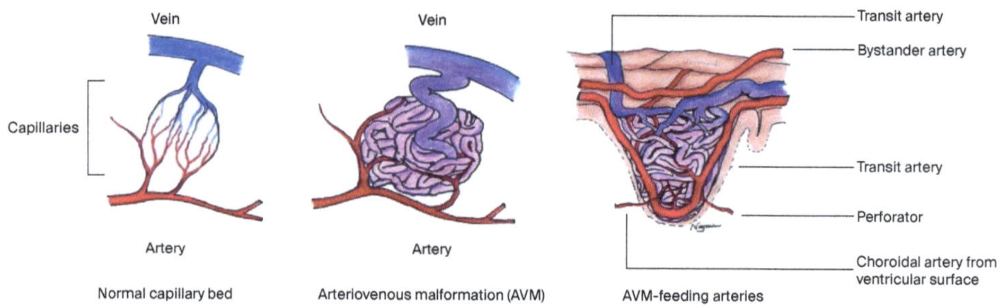

Figure 1. Schematic drawing of AVM. Source: Figure by authors.

4. Classification of AVMs

1. Pure dural AVM.
2. Parenchymal AVMs (discussed below) subclassified as:
   (i) Pial;
   (ii) Subcortical;
   (iii) Paraventricular;
   (iv) Combined.
3. Mixed parenchymal and dural (rare) (Spetzler et al. 2015).

Compact AVMs: The nidus of an AVM may be twisted tightly or loosely, according to preference. A compact AVM (Figure 2) has defined boundaries, no intermingled brain parenchyma, and is well apart from the surrounding brain, all of which help in defining a parenchymal dissection. Compact AVMs are simple to understand and follow.

Diffuse AVMs: With ambiguous boundaries, intermingled brain and poor distinctiveness, a diffuse AVM is twisted loosely, as if torn apart or unraveled, complicating parenchymal dissection. The neurosurgeon must determine the plane of demarcation between the AVM as well as the brain while dealing with diffuse AVMs. A diffuse AVM's border may be an uncontrolled periphery which has to be surrounded either broadly at the cost of the adjacent cerebral parenchyma, or narrowly enough to cross more of this vascular fringe. The interaction of eloquence as well as hemostasis pulls in and pushes back the circum-dissection, presenting a problem to the vascular neurosurgeon in determining the proper dissection distance. This decision may invite the dissection too near to the nidus, causing hemorrhage or leaving an aberrant piece of the nidus behind. Conversely, this decision may push the dissection much far away from the nidus, culminating in a full and simpler AVM excision, although more cerebral parenchyma removal than required (Spetzler et al. 2015).

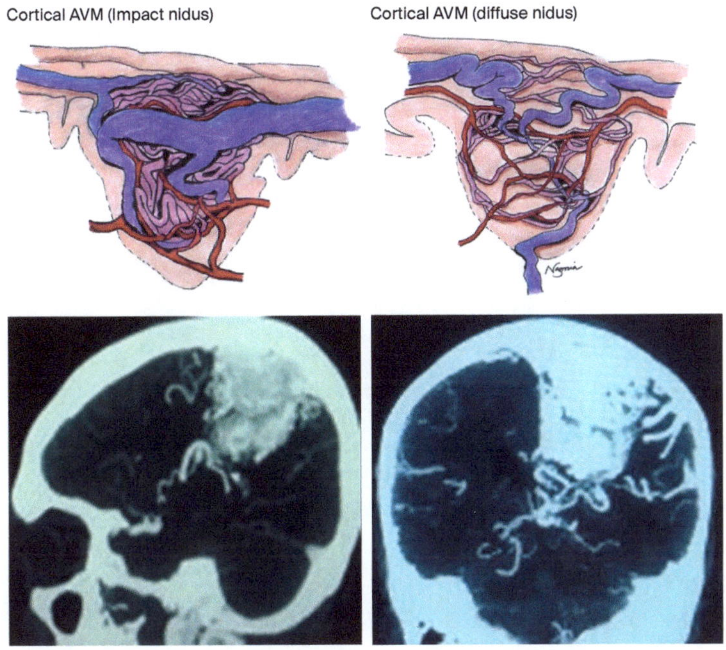

Figure 2. Image showing the compactness of an AVM. Source: Figure by authors.

5. Clinical Presentation

- Hemorrhage (50%):
    - Intracerebral (82%);
    - SAH;
    - Intraventricular;
    - Subdural.
- Seizure.
- Progressive neurological deficit (cerebral steal syndrome).
- Mass effect.
- Headaches.
- Hydrocephalus.

Of AVMs, 90% are supratentorial. The annual hemorrhage risk is 2–4%. If present with intracranial hemorrhage, then the annual hemorrhagic risk is 50% and epileptic seizure risk is 10–30% (Greenberg 2010; Nader et al. 2014; Knopman and Stieg 2014).

6. Natural History of Diseases

AVMs are associated with a 2.4% risk of bleeding per annum. The risk was the greatest in the 1st five years following diagnosis of an AVM and gradually reduced after that. Young age, past rupture, deep and infratentorial placements, and predominantly deep venous drainage are all possible causes for a recurrent AVM hemorrhage. Previous rupture, a big AVM, and infratentorial and deep placements are all risk factors on their own (Spetzler et al. 2015).

7. Radiological Assessment and Classification

- CT scan (Figure 3);
- CT angiogram;
- MR scan;
- Cerebral DSA (Figure 4);
- MR angiogram (Figure 5);
- MR tractography;

- Functional MRI (fMRI) (Greenberg 2010).

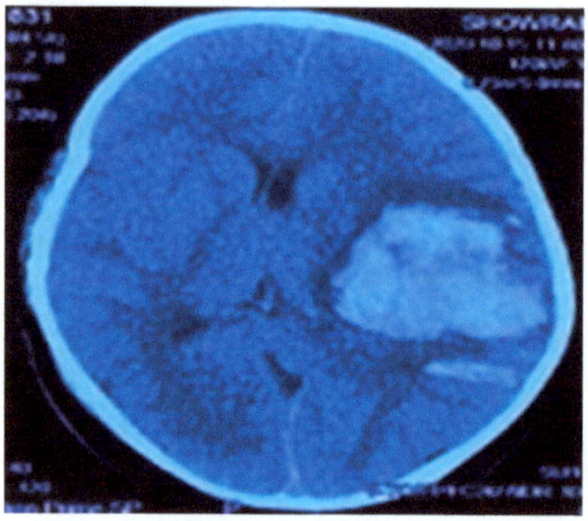

Figure 3. CT scan showing a lobar hematoma from a ruptured AVM. Multimodality imaging is needed in a cerebral AVM for the diagnosis, flow, feeders, drainage, location, size and compactness. Source: Figure by authors.

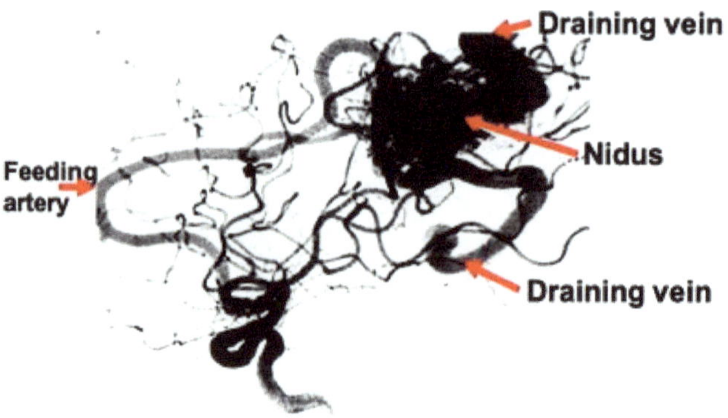

Figure 4. Angiography showing a compact nidus feed by the pericallosal artery and draining toward the deep venous system. Source: Figure by authors.

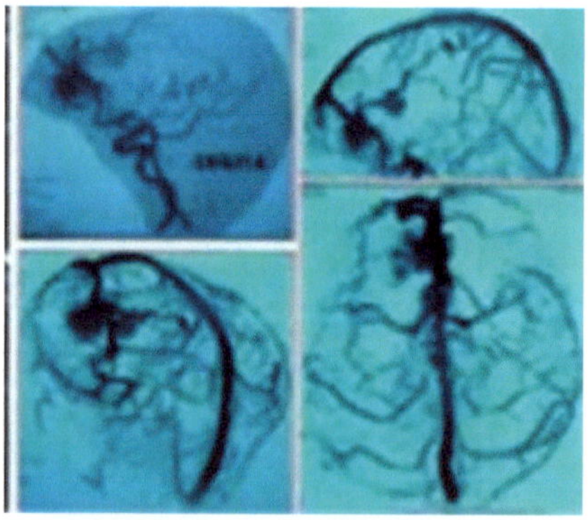

Figure 5. MRA showing a right frontal AVM feed by anterior circulation arteries and multiple drainages toward the superior sagittal sinus. Source: Figure by authors.

Yasargil classification of AVMs:

- Convexity (pallial);
- Central AVMs.

Limbic AVMs:

- Amygdalohippocampal;
- Parasplenial;
- Cingular;
- Callosal.

Medio-basal temporal AVMs:

- Amygdala;
- Anterior;
- Middle;
- Posterior;

Surgical exposure of different AVMs are shown in Table 1. Free surface of AVM is important for surgical resection (Table 2).

Table 1. Summary of the exposures to AVMs.

Type	Subtype	Craniotomy
Frontal AVM	Medial frontal	Bifrontal
	Lateral frontal	Frontal
	Paramedian frontal	Bifrontal
	Basal frontal	Orbital pterional
	Sylvian frontal	Pterional
Temporal AVM	Basal temporal	Temporal
	Lateral Temporal	Temporal
	Medial temporal	Orbitozygomatic
	Sylvian temporal	Pterional
Pareto-occipital AVM	Lateral parieto-occipital	Parieto-occipital
	Medial parieto-occipital	Torcular
	Paramedian parieto-occipital	Biparieto-occipital
	Basal occipital	Torcular
Ventricular/periventricular AVM	Callosal	Bifrontal
	Atrial	Parietal
	Ventricular body	Bifrontal
	Temporal horn	Temporal
Deep AVM	Anterior Midbrain	Orbito-zygomatic
	Posterior midbrain	Torcular
	Lateral pontine	Retrosigmoid
	Anterior Pontine	Retrosigmoid
	Anterior medullary	Suboccipital
	Lateral medullary	Far lateral
Cerebellar AVM	Suboccipital cerebellar	Suboccipital
	Vermian cerebellar	Torcular
	Tentorial cerebellar	Torcular
	Tonsillar cerebellar	Suboccipital
	Petrosal cerebellar	Retrosigmoid

Source: Authors' compilation based on data from Spetzler et al. (2015).

Table 2. Free surfaces of an AVM.

Free Surface on Convexity	AVM Subtype
Supratentorial	
Frontal convexity	Lateral frontal AVM, paramedian frontal AVM
Temporal convexity	Lateral temporal AVM
Parieto-occipital convexity	Lateral parieto-occipital AVM, paramedian parieto-occipital AVM
Infratentorial	
Cerebellar convexity	Suboccipital cerebellar AVM
Free Fissure surface	**AVM subtype**
Supratentorial	
Subfrontal plane	Basal frontal AVM
Subtemporal plane	Basal temporal AVM
	Medial temporal AVM (posterior)
Sylvian fissure	Frontal Sylvian AVM, temporal sylvian AVM, pure Sylvian AVM, insular AVM
Interhemispheric fissure	Medial frontal AVM, paramedian frontal AVM Medial parieto-occipital AVM
	Paramedian parieto-occipital AVM, callosal AVM
	Ventricular body AVM, basal ganglion AVM
Choroidal fissure	Ventricular body AVM Thalamic AVM
Supratentorial–infraoccipital	Basal occipital AVM
Infratentorial	
Sylvian fissure	Anterior midbrain AVM
Supracerebellar–infratentorial fissure	Tentorial cerebellar AVM, vermian cerebellar AVM, posterior midbrain AVM
Cerebello-mesencephalic fissure	Tentorial cerebellar AVM
	Posterior midbrain AVM
Cerebellopontine fissure	Petrosal cerebellar AVM, anterior pontine AVM, lateral pontine AVM
Cerebello-medullary fissure	Tonsillar cerebellar AVM, lateral medullary AVM

Source: Authors' compilation based on data from Spetzler et al. (2015).

Figure 6 are showing frontal convexity AVM.

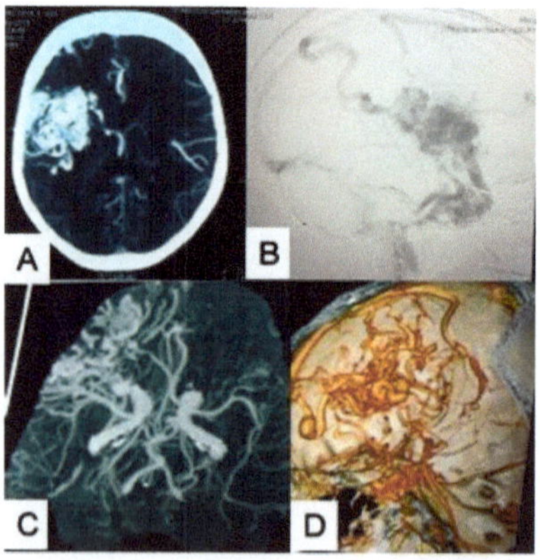

Figure 6. (**A**,**B**) CT angiogram showing a compact AVM of the lateral frontoparietal region fed by an MCA and venous drainage toward the superior sagittal sinus. (**C**,**D**) CT angiogram showing the right frontal diffuse AVM fed by branches from the middle cerebral artery and venous drainage toward the superior sagittal sinus. Source: Figure by authors.

The mesial parietal AVM is depicted in Figure 7.

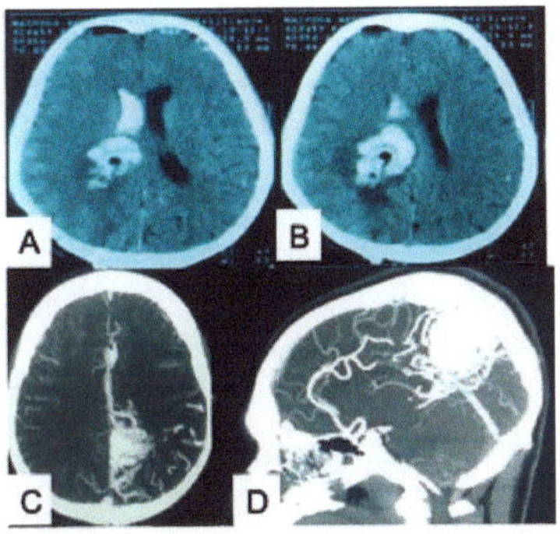

Figure 7. (**A**,**B**) CT scan of the brain showing an intraventricular along with a medial parietal bleed. (**C**,**D**) CT angiogram revealed a compact medial parietal (paracentral lobule) AVM fed by branches from the pericallosal artery and venous draining toward the superior sagittal sinus. Source: Figure by authors.

The posterior medial temporal AVM and Sylvian fissure AVM are demonstrated in Figures 8 and 9, respectively.

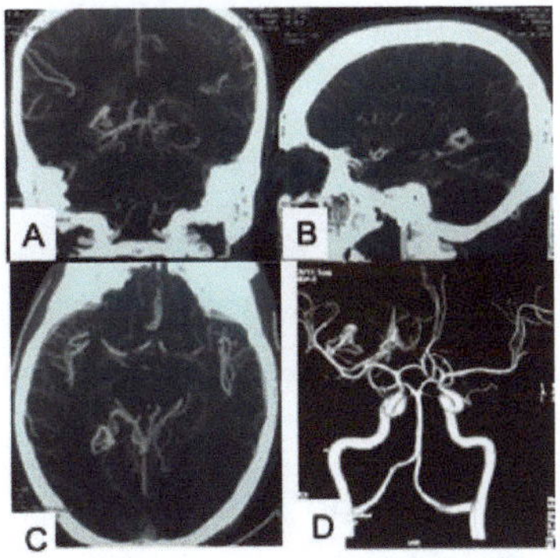

Figure 8. (**A**–**D**) CT angiogram showing a posterior medial temporal AVM fed by branches from the posterior cerebral artery and venous drainage toward the deep venous system. Source: Figure by authors.

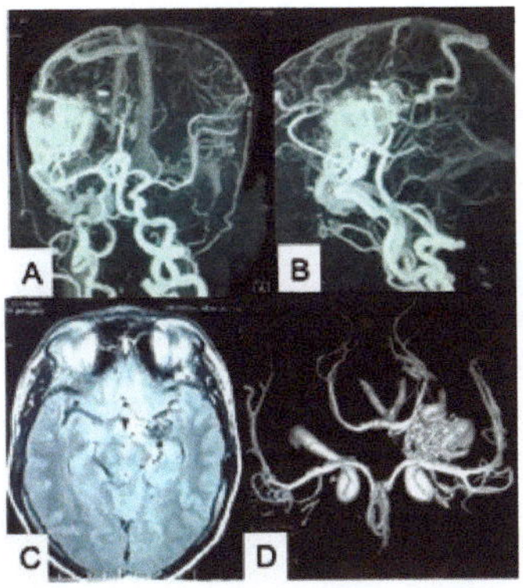

Figure 9. (**A**,**B**) CT angiogram showing a compact Sylvian fissure AVM fed by branches from the MCA and venous drainage toward the superior sagittal sinus. (**C**,**D**) MRA revealing a mesial temporal AVM fed by branches from the PCOM and anterior choroidal artery. Source: Figure by authors.

Spetzler–Martin Grading of AVM is shown in Table 3.

Table 3. Grading of AVMs.

Spetzler–Martin Grading	Points	Supplementary Grading
Size		Age, years
<3 cm	1	Less than 20
3–6 cm	2	20–40
>6 cm	3	More than 40
Venous drainage		**Hemorrhage**
Superficial	0	Yes
Deep	1	No
Eloquent brain		**Compactness**
Non-eloquent	0	Yes
Eloquent	1	No
Total Grade	5	

Note: Sensorimotor, language, visual cortex, hypothalamus, thalamus, internal capsule, brain stem, cerebellar nuclei, cerebellar peduncles or regions directly adjacent to these structures are eloquent brain. Source: Authors' compilation based on data from Spetzler et al. (2015) and Spetzler and Martin (1986).

A three-tier classification of brain AVMs was proposed, along with a management paradigm (Table 4).

Table 4. Three-tier classification of cerebral AVMs with management options.

Class	Spetzler-Martin Grade	Management
A	I and II	Resection
B	III	Multimodality treatment
C	IV and V	No treatment

Source: Authors' compilation based on data from Spetzler and Ponce (2011).

8. Treatment

There are various ways of treatment for AVMs depending on the Spetzler–Martin grading (Greenberg 2010; Spetzler et al. 2015; Nader et al. 2014; Knopman and Stieg 2014; Spetzler and Martin 1986; Feghali and Huang 2020; Flemming and Lanzino 2017; Pezeshkpour et al. 2020; van Beijnum et al. 2011; Ding et al. 2013).

The treatment options for AVMs are as follows:

- Observation;
- Embolization;
- Radio surgery;
- Microneurosurgery.

8.1. Microneurosurgical Treatment

8.1.1. The Fundamental Principles of AVM Surgery

1. Find, coagulate and divide arterial feeders;
2. Dissect the nidus of the AVM circumferentially;
3. Divide the main drainage vein or veins.

It is critical to keep the primary venous drainage open until the very end to avoid the AVM expanding and causing spontaneous bleeding.

The aim is to excise the AVM without damaging the normal parenchyma and its blood supply (Nader et al. 2014).

8.1.2. General Technique

Large craniotomy:

- To inspect the cortical vascular anatomy;
- To inspect the gyral and sulcal anatomy;
- To compare the location of feeder arteries, as well as draining vein/s with an angiogram.

Craniotomy with a margin of a few cm around the AVM.

- Be aware of trans-osseous feeders.

Just enough dural opening.
Exercise extreme caution when reflecting the dura;

- Inspect and coagulate dural feeders in large and giant AVMs;
- Careful reflection over large draining veins.

Identify as many feeders as possible on the surface;
Begin dissection to open the arachnoid adjacent to arteries and veins;
Open sulci to find feeders and relax the brain;
Follow feeders to the AVM nidus through the sulcus where they usually hide before reaching the AVM.
Differentiate feeding arteries from draining veins (veins that are larger and more delicate, and have thinner walls).
Systematically open every sulcus around the AVM to identify smaller feeders (Nader et al. 2014).

8.1.3. Surgical Outcomes

The surgical outcomes depend on the following:

- Approach with multimodal options;
- Intraoperative imaging technologies with guidance;
- Appropriate microsurgical planning;
- Rigorous training as well as expertise in microsurgery;
- Comprehensive micro-anatomical knowledge.

The majority of the scientific literature reports positive outcomes with microsurgical treatment of temporal AVMs (mortality 0–5%, morbidity 5–25%).

Complete obliteration should be 100%.

Regarding micro-neurosurgery, we need to carry out a wide craniotomy to expose the AVM generously. A frontal craniotomy, parietal craniotomy, temporal craniotomy or occipital craniotomy commonly is required according to the location of the AVM.

The initial aim is to find the feeding artery with preservation of the draining vein. We need to perform a pial incision (Figure 10) by insulin syringe or a 3 cc hypodermic syringe.

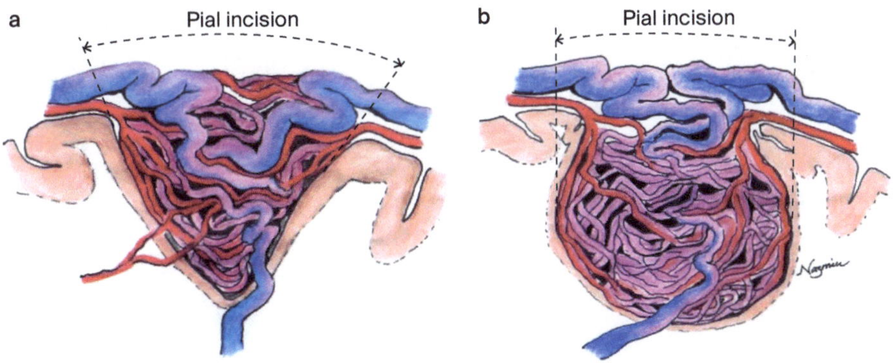

Figure 10. Pial incisions should optimize parallel exposure of AVM sides, (**a**) with tight incisions around conical AVMs and (**b**) wide incisions around spherical AVMs that optimize the visualization of deeper planes by resecting some of the overlying cortex (shaded areas). Source: Figure by authors.

Application of AVM clips or cautery of the feeding artery for proper hemostasis (Nader et al. 2014).

Circumferential dissection of the AVM nidus performed with nonstick irrigating or nonirrigating bipolar cautey. Usually, the nidus is conical in shape and the cone is directed toward the ventricle. The vessels become thinner and more fragile, so it is very difficult to carry out cautery and control bleeding.

Silver clips or AVM clips are useful in such a situation (Figures 11 and 12).

When using bipolar cautery, shrinkage of the feeding vessels is caused. Failure of proper hemostasis will cause hematoma formation as brain swelling. Thus, whenever there is brain swelling, we must check the cleavage between the brain parenchyma and AVM nidus by removal of the cottonoid. At the end, the draining vein needs to coagulate and cauterization is performed for the resection of the AVM nidus (Nader et al. 2014). Proper hemostasis must be carried out before closure of the dura by raising the blood pressure plus/minus Valsalva mechanism.

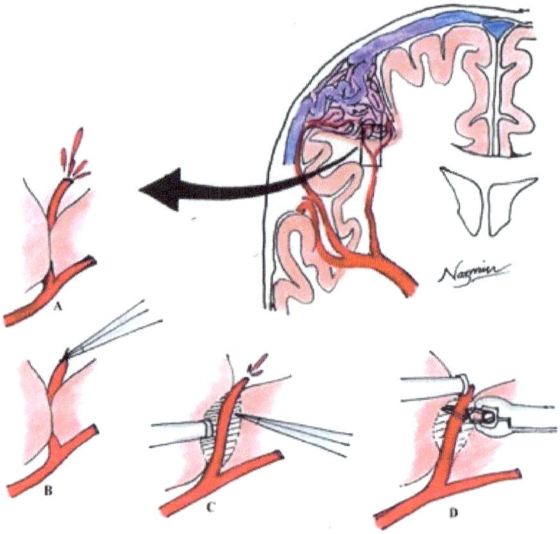

Figure 11. Controlling a deep perforating artery: (**A**) drying the area on a thin cottonoid; (**B**) attempting to coagulate it with bipolar cautery; (**C**) proximal dissection into white matter to free a segment of the artery proximal to the bleeding point, sometimes dissecting it into the sucker; and (**D**) applying the microclip. Source: Figure by authors.

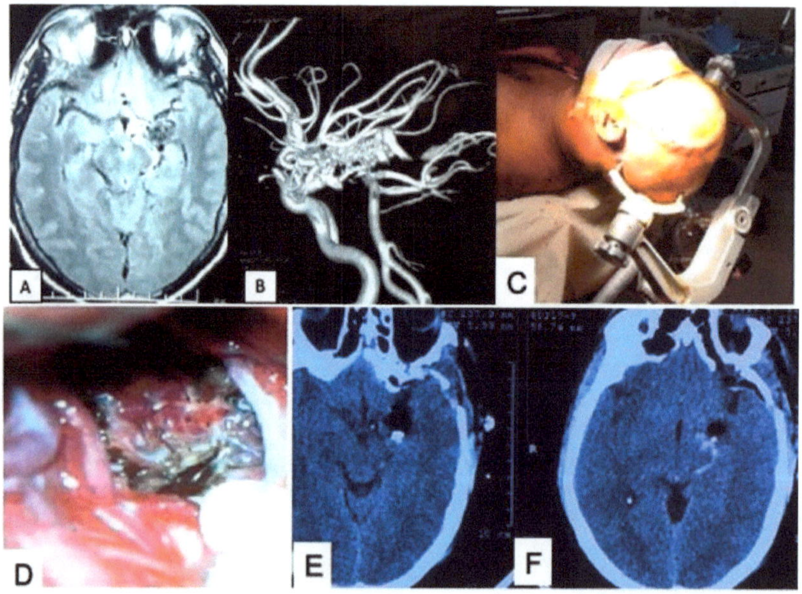

Figure 12. (**A**,**B**) MRI and MRA, respectively, showing a left mesial temporal AVM. (**C**) Patient was in a supine position, with the head end raised and tilting toward the contralateral side. (**D**) Preoperative picture showing an AVM in the mesial temporal area following the trans-Sylvian approach. (**E**,**F**) Postoperative picture showing a resection AVM from the mesial temporal area with a small amount hemorrhage in the temporal lobe. Source: Figure by authors.

8.1.4. Complications

Bleeding during surgery and brain swelling are the most common complications of an AVM resection.

An intraventricular bleed and subsequent hydrocephalus are other complications.

Seizure and impaired consciousness are not uncommon compilations.

Postoperative meningitis and late post-op hydrocephalus have to be kept in mind for some patients.

Hemiparesis or hemiplegia is another known complication of an AVM resection.

Intra-operative:

- Too wide margin of the resection;
- Parenchymal hemorrhage;
- Unrecognized intraventricular hemorrhage;
- Early occlusion of venous drainage;
- Occlusion of normal venous drainage;
- Retraction damage;
- Parenchymal damage from deep bleeding.

Postoperative:

- Hemorrhage from a residual AVM;
- Perfusion breakthrough;
- Seizures;
- Retrograde venous thrombosis;
- Retrograde arterial thrombosis;
- Vasospasm;
- Shocked brain (Nader et al. 2014).

9. Conclusions

Grade V and some grade IV AVMs should generally be treated conservatively.

Preoperative embolization should be used only to reduce the risk of the overall treatment.

Preoperative embolization should be guided by surgical considerations.

Indication for curative, palliative or pre-radiosurgery embolization is very limited.

Radiosurgery has a major role in AVM treatment and small AVMs with an unacceptable surgical risk (Spetzler et al. 2015).

Author Contributions: Conceptualization, methodology, validation, formal analysis, investigation, resources, data curation, S.A., F.H.C. and N.A.; writing—original draft preparation, S.A.; writing—review and editing, F.H.C.; visualization, supervision, M.H.S. All authors have read and agreed to the published version of the manuscript.

Funding: This research received no external funding.

Conflicts of Interest: The authors declare no conflicts of interest.

References

Ding, Dale, Chun-Po Yen, ZhiYuan Xu, Robert M. Starke, and Jason P. Sheehan. 2013. Radiosurgery for patients with unruptured intracranial arteriovenous malformations. *Journal of Neurosurgery* 118: 958–66. [CrossRef] [PubMed]

Feghali, James, and Judy Huang. 2020. Updates in arteriovenous malformation management: The post-ARUBA era. *Stroke & Vascular Neurology* 5: e000248. [CrossRef]

Flemming, Kelly D., and Giuseppe Lanzino. 2017. Management of Unruptured Intracranial Aneurysms and Cerebrovascular Malformations. *Continuum* 23: 181–210. [CrossRef] [PubMed]

Greenberg, Mark S. 2010. *Handbook of Neurosurgery*. New York: Thieme.

July, Julius, and Eka J. Wahjoepramono. 2019. *Neurovascular Surgery*. Singapore: Springer Nature.

Knopman, Jared, and Philip E. Stieg. 2014. Management of unruptured brain arteriovenous malformations. *Lancet* 383: 581–83. [CrossRef] [PubMed]

McCormick, William F. 1966. The pathology of vascular ("arteriovenous") malformations. *Journal of Neurosurgery* 24: 807–16. [CrossRef] [PubMed]

Nader, Remi, Cristian Gragnaniello, Michael L. Levy, Scott C. Berta, and Abdulrahman J. Sabbagh. 2014. *Neurosurgery Tricks of the Trade*. New York: Thieme.

Pezeshkpour, Parneyan, Adam A. Dmytriw, Kevin Phan, Manohar M. Shroff, Peter Dirks, Abhaya V. Kulkarni, and Prakash Muthusami. 2020. Treatment strategies and related outcomes for brain arteriovenous malformations in children: A systematic review and meta-analysis. *American Journal of Roentgenology* 215: 472–87. [CrossRef] [PubMed]

Spetzler, Robert F., and Neil A. Martin. 1986. A proposed grading system for arteriovenous malformations. *Journal of Neurosurgery* 65: 476–83. [CrossRef] [PubMed]

Spetzler, Robrt F., and Francisco A. Ponce. 2011. A 3-tier classification of cerebral arteriovenous malformations. *Journal of Neurosurgery JNS* 114: 842–49. [CrossRef] [PubMed]

Spetzler, Robert F., M. Yashar S. Kalani, and Peter Nakaji. 2015. *Neurovascular Surgery*. New York: Thieme.

van Beijnum, Janneke, H. Bart van der Worp, Dennis R. Buis, Rustam Al-Shahi Salman, L. Jaap Kappelle, Gabriël J. E. Rinkel, Jan Willem Berkelbach van der Sprenkel, W. Peter Vandertop, Ale Algra, and Catharina J. M. Klijn. 2011. Treatment of brain arteriovenous malformations: A systematic review and meta-analysis. *JAMA* 306: 2011–19. [CrossRef] [PubMed]

Cerebral Arteriovenous (AV) Fistula

Forhad H. Chowdhury, Shamshul Alam, Nazmin Ahmed and Mohammod Raziul Haque

Abstract: A cerebral arteriovenous fistula (AVF) is an abnormal direct connection of intracranial arteries and vein without intervening capillaries. Cerebral AV fistulas include dural AVFs, caroticocavernous fistulas (CCFs), vein of Galen malformations and pial AVFs. The clinical presentation of a cerebral AVF varies according to the site and magnitude of the fistula. A CT scan, MRI, CTA, MRA and DSA are the necessary investigation methods for diagnosis, classification and management purposes. The mainstay of treatment is an endovascular occlusion. A microsurgical occlusion or excision is needed when the endovascular procedure fails or is not possible. Here, the pathology, classification, clinical presentation and management of dural AVFs, vein of Galen malformations and pial AVFs are discussed. CCFs will be discussed in Chapter 15.

Abbreviations

ACA	anterior cerebral artery	AV	Arteriovenous
AVF	arteriovenous fistula	CT	computed tomography
CTA	computed tomographic angiogram	CVR	cortical venous reflux
DAVF/dAVF	dural arteriovenous fistula	DSA	digital subtraction angiogram
ECA	external carotid artery	ICA	internal carotid artery
ICH	intracranial hematoma	MHT	meningohypophyseal trunk
MMA	middle meningeal artery	MRI	magnetic resonance imaging
MRA	magnetic resonance angiogram	NBCA	n-butyl cyanoacrylate
PCA	posterior cerebral artery	PICA	posterior inferior cerebellar artery
SCA	superior cerebellar artery	SPS	superior petrosal sinus
SS	sigmoid sinus	SSS	superior sagittal sinus
TS	transverse sinus	VOG	vein of Galen
PAVF	pial arteriovenous angiogram		

1. Introduction

An arteriovenous fistula (AVF) is a pathological connection of vessels in the brain or the spinal cord, where one or more arteries directly drain into one or more veins or venous sinuses (Figure 1). If a fistula is formed, there is communication between the intracranial artery and vein that leads the venous system to become arterialized, resulting in a mass effect or brain hemorrhage (Gupta and Periakaruppan 2009; Reynolds et al. 2017).

Cerebral arteriovenous (AV) fistulas are discussed here in three groups:

1. Dural AV fistula;
2. Vein of Galen (VOG) malformation;
3. Pial AV fistula.

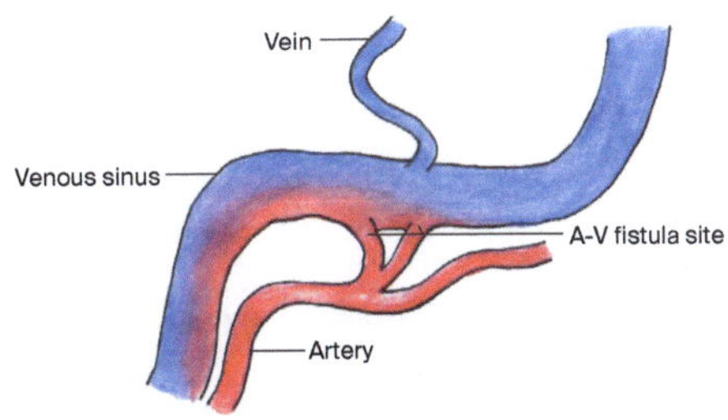

Figure 1. Schematic diagram of the arteriovenous fistula. Source: Figure by authors.

2. Dural AV Fistula (DAVF)

2.1. Epidemiology

Of intracranial vascular malformations, 10–15% are DAVFs (Luciani et al. 2001), typically encountered in middle-aged adults (acquired disease).

2.2. Distribution of Dural Supply

Group A: entire cerebral convexity, lateral segment of the cerebellar convexity and falx cerebri, supplied by the middle meningeal artery (MMA) convexity branch.

Group B: the cranial base perfused by external as well as internal carotid arteries.

Group C: the medial cerebellar convexity supplied by the vertebrobasilar system (mainly posterior meningeal).

The incidence of DAVFs at various locations is as follows (Lasjaunias et al. 1986):

- Transverse sinus (TS), 50% of cases;
- Cavernous sinus (CS), 16% of cases;
- Tentorium cerebelli, 12% of cases;
- Superior sagittal sinus (SSS), 8% of cases.

2.3. Classification of DAVFs

Before classification, the diagnosis and all information are collected by neuro-imaging. The essential modalities of investigations are a CT scan with a CTA, MRI with an MRA and gold standard cerebral DSA.

2.3.1. Cognard Classification

I	Antegrade meningeal vein or dural venous sinus
IIa	Retrograde into the dural venous sinus/meningeal vein
IIb	Antegrade and cortical venous reflux (CVR) (10–20% hemorrhage)
III	CVR no ectasia (40% hemorrhage)
IV	CVR with ectasia (65% hemorrhage)
V	Spinal venous drainage (Cognard et al. 1995)

2.3.2. Simplified Borden Classification

Lesion type	Definition
I	Draining is directly anterograde to the major sinus of the vein
II	Drains to the vein sinus, then back to the subarachnoid veins via retrograde drainage
III	Drains directly to subarachnoid veins (Figure 2) (Borden et al. 1995; Nader et al. 2014)

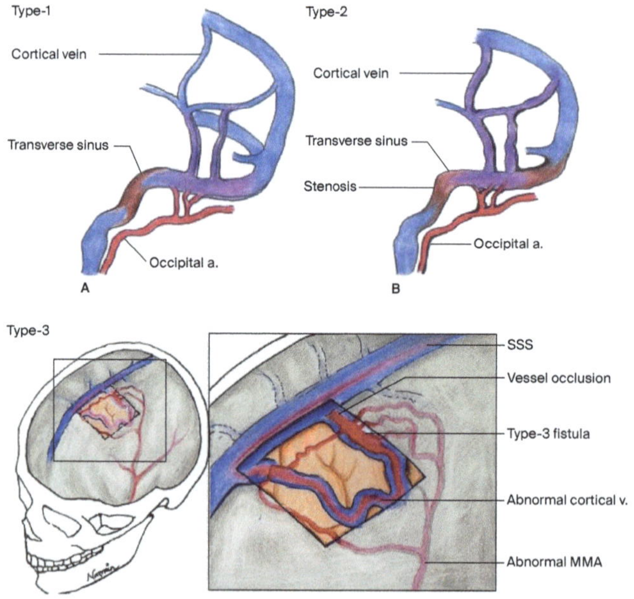

Figure 2. (**A–C**) Schematic sequential overview of the Borden classification of DAVFs. Source: Figure by authors.

2.4. *Signs and Symptoms*

People with DAVFs may experience no symptoms at all. When symptoms are present, they might range from minor discomfort to serious hemorrhage.

- Tinnitus (pulsatile)
- Headache
- Visual impairment
- Bruit (sound heard due to unusual blood flow)
- Seizure (Gupta and Periakaruppan 2009; Reynolds et al. 2017)

DAVF presentation is defined by its site, as well as pattern of venous drainage (Tables 1 and 2).

Table 1. Clinical features according to anatomical type of DAVF.

DAVF	Clinical Features
Transverse–sigmoid sinus DAVFs	Pulsatile tinnitus.
Cavernous sinus DAVFs	Exophthalmos, chemosis and blindness.
Superior sagittal sinus DAVFs	Hemorrhage, local venous congestion, cerebral edema and cerebral ischemia.
DAVFs with a premedullary draining vein	Myelopathy and progressive tetraplegia.

Source: Authors' compilation based on data from Gupta and Periakaruppan (2009), Reynolds et al. (2017) and Greenberg (2010).

Table 2. Clinical manifestations of DAVFs.

Clinical Features
Clinical features of an intracerebral hemorrhage (ICH)
Focal neurological deficit (such as limb weakness, dysphasia, cerebellar features, myelopathy) Generalized neurological deficit (such as dementia)
Tinnitus (pulsatile) and bruit (Objective)
Chemosis, conjunctival injection, proptosis, ophthalmoplegia
Visual impairment (due to increased intraocular pressure, orbital congestion, optic neuropathy or retinal hemorrhages)
Papilledema (due to pseudotumor cerebri or hydrocephalus induced by disturbed venous drainage)
Glaucoma
Facial pain (for compression of the 1st and 2nd division of the 5th nerve in the lateral wall of the cavernous sinus)
Headache
Pulsatile mass (palpated behind the mastoid process in the course of the occipital artery), seizure (focal or generalized)

Source: Authors' compilation based on data from Gupta and Periakaruppan (2009), Reynolds et al. (2017) and Greenberg (2010).

2.5. *Risk Factors*

Those predisposed to vein thrombosis, such as coagulation disorders that enhance the probability of a venous sinus occlusion, have genetic risk factors for DAVFs.

Persons in their late middle age (50–60 years) are the most commonly affected by DAVFs. DAVFs, on the other hand, can affect people of all ages, including youngsters.

Benign meningeal tumors have been linked to the development of DAVFs according to new research (Gupta and Periakaruppan 2009; Reynolds et al. 2017; Greenberg 2010).

2.6. *Treatment of Arteriovenous Fistulas (DAVFs)*

- Endovascular embolization—Embolization is the choice of treatment for most DAVFs. During this surgery, the neurosurgeon inserts a catheter into the arteries leading to the DAVF in the brain and injects liquid embolizing agents like NBCA, Onyx or glue into the feeding arteries. The injection blocks that artery, reducing blood flow via the DAVF.

- Microsurgical excision—This is used to close DAVFs that are not closed with endovascular treatment. We perform a craniotomy and separate the DAVF from the tissues surrounding the brain/spinal cord utilizing microsurgical techniques.

2.6.1. Surgical Technique

Two general approaches can be considered surgically. The first is the disconnection of the retrograde cortical venous drainage from the DAVF, leaving the DAVF intact but without any cortical venous reflux. This removes the danger from hemorrhage. The second approach is to remove the DAVF itself. In this procedure, it is critical that the sinus resection does not impair the normal cortical venous drainage.

1. Disconnection of cortical venous drainage: This is applied for all locations providing retrograde flow. The smallest approach possible with a clip is applied as close to the entry of the vein to the dura as possible.
2. Venous sinus resection involved in the DAVF: This approach is rarely required due to the introduction of liquid embolic agents and intravenous sinus temporary balloon protection of the venous sinus lumen. If the involved venous sinus is no longer functioning with normal venous drainage (thrombosed sinus, no important tributaries from the brain with collateral venous drainage exists), the DAVF with the venous sinus can be excised (Gupta and Periakaruppan 2009; Reynolds et al. 2017).

2.6.2. Endovascular Treatment

An Onyx trans-arterial embolization (TAE) is simple and effective therapy for DAVFs.

MMAs are the most feasible targets of Onyx TAEs except for skull base DAVFs.

Excessive Onyx migration into intact veins, as well as dangerous anastomoses among dural arteries should be avoided (Gupta and Periakaruppan 2009; Reynolds et al. 2017).

2.6.3. Gama-Knife Surgery

Gamma-knife surgery may be utilized to attack and shut the fistula. Radiation therapies take time to work (months–years), but they can be extremely effective at closing exceedingly difficult fistulas that have no other therapy options and when embolization or surgery is not possible.

2.7. Types of AV Fistulas (According to the Location) and Their Surgical Approach

a. **Transverse sinus and sigmoid sinus (SS) DAVFs:** The TS and SS have abnormal connections with several dural arterial branches arising from the MMA and the transmastoid branch originating from the occipital artery. A lateral suboccipital approach can be used to reach and treat it (Nader et al. 2014).
b. **Superior petrosal sinus AV fistula:** These can be exposed by a retro-sigmoid approach. Superior petrosal sinus (SPS) DAVFs are a subgroup of tentorial DAVFs that are situated at the petro-tentorial junction (Figures 3 and 4) and get internal carotid artery (ICA) perfusion from the meningohypophyseal trunk (MHT) and venous drainage into the petrosal vein, Rosenthal vein, lateral mesencephalic vein or cerebellar hemispheric veins (Luciani et al. 2001).

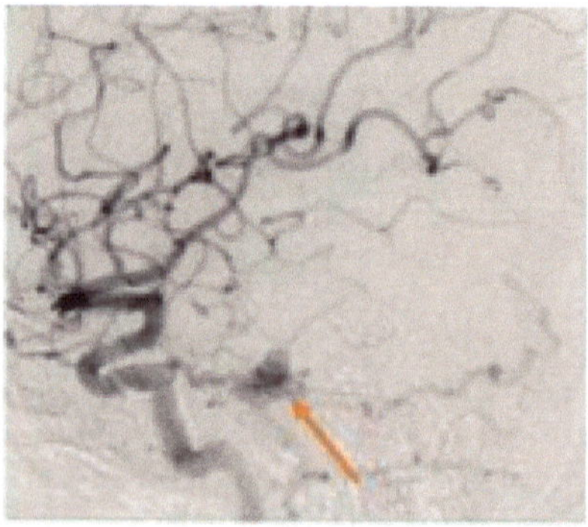

Figure 3. Superior petrosal sinus DAVF. Source: Figure by authors.

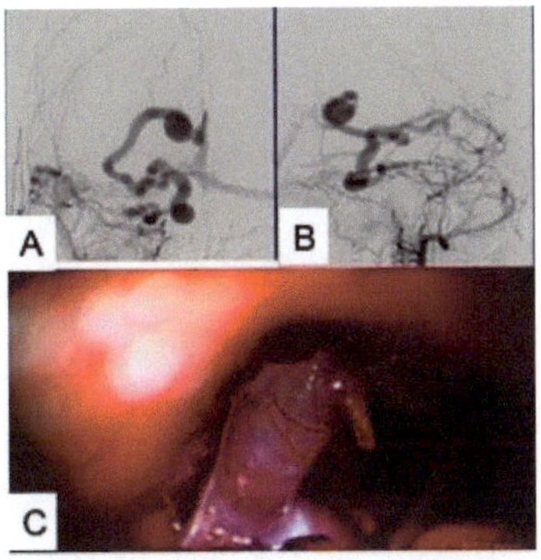

Figure 4. (**A**,**B**) DSA showing a right-sided superior petrosal sinus dural AVF. (**C**) Right extended retrosigmoid craniotomy and clipping of a superior petrosal sinus dural AVF. Source: Figure by authors.

c. **Middle fossa and cavernous sinus DAVFs:** These can be exposed via the middle fossa approach or lateral supraorbital approach.

d. **Tentorial DAVFs (Figure 5):** The arterial supply demonstrated on DSA is usually complex, multiple and in combination form. The feeders are from the following:

- ICA through tentorial branches of the ICA
  - The MHT (usually);
  - The inferolateral trunk.
- External carotid artery (ECA)
  - The MMA (usually);
  - The occipital artery (commonly);
  - The ascending pharyngeal artery.
- Vertebral artery
  - The musculospiral (extradural) artery;
  - The posterior meningeal artery.
- Basilar artery
  - The posterior inferior cerebellar artery (PICA);
  - Anterior inferior cerebellar artery;
  - Medial dural–tentorial branch of the superior cerebellar artery (SCA) (previously underrecognized);
  - The tentorial branch of the posterior cerebral artery (also known as the artery of Davidoff and Schechter).

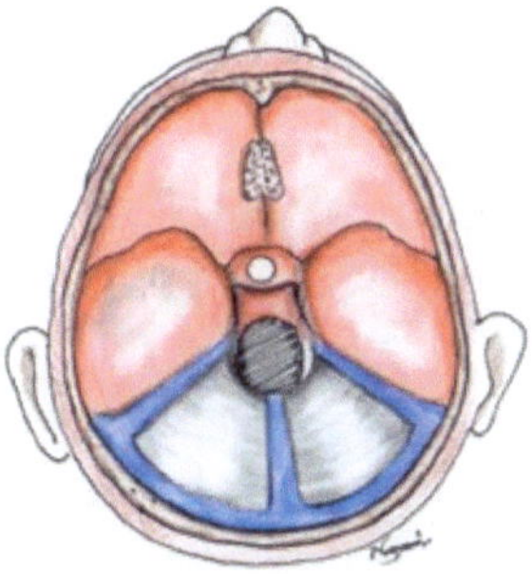

Figure 5. Location of different types of tentorial DAVFs such as-1: falx cerebellum, 2: torcular, and 3: petrotentorial on the right or left. Source: Figure by authors.

In these patients, a flow-related aneurysm can arise from a feeding PICA. There may be a bilateral fistulous supply, mainly involving the posterior division of the MMA and occipital arteries (Byrne and Garcia 2013; Nader et al. 2014).

Approach: The approach depends on the location. It can be exposed through the subtemporal approach in a park bench position.

e. Frontobasal DAVFs (Figures 6 and 7): Feeders are from the following:

- Bilateral ophthalmic arteries
  - Anterior ethmoidal arteries;
  - Posterior ethmoidal arteries.
- Bilateral external carotid arteries
  - From the ethmoidal and cavity branches of the internal maxillary arteries.
- Anterior cerebral arteries (ACA) (rare)
  - Frontopolar artery;
  - Orbitofrontal artery.

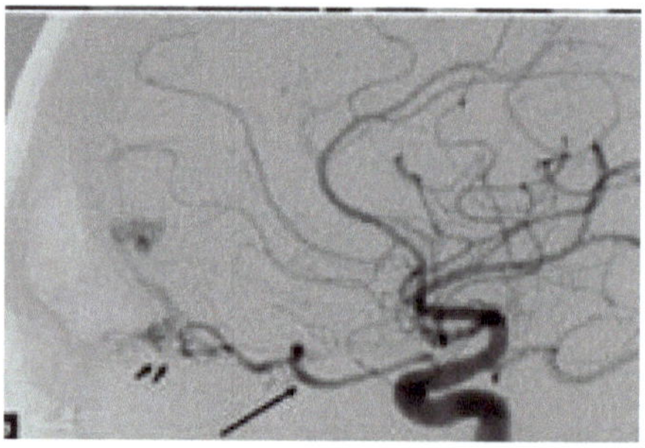

Figure 6. Frontobasal DAVF. Source: Figure by authors.

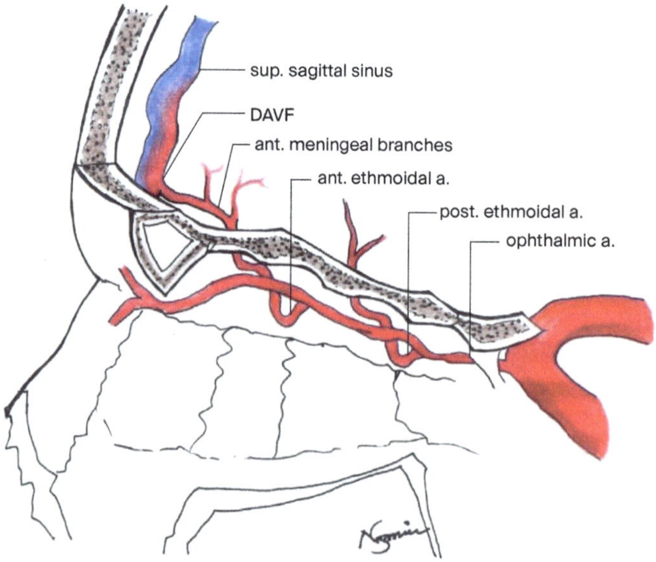

Figure 7. Diagram of a superior sagittal sinus fistula drained by feeders of the ophthalmic artery that was treated via the endoscopic endonasal approach for obliteration. Relevant branches of the ophthalmic artery are displayed. Source: Figure by authors.

Venous drainage is usually occurs in the rostral part of the SSS. It can be exposed through the anterior inter-hemispheric approach.

f. **Superior sagittal sinus DAVFs**: Arterial supply comes from the MMA. It can be approached through the midline frontal or parietal craniotomy approach (Figure 8).

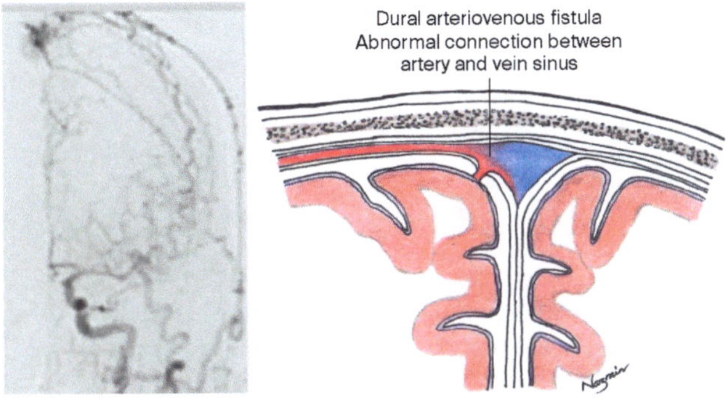

Figure 8. Superior sagittal sinus DAVF. Source: Figure by authors.

g. **Posterior fossa dural AV fistula**: Its arterial supply comes from the posterior meningeal artery, MMA and occipital artery. It can be approached by suboccipital craniotomy (Figure 9).

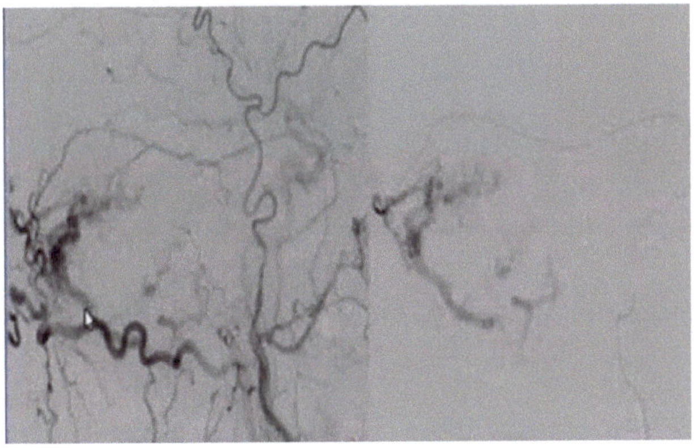

Figure 9. Posterior fossa DAVF. Source: Figure by authors.

h. **Spinal AV fistula** (also discussed in Chapter 16): When a fistula is formed, blood from an artery with high pressure flows directly into a low-pressure vein of low-flow anatomical structure. Hence, it causes venous congestion and spinal cord swelling. As the spinal cord swells, most patients begin to experience leg paralysis, back and leg pain, and bladder and bowel abnormalities. The patient may feel stiffness in the legs, shakiness or any other descriptive adjectives depending on what type of weakness (upper vs. lower motor neuron or both). The symptoms of bowel and bladder disorders might be vague: a person may feel unable to begin peeing, they may feel unable to control their bladder as they should or they may sense the urge to urinate and thus have incontinence. Fecal incontinence or constipation are also possible side effects. Male patients can also have impotency.

2.7.1. Diagnosis

1. Carried out by a spinal digital subtraction angiogram (DSA);
2. An MRI scan does not demonstrate the fistula site but shows the evidence of signal changes and probable location of the fistula, and a spinal MRA can show the fistula;
3. A spinal CTA is very helpful for surgery.

2.7.2. Treatment

The aim of management is to shut the fistula either by plugging it with endovascular embolization or by microsurgical disconnection by laminectomy.

It is approached by laminectomy and resection of the fistula.

2.7.3. Complication of Microsurgery

- Sever bleeding: >1000 mL;
- Ischemic complication: postoperative infarction;
- Hemorrhagic complication: ICH, epidural hematoma.

3. Vein of Galen Malformation

3.1. Introduction

A VOG malformation is a congenital abnormal formation of cerebral vessels that happens before birth. In this malformation, blood flows directly from cerebral arteries to a dilated great cerebral VOG.

The pressure, either directly from an artery through an AVF or by a tributary vein that gets flow directly from an artery, causes enlargement of the VOG.

3.2. Clinical Features

In neonates, malformations frequently cause heart failure, hydrocephalus and cranial bruits, as well as subarachnoid hemorrhage. Cardiac failure is caused by a magnitude of the arteriovenous shunt, which can steal up to 80% of the cardiac output by returning huge amount of blood under high pressure to the right side of heart, as well as pulmonary circulation, and the presence of a sinus venosus atrial septal defect. It is also the leading mode of death in these patients.

3.3. Classifications

Four types of vein of Galen malformations have been demonstrated:

- **Type I:** small pure cisternal fistula between the vein of Galen (voG) and either the pericallosal arteries (anterior or posterior) or posterior cerebral artery
- **Type II:** multiple fistulous communications between the vein of Galen and the thalamoperforating vessels
- **Type III:** high flow mixed type I and II
- **Type IV:** parenchymal arteriovenous malformation (AVM) with drainage into the vein of Galen
    - IVA: thalamic AVM
    - IVB: mesencephalic AVM
    - IVC: mesodiencephalic and cisternal AVM

3.4. Treatment: Options

a. Microsurgery;
b. Endovascular treatment by:
    - the arterial route or
    - venous route.

3.5. Outcomes

Babies often die either during the neonatal period or early infancy. In most patients, a VOG malformation cannot be corrected. Most die from an intracranial hemorrhage (Nader et al. 2014; Greenberg 2010; Gupta and Varma 2004).

4. Pial AV Fistula

Pial arteriovenous fistulas (PAVFs) are a type of cerebral vascular malformation that accounts for just 1.6% of all intracranial vascular abnormalities (Alurkar et al. 2016; Halbach et al. 1989). A brain AV venous malformation, on the other hand, has a nidus between the artery and the draining vein. Because there is no tangle of veins between the artery and the vein in a pial fistula, there is a greater pressure gradient, making the lesion more sensitive to rupture and causing symptoms, resulting in a worse prognosis for individuals with a PAVF. It usually presents with hemorrhage and rarely with pressure symptoms. The essential modalities of investigations are a CT scan with a CTA, MRI with an MRA and gold standard cerebral DSA (Alurkar et al. 2016).

Because of the high mortality rate associated with untreated instances, these lesions should be carefully diagnosed and treated as soon as possible, either via endovascular or microsurgical means (Alurkar et al. 2016; Nelson et al. 1992).

Author Contributions: Conceptualization, methodology, validation, formal analysis, investigation, resources, data curation, F.H.C., S.A. and N.A.; writing—original draft preparation, F.H.C. and S.A.; writing—review and editing, F.H.C.; visualization, supervision, N.A. and M.R.H. All authors have read and agreed to the published version of the manuscript.

Funding: This research received no external funding.

Conflicts of Interest: The authors declare no conflicts of interest.

References

Alurkar, Anand, Lakshmi Sudha Prasanna Karanam, Suresh Nayak, and Rajesh Kumar Ghanta. 2016. Intracranial Pial Arteriovenous Fistulae: Diagnosis and Treatment Techniques in Pediatric Patients with Review of Literature. *Journal of Clinical Imaging Science* 6: 2. [CrossRef] [PubMed]

Borden, Jonathan A., Julian K. Wu, and William A. Shucart. 1995. A proposed classification for spinal and cranial dural arteriovenous fistulous malformations and implications for treatment. *Journal of Neurosurgery* 82: 166–79. [CrossRef] [PubMed]

Byrne, J. V., and M. Garcia. 2013. Tentorial Dural Fistulas: Endovascular Management and Description of the Medial Dural-Tentorial Branch of the Superior Cerebellar Artery. *American Journal of Neuroradiology* 34: 1798–804. [CrossRef] [PubMed]

Cognard, Christophe, Yves P. Gobin, Laurent Pierot, Anne-Laure Bailly, Emmanuel Houdart, Alfredo Casasco, Jacques Chiras, and Jean-Jacques Merland. 1995. Cerebral dural arteriovenous fistulas: Clinical and angiographic correlation with a revised classification of venous drainage. *Radiology* 194: 671–80. [CrossRef] [PubMed]

Greenberg, Mark S. 2010. *Handbook of Neurosurgery*. New York: Thieme.

Gupta, A. K., and A. L. Periakaruppan. 2009. Intracranial dural arteriovenous fistulas: A Review. *Indian Journal of Radiology and Imaging* 19: 43–48. [CrossRef] [PubMed]

Gupta, A. K., and D. R. Varma. 2004. Vein of Galen malformations: Review. *Neurology India* 52: 43–53. [PubMed]

Halbach, Van V., Randall T. Higashida, Grant B. Hieshima, Carl W. Hardin, Christopher F. Dowd, and Stanley L. Barnwell. 1989. Transarterial occlusion of solitary intracerebral arteriovenous fistulas. *American Journal of Neuroradiology* 10: 747–52. [PubMed]

Lasjaunias, Pierre, Ming Chiu, Karel Ter Brugge, Atul Tolia, Michel Hurth, and Mark Bernstein. 1986. Neurological manifestations of intracranial dural arteriovenous malformations. *Journal of Neurosurgery* 64: 724–30. [CrossRef] [PubMed]

Luciani, Alain, Emmanuel Houdart, Charbel Mounayer, Jean-Pierre Saint Maurice, and Jean-Jacques Merland. 2001. Spontaneous closure of dural arteriovenous fistulas: Report of three cases and review of the literature. *American Journal of Neuroradiology* 22: 992–96. [PubMed]

Nader, Remi, Cristian Gragnaniello, Scott C. Berta, Abdulrahman J. Sabbagh, and Michael L. Levy. 2014. *Neurosurgery Tricks of the Trade-Cranial: Cranial*. New York: Thieme.

Nelson, K., Y. Nimi, P. Lasjaunias, and A. Berenstein. 1992. Endovascular embolization of congenital intracranial pial arteriovenous fistulas. *Neuroimaging Clinics of North America* 2: 309–17.

Reynolds, Matthew R., Giuseppe Lanzino, and Gregory J. Zipfel. 2017. Intracranial Dural Arteriovenous Fistulae. *Stroke* 48: 1424–31. [CrossRef] [PubMed]

Caroticocavernous Fistula (CCF)

Forhad H. Chowdhury, Shamshul Alam, Nazmin Ahmed and Mohammod Raziul Haque

Abstract: A carotid cavernous fistula (CCF) is a relatively common intracranial arteriovenous fistula, usually traumatic and spontaneous in origin. A CCF may be of direct or indirect variety, and clinically presents with pulsatile proptosis, chemosis and red eye. Investigations include a CT of the head, an MRI of the head, and a CTA, MRA and DSA of the brain. Endovascular therapy comes first in line, but microsurgical treatment is needed where endovascular therapy is not possible or fails. Here, the etiopathogenesis, classification and management of a CCF are discussed concisely.

Abbreviations

AV	Arteriovenous	CCF	caroticocavernous fistula
CT	computed tomography	CTA	computed tomographic angiogram
CS	cavernous sinus	DAVF	dural arteriovenous fistula
DSA	digital subtraction angiography	ECA	external carotid artery
ICA	internal carotid artery	IPS	inferior petrosal sinus
MRA	magnetic resonance angiogram	MRI	magnetic resonance imaging
RTA	road traffic accident		

1. Introduction

A carotid cavernous fistula (CCF) is commonly traumatic in origin, following road traffic accidents (RTAs) due to the avulsion or tear of the cavernous carotid artery. Hence, blood goes to the cavernous sinus (CS) of the same side, followed by the opposite CS and the superior ophthalmic vein (Greenberg 2010).

2. Anatomy of the Cavernous Sinus

The CS is a complicated venous region that runs from the sphenoid bone to the periosteal, as well as the meningeal layers of the dura. On both sides of the sellae turcica, there is a twin venous space. The superior and inferior intercavernous sinuses provide open communication between the two regions. From the superior orbital fissure (SOF) to the petrous apex, the CS extends anteriorly. The diaphragm sellae are located cranially, and the larger wing of the sphenoid is located caudally. The dura forms a lateral boundary for the sinus (Figure 1). The ICA, with its periarterial sympathetic plexus, is located medially within the CS, and its involvement may produce Horner's syndrome. The sixth nerve is located to the lateral of the ICA. The ophthalmic and maxillary divisions of the trigeminal nerve, oculomotor nerve and trochlear nerve are located within the lateral dural boundary of the CS. Chemosis and proptosis can occur when venous drainage is compromised. The venous linkages in the CS are complicated and valveless. It communicates with practically every key venous component in the head and neck, either directly or indirectly. The superior and inferior ophthalmic veins, the sphenoparietal sinuses, and the middle meningeal vein all drain the CS. The superior and inferior ophthalmic veins connect the CS to the facial vein and pterygoid venous plexus. The CS drains into the superior and inferior petrosal sinuses, which then flow into the sigmoid sinus and internal jugular vein (Chowdhury et al. 2012; Tang et al. 2010; Barrow et al. 1985).

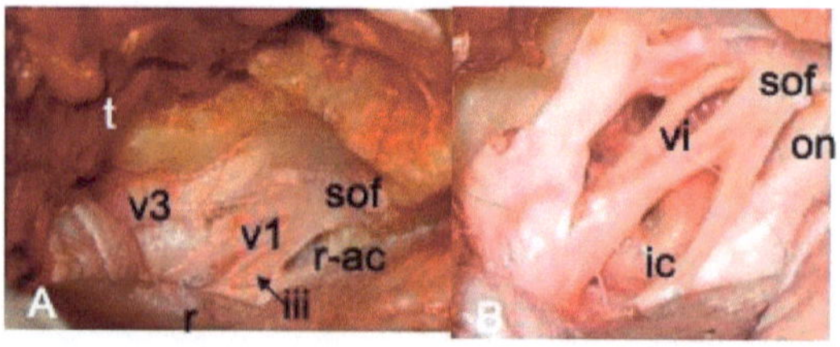

Figure 1. (**A**,**B**) Cadaveric dissection of the left CS after peeling of the dura from the CS with retraction of the temporal lobe extraduraly. (r—retractor, t—temporalis muscle, V3—mandibular nerve, V1—ophthalmic nerve, sof—superior orbital fissure, iii—oculomotor nerve, r-ac—root of anterior clinoid process (after drilling), vi—abducent nerve, ic—internal carotid artery and on—optic nerve). Source: Figure by authors.

3. Classification of the CCF

The CCF is generally classified depending on the arterial supply (Table 1, Figure 2). The clinical features and management approach are, however, mainly based on venous drainage.

Table 1. Barrow Classification.

Type	Pathogenesis	Arterial Supply	Hemodynamics
A	Head trauma/aneurysm rupture	ICA	High flow
B	Spontaneous	Dural branches of the ICA	Low flow
C	Spontaneous	Dural branches of the ECA	Low flow
D	Spontaneous	Dural branches of the ICA and ECA	Low flow

ICA: internal carotid artery, ECA: external carotid artery. Source: Authors' compilation based on data from Barrow et al. 1985; Cruz 1998.

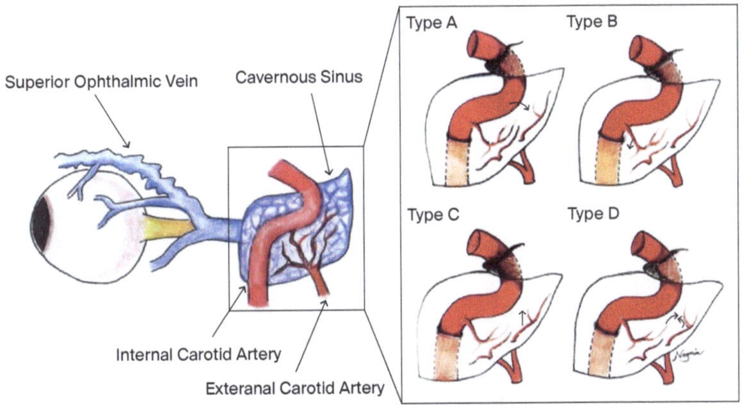

Figure 2. Types of carotid cavernous fistulas. Source: Figure by authors.

4. Pathophysiology

The underpinning pathophysiology (Greenberg 2010; Korkmazer et al. 2013; Ertl et al. 2019) for the clinical consequences of all caroticocavernous fistulas (CCFs) is characterized by elevated intracavernous venous sinus pressure. This is also likely to lead to retrograde venous drainage to the eye by the superior ophthalmic vein. Because of the interconnections between the two cavernous sinuses, contralateral eye involvement is common. Occasionally, due to occlusion of the superior ophthalmic vein by anterior intracavernous thrombosis, the clinical presentation may only occur contralateral to the fistula.

5. Natural History of CCFs

The natural history for the eye and vision is poor in extreme cases. Threats to vision can arise from a secondary glaucoma and extreme exophthalmos with consequent corneal damage. In the case of indirect CCFs, the clinical manifestations may be due to the combination of cavernous sinus thrombosis and a DAVF. In such cases, an extremely small DAVF may be responsible for extreme clinical manifestation. In the case of a direct CCF, retrograde flow in the ophthalmic artery may occur, contributing to retinal ischemia that, when combined with the high venous pressure, may lead to immediate permanent loss of vision.

Problems other than those with the eye can occur. Retrograde cortical venous drainage may be present (middle cerebral veins or pontine venous tributaries to the inferior petrosal sinus). When present, the considerations discussed relating to DAVFs need to be taken into account (Greenberg 2010; Macdonald 2008).

6. Etiology

Head or orbital injury;
Rupture of a cavernous ICA aneurysm;
ICA dissection (Greenberg 2010; Korkmazer et al. 2013; Ertl et al. 2019).

7. Clinical Presentation

7.1. *Symptoms*

Headache
Impaired vision
Double vision
Tinnitus (pulsatile)

7.2. *Signs*

Proptosis
Chemosis
Orbital bruit
Cranial nerve palsy
Corkscrew vessels of the conjunctiva
Increased intraocular pressure
Ophthalmoplegia
Ptosis
Venous pulsations
Heme in Schlemm's canal on gonioscopy (Greenberg 2010; Korkmazer et al. 2013; Ertl et al. 2019; Macdonald 2008; Kalangu et al. 2009; Bennett et al. n.d.).

8. Radiological Assessment

Besides a CT scan with a CTA (Figure 3) and MRI of the brain with an MRA (Figure 4), the definitive investigation method is a DSA of the brain to identify the feeding artery, draining vein and location of the AV fistula.

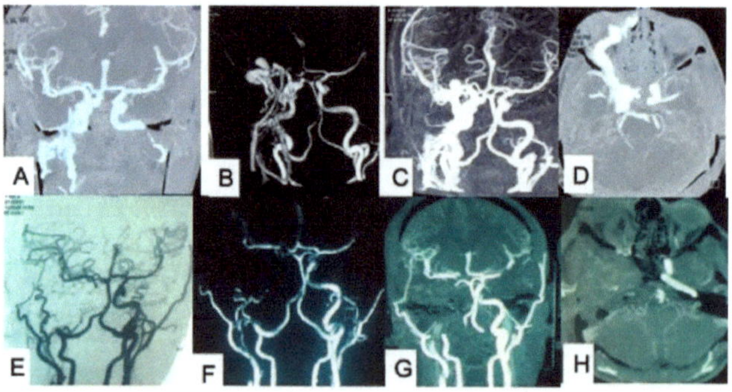

Figure 3. (**A–D**) Preoperative CTA showing a right-sided direct CCF. (**E–H**) CTA on the first POD after an STA–MCA bypass and ICA trapping. Source: Figure by authors.

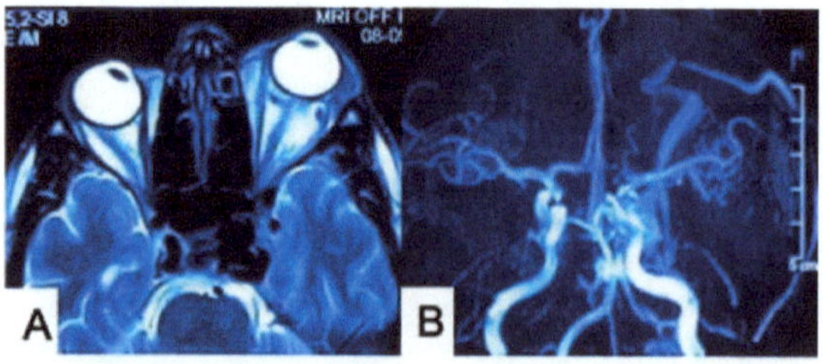

Figure 4. (**A**) MRI of the brain with an orbit showing the proptosis of the left eyeball, along with some irregularities in the cavernous sinus (left); (**B**) MRA showing the same constriction in the cavernous carotid artery, along with left-sided cavernous sinus dilatation and cortical venous drainage. Source: Figure by authors.

Proposed venous drainage-based classification system for CCFs;

Type	Venous drainage
I	Only posterior/inferior drainage
II	Posterior/inferior, as well as anterior drainage
III	Only anterior drainage
IV	Retrograde drainage into cortical veins ± other routes of venous drainage
V	High-flow direct shunt between a cavernous ICA and CS (Barrow type A) ± multiple routes of venous drainage (Kalangu et al. 2009).

9. Treatment of CCFs

Some traumatic CCFs may undergo spontaneous closure. There are various treatments for a CCF (Greenberg 2010; Cruz 1998; Korkmazer et al. 2013; Ertl et al. 2019; Macdonald 2008; Kalangu et al. 2009; Bennett et al. n.d.).

9.1. Carotid Compression

Carotid compression treatment may be successful in the closure of 17% of direct and 30% of dural CCFs.

9.2. Endovascular Management Is the Main Stay of Management

Approaches to carotid cavernous fistulas:

Transvenous routes via the following:

(a) Inferior petrosal sinus (IPS);
(b) Superior ophthalmic vein via the transfemoral route or direct surgical exposure;
(c) Facial vein via the transfemoral route;
(d) Transarterial route:

1. Direct CCFs are best managed with a detachable silicon balloon via an endo- arterial route;
2. Stent-assisted coil closure of a fistula may offer safe and effective management;
3. Onyx embolization by a transvenous route;
4. Microcoil embolization by a transvenous route;
5. Combination of Onyx and detachable coils through a transvenous route.

9.3. Surgical Trapping with or Without an STA–MCA Bypass

We commonly do surgical trapping of an ICA after thorough evaluation of the CCF by a DSA of cerebral vessels, cross-circulation study and balloon test occlusion (Figure 5).

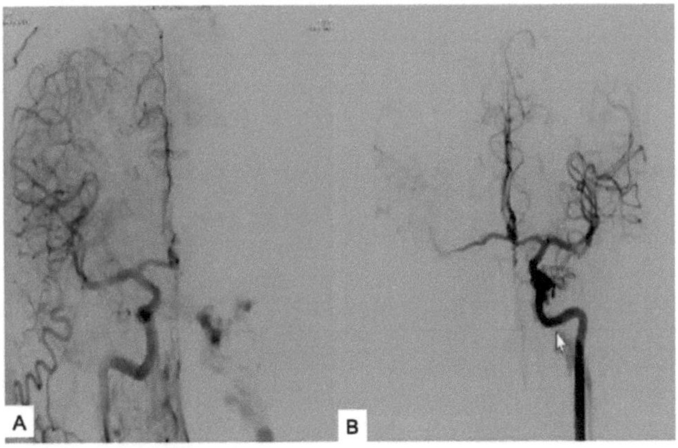

Figure 5. (**A**,**B**) Left and right cerebral ICA DSA, respectively, with a contralateral carotid occlusion in patients with a CCF. Source: Figure by authors.

We perform surgical trapping of the ICA by exposure and ligation at the high neck or Glasscock triangle in the middle fossa base, and ligation of a supraclinoidal ICA proximal to ophthalmic artery after anterior clinoidectomy. Some surgeons also use CS packing with trapping of the ICA.

[Balloon test occlusion: Before going to the occlusion or entrapment of an ICA, we need to evaluate the patency of the circle of Willis by performing a balloon test occlusion for half an hour.]

9.4. Gama-Knife Radiosurgery

In patients who fail or are unable to have an endovascular intervention, radiosurgical therapy of indirect CCFs has been advocated as a viable, non-invasive adjunct or primary treatment (Cruz 1998).

Author Contributions: Conceptualization, methodology, validation, formal analysis, investigation, resources, data curation, F.H.C., S.A. and N.A.; writing—original draft preparation, F.H.C. and S.A.; writing—review and editing, F.H.C.; visualization, supervision, N.A. and M.R.H. All authors have read and agreed to the published version of the manuscript.

Funding: This research received no external funding.

Conflicts of Interest: The authors declare no conflicts of interest.

References

Barrow, Daniel L., Robert H. Spector, Ira F. Braun, Jeffrey A. Landman, Suzie C. Tindall, and George T. Tindall. 1985. Classification and treatment of spontaneous carotid-cavernous sinus fistulas. *Journal of Neurosurgery* 62: 248–56. [CrossRef] [PubMed]

Bennett, Jeffrey L., Mithra O. Gonzalez, and Vikram Durairaj. n.d. Carotid-Cavernous Fistulas. Available online: https://www.uptodate.com/contents/carotid-cavernous-fistulas (accessed on 31 January 2021).

Chowdhury, Forhad, Mohammod Haque, Khandkar Kawsar, Shamim Ara, Quazi Mohammod, Mainul Sarker, and Atul Goel. 2012. Transcranial Microsurgical and Endoscopic Endonasal Cavernous Sinus (CS) Anatomy: A Cadaveric Study. *Journal of Neurological Surgery* A73: 296–306. [CrossRef] [PubMed]

Cruz, Julio. 1998. *Neurologic and Neurosurgical Emergencies*. Philadelphia: WB Saunders Company.

Ertl, Lorenz, Hartmut Brückmann, Maximilian Patzig, and Gunther Fesl. 2019. Endovascular therapy of direct dural carotid cavernous fistulas—A therapy assessment study including long-term follow-up patient interviews. *PLoS ONE* 14: e0223488. [CrossRef] [PubMed]

Greenberg, Mark S. 2010. *Handbook of Neurosurgery*. New York: Thieme.

Kalangu, Kazadi, Yoko Kato, Gilbert Dechambenoit, and Hirotoshi Sano. 2009. *Essential Practice of Neurosurgery*. Nagoya: Access Publishing Co., Ltd.

Korkmazer, Bora, Burak Kocak, Ercan Tureci, Civan Islak, Naci Kocer, and Osman Kizilkilic. 2013. Endovascular treatment of carotid cavernous sinus fistula: A systematic review. *World Journal of Radiology* 5: 143–55. [CrossRef] [PubMed]

Macdonald, R. Loch. 2008. *Neurosurgical Operative Atlas: Vascular Neurosurgery*. New York: Thieme.

Tang, Yen Zhi, Thomas Booth, Michael Steward, T. Solbach, and Thomas Wilhelm. 2010. The imaging of conditions affecting the cavernous sinus. *Clinical Radiology* 65: 937–45. [CrossRef] [PubMed]

Cerebral Cavernous Malformation (CCM)

Shamshul Alam, Forhad H. Chowdhury, Nazmin Ahmed and Mainul Haque Sarker

Abstract: A cavernous malformation is relatively rare in the brain. The dilated capillaries conglomerate together to form a nidus and the cavernoma (CM) within the brain. Usually, a cavernoma is silent, but it can present with bleeding and a seizure. It can occur in any area of the brain, but it has a higher tendency in the brainstem, deep structure of the brain and temporal lobe. MRI GRE and SW images are diagnostic for a CM. A symptomatic or ruptured CM demands surgical removal. In this chapter, the pathology, distribution and management of cavernomas are mentioned.

Abbreviations

CCM	cerebral cavernous malformation	CM	cavernous malformation
CT	computed tomography	DT	diffusion tensor
DSA	digital subtraction angiogram	DVA	dural venous anomaly
fMRI	functional magnetic resonance imaging	GRE	gradient recall echo
MRI	magnetic resonance	MVM	mixed vascular malformation
SEZ	safe entry zone	SW	susceptibility-weighted

1. Introduction

A cerebral cavernous malformations is one variety of an arteriovenous malformation where the dilated capillaries conglomerate together to form a nidus and the cavernoma (CM) within the brain. Usually, a cavernoma is silent, but it can manifest when there is bleeding or when present with a seizure. It can occur in any area of the brain but has a higher tendency in the brainstem, deep structure of the brain and temporal lobe (Greenberg 2010).

2. Natural History of Cavernoma

The incidence of a CCM varies from 0.17 to 0.56 per 100,000 per population per year (Al-Shahi et al. 2003). A CCM frequently presents in the fourth and fifth decade, and there is small female preponderance (58%). Roughly 50% of CCM patients remain asymptomatic, whereas about 25% present with single or multiple attacks of seizure. Additionally, patients can present with either hemorrhage (Figure 1A) (~12%) or focal neurological deficits (~15%) (Salman et al. 2012). Overall, the annual risk of a first-time cavernoma-related hemorrhage is low (0.4–0.6% per year) and the risk of subsequent hemorrhage is much higher (3.8–23% per year). The risk gradually decreases over time. It can present as multiple cavernoma (cavernomatosis) (Figure 1B) and can be familial.

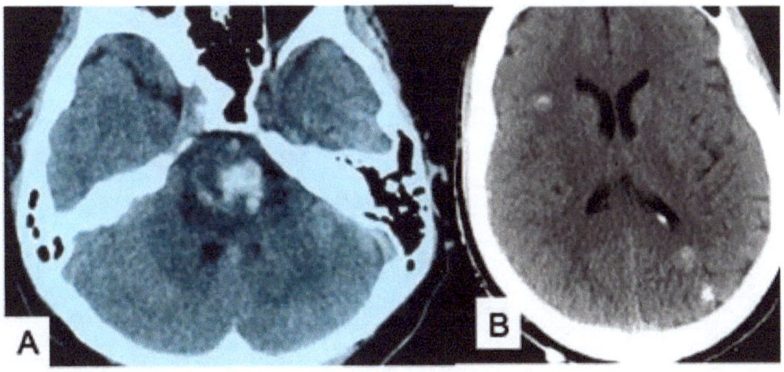

Figure 1. (**A**) CT scan showing bleeding in the pontine cavernoma. (**B**) CT scan showing multiple cavernoma. Source: Figure by authors.

3. Location

The distribution (locations) of CMs in a published series is shown in Table 1.

Table 1. Locations of cavernomas.

Location	Cavernoma	Percentage %
Cerebrum	84	69.4
Occipital	4	
Frontal	36	
Parietal	16	
Temporal	28	
Brainstem	17	14.0
Medulla	1	
Midbrain	2	
Pontomesencephalon	4	
Pons	8	
Pontomedullary	2	
Cerebellum	8	6.6
Cranial nerves	4	3.3
Spinal cord	8	6.6
Cervical	3	
Cervicomedullary	2	
Lumbar	1	
Thoracic	2	
Total CMs	121	99.9

Source: Authors' compilation based on data from Kirollos et al. (2019).

4. Developmental Venous Anomaly (DVA)

Developmental venous abnormalities (DVAs), also called venous malformations or venous angiomas, are frequently related to cavernomas. A DVA is a vascular abnormality that does not create any clinical signs on its own. In the proximity of a DVA, at least 40% of isolated cavernomas can occur.

The caput medusae indication of veins emptying into a solitary bigger collecting vein that then drains into either a dural venous sinus or a deep ependymal vein characterizes a DVA (Figure 2). The image has been compared to that of a palm tree. DVAs, on the other hand, can be found in any place, draining either superficially or deeply.

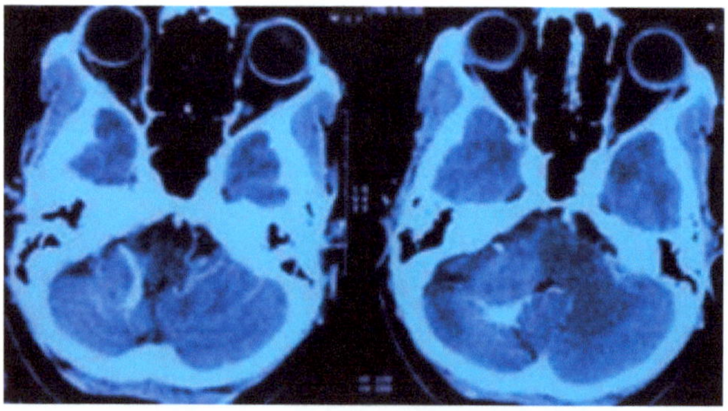

Figure 2. CT scan showing deep venous anomalies (DVAs), along with a cavernoma. Source: Figure by authors.

4.1. Associations

With the exception of the blue rubber bleb nevus syndrome, lesions are generally isolated (75%);

Mixed vascular malformations are found in 20% of cases (range: 8–33%) and are related to cavernous malformations (MVM)s;

Malformations of the venous system in the neck and head.

4.2. Classification Based on the Location

The most common locations (Figure 3) are as follows:

Fronto-parietal CM (36–64%), generally draining toward the lateral ventricle's frontal horn (Figure 3A,B);
Cerebellar hemispheric CM (14–27%), draining toward the 4th ventricle (Figure 3C);
Brainstem cavernoma (Figure 3D);
Spinal cavernoma (Figure 4).

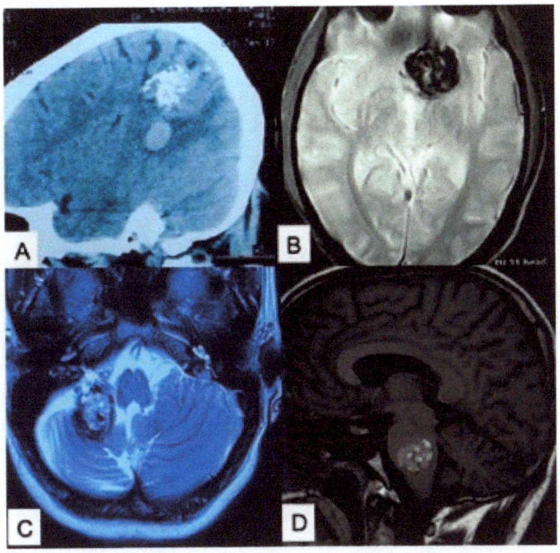

Figure 3. (**A**) CT scan showing a parietal cavernoma. (**B**) MRI showing a left basal frontal cavernoma. (**C**) MRI showing an rt cerebellar cavernoma. (**D**) MRI showing a pontine cavernoma. Source: Figure by authors.

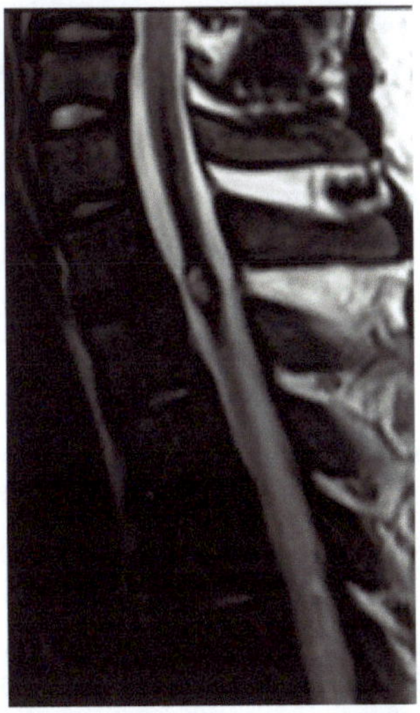

Figure 4. MRI showing a cervical spinal cord cavernoma. Source: Figure by authors.

5. Radiological Features of Cavernomas

State-of-the-art brain neuro-imaging techniques (called diffusion tensor tractography (DTI), gradient echo (GRE), as well as susceptibility-weighted (SW) sequences are used to permit for computational and noninvasive management planning (Table 2, Figure 5). Most cavernomas solely warrant observation with routine brain imaging to look for changes, recent bleeding ("hemorrhage") or new cavernoma/s.

Table 2. Imaging appearance of CMs.

CT	MRI	Angiography
Hyperdense	T2 bright areas with the susceptibility effect	Occult
	T1 can have bright areas, no appreciable enhancement, small adjacent DVA, if present strengthens the diagnosis	

Source: Table by authors.

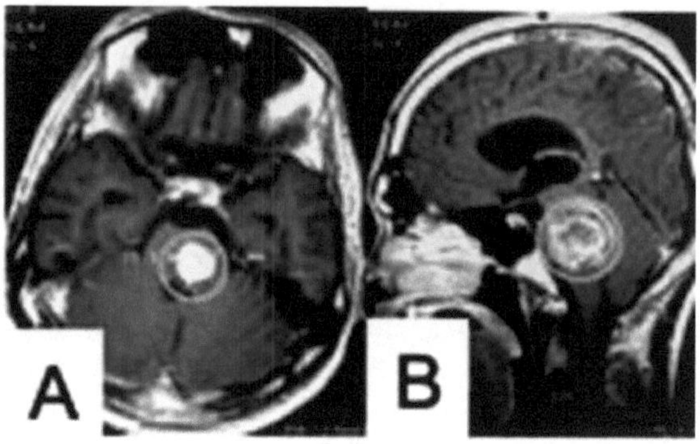

Figure 5. MRI of brain axial (**A**) and sagital (**B**) view showing a CM in the posterolateral pons with a halo sign. Source: Figure by authors.

A "popcorn" lesion is characterized by a center with a mixed signal in T1- and T2-weighted scans, that is bordered by a full hemosiderin ring with decreased signal intensity in T2W images. The severity of the hemorrhage affects the appearance of a CM. CMs have a tendency to expand with time. The common coexistence of a CM and DVA is thought to be the result of repetitive minor hemorrhages (D'Souza and Vadera 2022).

a. Zabramski classification of cerebral cavernous malformations (Zabramski et al. 1994):

   Type I: Subacute hemorrhage. T1—hyperintense. T2—hyper- or hypointense.

   Type II: The most common type—classic "popcorn" appearance. T1—heterogenous signal intensity at the center.

   Type III: Chronic hemorrhage. T1—isointense to hypointense at the center.

   Type IV: Numerous punctate micro-hemorrhages. T1—Hard to identify.

b. T 1 (Figure 6A): Variable signal based on the duration of the hemorrhage; Minimum fluid–fluid levels may be seen.

c. T 2 (Figure 6B):

   - Rim is hypointense;
   - Variable internal signal based on the duration of the blood products;
   - In a recent hemorrhage, an adjacent edema may be observed.

d. Gradient Recalled Echo (GRE) MRI:
   GRE T2/SWI (Figure 6C)

   - Blooming is prominent;
   - Helpful for finding tiny lesions that would otherwise go undetected by traditional spin echo sequences, particularly in individuals with familial or multiple cavernous malformations.

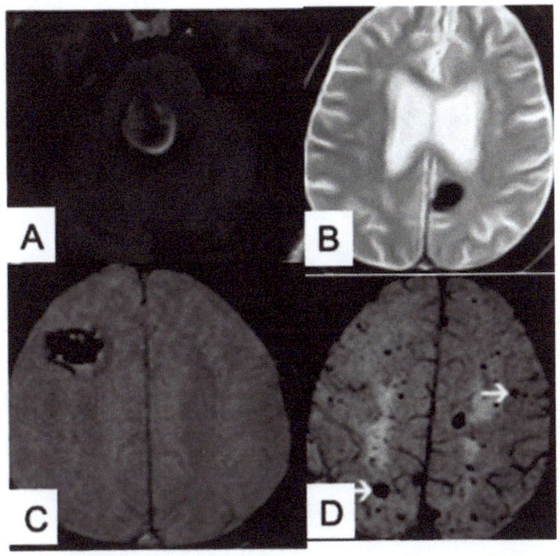

Figure 6. (**A**) MRI T1W image showing a high-signal hemosiderin ring. (**B**) MRI T2W image showing a hypointense lesion. (**C**) SW MRI showing an rt frontal cavernoma. (**D**) MRI showing multiple cavernomas. Source: Figure by authors.

With its capacity to show hemosiderin-filled cerebral parenchyma with a highly identifiable low intensity, a GRE MRI scan is a significant tool for diagnosing CMs. Traditional MRIs reveal an average of five lesions per patient in studies on familial CMs, whereas a T2W GRE MRI discovers a mean of sixteen pathologies per person. A GRE MRI is capable of not only identifying all existing lesions, but also delineating them more accurately. While a GRE MRI provides various advantages, it is vital to keep in mind that it increases the relative size of the CM. GRE MR imaging may also reveal multifocal CMs in older persons with hypertension, as well as a history of stroke, but these should not be confused with familial CMs; hypertensive angiopathy causes them.

e. Susceptibility-Weighted MR Imaging (Figure 6D): Since it reliably distinguishes deoxyhemoglobin and hemosiderin, susceptibility-weighted (SW) scanning is highly useful for identifying CMs. SW imaging is also the only approach for differentiating CMs and telangiectasias that do not bleed. It has been demonstrated to outline CMs more precisely, as well as discover additional CMs that are not seen with traditional imaging modalities.
f. Diffusion Tensor (DT) Imaging (Figure 7): Even though CMs are deeply placed in certain areas, DTI and fMRI are utilized preoperatively for better visualization of the lesions and nearby parenchyma in terms of improving the surgical success. The surgeon can see the white matter tracts that regularly pass over the hemosiderin rim of the CM using DT tractography. When removing CMs in the brain, an fMRI captures activity-dependent variations in cerebral blood flow, which is highly beneficial.

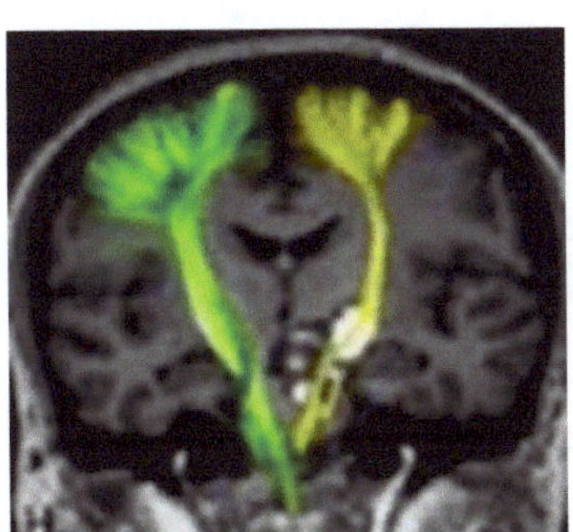

Figure 7. MR showing tractography in a cavernoma patient. Source: Figure by authors.

g. Angiography (DSA): CMs are angiographically occult and they do not have arteriovenous shunting.
h. CT scan of brain (Figure 8)

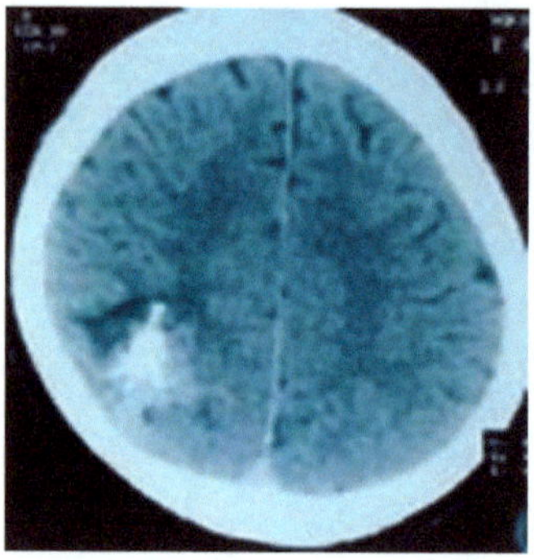

Figure 8. CT scan showing a calcified cavernoma. Source: Figure by authors.

6. Clinical Presentation

Seizures, headaches, neurologic deficits and asymptomatic presence are the four major kinds of clinical presentation. The most common presenting symptom is seizure, which affects 35–55% of patients. Several symptoms are found in many people. A bleed into the neighboring brain parenchyma occurs in some patients in each of the clinical groups. The hemorrhages are normally tiny, but they might be significant on rare occasions, causing the patient to rapidly deteriorate (Greenberg 2010).

7. Treatment

7.1. Microsurgery

Indications of surgery include a ruptured CM, CM with a mass affect, cranial nerve palsy and epilepsy. For a ruptured and symptomatic CM, it is the standard treatment (Greenberg 2010; D'Souza and Vadera 2022; Spetzler et al. 2020; Spetzler et al. 2017; Macdonald 2008; Mouchtouris et al. 2015).

7.1.1. Microsurgical Treatment of a Brainstem CM: Surgical Approaches

a. Brainstem anatomy: The diencephalon, midbrain, pons and medulla oblongata are the four components of the brainstem, which have an ectodermal origin. The brainstem links the cerebral hemispheres well with the spinal cord as well as the cerebellum. It is responsible for mandatory vital functions like respiration, cardiac pulsation, blood pressure, consciousness control and sleep. White and gray matter coexist in the brainstem.

Although complex, the internal anatomy of the brainstem is structured in three laminae (tectum, tegmentum and basis) that run the length of the brainstem (Spetzler et al. 2020).

b. Approaches to CMs in the brainstem

Microsurgical approaches to brain stem CMs are shown in Table 3.

c. Approaches to the midbrain
Supra cerebellar infratentorial approaches:

1. Midline;
2. Lateral;
3. Far lateral:

- Supracerebellar transtentorial approach;
- Occipital transtentorial approach.

The dorsal midbrain, pineal region and upper pons can also be approached by the occipital transtentorial approach:

d. Ventral midbrain approaches (shown Table 4);

e. For lateral midbrain and upper pons (shown Table 4).

Table 3. Surgical approaches to CMs in the brainstem.

Lesion location	Anterior	Lateral	Posterior
Midbrain	Pterional, orbitozygomatic (OZ) subtemporal	Lateral infratentorial supracerebellar (LIS)	LIS
Pons	Pterional, OZ subtemporal	Far lateral suboccipital retrosigmoid	Median suboccipital/4th ventricular
Medulla	Subtemporal, far lateral suboccipital transcondylar	Lateral suboccipital retrosigmoid	Median suboccipital/4th ventricular

Source: Authors' compilation based on data from Spetzler et al. (2017).

7.1.2. Safe Entry Zone (SEZ) to the Brainstem

A. Pons

Safe entry zones (SEZ) to the Brainstem are shown in Figure 9, and in pons are shown in Table 4.

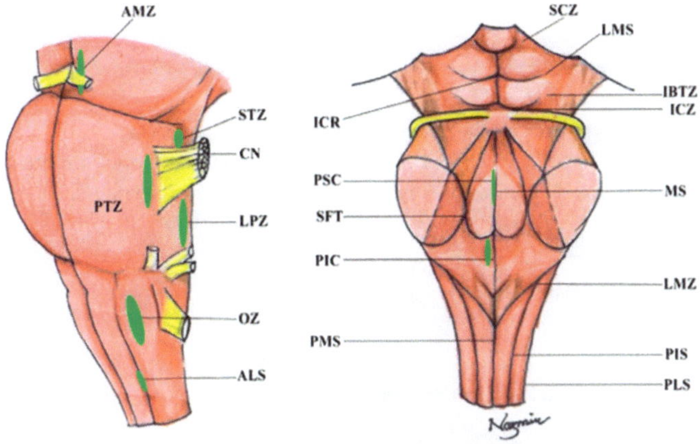

Figure 9. Principles of SEZs to the brainstem. The colored ellipses represent areas where petit neurotomies can be carried out to avoid minuscule perforators, prime nerve tracts and nuclei. (**Left**) Antero-lateral surface of the brainstem demonstrating some anterior and anterolateral SEZs. (**Right**) View of the dorsal surface of the brainstem demonstrating SEZs on the surface of the quadrigeminal plate, floor of the fourth ventricle. (ALS—anterolateral sulcus; AMZ—anterior mesencephalic zone; CN—cranial nerve; IBTZ—inferior brachium triangular zone; ICR—intercollicular region; ICZ—infracollicular zone; LMS—lateral mesencephalic sulcus; LMZ—lateral medullary zone; LPZ—lateral pontine zone; MS—median sulcus of fourth ventricle; OZ—olivary zone; PIC—paramedian infracollicular; PIS—posterior intermediatesulcus; PLS—posterior lateral sulcus; PMS—posterior median sulcus; PSC—paramedian supracollicular; PTZ—peritrieminal zone; SCZ—supracollicular zone; SFT—superior fovea triangle; STZ—supratigeminal zone). Source: Figure by authors.

Table 4. Pontine SEZ.

Approach	SEZ
Subtemporal transtentorial	Supratrigeminal
Anterior petrosectomy	Supratrigeminal, peritrigeminal
Suboccipital telovelar	Median sulcus of the 4th ventricle, paramedian infracollicular, superior fovea triangular
Retrosigmoid	Supratrigeminal, peritrigeminal lateral pontine
Retrolabrynthine	Supratrigeminal, peritrigeminal lateral pontine

Source: Authors' compilation based on data from Spetzler et al. (2017).

In the posterior pons/floor of the 4th ventricle, safe areas are the suprafacial triangle and infrafacial triangle (Spetzler et al. 2017). These areas are approached by a suboccipital teloveloar approach.

In the lateral pons, the safe areas are as follows:

- Supratrigeminal area;
- Peritrigeminal area;
- Infratrigeminal area (between 5th and 7th nerve);

The lateral pontine zone can be reached by a retrosigmoid approach.

To reach betel, more wide exposure is required and then we need to utilize a presigmoid approach.

B. Medulla Oblongata

Medullary safe entry zone: In the anterior medulla, the safe zone is the olivary area. The olive is a small elevation formed by the location of the inferior olivary nucleus.

Olivary zone: The olivary zone can be reached by the far lateral approach.

Dorsal medullary safe zone: The dorsal lateral medullary zone is a posterior midline sulcus and laterally medullary zone, respectively. This area is approached by midline suboccipital craniotomy.

7.2. *Conservative Treatment*

Conservative treatment is utilized for incidental CMs.

7.3. *Stereotactic Radiosurgery*

Stereotactic radiosurgery is usually not recommended.

Author Contributions: Conceptualization, methodology, validation, formal analysis, investigation, resources, data curation, S.A., F.H.C. and N.A.; writing—original draft preparation, S.A. and F.H.C.; writing—review and editing, F.H.C., visualization, supervision, M.H.S. All authors have read and agreed to the published version of the manuscript.

Funding: This research received no external funding.

Conflicts of Interest: The authors declare no conflicts of interest.

References

Al-Shahi, Rustam, Jo J. Bhattacharya, David G. Currie, Vakis Papanastassiou, Vaughn Ritchie, Richard C. Roberts, Robin J. Sellar, and Charles P. Warlow. 2003. Prospective, population- based detection of intracranial vascular malformations in adults: The Scottish Intracranial Vascular Malformation Study (SIVMS). *Stroke* 34: 1163–69. [CrossRef] [PubMed]

D'Souza, D., and S. Vadera. 2022. Cerebral Cavernous Venous Malformation. Reference Article, Radiopaedia.org. Available online: https://doi.org/10.53347/rID-1064 (accessed on 4 April 2022).

Greenberg, Mark S. 2010. *Handbook of Neurosurgery*. New York: Thieme.

Kirollos, Ramez, Adel Helmy, Simon Thomson, and Peter Hutchinson. 2019. *Oxford Textbook of Neurological Surgery*. Oxford: Oxford University Press.

Macdonald, R. Loch. 2008. *Neurosurgical Operative Atlas: Vascular Neurosurgery*. New York: Thieme.

Mouchtouris, Nikolaos, Nohra Chalouhi, Ameet Chitale, Robert M. Starke, Stavropoula I. Tjoumakaris, Robert H. Rosenwasser, and Pascal M. Jabbour. 2015. Management of cerebral cavernous malformations: From diagnosis to treatment. *Scientific World Journal* 2015: 808314. [CrossRef] [PubMed]

Salman, Rustam Al-Shahi, Julie M. Hall, Margaret A. Horne, Fiona Moultrie, Colin B. Josephson, Jo J. Bhattacharya, Carl E. Counsell, Gordon D. Murray, Vakis Papanastassiou, Vaughn Ritchie, and et al. 2012. Untreated clinical course of cerebral cavernous malformations: A prospective, population-based cohort study. *The Lancet Neurology* 11: 217–24. [CrossRef] [PubMed]

Spetzler, Robert F., M. Yashar S. Kalani, and Michael T. Lawton. 2020. *Surgery of the Brainstem*. New York: Thieme.

Spetzler, Robert F., M. Yashar S. Kalani, and Peter Nakaji. 2017. *Color Atlas of Brainstem Surgery*. New York: Thieme.

Zabramski, Joseph M., Thomas M. Wascher, Robert F. Spetzler, Blake Johnson, John Golfinos, Burton P. Drayer, Ben Brown, Daniel Rigamonti, and Geraldine Brown. 1994. The natural history of familial cavernous malformations: Results of an ongoing study. *Journal of Neurosurgery* 80: 422–32. [CrossRef] [PubMed]

Moyamoya Disease (MMD)

Shamshul Alam, Forhad H. Chowdhury, Nazmin Ahmed and Mohammod Raziul Haque

Abstract: Moyamoya disease (MMD) is a progressive occluding intracranial carotid artery disease, which can be either unilateral or bilateral. Here, the anterior circulation is commonly involved. In the center core, there is development of a profuse thin wall capillary known as moyamoya vessels. MMD is among the most common causes of neurological morbidity and disability in children. In children, it usually presents with ischemia and infarct, whereas in adults, it presents with hemorrhage. A CT scan of the head, an MRI of the brain, CTA and MRA are the necessary investigation methods, whereas a cerebral DSA is the gold standard. Perfusion images are important for follow up. Treatment includes cerebral revascularization by a direct or indirect bypass, or in combination. In this chapter, the etiopathogenesis, clinical features, investigation methods and management of MMD will be discussed.

Abbreviations

ACA	anterior cerebral artery	CBF	cerebral blood flow
CVR	cerebrovascular reservoir	ECA	external carotid artery
EDAS	Encephaloduroarterio synangiosis	EDMAS	encephaloduromyoarterio synangiosis
EDMAPS	encephaloduromyoarteriopial synangiosis	EMS	encephalomyosynangiosis
EGS	Encephalogaleosynangiosis	ICA	internal carotid artery
ICH	intracerebral hemorrhage	ICP	intracranial pressure
MCA	middle cerebral artery	MMD	moyamoya disease
NF	Neurofibromatosis	OA	occipital artery
PCA	posterior cerebral artery	STA	superficial temporal artery
TIA	transient ischemic attack		

1. Introduction

Moyamoya disease (MMD) is a rare variety of congenital vascular abnormalities where there is progressive occlusion of the intracranial carotid artery, which is either unilateral or bilateral. The progressive bilateral spontaneous occlusion of ICAs with compensatory capillary collaterals look like a "puff of smoke" (Japanese: moyamoya) on angiogram (Figure 1). It is a progressive disease where the anterior circulation, such as the supraclinoidal carotid artery, is usually involved. Hence, the large area becomes ischemic. In the center core, there is development of a profuse thin wall capillary known as moyamoya vessels. MMD is among the most common causes of neurological morbidity and disability in children due to cerebrovascular illness, such as cognitive and motor dysfunctions. According to previous research, infants have a higher frequency of ischemia pathophysiology due to insufficient perfusion, whereas adults have a higher prevalence of bleeding due to the fragility of neovessels (Kirollos et al. 2019).

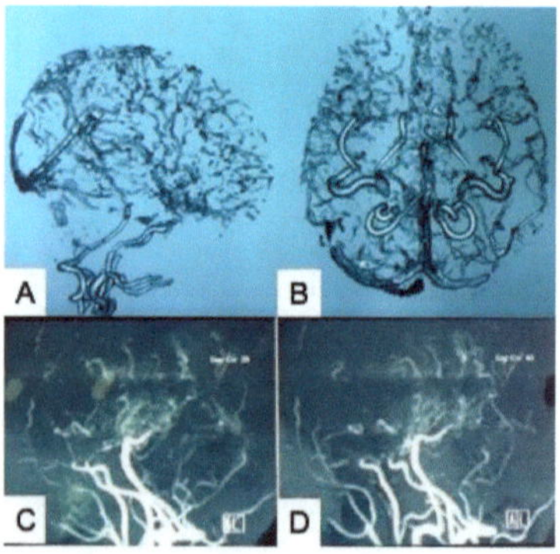

Figure 1. (**A**,**B**) CTA showing moyamoya vessels; (**C**,**D**) MRA showing moyamoya vessels. Source: Figure by authors.

2. Moyamoya Syndrome-Associated Diseases

- Sickle cell anemia
- Neurofibromatosis type I
- Past cranial radiation therapy
- Trisomy 21
- Primary dwarfism
- Congenital cardiac diseases
- Giant cervicofacial hemangiomas and PHACE syndrome
- Renal artery stenosis
- Alagille syndrome
- Hyperthyroidism
- (PHACE—posterior fossa abnormalities, hemangioma, arterial lesion, cardiac abnormalities and/or artic coarctation and eye abnormalities) (Greenberg 2010).

3. Epidemiology

MMD was first discovered in Asian patients, although it has now been observed in people of various races and ethnicities. The precise number of incidents is unknown. According to Japanese studies, the yearly incidence is between 0.35 and 0.94 per 100,000 people, and the yearly prevelence is 3.16–10.5 per 100,000 people. In comparison to males, females have a twice-as-high rate (July and Wahjoepramono 2019).

3.1. Types

The Ministry of Health and Welfare of Japan categorized MMD according to its manifestation into four types:

a. Ischemic;
b. Hemorrhagic;
c. Epileptic;
d. Others.

At a pediatric age, the ischemic type is the most common, and in adults, the hemorrhagic type is the most common.

3.2. The Suzuki Stages

The Suzuki stage (July and Wahjoepramono 2019) appears to correlate with collateralization in children, but not in adults.

Stage I

- "Narrowing of the ICA fork"
- Narrowed ICA termination.

Stage II

- "Beginning of the moyamoya";
- Dilated MCA and ACA, as well as narrowed ICA termination with moyamoya alteration.

Stage III

- "Intensification of the moyamoya";
- Further increases in moyamoya change of the ICA termination with a narrowed ACA and MCA.

Stage IV

- "Minimization of moyamoya";
- Moyamoya change decreasing with occlusive alterations in the ICA with a tenuous ACA and MCA.

Stage V

- "Decreasing of moyamoya";
- Further decreases in moyamoya change with occlusion of the ICA, ACA and MCA.

Stage VI

- "Disappearance (lost) of moyamoya";
- ICA essentially disappears and the brain is supplied by the ECA.

Posterior circulation is usually not affected by MMD; however, it can be affected, too. Usually, the development of MMD peaks at two ages: childhood and adulthood; often it presents as either ischemic features or hemorrhagic manifestation, and sometimes seizure disorder. Often, patients suffer for a long period of time before arriving to seek medical attention. Any form of an angiogram is the diagnostic method for MMD. We usually employ a CT angiogram or MR angiogram as the first-line investigation method for MMD (Kirollos et al. 2019).

Because juvenile MMD is more likely to advance than adult MMD, revascularization surgery is recommended for the majority of children with MMD. As a result, in order to attain a positive clinical result in children, an early diagnosis and active intervention are critically needed before irreparable brain damage (Figure 2) happens. As previously stated, the risk of stroke in silent MMD patients or those with MMD who have a relatively stable circulatory condition appears to be high (Kirollos et al. 2019; Zhang et al. 2021).

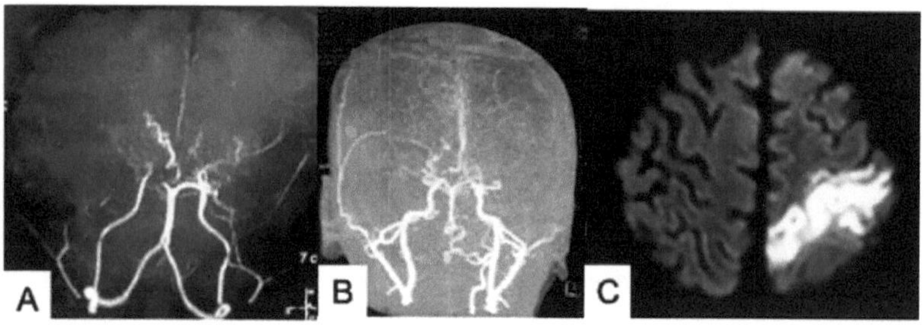

Figure 2. Bilateral supranclinoidal carotid artery occlusion (**A**,**B**) and high signal intensity along the motor strip due to ischemia (**C**). Source: Figure by authors.

4. Treatment

4.1. Surgical Revascularization

- Direct revascularization
- Indirect revascularization
- In combination

4.1.1. Indication of Surgery

- ICH;
- Symptomatic ischemia or transient ischemic attack (TIA);
- Cognitive impairment;
- Decreased CBF and/or CVR;
- Selective asymptomatic cases (ivy sign on MRI) (50% progress within 5 years).

One of the common indications of surgery is multiple episodes of a TIA. The aim of surgery is to preclude further events by re-establishing enough blood supply to the involved brain (Kirollos et al. 2019; Zhang et al. 2021; Katsumi 2019; Macdonald 2008; Nader et al. 2013).

Perioperative management principles in MMD patients are listed in Table 1.

Table 1. Perioperative management guidelines for moyamoya patients.

Time	Guidelines
At 1 day before operation	Continuation of aspirin therapy (generally 81 mg daily per oral if weight <70 kg and 325 mg daily per oral if weight $\geq$70 kg);
	Admission of patient for overnight intravenous fluid hydration (isotonic saline 1.25–1.5$\times$ maintenance).

Table 1. *Cont.*

Time	Guidelines
At induction of anesthesia	Commencement of EEG monitoring;
	Maintenance of normal BP during induction of anesthesia and normal temperature (particularly in smaller children), normal PCO2 (eliminate hyperventilation to reduce vasoconstriction, PCO2 > 35 mm Hg) and normal blood PH;
	Installment of extra intravenous channels, arterial channel, urinary catheter and a pulse oximeter;
	Placement of precordial Doppler (for venous air embolus surveillance).
During surgery	Maintenance of normocarbia, normotension, normothermia, normal pH, enough hydration and adequate oxygenation;
	Slowing of EEG tracing may respond to sequential BP increases or other techniques to improve the CBF.
Postoperatively	Avoidance of hyperventilation (equivalent with crying in pediatric age), analgesia is vital; Maintenance of aspirin on postoperative day 1;
	Maintenance of intravenous fluid at 1.25–1.5× maintenance until the patient is completely recovered and drinking enough (frequently from 48 to 72 h).

Source: Authors' compilation based on data from Kirollos et al. (2019).

4.1.2. Surgical Methods

A. Direct arterial bypass:

- STA–MCA;
- STA–ACA;
- OA–PCA.

B. Indirect:

- EDAS;
- EDAMS;
- EMS;
- EDMAPS;
- Pial synangiosis;
- Omental synangiosis;
- Multiple burr hole.

Different techniques that are used for indirect revascularizations in MMD are listed in Table 2.

Table 2. Different tissues (techniques) that are used for indirect revascularizations.

Different Tissues
1. Techniques utilizing the galea
2. Techniques utilizing the scalp artery
3. Techniques utilizing the temporal or other muscles
4. Techniques utilizing the dura mater
5. Techniques utilizing a combination of the above
6. Techniques utilizing the omentum
7. Direct and indirect anastomoses (combined)

Source: Table by authors.

C. Both direct and indirect methods: We commonly employ both direct and indirect methods of a brain bypass for moyamoya disease for both ischemic and hemorrhagic cases. A direct bypass is performed with the STA and MCA M4 branch. It is better to perform a more direct bypass, preferably two bypasses via the frontal and parietal branches.

4.1.3. Bypass Surgery in MMD for Cerebral Revascularization

Cerebral bypass surgery involves the use of grafts to revascularize either an extracranial vessel and an intracranial vessel or an intracranial artery, as well as another intracranial artery (radial artery, saphenous vein, etc.). The goal of a bypass is to restore or redirect blood flow from a restricted, obstructed or damaged channel to the distal portion of the artery. It is fairly typical to simply use the natural supplied artery, such as the STA, and bypass it entirely to reach the MCA (Katsumi 2019).

Direct Cerebral Bypass for MMD

The term "direct bypass" refers to an anastomosis of the superficial temporal artery (STA) to the middle cerebral artery (MCA), which can enhance cerebral perfusion in surgical areas almost instantly (Figures 3 and 4). Other direct methods are STA–ACA and OA–PCA bypasses.

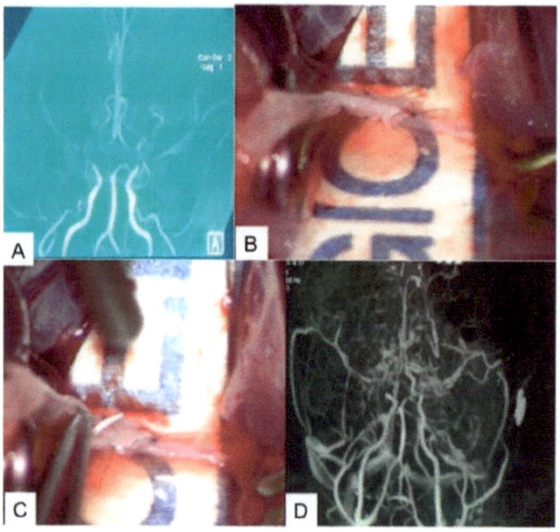

Figure 3. (**A**) MRA of the brain showing bilateral MMD in a 4-year-old child; (**B**,**C**) preoperative pictures of a direct STA–MCA bypass; (**D**) postoperative CTA on the first POD of the brain showing increased vascularity of the brain. Source: Figure by authors.

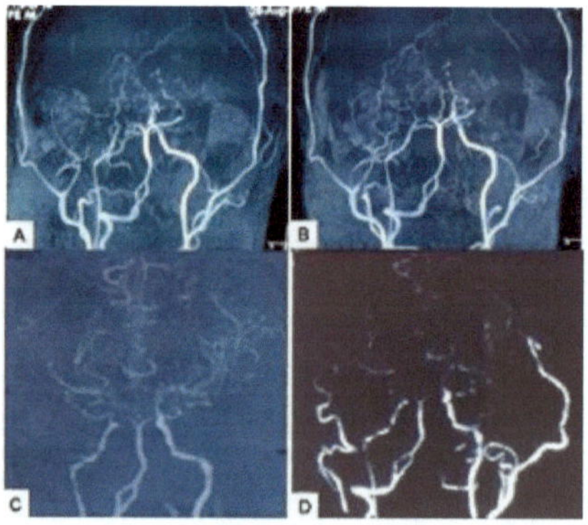

Figure 4. (**A**,**B**) Preoperative CTA of the brain in an adult with bilateral symptomatic MMD; (**C**,**D**) postoperative CTA on the first POD showing a direct STA–MCA bypass with increased parenchymal vascularity. Source: Figure by authors.

Indirect Cerebral Bypass for MMD

There are verities of indirect cerebral bypasses that include encephalomyosynangiosis, encephaloduroarteriosynangiosis, ribbon encephaloduroarteriomyosynangiosis, the multiple burr hole surgery technique, encephaloduromyoarteriopericraniosynangiosis, omentum transplantation, etc.

a. EDAS (Encephaloduroarteriosynangiosis): EDAS surgery is an indirect way of establishing new arterialization in the brain. It uses the STA which is dissected free from the adjacent soft tissue and then put directly on the cortical surface.
b. Encephalogaleo synangiosis (EGS): In the ACA region, a bifrontal EGS with a craniotomy showed better angiogenesis and an improved CBF. It is thought to be a straightforward, safe and successful surgical treatment for improving ischemia in the ACA area in pediatric patients.
c. Encephalomyosynangiosis (EMS): The encephalomyosynangiosis (EMS) operation is an indirect revascularization technique where the temporalis muscle is divided and transferred onto the surface of the brain through a hole in the skull. Between blood-rich muscle and the brain, new veins emerge throughout time.
d. Encephaloduroarteriomyosynangiosis (EDAMS): EDAMS surgery is a summation of simultaneous EDAS and EMS.
e. Multiple burr hole: In the management of MMD in children, many burr holes and arachnoid apertures are formed over both cerebral hemispheres (Figure 5).

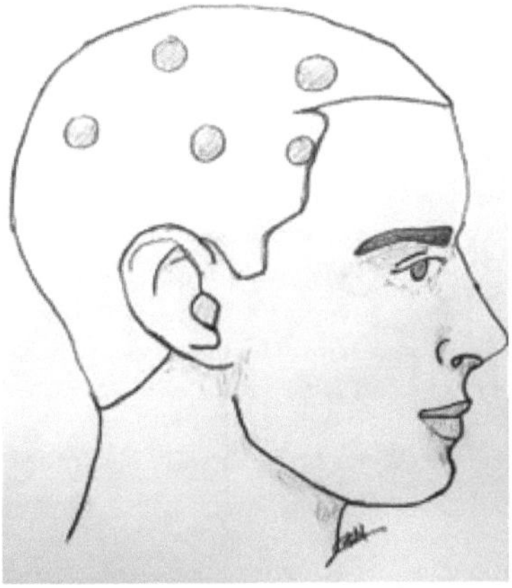

Figure 5. Revascularization through burr holes. Outline of the burr hole sites (2-to-4) to achieve indirect revascularization. Source: Figure by authors.

The most favorable feature of direct revascularization is the immediate increase in blood flow. Delayed synangiosis is also a possibility. Direct cerebral revascularization, on the other hand, is a more difficult technique with a lengthier learning curve than indirect cerebral revascularization.

4.1.4. Complications of Cerebral Revascularization in MMD

Scalp avascular necrosis is not an uncommon complication. When the STA and its branches are taken for a bypass, it may affect scalp blood supply due to rough dissection during the harvesting of the STA. Increased intracranial pressure (ICP) is a sign of hyperperfusion syndrome, which is caused by a rapid increase in cerebral blood flow. The complication of hyperperfusion syndrome has been described in patients managed for MMD, mostly adults and those managed with the direct cerebral revascularization method.

This necrosis usually needs regular dressing and sometimes plastic surgical intervention for correction.

Failed direct (i.e., STA–MCA) bypass which may have manifested in the form of increased weakness of the limbs or new development of hemiparesis.

Failure of an indirect bypass.

Intracerebral hemorrhage.

Surgical therapy for MMD should be explored for symptomatic patients due to the disease's progressive nature. An early diagnosis and prompt treatments are required for young patients before irreparable brain damage occurs. Surgical revascularization is an efficacious therapy for ischemic or hemorrhagic stroke prevention.

4.2. Conservative Treatment

Conservative treatments is used in incidental cases, with follow up to see any progression.

Drug therapy for moyamoya disease (efficacy is not known):

- Aspirin;
- Beta blocker;
- Ca chanel blocker (amlodipine).

Author Contributions: Conceptualization, methodology, validation, formal analysis, investigation, resources, data curation, S.A., F.H.C. and N.A.; writing—original draft preparation, S.A. and F.H.C.; writing—review and editing, F.H.C.; visualization, supervision, M.R.H. All authors have read and agreed to the published version of the manuscript.

Funding: This research received no external funding.

Conflicts of Interest: The authors declare no conflicts of interest.

References

Greenberg, Mark S. 2010. *Handbook of Neurosurgery*. New York: Thieme.

July, Julius, and Eka J. Wahjoepramono. 2019. *Neurovascular Surgery*. Singapore: Springer Open.

Katsumi, Takizawa. 2019. Superficial temporal artery (STA) to middle cerebral artery (MCA) bypass. Paper presented at 5th Winter Seminar of Cerebrovascular Diseases, Nagoya, Japan, January 21–24; p. 128.

Kirollos, Ramez, Adel Helmy, Simon Thomson, and Peter Hutchinson. 2019. *Oxford Textbook of Neurological Surgery*. Oxford: Oxford University Press.

Macdonald, R. Loch. 2008. *Neurosurgical Operative Atlas: Vascular Neurosurgery*. New York: Thieme.

Nader, Remi, Cristian Gragnaniello, Scott C. Berta, Abdulrahman J. Sabbagh, and Michael L. Levy. 2013. *Neurosurgery Tricks of the Trade-Cranial: Cranial*. New York: Thieme.

Zhang, Angie, Nolan Brown, Barry Cheaney II, Jessica K. Campos, R. Chase Ransom, and Frank P. K. Hsu. 2021. Updates in the management of moyamoya disease. *Interdisciplinary Neurosurgery* 23: 100976. [CrossRef]

Endovascular Neurosurgery

Sharif Uddin Khan, Forhad H. Chowdhury, Patwary Mohammod Faruque, Shirazi Shafiqul Islam and Kazi Mohibur Rahman

Abstract: There are two pathways for the surgical management of neurovascular diseases: one is microvascular neurosurgery and the other is endovascular neurosurgery. Nearly three decades have passed since the introduction of endovascular neurosurgery, and now it has taken its shape and definitive role in the management of neurovascular diseases such as intracranial aneurysms, arteriovenous fistulas of the brain and spinal cord, arterial stenosis, and intracranial and spinal AVMs. It can be used for curative or palliative purposes. It can also be used in combination with microsurgery and radiosurgery. This chapter will discuss the endovascular management of brain aneurysms, carotid and vertebral system arterial stenosis, intracranial and spinal AVMs, and dural AV fistulas (head and spine).

Abbreviations

ADC	afferent diffusion coefficient	ASA	anterior spinal artery
AVF	arteriovenous fistula	AVM	arteriovenous malformation
BAC	balloon-assisted coiling	BMT	best medical therapy
CARAT	cerebral aneurysm re-rupture after treatment	CAS	carotid artery stenting
CCA	common carotid artery	CCF	caroticocavernous fistula
CEA	carotid endarterectomy	CPA	cerebello-pontine angle
CT	computed tomography	CTA	computed tomographic arteriogram
CVR	cortical venous reflux	DAVF	dural arteriovenous fistula
DCCF	direct CCF	DSA	digital subtraction angiography
DW	diffusion-weighted	ECA	external carotid artery
EVT	endovascular therapy	FD	flow diverter
fMRI	functional magnetic resonance imaging	GRAS	gradient echo sequences
IA	intracranial aneurysm	ICA	internal carotid artery
ICCF	indirect CCF	ICG	indocyanine green
ICH	intracranial hematoma	ICP	intracranial pressure
MMA	middle meningeal artery	MRA	magnetic resonance angiography
MRI	magnetic resonance imaging	*n*-BCA	*n*-butyl 2-cyanoacrylate
PSA	posterior spinal artery	PVA	polyvinyl alcohol
PW	perfusion-weighted	SAC	stent-assisted coiling
SAH	subarachnoid hemorrhage	SDH	subdural hematoma
SVM	spinal vascular malformation	TIA	transient ischemic attack
TOF	time of flight	VA	vertebral artery

1. History of Endovascular Neurosurgery

Morgagni of Padua recorded dilatation of the posterior division of right and left carotid arteries in 1761. An aneurysm with a rupture was first noticed by Biumi of Milan in 1765. Blackall reported the case report of a subarachnoid hemorrhage (SAH) linked to a cerebral aneurysm in 1814. Earlier than the invention of angiography, only few aneurysms could be identified before an SAH. Sometimes, they may present as a space-occupying lesion that might be noticed on a pneumoencephalogram. Keen published Victor Horsley's surgery on a case with a big pulsatile blood cyst in 1890. Harvey Cushing discovered a brain aneurysm in managing a lesion that he believed to be a pituitary tumor. In his assertation of the pituitary body and its disorders, he compiled the case of a patient with a bitemporal visual deficit, hypopituitarism and a possible interpeduncular space aneurysm. In 1917, Cushing ligated an internal carotid artery (ICA) intracranially following an aneurysm rupture during operation, and the patient died. In 1926, Cushing wrapped an ICA aneurysm with muscle where hemiplegia had developed; the patient died later. However, post-mortem, the aneurysm was found to be thrombosed. The clinical diagnosis was an intracranial cyst (Smith et al. 1994).

Norman Dott conducted the first direct surgery on a cerebral aneurysm in 1933, wrapping a burst aneurysm, while Walter Dandy executed the first clipping of an aneurysm in 1938. When microsurgery was established in the 1960s, the surgical outcomes improved considerably (Maurice-Williams and Lafuente 2003).

Injecting iodinated contrast media into the carotid artery (direct puncture) and then utilizing Roentgen rays was the first experience with a cerebral angiogram, which was invented by Portuguese physician Egas Moniz at the University of Lisbon in 1927 (Lowis and Minagar 2003).

Per Amudsen, a Norwegian radiologist, was the first to conduct total cerebral angiography using a transfemoral technique in 1964. In 1964, Charles Dotter, the pioneer of angioplasty and interventional radiology, was the first to perform an endovascular operation, conducting a therapeutic angioplasty of the femoral artery in a female of 82 years with an ischemic lower limb who rejected amputation (Payne 2001).

Fedor Serbinenko devised a technique for the treatment of aneurysms in the ICA by occluding the light with balloons deployed into the vessel. The first treatment was performed in Moscow in 1970, when an internal carotid artery was occluded to manage a carotid–cavernous fistula (CCF). As such, he can be called the first interventional neuroradiologist, interventionist and endovascular neurosurgeon (Teitelbaum et al. 2000). Neuroradiologists all across the world perfected this technique, with Jacques Moret in Paris, Grant Hieshima in San Francisco and Gerard Debrun in Canada being the first and most outstanding. Image technology in radiology and neuroradiology units improved dramatically in tandem with the development of catheters. The technique of digital subtraction angiography (DSA) was pioneered by Charles Mistretta in 1979 (Celesia et al. 1983).

The work of two Italian physicians, Guido Guglielmi and Cesare Gianturco, revolutionized endovascular surgery by the end of the 1980s and the beginning of the 1990s. The first one had a strong understanding of diagnostic radiology, as well as a strong capacity to tackle technical and manual issues. He devised Gianturco's coils, which he utilized to embolize arteries, including aneurysms, for the first time. Gianturco also designed the first endovascular stent recognized by the American Food and Drug Administration, a device that has a long history. Hilal was the first at Columbia University to utilize coils to manage cerebral aneurysms in the late 1980s, but his technique was ineffective and risky since the coils were deployed with minimal control, putting the parent vessel at the risk of an occlusion. Guido Guglielmi's work at UCLA redefined coil embolization when he learned that electricity could be used to control the release of coils; in 1991, he described the embolization of cerebral aneurysms using detachable platinum coils (Guglielmi's coils). Aneurysm therapy has thus become more affordable and safe (Vaidya et al. 2008).

For decades, clipping a burst aneurysm was thought to be the only option; however, the invention of the GDC coil in 1990 provided an option that avoided the open surgery (Maurice-Williams and Lafuente 2003).

2. SAH and Intracranial Aneurysms

An intracranial aneurysm (IA) rupture is a dangerous and often fatal clinical emergency that necessitates prompt surgery. Approximately 12% of patients die before entering the hospital, 33% within 48 h and 50% within 30 days of the rupture, with 50% of survivors suffering from chronic disability and reliance (Taheri et al. 2015; Sehba et al. 2012). Therefore, it is advised that patients with a burst intracranial aneurysm should receive surgical treatment before dawn or sunset, whichever occurs first.

The approximate incidence of unruptured IAs is nearly 3.2% (Pierot and Wakhloo 2013; Vlak et al. 2011). Most IAs are usually symptomless until rupture, leading to an SAH. The mortality of IA rupture is very high (from 27% to 44%) (Nieuwkamp et al. 2009). Even though the management of a ruptured IA is direly an emergency, indication for the management of incidental IAs is still controversial. Management of the patients with IAs depends on aneurysm shape (saccular versus fusiform) and location (geometry), size (large/small/giant), neck size (large/small), location (posterior versus anterior circulation) and other factors. The heterogeneity suggests that EVTs must use diverse ways to treat all types of IAs. Various therapy strategies for an EVT of IAs have been developed over the previous three decades (Pierot et al. 2012a; Pierot and Wakhloo 2013).

2.1. Endovascular Coiling

The evolution of coils with a controlled deployable system (Figures 1–3) was definitely the first key step for the generalized utilization of endovascular therapy (EVT) (Guglielmi et al. 1991a, part 1; Guglielmi et al. 1991b, part 2).

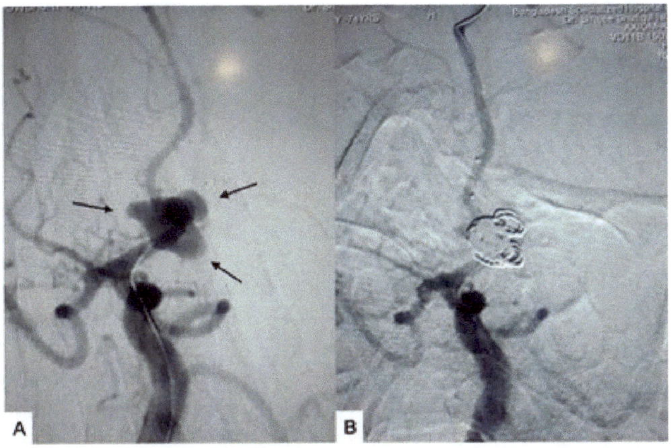

Figure 1. (**A**) DSA showing the pre-embolization state of an ACOM aneurysm; (**B**) DSA after coil embolization of an ACOM aneurysm. Source: Figure by authors.

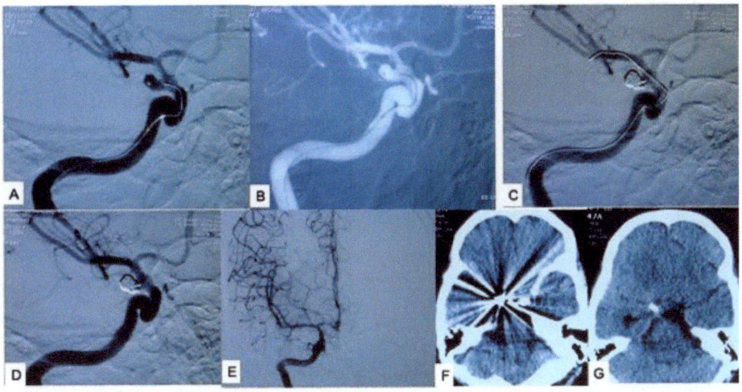

Figure 2. Preoperative pictures of a coil of a right PCOM aneurysm. (**A**) Microcatheter at the neck of the aneurysm; (**B**) road map; (**C**,**D**) coils inside the aneurysm; (**E**) post-coiling DSA; (**F**,**G**) postoperative CT scan after coiling. Source: Figure by authors.

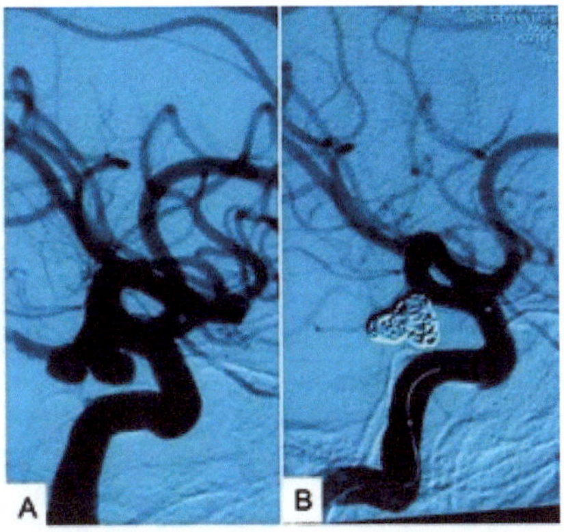

Figure 3. Bilobed PCOM aneurysm. (**A**) Before coiling; (**B**) after coiling. Source: Figure by authors.

The two most common hazards of coiling are thromboembolic hazards and intraprocedural rupture (Pierot et al. 2008a; Cognard et al. 2011). The incidence of thromboembolic complications and intraoperative ruptures linked with coiling was found to be 7.3% and 2.0% in unruptured aneurysms, respectively. An intraoperative rupture was associated with a greater death rate (16.7%) than thromboembolic complications (4.1%). An intraprocedural ruptured aneurysm and thromboembolism were more common in ruptured aneurysms, with 13.3% and 3.7%, respectively (Cognard et al. 2011). Thus, the perioperative use of intravenous heparin and aspirin for incidental, and in few cases, for ruptured aneurysms as well, is adopted (Ries et al. 2006). The two main hurdles for coiling are as follows (Pierot and Wakhloo 2013):

(1) Difficult coiling due to their shape (giant and large aneurysms, fusiform types of aneurysms, wide neck aneurysms, aneurysms with an unaffordable size, relationship between aneurysm neck, dome and parent artery)—This resulted in the introduction of new technologies and techniques, incorporating balloon-assisted aneurysm coiling, stent abetting coiling and flow diversion (FD)/flow disruption.
(2) The decreased durability of coiling (Cognard et al. 1999; Raymond et al. 2003)— Reopening of an aneurysm occurs in 20.8% of cases, necessitating retreatment in 10.3%, according to a systematic study (Ferns et al. 2009). Recent burst, hypertension, smoking, neck size and aneurysm diameter, as well as the quality of early postoperative aneurysm occlusion are all related to a greater risk of recanalization and recurrence (coil packing density) (Hope et al. 1999; Vallée et al. 2004; Ortiz et al. 2008; Choi et al. 2010; Songsaeng et al. 2011; Gallas et al. 2005; Wakhloo et al. 2007; Willinsky et al. 2009; Pierot et al. 2012c). Surface-modified coils, such as polyglycolic–lactic acid coils, as well as hydrocoils, were created to address the recanalization rate, but they are no more effective than bare platinum coils (Pierot et al. 2008b; White et al. 2011). Aneurysm recanalization's clinical importance isn't well understood. The Cerebral Aneurysm Re-rupture After Treatment (CARAT) study found that the extent of aneurysm occlusion following initial therapy was a robust predictor of the probability of future rupture in SAH cases (Johnston et al. 2008). Because aneurysm recanalization is a probability, a DSA and MRA follow-up is required (Johnston et al. 2008; Pierot et al. 2006, 2012d, 2012f).

2.2. Balloon-Assisted Coiling

Moret et al. were the first to introduce balloon-assisted coiling (BAC, remodeling approach) for expanding EVT to broad-neck IAs (Moret et al. 1997). During each coil installation, a nondetachable balloon is momentarily inflated anterior to the aneurysm's neck (Figure 4) (Pierot et al. 2012b). The balloon is basically kept in the main anterior to the aneurysm neck in sidewall aneurysms. The procedure for bifurcation aneurysms is more difficult. There are several options available, including using two balloons, a round-shaped balloon, a hyper-compliant balloon or a double-lumen balloon. The balloon is deflated and withdrawn at the end of the intervention, and so no device is kept in situ unless a stenting is to be kept in place later.

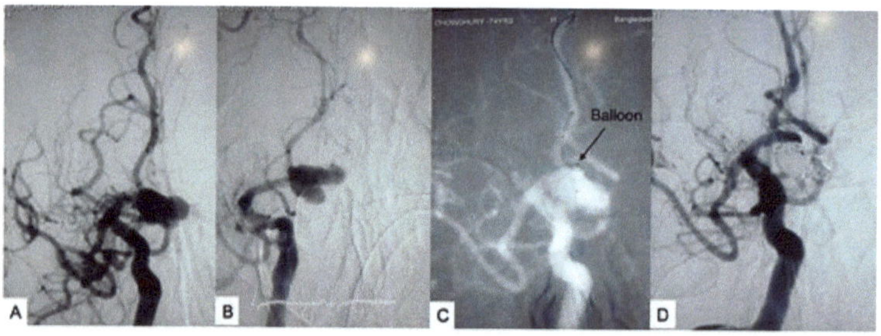

Figure 4. Balloon-assisted coiling of an ACOM aneurysm. (**A**,**B**) DAS before coiling showing a complex ACOM aneurysm and ACOM complex; (**C**) road map after the placement of a balloon, (**D**) after coil embolization. Source: Figure by authors.

When compared to standard coiling, BAC has more procedural complications (Sluzewski et al. 2006). This group had greater rates of thromboembolic events, including intraoperative rupture, 9.8% and 4.0%, respectively, than the coiling alone subgroup, which had 2.2% and 0.8%, respectively (Pierot et al. 2009; Pierot et al. 2011). Treatment morbidity in the coiling group was 3.9% compared to 2.5% in the BAC group, while treatment mortality was 1.2% in the coiling group and 1.3% in the BAC group. The impact of BAC on anatomic outcomes is still unknown (Pierot and Wakhloo 2013).

BAC has a higher incidence of incomplete aneurysm occlusion (27.7%) than normal coiling (16.9%); retreatment is also more common in BAC (16.9% versus 9.0% for standard coiling) (Sluzewski et al. 2006). In one series, 73% of cases in the BAC group and 49% of those managed with coiling alone had complete blockage (Pierot and Wakhloo 2013; Shapiro et al. 2008). Balloon-assisted coil embolization was originally designed to treat wide-neck aneurysms; however, it can also be employed in cases of an intraoperative burst, where the balloon aid may be linked to a higher likelihood of a similar or better clinical result than traditional coiling (Santillan et al. 2012). A balloon aid should be utilized not only to facilitate coiling, but also as a sentinel in the event of a preoperative rupture. The balloon remains deflated over the aneurysm's neck; it is solely inflated in the event of an intraprocedural rupture (Pierot and Wakhloo 2013).

2.3. *Stent-Assisted Coiling*

Some difficult aneurysms, such as broad-neck aneurysms, massive and giant aneurysms, as well as fusiform aneurysms, are managed by stent-assisted coiling (SAC) (Figure 5) (Wakhloo et al. 1998, 2008; Mericle et al. 1998; Lanzino et al. 1998).

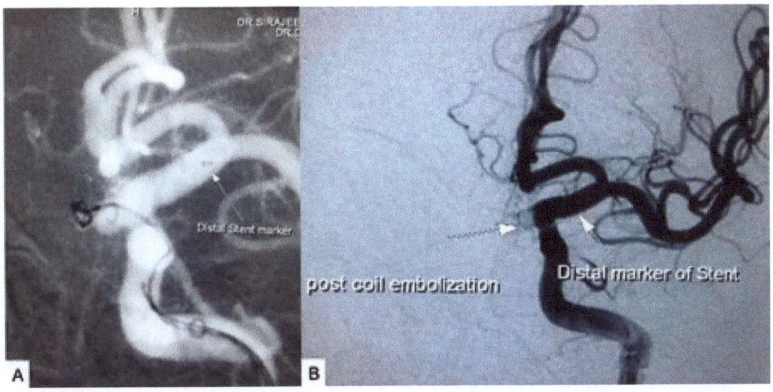

Figure 5. Stent-assisted coiling of an ICA aneurysm. (**A**) Stent-assisted placement of the coil in an aneurysm; (**B**) after coil embolization. Source: Figure by authors.

In the beginning, due to the unavailability of stents definably devised for the endovascular therapy, tough coronary stents were utilized. Eventually, numerous stents devoted to the management of IAs became accessible, making treatment much more effective. Another intriguing advance is the creation of low-profile stents, which allow for BAC and SAC to be combined (Kadziolka et al. 2013).

SACs were also employed as a last resort in the event of coil herniation or coil migration into the main vascular lumen. As stents are used to bridge the aneurysm neck in the main artery, the chance of a stent thrombosis is more than with coiling alone. Antiplatelet therapy is therefore required both before and after surgery. SACs were first limited to aneurysms that had not ruptured. Despite this, stenting has been performed in burst aneurysms according to experience (Pierot and Wakhloo 2013).

An option for preventing aneurysm recanalization was stenting. This, in turn, contributed to an increase in the usage of SACs. The safety and effectiveness of SACs in comparison to normal coiling remain unknown. SACs were linked to a greater prevalence of irreversible neurological problems (7.4%) when compared to normal coiling (3.8%) in a study ($p = 0.644$). The procedure-related death rate was 4.6% in the stenting group versus 1.2% in the non-stenting group ($p = 0.006$). In 50% of the patients, follow-up was available, and angiographic reappearance was substantially higher in the non-stenting group (33.5%) than in the stenting group (14.9%; $p = 0.0001$) (Piotin et al. 2010).

According to a review by Shapiro et al. (2012), the total complication rate was 19%, with a fatality rate of 2.1%. In 10% and 2.2% of cases, respectively, thromboembolic and hemorrhagic consequences were found. In 9% of the instances, there were technical problems related to stenting. Of the aneurysms, 45% were quickly and totally occluded after stenting. The occlusion rate climbed to 61% on follow-up angiograms, with stent stenosis or stent occlusion occurring in 3.5% and 0.6% of cases, respectively. In spite of the increasing risk of thromboembolic events and hemorrhage, the literature analysis found that stents could be utilized in conjunction with coiling to enhance the speed of a full occlusion in a subset of more complicated aneurysms (Pierot and Wakhloo 2013). Complications associated with SACs are pre-procedural complications, death, recanalization, in-stent stenosis, stent migration and a delayed infarction (Pierot and Wakhloo 2013; Lee et al. 2013).

SACs are commonly used to treat ruptured aneurysms (Wakhloo et al. 2012). A literature review on SACs for ruptured IAs found that they had a greater technical success rate (93%) but also had a higher incidence of clinically significant cerebral bleeding (up to 11%) and thrombosis (6%). A total of 14% of patients had bad outcomes, with up to 19% of them dying (Pierot and Wakhloo 2013; Bodily et al. 2011).

SACs have made more difficult aneurysms more treatable, with a decreased rate of recanalization and retreatment. However, the risk of bleeding and thromboembolism during the procedure, particularly in ruptured aneurysms, is higher than with normal coiling (Pierot and Wakhloo 2013).

2.4. Flow Diversion

A new armamentarium for aneurysm treatment flow diverters (FDs) was introduced in 2007 (Pierot and Wakhloo 2013). FDs (Figure 6) are low-porosity tubular stent-like endovascular devices which have two principal mechanisms of function (Pierot and Wakhloo 2013):

1. Flow redirection: It covers the aneurysm neck that decreases flow into the aneurysm sac by enhancing the resistance caused by the implant's mesh, while still enabling blood to flow through nearby perforators as well as the side branches. As a result, the flow of blood is diverted away from the aneurysm sac and toward the distal parent artery. Aneurysmal thrombosis is caused by a decrease in blood flow within the aneurysm sac, which causes circulatory stagnation.
2. Tissue overgrowth: The FD acts as a scaffold or framework for the neo-endothelialization of the aneurysm neck.

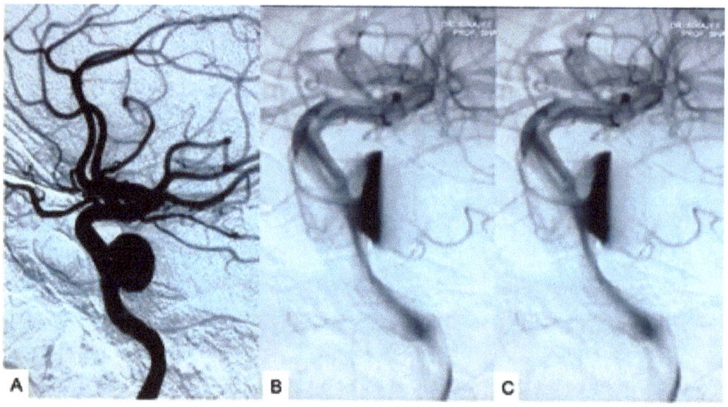

Figure 6. Flow diversion in a case of a cavernous segment ICA aneurysm. (**A**) Before the deployment of a flow diverter; (**B**,**C**) after the deployment of a flow diverter in a cavernous segment of the ICA. Source: Figure by authors.

FDs have been shown to be safe and efficacious in the management of aneurysms in preclinical investigations (Kallmes et al. 2007; Sadasivan et al. 2009).

The majority of preliminary clinical studies with FDs were described in small single-center or multicenter retrospective groups (Lylyk et al. 2009; Szikora et al. 2010; Byrne et al. 2010; Lubicz et al. 2010; Berge et al. 2012). The findings showed that treating a brain aneurysm is quite feasible, with tolerable periprocedural complications, low morbidity and fatality rates, and pleasing efficacy. These findings have recently been bolstered by substantial prospective and retrospective single-center and multicenter investigations (Kan et al. 2012; Piano et al. 2013; O'Kelly et al. 2013). Complex aneurysms, such as fusiform aneurysms, massive and giant aneurysms, broad-neck aneurysms and recurrent aneurysms after earlier coiling, are treated by flow diversion.

A recent prospective study employed in the management of complicated aneurysms found that FD has high effectiveness and a good safety profile. In 108 patients, this study treated massive and enormous, broad-necked aneurysms in the intracranial ICA. The procedure was technically possible in 99.1% of cases, with satisfactory safety, as well as high effectivity (73.6% of aneurysms fulfilled the study's combined primary efficacy end objective of full closure at day 180 sans severe constriction of the parent channel; no supplementary coils were utilized) (5.6% of cases had a major same-sided infarct or death, which was the primary safety limit point) (Pierot and Wakhloo 2013; Becske et al. 2013).

Although the indications for FDs are still being worked out, it appears that FDs are most commonly utilized in big and giant aneurysms (along with fusiform aneurysms), multiple aneurysms within a segmental sick artery, wide-neck aneurysms and recurring aneurysms. As double antiplatelet therapy is required, the majority of aneurysms managed are unruptured. Flow diversion treatment, on the other hand, is effective in aneurysms that are too small to be treated with traditional coiling, such as blister-like aneurysms (Kulcsár et al. 2010).

More patient information on potential problems is becoming accessible as the use of FDs becomes more popular. Thromboembolic events and intraprocedural bursts are possible with any EVT of aneurysms. Although there is a lower chance of intraprocedural rupture due to the absence of endosaccular manipulations, the chance of thromboembolism is higher than with normal coiling or BAC. Preoperative and postoperative dual (usually) antiplatelet therapy is recommended to prevent thromboembolic events (Pierot and Wakhloo 2013).

It is worth noting that the majority of FD-related problems have occurred in giant and large aneurysms with a high natural risk of hemorrhage, that are otherwise endovascularly untreatable. Aneurysms rupture close after FD deployment in 1.0% of patients (Kulcsár and Szikora 2012). To prevent late rupture in FDs, especially in giant and large aneurysms, a few coils can be placed in the aneurysm sac before deployment of an FD, and steroids can be used after aneurysm treatment. Delayed ipsilateral parenchymal hemorrhage is another potentially lethal complication. The incidence is not exactly known, but Cruz et al. reported an 8.5% incidence (Cruz et al. 2012). Another important concerning issue of FDs is the patency of the perforators and side arterial branches covered by the implant. The migration of FDs is another rare concern. After the application of FDs, perforators can be occluded, resulting in deep infraction contributing to mortality and morbidity (Kulcsár et al. 2010). Late thrombosis of FDs can occur during the post-treatment period, and so, long-term follow-up is necessary (Fiorella et al. 2010; Kulcsár and Szikora 2012). The long-term results of FDs are yet to be known.

2.5. *Flow Disruption*

Intrasaccular flow disruption is an endovascular implant similar to intraluminal flow disruption, except that the mesh of the flow disruptor is positioned within the aneurysm pouch, causing blood flow stagnation and thrombosis.

Preclinical trials demonstrated the technique's practicality, as well as its efficacy and safety (Ding et al. 2011). The technical success of the treatment was high (100.0%) in a retrospective, preliminary, multicenter small series managed with the flow disruption device, with no death and low morbidity (4.8%) (Pierot et al. 2012e). This can be utilized to treat the basilar artery, middle cerebral artery, anterior communicating artery and ICA bifurcation aneurysms with a wide neck (Pierot et al. 2013). Antiplatelet therapy is not required because the flow disruptor implant is put entirely within the aneurysm, although the risk of a intraoperative burst is increased (Pierot and Wakhloo 2013). There is still a lot to learn about flow disruption.

2.6. *Embolization with Liquid Embolic Agents*

Liquid embolic agents have been investigated as a therapy for IAs. Onyx (Covidien/EV3, Irvine, CA) was the product with the most significant development, as well as the most extensive clinical evaluation (Molyneux et al. 2004). The product is gradually administered into the aneurysm sac under the supervision of a remodeling balloon, filling the aneurysm from the fundus to the neck. The preliminary results with uncoilable IAs were satisfactory, with good effectiveness and safety (Molyneux et al. 2004). However, rising safety issues (mass effect of giant and big IAs grew following filling with Onyx, stenosis of the parent vessel due to Onyx leaks) stunted the technique's expansion (Carlson et al. 2013).

In summary, various endovascular alternatives for the management of IAs are now available, including normal coiling, SAC, BAC and flow diversion. To preclude re-hemorrhage and subsequent complications linked to an SAH-related hydrocephalus and vasospasm, ruptured aneurysms must be treated on an emergency basis. Standard coiling or BAC is still used to treat ruptured aneurysms. Currently, flow disruption has not been adequately tested for emergency use. These procedures should not be utilized in burst aneurysms, since antiplatelet is required following SAC and flow diversion. Unruptured aneurysm treatment indications should be explored and reviewed on a case-by-case approach, taking into account clinical presentation, patient age and comorbidities, as well as aneurysm size and location. Treatment with normal coiling or BAC is usually appropriate for minor aneurysms with small necks, while SAC and FDs are rarely used unless aneurysms are threatening to recur. Due to the possibly high rate of recanalization in giant and large, wide-neck and fusiform aneurysms, more comprehensive treatment, comprising SAC, flow diversion and flow disruption, should be used. More sophisticated devices and procedures have been developed as a result of scientific advancements in neuroimaging and device manufacturing, allowing for EVT to treat cerebral aneurysms that were previously believed to be untreatable by EVT. To assess the efficacy and safety of numerous upcoming new technologies, randomized trials will be required for the treatment of aneurysms in the brain (Pierot et al. 2012a; Pierot and Wakhloo 2013).

3. Carotid Atherosclerotic Stenosis and Stenting

The details of carotid artery stenosis are discussed in Chapter 10. Carotid artery stenting (CAS) (Figures 7–9) is an endovascular treatment that involves placing a stent within the artery's lumen to alleviate stenosis and minimize the risk of an ischemic stroke. When carotid endarterectomy (CEA) is deemed too dangerous, CAS is utilized to address the carotid artery stenosis in high-risk cases.

Carotid stenting is used to reduce the risk of an ischemic stroke caused by stenosis of the carotid artery. Carotid stenosis can be painless or cause symptoms (TIAs or strokes).

While CEA has traditionally been the treatment of choice for carotid stenosis, stenting provides an option for people who are not surgical candidates. When there are a lot of CEA risk factors, stenting is recommended instead. Medical comorbidities (severe lung disease, severe cardiac disease, cardiac failure) and anatomic attributes (opposite carotid occlusion, neck radiation therapy, prior same-sided carotid artery surgery, intracranial or intra-thoracic carotid disease) are all risk factors that can make CEA more difficult and dangerous (Gurm et al. 2008).

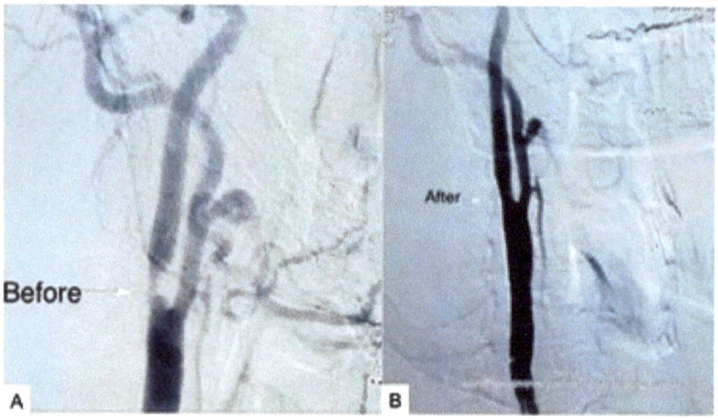

Figure 7. Initial segment of ICA stenting in severe carotid stenosis. (**A**) Before stenting; (**B**) after stenting. Source: Figure by authors.

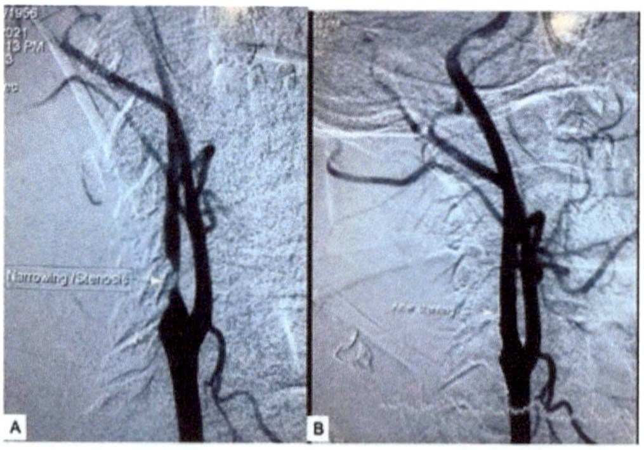

Figure 8. Initial segment of ICA stenting in severe carotid stenosis. (**A**) Before stenting; (**B**) after stenting. Source: Figure by authors.

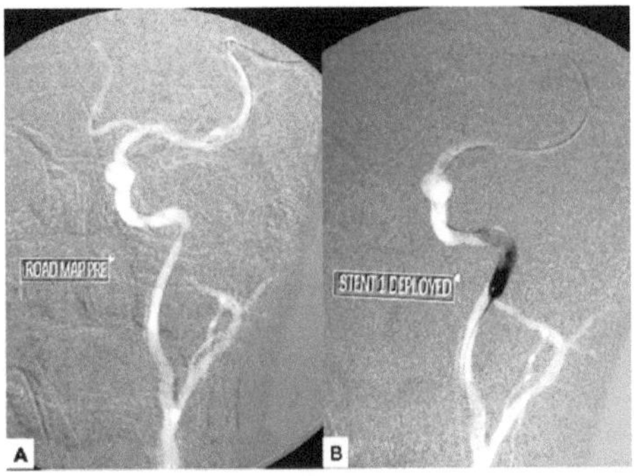

Figure 9. ICA stenting for stenosis at the junction of the cervical and petrous part of the ICA. (**A**) Road map of stent placement across the stenosis; (**B**) stent deployment with dilatation of stenosis. Source: Figure by authors.

Precaution: Although death and stroke following both CEA and CAS are low, the rates of death and stroke after a CAS may be higher than after a CEA, especially for a transfemoral route CAS in persons over 70 years of age (Bonati et al. 2012).

3.1. *Endovascular Techniques*

CAS is consistent with the placement of an intraarterial stent (https://en.wikipedia.org/wiki/Stent (accessed on 12 July 2021)) across arterial stenosis under general or local anesthesia.

CAS is commonly performed through the percutaneous femoral artery route. Critical steps include arterial access, passing of the guidewire across the stenosis, placing a stent across the stenosis and withdrawal of all the vascular access. The guide wire and sheath are progressed to the side to be treated through the femoral artery, external iliac artery, common iliac artery and the aorta. Other procedures, such as the utilization of a cerebral protection device (embolism protection device), pre/post-stent balloon angioplasty and cerebral DSA, may or may not be undertaken.

3.2. *Post-Procedural Outcomes*

Recovery after CAS is relatively simple provided there are no events. Patients typically stay in hospital for 0–1 day. The systolic blood pressure is kept under 140 mm of mercury. Reperfusion/hyperperfusion syndrome can be caused by high blood pressure in the early days after surgery.

The most concerning short-term consequence of any carotid artery stroke prevention operation is the occurrence of a stroke. Patients should be selected for CAS so that the procedure's "long-term risk prevention" is greater than the "short-term risk" of producing a stroke at the time of the surgery. Bleeding, infection and cardiac problems are among the other risks.

Recurrent stenosis/pseudoaneurysm development is a possible late consequence. It is necessary to follow up with a duplex ultrasonogram, CTA or MRA. When a patient has symptoms of carotid occlusive disease/stenosis (CEA/CAS), the risk reduction intervention is most effective—typically stroke or TIA (Paraskevas et al. 2009). For symptomatic individuals, there is inadequate evidence to say whether stenting or CEA is preferable. Asymptomatic carotid stenosis should only be treated in the background of randomized clinical trials (stenosis > 70%) (Derdeyn Colin 2007).

4. Intracranial Arterial Stenosis and Stenting

Intracranial arterial stenosis is a frequent etiology of ischemic strokes (middle cerebral artery, intradural ICA, anterior cerebral artery or intradural vertebrobasilar artery stenosis). At the end of 30 days, the stenting group had a 14.7% risk of an ischemic stroke or death compared to 5.8% in the medically managed group, and 23% in the stenting group compared to 15% in the medical group at a median follow-up of 32.4 months in the randomized multicenter study called Stenting and Aggressive Medical Management for the Prevention of Recurrent Stroke in Intracranial Stenosis (SAMMPRIS). The findings demonstrated that medical care is superior to endovascular stunting, and that intracranial arterial stenting has almost been phased out in recent years. In this series, 16 cases in the stenting group (7.1%) experienced a severe debilitating or fatal stroke within 30 days, primarily due to perioperative events, analogous to 4 cases in the medical group (1.8%). On the other hand, 5 cases (2.2%) in the stenting group, as well as 14 cases (6.2%) in the medical group experienced a debilitating or fatal stroke after 30 days, demonstrating that stenting has a significant advantage if periprocedural problems can be controlled or avoided. It is necessary to assess the role and result of intracranial stenting in the preclusion of debilitating or fatal stroke (Chimowitz et al. 2011; Yu and Jiang 2018).

5. Vertebral Artery (VA) Stenosis and Stenting

Patients with a recent symptomatic vertebrobasilar insufficiency/stenosis, similar to carotid artery stenosis, have a substantial risk of a recurrent ischemic stroke, with the risk being the highest in the first month (Payne 2001). Angioplasty and/or stenting can be used to treat stenosis of the vertebral artery (VA) (Figure 10). Stenting may be a good therapeutic approach according to one case series (Oshizumi et al. 2004; Eberhardt et al. 2006; Stayman et al. 2011). Stenting for extracranial VA stenosis has been linked with very few complication rates (1–1.5%) (Stayman et al. 2011), whereas intracranial stenosis is accompanied with higher hazards rates (7–10%) (Eberhardt et al. 2006). However, new randomized trial data have dampened the enthusiasm. In patients with an intracranial arteries stenosis, the Stenting and Aggressive Medical Management for Preventing Recurrent Stroke in Intracranial Stenosis (SAMMPRIS) trial found that stenting was worse than the best medical therapy (BMT) in preventing recurrent stroke (Chimowitz et al. 2011); there were, however, only a few patients with a VA stenosis (Lutsep et al. 2015).

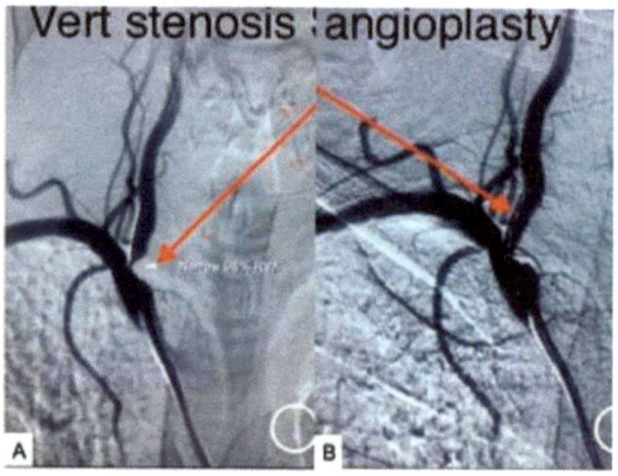

Figure 10. VA stenting at its origin. (**A**) Pre-stenting DSA; (**B**) after stent deployment. Source: Figure by authors.

6. Carotid–Cavernous Fistula (CCF)

The CCF (caroticocavernous fistula) (Figure 11) occurs due to a tear in the ICA, which permits it to develop a low-resistance, high-flow fistula with the cavernous sinus's venous system. A CCF can be direct or indirect (Barrow et al. 1985; Cohen and Rad 2004). Blood is diverted from the ICA into the cavernous sinus in a direct CCF (DCCF); in an indirect CCF (ICCF), there is a dural arteriovenous connection and a reduced flow rate. The details of a CCF are described in Chapter 15.

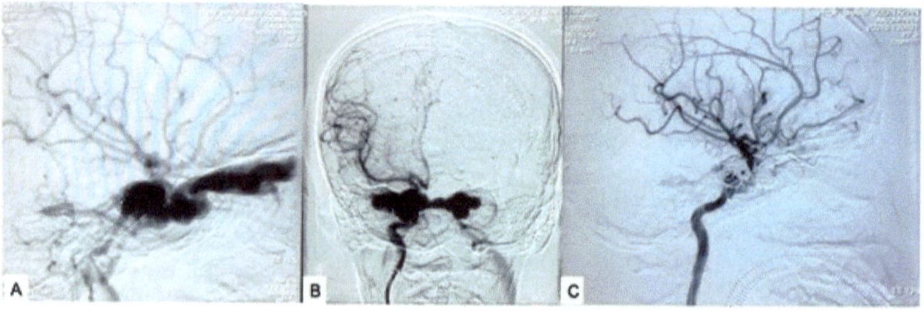

Figure 11. Direct CCF repair with endovascular coiling. (**A**,**B**) Pre-embolization; (**C**) after repair of the fistula with coils. Source: Figure by authors.

6.1. Classification

A CCF is divided into direct (Type A) or indirect (Types B–D) categories (Barrow et al. 1985; Cohen and Rad 2004; Henderson and Miller 2017):

Type A/direct: DCCF is a high-flow fistula between the ICA and cavernous sinus (CS):

(a) Traumatic (including iatrogenic): occurs in 0.2% of patients with traumatic head injury. Iatrogenic DCCF occurs following percutaneous trigeminal rhizotomy, an endovascular procedure.
(b) Spontaneous: ruptured cavernous sinus ICA aneurysm with connective tissue disorders.

Type B-D/Indirect: most ICCFs are shunts from dural arteries that are branches of the ICA/ECA:

Type B: from the dural branches of the ICA;
Type C: from the dural branches of the ECA;
Type D: from the dural branches of both the ICA and ECA.

6.2. Etiopathology with Mode of Presentation

The pressure difference in a DCCF causes flow reversal into the superior ophthalmic vein, as well as superficial middle cerebral vein and rapid diverting to the inferior petrosal sinus and pterygoid vein, resulting in a pulsating exophthalmos and orbital bruit, as well as visual changes, orbital pain and proptosis.

The majority of symptoms are unmistakably caused by arterialization of the CS with draining orbital veins. Venous congestion and hemorrhage coupled with headache, chemosis, vertigo, tinnitus and cranial nerve paralysis are some of the most prevalent complications.

In patients with a CCF, having arterial steal leads to cerebral hypoperfusion that causes focal neurological impairments.

6.3. Investigations: Evaluation

A CT–CTA or MRI–MRA of the head usually demonstrates proptosis, which is characterized by engorged and serpiginous intraorbital vessels, including the superior ophthalmic vein (best observed on T2WI coronals) and convexity of the lateral wall of the cavernous sinus.

A DSA shows diversion of blood from the ICA into the CS. Quick opacification of the petrosal sinus and/or ophthalmic vein may be seen.

Mehringer–Hieshima maneuver: injection of contrast at a rate of 2–3 mL/s into diseased carotid while compressing the cervical carotid artery (down to the catheter tip) to control flow to help demonstrate the fistula.

Huber maneuver: lateral view, inject VA and compress the affected carotid artery. It aids in detecting the upper limit of the fistula, many fistulous openings and the total transection of the ICA (Henderson and Miller 2017; Morris 2007).

6.4. Treatment

The patient's stability, the anatomy of the fistula and the hemodynamics of the system all play a role in CCF management. Management should ideally work on repairing or obliterating the tear or connection while maintaining flow through the ICA (Fiorella et al. 2008). Total blockage of the artery may be required in some cases. Because 20–50% of low-flow CCFs thrombose spontaneously, they can be observed as long as visual acuity is constant and intraocular pressure is less than 25. High-flow CCFs that are symptomatic (e.g., gradual vision degradation) seldom thrombose spontaneously, and therapy is generally required. Parkinson reported a straightforward surgical repair of a traumatic CCF while keeping the ICA intact in 1973. While any treatment in this anatomic area is difficult, open surgical repair in the acute environment amid probable polytrauma in patients carries a high risk of morbidity; hence, endovascular closure is the preferred option if the patient can tolerate it (Henderson and Miller 2017; Geibprasert et al. 2009).

6.4.1. Endovascular Treatment

The goal of treatment is eliminating the fistula.

A cerebral DSA is used to detect the precise size and location, as well as its venous drainage of the fistula. Angiography with 7.5 frames per second should be considered instead of the normal 2–4 frames per second to handle the excessive flow. Any vascular injuries/anomalies in addition to the CCF should be looked for. Both

ECAs and ICAs are catheterized selectively to measure their role in the CCF. To better measure the cross-flow from the contralateral side, angiography is conducted after physical compression of the CCA on the side of the fistula. The excessive blood circulation to the fistula will be reduced by digital compression, allowing for viewing of the fistula.

Rotational angiography with 3D reformatting may be performed to study the fistula and select proper working views for the interventional procedure. The CS, inferior and superior ophthalmic veins, sphenoparietal sinus, superior and inferior petrosal sinuses, and pterygoid plexus are all key venous involvements to be aware of.

The following routes may be utilized for managing CCFs: transarterial, transvenous and superior ophthalmic vein.

Coils: The ideal route is the transarterial coil embolization of CCFs. Utilizing road mapping, the microcatheter is moved over the microware into the CS via the fistula. Coils are then deployed and detached. Periodic angiography is performed and further coils placed. Complete occlusion is indicated by no further contrast entering the CS.

Onyx: In case of a high-flow fistula, prior to Onyx deposition, it may be recommended to deposit coils into the CS initially to slow down the blood flow. A balloon can be inflated within the parent ICA to protect it.

NBCA: To prevent undesired deposits in the venous sinuses, an NBCA should be used with extreme caution, especially after slowing the flow through the CCF. A balloon may be placed in the parent artery to safeguard it.

Stents: Stents provide the required parent vessel protection by acting as a non-occlusive scaffold along the ostium of the fistula. A self-expanding, flexible stent is utilized in the pipeline embolization procedure. Covered stents can be utilized instead of coils and balloon-assisted or stent insertion. The possible tortuosity of the vasculature plus the stiffness of the stent occludes any small arteries in the vicinity, which is one of the key obstacles in the proper delivery as well as deployment of covered stents.

Balloons: Type A CCFs can be repaired using a removable balloon occlusion. Low cost, easy navigation to the fistula, and the capability to intermittently inflate and deflate the balloon permit for the constant appraisal of the fistula anatomy as advantages of the balloon.

Choice of Technique

With indirect fistulas, it is mandatory to place coils on the side of venous (otherwise new feeders will be recruited). Coils or clips may be used to occlude direct fistulas (Henderson and Miller 2017; Fiorella et al. 2008; Geibprasert et al. 2009; Chalouhi et al. 2012).

7. Cranial Dural Arteriovenous Fistulas (DAVFs)

7.1. Introduction

A DAVF (Figure 12) is a vascular pathology in which an arterio-venous shunt is within the two layers of the dura mater. Multiple branches of the ICA/ECA or vertebral arteries create direct communication with the venous sinus and/ or cerebral veins. They are considered acquired rather than congenital lesions. Lesions leading the arterialization of intradural veins (leptomeningeal cortical vein) are linked with an ICH. Multiple fistulas may be found in up to 8% of cases. They are usually found adjacent to the dural venous sinuses. The details, including the Borden and Cognard classification of cranial AV fistula is discussed in Chapter 14.

7.2. Common Locations

- Transverse/sigmoid: the most common (63% of cases) with a slight left-sided predominance (Baharvahdat et al. 2020), with the epicenter of these almost invariably at the junctional site of the transverse and sigmoid sinuses (Figure 12);
- Tentorial/petrosal;
- Anterior fossa/ethmoidal;
- Middle fossa/Sylvian;
- Cavernous sinus (carotid–cavernous fistula—CCF);
- Superior sagittal sinus;
- Foramen magnum (Intracranial Dural Arteriovenous Fistula 2021).

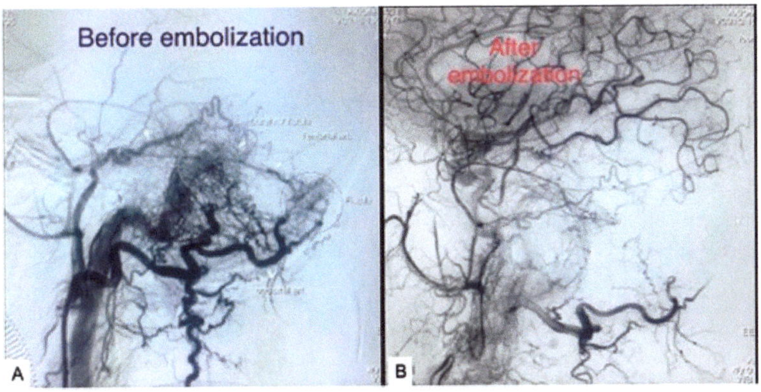

Figure 12. Sigmoid sinus dural AVF. (**A**) Before embolization; (**B**) after embolization. Source: Figure by authors.

7.3. Epidemiology

DAVFs constitute 10–15% of all intracranial AVMs. Of the patients, 61–66% occur in females, and patients are usually in their 40s or 50s. They can occur seldom in children. When they occur, they tend to be more complex, bilateral dural sinus malformations (Baharvahdat et al. 2020; Graeb and Dolman 1986; Arnautovic and Krisht 2000; Ashour et al. 2012).

7.4. Clinical Features

Pulsatile tinnitus is the most common presenting symptom of a DAVF. Cortical venous drainage with possible venous hypertension can produce IC-HTN, and this is the most common cause of mortality and morbidity, and thus the robust indication for DAVF management. DAVFs may also cause global cerebral edema or hydrocephalus due to impaired cerebral venous drainage or by disturbed function of the arachnoid granulations, respectively. Other DAVF symptoms/signs include headaches, seizures, cranial nerve palsies and orbital venous congestion (Intracranial Dural Arteriovenous Fistula 2021; Baharvahdat et al. 2020).

7.5. Natural History and Risk of Hemorrhage

The concept of a benign vs. aggressive DAVF behavior depends on the presence or absence of cortical venous drainage. Data reported by the University of Toronto group over a 3-year period show that 98% of benign lesions (no cortical venous drainage) remained benign (Intracranial Dural Arteriovenous Fistula 2021; Davies et al. 1997). On the other hand, over a 4-year period, the annual hemorrhage rates, non-hemorrhagic neuro-deficit and mortality were 8.1%, 6.9% and 10.4% for aggressive fistulas (with cortical venous drainage) (Intracranial Dural Arteriovenous Fistula 2021; van Dijk et al. 2002). In a meta-analysis of 377 cases (Ashour et al. 2012), three DAVF locations were associated with particularly aggressive behavior (aggressive: benign ratio): tentorial (31:1), middle fossa/Sylvian (2.5:1), anterior fossa/ethmoidal (2.1:1). Most Borden Type I lesions or Cognard Type I and IIa are benign lesion, whereas higher-grade fistulas are dangerous (Intracranial Dural Arteriovenous Fistula 2021).

7.6. Investigation: Evaluation

A brain CT or MRI without contrast is often normal.

A CTA may reveal dilated and tortuous vessels corresponding to enlarged arterial supplier or ectatic draining veins.

An MRA may show dilated and engorged pial vessels, early distinctive venous sinus filling, sinus engorgement or occlusion and white matter edema due to venous hypertension.

DSA: Full six-vessel cerebral angiography (bilateral ICAs, bilateral ECAs and bilateral vertebral arteries) is required to reach the diagnosis and plan the treatment.

DAVFs with angiographic findings include the following:

A selective DSA shows prolong cerebral circulation time. This occurs in venous congestive encephalopathy.

Pseudo phlebitis pattern: The cerebral surface shows the tortuous and dilated collateral veins in the venous phase of the DSA. This finding is connected with a higher risk of hemorrhage or neuro-deficits of non-hemorrhagic origin.

Cortical venous reflux (CVR): To confirm that this is not omitted, a selective (rather than non-selective, global) DSA should always be performed when investigating a DAVF. A venous obstruction or stenosis is frequently seen in patients with CVR.

Several classification systems have been published to characterize DAVFs.

The Borden and Cognard systems are the most commonly utilized grading systems. Cortical venous drainage is the definite angiographic feature that distinguishes benign (low-grade) from aggressive (high-grade) fistulas (Intracranial Dural Arteriovenous Fistula 2021; Baharvahdat et al. 2020). (Borden I, Cognard I and Cognard IIa are low-grade; all others are high-grade.)

7.7. *Treatments*

Management options:

Conservative;
Endovascular;
Microsurgery;
Radiosurgery;
Any combination of surgery, endovascular and radiosurgery.

An AVF with cortical venous drainage should usually be treated. Lesions without cortical venous drainage should be followed radiographically and clinically (2% may evolve to develop cortical venous drainage). An alteration in a bruit (either disappearance or worsening) should be reinvestigated. Here, endovascular options are discussed.

Indications for intervention:

1. Presence of cortical venous drainage;
2. Neurologic dysfunction;
3. Hemorrhage;
4. Orbital venous congestion;
5. Refractory symptoms (headache, pulsatile tinnitus) (Intracranial Dural Arteriovenous Fistula 2021; Baharvahdat et al. 2020; Arnautovic and Krisht 2000; Ashour et al. 2012; Davies et al. 1997).

7.7.1. DAVF Embolization

The approach (Figure 12) may be transvenous, transarterial or a combination. Whenever possible, a transvenous route is preferred, as the rate of fistula closures is higher through the transvenous route.

7.7.2. Transarterial Embolization

Transarterial embolization is classically utilized for (a) high-grade DAVFs, (b) direct cortical venous drainage, (c) situations where venous access is difficult or limited, (d) de novo DAVFs may occur at a secondary location after transvenous embolization, probably due to hypertension and (e) hazards related to the transvenous approach can be precluded (sixth nerve palsy from superior petrosal sinus catheterization).

7.7.3. Transvenous Embolization

The transvenous route is preferred when (a) the prime arterial supplier of a DAVF arises from the ICA or the vertebral artery, (b) possible extracranial-to-intracranial anastomoses sites are involved and (c) arterial supply to the cranial nerves is in danger.

Alternatively, in lieu of performing a total occlusion, partial treatment can be considered only such that CVR is ruled out, turning the fistula into the Borden type I (benign).

When utilizing the venous route, it should be ensured that the venous path is not tenuous (e.g., acute DAVF), making it vulnerable to rupture during catheter handling.

Coils: The right-sized coils according to the maximum diameter of the fistulous spot to be occluded should be selected. As many coils as necessary to close the fistula should be installed. A "combination" method may be performed, in which coils are deposited first to decrease the rapid blood circulation via the fistula, then a liquid embolic agent is used to close the fistula. A microcatheter compliant with the liquid embolic agent if this method is used should be used.

Onyx: During transarterial embolization with liquid embolic agents, the microcatheter should be kept as near as possible to the fistula. It is important to disrupt the fistulous connection to achieve cure. Therefore, Onyx must penetrate into the venous side of the DAVF.

nBCA: It is used less commonly after the availability of Onyx.

The other modalities of treatments are manual carotid self-compression, surgery and stereotactic radiosurgery.

The therapy of choice for DAVFs is endovascular management. A transarterial or transvenous technique is one of the many alternatives available. Coils, Onyx and n-BCA are just a few of the embolizing agents that can be used.

8. Cranial Arterio-Venous Malformation (AVM)

8.1. Introduction

An irregular grouping of blood vessels occurs when arterial blood travels straight into the draining veins passing through the typical capillary beds in between. No parenchyma remains within the nidus. AVMs are generally congenital lesions that tend to increase in size somewhat with age and frequently turn from low-flow juvenile lesions at birth to medium-to-high-flow high-pressure AVMs in adulthood (Frosting 2003). Cerebral AVMs are also discussed in Chapter 13.

8.2. Anatomy

They are made up of a tangled web of afferent feeding arteries, as well as draining veins connected by an irregular intervening capillary bed called the nidus that may or may not have straight arteriovenous shunts. A compact nidus, which forms a tumor-like well-circumscribed system, and diffuse nidus, which has sparse, aberrant AV channels scattered across normal brain tissue, can be more or less distinguished.

One or more feeding arteries are possible. They might be somewhat enlarged or have a nearly normal lumen. High flow can cause the following:

(a) Saccular aneurysms at the plane of the circle of Willis, the feeding arteries or the nidus.
(b) High-flow (angiopathy) with increasing stenosis and ultimate occlusion of the supplying arteries. Draining veins might be single or many, deep or cortical. The dilation and tortuosity of the affected veins are caused by direct shunting of blood at high pressure. High flow can also cause localized stenosis and secondary venous aneurysmal dilatation, especially when the veins pass through the dura to enter the sinus (Frosting 2003).

They may be divided as follows (Chaloupka and Huddle 1998):

1. Parenchymal AVMs (mentioned below). Sub-classified as:
    (a) Paraventricular;
    (b) Subcortical;
    (c) Pial;
    (d) Combined.
2. Pure dural AVM.
3. Mixed parenchymal and dural (rare).

AVM-related syndromes include Sturge–Weber, Rendu–Osler–Weber, Klippel–Trenaunay, Wyburn–Mason, Parks–Weber etc.

8.3. Etiopathogenesis

Congenital vascular abnormalities characterized by improper direct connections between venous and arterial systems are hypothesized to be the cause of cerebral AVMs (Mullan et al. 1996; van Beijnum et al. 2007).

Although the precise embryological genesis is uncertain, both the maintenance of a basic arteriovenous link and its development before or after delivery have been hypothesized (Fleetwood and Steinberg 2002).

8.4. Epidemiology

There is hardly any information in the published literature about the incidence of AVMs, or the percentage of a population with an AVM diagnosis at any given period. Because of the disease's rarity and the presence of symptomless patients, determining a real prevalence estimate is hard and unlikely. A retrospective investigation in a Scottish region reported an incidence of AVMs of 15 per 100,000 live persons over the age of 16 years in unselected populations (Al-Shahi et al. 2002). Because asymptomatic AVMs are not included in this study, the prevalence is clearly underestimated.

8.5. Pathology

Cerebral AVMs consist of (a) aggregations and unusually muscularized feeders that may also have modifications such as doubling or damage of the elasticity, segmental thinning of the wall and fibrosis of the media; (b) arterialized veins of various sizes and wall thicknesses; (c) anatomically ambiguous vessels consisting of fibrous tissue only or showing both venous and arterial criteria; and (d) intervening gliotic tissue. They connect to a regular cerebral vessel by anastomosis (Frosting 2003).

8.6. Physiopathology and Biology

The pathophysiology of cerebral AVMs is uncertain; however, new research suggests that abnormal vasculogenesis or angiogenesis may have a role in their genesis and progression. Protein ligands bind and modulate the actions of transmembrane receptor tyrosine kinases, form and remodel blood vessels in both processes (Frosting 2003).

8.7. Natural History

Cerebral AVMs are diseases that are unaffected by significant anatomic changes over time. But, because AVMs are dynamic, they are subject to ongoing anatomic and hemodynamic changes. When the patient's ability to properly adapt has attained its limit, an AVM becomes symptomatic. They are most commonly clinically obvious in young individuals, especially those under the age of 40 years. The evolutionary history of cerebral AVMs rarely includes expansion, reduction or regression anatomically. The spontaneous obliteration of AVMs in the brain is extremely unusual. The following factors aid in AVM thrombosis regression:

- The AVM's anatomy;
- Surgical treatment of the AVM;
- Squeezing of the AVM by a neighboring mass (such as a hematoma).

In most cases, an AVM nidus thrombosis is caused by an intracerebral or SAH. In this situation, the blood clot's mass effect may change the dynamic of the AVM and reduce blood circulation, most likely by compressing draining veins to the point of thrombosis. Surgical intervention, such as the removal of a blood clot or the implantation of a shunt, has been connected to the regression of AVMs, which is understandable given the compression of the veins caused by hemorrhage or edema. It is also possible that spontaneous regression occurs.

The presence of a sole draining vein (84% of instances of spontaneous occlusion), a single arterial feeder (30%) and a small AVM nidus (less than 3 cm in 50% of cases) are all linked to a spontaneous occlusion of brain AVMs (Frosting 2003).

8.8. Clinical Features

8.8.1. General Information of Presentation

Hemorrhage (most common);

Seizures;

The mass effect: for example, trigeminal pain caused by a CPA AVM;

Stealth ischemia;

H/A: extremely unusual. AVMs have been linked to migraines in the past. Visual impairment (usually hemianopsia/quadrantanopsia) and H/A that are identical from migraine can be symptoms of occipital AVMs;

Bruit: this is especially true for dural AVMs;

A higher ICP;

Almost exclusively found in children, frequently with big midline AVMs draining into an expanded vein of Galen:

(a) Hydrocephalus and macrocephaly: As a result of constriction of the Sylvian aqueduct by an enlarged Galen vein or elevated venous pressure;
(b) Cardiomegaly with congestive cardiac failure;
(c) Prominence of the frontal veins (due to raised venous pressure) (Drake 1979; Kupersmith et al. 1996).

8.8.2. Hemorrhage

The peak age for rupture of a brain AVM is between 15 and 20 years. The reported morbidity and mortality from an AVM hemorrhage varies extensively. Approximately, it is 10% mortality and 30–50% morbidity (neuro-deficit) from each rupture.

Hemorrhage Location with AVMs

ICH (intraparenchymal): 82% (the most common site of hemorrhage).

Intraventricular hemorrhage:

(a) Usually happens in combination with an ICH due to rupture of the ICH into the ventricle;
(b) An intraventricular AVM may be indicated by a pure IVH (without an ICH).

Subarachnoid: SAH can also occur by the burst of a feeding artery aneurysm, which is prevalent with AVMs.

Subdural: this is a rare occurrence. It is possible that this is the genesis of a spontaneous SDH (Perret and Nishioka 1966; Hartmann et al. 1998).

Hemorrhage Rate Related to AVM Size

Small AVMs have the tendency to bleed more than large ones.

Larger AVMs are associated with seizure more frequently as they are more likely to engage the cerebral cortex because of their size. Small AVMs, on the other hand, have substantially higher pressure in the supplying arteries. As a result, smaller AVMs are more deadly than larger ones (Crawford et al. 1986; Spetzler et al. 1992).

Hemorrhage Rate in Relation to Spetzler–Martin Grade (Controversial)

Some studies have demonstrate a higher risk with Spetzler–Martin (S-M) grade 4–5 AVMs, while others show the opposite:

S-M grade 1–3: annual risk of bleeding is 3.5%;

S-M grade 4–5: hemorrhage is a 2.5% annual risk in S-M grade 4–5 (Jayaraman et al. 2007).

Yearly and Lifetime Risk of Hemorrhage and Re-Hemorrhage

An AVM has a 2–4% chance of causing bleeding on average. The risk of rebleeding in the first year after a hemorrhage was 6–14%, which declines to 2% per year after 10 years (Kondziolka et al. 1995).

Factors increasing the risk of bleeding (Frosting 2003; Kondziolka et al. 1995):

Anatomic Factors

(a) Feeding Vessels:
    Arterial aneurysms;
    Feeders from the ECA;
    Feeders by perforators and the vertebra-basilar system.
(b) Nidus:
    Size;
    Location;
    Angiogenesis.
(c) Venous Drainage:
    Venous stenosis.
    Deep venous drainage.
    Venous reflux;
    Solitary draining vein;
    Venous ectasia.

Hemodynamic Factors

Feeding artery pressures;
Draining vein pressures.

Factors decreasing the risk of bleeding (Frosting 2003):

1. Nidus—reduction in the pressure into the nidus:

(a) Arterial stenosis;
(b) Arterial angioectasia.

2. Arteriovenous fistulas.

Severity of the Hemorrhage

The rupture of cerebral AVMs (Frosting 2003; Hartmann et al. 1998) is less serious in comparison with that of aneurysms, with fatality rates of 10 to 15%, as well as overall morbidity rates of less than 50%. Subarachnoidal (30%), intraventricular (16%), parenchymal (23%) and mixed sites (31%) are the most common locations for cerebral AVM hemorrhages. A neurological deficiency is generally accompanied by parenchymal hemorrhages (52%). In general, 47% of cases had a positive outcome following the hemorrhage, and another 37% of cases were self-sufficient in their daily lives.

In truth, an AVM rupture is just as destructive as an aneurysm rupture. While an aneurysm rupture is more fatal than an AVM rupture (21% versus 9%), AVM ruptures have a lower success rate (49% versus 56%) as a result of the increased risk of a parenchymal hematoma.

8.8.3. Seizures

The younger the patient, greater the chance of experiencing seizures at the time of detection. Patients who arrive with bleeding have a 22% chance of having epilepsy in the next 20 years. No AVM discovered by chance or presenting with a neurological impairment develops seizures. Seizures are usually partial or partially complex in nature. Between 27% and 35% of patients experience generalized seizures. Seizures are more commonly related to cortical AVMs. Antiepileptic medicines are effective in controlling seizures in a large majority of instances (Ding et al. 2015; Lv et al. 2010).

8.8.4. Headache

In 7–48% (mean: 31%) of cases, the first symptom is a chronic headache (Mast et al. 1995). There is no recognized link between headache, migraine and AVMs. There are no characteristics that point to the diagnosis of an AVM, such as incidence, duration or severity.

8.8.5. Focal Neuro-Deficits

In 1–40% of cases, focal neurological impairments without bleeding are the first symptom. Focal neuro-deficiencies can be gradual, persistent or reversible in nature. The cause of reversible focal neurologic impairments is unclear, as a post-ictal origin may not be ruled out. Different hypotheses for the evolution of neurologic deficits exist: the mass effect, venous hypertension or steal phenomena are all terms for the same thing (Frosting 2003; Mast et al. 1995).

8.9. AVMs and Aneurysms

About 7% of cases with cerebral AVMs have associated aneurysms (Frosting 2003). Seventy five percent of them are situated on the major supplying artery.

These AVM-associated aneurysms may be classified as the following five types:

Type	Aneurysm location
I	Proximal to the ipsilateral main artery that feeds the AVM;
IA	Proximal to a large artery but on the opposite side of an AVM;
II	The superficial feeding artery is situated at the distal end of the artery;
III	On the deep feeding artery, proximal or distal ("bizarre");
IV	On a non-AVM artery; on draining veins or within the nidus, aneurysms can occur.

Symptomatic AVMs or aneurysms are usually addressed first when treating AVMs and aneurysms (whenever feasible, both should be treated simultaneously). If it is not evident which one bled, the aneurysm is most likely to be accountable, though the majority of AVM-related aneurysms will regress after the AVM is removed (66%).

8.10. Investigations and Evaluation

8.10.1. Aims of Neuro-Imaging

1. To reach the diagnosis of cerebral AVMs;
2. For pre-treatment assessment of brain AVMs (to abet in decision-making);
3. To manage brain AVMs as a only therapy or in combination with radiosurgery or surgery;
4. For post-treatment follow-up and evaluation.

8.10.2. CT and CTA of the Head

A CT scan of the head is the best neuroimaging to exclude acute hemorrhage and its types, i.e., parenchymal, subarachnoid and intraventricular. It can also show the calcifications within the pathology. When the patient is young, the parenchymal hematoma is lobar. The calcifications or spontaneously highly dense serpiginous formations (Vessels voids) are present and should be discussed.

The changed appearances of the ventricular system can be visualized:

- Effacement of the ventricular system due to the mass effect generated by the AVM;
- Focal dilatation in the case of concomitant parenchymal atrophy;
- Hydrocephalus can occur as a result of a prior hemorrhage or when the ventricular cavity is squeezed by the AVM's engorged drainage veins;
- A contrast CT scan may reveal enhancement within the arteries, as well as a sharpening of the nidus (Frosting 2003; Chaloupka and Huddle 1998; Spetzler and Martin 1986; Peschillo et al. 2014).

8.10.3. MRI and MRA of the Head

In unruptured AVMs or lobar hematomas, an MRI is frequently used days or weeks following the hemorrhage to look for the underlying pathology. Three levels of evaluation of the AVM can be obtained using a separate sequence of MRI images:

- Analytical sequences for anatomical analysis;
- MR angiography for vascular analysis and fMRI for functional analysis.

8.10.4. Anatomic Analysis of AVMs

T1, T2 and T1 with a gadolinium MRI can completely define the anatomic location and the size of the nidus. An MRI always defines anatomic localization better than angiography. As a result of the flow void phenomenon, the circulating vessels have no signal on T1W and T2W imaging. With traditional imaging sequences, portrayal of arterial feeders as well as draining veins is frequently unclear. An MRI is also a superior tool for showing the specific location of parenchymal lesions produced by an AVM. A current and earler hematoma can be seen using magnetic resonance imaging. A recent hematoma, on the other hand, may obscure a minor AVM, resulting in a false negative MR. Perinidal signal anomalies, notably hypersignal on T2W imaging, can be a marker of perinidal ischemia in the absence of blood. An MR can detect AVM-induced morphological alterations, as well as their parenchymal and ventricular consequences:

- Ventricular system dilatation due to parenchymal atrophy;
- Hydrocephalus in the case of an earlier hemorrhage or if the ventricular cavity is squeezed by engorged draining veins;
- Hydrocephalus in the case of a previous hemorrhage or whether the ventricular system is squeezed by engorged draining veins.

8.10.5. Vascular Analysis of Cerebral AVMs

Three-dimensional depictions of AVM architecture can be obtained by phase contrast and time-of-flight (TOF) techniques. Anatomic coverage and preciseness are the limitations of these techniques. The accurate size of the nidus cannot be calculated, intranidal aneurysms are not commonly visible, portrayal of the draining veins is not consistent, and small-caliber vessels and areas of sluggish blood circulation cannot be reliably seen. In addition, dynamic information cannot be obtained by these sequences. New gadolinium-contrasted MRAs are better than TOF MRAs, but still less demonstrating than DSA images for picturesque components of AVMs, as both temporal and spatial resolution are not available.

8.10.6. Functional Analysis of Brain AVMs

A perfusion PWI and diffusion DWI, apparent diffusion coefficient (ADC) imaging and bold sequences are all part of a functional MRI (fMRI). The nidus normally has a weak signal with a big and uniform increase in ADC. In AVMs, DWI and PWI have a small impact. The functional sections of the brain in an eloquent area AVM, especially the visual, sensorimotor and language areas, can be visualized with an fMRI. The use of bold sequences helps identify hemodynamic alteration in the cortex while performing a certain activity. A change in the activated cortex with common interhemispheric transmission is noted in most where AVMs are situated in the eloquent cortex.

8.10.7. Characteristics of a Cerebral AVM on MRI

- Increased intensity on partial flip-angle T1WI or T2WI within the AVM;
- Flow void on T1WI or T2WI within the AVM;
- Increased intensity on partial flip-angle T1WI or T2WI within the AVM;
- Flow void on T1WI or T2WI within the AVM;
- A significant amount of edema around the lesion could indicate a bleeding tumor rather than an AVM;
- A complete ring of low density (as a result hemosiderin) around the lesion alludes to an AVM over neoplasm on gradient echo sequences (GRASs);
- An entire ring of low density (as a result of hemosiderin) around the lesion alludes to an AVM over neoplasm on gradient echo sequences (GRASs) (Frosting 2003; Chaloupka and Huddle 1998; Spetzler and Martin 1986; Peschillo et al. 2014).

8.10.8. CT Angiography (CTA)/MR Angiography (MRA) Findings in a Brain AVM

On angiography, AVMs have the following characteristics:

- Large feeding artery;
- Angle of vessels;
- Draining veins are shown in the same pictures as the arteries (arterial phase);
- Large draining veins.

Angiography can detect most AVMs, but not all (Frosting 2003; Chaloupka and Huddle 1998; Spetzler and Martin 1986; Peschillo et al. 2014).

8.10.9. Selective and Super-Selective DSA

CTA and MRA are not adequate for an accurate description of the anatomic and hemodynamic features of an AVM. Functional and anatomical information that is therapeutically important must still be obtained through angiography. Injecting into the ICA, ECA and vertebral arteries is required for selective angiography. Multiple projections are used to analyze and gather data on arterial feeders, nidus and venous drainage (anteroposterior, lateral and oblique). A 3D DSA (three-dimensional DSA) could be useful. However, even a perfect DSA is frequently insufficient for making precise therapy judgments. Large feeding arteries may have a hazy architecture, whereas small feeding arteries may not be apparent on a selective DSA. Intranidal aneurysms and straight intranidal AV fistulas are frequently ignored, despite the fact that the extent of the nidus is usually well demonstrated by selective angiography. The venous drainage of the brain AVM is usually well received by a selective DSA, but as the AVM is injected as a whole, the compartments of the AVM, as well as their venous drainage are frequently not well understood. Because of these factors, super-selective angiography is frequently required for a more complete investigation of AVMs and may become increasingly relevant in decision-making. The manual injection of each particular artery feeder is used in super-selective angiography. It is usually the first step in the therapeutic embolization procedure (Frosting 2003; Chaloupka and Huddle 1998; Spetzler and Martin 1986; Peschillo et al. 2014).

8.11. Grading of Cranial AVM

8.11.1. Spetzler–Martin Grade of AVMs

Grade = sum of points from Table 1 ranges from 1 to 5. Untreatable AVMs (by any means: surgery, SRS, etc.) are assigned a distinct grade 6, since excision would almost always result in a debilitating deficiency or death. This scale has been shown to have good prognostic predictability. It may not be applicable to pediatrics

(AVMs are immature and change with time; AVMs mature at ≈age 18 years and tend to become more compact). Spetzler–Martin Grading of AVM with Supplementary grading is shown in Table 1.

Table 1. Grading of AVMs.

Spetzler–Martin Grading	Points	Supplementary Grading
Size		**Age, years**
<3 cm	1	Less than 20
3–6 cm	2	20–40
>6 cm	3	More than 40
Venous drainage		**Hemorrhage**
Superficial	0	Yes
Deep	1	No
Eloquent brain		**Compactness**
Non-eloquent	0	Yes
Eloquent	1	No
Total Grade	5	

Note: Sensorimotor, language, visual cortex, hypothalamus, thalamus, internal capsule, brain stem, cerebellar nuclei, cerebellar peduncles or regions directly adjacent to these structures are eloquent brain. Source: Authors' compilation based on data from Spetzler et al. (2015) and Spetzler and Martin (1986).

Size: On non-magnified angiography, the largest nidus diameter measured is related to (and therefore implicitly includes other factors relating to) the hardship of AVM excision, e.g., number of feeders, severity of steal, etc.

Eloquence (eloquent brain): This includes the language, sensorimotor and visual areas; thalamus and hypothalamus; internal capsule; brainstem; deep cerebellar nuclei; cerebellar peduncles.

Venous Drainage: If all venous drainage occurs via the cortical venous system, it is called superficial; if any or all drainage is through deep veins, it is considered deep (e.g., internal cerebral vein (great cerebral vein), basal vein of Rosenthal or pre-central cerebellar vein).

8.11.2. Outcome Based on Spetzler–Martin Grade

Spetzler published a three-tiered management recommendation scheme as follows:

Class A (S–M Grade I & II): surgical excision;

Class B (S–M Grade III): multimodality management;

Class C (S–M Grades IV and V): follow clinically and repeat angiogram every 5 years.

Treatment is only for progressive neurologic deficit, steal-related symptoms or aneurysms identified on surveillance angiograms.

8.12. Treatments

8.12.1. Microsurgical Treatment

Whenever possible, the gold standard in cerebral AVM treatment is microsurgery. When microsurgery is accomplished by skilled vascular neurosurgeons, an angiographic recovery with lower rates of morbidity and mortality (from 1% to 10%) can be accomplished for smaller (nidus 3 cm) AVMs in 94–100% of patients. For larger AVMs located in crucial or eloquent brain regions, these percentages vary greatly. Only 22% and 17% of AVMs of the IV and V grades of the Spetzler and Martin classifications can be cured by angiography, respectively. In cases of microsurgery, permanent neurological impairments or mortality occur in 7.4% of cases (range: 0–40%). In this study, an effective AVM occlusion was accomplished in 96% of instances (range: 0–100%) (Spetzler and Martin 1986). Microsurgery may be used as part of a multimodal management plan that includes endovascular surgery to decrease the nidus volume and treatment or mitigation of future vascular abnormalities. In most cases, vascular neurosurgeons desire selective embolization of deep arterial feeders on the flip side of the surgical field from their neuro-interventional colleagues, ideally using Onyx instead of glue to enhance surgical removal (Peschillo et al. 2014).

In circumstances where an AVM appeared to be inoperable earlier, a combination of surgery plus radiosurgery (Sanchez-Mejia et al. 2009) may be used. First, radiosurgery is used to shrink the AVM. Radiosurgery can also be utilized as a follow-up treatment following microsurgery.

Unprecedented advancements in the armamentarium of vascular neurosurgeons have significantly broadened the therapeutic choices available. The utilization of indocyanine green (ICG) during microsurgery allows for the visualization of residual AVM sections, resulting in better surgical outcomes (Killory et al. 2009). Furthermore, the advent of non-stick bipolar forceps has resulted in a significant technological advancement. The recent groundbreaking 3D implementations in microsurgery permit the real-time merging of MRA or MRI images with the microsurgical operation field, resulting in an additive role with other imaging devices such as navigation, DTI and tractography, as well as fMRI to further accelerate progress toward an upgraded understanding of the brain AVM anatomy and, as a result, superior microsurgical results (Peschillo et al. 2014).

8.12.2. Endovascular Therapy

Although the ultimate target of cerebral AVM treatment is the total occlusion of its nidus, this is not achievable or feasible all the time. An endovascular treatment (Figure 13) may be utilized in the following scenarios:

1. Embolization may be accomplished either before to surgery or radiosurgery;
2. To manage vascular anomalies with an AVM;
3. As a curative treatment;
4. In a palliation target (i.e., mitigation of blood circulation in steal symptoms) (Fiorella et al. 2006).

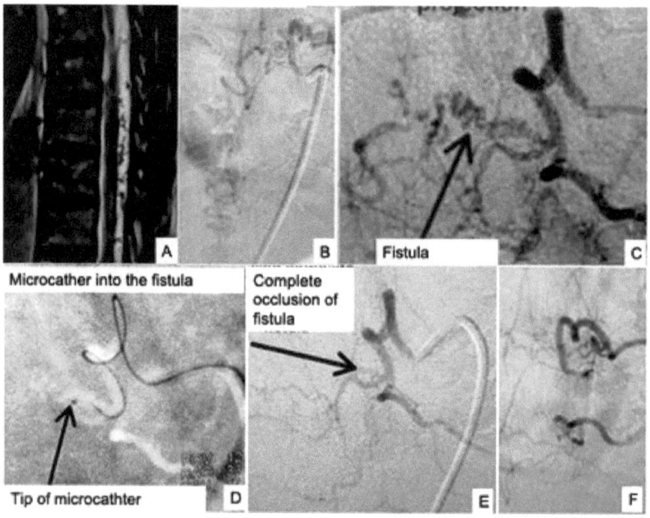

Figure 13. Endovascular closure of a dorsal spinal AVF. (**A**) MRI T2W image in sagittal view showing a suspected dorsal AVM. (**B**,**C**) Spinal DSA showing an AVF supplied by the left 8th intercostal artery; (**D**) road map microcatheter tip at the site of the fistula; (**E**) occlusion of the fistula; (**F**) DSA after occlusion of an AVF. Source: Figure by authors.

Embolic agents come in a variety of forms. n-Butyl cyanoacrylate (n-BCA), PVA/ Embospheres, ETOH, coils and, recently, Onyx (a biocompatible polymer of ethyl vinyl alcohol copolymer dissolved in an organic solvent (dimethyl sulfoxide) that promotes substantial AVM volume shrinkage and, in some cases, anatomic and angiographic cure) are all commonly used agents (Peschillo and Delfini 2012). The invention of microcatheters with detachable tips completely changed the techniques employed to inject embolic agents, since these microcatheters are significantly less prone to risks (due to microcatheter entrapment), resulting in improved endovascular therapy efficacy (Peschillo et al. 2014).

Despite the fact that the intra-arterial route is the most common, a transvenous technique has been developed in recent years with promising results (Consoli et al. 2013; Kessler et al. 2011). Due to the potential hemorrhagic consequences from any manipulation of the venous portion of a brain AVM while its core and nidus are still patent, endovascular neurosurgeons are frequently hesitant to employ the venous route. Only in exceptional circumstances should the transvenous technique be used (such as when it is impossible to negotiate the microcatheter through tortuous and small arteries to reach in the AVM nidus, in the case of high-flow venous-side aneurysm obliteration or when surgery/radiosurgery is not practical). The progressive and well-controlled deposition of Onyx within the draining vein, as well as the transvenous fast nidal closure with the backward filling of all its feeders can prevent hemorrhage (Massoud 2013).

In general, satisfactory Onyx injection results are achieved by first forming a plug in the vascular lumen just prior to the microcatheter tip and thereafter injecting. Chapot's "pressure-cooker" approach involves trapping the detachable component of an Onyx-compatible microcatheter with glue and coils to achieve wedge-flow situations, allowing for a better knowledge of macrofistulous cerebral AVMs and more thorough, forceful and well-controlled Onyx embolization (Chapot et al. 2014). In the same way, double-lumen balloons could help with endovascular therapy of brain AVMs (inflating a balloon at the Onyx injection site could eliminate the necessity for a plug and its hazards). However, the main issue with this technique is the difficulty in negotiating the dual-lumen balloon into distal arterial feeders, particularly small ones, as these vessels can often only be accessed with small microcatheters, or flow-directed microcatheters and overpenetration of the nidus, which has negative hemodynamic implications, particularly with venous penetration (Jagadeesan et al. 2013).

After the embolization of an AVM, 6.6% (range, 0–28%) experience permanent neurologic impairments or death. While embolization is successful, cerebral AVM obliteration is only achieved in 13% of cases (range: 0–94%) (Spetzler and Martin 1986).

8.12.3. Radiosurgery

In some situations of high-grade AVMs that are considered inoperable or have a significant risk of severe or even fatal consequences if managed with microsurgery or endovascular surgery, radiosurgery may be successful. The delay of postoperative effects and iatrogenic morbidity are two major drawbacks of radiosurgery. The average wait period for the results is two years (can be up to four years). Individuals with an AVM are regrettably exposed to hemorrhage dangers analogous to non-operated patients during the latency period. The second constraint is that radiation may harm structures close to the radiosurgical target volume, resulting in iatrogenic morbidity.

In 50–90% of cases, total obliteration is documented, and the incidence is inversely proportionate to the size of the AVM nidus in the brain. Even if a patient is thought to be cured after radiosurgery, a hemorrhagic episode can occur in less than 1% of cases (Peschillo et al. 2014). In 5.1% of instances (range, 0–21%), permanent neurological impairments or death occur (Spetzler and Martin 1986).

For achieving the greatest outcomes for AVMs, a multidisciplinary, case-by-case approaching technique should be used. Anatomical and biological individual-case unique aspects and natural history with a concentration on clinical symptoms should be addressed and kept in mind while developing treatment for brain AVMs on a case-by-case approach. A team of neuro-endovascular interventionists, vascular neurosurgeons and radiosurgery specialists should review all patients.

9. Spinal Vascular Malformation (SVM)

Spinal arteriovenous malformations (SVMs) are rarer pathologies to come across, with devastating consequences if left untreated. The improvement in and invention of endovascular embolization for these lesions has resulted from a growing understanding of the angioarchitecture and pathophysiology of SVMs. In the context of a multimodal management strategy, additional advancements in imaging, interventional and surgical procedures enable neurosurgeons to address these lesions more successfully and efficiently (Patsalides et al. 2011).

9.1. Classification

Early and initial classifications were absolutely descriptive and founded on histology, neglecting the essential realization of the pathophysiology of these different pathologies. There are two types of AVMs depending on hemodynamic attributes: 1) spinal AVFs with a direct shunt between the artery and vein, and 2) AVMs with a nidus (a network of aberrant arteries) between the artery and vein (Krings et al. 2005). Capillary telangiectasias and cavernous hemangiomas are vascular abnormalities that require surgery and cannot be treated with endovascular techniques (Barnwell et al. 1990).

9.1.1. Topographic Classification of SVMs

A. AVM

1. Intramedullary (also known as type II or glomus-type AVM);
2. Pial;
3. Epidural;
4. Intra- and extramedullary (also called type III, juvenile AVM, intradural– extradural or metameric AVM).

B. AVF

1. Pial AVF (also called type IV, ventral intradural AVF, spinal cord AVF or perimedullary AVF):

   a. Giant;
   b. Large;
   c. Small.

2. Dural AVF (also called dorsal intradural or type I AVF);
3. Epidural AVF (also called extradural AVF) (Patsalides et al. 2011).

9.2. Pathophysiology

Myelopathy (motor and sensory deficits, bowel and bladder dysfunction), back pain, radicular discomfort or deficit, or spinal column deformities can all be caused by spinal arteriovenous lesions. Bleeding, arterial steal, venous hypertension and mass effect are all potential causes of spinal cord injury, and their significance varies depending on the pathology. Acute neurologic impairments can result from a spinal cord parenchymal hemorrhage and/or spinal subarachnoid hemorrhage. In spinal AVMs, the risk of hemorrhage is higher. Hemorrhage can occur in giant and big spinal AVFs, cervical DAVFs and intracranial DAVFs with perimedullary venous drainage, although thoracic and lumbar DAVFs and small spinal cord AVFs are linked to less hemorrhage (Rosenblum et al. 1987; Mourier et al. 1993). Spinal artery aneurysms and intranidal aneurysms have a higher risk of rupture (Biondi et al. 1992).

Seldom, spinal AVMs along with intracranial venous drainage may have posterior fossa bleeding (Di Chiro and Doppman 1970). With arteriovenous lesions and perimedullary venous outflow, venous hypertension is typically severe.

A spinal DAVF is the most common etiology of venous hypertension, although it can also be caused by any lesion with perimedullary venous drainage like pial spinal AVFs or numerous intracranial dural AVFs. As a result of a lack of valves, the pressure in the perimedullary veins is unusually high, which is transferred to the intrinsic veins of the spinal cord, resulting in "arterialization" with tortuous and thickened walls. The reduced intramedullary arteriovenous pressure difference leads to reduced tissue perfusion, as well as spinal cord hypoxia (Hurst et al. 1995). The disruption and malfunction of the blood–cord barrier come from the lack of autoregulation of the intrinsic cord vessels, resulting in cord edema (Jellema et al. 2006). In the upright position, the conus is the lowest section of the spinal cord; therefore, venous hypertension predominates here, abated by a valveless venous system. Because the pressure in the draining veins differs from arterial pressure, exercise causes increased discomfort. Venous hypertension can be established with a DSA of the Adamkiewicz artery, which shows the prolonged severe venous phase (Merland et al. 1980). Pathologies involving high-flow arteriovenous shunts might cause arterial blood to be stolen from a normal spinal cord section nearby (Djindjian et al. 1978). Due to the poor possibility for collateral arterial supply to normal spinal cord tissue, lesions in the dorsal side of the spinal cord fed by the ASA are also vulnerable to arterial steal. Myelopathy caused by mass impact is a fairly uncommon occurrence. Large aneurysms (el Mahdi et al. 1989) and dilated veins/varices, like those found in huge spinal cord AVFs, can apply pressure on the spinal cord and nerve roots.

9.3. Clinical Manifestation

9.3.1. Spinal Cord AVMs

AVMs in the spinal cord comprise 20–30% of all SVMs (Krings et al. 2005). They are high-flow lesions with a distinct nidus that are fed by one branch of the ASA and/or PSA. They have a localized pattern of arteriovenous shunts which drain into the spinal veins, similar to brain AVMs. Aneurysms of the supplying arteries and the nidus are common complications (Biondi et al. 1992). AVMs in the spinal cord are evenly distributed along the long axis of the spinal cord and can possess a more complicated architecture, with both extramedullary and intramedullary components that disregard tissue planes. The conus medullaris AVM (Spetzler et al. 2002) is a separate kind that may extend along the filum terminale and is found on the cauda equina or conus medullaris. AVMs of the spinal cord usually appear in infancy or early adulthood, with clinical symptoms appearing suddenly due to bleeding or compression-related myelopathy. Patients may experience sensory and/or motor deficiencies, as well as bowel and bladder problems and pain. Following the initial incident, most patients have a partial improvement, but further occurrences are almost certain to occur, resulting in progressive cord function degradation. Venous hypertension and arterial steal are two possible sequences that might lead to progressive myelopathy; however, they are uncommon. AVMs of the conus medullaris commonly cause myelopathy and radiculopathy at the same time (Spetzler et al. 2002).

9.3.2. Pial AVFs

Pial AVFs (Figure 13) have a few or a single intradural direct arteriovenous shunts sans an intervening nidus as a hallmark. It is a condition of the cord's pial surface. The ASA or PSA supplies the feeder/s (one or more), and the shunt/s drain into the spinal cord veins. Based on the size and flow of the direct shunt, pial AVFs are categorized into three types: tiny (Type 1), large (Type 2) and giant (Type 3) (Gueguen et al. 1987).

AVFs of type 1 (small) have a low flow shunt between a branch of the ASA and a slightly dilated spinal vein. These are frequently seen on the filum terminale or the anterior surface of the conus medullaris. DAVFs and small AVFs on the conus medullaris are frequently mistaken. There may be a single or several shunts in Type 2 or large AVFs, with increased flow and ampullary dilatation of the draining vein. They are fed by one or more modestly dilated feeders from the PSA and normally lie on the posterolateral surface of the conus medullaris. Many arterial feeders converge on one or a few shunts in large AVFs. Type 3 AVFs have one or more high-flow shunts, as well as one or more dilated arterial supplies from the ASA and PSA. The arterial suppliers converge to form a single shunt that drains into dilated arterialized draining veins. Giant AVFs have a stronger affinity for the conus medullaris area and can be found in complex vascular malformation syndromes, although they may also be detected in other conditions (Nakstad et al. 1993).

AVFs of Type 2 and 3 are more common in childhood and adolescence. An SAH can cause symptoms to appear suddenly, although venous hypertension, vascular steal or pressure on the spinal cord and/or nerve roots are more likely to cause progressive sensory and motor degeneration, including sphincter dysfunction. SAHs are caused by venous rupture (Ricolfi et al. 1997).

Type 1 AVFs appear later in life, with progressive neuro-deficiencies caused by venous hypertension, whereas SAHs occur infrequently. Hematomyelia can occur when the anterior spinal vein, that is located subpially, ruptures (Rodesch et al. 2004). A spinal DSA is required for all of these illnesses in order to clinch the diagnosis, describe the shunt and choose the treatment strategy.

9.3.3. Epidural AVF

This kind of AVF is more uncommon and carries a higher risk of morbidity. The shunt is located between an artery and the epidural venous plexus. Presenting symptoms are mainly due to the mass effect and subsequent hematoma; venous hypertension or steal syndrome are uncommon unless the shunt drains into the spinal cord vein/s (Arnaud et al. 1994; Clarke et al. 2009; Weingrad et al. 1979; Kawabori et al. 2009; Willinsky et al. 1990). It is most common in the cervical region. Surgery or embolization are the two therapeutic choices, with the latter being preferred. Liquid embolic agents should be used to occlude the shunt and the proximal draining vein. It is also possible to use a transvenous route. When the spinal cord is not draining via the vein to be embolized, a transvenous route can be used to finish the embolization (Szajner et al. 1999; Willinsky et al. 1993).

9.3.4. Intramedullary–Extramedullary Spinal AVM

This is also called an intradural–intradural spinal AVM, and is the rarest form. This complex spinal AVM evolves along a discrete embryonic somatic level and involves more than one structure of spinal dura, cord, vertebra, paravertebral soft tissue or skin. Total somatic involvement occurs in Cobb syndrome. Incomplete somatic involvement is more common and may be associated with diffuse angiomatosis (e.g., Rendu–Osler–Weber disease). They typically present in childhood or in young adults, like manifestations of other spinal AVMs. Numerous arterial supplies from several vertebral levels are prevalent (Patsalides et al. 2011).

9.3.5. Intracranial DAVF with Cervical Perimedullary Venous Drainage

In the Djindjian–Merland classification, this is categorized as Type V (Houdart et al. 1993), where it represents a special type of intracranial lesion that manifests with spinal cord manifestations. It receives blood flow from the meningeal branches of the ECA, ICA and VA, and drains into veins around the brainstem and upper cervical spinal cord. It generally presents between the third and seventh decades of life due to venous hypertension (Ricolfi et al. 1999). These lesions demand the need for catheter angiographic evaluation from the cranium to the sacrum.

9.4. Spinal DSA and ITS Techniques

Despite major advancements in non-invasive spine vascular imaging, the spinal DSA is the gold standard test for diagnosing and classifying SVMs. For patient comfort and needed apnea during thoracic spine examination, a general anesthetic is preferred. The 5F sheath is inserted through the femoral route into the common femoral artery. Power injection with a pig-tail high-flow catheter put in the descending thoracic aorta at the mid-dorsal level can be used to obtain an aortogram. Each dorsal and lumbar artery should be examined on both sides. For cervical spinal DSA, the vertebral, deep cervical arteries and ascending cervical arteries must be canulated and examined. For lumbo-sacral spinal locations, internal iliac and iliolumbar arteries should be investigated. The examination of venous drainage should be included in spinal angiography, especially following injection in the Adamkiewicz artery. Venous drainage is protracted or nonexistent in severe venous hypertension and myelopathy involving the dorso-lumbar spine. The cause (typically a DAVF) must be present if venous hypertension is discovered. After therapy, an elevated venous outflow is a positive predictive sign (Gobin et al. 1992).

9.5. Endovascular Therapy for SVMs

The hemodynamics of SVMs, their position in the longitudinal and axial planes, and the angioarchitecture of the pathology all have a role in the management of spinal vascular lesions. For many arteriovenous malformations, endovascular treatment may be the preferred treatment. Nonetheless, microsurgery plays an important role, and a comprehensive therapeutic approach is required. One of the most crucial factors to examine before any neuro-intervention is the patient's preoperative neurologic condition. Because postoperative functional success is strongly linked to the preoperative neuro-status, maximum functional restoration can be attained by treating patients early before serious neuro-deterioration sets in. In patients with severe neuro-deficiencies, partial results may still be attainable (Patsalides et al. 2011).

9.5.1. General Principles for Embolization

To reduce the chance of a vascular attack on the spinal cord, the vascular anatomy must be clearly defined prior to operation. PSAs have many more arterial anastomoses than ASAs, implying that sufficient collateral flow is more likely following an occlusion of the PSA rather than the ASA. As a result, an occlusion of the posterior radiculomedullary artery supplying, the PSA may occur without any clinical effects. The obstruction of an anterior radiculomedullary artery that supplies the ASA, on the other hand, is linked to a substantial risk of spinal cord infarction/ischemia (Patsalides et al. 2011).

It refers to the levels below and above for anastomoses that would supply the ASA region prior to embolization. When embolizing a vascular abnormality with arterial steal, extra caution is required because partial obstruction of the feeding artery would result in diminished arterial steal, as well as the possible emergence of normal spinal arteries; unintentional embolization of these arteries should be avoided (Patsalides et al. 2011).

The rich pial perimedullary anastomoses joining the ASA and PSA are also a matter for worry, as they may result in the unintentional embolization of the ASA while embolizing a posterior radiculomedullary artery. This embolization in wedge flow can alter normal flow patterns, allowing for the embolic agent to reach arteries that were not visible on the pre-embolization DSA. In an AVM, obstruction of the venous drainage of a big arteriovenous shunt can cause nidus rupture and rupture, while in an AVF, it can produce increased venous hypertension. Last but not least, an occlusion of a feeding artery to an arteriovenous shunt too close to the shunt is usually ineffectual since alternative arterial connections may be recruited and expanded to supply the shunt;

however, because more blood is diverted to the shunt, there may be greater arterial theft. At the same time, access to the shunt for additional embolization is limited (Patsalides et al. 2011).

9.5.2. Malformation-Specific Therapy

Intramedullary AVM

Intramedullary AVMs should be managed to change the course of the disease and lower the risk of bleeding. The outcome of untreated spinal AVMs is bleak (Aminoff and Logue 1974; Hurth et al. 1978). Microsurgery, embolization or a combination of the two is currently a possible treatment. When a long endovascular approach or an unstable catheter location make catheter access problematic, surgery is the only choice. A lesion that is superficially placed in the back is more appealing for a safe resection. Surgical treatment of anteriorly placed lesions is still possible, particularly in the cervical area, where collateral circulation to the spinal cord might develop caudally. Filum terminale AVMs can also be treated surgically.

Embolization can be used as a main treatment or as a supplement for microsurgery in the treatment of intramedullary spinal AVMs (Djindjian et al. 1973; Doppman et al. 1968). Modern microcatheters allow for the selective catheterization of the anterior and posterior spinal arteries supplying the AVM; therefore, embolization with a liquid or particle embolic agent is possible. These AVMs do not use coils as they need relatively rigid microcatheters that are dangerous to maneuver. As a result, coils can only be utilized for proximal embolization, which might cause collateral circulation to the nidus to develop, preventing future safe interventional access.

The advantages of particle embolic agents include sequential embolization and the capability to monitor the result clinically as well as angiographically during the intervention. However, recanalization has a long-term negative impact. Particle embolization necessitates angiographic monitoring every year, as well as further embolization in the event of recanalization.

Multiple embolizations may be required as the AVM recanalization rate is as high as 80% (Biondi et al. 1990). Essentially, particle embolization is a palliative procedure that affects the natural history, and it may produce a positive clinical result rather than a definitive solution.

Liquid embolic agents have the advantage of providing a more lasting occlusion that is less likely to recanalize, but they also carry the danger of unintentional embolization of normal perforating arteries which are not shown on DSA. When possible, a liquid embolic agent should be utilized, particularly if embolization is the primary or exclusive treatment. The liquid embolic agent should be injected into the nidus or as close to it as possible. The use of n-BCA, (Rodesch et al. 2003) for spinal AVF embolizations had the satisfactory clinical outcome of up to 83%. Thirteen percent of individuals get permanent morbidity as a result of embolization. A severe deficit occurs in cases where embolization is performed through the ASA. Nowadays, Onyx (ev3, Irvine, California) is also utilized to manage spinal cord AVMs.

Embolization for Intramedullary AVMs

Embolization of an intramedullary AVM is generally accomplished while the patient is sedated and receiving systemic heparin. A microcatheter is inserted into the radiculomedullary branch that nourishes the AVM, and a 5F guide catheter is implanted at the ostium of the segmental artery. In most cases, flow-directed microcatheters are preferable to tougher braided microcatheters. The microcatheter should be placed inside or as near to the nidus as possible for lesions fed by the ASA, particularly in a sulcal artery beyond the ASA's longitudinal axis. This reduces the risk of embolization of a normal ASA branch by accident. Although the implications of unintentionally occluding typical PSA branches are not as severe, similar concepts apply to lesions fed by a feeder from the PSA. Because of the lower procedure-related risk, AVMs fed by both ASA and PSA feeders should be treated initially. Embolization is commonly carried out with a 1:2 to 1:3 mixture of n-BCA and ethiodized oil, with tantalum powder added to boost the embolic material's radiodensity. A larger concentration of n-BCA can be employed for high-flow shunts. To avoid recurrent hemorrhage, it is critical to embolize false and flow-related aneurysms (Konan et al. 1999). For the next 24–48 h, the patient should be observed in a neurologic critical care unit. To preclude thrombosis of the normal spinal arteries, systemic heparin is maintained for 24 h (low-dose regimen with a target-activated partial thromboplastin time of 50 to 60 s) (Patsalides et al. 2011).

Intramedullary–Extramedullary AVM and Complex Angiomatosis

Due to the complex architecture and the real fact of the intermingling of the cord parenchyma in an actual AVM, the treatment of these lesions is very difficult. Although there is no known optimal treatment for these lesions, microsurgery and embolization may be carried out alone or in combination. In reality, treatment should be palliative, with the goal of alleviating symptoms produced by a hematoma, arterial steal, venous hypertension or direct mass effect. The closure of a feeding artery (Mourier et al. 1993) and decompressive laminectomy are two simple procedures (Biondi et al. 1992; Di Chiro and Doppman 1970; Hurst et al. 1995). When utilized preoperatively, embolization can be utilized with particles.

Pial AVFs

Pial AVFs are a diverse set of vascular pathologies, with treatment options based mostly on the angioarchitecture of the lesion. Surgical or endovascular treatment should be used as soon as possible. Embolization can also be used in conjunction with microsurgery (Hida et al. 1999). The only approach to prevent long-term recurrence is to obliterate the pial fistula completely and permanently. Liquid embolic agents are the favored materials for embolization, while PVA particles should only be utilized for pre-microsurgical embolization. As the feeder is a distal branch of a thin ASA, super-selective catheterization and retaining the microcatheter in the fistula for efficient embolization is problematic in small pial fistulas (Riche et al. 1983). Because there are several feeding arteries, some of which are perimedullary or transmedullary branches that cannot be catheterized safely, embolization alone is rarely helpful for larger AVFs. Embolization has been documented in a few occurrences, with some cases being partially embolized and recurrence (Oran et al. 2005; Cho et al. 2005). Microsurgical management, on the other hand, is curative, particularly in lesions of the dorsal/dorsolateral cord. The purpose of the surgery is to cut off the junction between the venous and arterial systems while leaving the ASA branches intact. Because of their bigger diameter and rapid flow through the shunt, super-selective arterial feeder catheterization is more practicable in huge fistulas. The enlarged draining veins raise the chances of an intraoperative rupture, making surgical therapy more difficult. As a result, embolization is the preferred treatment for these kinds of lesions. The most difficult aspect of embolization is getting the embolization agent into the right spot without causing venous migration (Mourier et al. 1993; Ricolfi et al. 1997).

As the particles can pass past the shunt and into the venous circulation, causing thrombosis or pulmonary embolism, they should not be used alone. Instead, coils should be utilized alone or in combination with liquid embolic materials. Coils can be inserted in huge AVFs to act as a template for the liquid embolic agent, preventing it from passing through the shunt and onto the venous side. This approach necessitates the utilization of a microcatheter with a big enough inner diameter to facilitate coil deployment. For recurrence prevention, the fistula and proximal draining veins should be embolized. Transient worsening of symptoms may be due to progressive backward thrombosis of the draining veins. Systemic heparin can prevent this for 24–48 h after embolization (Patsalides et al. 2011).

Author Contributions: Conceptualization, methodology, validation, formal analysis, investigation, resources, data curation, S.U.K., F.H.C. and P.M.F.; writing—original draft preparation, F.H.C. and P.M.F.; writing—review and editing, F.H.C.; visualization, supervision, S.S.I. and K.M.R. All authors have read and agreed to the published version of the manuscript.

Funding: This research received no external funding.

Conflicts of Interest: The authors declare no conflicts of interest.

References

Al-Shahi, Rustam, J. S. Y. Fang, S. C. Lewis, and Charles P. Warlow. 2002. Prevalence of adults with brain arteriovenousmalformations: A community-based study in Scotlandusing capture-recapture analysis. *Journal of Neurology, Neurosurgery & Psychiatry* 73: 547–51.

Aminoff, M. J., and Valentine Logue. 1974. The prognosis of patients with spinal vascular malformations. *Brain* 97: 211–18. [CrossRef] [PubMed]

Arnaud, O., F. Bille, J. Pouget, G. Serratrice, and G. Salamon. 1994. Epidural arteriovenous fistula with perimedullary venous drainage: Case report. *Neuroradiology* 36: 490–91. [CrossRef]

Arnautovic, Kenan I., and Ali F. Krisht. 2000. Transverse-Sigmoid Sinus Dural Arteriovenous Malformations. *Contemporary Neurosurgery* 21: 1–6. [CrossRef]

Ashour, Ramsey, Mohammad Ali Aziz-Sultan, Maryam Soltanolkotabi, Samantha E. Schoeneman, Tord D. Alden, Michael C. Hurley, Arthur J. Dipatri, Tadanori Tomita, Mohamed Samy Elhammady, and Ali Shaibani. 2012. Safety an decacy of onyx embolization for pediatric cranial and spinal vascular lesions and tumors. *Neurosurgery* 71: 773–84. [CrossRef]

Baharvahdat, Humain, Yinn Cher Ooi, Wi Jin Kim, Ashkan Mowla, Alexander L. Coon, and Geoffrey P. Colby. 2020. Updates in the management of cranial dural arteriovenous fistula. *Stroke and Vascular Neurology* 5: 50–58. [CrossRef]

Barnwell, Stanley L., Christopher F. Dowd, Richard L. Davis, Michael S. B. Edwards, Philip H. Gutin, and Charles B. Wilson. 1990. Cryptic vascular malformations of the spinal cord: Diagnosis by magnetic resonance imaging and outcome of surgery. *Journal of Neurosurgery* 72: 403–7. [CrossRef]

Barrow, Daniel L., Robert H. Spector, Ira F. Braun, Jeffrey A. Landman, Suzie C. Tindall, and George T. Tindall. 1985. Classification and treatment of spontaneous carotid-cavernous sinus fistulas. *Journal of Neurosurgery* 62: 248–56. [CrossRef]

Becske, Tibor, David F. Kallmes, Isil Saatci, Cameron G. McDougall, István Szikora, Giuseppe Lanzino, Christopher J. Moran, Henry H.Woo, Demetrius K. Lopes, Aaron L. Berez, and et al. 2013. Pipeline for uncoilable or failed aneurysms: Results from a multicenter clinical trial. *Radiology* 267: 858–68. Available online: http://radiology.rsna.org/ (accessed on 26 February 2013). [CrossRef]

Berge, J., A. Biondi, P. Machi, H. Brunel, L. Pierot, J. Gabrillargues, K. Kadziolka, X. Barreau, V. Dousset, and A. Bonafé. 2012. Flow-diverter silk stent for the treatment of intracranial aneurysms: 1-year follow-up in a multicenter study. *American Journal of Neuroradiology* 33: 1150–55. [CrossRef]

Biondi, Alessandra, J. J. Merland, J. E. Hodes, J. P. Pruvo, and D. Reizine. 1992. Aneurysms of spinal arteries associated with intramedullary arteriovenous malformations. I. Angiographic and clinical aspects. *American Journal of Neuroradiology* 13: 913–22.

Biondi, Alessandra, Jean-Jacques Merland, Daniel Reizine, A. Aymard, J. E. Hodes, P. Lecoz, and A. Rey. 1990. Embolization with particles in thoracic intramedullary arteriovenous malformations: Long-term angiographic and clinical results. *Radiology* 177: 651–58. [CrossRef]

Bodily, K. D., H. J. Cloft, G. Lanzino, D. J. Fiorella, P. M. White, and David F. Kallmes. 2011. Stent-assisted coiling in acutely ruptured intracranial aneurysms: A qualitative, systematic review of the literature. *American Journal of Neuroradiology* 32: 1232–36. [CrossRef] [PubMed]

Bonati, Leo H., Philippe Lyrer, Joerg Ederle, Roland Featherstone, and Martin M. Brown. 2012. Percutaneous transluminal balloon angioplasty and stenting for carotid artery stenosis. *The Cochrane Database of Systematic Reviews* 9: CD000515. [CrossRef] [PubMed]

Byrne, James V., Radu Beltechi, Julia A. Yarnold, Jacqueline Birks, and Mudassar Kamran. 2010. Early experience in the treatment of intra-cranial aneurysms by endovascular flow diversion: A multicentre prospective study. *PLoS ONE* 5: e12492. [CrossRef] [PubMed]

Carlson, Andrew P., Ali Alaraj, Sepideh Amin-Hanjani, Fady T. Charbel, and Victor A. Aletich. 2013. Continued concern about parent vessel steno-occlusive progression with Onyx HD-500 and the utility of quantitative magnetic resonance imaging in serial assessment. *Neurosurgery* 72: 341–52. [CrossRef]

Celesia, Gastone G., Charles M. Strother, Patrick A. Turski, Michael F. Stieghorst, Joseph F. Sackett, and Charles A. Mistretta. 1983. Digital Subtraction Arteriography. A New Method for Evaluation of Extracranial Occlusive Disease. *Archives of Neurology* 40: 70–74. [CrossRef]

Chalouhi, Nohra, Aaron S. Dumont, Stavropoula Tjoumakaris, L. Fernando Gonzalez, Jurij R. Bilyk, Ciro Randazzo, David Hasan, Richard T. Dalyai, Robert Rosenwasser, and Pascal Jabbour. 2012. The superior ophthalmic vein approach for the treatment of carotid-cavernous fistulas: A novel technique using Onyx. *Neurosurgical Focus* 32: E13. [CrossRef] [PubMed]

Chaloupka, John C., and Daniel C. Huddle. 1998. Classification of vascular malformations of the central nervous system. *Neuroimaging clinics of North America* 8: 295–321.

Chapot, René, Paul Stracke, Aglaé Velasco, Hannes Nordmeyer, Markus Heddier, Michael Stauder, Petra Schooss, and Pascal J. Mosimann. 2014. The pressure cooker technique for the treatment of brain AVMs. *Journal of Neuroradiology* 41: 87–91. [CrossRef] [PubMed]

Chimowitz, Marc I., Michael J. Lynn, Colin P. Derdeyn, Tanya N. Turan, David Fiorella, Bethany F. Lane, L. Scott Janis, Helmi L. Lutsep, Stanley L. Barnwell, Michael F. Waters, and et al. 2011. Stenting versus aggressive medical therapy for intracranial arterial stenosis. *New England Journal of Medicine* 365: 993–1003. [CrossRef] [PubMed]

Cho, Keun Tae, Dong Yeob Lee, Chun Kee Chung, Moon Hee Han, and Hyun Jib Kim. 2005. Treatment of spinal cord perimedullary arteriovenous fistula: Embolization versus surgery. *Neurosurgery* 56: 232–41. [CrossRef] [PubMed]

Choi, Dae Seob, Mun Chul Kim, Seon Kyu Lee, Robert A. Willinsky, and Karel G. Terbrugge. 2010. Clinical and angiographic long-term follow-up of completely coiled aneurysms using endovascular technique. *Journal of Neurosurgery* 112: 575–81. [CrossRef] [PubMed]

Clarke, Michelle J., Todd A. Patrick, J. Bradley White, Harry J. Cloft, William E. Krauss, E. P. Lindell, and David G. Piepgras. 2009. Spinal extradural arteriovenous malformations with parenchymal drainage: Venous drainage variability and implications in clinical manifestations. *Neurosurgical Focus* 26: E5. [CrossRef]

Cognard, Christophe, Alain Weill, Laurent Spelle, Michel Piotin, Lina Castaings, Alain Rey, and Jacques Moret. 1999. Long-term angiographic follow-up of 169 intracranial berry aneurysms occluded with detachable coils. *Radiology* 212: 348–56. [CrossRef]

Cognard, Christophe, Laurent Pierot, René Anxionnat, Frédéric Ricolfi, and Clarity Study Group. 2011. Results of embolization used as the first treatment choice in a consecutive nonselected population of ruptured aneurysms: Clinical results of the Clarity GDC study. *Neurosurgery* 69: 837–41. [CrossRef]

Cohen, James, and Ionel Rad. 2004. Contemporary management of carotid blowout. *Current Opinion in Otolaryngology & Head and Neck Surgery* 12: 110–15.

Consoli, A., L. Renieri, S. Nappini, N. Limbucci, and S. Mangiafico. 2013. Endovascular treatment of deep hemorrhagic brain arteriovenous malformations with transvenous onyx embolization. *The American Journal of Neuroradiology* 34: 1805–11. [CrossRef]

Crawford, P. M., C. R. West, D. W. Chadwick, and M. D. Shaw. 1986. Arteriovenous Malformations of the Brain: Natural History in Unoperated Patients. *Journal of Neurology, Neurosurgery & Psychiatry* 49: 1–10.

Cruz, J. P., M. Chow, C. O'Kelly, B. Marotta, J. Spears, W. Montanera, D. Fiorella, and T. Marotta. 2012. Delayed ipsilateral parenchymal hemorrhage following flow diversion for the treatment of anterior circulation aneurysms. *American Journal of Neuroradiology* 33: 603–8. [CrossRef]

Davies, M. A., J. Saleh, K. Ter Brugge, R. Willinsky, and M. C. Wallace. 1997. The natural history and management of in tracranial dural arteriovenous fistulae. Part 1: Benign lesions. *Interventional Neuroradiology* 3: 295–302. [CrossRef] [PubMed]

Derdeyn Colin, P. 2007. Carotid Stenting for Asymptomatic carotid. *Stroke* 38: 715–20. [CrossRef] [PubMed]

Di Chiro, Giovanni, and John L. Doppman. 1970. Endocranial drainage of spinal cord veins. *Radiology* 95: 555–60. [CrossRef] [PubMed]

Ding, Dale, Robert M. Starke, Mark Quigg, Chun-Po Yen, Colin J. Przybylowski, Blair K. Dodson, and Jason P. Sheehan. 2015. Cerebral Arteriovenous Malformations and Epilepsy, Part 1: Predictors of Seizure Presentation. *World Neurosurgery* 84: 645–52. [CrossRef]

Ding, Yong H., Debra A. Lewis, Ram Kadirvel, D. Dai, and David F. Kallmes. 2011. The Wowen EndoBridge: A new occlusion device. *American Journal of Neuroradiology* 32: 607–11. [CrossRef]

Djindjian, M., R. Djindjian, M. Hurth, R. Houdart, and A. Rey. 1978. Steal phenomena in spinal arteriovenous malformations. *Journal of Neuroradiology* 5: 187–201.

Djindjian, R., J. Cophignon, A. Rey, J. Theron, J. J. Merland, and R. Houdart. 1973. Superselective arteriographic embolization by the femoral route in neuroradiology: Study of 50 cases. II. Embolization in vertebromedullary pathology. *Neuroradiology* 6: 132–42.

Doppman, JohnL, GiovanniDi Chiro, and Ayub Ommaya. 1968. Obliteration of spinal-cord arteriovenous malformation by percutaneous embolisation. *Lancet* 1: 477. [CrossRef]

Drake, Charles G. 1979. Cerebral AVMs: Considerations for and Experience with Surgical Treatment in 166 Cases. *Clinical Neurosurgery* 26: 145–208. [CrossRef]

Eberhardt, Olaf, Thomas Naegele, Sabine Raygrotzki, Michael Weller, and Ulrike Ernemann. 2006. Stenting of vertebrobasilar arteries in symptomatic atherosclerotic disease and acute occlusion: Case series and review of the literature. *Journal of Vascular Surgery* 43: 1145–54. [CrossRef] [PubMed]

el Mahdi, Mokhtar A., Mohamed A. Rudwan, Salah M. Khaffaji, and F. A. Jadallah. 1989. A giant spinal aneurysm with cord and root compression. *Journal of Neurology, Neurosurgery & Psychiatry* 52: 532–35.

Ferns, Sandra P., Marieke E. S. Sprengers, Willem Jan van Rooij, Gabriel J. E. Rinkel, Jeroen C. van Rijn, Shandra Bipat, Menno Sluzewski, and Charles B. L. M. Majoie. 2009. Coiling of intracranial aneurysms: A systematic review on initial occlusion and reopening and retreatment rates. *Stroke* 40: e523–29. [CrossRef] [PubMed]

Fiorella, David, Daniel Hsu, Henry H. Woo, Robert W. Tarr, and Peter Kim Nelson. 2010. Very late thrombosis of a pipeline embolization device construct: Case report. *Neurosurgery* 67: onsE313–14; discussion on E314. [CrossRef] [PubMed]

Fiorella, David, Felipe C. Albuquerque, Henry H. Woo, Cameron G. McDougall, and Peter A. Rasmussen. 2006. The role of neuroendovascular therapy for the treatment of brain arteriovenous malformations. *Neurosurgery* 59: S3-163–S3-177. [CrossRef] [PubMed]

Fiorella, David, Henry H. Woo, Felipe C. Albuquerque, and Peter K. Nelson. 2008. Definitive reconstruction of circumferential, fusiform intracranial aneurysms with the pipeline embolization device. *Neurosurgery* 62: 1115–20. [CrossRef] [PubMed]

Fleetwood, Ian G., and Gary K. Steinberg. 2002. Arteriovenous malformations. *Lancet* 359: 863–73. [CrossRef]

Frosting, M. 2003. *Intracranial Vascular Malformation and Aneurysm. From Diagnostic Work-Up to Endovascular Therapy*. Berlin/Heidelberg and New York: Springer.

Gallas, Sophie, Anne Pasco, Jean-Philippe Cottier, Jean Gabrillargues, Jacques Drouineau, Christophe Cognard, and Denis Herbreteau. 2005. A multicenter study of 705 ruptured intracranial aneurysms treated with Guglielmi detachable coils. *American Journal of Neuroradiology* 26: 1723–31.

Geibprasert, S., S. Pongpech, D. Armstrong, and T. Krings. 2009. Dangerous Extracranial– Intracranial Anastomoses and Supply to the Cranial Nerves: Vessels the Neuro- interventionalist Needs to Know. *American Journal of Neuroradiology* 30: 1459–68. [CrossRef]

Gobin, Y. Pierre, Andre Rogopoulos, Armand Aymard, Mazen Khayata, Daniel Reizine, Jacques Chiras, and Jean-Jacques Merland. 1992. Endovascular treatment of intracranial dural arteriovenous fistulas with spinal perimedullary venous drainage. *Journal of Neurosurgery* 77: 718–23.

Graeb, Douglas A., and Clarisse L. Dolman. 1986. Radiological and Pathological Aspects of Dural Arteriovenous Fistulas. *Journal of Neurosurgery* 64: 962–7. [CrossRef] [PubMed]

Gueguen, B., J. J. Merland, M. C. Riche, and A. Rey. 1987. Vascular malformations of the spinal cord: Intrathecal perimedullary arteriovenous fistulas fed by medullary arteries. *Neurology* 37: 969–79.

Guglielmi, Guido, Fernando Vinuela, Ivan Sepetka, and Velio Macellari. 1991a. Electrothrombosis of saccular aneurysms via endovascular approach. Part 1: Electrochemical basis, technique, and experimental results. *Journal of Neurosurgery* 75: 1–7. [CrossRef] [PubMed]

Guglielmi, Guido, Fernando Vinuela, Ivan Sepetka, and Velio Macellari. 1991b. Electrothrombosis of saccular aneurysms via endovascular approach. Part 2: Preliminary clinical experience. *Journal of Neurosurgery* 75: 8–14. [CrossRef]

Gurm, Hitinder S., Jay S. Yadav, Pierre Fayad, Barry T. Katzen, Gregory J. Mishkel, Tanvir K. Bajwa, Gary Ansel, Neil E. Strickman, Hong Wang, Sidney A. Cohen, and et al. 2008. Long-term results of carotid stenting versus endarterectomy in high-risk patients. *New England Journal of Medicine* 358: 1572–79. [CrossRef] [PubMed]

Hartmann, Andreas, Henning Mast, J. P. Mohr, Hans-Christian Koennecke, Andrei Osipov, John Pile-Spellman, D. Hoang Duong, and William L. Young. 1998. Morbidity of intracranial hemorrhage in patients with cerebral arteriovenous malformation. *Stroke* 29: 931–34. [CrossRef] [PubMed]

Henderson, A. D., and N. R. Miller. 2017. Carotid-cavernous fistula: Current concept of aetiology, investigation, management. *Eye* 32: 164–72. [CrossRef] [PubMed]

Hida, Kazutoshi, Yoshinobu Iwasaki, Katsuya Goto, Kazuo Miyasaka, and Hiroshi Abe. 1999. Results of the surgical treatment of perimedullary arteriovenous fistulas with special reference to embolization. *Journal of Neurosurgery* 90: 198–205.

Hope, J. K. Ayton, James V. Byrne, and Andrew J. Molyneux. 1999. Factors influencing successful angiographic occlusion of aneurysms treated by coil occlusion. *American Journal of Neuroradiology* 20: 391–99.

Houdart, E., Y. P. Gobin, A. Casasco, A. Aymard, D. Herbreteau, and J. J. Merland. 1993. A proposed angiographic classification of intracranial arteriovenous fistulae and malformations. *Neuroradiology* 35: 381–85. [CrossRef]

Hurst, R. W., L. C. Kenyon, E. Lavi, E. C. Raps, and P. Marcotte. 1995. Spinal dural arteriovenous fistula: The pathology of venous hypertensive myelopathy. *Neurology* 45: 1309–13. [CrossRef]

Hurth, M., R. Houdart, R. Djindjian, A. Rey, and M. Djindjian. 1978. Arteriovenous malformations of the spinal cord: Clinical, anatomical and therapeutic consideration: A series of 150 cases. *Progress in Neurological Surgery* 9: 238–66.

Intracranial Dural Arteriovenous Fistula. 2021. Available online: https://operativeneurosurgery.com/doku.php?id=intr acranial_dural_arteriovenousfistula (accessed on 21 April 2021).

Jagadeesan, Bharathi D., Mikayel Grigoryan, Ameer E. Hassan, Andrew W. Grande, and Ramachandra P. Tummala. 2013. Endovascular balloon-assisted embolization of intracranial and cervical arteriovenous malformations using dual-lumen coaxial balloon microcatheters and onyx. *Neurosurgery* 73: 238–43. [CrossRef] [PubMed]

Jayaraman, M. V., M. L. Marcellus, H. M. Do, S. D. Chang, J. K. Rosen berg, G. K. Stein berg, and M. P. Marks. 2007. Hemorrhage rate in patients with Spetzler-Martin grades IV and V arteriovenous malformations: Is treatment justified? *Stroke* 38: 325–29. [CrossRef]

Jellema, K., C. C. Tijssen, and J. van Gijn. 2006. Spinal dural arteriovenous fistulas: A congestive myelopathy that initially mimics a peripheral nerve disorder. *Brain* 129: 3150–64. [CrossRef]

Johnston, S. Claiborne, Christopher F. Dowd, Randall T. Higashida, Michael T. Lawton, Gary R. Duckwiler, and Daryl R. Gress. 2008. Predictors of rehemorrhage after treatment of ruptured intracranial aneurysms: The Cerebral Aneurysm Rerupture after Treatment (CARAT) study. *Stroke* 39: 120–25. [CrossRef]

Kadziolka, Krzysztof, Catherine Tomas, Georges Robin, and Laurent Pierot. 2013. Combined use of a double-lumen remodeling balloon and a low-profile stent in the treatment of intracranial aneurysms ('remostent' technique): A technical note. *Journal of Neuroradiology* 40: 50–53. [CrossRef] [PubMed]

Kallmes, David F., Yong Hong Ding, Daying Dai, Ramanathan Kadirvel, Debra A. Lewis, and Harry J. Cloft. 2007. A new endoluminal, flow-disrupting device for treatment of saccular aneurysms. *Stroke* 38: 2346–52. [CrossRef]

Kan, Peter, Adnan H. Siddiqui, Erol Veznedaroglu, Kenneth M. Liebman, Mandy J. Binning, Travis M. Dumont, Christopher S. Ogilvy, J. R. Gaughen, Jr., J. Mocco, G. J. Velat, and et al. 2012. Early post-market results after treatment of intracranial aneurysms with the Pipeline Embolization device: A US multicenter experience. *Neurosurgery* 71: 1080–87. [CrossRef] [PubMed]

Kawabori, Masahito, Kazutoshi Hida, Shunsuke Yano, Takeshi Asano, and Yoshinobu Iwasaki. 2009. Cervical epidural arteriovenous fistula with radiculopathy mimicking cervical spondylosis. *Neurologia Medico-Chirurgica* 49: 108–13. [CrossRef]

Kessler, Iruena, Roberto Riva, Maria Ruggiero, Monica Manisor, Maher Al-Khawaldeh, and Charbel Mounayer. 2011. Successful transvenous embolization of brain arteriovenous malformations using onyx in five consecutive patients. *Neurosurgery* 69: 184–93. [CrossRef]

Killory, Brendan D., Peter Nakaji, L. Fernando Gonzales, Francisco A. Ponce, Scott D. Wait, and Robert F. Spetzler. 2009. Prospective evaluation of surgical microscope-integrated intraoperative near-infrared indocyanine green angiography during cerebral arteriovenous malformation surgery. *Neurosurgery* 65: 456–62. [CrossRef] [PubMed]

Konan, Alexis Victorien, Jean Raymond, and Daniel Roy. 1999. Transarterial embolization of aneurysms associated with spinal cord arteriovenous malformations: Report of four cases. *Journal of Neurosurgery* 90: 148–54. [CrossRef] [PubMed]

Kondziolka, Douglas, Mark R. McLaughlin, and John RW Kestle. 1995. Simple Risk Predictions for Arteriovenous Malformation Hemorrhage. *Neurosurgery* 37: 851–55. [CrossRef] [PubMed]

Krings, Timo, Michael Mull, Joachim M. Gilsbach, and Armin Thron. 2005. Spinal vascular malformations. *European Radiology* 15: 267–78. [CrossRef]

Kulcsár, Zsolt, and István Szikora. 2012. The ESMINT Retrospective Analysis of Delayed Aneurysm Ruptures after flow diversion (RADAR) study. *EJMINT* 2012: 1244000088. Available online: http://www.ejmint.org/ (accessed on 26 February 2010).

Kulcsár, Zsolt, Stephan G. Wetzel, Luca Augsburger, Andreas Gruber, Isabel Wanke, and Daniel Andre Rüfenacht. 2010. Effect of flow diversion treatment on very small ruptured aneurysms. *Neurosurgery* 67: 789–93. [CrossRef]

Kupersmith, M. J., M. E. Vargas, A. Yashar, M. Madrid, K. Nelson, A. Seton, and A. Berenstein. 1996. Occipital arteriovenous malformations: Visual disturbances and presentation. *Neurology* 46: 953–57. [CrossRef]

Lanzino, G., A. K. Wakhloo, R. D. Fessler, M. L. Hartney, L.R. Guterman, and L. N. Hopkins. 1998. Efficacy and current limitations of intravascular stents for intracranial internal carotid, vertebral, and basilar artery aneurysms. *Journal of neurosurgery* 91: 538–46. [CrossRef]

Lee, S. J., Y. D. Cho, H.-S. Kang, J. E. Kim, and M. H. Han. 2013. Coil embolization using the self-expandable closed-cell stent for intracranial saccular aneurysm: A single-center experience of 289 consecutive aneurysms. *Clinical Radiology* 68: 256–63. [CrossRef]

Lowis, George W., and Alireza Minagar. 2003. The neglected research of Egas Moniz of internal carotid artery (ICA) occlusion. *Journal of the History of the Neurosciences* 12: 286–91. [CrossRef]

Lubicz, Boris, Laurent Collignon, Gaï Raphaeli, Jean-Pierre Pruvo, Michael Bruneau, Olivier De Witte, and Xavier Leclerc. 2010. Flow-diverter stent for the endovascular treatment of intracranial aneurysms: A prospective study in 29 patients with 34 aneurysms. *Stroke* 41: 2247–53. [CrossRef]

Lutsep, Helmi L., Michael J. Lynn, George A. Cotsonis, Colin P. Derdeyn, Tanya N. Turan, David Fiorella, L. Scott Janis, Bethany F. Lane, Jean Montgomery, Marc I. Chimowitz, and et al. 2015. Does the Stenting Versus Aggressive Medical Therapy Trial Support Stenting for Subgroups With Intracranial Stenosis? *Stroke* 46: 3282–84. [CrossRef]

Lv, X., Y. Li, C. Jiang, X. Yang, and Z. Wu. 2010. Brain arteriovenous malformations and endovascular treatment: Effect on seizures. *Interventional Neuroradiology* 16: 39–45. [CrossRef] [PubMed]

Lylyk, Pedro, Carlos Miranda, Rosana Ceratto, Angel Ferrario, Esteban Scrivano, Hugh Ramirez Luna, Aaron L. Berez, Quang Tran, Peter K. Nelson, and David Fiorella. 2009. Curative endovascular reconstruction of cerebral aneurysms with the pipeline embolization device: The Buenos Aires experience. *Neurosurgery* 64: 632–42. [CrossRef] [PubMed]

Massoud, Tarik F. 2013. Transvenous retrograde nidus sclerotherapy under controlled hypotension (TRENSH): Hemodynamic analysis and concept validation in a pig arteriovenous malformation model. *Neurosurgery* 73: 332–42. [CrossRef] [PubMed]

Mast, Henning, J. P. Mohr, Andrei Osipov, John Pile-Spellman, Randolph S. Marshall, Ronald M. Lazar, Bennett M. Stein, and William L. Young. 1995. 'Steal' Is an Unestablished Mechanism for the Clinical Presentation of Cerebral Arteriovenous Malformations. *Stroke* 26: 1215–20. [CrossRef] [PubMed]

Maurice-Williams, R. S., and J. Lafuente. 2003. Intracranial aneurysm surgery and its future. *Journal of the Royal Society of Medicine* 96: 540–43. [CrossRef]

Mericle, Robert A., Giuseppe Lanzino, Ajay K. Wakhloo, Lee R. Guterman, and L. Nelson Hopkins. 1998. Stenting and secondary coiling of internal carotid artery aneurysm: Technical case report. *Neurosurgery* 43: 1229–34. [CrossRef]

Merland, J. J., M. C. Riche, and J. Chiras. 1980. Intraspinal extramedullary arteriovenous fistulae draining into the medullary veins. *Journal of Neuroradiology* 7: 271–320.

Molyneux, Andrew J., Saruhan Cekirge, Isil Saatci, and Gyula Gál. 2004. Cerebral Aneurysm Multicenter European Onyx (CAMEO) trial: Results of a prospective observational study in 20 European centers. *American Journal of Neuroradiology* 25: 39–51.

Moret, J., C. Cognard, A. Weill, L. Castaings, and A. Rey. 1997. The "remodelling technique" in the treatment of wide neck intracranial aneurysms. *Interventional Neuroradiology* 3: 21–35. [CrossRef] [PubMed]

Morris, Pearse. 2007. *Practical Neuroangiography*. Philadelphia: Lippincott, pp. 498–99.

Mourier, K. L., Y. P. Gobin, B. George, G. Lot, and J. J. Merland. 1993. Intradural perimedullary arteriovenous fistulae: Results of surgical and endovascular treatment in a series of 35 cases. *Neurosurgery* 32: 885–91. [CrossRef] [PubMed]

Mullan, Sean, Saeid Mojtahedi, Douglas L. Johnson, and R. Loch Macdonald. 1996. Embryological basis of some aspectsof cerebral vascular fistulas and malformations. *Journal of Neurosurgery* 85: 1–8. [CrossRef] [PubMed]

Nakstad, P. H., J. K. Hald, and S. J. Bakke. 1993. Multiple spinal arteriovenous fistulas in Klippel-Trenaunay-Weber syndrome treated with platinum fibre coils. *Neuroradiology* 35: 163–65. [CrossRef]

Nieuwkamp, Dennis J., Larissa E. Setz, Ale Algra, Francisca H. H. Linn, Nicolien K. de Rooij, and Gabriël J. E. Rinkel. 2009. Changes in case fatality of aneurysmal subarachnoid haemorrhage over time, according to age, sex, and region: A meta-analysis. *The Lancet Neurology* 8: 635–42. [CrossRef] [PubMed]

O'Kelly, C. J., J. Spears, M. Chow, J. Wong, M. Boulton, A. Weill, R. A. Willinsky, M. Kelly, and T. R. Marotta. 2013. Canadian experience with the pipeline embolization device for repair of unruptured intracranial aneurysms. *American Journal of Neuroradiology* 34: 381–87. [CrossRef] [PubMed]

Oran, Ismail, Mustafa Parildar, and Abdurrahim Derbent. 2005. Treatment of slow-flow (type I) perimedullary spinal arteriovenous fistulas with special reference to embolization. *American Journal of Neuroradiology* 26: 2582–86.

Ortiz, Rafael, Michael Stefanski, Robert Rosenwasser, and Erol Veznedaroglu. 2008. Cigarette smoking as a risk factor for recurrence of aneurysms treated by endosaccular occlusion. *Journal of Neurosurgery* 108: 672–75. [CrossRef] [PubMed]

Oshizumi, H., H. Inoya, H. Masuzawa, K. Sato, and S. Nakamura. 2004. Stent-assisted percutaneous transluminal angioplasty for intracranial vertebral and basilar artery stenosis: Two case reports. *No Shinkei Geka* 32: 627–34. (In Japanese). [PubMed]

Paraskevas, Kosmas I., Dimitri P. Mikhailidis, and Frank J. Veith. 2009. Carotid artery stenting may be losing the battle against carotid endarterectomy for the management of symptomatic carotid artery stenosis, but the jury is still out. *Vascular* 17: 183–89. [CrossRef]

Patsalides, A., J. Knopman, A. Santillan, A. J. Tsiouris, H. Riina, and Y. P. Gobin. 2011. Endovascular Treatment of Spinal Arteriovenous Lesions: Beyond the Dural Fistula. *American Journal of Neuroradiology* 32: 798–808. [CrossRef]

Payne, Misty M. 2001. Charles Theodore Dotter: The Father of Intervention. *Texas Heart Institute Journal* 28: 28–38. [PubMed]

Perret, George, and Hiro Nishioka. 1966. Report on the Cooperative Study of Intracranial Aneurysms and Subarachnoid Hemorrhage: Arteriovenous Malformations. *Journal of Neurosurgery* 25: 467–90. [CrossRef] [PubMed]

Peschillo, Simone, Alessandro Caporlingua, Claudio Colonnese, and Giulio Guidetti. 2014. Brain AVMs: An Endovascular, Surgical, and Radiosurgical Update. *The Scientific World Journal* 2014: 834931. [CrossRef] [PubMed]

Peschillo, Simone, and Roberto Delfini. 2012. Endovascular neurosurgery in Europe and in Italy: What is in the future? *World Neurosurgery* 77: 248–51. [CrossRef]

Piano, Mariangela, Luca Valvassori, Luca Quilici, Guglielmo Pero, and Edoardo Boccardi. 2013. Midterm and long-term follow-up of cerebral aneurysms treated with flow diverter devices: A single-center experience. *Journal of Neurosurgery* 118: 408–16. [CrossRef]

Pierot, Laurent, and Ajay K. Wakhloo. 2013. Endovascular Treatment of Intracranial Aneurysms: Current Status. *Stroke* 44: 2046–54. [CrossRef]

Pierot, Laurent, C. Delcourt, F. Bouquigny, D. Breidt, B. Feuillet, O. Lanoix, and S. Gallas. 2006. Follow-up of intracranial aneurysms selectively treated with coils: Prospective evaluation of contrast-enhanced MR angiography. *American Journal of Neuroradiology* 27: 744–49.

Pierot, Laurent, X. Leclerc, A. Bonafé, S. Bracard, and French Matrix Registry Investigators. 2008a. Endovascular treatment of intracranial aneurysms with matrix detachable coils: Midterm anatomic follow-up from a prospective multicenter registry. *American Journal of Neuroradiology* 29: 57–61. [CrossRef]

Pierot, Laurent, Laurent Spelle, Fabien Vitry, and ATENA Investigators. 2008b. Clinical outcome of patients harbouring unruptured intracranial aneurysms treated by endovascular approach: Results of the ATENA trial. *Stroke* 39: 2497–504. [CrossRef]

Pierot, Laurent, Laurent Spelle, Xavier Leclerc, Christophe Cognard, Alain Bonafé, and Jacques Moret. 2009. Endovascular treatment of unruptured intracranial aneurysms: Comparison of safety of remodeling technique and standard treatment with coils. *Radiology* 251: 846–55. [CrossRef]

Pierot, Laurent, C. Cognard, L. Spelle, J. Moret, and CLARITY group. 2011. The remodelling technique for endovascular treatment of ruptured intracranial aneurysms is more efficacious than standard coiling with a similar safety. *Radiology* 258: 546–53. [CrossRef] [PubMed]

Pierot, Laurent, C. Cognard, F. Ricolfi, R. Anxionnat, and on behalf of CLARITY Group. 2012a. Mid-term anatomical results after endovascular treatment of ruptured intracranial aneurysms with GDC™ and Matrix™ coils: Analysis of the CLARITY series. *American Journal of Neuroradiology* 33: 469–73. [CrossRef] [PubMed]

Pierot, Laurent, C. Cognard, L. Spelle, and J. Moret. 2012b. Safety and efficacy of balloon remodeling technique during endovascular treatment of intracranial aneurysms: Critical review of the literature. *American Journal of Neuroradiology* 33: 12–15. [CrossRef] [PubMed]

Pierot, Laurent, C. Cognard, R. Anxionnat, F. Ricolfi, and CLARITY Investigators. 2012c. Endovascular treatment of ruptured intracranial aneurysms: Factors affecting midterm quality anatomic results: Analysis in a prospective, multicenter series of patients (CLARITY). *American Journal of Neuroradiology* 33: 1475–80. [CrossRef] [PubMed]

Pierot, Laurent, C. Portefaix, J.-Y. Gauvrit, and A. Boulin. 2012d. Follow-up of coiled intracranial aneurysms: Comparison of 3DTOF at 3T and 1.5T in a large, prospective series. *American Journal of Neuroradiology* 33: 2162–66. [CrossRef]

Pierot, Laurent, T. Liebig, V. Sychra, K. Kadziolka, F. Dorn, and C. Strasilla. 2012e. Intrasaccular flow disruption: A new endovascular approach for the treatment of intracranial aneurysms. Results of a preliminary clinical evaluation in a multicenter series. *American Journal of Neuroradiology* 33: 1232–38. [CrossRef]

Pierot, Laurent, Christophe Portefaix, Anne Boulin, and Jean-Yves Gauvrit. 2012f. Follow-up of coiled intracranial aneurysms: Comparison of 3D time-of-flight and contrast-enhanced magnetic resonance angiography at 3T in a large, prospective series. *European Radiology* 22: 2255–63. [CrossRef]

Pierot, Laurent, Joachim Klisch, Christophe Cognard, Istvan Szikora, Benjamin Mine, Krzysztof Kadziolka, Vojtech Sychra, Istvan Gubucz, Anne-Christine Januel, and Boris Lubicz. 2013. Endovascular WEB flow disruption in middle cerebral artery aneurysms: Preliminary feasibility, clinical, and anatomical results in a multicenter study. *Neurosurgery* 73: 27–34. [CrossRef]

Piotin, Michel, Raphaël Blanc, Laurent Spelle, Charbel Mounayer, Rhelen Piantino, Paul J. Schmidt, and Jacques Moret. 2010. Stent-assisted coiling of intracranial aneurysms: Clinical and angiographic results in 216 consecutive aneurysms. *Stroke* 41: 110–15. [CrossRef]

Raymond, Jean, François Guilbert, Alain Weill, Stavros A. Georganos, Louis Juravsky, Anick Lambert, Julie Lamoureux, Miguel Chagnon, and Daniel Roy. 2003. Long-term angiographic recurrences after selective endovascular treatment of aneurysms with detachable coils. *Stroke* 34: 1398–403. [CrossRef]

Riche, M. C., J. P. Melki, and J. J. Merland. 1983. Embolization of spinal cord vascular malformations via the anterior spinal artery. *American Journal of Neuroradiology* 4: 378–81. [PubMed]

Ricolfi, F., C. Manelfe, J. F. Meder, P. Arrué, P. Decq, P. Brugieres, C. Cognard, and A. Gaston. 1999. Intracranial dural arteriovenous fistulae with perimedullary venous drainage: Anatomical, clinical and therapeutic considerations. *Neuroradiology* 41: 803–12. [CrossRef] [PubMed]

Ricolfi, F., P. Y. Gobin, A. Aymard, F. Brunelle, A. Gaston, and J. J. Merland. 1997. Giant perimedullary arteriovenous fistulas of the spine: Clinical and radiologic features and endovascular treatment. *American Journal of Neuroradiology* 18: 677–87.

Ries, Thorsten, Jan-Hendrik Buhk, Thomas Kucinski, Einar Goebell, Ulrich Grzyska, Hermann Zeumer, and Jens Fiehler. 2006. Intravenous administration of acetylsalicylic acid during endovascular treatment of cerebral aneurysms reduces the rate of thromboembolic events. *Stroke* 37: 1816–21. [CrossRef] [PubMed]

Rodesch, G., M. Hurth, H. Alvarez, B. Ducot, M. Tadie, and P. Lasjaunias. 2004. Angio- architecture of spinal cord arteriovenous shunts at presentation: Clinical correlations in adults and children—The Bicetre experience on 155 consecutive patients seen between 1981–1999. *Acta Neurochirurgica* 146: 217–26. [CrossRef]

Rodesch, Georges, Michel Hurth, Beatrice Ducot, Hortensia Alvarez, Philippe David, Marc Tadie, and Pierre Lasjaunias. 2003. Embolization of spinal cord arteriovenous shunts: Morphological and clinical follow-up and results—Review of 69 consecutive cases. *Neurosurgery* 53: 40–49.

Rosenblum, Bruce, Edward H. Oldfield, John L. Doppman, and Giovanni Di Chiro. 1987. Spinal arteriovenous malformations: A comparison of dural arteriovenous fistulas and intradural AVM's in 81 patients. *Journal of Neurosurgery* 67: 795–802. [CrossRef]

Sadasivan, Chander, Liliana Cesar, Jaehoon Seong, Audrey Rakian, Qing Hao, Fermin O. Tio, Ajay K. Wakhloo, and Baruch B. Lieber. 2009. An original flow diversion device for the treatment of intracranial aneurysms: Evaluation in the rabbit elastase-induced model. *Stroke* 40: 952–8. [CrossRef]

Sanchez-Mejia, Rene O., Michael W. McDermott, Jeffery Tan, Helen Kim, William L. Young, and Michael T. Lawton. 2009. Radiosurgery facilitates resection of brain arteriovenous malformations and reduces surgical morbidity. *Neurosurgery* 64: 231–28. [CrossRef]

Santillan, A., Y. P. Gobin, E. D. Greenberg, L. Z. Leng, H. A. Riina, P. E. Stieg, and A. Patsalides. 2012. Intraprocedural aneurysmal rupture during coil embolization of brain aneurysms: Role of balloon-assisted coiling. *American Journal of Neuroradiology* 33: 2017–21. [CrossRef]

Sehba, Fatima A., Jack Hou, Ryszard M. Pluta, and John H. Zhang. 2012. The importance of early brain injury after subarachnoid hemorrhage. *Progress in Neurobiology* 97: 14–37. [CrossRef] [PubMed]

Shapiro, M., J. Babb, T. Becske, and P. K. Nelson. 2008. Safety and efficacy of adjunctive balloon remodeling during endovascular treatment of intracranial aneurysms: A literature review. *American Journal of Neuroradiology* 29: 1777–81. [CrossRef] [PubMed]

Shapiro, M., T. Becske, D. Sahlein, J. Babb, and Peter Kim Nelson. 2012. Stent-supported aneurysm coiling: A literature survey of treatment and follow-up. *American Journal of Neuroradiology* 33: 159–63. [CrossRef] [PubMed]

Sluzewski, Menno, Willem Jan Van Rooij, Guus N. Beute, and Peter C. Nijssen. 2006. Balloon-assisted coil embolization of intracranial aneurysms: Incidence, complications, and angiography results. *Journal of Neurosurgery* 105: 396–99. [CrossRef] [PubMed]

Smith, Robert R., Yuri N. Zubkov, Yahgoub Tarassoli, Robert R. Smith, Yuri N. Zubkov, and Yahgoub Tarassoli. 1994. The History of Aneurysm Surgery. In *Cerebral Aneurysms*. New York: Springer, pp. 1–9. [CrossRef]

Songsaeng, Dittapong, Sasikhan Geibprasert, Karel G. Ter Brugge, Robert Willinsky, Michael Tymianski, and Timo Krings. 2011. Impact of individual intracranial arterial aneurysm morphology on initial obliteration and recurrence rates of endovascular treatments: A multivariate analysis. *Journal of Neurosurgery* 114: 994–1002. [CrossRef]

Spetzler, Robert F., and Neil A. Martin. 1986. A proposed grading system for arteriovenous malformations. *Journal of Neurosurgery* 65: 476–83. [CrossRef]

Spetzler, Robert F., M. Yashar S. Kalani, and Peter Nakaji. 2015. *Neurovascular Surgery*. New York: Thieme.

Spetzler, Robert F., Paul W. Detwiler, Howard A. Riina, and Randall W. Porter. 2002. Modified classification of spinal cord vascular lesions. *Journal of Neurosurgery* 96: 145–56. [CrossRef]

Spetzler, Robert F., Ronald W. Hargraves, Patrick W. McCormick, Joseph M. Zabramski, Richard A. Flom, and Richard S. Zimmerman. 1992. Relationship of Perfusion Pressureand Size to Risk of Hemorrhage from Arteriovenous Malformations. *Journal of Neurosurgery* 76: 918–23. [CrossRef]

Stayman, Aaron N., Raul G. Nogueira, and Rishi Gupta. 2011. A systematic review of stenting and angioplasty of symptomatic extracranial vertebral artery stenosis. *Stroke* 42: 2212–26. [CrossRef]

Szajner, Maciej, Alain Weill, Michel Piotin, and Jacques Moret. 1999. Endovascular treatment of a cervical paraspinal arteriovenous malformation via arterial and venous approaches. *American Journal of Neuroradiology* 20: 1097–99.

Szikora, I., Z. Berentei, Z. Kulcsar, M. Marosfoi, Z. S. Vajda, W. Lee, A. Berez, and Peter Kim Nelson. 2010. Treatment of intracranial aneurysms by functional reconstruction of the parent artery: The Budapest experience with the pipeline embolization device. *American Journal of Neuroradiology* 31: 1139–47. [CrossRef] [PubMed]

Taheri, Zeinab, Mohammad Hosein Harirchian, Hosein Ghanaati, Alireza Khoshnevisan, Payman Salamati, Mojtaba Miri, Kavous Firouznia, Mina Saeednejad, Madjid Shakiba, and Vafa Rahimi-Movaghar. 2015. Comparison of endovascular coiling and surgical clipping for the treatment of intracranial aneurysms: A prospective study. *Iranian Journal of Neurology* 14: 22–28. [PubMed]

Teitelbaum, George P., Donald W. Larsen, Vladimir Zelman, Anatolii G. Lysachev, and Leonid B. Likhterman. 2000. A tribute to Dr. Fedor A. Serbinenko, founder of endovascular neurosurgery. *Neurosurgery* 46: 462–70. [CrossRef] [PubMed]

Vaidya, Sandeep, Kathleen R. Tozer, and Jarvis Chen. 2008. An Overview of Embolic Agents. *Seminars in Interventional Radiology* 25: 204–15. [CrossRef] [PubMed]

Vallée, Jean-Noël, Laurent Pierot, Alain Bonafé, Francis Turjman, Pierre Flandroy, Jérôme Berge, Georges Rodesch, and Serge Bracard. 2004. Endovascular treatment of intracranial wide-necked aneurysms using three-dimensional coils: Predictors of immediate anatomic and clinical results. *American Journal of Neuroradiology* 25: 298–306.

van Beijnum, J., H. B. Van der Worp, H. M. Schippers, O. Van Nieuwenhuizen, L. J. Kappelle, G. J. E. Rinkel, J. W. Berkelbach van der Sprenkel, and C. J. M. Klijn. 2007. Familial occurrence of brain arteriovenous malformations: A systematic review. *Journal of Neurology, Neurosurgery & Psychiatry* 78: 1213–17.

van Dijk, J. Marc C., Karel G. terBrugge, Robert A. Willinsky, and M. Christopher Wallace. 2002. Clinical course of cranial dural arteriovenous fistulas with long-term persistent cortical venous reflux. *Stroke* 33: 1233–36. [CrossRef]

Vlak, Monique H. M., Ale Algra, Raya Brandenburg, and Gabriël J. E. Rinkel. 2011. Prevalence of unruptured intracranial aneurysms, with emphasis on sex, age, comorbidity, country, and time period: A systematic review and meta-analysis. *The Lancet Neurology* 10: 626–36. [CrossRef]

Wakhloo, Ajay K., Giuseppe Lanzino, Baruch B. Lieber, and L. Nelson Hopkins. 1998. Stents for intracranial aneurysms: The beginning of a new endovascular era [Editorial comment]? *Neurosurgery* 43: 377–79. [CrossRef]

Wakhloo, Ajay K., I. Linfante, C. F. Silva, E. A. Samaniego, G. Dabus, V. Etezadi, Gabriela Spilberg, and Matthew J. Gounis. 2012. Closed-cell stent for coil embolization of intracranial aneurysms: Clinical and angiographic results. *American Journal of Neuroradiology* 33: 1651–56. [CrossRef]

Wakhloo, Ajay K., Jake Mandell, Matthew J. Gounis, Christopher Brooks, Italo Linfante, Jesse Winer, and John P. Weaver. 2008. Stent-assisted reconstructive endovascular repair of cranial fusiform atherosclerotic and dissecting aneurysms: Long-term clinical and angiographic follow-up. *Stroke* 39: 3288–96.

Wakhloo, AK, J Gounis, JS Sandhu, N Akkawi, A Schenck, and I Linfante. 2007. Complex- shaped platinum coils for intracranial aneurysms—Higher packing density and improved mid-term angiographic outcome. *American Journal of Neuroradiology* 28: 1395–1400. [CrossRef]

Weingrad, Daniel N., John L. Doppman, Paul B. Chretien, and Giovanni Di Chiro. 1979. Paraplegia due to posttraumatic pelvic arteriovenous fistula treated by surgery and embolization: Case report. *Journal of Neurosurgery* 50: 805–10. [CrossRef]

White, Philip M., Stephanie C. Lewis, Anil Gholkar, Robin J. Sellar, Hans Nahser, Christophe Cognard, Lynn Forrester, Joanna M. Wardlaw, and HELPS Trial Collaborators. 2011. Hydrogel-coated coils versus bare platinum coils for the endovascular treatment of intracranial aneurysms (HELPS): A randomised controlled trial. *The Lancet* 377: 1655–62. [CrossRef] [PubMed]

Willinsky, R. A., J. Peltz, L. Da Costa, R. Agid, and R. I. Farb. 2009. Clinical and angiographic follow-up of ruptured intracranial aneurysms treated with endovascular embolization. *American Journal of Neuroradiology* 30: 1035–40. [CrossRef] [PubMed]

Willinsky, R., W. Montanera, M. C. Wallace, and F. Gentili. 1993. Spinal epidural arteriovenous fistulas: Arterial and venous approaches to embolization. *American Journal of Neuroradiology* 14: 812–17. [PubMed]

Willinsky, Robert, Karel Terbrugge, Pierre Lasjaunias, and Walter Montanera. 1990. The variable presentations of craniocervical and cervical dural arteriovenous malformations. *Surgical Neurology* 34: 118–23. [CrossRef] [PubMed]

Yu, Wengui, and Wei-Jian Jiang. 2018. Stenting for intracranial stenosis: Potential future for the prevention of disabling or fatal stroke. *Stroke and Vascular Neurology* 3: e000158. [CrossRef]

Section VIII: Cranial Infection

Cerebral Infection and Parasitic Infestation

Mohammod Zahed Hossain, Forhad H. Chowdhury and Mohammod Hossain

Abstract: Cerebral infection and infestation are devastating events that can invite many life-threatening complications. The management of such complications may need neurosurgical intervention. Common cerebral infections include acute bacterial meningitis, tubercular and fungal infection. Common complications of acute bacterial meningitis that need neurosurgical intervention are hydrocephalus, brain abscess and subdural empyema. Tubercular and fungal infection usually complicate with granuloma or abscess formation, especially in immunocompromised or diabetic patients; however, hydrocephalus is also frequent in tubercular infection. Neurocysticercosis and hydatidosis are common parasitic infestations of the CNS. In this chapter, acute bacterial meningitis, viral meningitis, brain abscess, subdural empyema, fungal and tubercular infections are discussed, including their neurosurgical management. Parasitic infestations, neurocysticercosis, hydatidosis and cerebral malaria are discussed in brief. Finally, an important neurosurgical infection "shunt infection" is discussed in the last part of the chapter.

Abbreviations

ABM	acute bacterial meningitis	ADA	adenosine deaminase
AFB	acid-fast bacillus	AIDS	acquired immunodeficiency syndrome
ATT	anti-tubercular therapy	BCG	bacillus Calmette–Guerin
CD	Chagas disease	CFP	culture filtrate protein
CT	computed tomography	GIT	gastrointestinal tract
ELISA	enzyme-linked immunosorbant assay	EMB	ethambutol
ESAT6	early secreted antigenic target 6	FLAIR	fluid-attenuated inverse-recovery
HCP	Hydrocephalus	^{1}H-MRS	proton magnetic resonance spectroscopy
HAT	human African trypanosomiasis	HIV	human immunodeficiency virus
HSV	herpes simplex virus	ICSOL	intracranial space occupying lesion
INH	Isoniazid	IT	intrathecal
IVT	Intraventricular	IFN	interferon
ICP	intracranial pressure	IICP	increased intracranial pressure
IGRA	interferon-γ release assays	MRI	magnetic resonance imaging
MRS	magnetic resonance spectroscopy	MTB	mycobacterium tuberculosis
NAA	n-acetyl acetic acid	NCC	neurocysticercosis
NHL	non-Hodgkin's lymphoma	PCO2	partial pressure of oxygen
PCR	polymerase chain reaction	PPD	purified protein derivative
PZA	Pyrazinamide	RIF	rifampicin
SOL	space-occupying lesion	SDE	subdural empyema
SIADH	syndrome of inappropriate antidiuretic hormone	TOF	Tetrology of Fallot
TB	Tuberculosis	TIWI	T1-weighted image
T2WI	T2-weighted image	TBA	tubercular brain abscess
TBM	tubercular meningitis	WHO	World Health Organization
WNV	West Nile virus	VZV	varicella-zoster virus

1. Introduction

A cerebral infection is a common condition encountered in neurological and neurosurgical practice. Because of the protective barrier of its bony components (skull and spinal column), the meninges, as well as the blood–brain barrier (BBB), the central nervous system (CNS) is particularly resistant to infection by bacteria and other pathogens. The CNS, on the other hand, is more vulnerable to infections than most other tissues once infection has begun. In the CNS, host defensive systems that are ordinarily observed in other parts of the body are insufficient to prevent bacterial reproduction and disease progression (Beatriz and Lopez 2019). The intensity of a bacterial CNS infection is heavily influenced by preexisting and/or predisposing factors. Respiratory and systemic infections, head trauma, past neurosurgical surgeries, cancer, alcoholism and other immunodeficiency conditions are also examples (Beatriz and Lopez 2019).

An intracranial infection affects the brain and meninges, and intraspinal infection affects the spinal cord and its meninges. Infections of the CNS are caused by viral, bacterial, fungal, protozoal and prionic agents.

Bacterial infections can affect diverse parts of the CNS, leading to a variety of clinical and pathologic symptoms. Meningitis, encephalitis and abscess are the three major infectious disorders based on the location and form of the inflammatory reaction. TB meningitis, tubercular abscess and tuberculoma are examples of tuberculous infection lesions.

2. Acute Bacterial Meningitis

Acute bacterial meningitis (ABM) is an emergency condition in neurology that can be fatal. It is characterized by a purulent infection in the subarachnoid spaces, which is frequently accompanied by meningeal inflammation, inflammation of the cerebral tissue and cerebral vasculature (LaPenna and Roos 2019). It affects the brain's leptomeninges. The term "meningitis" points to inflammation of the meninges in general. Meningitis can be due to a wide range of infectious as well as noninfectious diseases (Dorsett and Liang 2016). Acute bacterial meningitis, often known as purulent meningitis, is a serious sickness marked by purulent cerebrospinal fluid (CSF); it progresses quickly and is lethal if left untreated (Beatriz and Lopez 2019). The complication and mortality rates are both extremely high. As a result, early detection of clinical symptoms, early initiation of empiric antibiotic/s, correct diagnostic investigations and awareness of typical consequences are critical in the treatment of bacterial meningitis patients (LaPenna and Roos 2019). ABM occurs when bacteria reach the subarachnoid spaces via bacteremia (typically from an upper respiratory tract source), contiguous extension from dental or paranasal sinus infections, traumatic or congenital external communications or neurosurgical treatment (Dorsett and Liang 2016; Tintinalli and Stapczynski 2011).

2.1. Epidemiology

The most frequent purulent CNS illness is bacterial meningitis. Because of the introduction of conjugate vaccinations in the 1990s, occurrences of community-acquired bacterial meningitis have decreased significantly, although the fatality rates remain high (LaPenna and Roos 2019; Thigpen et al. 2011). Bacterial meningitis is much more common in developing nations, particularly in Sub-Saharan Africa, than it is in developed countries (LaPenna and Roos 2019).

Prior to the introduction of vaccines, the most common causes of ABM were reported to be Hemophilus influenza type b (Hib), Streptococcus pneumoniae and Neisseria meningitides, with their relative contributions differing by location, time and age group in different regions of the Earth (Jayaraman et al. 2018; McIntyre et al. 2012; Ramakrishnan et al. 2009). Since the 1980s, the frequency of community-acquired bacterial meningitis among American children has decreased dramatically because of the introduction of efficient vaccines against Hemophilus influenzae type b and Streptococcus pneumoniae (Honda and Warren 2009; Adams et al. 1993; Centers for Disease Control and Prevention 2005). The incidence rate of community-onset bacterial meningitis (3–6 cases per 100,000 people) among adults, on the other hand, has remained constant over the last decade (Honda and Warren 2009; Choi 2001; Short and Tunkel 2000).

2.2. Etiology and Pathophysiology

Bacteria enter the CNS after direct introduction of the cerebral tissue or from an infective focus external to the CNS. The route of entry of the microorganisms is (1) hematogenous, (2) direct spread from adjacent area infection, (3) direct inoculation by penetrating wound or during operation. The most prevalent route of infection is hematogenous transmission, and the upper respiratory tract is the most common entry point for microorganisms (Beatriz and Lopez 2019).

When the pathogenic bacteria settle and colonize the nasopharyngeal mucosa and enter the bloodstream through epithelial cells, meningitis develops. The bacteria must replicate and survive the host's defenses in the bloodstream in order to get direct entry to the CNS via the choroid plexus or microvasculature; pass the BBB; and survive and grow in the CSF (Beatriz and Lopez 2019; Kim 2003). Most bacteria get entrance to the CSF through mechanisms that are nor totally understood. Because the CSF lacks key host defense mechanisms, including lower concentrations of immunoglobulins and complement, bacterial proliferation is aided once the bacteria are present. The immune condition of the host, as well as the virulence of the bacteria, will undoubtedly play a part in the infection's development (Beatriz and Lopez 2019; Kim 2003). Once bacteria enter the CSF fluid, their multiplication causes the BBB to become more permeable by releasing proinflammatory and toxic chemicals (Kim 2003).

Meningitis can also be caused by germs being transmitted directly from neighboring tissues to the brain, such as the (a) paranasal air sinuses, (b) middle ear cavity and mastoid sinuses, or (c) via an emissary vein from the scalp and face. Pathogen inoculation can also occur as a result of direct trauma implantation in penetrating traumas and compound skull fractures, as well as subsequent surgical operations and invasive investigation and therapeutic interventions, including due to congenital abnormalities like myelomeningoceles (Beatriz and Lopez 2019).

The three primary agents that cause ABM are N meningitides, S pneumoniae and H influenzae (Thigpen et al. 2011). Most surveillance studies in the USA revealed that S pneumoniae (61%), N meningitides (16%), group B streptococcus (14%), H influenzae (7%), and Listeria monocytogenes were the most common causative pathogens of bacterial meningitis (2%) (Dery and Hasbun 2007). A study conducted in Bangladesh revealed a similar picture (Gurley et al. 2009). Pneumococcal meningitis is caused by immune deficiencies (such as asplenia or agammaglobulinemia). Meningococcal meningitis is more likely in people who have asplenia or terminal complement insufficiency (Honda and Warren 2009; Overturf 2003). Escherichia coli, Streptococcus, Staphylococcus aureus and Moraxella were among the less frequent organisms discovered (Gurley et al. 2009).

Those who have recently undergone neurosurgical surgery, suffered head trauma or had endocarditis should be tested for Staphylococcus aureus species. Gram-negative bacilli can generate meningitis in persons who have had neurosurgery. Streptococci species and Gram-negative anaerobic organisms can cause meningitis in patients with otitis, sinusitis or mastoiditis (Beatriz and Lopez 2019; LaPenna and Roos 2019).

Purulent exudates might be detected in the subarachnoid space during the acute phase of the disease. There may be significant congestion of the leptomeningeal arteries, as well as cerebral edema. The meninges have an abundance of cellular infiltrates made up of neutrophils, as well as fibrin exudate. Bacteria can be found both within and outside the cell. Subacute and chronic stages may begin with a shift in cellular inflammatory infiltrates to mononuclear cells, such as lymphocytes, plasma cells and macrophages, once the infectious sequences have been brought under control by therapy (Beatriz and Lopez 2019). Fibroblast growth can be variable, resulting in leptomeningeal fibrosis. Inflammatory vasculitis with microthrombosis and cortical infarctions can be found in this stage of the disease. Purulent ventriculitis develops when an infection spreads into the ventricles, resulting in purulent collections that obstruct the ventricular system's foramina, preventing CSF passage and causing obstructive hydrocephalus. Communicating hydrocephalus can also be caused by leptomeningeal fibrosis, which causes poor CSF reabsorption (Beatriz and Lopez 2019). The infected process can spread to the cranial nerves, particularly the cochlear nerves, resulting in hearing impairment, which is one of the most common meningitis complications in children (Beatriz and Lopez 2019; Edwards and Baker 1981). Other cranial nerve palsies can result from basal meningitis.

2.3. *Clinical Features*

The classical triad of ABM is fever, headache and a stiff neck (LaPenna and Roos 2019). Some authors have included an altered state of consciousness instead of a headache in the classic triad. Although each of these signs/symptoms is common, the trio may not be present. Vomiting, a lowered degree of consciousness and photophobia are some of the other indications and symptoms. Temperatures greater than or equal to 37.7 °C/100 °F are the most sensitive of these symptoms, appearing in 95% of individuals at presentation and 99% within 24 h (LaPenna and Roos 2019; Durand et al. 1933). Headache, fever, altered sensorium and neck stiffness are symptoms that nearly all individuals with ABM will have (LaPenna and Roos 2019; van de Beek et al. 2004). Seizures were identified in 15% of adult cases (Weisfelt et al. 2006). In extreme cases, ABM can cause coma, seizures and focal neurologic impairments, all of which are linked to a poor prognosis (Honda and Warren 2009; Aronin et al. 1998; Flores-Cordero et al. 2003). Age, anatomic anomalies, concurrent illness, immunological function and the causative agent can all influence the severity of symptoms (Honda and Warren 2009). A full neurologic examination, as well as a general examination with a focus on the head, nose, ear and nasopharynx, should be performed on a suspected meningitis patient. Meningitis-specific movements, including Kernig's sign, jolt accentuation of headache and Brudzinski's sign can all indicate the existence of meningeal irritation (Honda and Warren 2009). Nuchal stiffness, which affects about 80% of people, should be tested during physical examination (LaPenna and Roos 2019; van de Beek et al. 2004; Weisfelt et al. 2006). Kernig's and Brudzinski's signs are traditional signs; however, their sensitivity is limited and their diagnostic value is dubious (LaPenna and Roos 2019; Thomas et al. 2002). A petechial rash, which is very symptomatic of meningococcemia, should be evaluated on the skin of patients (LaPenna and Roos 2019). The anterior fontanelle bulges in babies. Papilledema may be present in some patients. When tapping your lumbar region, it will be noticed that the opening pressure is higher.

Based on the seriousness of the disease, signs of brain dysfunction such as confusion, delirium and lethargy might progress to a coma. Clinical signs can differ depending on the individual's age. For example, newborns rarely show signs of meningismus and are more prone to septicemia-like symptoms. Acute meningitis in the elderly can have a more subtle beginning, manifesting as tiredness and disorientation rather than the symptoms of a more severe feverish infection. Clinical signs and symptoms (Table 1) differ depending on the bacterial pathogen. For example, meningococcus meningitis is often grave, and even when the condition is detected early and appropriate treatment is administered, 5 to 10% of people die within 24 to 48 h of the start of symptom (Beatriz and Lopez 2019; Bilukha and Rosenstein 2005).

Table 1. Presenting clinical features of cases with ABM.

Sign or Symptom	Approximate Frequency (%)
Fever	>90
Headache	>90
Altered level of consciousness	>80
Meningismus	>85
Convulsion/seizures	~30
Vomiting	~35
Focal neurological deficit/s	10~20
Papilledema	<5

Source: Authors' compilation based on data from Honda and Warren (2009).

2.4. *Laboratory Investigations*

2.4.1. CSF: Opening Pressure, Chemistries and Cell Count

Meningitis is diagnosed by analyzing the cerebrospinal fluid because there may be no identifiable symptoms or physical signs. To avoid a misdiagnosis, the CSF must be interpreted carefully, the opening pressure is generally higher, in ABM, but the range might vary. For cryptococcal meningitis, measuring the opening pressure is very crucial because a high opening pressure (>250 mm Hg) is a poor prognostic sign (Honda and Warren 2009; Saag et al. 2000). Pleocytosis (100 cells/mm^3 to 10,000 cells/mm^3) is commonly detected in individuals with ABM, with neutrophil-predominant pleocytosis accounting for 80 to 95% of cases (Honda and Warren 2009; van de Beek et al. 2004; van de Beek et al. 2006). Up to 10% of patients with ABM have a normal or modestly raised CSF leukocyte count, which indicates a bad prognosis (Honda and Warren 2009; van de Beek et al. 2004). Although lymphocyte-predominant pleocytosis is common in viral, tuberculous or fungal meningitis, the presence of lymphocytes in the CSF does not exclude the potential of ABM. Almost all cases with bacterial meningitis have an increase in protein (Honda and Warren 2009; Tunkel et al. 2004). A lower glucose level in the CSF (less than 40 mg/dL) suggests the diagnosis of bacterial meningitis (Honda and Warren 2009; Tunkel et al. 2004). Other biochemical indicators, such as a high amount of lactate in the CSF or a high level of serum procalcitonin may help identify ABM from other causes of meningeal inflammation/irritation (Honda and Warren 2009; Genton and Berger 1990; Viallon et al. 1999).

2.4.2. Gram Stain and Cultures

As the sterilization of CSF may occur as early as 15 min following parenteral antibiotic therapy, a rapid Gram stain of the CSF can produce the rapid detection of the causal bacteria (Honda and Warren 2009; Kanegaye et al. 2001). A Gram stain of the CSF may show the pathogenic bacterium even if the CSF culture is negative. In bacterial meningitis, the sensitivity of a Gram stain varies from 60 to 90%, based on the number of bacteria in the CSF (Honda and Warren 2009; van de Beek et al. 2004). A positive Gram stain for bacterial meningitis is extremely specific. The yield of a Gram stain may be increased by centrifuging the samples. The culture of the CSF is crucial in the diagnosis of ABM (Honda and Warren 2009).

2.4.3. Serology, PCR and Latex Agglutination

The use of PCR assays in the detection of viral meningitis has been very beneficial (Honda and Warren 2009; Kupila et al. 2006). For both bacterial (N meningitidis, S pneumoniae and H influenzae) and viral (HSV, VZV and enteroviruses) meningitis, PCR has a specificity and sensitivity of above 90% (Honda and Warren 2009; Radstrom et al. 1994; DeBiasi and Tyler 1999). Despite the fact that PCR assays are the gold standard for detecting viral meningitis, clinical matching is always recommended because false positive/negative results are possible (Honda and Warren 2009).

2.4.4. Cranial Imaging

Despite the low incidence (2%) of the existence of space-occupying lesions or mass effect in the common patient population, a CT scan is routinely conducted before lumbar puncture (Honda and Warren 2009; Hasbun et al. 2001). Prior to lumbar puncture, defined clinical criteria can help eliminate unnecessary cranial imaging. When a CT scan is recommended, the first dose of antimicrobials should be given before the cranial imaging (Honda and Warren 2009; Tunkel et al. 2004).

The findings of neuroimaging in acute meningitis differ according to the stage of the meningitis. In the early stages, imaging findings may be normal. On MRI, diffuse meningeal enhancement is seen with infrequent involvement of the perivascular Virchow–Robin spaces in the course of more advanced disease. Cerebral edema is also present, along with communicating hydrocephalus. On T2W or fluid attenuation inversion recovery (FLAIR) scans, hyperintensity of the cortical ribbon, most commonly representing an incipient infarction secondary to localized vasculitis, can be detected (Beatriz and Lopez 2019; Grossman and Yousem 2003).

2.4.5. Hematology

Neutrophilic leukocytosis with a high ESR is found in bacterial meningitis. Viral and fungal meningitis shows non-specific findings.

Investigations should also be carried out for evaluation of the source of infection.

2.5. Treatment

2.5.1. Antimicrobial Therapy

Though the management of meningitis patients is akin to that of other infectious disorders, empiric antibiotic therapy should be initiated soon after clinical diagnosis. Antimicrobials should be chosen empirically based on their action against the most possible pathogens, age, epidemiologic information, patient immunological status or other predisposing variables (e.g., history of the base of skull fracture or penetrating injury). Because the concentration of antimicrobials in the CSF is changeable, a bactericidal antibiotic is significantly preferred over one with bacteriostatic activity. Because S pneumoniae and N meningitidis cause nearly 80% of community-onset meningitis, third-generation cephalosporins (e.g., ceftriaxone, cefotaxime) have been utilized as first-line medicines (Honda and Warren 2009; van de Beek et al. 2004; Schuchat et al. 1997).

Antibiotic treatment should be adjusted once a causal bacterium has been detected. The selection of pathogen-targeted treatment is based on antimicrobial susceptibility in vitro and antimicrobial agent penetration into the cerebrospinal fluid (Honda and Warren 2009). However, if clinical improvement with an empiric antimicrobial agent has been demonstrated at this time, the empiric treatment that has already been provided should be continued.

Antimicrobial treatment should be prescribed for at least 5 days following the start of symptoms, including fever. Some authors advised that all patients receive treatment for at least 14 days (Greenberg 2010).

Antimicrobial agents should be administered intravenously. Antimicrobial drugs can be given intraventricularly or intrathecally in the case of postsurgical meningitis or ventriculitis (Remeš et al. 2013). In post-surgical individuals with meningitis and ventriculitis, intraventricular (IVT) or lumbar intrathecal (IT) antibiotics can result in very rapid CSF sterilization. Individuals treated with IVT/IT antibiotics have a very low relapse incidence of meningitis and/or ventriculitis. Antibiotics administered intraventricularly/lumbar intrathecally appear to be an efficacious and safe therapy for CNS infections produced by multidrug-resistant bacteria (Remeš et al. 2013).

Because the etiologic organisms vary from those shown in community-onset meningitis, broader-spectrum antibiotic drugs are necessary to treat nosocomial meningitis. Vancomycin in combination with 3rd or 4th cephalosporins or a carbapenem is an effective empiric antimicrobial treatment. Newer antistaphylococcal medicines (e.g., linezolid or daptomycin) were seen to be efficacious in the treatment of staphylococcal meningitis

(Honda and Warren 2009). In situations of nosocomial meningitis, removal of retained foreign bodies (e.g., contaminated bone fragment, intraventricular catheter, dirty debris in compound depressed fracture) is indicated.

Sinusitis, upper respiratory tract, CSOM, endocarditis and other causative factors should be treated.

2.5.2. Adjuvant Therapy

Corticosteroids have been utilized for ABM in pediatric cases, according to a controlled, randomized study in the 1980s. Dexamethasone treatment in the pediatric patient with ABM is accompanied with a lower death rate, as well as reduced frequency of neurological or audiological sequelae dues to a decrease in the host inflammatory reaction in the subarachnoid spaces (Honda and Warren 2009; Lebel et al. 1988; Odio et al. 1991; Schaad et al. 1993).

2.5.3. Supportive Care

In the treatment of meningitis, extensive supportive care is essential. It is critical to provide appropriate circulatory resuscitation. To avoid negative neurologic outcomes caused by dehydration, many specialists suggest euvolemic states over restricted volume states (Honda and Warren 2009; Maconochie et al. 2008). Periodic mental status evaluations are beneficial for assessing the recovery and early detection of fresh focal neurological abnormalities or seizures. Aggravation of meningeal inflammation, cerebral abscess with adjoining edema, hyponatremia and fever due to the syndrome of inappropriate antidiuretic hormone (SIADH), or toxicity due to high doses of antibiotics, particularly beta-lactams or carbapenems, can all cause mental status changes in individuals with meningitis (Honda and Warren 2009).

2.6. Complications and Treatment

The frequent complications of bacterial meningitis include the following:

1. Raised intracranial pressure is a frequent complication of bacterial meningitis;
2. Hyponatremia is a condition in which there is a lack of sodium (25%);
3. Affliction of a seizure (13–15%);
4. Hydrocephalus (acute) (3–8%);
5. Encephalitis is a disease that affects the brain and hearing loss is the most prevalent symptom of cranial nerve palsy;
6. Cortical insufficiency;
7. Effusion of the subdural space;
8. Abscess in the brain;
9. Dystonia;
10. Paralysis in a specific area;
11. Mental retardation, etc. (Honda and Warren 2009; Vasudeva 2019).

Increased intercranial pressure is seen in more than half of cryptococcal meningitis patients (Honda and Warren 2009; Saag et al. 2000). To manage acute hydrocephalus or increased intracranial pressure, repeated lumbar punctures, ventriculostomy, lumbar CSF drain or ventricular shunt insertion should be explored (Honda and Warren 2009; Saag et al. 2000).

The most common consequences of meningitis are hyponatremia and seizures. Hyponatremia affects about 25% of cases of bacterial meningitis (Honda and Warren 2009; Genton and Berger 1990). Hyponatremia can be caused by different factors, including salt depletion, SIADH, vigorous hydration or hypoadrenalism. Serial electrolyte monitoring should be used to ensure that serum electrolytes are properly adjusted. Seizures occur in 13–15% of ABM cases (Honda and Warren 2009; van de Beek et al. 2004; Aronin et al. 1998). Electroencephalographic monitoring should be undertaken in individuals with a history of seizure or variable mental status (Honda and Warren 2009; van de Beek et al. 2006). Seizures should be managed with IV anticonvulsants like lorazepam, midazolam, barbiturate or phenytoin as soon as possible. Though the necessity for anticonvulsants as a seizure prophylaxis in all cases of ABM is unclear, anticonvulsants should be used whenever clinical proof of seizure or a mass lesion is discovered (Honda and Warren 2009). In the condition of severe encephalitis, cerebral edema can occur, requiring ICP control with mannitol (1 g/kg first dose, 0.25–0.5 g/kg q6h), IV dexamethasone, or endotracheal intubation and mild hyperventilation, with arterial PCO2 of about 28–30 mm Hg. In these circumstances, an ICP monitor with transduced intraparenchymal pressure should be placed (Wan 2018).

3. Viral Meningitis

Meningitis, encephalitis and myelitis are frequent viral infections of the CNS found in clinical practice around the world (Abid et al. 2018; Big et al. 2009). Aseptic meningitis is a kind of viral meningitis. In adults, enteroviruses like coxsackieviruses and echoviruses are the most common etiology of viral meningitis (Honda and Warren 2009; Connolly and Hammer 1990). In western and south Asian countries, enteroviruses are by far the most common pathogens associated in viral meningitis (from 85 to 90% from all viral etiologies) (Abid et al. 2018; Rotbart et al. 1998; Caballero et al. 2011). Herpes viruses, such as HSV1/HSV2 and varicella-zoster virus, are infamous globally as the causes of viral encephalitis and meningitis (Abid et al. 2018; Tan et al. 2014). HSV-1 causes herpes simplex virus (HSV) encephalitis, which has an occurrence rate of 1 case per 250,000 people in the USA (van de Beek et al. 2006). HSV encephalitis has a bimodal age distribution, with cases younger than 20 years and older than 50 years of age being the most prevalent. HSV-2 is a common etiologic agent of meningitis, responsible for 17% of aseptic meningitis cases. In the USA (Honda and Warren 2009; Kupila et al. 2006), arboviruses, including the West Nile virus (WNV), have emerged as common causes of meningoencephalitis (Honda and Warren 2009). Aseptic meningoencephalitis is a complication of acute HIV infection (Honda and Warren 2009; Newton et al. 2002).

The clinical features of viral meningitis are akin to those of bacterial meningitis.

In viral, tuberculous, fungal meningitis, lymphocyte-predominant pleocytosis is common (Honda and Warren 2009).

The management of viral meningitis treatment is mainly supportive. Rest, fluids, antipyretics and analgesic or NSAID drugs can be administered as necessary. The most important decision is whether or not to initiate antibiotic treatment for bacterial meningitis on an empirical basis while waiting for the causes to be detected. If bacterial meningitis is suspected, intravenous (IV) antibiotics should be initiated as soon as possible (Wan 2018; Nigrovic et al. 2013). Several antiviral drugs are currently being evaluated in the general population; however, their effectiveness in precluding the potentially fatal complications of viral meningitis is yet to be determined. In herpetic viral infections, acyclovir is remarkedly beneficial solely if given very early in the course of the illness (Wan 2018). Seizure and encephalitis should be treated accordingly.

4. Fungal Infections

Fungal infections of the CNS can be fatal, and they are virtually often a clinical surprise. They have a mild presentation with few diagnostic features, and they are frequently misdiagnosed as pyogenic abscess, tuberculous meningitis or brain neoplasms (Sheikh and Amr 2010).

There are two types of fungal species that can harm the central nervous system (Sheikh and Amr 2010):

I. Pathogenic fungi: Infectious fungus that can infect healthy hosts.

(i) Cryptococcus neoformans is a kind of cryptococcus. (ii) Histoplasma capsulatum is the second kind of histoplasma. (iii) Coccidioides immitis is a kind of coccidioid. (iv) Paracoccidioides Braziliensis, (v) Sporothrix schenckii is a species of Sporothrix. (vi) Blastomyces dermatides is the sixth species in the Blastomyces genus.

II. Opportunistic fungi: Commonly generate infections in immunocompromised people.

1. Aspergillosis 2. Zygomycosis (Mucormycosis) 3. Cerebral Phaeohyphomycoses 4. Candidiasis (*C. albicans, C. tropicalis, C. lusitaniae, C. viswathii*) 5. Penicillioses

Meningitis can be caused by any of the major fungal infections. Meningitis can be due to a variety of fungi, ranging from relatively frequent cryptococcal meningitis to uncommon meningitis caused by filamentous or dimorphic fungi. CNS infections can be caused by Cryptococcus, Aspergillus, Candida and a variety of molds. Brain abscesses can be caused by many of the etiologic pathogens of fungal meningitis. *Candida* spp. are the most common etiologic pathogen, followed by *Aspergillus* spp.; however, Cryptococcus neoformans and other fungi can also be responsible for meningitis (Sheikh and Amr 2010).

Generally, a fungal infection of the CNS can result in one or more of the symptoms listed below (Sheikh and Amr 2010):

- Encephalitis;
- Chronic and sub-acute meningitis;
- Granulomas parenchymal or brain abscesses;
- Vascular thrombosis resulting in stroke, infarction or myelopathy;
- Vasculitis.

The most common variety of the disease is intraparenchymal abscesses or basal meningitis caused by fungal pathogens.

Clinical manifestations of fungal infection lack specific findings but present as other meningitis of more insidious onset, not responding to usual antibiotics. A CSF culture and PCR provide the diagnosis. The detection of cryptococcal meningitis and cryptococcal antigen latex agglutination of the CSF show excellent sensitivity and specificity (sensitivity: 93–100%; specificity: 93–98%) (Honda and Warren 2009). When present with a fungal granuloma, it mimics ICSOL or brain abscesses. It presents with features of the site of involvement. Cavernous sinus syndrome, cranial nerve palsy, hemiparesis and seizure may be the clinically presenting feature. Cranial imaging by a CT or an MRI is not specific. Postoperative histopathology can provide an answer. Specific antifungal agents, excision of the granuloma and reversal of immunosuppression, and immunomodulation state are the treatments (Sheikh and Amr 2010). Polyenes (amphotericin B), triazoles (itraconazole, voriconazole, isavuconazole and posaconazole), echinocandins (micafungin, caspofungin and anidulafungin) and flucytosine are four primary types of antifungal drugs that can be used to treat CNS infections (5-FC) (Sheikh and Amr 2010).

5. Brain Abscess

The localized intraparenchymal collection of pus in any part of the brain, e.g., cerebrum, cerebellum or brainstem, is called a brain abscess.

Brain abscesses are widespread in affluent countries and considerably more so in impoverished countries (Chowdhury et al. 2015; Bernardini 2004). Despite the introduction of modern neurosurgical innovation such as stereotactic aspiration and biopsy, improved culturing methods for detecting the infectious agent and new antibiotics, as well as noninvasive imaging methods, brain abscesses remain a public health concern, particularly in underdeveloped countries (Chowdhury et al. 2015). In impoverished countries, brain abscesses account for roughly 8% of intracranial space-occupying lesions, but in Western countries, the figure is closer to 2% (Chowdhury et al. 2015; Bernardini 2004; Zhang et al. 2014; Loftus et al. 1996; Sharma et al. 2000).

5.1. Etiology and Pathogenesis

The risk factors for brain abscess formation are multifactorial, including (a) pulmonary abnormalities (infection, A–V fistula, etc.), (b) cardiac pathology (congenital cyanotic heart disease, bacterial endocarditis, etc.), (c) nearby infections (CSOM, sinusitis, etc.), (d) penetrating head trauma, (e) AIDS, etc.

Brain abscesses are generally the outcome of a secondary infection from an extracerebral original source that disseminates to the CNS via (1) hematogenous spread or (2) contiguous extend from nearby structures (Beatriz and Lopez 2019).

Abscesses caused by hematogenous dissemination from a distant focus, responsible for roughly 20% to 25% of all cases (Beatriz and Lopez 2019; Brown and Gray 2009). Pulmonary infections, like bronchiectasis and lung abscesses, are the most prevalent primary causes in adults, followed by dental infections. Infections of the pelvis and abdomen, septicemia and bacterial endocarditis are some of the other causes. Congenital heart disorders with a right-to-left shunt owing to paradoxical emboli are the most prevalent primary causes in children (Beatriz and Lopez 2019; Frazier et al. 2008). About 20% of patients have abscesses caused by the contiguous extension of a local infection into the brain (Carpenter et al. 2007). Sinusitis, chronic and acute otitis, and mastoiditis are all common causes of an infection in children. Sinusitis and osteomyelitis of neighboring skull anatomical structures are the typical causes of an infection in adults. The direct insertion of germs in penetrating head injuries and postsurgical treatments can also cause brain abscesses. Certain abscesses can occur anywhere from 2 to 37% of the time in these situations (Beatriz and Lopez 2019; Honda and Warren 2009; Carpenter et al. 2007). In roughly 25% of brain abscesses, the cause of infection is idiopathic; a comprehensive work-up for cardiac shunts is required in the case of cryptogenic abscesses. Most brain abscesses are single lesions that develop in areas near the infection's initial source. Abscesses caused by direct extension from the odontogenic foci or frontal sinuses are mainly seen in the frontal lobe; abscesses caused by otogenic infections, on the other hand, are generally cerebellar or temporal. Multiple abscesses are caused by hematogenous dissemination and while they can occur anywhere in the brain, most are frequently seen in the region of the middle cerebral artery.

Regarding their spread from the nasopharynx and oropharynx, streptococci are the most common etiology of pyogenic brain abscesses. Another common reason for brain abscesses is anaerobic bacteria, which commonly occur as part of a multi-microbial infection. Brain abscess microbiology is influenced by the initial location of the infection.

In individuals with lung abscesses, *Streptococcus* spp. and anaerobic microbes are frequently isolated. Individuals with brain abscesses caused by endocarditis frequently have Staphylococcus aureus or viridians-group streptococci (Honda and Warren 2009). Gram-negative enteric bacilli are frequently seen in conjunction with a genitourinary or intra-abdominal source. Brain abscesses due to otitis externa or otitis media can contain *Pseudomonas* spp. (Honda and Warren 2009; Mathisen and Johnson 1997). Brain abscesses that result from neurosurgical treatments or head trauma typically contain *Staphylococcus* spp. and aerobic Gram-negative bacilli (Honda and Warren 2009). Bacterial agent and sources in bacterial brain abscess are shown in Table 2.

Table 2. Bacterial brain abscess: bacterial agent and source.

Location of the Primary Infection	Bacterial Pathogen(s)
Hematogenous Spread	
Congenital cyanotic cardiac disease	*Haemophilus* spp., *Streptococcus* spp., *S. aureus*
Bacteremia and endocarditis	*Streptococcus* spp., *S. aureus*
Lung infections	*Streptococcus* spp., anaerobic Gram-negative, *Fusobacterium, Nocardia, Actinomyces*
Genitourinary and intra-abdominal infection	Enteric Gram-negative bacilli
Spread of Contiguous Infection	
Odontogenic and sinuses infections	*Streptococcus* spp., *S. aureus, Bacteroides, Enterobacteriaceae, Haemophilus* spp.
Mastoid and ear infections	*Streptococcus* spp., *Enterobacteriaceae, Pseudomonas, Bacteroides* spp.
Penetrating head trauma	Staphylococci, *Bacteroides* spp., *Enterobacteriaceae, Clostridium*
Post-surgical procedures	*S. aureus, Pseudomonas*

Source: Authors' compilation based on data from Honda and Warren (2009).

5.1.1. Stages of Cerebral Abscess

There are four well-recognized stages of a cerebral abscess (Table 3).

Table 3. Histologic staging of cerebral abscesses.

Stage	Pathology	Resistant to Inserting a Needle
Stage 1: Early cerebritis Days: 1–3	Early infection, perivascular infiltration of inflammatory cells around the central core of coagulation necrosis, poorly demarcated from the surrounding brain.	Intermediate resistance
Stage 2: Late cerebritis Days: 4–9	Pus generation in necrotic center which is encircled by inflammatory cells, a fibroblast.	No resistance
Stage 3: Early capsule development Days: 10–13	Neovascularity, necrotic center, a capsule is better formed on the cortical side than on the ventricular side of the lesion.	No resistance
Stage 4: Late capsule formation Days: >14	Dense collagenous capsule with well-defined necrotic center, gliosis around the capsule.	Firm resistance, "pop" on entering

Source: Authors' compilation based on data from Greenberg (2010).

5.2. *Clinical Features and Diagnosis*

None of the symptoms are specific (Greenberg 2010). The clinical signs of people with brain abscesses differ depending on where the abscess is located and how virulent the germs are. Fever, headaches and altered mental status are the most classical symptoms (Beatriz and Lopez 2019). Focal neurological impairments and other features of a space-occupying mass (hemiparesis, seizure, etc.) may also be present based on the site of the abscess, as well as clinical features of a raised ICP (vomiting/nausea, headache, lethargy, etc.) (Beatriz and Lopez 2019).

5.3. Imaging

The widespread availability of imaging tests has assisted in the detection of brain abscesses. In the case of a well-developed or chronic brain abscess, a contrast CT scan may show single- or multiple-ring-enhanced lesions (Figure 1). To identify a brain abscess, a contrast MRI is more specific and sensitive than a contrast CT scan (Figure 2) (Honda and Warren 2009).

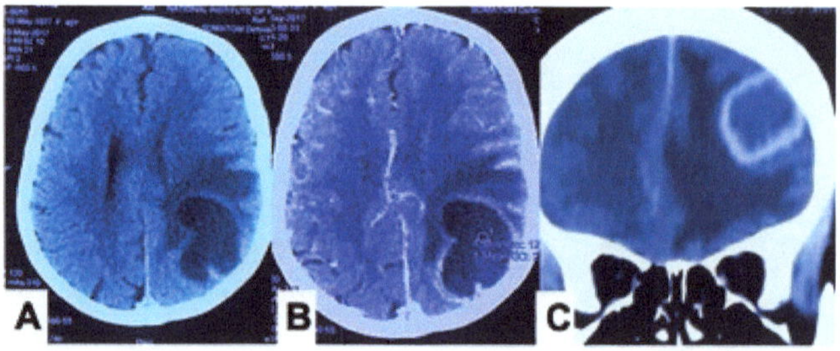

Figure 1. Plane (**A**) and contrast (**B**,**C**) CT scan of a head with a parieto-occipital brain abscess. Source: Figure by authors.

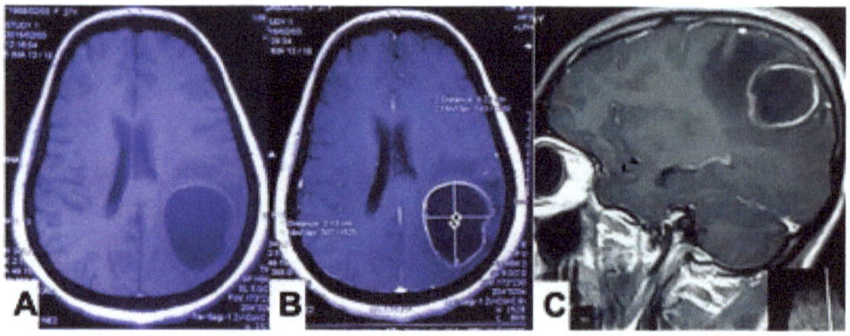

Figure 2. Plane (**A**) and contrast (**B**,**C**) MRI of a brain with parieto-occipital abscess. Source: Figure by authors.

MR spectroscopy is helpful for differentiating from other SOL-like metastases, GBM, etc. Lactate and acetate are increased in abscess. On in vivo MR spectroscopy, pyogenic and tuberculous abscesses can be distinguished by their distinct metabolite patterns, with detection of amino acids, succinate and acetate in pyogenic abscesses and a lipid peak in tuberculous abscesses (Figure 3) (Mohindra et al. 2016).

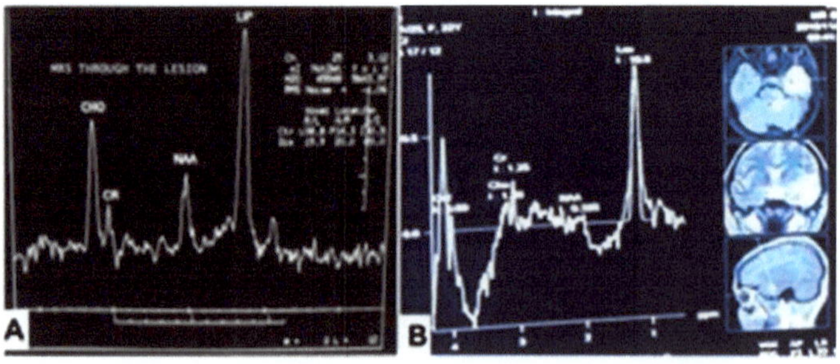

Figure 3. (**A**,**B**) MRS through a tuberculous brain abscess showing increased lipid and lactate peaks. Source: Figure by authors.

The differential diagnosis of brain abscesses is necrotic neoplasms such as glioblastomas multiforme and metastasis, which are sometimes hard to differentiate by a conventional CT scan and MRI. Combined proton magnetic resonance spectroscopy (^{1}H-MRS) and diffusion-weighted magnetic resonance imaging (DWI) are utilized for the diagnosis of brain abscesses and glioblastoma. DWI shows the brain abscess as a homogeneous hyperintense mass and ^{1}H-MRS shows the presence of acetate, lactate and amino acids, as well as the absence of normal brain elements. DWI sometimes shows glioblastoma multiforme as a hyperintense mass; however, ^{1}H-MRS shows a significantly elevated lactate and reduced N-acetyl-aspartate. A combination of the findings of DWI and ^{1}H-MRS can differentiate brain abscessse and glioblastomas (Nakaiso et al. 2002).

Hematological studies are non-specific and may be normal. Investigations for the primary source of infection should be carried out.

5.4. *Treatment*

The successful care of a brain abscess necessitates a comprehensive approach. The management team's nucleus is a neurosurgeon who collaborates closely with an infectious disease specialist, a neurologist and a neuroradiologist. Neuroradiological examination, surgical intervention, antibiotic usage and elimination of primary infected foci are all part of this strategy (Alvis Miranda et al. 2013). There is no one-size-fits-all approach to treating a brain abscess. It involves long-term antimicrobial treatment, surgical drainage or excision, and correction of the primary source of infection (Greenberg 2010).

5.4.1. Medical Therapy

While empiric antibiotic therapy should be initiated, particularly in cases with sepsis or eminent herniation, effort should be employed to obtain a tissue or microbiologic diagnosis as soon as possible (Honda and Warren 2009; Cunha 2001). Empiric antibiotics should cover Gram-negative, Gram-positive and anaerobic germs, since brain abscesses are typically polymicrobial (Honda and Warren 2009). In general, an empiric antibiotic combination includes the following (Greenberg 2010):

(1) Third- or fourth-generation cephalosporin;
(2) Vancomycin;
(3) Metronidazole.

Carbapenems may be used instead of cephalosporins and metronidazole in some cases (Honda and Warren 2009).

Antibiotic therapy can be adjusted if a causal bacterium has been identified. But if clinical improvement is shown with empiric treatment, it should be continued.

Antibiotics should be administered by an intravenous route and continued for at least 6–8 weeks (Greenberg 2010).

Sole medical management is indicated in the following conditions:

Early stage (cerebritis) of the disease before encapsulation;
Small lesion (<2.5 cm);
Multiple lesions;
Abscess in critical location (deep-seated, dominant hemisphere and eloquent area, brain abscess);
Poor surgical candidate;
Concomitant meningitis/or encephalitis;
Duration of symptoms <2 weeks;
Patient showing definite improvement within the first week of initiation of antibiotics.

In cases with brain abscesses, seizures are a common consequence which occur in 13 to 25% of cases. Though seizures may have little effect on the overall mortality, an anticonvulsant should be provided at an early stage of treatment to preclude seizures (Honda and Warren 2009). Dexamethasone has been utilized to lower intracranial pressure in patients who are at the risk of brain herniation. The effectiveness of steroids in the management of a brain abscess is unknown (Honda and Warren 2009).

5.4.2. Surgical Treatment

The indications for surgical treatment include the following (Greenberg 2010):

(1) Remarkable mass effect produced by the abscess seen on CT or MRI;
(2) Diagnostic dilemma;
(3) Near the ventricle (likelihood of an intraventricular rupture);
(4) Signs of remarkedly raised intracranial pressure;
(5) Grave neurologic status;
(6) Traumatic brain abscess accompanied by foreign material;

(7) Multiloculated abscess;
(8) Fungal abscess;
(9) Failure of medical treatment (neuro-deterioration increasing in size after 2 weeks of treatment, progressing toward the ventricle and no reduction in size after 4 weeks of treatment);
(10) No facility for follow-up by a CT scan every 1–2 weeks.

The following are the guiding principles for surgical care according to the British Society for Antimicrobial Chemotherapy's "Infection in Neurosurgery" Working Party (Alvis Miranda et al. 2013; Infection in Neurosurgery Working Party of the British Society for Antimicrobial Chemotherapy 2000):

- To reduce raised intracranial pressure urgently;
- Diagnosis confirmation;
- To get pus for microbiological studies;
- To potentiate the effectivity of antibiotic therapy;
- To preclude the ventricular extension of an infection iatrogenically.

The surgical procedures utilized are (1) needle aspiration via a bur hole, (2) total resection after craniotomy and (3) stereotactic aspiration.

Most surgical treatment is needle aspiration. If necessary, it can be carried out under local anesthetic. Irrigation with antibiotics and regular saline can be combined. In roughly 70% of cases, it is needed to repeat the procedure. Surgical excision may be required in some cases (Greenberg 2010).

Abscesses that expand after 2 weeks of antibiotic medication or fail to diminish after 3 to 4 weeks of antibiotics are usually treated with craniotomy and excision. Multiloculated abscesses and bigger lesions with a noticeable effect which are superficial and situated in non-eloquent areas of the brain are also candidates for a craniotomy (Figure 4) (Moorthy and Rajshekhar 2008). Repeated pus collection following aspiration can result in abrupt neurological deterioration; hence, the removal of abscesses in the cerebellum is also suggested (Moorthy and Rajshekhar 2008). A craniotomy may be required to remove bone chips or foreign material from a traumatic brain abscess (Honda and Warren 2009).

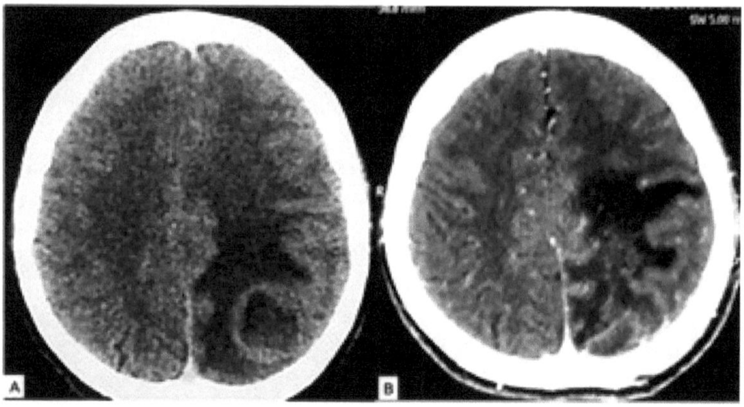

Figure 4. Pre- (**A**) and (**B**) postoperative (craniotomy) CT of a brain abscess. Source: Figure by authors.

There are some advantages in removing a brain abscess in a patient who is otherwise neurologically sound. As a result, the risk of recurring pus collection is virtually completely minimized, and the cost of repeated imaging is reduced. The length of stay in the hospital is also shortened (Moorthy and Rajshekhar 2008). As the capsule is frequently attached to the neighboring white matter, the neurosurgical procedure may inflict an unintentional extensive injury to adjacent viable brain tissue. Primary resection of a brain abscess carries the risk of severe damage to the adjacent brain, with a greater probability for neurological impairment and epilepsy (Alvis Miranda et al. 2013).

Stereotactic aspiration is used to treat deep-seated abscesses and lesions of the brainstem that do not respond to antibiotics alone.

Multiple abscesses are effectively treated by aspirating the largest one and then starting antibiotic therapy which may be needed for up to 3–6 months (Moorthy and Rajshekhar 2008).

Ventricular drainage is utilized to manage brain abscesses that burst into the ventricles, along with intravenous and/or intrathecal antimicrobials (Brook 2017).

5.4.3. Treatment of the Primary Source of Infection

A middle ear infection can be surgically managed at the same time or shortly after an otogenic brain abscess is treated (Moorthy and Rajshekhar 2008). Tetralogy of Fallot (TOF) should be corrected as soon as possible. Other sources should be treated according to their merit.

6. Subdural Empyema

Despite rigorous neurosurgery therapy, the subdural empyema (SDE), i.e., a purulent infection of the area between the cerebral dura and the arachnoid mater, is a neurosurgical emergency with a 10–13% fatality rate (Honda and Warren 2009). Subdural abscess, circumscript meningitis and pachymeningitis interna are all terms used to describe this condition (Agrawal et al. 2007). It is generally unilateral and spreads quickly through the subdural area until it is stopped by particular restrictions (e.g., tentorium cerebelli, falx cerebri, base of the brain and the foramen magnum). It accounts for 20% of all intracranial abscess cases. Men are more likely to contract the infection, accounting for up to 80% of the cases (Agrawal et al. 2007).

Subdural empyema has a pathophysiology that is akin to that of a cerebral abscess: direct spread from a nearby focus (e.g., paranasal air sinus infections, otitis media, cranial trauma or cranial osteomyelitis) or hematogenous dissemination from distant foci (Honda and Warren 2009; Agrawal et al. 2007). SDE is usually a consequence of purulent meningitis in babies (Greenberg 2010; Agrawal et al. 2007; Segun 2017; Rich et al. 2000; Barkovich 2000). Hematogenous dissemination from a distant target, especially the lungs, is rare (Honda and Warren 2009). An SDE can develop following cranial trauma or surgery, especially if there is an open depressed fracture with penetrating injuries (Greenberg 2010; Agrawal et al. 2007). Retrograde septic thrombophlebitis can potentially spread the illness (Agrawal et al. 2007; Tewari et al. 2004). Subdural empyema, which is linked to thrombophlebitis and venous sinus thrombosis, may result in a cerebral abscess or an infarction (Agrawal et al. 2007).

Subdural empyema has a microbiology profile that is similar to that of brain abscesses. Staphylococci, anaerobes and aerobic streptococci, Streptococcus pneumoniae, Hemophilus influenzae and other Gram-negative bacteria are common causal organisms (French et al. 2014).

6.1. Presentation

The most frequent clinical presentation features are a triad of sinusitis, fever and neuro-deficits, with a fulminant, as well as a swift downhill course (Agrawal et al. 2007). The common clinical features are summarized in Table 4.

Table 4. Clinical features of SDEs.

History	Physical Examination
Fever	Altered mental status: drowsiness, confusion, stupor and coma
Headache	Meningeal irritation signs or meningismus
Recent history (<2 week) of sinusitis, mastoiditis, meningitis, otitis media, cranial trauma or surgery, sinus surgery or respiratory infection	Hemiparesis or hemisensory deficits
Drowsiness, confusion, stupor or coma	Aphasia or dysarthria
Hemiparesis or hemiplegia	Seizure
Seizure-generalized or focal	Swelling, sinus tenderness or inflammation
Nausea or vomiting	Papilledema and other features of a raised ICP like vomiting/nausea, gait disturbance and altered mental status
Blurring of vision (amblyopia)	Homonymous hemianopsia

Table 4. *Cont.*

History	Physical Examination
Dysphasia	III, V or VI cranial nerves palsies; particularly if the abscess is close to the petrous portion of the temporal bone, generating facial pain and 6th nerve palsy
Recent H/O brain abscess	Fixed and dilated pupil on the same side as a result of compression of the oculomotor nerve

Source: Authors' compilation based on data from Agrawal et al. (2007).

6.2. Evaluation

As clinical findings are nonspecific for the diagnosis, laboratory data and neuro-imaging studies are helpful to reach the diagnosis.

6.2.1. Laboratory Data

The WBC count, ESR and C-reactive protein level can all be significantly high, and these tests can help determine which patients should be scanned (Agrawal et al. 2007).

Regarding the risk of cerebral herniation, lumbar puncture is not recommended if intracranial pressure is elevated. When increased intracranial pressure has been ruled out, lumbar puncture will be useful in ruling out meningitis. Findings in the CSF may indicate the existence of infection (Agrawal et al. 2007).

6.2.2. Imaging

The neuroimaging diagnosis of an SDE has traditionally relied on CT and MRI. The primary procedure for the rapid and noninvasive detection of an SDE is carried out via high-resolution, contrast CT scanning. A lenticular or crescentic extracerebral hypodense region over the hemisphere or along the falx can be seen on a contrast CT of the head in the coronal and axial planes. The infusion of contrast material improves the delineation of the edges (Figure 5) (Greenberg 2010; Agrawal et al. 2007).

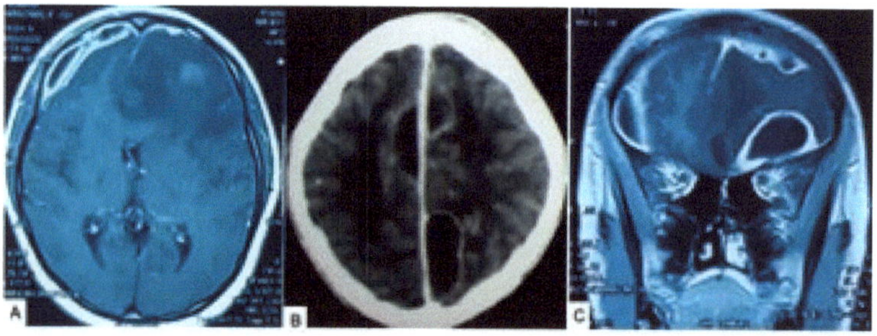

Figure 5. Subdural empyema; (**A**) interhemispheric; (**B**) convexity; (**C**) subfrontal and convexity. Source: Figure by authors.

MRI with gadolinium contrast is the preferred diagnostic technique for an intracranial SDE. SDEs are characterized by fluid collection encircled by a contrast-enhancing rim. Extra-axial fluid and its rim enhancement are better visualized with an MRI than with a CT. T1WI exhibits a modest signal, while T2WI shows a reasonably high signal (Agrawal et al. 2007).

6.3. Treatment

The keys to better clinical results are early and correct diagnosis, quick neurosurgical intervention and adequate antibiotic medication. Surgical drainage and antibiotic treatment are the principal forms of treatment. SDE pus should always be sent to the lab for anaerobic and aerobic culturing. Wide craniotomy with irrigation improvises the result in an SDE by permitting wide exposure, satisfactory exploration and better drainage of subdural pus material. Neuroimaging can precisely localize the pus which can be removed through a burr hole; however, wide craniotomy, evacuation and irrigation are the methods of choice, as they allows for wide exposure, appropriate exploration and better evacuation of subdural pus (debride and drain). The goal of therapy is to completely drain the pus and eliminate the source of illness (Greenberg 2010; Agrawal et al. 2007). Another technique is drainage and irrigation through stereotactic burr hole implantation, but this is less preferable due to reduced exposure and the possibility of incomplete purulent material evacuation (French et al. 2014). In critically unwell patients, bur hole evacuation is recommended.

Antibiotics should be initiated as soon as possible and changed as needed based on the culture, with sensitivity assessment.

7. Tuberculosis

Tuberculosis is generated by mycobacterium tuberculosis. It is highly prevalent in underdeveloped countries, but it is growingly threatening public health in advanced nations due to rising HIV epidemics, as well as migration from third-world countries (Hossain et al. 2017; Ertem et al. 2010). Tuberculosis persists as a serious global health issue. Globally, an estimated 10.4 million new cases of tuberculosis were notified in 2015. By 2030, 15 years after its declaration, the World Health Organization's "End TB Strategy" aims to a 90% decrease in TB-related mortality and an 80% decrease in TB occurrence (Davis et al. 2018). One of the most dangerous clinical presentations of tuberculosis is CNS involvement, which occurs in 5–10% of extrapulmonary tuberculosis cases and accounts for about 1% of all TB cases (Hossain et al. 2017; Cherian and Thomas 2011). Immunosuppression, whether caused by solid organ transplantation or HIV infection, increases the danger of contracting or reactivating tuberculosis which complicates the management of underlying immunosuppression, as well as CNS tuberculosis (Hossain et al. 2017; Nelson and Zunt 2011). HIV infection increases the likelihood of contracting tuberculosis, the rate at which the illness progresses from latent to active, and TB-related mortality and morbidity (Hossain et al. 2017; Nelson and Zunt 2011). HIV-positive people with tuberculosis are five times more likely than HIV-negative people to have CNS involvement (Nelson and Zunt 2011). Tubercular meningitis (TBM), tubercular abscesses and intracranial tuberculomas are all symptoms of CNS tuberculoma, the most serious form of extrapulmonary tuberculoma (Chou et al. 2012). Meningitis or no meningeal involvement can accompany intracranial tuberculoma. Tuberculomas are more commonly detected in the supratentorial space in adults, and multiple tuberculomas are more common than single tuberculoma (Chou et al. 2012; Bayındır et al. 2006).

7.1. Epidemiology

Although TB usually involves the lungs, it can occur in any organ or tissue. Extrapulmonary TB accounts for 20–25% of reported cases in countries with comprehensive diagnostic and reporting systems. Extrapulmonary cases (without concomitant pulmonary disease) accounted for 14% of all notified cases (new and relapse) worldwide in 2007 (WHO 2010). According to the WHO, 8.8 million new cases of active tuberculosis were reported per year in 2005, resulting in 1.6 million fatalities (Rock et al. 2008; WHO 2007). According to the WHO, 9.27 million new cases of tuberculosis (139/100,000 population) occurred in 2007, similar to the 9.24 million new cases (140/100,000 population) in 2006 (Cherian and Thomas 2011). Tuberculosis continues to be a global problem, with most new active tuberculosis infections occurring in emerging and poor countries (Rock et al. 2008; WHO 2007). Demographic factors like poverty, congestion, malnutrition and a weakened immune system account for 80% of new tuberculosis cases worldwide, whereas HIV accounts for the rest of the 20% tuberculosis cases in Sub-Saharan Africa (Rock et al. 2008; WHO 2007; Waaler 2002).

7.2. Pathogenesis

M. tuberculosis is an acid-fast bacillus (AFB) which infects predominantly humans and is aerobic, nonmotile and non-spore-forming. It has a sluggish doubling period (from 15 to 20 h) and takes many weeks to develop on traditional Löwenstein–Jensen media, where it usually grows in parallel groups, generating serpentine cording's colonial characteristic (Rock et al. 2008). CNS tuberculosis can also be caused by *Mycobacterium bovis* and atypical *Mycobacterium* spp. (Chowdhury et al. 2017).

The inhalation of droplet nuclei carrying *Mycobacterium tuberculosis* bacteria causes infection, which results in bacillus seeding in the respiratory unit of the lungs. The bacilli engage with alveolar macrophages through a variety of receptors once they reach the alveoli (Rock et al. 2008). Ingestion and direct contact with eroded mucosa or skin can potentially lead to infection. When these innate immune cells are activated, a cascade of chemokines and cytokines is produced, a type 1 T-helper cell-mediated immune response is triggered and a granuloma form (Hossain et al. 2017). CNS tuberculosis is always a secondary infection that enters the CNS by a hematogenous pathway from a primary or secondary location.

7.3. *Pathology*

Tuberculosis is characterized by chronic granulomatous inflammation that results in a caseating granuloma, a foreign body variety of giant cell granuloma. The disease starts with the formation of tiny tuberculous foci (rich foci) inside the spinal cord, brain or meninges in CNS tuberculosis. The site of these foci, as well as the ability to regulate them, decides which type of CNS TB develops. Tuberculous meningitis (TBM) is the most prevalent form of CNS tuberculosis, followed by tubercular encephalitis, intracranial tuberculoma and a tuberculous brain abscess (Hossain et al. 2017; Rock et al. 2008).

7.3.1. TB Meningitis

The most prevalent symptom of neuro-tuberculosis is tuberculous meningitis (Beatriz and Lopez 2019). A dense gelatinous exudate arises after tubercle bacilli form a granuloma and is released into the subarachnoid space; it is most prominent anteriorly in the suprasellar area and interpeduncular fossa (Figure 6), and it may extend across the prepontine cistern and around the spinal cord. This exudate surrounds arteries and cranial nerves, causing a bottleneck in the circulation of the CSF at the tentorial aperture, resulting in hydrocephalus. RBC, neutrophils and macrophages are seen in the exudate, preceded by lymphocytes in more developed exudates. Rich foci are found in both the meninges and the brain, and they usually follow a vascular pattern (Rock et al. 2008). The genesis of vasculitis in the vessels of the circulus arteriosus, the vertebrobasilar system and the perforators of the middle cerebral artery, leading in infarctions in the supplying areas of these vessels, is the most significant consequence of TBM (Rock et al. 2008).

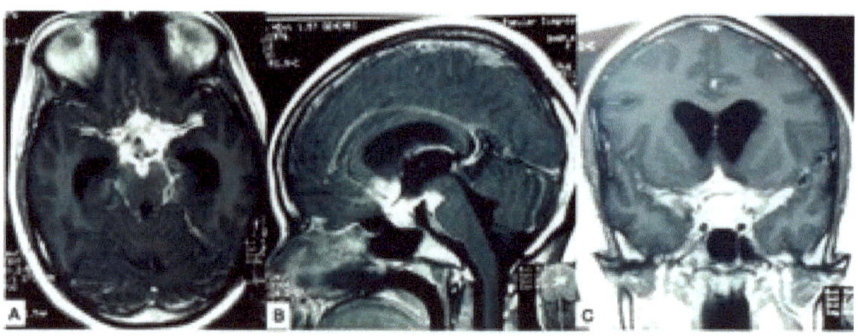

Figure 6. **(A–C)** Contrast MRI axial, sagittal and coronal image showing basal tubercular meningitis with a granuloma. Source: Figure by authors.

7.3.2. Tuberculoma

When tubercles in the tissue expand sans bursting into the subarachnoid space, tuberculomas form. As a result, they frequently take place in the absence of TBM, but they can also develop in the presence of TBM. Multiple tuberculomas are seen more frequently than solitary lesions. Around a central area of caseating necrosis, tuberculomas of the cerebrum show classic granulomatous responses composed of epithelioid cells and giant cells mixed with mainly lymphocytes. In contrast to pus, any liquefaction of the center area of necrosis produces straw-colored or clear fluid (Rock et al. 2008). Three forms of intracranial tuberculoma have been identified based on MRI findings: caseating or noncaseating with a solid core, and caseating with a liquid center (Hossain et al. 2017; Chou et al. 2012). Lesions in children are often infratentorial, but lesions in adults are typically supratentorial. Tuberculomas of the cerebrum, cerebellum and brainstem can arise in both infratentorial and supratentorial locations.

7.3.3. Tubercular Brain Abscess (TBA)

Abscess development is a rare symptom of CNS tuberculosis. TBA is identified by an encapsulated collection of pus containing alive bacilli, without indications of a characteristic tubercular granuloma, and must be recognized from granulomas with central caseation, as well as liquefaction-imitating pus. TBAs can appear as single or numerous lesions (Hossain et al. 2017; Rock et al. 2008; Chowdhury et al. 2017; Kumar et al. 2002). TBA might be monocular or multilocular in nature (Kumar et al. 2002). Tuberculous abscesses are larger than tuberculomas, often measuring more than 3 cm in diameter. Fever, headache and focal neurologic impairments are common symptoms of tuberculous abscesses, which are more severe than tuberculomas (Nelson and Zunt 2011). Patients with defective cell-mediated immunity, such as AIDS and other immunodeficiencies which prevent a granulomatous inflammatory response, are more likely to develop this lesion. Tuberculous abscess patients have a more grievous clinical presentation than tuberculomas patients (Beatriz and Lopez 2019).

7.4. Clinical Features

Most individuals with tubercular meningitis (TBM) have a history of vague ill health that lasts 2 to 8 weeks before meningeal irritation develops. Malaise, anorexia, weariness, fever, myalgias and headache are some of the nonspecific symptoms (Cherian and Thomas 2011). Adults with TBM frequently exhibit conventional meningitis symptoms like fever, headache and meningismus (stiff neck), as well as localized neurological impairments, behavioral abnormalities and changes in consciousness. Fever, convulsions, stiff neck and gastrointestinal symptoms like vomiting and nausea are frequent in children with TBM (Rock et al. 2008). In children, headaches are less frequent than in adults. Furthermore, because the meninges at the base of the brain are more likely to be involved, symptoms associated with cranial nerve dysfunction may be noted in a substantial proportion of individuals (up to 70%) (Beatriz and Lopez 2019). Usually, the most afflicted nerve is the sixth cranial nerve. When the optic nerve is involved, vision loss might be a dominant clinical manifestation. Vision loss in these patients could be caused by optochiasmatic arachnoiditis, 3rd ventricle compression of the optic chiasma (if hydrocephalus occurs) or an optic nerve granuloma. Papilloedema may be discovered through ophthalmoscopic examination. Choroid tubercles are yellow lesions with vague edges that can be found singly or in clusters on funduscopy (Cherian and Thomas 2011).

Patients with a tuberculoma or TBA frequently present with headaches, papilledema, seizures or other symptoms of increased intracranial pressure (IICP), depending on their site. With tuberculomas, the onset of symptoms is commonly measured in weeks or months.

TBA has a shorter incubation period (1–3 months) than tuberculoma, but a longer incubation period than pyogenic cerebral abscesses. It is characterized by headaches, fever and localized neurological impairments (Rock et al. 2008; Kumar et al. 2002). The involvement of long white fiber tracts can cause hemisensory deficit or hemiplegia, and engagement of cranial nerve nuclei result to cranial nerve palsy such as diplopia, facial palsy, gaze palsy, dysphagia, etc. The patient may have a low degree of consciousness as a result of the involvement of or pressure on the reticular activating system. Tuberculoma of the upper brainstem, primarily in the midbrain, obstructs CSF flow and results in hydrocephalus, with nausea, vomiting, headache, visual disturbances, papilledema and reduced awareness as the symptoms (Kumar et al. 2002; Sutlas et al. 2003). Different disorders can accompany a midbrain lesion. Weber's syndrome (Warembourg et al. 1960) is characterized by oculomotor nerve palsy and hemiparesis on the contralateral side. When the TBA affects the tegmentum of the midbrain with a red nucleus, Benedict's syndrome manifests as 3rd nerve palsy with contralateral hemiparesis, except for the arm, which displays ataxia, hyperkinesia and coarse intention tremor (Greenberg 2010).

Movement disorders such as parkinsonism, tremor, extrapyramidal syndrome, chorea, dystonia, myoclonus and hemiballismus can arise when the basal ganglia are involved. Behavioral abnormalities, cognitive impairment, pituitary hypofunction, cachexia, diabetes insipidus, precocious puberty and other symptoms of diencephalic involvement may occur (Chowdhury et al. 2017).

7.5. *Diagnosis*

7.5.1. Traditional CSF Analysis

Cytology

A typical CSF examination can reveal moderate lymphocytic pleocytosis, moderately increased protein levels and hypoglycorrhachia in cases with CNS TB (low glucose) (Rock et al. 2008).

The presence of tubercular bacilli in the CSF, either by smear examination or tubercular culture, is essential for a definitive diagnosis of TBM. Standard staining procedures applied to CSF samples, such as Ziehl–Neelsen, Kinyoun or auramine-rhodamine, have been reported to detect about 100 AFB/mL of the CSF. It has been proposed that if remarkable volumes of the CSF are studied arduously, the organism can be identified in over 90% of centrifuged CSF specimens, along with ventricular CSF, producing the greatest identification rates. CSF culture positivity rates for clinically confirmed cases range between 25% and 70% (Cherian and Thomas 2011).

Molecular and Biochemical Analysis

Commercially obtainable nucleic acid amplification (NAA) techniques and other polymerase chain reaction (PCR)-based techniques, antibody and antigen detection or chemical assays like adenosine deaminase (ADA), as well as tuberculostearic acid measurements are currently available molecular-based techniques (Cherian and Thomas 2011; Rock et al. 2008). Commercial nucleic acid amplification (NAA) assays (PCR) for the diagnosis of tubercular meningitis are 56% sensitive and 98% specific, and when significant volumes of the CSF are studied, the diagnostic yield of NAA increases (Cherian and Thomas 2011; Pai et al. 2003).

Skin tests that are positive for CNS TB have a diagnostic value of 10–20% (Cherian and Thomas 2011; Kilpatrick et al. 1996) to 50% (Cherian and Thomas 2011; Mahadevan et al. 2005). The efficiency of the tuberculin test for the diagnosis of tuberculosis varies depending on age, BCG vaccination, nutritional state, HIV infection and administration manner (Cherian and Thomas 2011; Joos et al. 2006).

ADA (adenosine deaminase) is a cell-mediated immune marker that is mostly associated with lymphocyte proliferation and differentiation (Cherian and Thomas 2011; Kashyap et al. 2006). The sensitivities and specificities of ADA in the CSF were measured to be between 44 and 100%, and 71 and 100%, respectively (Cherian and Thomas 2011; Rock et al. 2008). The development of T-cell-based interferon release assays have been a significant advancement in recent years (IGRAs). IGRAs are in vitro tests that rely on the release of interferon (IFN) after T-cell activation by antigens that are more specific to MTB than pure protein derivatives (PPD) (like early secreted antigenic target 6 (ESAT6) and culture filtrate protein 10 (CFP10)) (Cherian and Thomas 2011).

7.5.2. Imaging

Before starting or within the first 48 h of treatment, every case with tubercular meningitis should be examined using contrast CT imaging (Cherian and Thomas 2011; Thwaites et al. 2009). An early brain CT scan aids in the diagnosis of TBM and can offer crucial baseline information for surgical hydrocephalus treatments (Cherian and Thomas 2011). Hydrocephalus, contrast enhancement of basal meninges and infarctions in the cerebral hemisphere and brain stem are common neuroradiological findings in tuberculous meningitis (Beatriz and Lopez 2019) (Figure 6). In terms of identifying and assessing CNS TB, a contrast MRI is widely thought to be better than a CT. While an MRI is undoubtedly superior to a CT for detecting parenchymal and meningeal irregularities, its limited availability globally and the need for general anesthesia in youngsters imply that it may have a minimal influence on TBM detection globally (Rock et al. 2008).

Tuberculomas are low-density, lobulated or spherical masses with uneven walls that display homogeneous or ring-enhancing uptake following contrast injection (Figures 7–9). They might appear as single or numerous nodules (Rock et al. 2008; Katti 2004). The extent of edema around the tuberculoma is assumed to be inversely proportional to the age of the tubercular lesion; the radiographic appearance of tuberculomas depends largely on whether the TB lesion is caseating, noncaseating, with a solid center or caseating with a liquid center (Rock et al. 2008; Bernaerts et al. 2003). T1-weighted images of tuberculoma are isointense to modestly hyperintense, while T2-weighted images are hypointense (Sanei Taheri et al. 2015; Sharma et al. 2008) (Figure 10). The gray–white matter interface is where most tuberculomas are found (Beatriz and Lopez 2019).

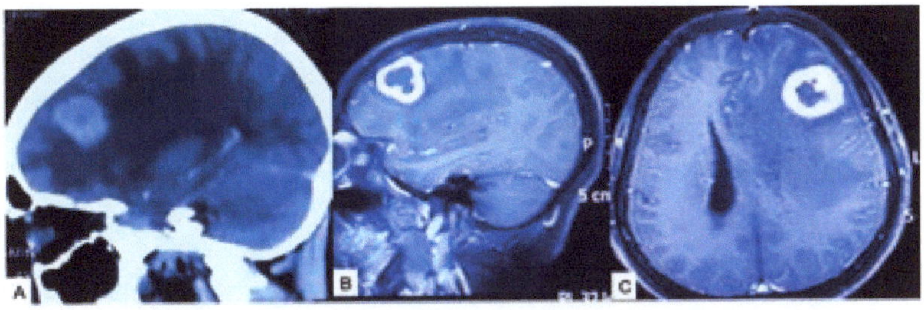

Figure 7. Contrast-enhanced CT (**A**) and MRI (**B**,**C**) showing lt. frontal tuberculoma. Source: Figure by authors.

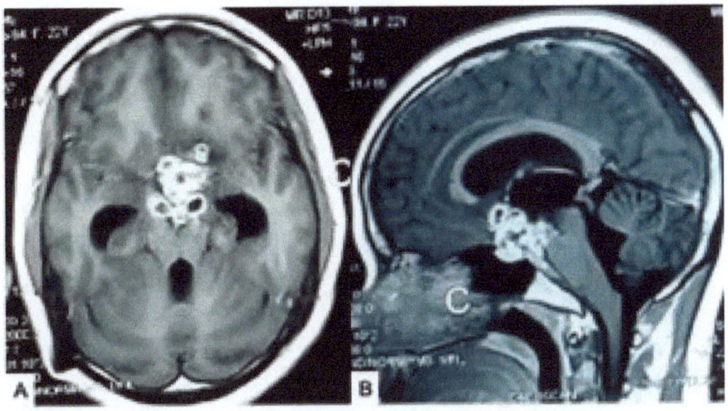

Figure 8. Multiloculated tuberculoma on a contrast-enhanced MRI (**A**,**B**). Source: Figure by authors.

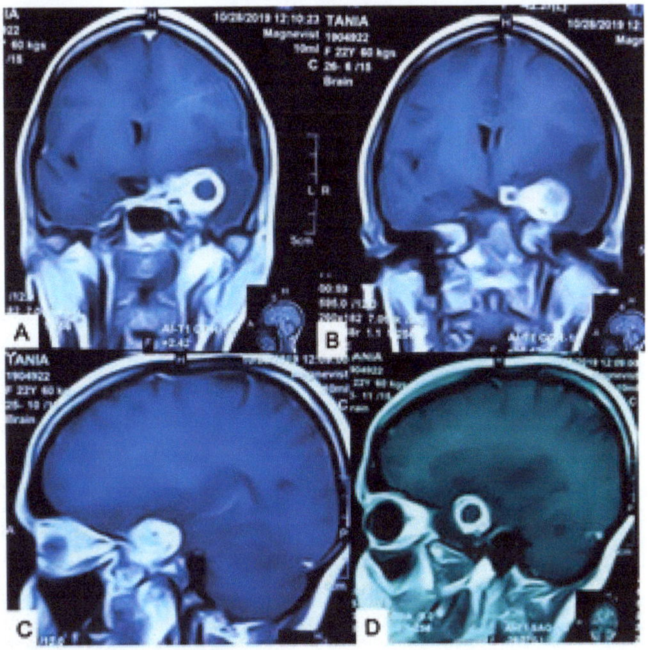

Figure 9. Tuberculoma in the medial temporal region on a contrast-enhanced MRI (**A–D**). Source: Figure by authors.

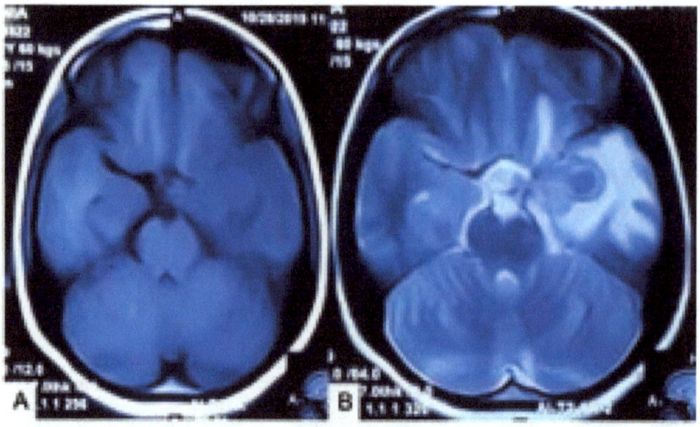

Figure 10. Tuberculoma on an MRI: (**A**) T1WI isointense; (**B**) T2WI hypointense. Source: Figure by authors.

A tuberculous abscess is a rare condition marked by liquefaction and pus in the center. It is often multiloculated and can be solitary or multiple. Tuberculous abscesses are distinct from tuberculomas, which include central caseation and liquefaction that resemble pus. On a CT scan, the tubercular abscess has a hypodense appearance with peripheral edema, as well as a mass effect. The central necrotic area exhibits increased signal strength on T2W imaging. Ring enhancement can be seen on postcontrast pictures, which is usually thin and consistent (Sanei Taheri et al. 2015). Other radiographic techniques, like magnetic resonance spectroscopy (MRS), have been found to differentiate tuberculomas from cysticercosis but not from CNS non-Hodgkin lymphoma (NHL). In tuberculoma (Hossain et al. 2017; Rock et al. 2008), an MRS indicates a higher lipid peak with lower N-acetyleaspartate and choline levels (Hossain et al. 2017; Sharma et al. 2008). An MRS uses a big lipid lactate peak to selectively identify tuberculomas (Cherian and Thomas 2011; Kingsley et al. 2006) (Figure 3).

7.6. Complications

Cortical infarcts and hydrocephalus are two significant consequences of tuberculous meningitis. The infarcts are caused by endarteritis obliterans, which causes severe vascular alterations. Because the basal perforating arteries are involved, the majority of the infarcts occur in the corpus striatum and internal capsule. The inflammatory exudate transforms to a more fibroblastic response as the disease and treatment proceed, which can result in meningeal fibrosis, CSF blockage and communicative hydrocephalus. Due to granulomatous ependymitis, obstructive hydrocephalus can be due to a focal blockage of the cerebral aqueduct or ventricular foramen (Beatriz and Lopez 2019).

7.7. Treatment

Tuberculosis is a systemic disease. Anti-tubercular chemotherapy is the treatment for TB according to the WHO guidelines. Along with anti-tubercular chemotherapy, other forms of treatment may be needed according to the site of involvement and type of pathology. The WHO categorizes the drugs according to different combinations of drugs. WHO-recommended anti-TB medication formulations and fixed-dose drug combinations have recently been included on the WHO Model List of Essential Medicines (WHO 2010). Isoniazide (INH), rifampicin (RIF), pyrizinamide (PZA), ethambutol (EMB) and streptomycin are the first-line anti-TB medications recommended. For all instances of tuberculosis (pulmonary and extrapulmonary), the WHO recommends a 6-month treatment program. Some specialists, however, advocate for a therapy period of 9–12 months (WHO 2010).

The present WHO recommendations for TBM depend on those used to treat pulmonary TB and recommend that all patients be treated with two months of rifampicin (RMP), isoniazid (INH), pyrazinamide (PZE) and ethambutol (ETB), followed by up to ten months of RMP and INH (Davis et al. 2018; WHO 2010). Although starting this regimen before the commencement of coma is the best predictor of survival from TB meningitis (Prasad et al. 2016), this regimen ignores the anti-tuberculosis medications' varied capacity to permeate the brain (Davis et al. 2018; Donald 2010).

The utilization of steroids as an additional therapy in the management of CNS tuberculosis dates back to the 1950s and is still a contentious topic today (Hossain et al. 2017; Rock et al. 2008). According to Prasad et al.'s meta-analysis, steroid use is linked to fewer deaths (Rock et al. 2008; Prasad et al. 2000). In cases of CNS TB, the current guidelines from the Infectious Diseases Society of America, the Centers for Disease Control and Prevention, and the American Thoracic Society recommend steroid therapy as an adjuvant therapy to regular anti-TB chemotherapy.

Dexamethasone, at a starting dose of 8 mg/day for children weighing less than 25 kg and 12 mg/day for children weighing 25 kg or more and adults, is the standard treatment. The starting dose is given for three weeks, then gradually reduced over the next three weeks (Hossain et al. 2017; Rock et al. 2008).

Since the discovery of efficient anti-TB chemotherapy, the main functions of surgery have been to treat serious complications, including hydrocephalus, the mass effect of tuberculomas and brain abscesses (Rock et al. 2008). Tuberculomas respond to anti-TB chemotherapy in the majority of cases, and surgery is not required. However, a huge tuberculoma that is having a significant mass effect, a tuberculoma that is enlarging paradoxically or a diagnostic difficulty necessitates surgical intervention. When a tuberculoma is superficial and easily accessible, surgical removal is also advised as a first-line treatment (Demetriou 2013).

Surgical draining or excision is required for large and chronic abscesses. In the case of smaller and more perplexing lesions, stereotactic biopsy may be used for tissue diagnosis (Hossain et al. 2017). TBA surgical intervention has three goals: (1) to lower the size of the space-occupying mass and relieve the elevated ICP; (2) to minimize the bacterial load; (3) to histopathologically investigate the TBA's wall to confirm the diagnosis of a TBA (Mohindra et al. 2016). Simple aspiration (one time), repeated aspiration via a burr hole, continuous drainage, fractional drainage, stereotactic aspiration and craniotomy followed by excision are some of the treatment possibilities. There are reports describing the complete cure of tuberculous abscesses with multiple aspirations and chemotherapy, but based on the results of Mohindra et al.'s series, large-sized (more than 3 cm in diameter) lesions invariably require excision and smaller ones resolve completely with adequate duration of appropriate ATT regimen (Mohindra et al. 2016).

8. Parasitic Infestations

Parasitic illnesses of the CNS persist to be a major etiology of morbidity, as well as mortality around the world. Millions of adults and children in low- and middle-income nations suffer from cognitive, neurological and mental health disorders caused by parasite infections (Carpio et al. 2016).

The CNS can be affected by any parasite that affects humans; nevertheless, cysticercosis is the most prevalent parasitic infestation of the CNS. Toxoplasmosis, echinococcosis and schistosomiasis are some of the less common illnesses. Paragonimiasis, toxocariasis, malaria, onchocerciasis, human African trypanosomiasis (HAT) and American trypanosomiasis (Chagas disease (CD)), as well as angiostrongyliasis are all rare parasitic disorders that involve the CNS. The causative parasites, vector or intermediary hosts, routes of transmission and endemic areas or geographic distributions of these diseases are all different (Carpio et al. 2016).

8.1. Neurocysticercosis

Cysticercosis is the most common parasitic infestation of the brain and spinal cord. Cysticercosis is caused by the larval stage of pork tape worm Taenia solium, which has marked predilection for neural tissue. The human GIT is the sole habitat for adult worms. When humans ingest food contaminated with viable eggs, the eggs hatch into a larva in the duodenum, enter into the circulation and gain access to the brain.

There are two types of cysts that develop in the brain: (1) cystercercus cellulosae are regular, round or oval, thin-walled, 3–20 mm size, and tend to develop in the parenchyma or subarachnoid space, producing mild inflammation; (2) cystercercus racemosus is larger (4–24 mm size), grows actively in a grape shape as clusters in the basal subarachnoid space, producing intense inflammation (Greenberg 2010).

The locations of cysts tend to fall in the following four groups: (a) meningeal, (b) parenchymal, (c) ventricular, and (d) mixed (Greenberg 2010). NCC has a wide variety of clinical symptoms that are largely influenced by the site of cysts and the host's immunological response. The most common signs of cysts in the brain parenchyma include seizures, headaches, focal impairments and cognitive problems, all of which are associated with an elevated ICP (Greenberg 2010; Carpio et al. 2016). The most common causes of this illness are acute hydrocephalus caused by intraventricular cysts, or persistent hydrocephalus caused by arachnoiditis or ependymitis (Carpio et al. 2016). Cranial nerve palsies can occur with basal arachnoiditis (Greenberg 2010).

8.1.1. Diagnosis

Cysticercosis antibody titers determined by ELISA are considered significant at 1:64 in serum and 1:8 in the CSF. Mild peripheral eosinophilia and eosinophils in the CSF may be an indication (Schaad et al. 1993). The best option would be to look for parasite DNA in the CSF. The identification of parasite DNA using PCR is a relatively straightforward experimental method that is now garnering far more interest than the serological detection of viable parasite-released products (Carpio et al. 2016).

Neuroimaging is helpful in the detection of NCC because it allows for the identification of the parasite's stages of evolution, as well as the quantity and location of the lesions. Neuroimaging techniques enable observation of the parasite's vesicular, granular–nodular, colloidal and calcified phases in the CNS. For the identification of the scolex and the detection of extraparenchymal NCC, an MRI scan is more sensitive than a CT (Carpio et al. 2016). Ring-enhancing cystic lesions of various sizes in a parenchymal or extraparenchymal lesion with mild inflammatory change (edema) are present on MRI. Intraparenchymal punctate calcification can be seen on CT. Hydrocephalus can be seen in intraventricular cysts. A skull X-ray may show calcification in 13–15% of cases (Greenberg 2010).

8.1.2. Treatment

Medical treatment is the mainstay of treatment.

Antihelminthic drugs include the following:

- Albendazole, 15 mg/kg/d in 2–3 divided doses with corticosteroids, 16 mg/d for 3 months;
- Praziquantel, 50 mg/kg/d in 3 divided doses, with corticosteroids for 15 days;
- Albendazole/praziquantel plus corticosteroids if >2 active parenchymal cysts.

Surgery is sometimes needed for establishing the diagnosis. CSF diversion is needed in the HCP.

8.2. Hydatidosis

The parasite Echinococcus granulosus causes cystic echinococcosis or hydatid disease (cyst). Men are the intermediate host and are infected either by ingesting food contaminated with the ova or by direct contact with an infected dog. Ova hatches into a larva in the stomach; it then disseminates through systemic circulation from the stomach mucosa to the brain (few larvae bypass hepatic and pulmonary filtration). The infestation may be primary or subsequent to the burst of a primary cerebral cyst, either spontaneously or traumatically, or to the embolization of cardiac cysts (Carpio et al. 2016). Primary cysts are usually solitary and secondary cysts are multiple (Greenberg 2010).

Cysts may go unnoticed until they reach a size that causes a mass effect. Brain lesions affect 1 to 4% of cystic echinococcosis patients, with nonspecific clinical symptoms such as a raised ICP and seizure activities, similar to those of a space-occupying mass. There is one record of an infected cranial hydatid cyst in the literature reported by the author in 2010 (Hossain et al. 2010).

The detection of cerebral hydatid cysts relies heavily on imaging techniques like CT and MRI (Limaiem and Kchir 2014). In imaging examinations, hydatid cysts may appear as big, well-marked, smooth and thin-walled cystic lesions with a spherical or oval form and no edema. On CT, the cyst contents exhibit a CSF-like density, and all MR sequences show CSF-like signal patterns. A tiny rim of enhancement can be noticed on post-contrast photos. The existence of a daughter cyst within a cystic lesion is regarded as an echinococcus cyst that is pathognomonic (Carpio et al. 2016). Serological tests (ELISA or CFT) for the detection of antibodies can help in the diagnosis.

Treatment is surgical removal of an intact cyst by craniotomy, along with Albebdazole 400 mg bid for 28 days (Greenberg 2010).

8.3. Cerebral Malaria

Malaria is the most common parasite infection on the planet. It primarily affects African children, as well as Asian adults, with the overwhelming majority of instances (>90%) occurring in children aged 5 years and less. Plasmodium falciparum causes cerebral malaria, which can produce acute encephalopathy (fever and convulsions), which can be deadly or progress to diverse neurological sequelae. Headache, weakness, abdominal discomfort, muscle aches and erratic fever are among the earliest symptoms of malaria. Nausea, vomiting and orthostatic hypotension are other common side effects. They can later develop into a severe headache followed by drowsiness, confusion, generalized seizures and coma. Residual neurologic impairments are typical in persons who survive cerebral malaria. Microscopy detection of the parasite is the gold standard for diagnosing malaria (Idro et al. 2010; Mohamed and Mansour 2017).

The treatment of cerebral malaria according to the WHO guidelines should be carried out by IV artesunate (2.4 mg/kg/dose) at 0, 12, 24 and 48 h.

9. Shunt Infection

Infection and malfunction are the most common complications of a ventricular shunt system, and both are interrelated. Because of the foreign bodies and direct communication with the CNS, shunt infections are difficult to treat. Infection is recorded in 4–30% of cases, depending on the patient's history, the presence of an external drainage and previous infection history (Stadler et al. 2019). Shunt infection rates per case range from 10–22% and roughly 6.0% every procedure, with 90% of infections happening within 30 days of surgery (Gutierrez-Murgas and Snowden 2014). Children with shunt infection have a higher rate of mortality and morbidity, with an increased risk of seizure. The time between surgery and infection presentation varies from 15 to 12 months (Stadler et al. 2019).

9.1. *Etiology and Pathogenesis*

The risk factors for shunt infection are as follows (Greenberg 2010; Gutierrez-Murgas and Snowden 2014; Stadler et al. 2019):

(1) Young age;
(2) Length of the procedure;
(3) Open neural tube defect;
(4) Timing of operation—early timing of the day decreases the chance of an infection;
(5) Failure to maintain adequate asepsis;
(6) Postoperative other site infection like RTI, abdominal infection, UTI, etc.;
(7) Low birth weight and prematurity;
(8) Relative immunosuppression;
(9) Number of aspirations or revisions;
(10) Length of hospital stay;
(11) Neurosurgeon's experience, skills and neurosurgical technique;
(12) Manipulation of the indwelling shunt tube during surgery.

The majority of shunt infections are due to Gram-positive bacteria, with coagulase- negative staphylococci (Staph epidermidis) detected in 17 to 78% of cases, and Staphylococcus aureus found in 4% to 30% of cases (Gutierrez-Murgas and Snowden 2014; Stadler et al. 2019).

Biofilm formation is an important issue in shunt infection and antibiotic resistance. Biofilms are self-contained populations of bacteria or fungi that develop a heterogeneous structure made of biological parts and a complicated self-produced matrix to cling to surfaces (Scherr et al. 2014). The first adhesion of an organism to an artificial or host surface is the first step in the development of a biofilm. Bacteria concentrate and grow on the bacterial device or host surface after attachment. This is a serious issue since biofilms can evade the immune system of the host and are more resistant to antimicrobial therapy (Gutierrez-Murgas and Snowden 2014; Hess et al. 2012). Maturation and detachment occur when bacteria attach and replicate on the medical device, allowing for biofilm-related illnesses and sepsis to develop and spread (Gutierrez-Murgas and Snowden 2014).

9.2. *Clinical Manifestations*

The range of clinical features include the following (Stadler et al. 2019):

(1) Wound infection: symptoms of inflammation and purulent discharge, with organisms identified by Gram stain or culture in an incision or shunt tract. Shunt infections should be managed as wound breakdown with exposed shunt tubing.
(2) Meningitis: meningismus, fever, CSF leukocytosis and organisms identified on Gram stain or culture are all symptoms of meningitis.

(3) Peritonitis: fever, abdominal rigidity and tenderness (abdominal pseudocyst and abscesses can both present with a mass and a fever), and organisms identified by Gram stain or culture. Fever, leukocytosis and a positive blood culture are all signs of vascular shunts, with or without shunt nephritis or cor pulmonale.
(4) Minimal evidence of CSF contamination with bacteria collected from purulent exudate in or on shunt material, Gram stain of CSF extracted from the shunt or positive culture on fluid aspirated from the shunt under sterile conditions are all signs of an infected shunt apparatus. Any end of the shunt tube can become clogged, resulting in symptoms of an elevated ICP.

9.3. Laboratory Data

Leucocytosis with a high ESR. Blood culture is positive in less than one third of the cases. Shunt tap and CSF study, including culture, are very important. Culture of the shunt device after removal is positive in >90% of cases.

9.4. Treatment

Shunt infections are currently treated by shunt removal, as well as systemic or intraventricular antibiotics. Shunt removal, along with antibiotic treatment and external ventricular drainage, was determined to be the most efficient method of eradicating shunt infection in children (Gutierrez-Murgas and Snowden 2014; Schreffler et al. 2002). Vancomycin for the wide spectrum coverage of staphylococci and other Gram-positive organisms, and cefepime, ceftazidime or meropenem for the coverage of Gram-negative bacteria are two empiric antibiotics advised by the Infectious Diseases Society of America (Gutierrez-Murgas and Snowden 2014; Prusseit et al. 2009). Rifampicin may be added for increased coverage (Greenberg 2010). After obtaining the culture report, antibiotics may be modified. Antibiotics should be continued 10–14 days after the CSF becomes sterile (Greenberg 2010).

Author Contributions: Conceptualization, methodology, validation, formal analysis, investigation, resources, data curation, M.Z.H. and F.H.C.; writing—original draft preparation, M.Z.H.; writing—review and editing, F.H.C.; visualization, supervision, M.H. All authors have read and agreed to the published version of the manuscript.

Funding: This research received no external funding.

Conflicts of Interest: The authors declare no conflicts of interest.

References

Abid, Fatma Ben, Mohammed Abukhattab, Hafedh Ghazouani, Obada Khalil, Ahmed Gohar, Hussam Al Soub, Muna Al Maslamani, Abdullatif Al Khal, Eman Al Masalamani, Said Al Dhahry, and et al. 2018. Epidemiology and clinical outcomes of viral central nervous system infections. *International Journal of Infectious Diseases* 73: 85–90. [CrossRef] [PubMed]

Adams, William G., Katherine A. Deaver, Stephen L. Cochi, Brian D. Plikaytis, Elizabeth R. Zell, Claire V. Broome, and Jay D. Wenger. 1993. Decline of childhood Haemophilus influenza type b (Hib) disease in the Hib vaccine era. *JAMA* 269: 221–26. [CrossRef] [PubMed]

Agrawal, Amit, Jake Timothy, Lekha Pandit, Lathika Shetty, and J. P. Shetty. 2007. A Review of Subdural Empyema and Its Management. *Infectious Diseases in Clinical Practice* 15: 149–53. [CrossRef]

Alvis Miranda, Hernando, Sandra Milena Castellar-Leones, Mohammed Awad Elzain, and Luis Rafael Moscote-Salazar. 2013. Brain abscess: Current management. *Journal of Neurosciences in Rural Practice* 4: S67–S81. [CrossRef]

Aronin, Steven I., Peter Peduzzi, and Vincent J. Quagliarello. 1998. Community-acquired bacterial meningitis: Risk stratification for adverse clinical outcome and effect of antibiotic timing. *Annals of Internal Medicine* 129: 862–69. [CrossRef]

Barkovich, A. James. 2000. *Pediatric Neuroimaging*. Philadelphia: Lippincott Williams & Wilkins, pp. 715–70.

Bayındır, Cicek, Özgür Mete, and Bilge Bilgic. 2006. Retrospective study of 23 pathologically proven cases of central nervous system tuberculomas. *Clinical Neurology and Neurosurgery* 108: 353–57. [CrossRef]

Beatriz, M., and S. Lopez. 2019. Pathology of Bacterial CNS Infections. Available online: https://emedicine.medscape.com/article/1806579-overview?form=fpf (accessed on 30 May 2022).

Bernaerts, A., F. M. Vanhoenacker, P. M. Parizel, J. W. M. Van Goethem, R. Van Altena, A. Laridon, J. De Roeck, V. Coeman, and A. M. De Schepper. 2003. Tuberculosis of the central nervous system: Overview of neuroradiological findings. *European Radiology* 13: 1876–90. [CrossRef]

Bernardini, Gary L. 2004. Diagnosis and management of brain abscess and subdural empyema. *Current Neurology and Neuroscience Reports* 4: 448–56. [CrossRef]

Big, Cecilia, Lora A. Reineck, and David M. Aronoff. 2009. Viral infections of the central nervous system: A case-based review. *Clinical Medicine & Research* 7: 142–46.

Bilukha, Oleg O., and Nancy Rosenstein. 2005. Prevention and control of meningococcal disease. Recommendations of the Advisory Committee on Immunization Practices (ACIP). *MMWR Recommendations Report* 54: 1–21.

Brook, Itzhak. 2017. Brain Abscess Treatment & Management. Available online: https://reference.medscape.com/article/212946-treatment (accessed on 30 May 2022).

Brown, E., and F. Gray. 2009. Bacterial infections. In *Greenfield's Neuropathology*. Edited by S. Love, D. N. Louis and D. W. Ellison. London: Hodder Arnold.

Caballero, P. E. Jiménez, F. Munoz Escudero, S. Murcia Carretero, and A. Verdú Pérez. 2011. Descriptive analysis of viral meningitis in a general hospital: Differences in the characteristics between children and adults. *Neurología (English Edition)* 26: 468–73. [CrossRef]

Carpenter, J., S. Stapleton, and R. Holliman. 2007. Retrospective analysis of 49 cases of brain abscess and review of the literature. *European Journal of Clinical Microbiology & Infectious Diseases* 26: 1–11.

Carpio, Arturo, Matthew L. Romo, R. M. E. Parkhouse, Brooke Short, and Tarun Dua. 2016. Parasitic diseases of the central nervous system: Lessons for clinicians and policy makers. *Expert Review of Neurotherapeutics* 16: 401–14. [CrossRef] [PubMed]

Centers for Disease Control and Prevention. 2005. Direct and indirect effects of routine vaccination of children with 7-valent pneumococcal conjugate vaccine on incidence of invasive pneumococcal disease–United States, 1998–2003. *Morbidity and Mortality Weekly Report* 54: 893–97.

Cherian, A., and S. V. Thomas. 2011. Central nervous system tuberculosis. *African Health Sciences* 11: 116–27. [PubMed]

Choi, Chester. 2001. Bacterial meningitis in aging adults. *Clinical Infectious Diseases* 33: 1380–85. [CrossRef] [PubMed]

Chou, Ping-Song, Ching-Kuan Liu, Ruey-Tay Lin, Chiou-Lian Lai, and A-Ching Chao. 2012. Central nervous system tuberculosis: A forgotten diagnosis. *The Neurologist* 18: 219–22. [CrossRef]

Chowdhury, Forhad Hossain, Md Raziul Haque, Mainul Haque Sarkar, S. M. Noman Khaled Chowdhury, Zahed Hossain, and Shisir Ranjan. 2015. Brain abscess: Surgical experiences of 162 cases. *Neuroimmunology and Neuroinflammation* 2: 153–61. [CrossRef]

Chowdhury, Forhad Hossain, Mohammod Raziul Haque, and Mainul Haque Sarker. 2017. Cerebrum, Cerebellum and deep structures of the brain. In *Tuberculosis (ch-8) in Tuberculosis of the Central Nervous System*. Edited by Mehmet Turgut Mehmet, Akhaddar Akhaddar, Ahmet T. Turgut and Ravindra K. Garg. Cham: Springer, pp. 79–102. [CrossRef]

Connolly, Kevin J., and Scott M. Hammer. 1990. The acute aseptic meningitis syndrome. *Infectious Disease Clinics of North America* 4: 599–622. [CrossRef]

Cunha, Burke A. 2001. Central nervous system infections in the compromised host: A diagnostic approach. *Infectious Disease Clinics of North America* 15: 567–90. [CrossRef]

Davis, Angharad, Graeme Meintjes, and Robert J. Wilkinson. 2018. Treatment of Tuberculous Meningitis and Its Complications in Adults. *Current Treatment Options in Neurology* 20: 1–15. [CrossRef] [PubMed]

DeBiasi, Roberta L., and Kenneth L. Tyler. 1999. Polymerase chain reaction in the diagnosis and management of central nervous system infections. *Archives of Neurology* 56: 1215–19. [CrossRef] [PubMed]

Demetriou, George A. 2013. Brainstem tuberculosis. *BMJ Case Reports* 2013: bcr2013010359. [CrossRef] [PubMed]

Dery, MarkAlain, and Rodrigo Hasbun. 2007. Changing epidemiology of bacterial meningitis. *Current Infectious Disease Reports* 9: 301–7. [CrossRef]

Donald, P. R. 2010. Cerebrospinal fluid concentrations of antituberculosis agents in adults and children. *Tuberculosis* 90: 279–92. [CrossRef]

Dorsett, Maia, and Stephen Y. Liang. 2016. Diagnosis and Treatment of Central Nervous System Infections in the Emergency Department. *Emergency Medicine Clinics of North America* 34: 917–42. [CrossRef]

Durand, Marlene L., Stephen B. Calderwood, David J. Weber, Samuel I. Miller, Frederick S. Southwick, Verne S. Caviness, Jr., and Morton N. Swartz. 1933. Acute bacterial meningitis in adults. A review of 493 episodes. *New England Journal of Medicine* 328: 21–28. [CrossRef]

Edwards, Morven S., and Carol J. Baker. 1981. Complications and sequelae of meningococcal infections in children. *The Journal of Pediatrics* 99: 540–45. [CrossRef]

Ertem, Devrimsel Harika, Nurhak Demir Aslan, Yavuz Altunkaynak, Didem Sayın Yıldız, and Sevim Baybaş. 2010. Isolated Brain Stem Tuberculoma: A Case Report and Review of The Literature. *Düşünen Adam The Journal of Psychiatry and Neurological Sciences* 23: 288–92. [CrossRef]

Flores-Cordero, Juan M., Rosario Amaya-Villar, Maria D. Rincón-Ferrari, Santiago R. Leal-Noval, José Garnacho-Montero, Ana C. Llanos-Rodríguez, and Francisco Murillo- Cabezas. 2003. Acute community acquired bacterial meningitis in adults admitted to the intensive care unit: Clinical manifestations, management and prognostic factors. *Intensive Care Medicine* 29: 1967–73. [CrossRef]

Frazier, James L., Edward S. Ahn, and George I. Jallo. 2008. Management of brain abscesses in children. *Neurosurgical Focus* 24: E8. [CrossRef] [PubMed]

French, Heath, Nathan Schaefer, Gerben Keijzers, David Barison, and Sarah Olson. 2014. Intracranial subdural empyema: A 10-year case series. *Ochsner Journal* 14: 188–94. [PubMed]

Genton, B., and J. P. Berger. 1990. Cerebrospinal fluid lactate in 78 cases of adult meningitis. *Intensive Care Medicine* 16: 196–200. [CrossRef] [PubMed]

Greenberg, Mark S. 2010. *Handbook of Neurosurgery*. New York: Thieme Medical Publishers, pp. 208–55.

Grossman, R. I., and D. M. Yousem. 2003. Infectious and noninfectious inflammatory diseases of the brain. In *Neuroradiology: The Requisites*. Edited by Robert I. Grossman and D. M. Yousem. Philadelphia: Mosby.

Gurley, Emily S., M. Jahangir Hossain, Susan P. Montgomery, Lyle R. Petersen, James J. Sejvar, Leonard W. Mayer, Anne Whitney, Dull Peter, Nahar Nazmun, Uddin A. K. M. Rafique, and et al. 2009. Etiologies of Bacterial Meningitis in Bangladesh: Results from a Hospital- Based Study. *The American Journal of Tropical Medicine and Hygiene* 81: 475–83. [CrossRef] [PubMed]

Gutierrez-Murgas, Yenis, and Jessica N. Snowden. 2014. Ventricular shunt infections: Immunopathogenesis and clinical management. *Journal of Neuroimmunology* 276: 1–8. [CrossRef] [PubMed]

Hasbun, Rodrigo, James Abrahams, James Jekel, and Vincent J. Quagliarello. 2001. Computed tomography of the head before lumbar puncture in adults with suspected meningitis. *New England Journal of Medicine* 345: 1727–33. [CrossRef]

Hess, Donavon J., Michelle J. Henry-Stanley, and Carol L. Wells. 2012. Interplay of antibiotics and bacterial inoculum on suture-associated biofilms. *Journal of Surgical Research* 177: 334–40. [CrossRef]

Honda, Hitoshi, and David K. Warren. 2009. Central Nervous System Infections: Meningitis and Brain Abscess. *Infectious Disease Clinics of North America* 23: 609–23. [CrossRef]

Hossain, Md Zahed, Md M. Rahman, and Shah M. Badruddoza. 2010. Cranial hydatid abscess. *Tropical Doctor* 40: 255–56. [CrossRef]

Hossain, Md Zahed, Ali Akhaddar, Ahmet T. Turgut, and Forhad H. Chowdhury. 2017. Brain stem tuberculosis. In *Tuberculosis of the Central Nervous System*. Edited by Mehmet Turgut, Ali Akhaddar, Ahmet T. Turgut and Ravindra K. Garg. Cham: Springer, pp. 103–18. [CrossRef]

Idro, Richard, Kevin Marsh, Chandy C. John, and Charles R. J. Newton. 2010. Cerebral Malaria; Mechanisms of Brain Injury And Strategies for Improved Neuro-Cognitive Outcome. *Pediatric Research* 68: 267–64. [CrossRef]

Infection in Neurosurgery Working Party of the British Society for Antimicrobial Chemotherapy. 2000. The rational use of antibiotics in the treatment of brain abscess. *British Journal of Neurosurgery* 14: 525–30. [CrossRef] [PubMed]

Jayaraman, Yuvaraj, Balaji Veeraraghavan, Girish Kumar Chethrapilly Purushothaman, Bharathy Sukumar, Boopathi Kangusamy, Ambujam Nair Kapoor, Nivedita Gupta, Sanjay Madhav Mehendale, and Hospital Based Sentinel Surveillance of Bacterial Meningitis (HBSSBM) Network Team. 2018. Burden of bacterial meningitis in India: Preliminary data from a hospital-based sentinel surveillance network. *PLoS ONE* 13: e0197198. [CrossRef] [PubMed]

Joos, T. J., W. C. Miller, and D. M. Murdoch. 2006. Tuberculin reactivity in bacille Calmette- Guerin vaccinated populations: A compilation of international data. *The International Journal of Tuberculosis and Lung Disease* 10: 883–91. [PubMed]

Kanegaye, John T., Peyman Soliemanzadeh, and John S. Bradley. 2001. Lumbar puncture in pediatric bacterial meningitis: Defining the time interval for recovery of cerebrospinal fluid pathogens after parenteral antibiotic pretreatment. *Pediatrics* 108: 1169–74. [CrossRef] [PubMed]

Kashyap, Rajpal S., Rani P. Kainthla, Anju V. Mudaliar, Hemant J. Purohit, Girdhar M. Taori, and Hatim F. Daginawala. 2006. Cerebrospinal fluid adenosine deaminase activity: A complementary tool in the early diagnosis of tuberculous meningitis. *Cerebrospinal Fluid Research* 30: 1–6. [CrossRef]

Katti, Muralidhar K. 2004. Pathogenesis, diagnosis, treatment, and outcome aspects of cerebral tuberculosis. *Medical Science Monitor* 10: RA215–29.

Kilpatrick, Michael E., N. I. Girgis, D. Tribble, and Z. Farid. 1996. The value of the tuberculin skin test in patients with tuberculous meningitis. *The Journal of the Egyptian Public Health Association* 71: 1–8.

Kim, Kwang Sik. 2003. Pathogenesis of bacterial meningitis: From bacteraemia to neuronal injury. *Nature Reviews Neuroscience* 4: 376–85. [CrossRef]

Kingsley, Peter B., Tanmaya C. Shah, and Rona Woldenberg. 2006. Identification of diffuse and focal brain lesions by clinical magnetic resonance spectroscopy. *NMR in Biomedicine* 19: 435–62. [CrossRef]

Kumar, Raj, C. Pandey, Neeta Bose, and Surabhi Sahay. 2002. Tuberculous brain abscess: Clinical presentation, pathophysiology and treatment (in children). *Child's Nervous System* 18: 118–23. [CrossRef]

Kupila, L., T. Vuorinen, R. Vainionpaa, V. Hukkanen, R. J. Marttila, and P. Kotilainen. 2006. Etiology of aseptic meningitis and encephalitis in an adult population. *Neurology* 66: 75–80. [CrossRef] [PubMed]

LaPenna, Paul A., and Karen L. Roos. 2019. Bacterial Infections of the Central Nervous System. *Seminars in Neurology* 39: 334–42. [CrossRef] [PubMed]

Lebel, Marc H., Bishara J. Freij, George A. Syrogiannopoulos, Dale F. Chrane, M. Jean Hoyt, Sunita M. Stewart, Betsy D. Kennard, Kurt D. Olsen, and George H. McCracken, Jr. 1988. Dexamethasone therapy for bacterial meningitis. Results of two double-blind, placebo-controlled trials. *New England Journal of Medicine* 319: 964–71. [CrossRef] [PubMed]

Limaiem, Faten, and Nidhameddine Kchir. 2014. Hydatidosis of brain. In *Hydatidosis of the Central Nervous System Diagnosis and Treatment*. Edited by Mehmet Turgut. Berlin/Heidelberg: Springer, pp. 61–70.

Loftus, C. M., R. K. Osenbach, and J. Biller. 1996. Diagnosis and management of brain abscess. In *Neurosurgery*, 2nd ed. Edited by R. H. Wilkins and S. S. Rengachary. New York: McGraw Hill, pp. 3285–98.

Maconochie, I. K., J. H. Baumer, and M. Stewart. 2008. Fluid therapy for acute bacterial meningitis. *The Cochrane Database of Systematic Reviews* 5: CD004786.

Mahadevan, B., S. Mahadevan, V. Tiroumourougane Serane, and R. Narasimhan. 2005. Tuberculin reactivity in tuberculous meningitis. *Indian Journal of Pediatrics* 72: 213–15. [CrossRef]

Mathisen, Glenn E., and J. Patrick Johnson. 1997. Brain abscess. *Clinical Infectious Diseases* 25: 763–79. [CrossRef]

McIntyre, Peter B., Katherine L. O'Brien, Brian Greenwood, and Diederik Van De Beek. 2012. Effect of vaccine on bacterial meningitis worldwide. *The Lancet* 380: 1703–11. [CrossRef] [PubMed]

Mohamed, Amal, and Asmaa Mansour. 2017. Parasites in central nervous system. *International Journal of Medicine in Developing Countries* 1: 72–77. [CrossRef]

Mohindra, Sandeep, Amey Savardekar, Rahul Gupta, Manjul Tripathi, and Swapnil Rane. 2016. Tuberculous brain abscesses in immunocompetent patients: A decade long experience with nine patients. *Neurology India* 64: 66–74. [CrossRef]

Moorthy, Ranjith K., and Vedantam Rajshekhar. 2008. Management of brain abscess: An overview. *Neurosurgical Focus* 24: E3. [CrossRef]

Nakaiso, Mami, Masaaki Uno, Masafumi Harada, Teruyoshi Kageji, Osamu Takimoto, and Shinji Nagahiro. 2002. Brain Abscess and Glioblastoma Identified by Combined Proton Magnetic Resonance Spectroscopy and Diffusion-Weighted Magnetic Resonance Imaging. *Neurologia Medico-Chirurgica* 42: 346–48. [CrossRef] [PubMed]

Nelson, Christina A., and Joseph R. Zunt. 2011. Tuberculosis of the Central Nervous System in Immunocompromised Patients: HIV Infection and Solid Organ Transplant Recipients. *Clinical Infectious Diseases* 53: 915–26. [CrossRef] [PubMed]

Newton, P. J., W. Newsholme, N. S. Brink, H. Manji, I. G. Williams, and R. F. Miller. 2002. Acute meningoencephalitis and meningitis due to primary HIV infection. *BMJ* 325: 1225–27. [CrossRef] [PubMed]

Nigrovic, Lise E., Andrew M. Fine, Michael C. Monuteaux, Samir S. Shah, and Mark I. Neuman. 2013. Trends in the management of viral meningitis in United States Children's Hospitals. *Pediatrics* 131: 670–76. [CrossRef] [PubMed]

Odio, Carla M., Idis Faingezicht, Maria Paris, Martin Nassar, Aristides Baltodano, Jodi Rogers, Xavier Sáez-Llorens, Kurt D. Olsen, and George H. McCragken, Jr. 1991. The beneficial effects of early dexamethasone administration in infants and children with bacterial meningitis. *New England Journal of Medicine* 324: 1525–31. [CrossRef]

Overturf, Gary D. 2003. Indications for the immunological evaluation of patients with meningitis. *Clinical Infectious Diseases* 36: 189–94. [CrossRef]

Pai, Madhukar, Laura L. Flores, Nitika Pai, Alan Hubbard, Lee W. Riley, and John M. Colford. 2003. Diagnostic accuracy of nucleic acid amplification tests for tuberculous meningitis: A systematic review and meta-analysis. *The Lancet Infectious Diseases* 3: 633–43. [CrossRef]

Prasad, K., J. Volmink, and G. R. Menon. 2000. Steroids for treating tuberculous meningitis. *The Cochrane Database of Systematic Reviews* 3: CD002244.

Prasad, Kameshwar, Mamta B. Singh, and Hannah Ryan. 2016. Corticosteroids for managing tuberculous meningitis. *Cochrane Database of Systematic Reviews* 2016: CD002244. [CrossRef]

Prusseit, Julia, Matthias Simon, Christian Von der Brelie, Axel Heep, Ernst Molitor, Sebastian Völz, and Arne Simon. 2009. Epidemiology, prevention and management of ventriculoperitoneal shunt infections in children. *Pediatric Neurosurgery* 45: 325–36. [CrossRef]

Radstrom, P., A. Bäckman, N. Y. Qian, Peter Kragsbjerg, C. Påhlson, and Per Olcén. 1994. Detection of bacterial DNA in cerebrospinal fluid by an assay for simultaneous detection of Neisseria meningitidis, Haemophilus influenzae, and streptococci using a seminested PCR strategy. *Journal of Clinical Microbiology* 32: 2738–44. [CrossRef] [PubMed]

Ramakrishnan, Meenakshi, Aaron J. Ulland, Laura C. Steinhardt, Jennifer C. Moïsi, Fred Were, and Orin S. Levine. 2009. Sequelae due to bacterial meningitis among African children: A systematic literature review. *BMC Medicine* 7: 47. [CrossRef] [PubMed]

Remeš, František, Robert Tomáš, Vlastimil Jindrák, Václav Vaniš, and Michal Šetlík. 2013. Intraventricular and lumbar intrathecal administration of antibiotics in postneurosurgical patients with meningitis and/or ventriculitis in a serious clinical state. *Journal of Neurosurgery* 119: 1596–602. [CrossRef] [PubMed]

Rich, P. M., N. P. Deasy, and J. M. Jarosz. 2000. Intracranial dural empyema. *The British Journal of Radiology* 73: 1329–36. [CrossRef] [PubMed]

Rock, R. Bryan, Michael Olin, Cristina A. Baker, Thomas W. Molitor, and Phillip K. Peterson. 2008. Central nervous system tuberculosis: Pathogenesis and clinical aspects. *Clinical Microbiology Reviews* 21: 243–61. [CrossRef]

Rotbart, Harley A., P. J. Brennan, Kenneth H. Fife, Jose R. Romero, Johanna A. Griffin, Mark A. McKinlay, and Frederick G. Hayden. 1998. Enterovirus meningitis in adults. *Clinical Infectious Diseases* 27: 896–98. [CrossRef]

Saag, Michael S., Richard J. Graybill, Robert A. Larsen, Peter G. Pappas, John R. Perfect, William G. Powderly, Jack D. Sobel, and William E. Dismukes. 2000. Practice guidelines for the management of cryptococcal disease. Infectious Diseases Society of America. *Clinical Infectious Diseases* 30: 710–18. [CrossRef]

Sanei Taheri, Morteza, Mohammad Ali Karimi, Hamidreza Haghighatkhah, Ramin Pourghorban, Mohammad Samadian, and Hosein Delavar Kasmaei. 2015. Central nervous system tuberculosis: An imaging-focused review of a reemerging disease. *Radiology Research and Practice* 2015: 202806. [CrossRef]

Schaad, Urs B., J. Wedgwood, U. Lips, H. E. Gnehm, Ivo Heinzer, and A. Blumberg. 1993. Dexamethasone therapy for bacterial meningitis in children. Swiss Meningitis Study Group. *The Lancet* 342: 457–61. [CrossRef]

Scherr, Tyler D., Cortney E. Heim, John M. Morrison, and Tammy Kielian. 2014. Hiding in Plain Sight: Interplay between Staphylococcal Biofilms and Host Immunity. *Frontiers in Immunology* 5: 37. [CrossRef]

Schreffler, Rachel T., Andrew J. Schreffler, and Robert R. Wittler. 2002. Treatment of cerebrospinal fluid shunt infections: A decision analysis. *The Pediatric Infectious Disease Journal* 21: 632–36. [CrossRef] [PubMed]

Schuchat, Anne, Katherine Robinson, Jay D. Wenger, Lee H. Harrison, Monica Farley, Arthur L. Reingold, Lewis Lefkowitz, and Bradley A. Perkins. 1997. Bacterial meningitis in the United States in 1995. Active Surveillance Team. *New England Journal of Medicine* 337: 970–76. [CrossRef] [PubMed]

Segun, Toyin Dawodu. 2017. Subdural Empyema Clinical Presentation. Available online: https://emedicine.medscape.com/article/1168415-clinical (accessed on 30 May 2022).

Sharma, B. S., S. K. Gupta, and V. K. Khosla. 2000. Current concepts in the management of pyogenic brain abscess. *Neurology India* 48: 105–11. [PubMed]

Sharma, C., B. Kumawat, G. Tripathi, and S. Dixit. 2008. Isolated sensory trigeminal neuropathy-a rare clinical presentation of brain stem tuberculoma. Case report. *The Internet Journal of Neurology* 11: 1–3.

Sheikh, Salwa S., and Samir S. Amr. 2010. Fungal Infections of the Central Nervous System. In *Progress in Mycology*. Edited by Mahendra Rai and György Kövics. Dordrecht: Springer. [CrossRef]

Short, William R., and Allan R. Tunkel. 2000. Changing epidemiology of bacterial meningitis in the United States. *Current Infectious Disease Reports* 2: 327–31. [CrossRef]

Stadler, James A., II, Hamidreza R. Aliabadi, and Gerald A. Grant. 2019. Complications Associated With Cerebrospinal Fluid Diversion. In *Complications in Neurosurgery*. Amsterdam: Elsevier. [CrossRef]

Sutlas, P. N., A. Ünal, H. Forta, S. Şenol, and D. Kırbaş. 2003. Tuberculous meningitis in adults: Review of 61 cases. *Infection* 31: 387–91. [CrossRef]

Tan, Le Van, Le Hong Thai, Nguyen Hoan Phu, Ho Dang Trung Nghia, Ly Van Chuong, Dinh Xuan Sinh, Nguyen Duy Phong, Nguyen Thi Hoang Mai, Dinh Nguyen Huy Man, Vo Minh Hien, and et al. 2014. Viral aetiology of central nervous system infections in adults admitted to a tertiary referral hospital in southern Vietnam over 12 years. *PLoS Neglected Tropical Diseases* 8: e3127. [CrossRef]

Tewari, Manoj K., Rewati R. Sharma, Vinod K. Shiv, and Santosh D. Lad. 2004. Spectrum of intracranial subdural empyemas in a series of 45 patients: Current surgical options and outcome. *Neurol India* 52: 346–49.

Thigpen, Michael C., Cynthia G. Whitney, Nancy E. Messonnier, Elizabeth R. Zell, Ruth Lynfield, James L. Hadler, Lee H. Harrison, Monica M. Farley, Arthur Reingold, Nancy M. Bennett, and et al. 2011. Emerging Infections Programs Network. Bacterial meningitis in the United States, 1998–2007. *New England Journal of Medicine* 364: 2016–25. [CrossRef]

Thomas, Karen E., Rodrigo Hasbun, James Jekel, and Vincent J. Quagliarello. 2002. The diagnostic accuracy of Kernig's sign, Brudzinski's sign, and nuchal rigidity in adults with suspected meningitis. *Clinical Infectious Diseases* 35: 46–52. [CrossRef]

Thwaites, Guy, Martin Fisher, Cheryl Hemingway, Geoff Scott, Tom Solomon, and John Innes. 2009. British Infection Society guidelines for the diagnosis and treatment of tuberculosis of the central nervous system in adults and children. *Journal of Infection* 59: 167–87. [CrossRef] [PubMed]

Tintinalli, Judith E., and J. Stephan Stapczynski. 2011. *Tintinalli's Emergency Medicine: A Comprehensive Study Guide*. New York: McGraw-Hill.

Tunkel, Allan R., Barry J. Hartman, Sheldon L. Kaplan, Bruce A. Kaufman, Karen L. Roos, W. Michael Scheld, and Richard J. Whitley. 2004. Practice guidelines for the management of bacterial meningitis. *Clinical Infectious Diseases* 39: 1267–84. [CrossRef] [PubMed]

van de Beek, Diederik, Jan de Gans, Allan R. Tunkel, and Eelco F. M. Wijdicks. 2006. Community-acquired bacterial meningitis in adults. *New England Journal of Medicine* 354: 44–53. [CrossRef] [PubMed]

van de Beek, Diederik, Jan De Gans, Lodewijk Spanjaard, Martijn Weisfelt, Johannes B. Reitsma, and Marinus Vermeulen. 2004. Clinical features and prognostic factors in adults with bacterial meningitis. *New England Journal of Medicine* 351: 1849–59. [CrossRef]

Vasudeva, Shikha S. 2019. Meningitis. Medscape. Available online: https://emedicine.medscape.com/article/232915-overview (accessed on 31 May 2022).

Viallon, Alain, Fabrice Zeni, Claude Lambert, Bruno Pozzetto, Bernard Tardy, Christophe Venet, and Jean-Claude Bertrand. 1999. High sensitivity and specificity of serum procalcitonin levels in adults with bacterial meningitis. *Clinical Infectious Diseases* 28: 1313–16. [CrossRef] [PubMed]

Waaler, H. T. 2002. Tuberculosis and poverty. *International Journal of Infectious Diseases* 6: 745–46.

Wan, Cordia. 2018. Viral Meningitis Treatment & Management. Available online: https://emedicine.medscape.com/article/1168529-treatment (accessed on 30 May 2022).

Warembourg, H., G. Niquet, J. Lekieffre, M. Thoreux, and J. Coupin. 1960. Onset of meningeal tuberculosis with Weber's syndrome. *Lille Medical* 5: 3.

Weisfelt, Martijn, Diederik van de Beek, Lodewijk Spanjaard, Johannes B. Reitsma, and Jan de Gans. 2006. Clinical features, complications, and outcome in adults with pneumococcal meningitis: A prospective case series. *The Lancet Neurology* 5: 123–29. [CrossRef]

WHO. 2007. *Global Tuberculosis Control: Surveillance, Planning, Financing*. WHO Report. WHO/ HTM/TB/2007.376. Geneva: WHO, pp. 1–70.

WHO. 2010. *Treatment of Extrapulmonary TB and of TB in Special Situation. Treatment of Tuberculosis Guidelines*, 4th ed. WHO/HTM/TB/2009.420. Geneva: Stop TB Department, WHO, pp. 95–99.

Zhang, Chenran, Liuhua Hu, Xiaojun Wu, Guohan Hu, Xuehua Ding, and Yicheng Lu. 2014. A retrospective study on the aetiology, management, and outcome of brain abscess in an 11 year, single centre study from China. *BMC Infectious Diseases* 14: 311. [CrossRef]

Section IX: Cranial Neoplasms

Brain Tumours

Mohammod Raziul Haque, Robert Ahmed Khan, S.I.M. Khairun Nabi Khan and Forhad H. Chowdhury

Abstract: Primary brain neoplasms can be benign or malignant. Primary neoplasms can originate from the brain parenchyma (intrinsic), meninges, cranial nerves, pituitary gland, choroid plexus, and from the ventricles. Primary malignant brain tumours have an annual global age-standardized incidence of 3.7/100,000 for men and 2.6/100,000 for women, with mortality rates of 2.8 per 100,000 for men and 2.0 per 100,000 for women. Common intracranial malignant tumours are glioma, ependymoma, medulloblastoma, and secondary metastatic tumours, whereas common benign tumours are meningioma, schwannoma, and sellar and suprasellar tumours. Clinical presentation depends on site, size, and on the age of the patient. The most common presentations include headache, seizure, features of raised ICP, and focal neuro-deficit/s. A CT scan and an MRI of the head with contrast are enough for diagnosing most brain tumours. Surgery is the primary modality of management. Surgical approaches differ according to size, site, age, nature of neoplasm, and operator experience and expertise as well. Prognosis depends on histological type, extent of resection, and postoperative therapy (where needed) as well. In this chapter, we will briefly discuss the surgical management of the most common brain tumours.

Abbreviations

ACTH	adrenocorticotrophin hormone	ADC	afferent diffusion co-efficient
AVM	arteriovenous malformation	BAER	brainstem auditory evoked response
BBB	blood–brain barrier	BCNU	biodegradable carmustine
CNS	central nervous system	CTV	clinical target volume
CT	computed tomography	CSF	cerebrospinal fluid
CUSA	Cavitron ultrasonic aspirator	DI	diabetes insipidus
DEBS	direct electrical brain stimulation	DTI	diffusion tensor imaging
DSA	digital subtraction angiogram	ECoG	Electrocorticogram
DW	diffusion-weighted	EEG	electroencephalogram
FIEST	fast imaging employing steady-state acquisition	ETV	endoscopic third ventriculostomy
EOR	extent of resection	FDG-PET	flurodeoxyglucose PET
EVD	external ventricular drainage	FSH	follicle-stimulating hormone
fMRI	functional magnetic resonance imaging	GTV	gross tumour volume
GTR	gross total resection	HGG	high-grade glioma
HCG	human chorionic gonadotrophin	ICG	indocyanine green
HPC	Hemangiopericytoma	iMRI	intraoperative MRI
ICP	intracranial pressure	IPS	inferior petrosal sinus
IDH	isocitrate dehydrogenase	KPS	Karnofsky performance status
IMRT	intensity-modulated radiotherapy	LH	luteinizing hormone
LGG	low-grade glioma	MB	Medulloblastoma
LINAC	linear accelerator	MEG	magneto encephalography
MRI	magnetic resonance imaging	MEP	motor evoked potential
MRA	magnetic resonance angiogram	NAA	N-acetyl aspartate
MRS	magnetic resonance spectroscopy	OS	overall survival
PET	positron emission tomography	PFS	progression-free survival
PTV	planning target volume	SPECT	single-photon emission computed tomography
SEP	sensory evoked potential	SFT	solitary fibrous tumour
SSS	superior sagittal sinus	SRS	stereotactic radiotherapy
TCD	transcranial doppler	TMZ	Temozolomide
TSH	thyroid-stimulating hormone	USG	Ultrasonogram
VEP	visual evoked potential	VDE	velocity of diametric expression
VPS	ventriculoperitoneal shunt	WBRT	whole-brain radiotherapy
XRT	X-ray radiotherapy		

1. Incidence/Epidemiology

Primary malignant brain tumours have an annual global age-standardized incidence of 3.7/100,000 for men and 2.6/100,000 for women, with mortality rates of 2.8 and 2.0 per 100,000 for men and for women (GLOBOCAN 2002). In the USA, the incidence of both non-malignant and primary malignant brain tumours is 14.8/100,000 per year, with 6–8/100,000 having a high-grade neoplasm. The annual incidence rate of metastatic brain tumours is estimated to be 8.3–11/100,000 people. Tumour types are distributed differently by age. According to the Swedish Cancer Registry, the commonest types of tumours in paediatric cases aged 15 years and younger are medulloblastoma (23.5%) and low-grade glioma (31.7%); this is in stark contrast to adult cases, where high-grade glioma (30.5%) and meningioma (29.4%) are the commonest types of adult primary brain neoplasms. The 5- and 10-year survival rates are 29.1% and 25.3%, respectively, according to the American Cancer Society (ACS; www.cancer.org), and vary greatly by age and histology. Glioblastoma multiforme (GBM) has a 5-year survival rate of 3.3%, while lower-grade gliomas like oligodendroglioma, pilocytic astrocytoma, and ependymoma have 5-year survival rates of over 70%. Astrocytoma (not otherwise specified), malignant glioma, anaplastic astrocytoma, and lymphoma have comparable overall survival rates. For the majority of histologies, five-year survival rates drop as people get older (www.cbtrus.org). However, some histologic categories (e.g., ependymoma and GBM) have a lower survival rate in paediatric patients and in the elderly. The disparity in incidence rates between men and women is one of the most constant findings in the epidemiology of brain tumours; glioma is more prevalent in men, while meningioma is more common in women (Newton 2016; Bondy et al. 2008).

In both population registry data and clinical trials, histologic grade and type, age, extent of resection, tumour site, radiation therapy, and various chemotherapy regimens have been consistently and conclusively associated with survival. GBM and anaplastic astrocytoma patients' survival is also predicted by their Karnofsky performance status (KPS) at diagnosis, as well as other measures of physical and mental capability (Levin et al. 2001).

2. Classification

In the 2016 update, molecular markers were incorporated into the histological classification of brain tumours for the first time. The main changes were in the glioma and medulloblastoma groups. In the context of glioma, "genotype trumps over phenotype", and classification is based on the assessment of IDH mutations as well as 1p/19q status in diffuse glioma (van den Bent et al. 2017). Diffuse midline glioma, H3 K27M-mutant, RELA fusion-positive ependymoma, embryonal tumour with multi-layered rosettes, C19MC-altered, and hybrid nerve sheath tumours are among the new additions. Protoplasmic and fibrillary astrocytoma, glioblastoma cerebri, and cellular ependymoma are among the variants and patterns that have been removed because they no longer have biological or diagnostic significance. Other changes include the removal of the term "primitive neuroectodermal tumour", the addition of a criterion for brain invasion in atypical meningioma, the distinction of melanotic schwannoma from other types of schwannoma, and the grouping of solitary fibrous tumours and haemangiopericytoma as a single entity. There is also an increase in the number of entities in nerve sheath tumours and CNS haematopoietic/lymphoid cancers (Gupta and Dwivedi 2017).

The sixth iteration of the global standard for the categorization of brain and spinal cord malignancies is the WHO Classification of Malignancies of the Central Nervous System (CNS), which was released in 2021. This is the fifth edition of this classification, updated in 2021 (Table 1), and it adds significant modifications that enhance the use of molecular diagnostics in CNS tumour classification, building on the work of the Consortium to Inform Molecular and Practical Approaches to CNS Tumor Taxonomy and on the fourth edition, published in 2016. However, it continues to be allied with other well-established methods of tumour diagnosis, like immunohistochemistry and histology. In doing so, the fifth edition highlights the significance of integrated diagnostics and layered reports while establishing some distinct approaches to CNS tumour nomenclature and grading. There is an introduction of new tumour kinds and subtypes, some of which are based on cutting-edge diagnostic tools like DNA methylome analysis. The main changes to tumour taxonomy introduced in the 2021 edition are outlined in this section, along with particular modifications to each taxonomic group (Louis et al. 2021).

Table 1. WHO classification of CNS tumours of 2021 is shown below.

1. Gliomas, Glioneuronal Tumours, and Neuronal Tumours
1.1 Adult-type diffuse gliomas
1.1.1 Astrocytoma, IDH-mutant
1.1.2 Oligodendroglioma, IDH-mutant, and 1p/19q-codeleted
1.1.3 Glioblastoma, IDH-wildtype
1.2 Paediatric-type diffuse low-grade gliomas
1.2.1 Diffuse astrocytoma, MYB- or MYBL1-altered
1.2.2 Angiocentric glioma
1.2.3 Polymorphous low-grade neuroepithelial tumour of the young (PLNTY)
1.2.4 Diffuse low-grade glioma, MAPK pathway-altered
1.3 Paediatric-type diffuse high-grade gliomas
1.3.1 Diffuse midline glioma, H3 K27-altered
1.3.2 Diffuse hemispheric glioma, H3 G34-mutant
1.3.3 Diffuse paediatric-type high-grade glioma, H3-wildtype and IDH-wildtype
1.3.4 Infant-type hemispheric glioma
1.4 Circumscribed astrocytic gliomas
1.4.1 Pilocytic astrocytoma
1.4.2 High-grade astrocytoma with piloid features
1.4.3 Pleomorphic xanthoastrocytoma
1.4.4 Subependymal giant-cell astrocytoma
1.4.5 Chordoid glioma
1.4.6 Astroblastoma, MN1-altered
1.5 Glioneuronal and neuronal tumours
1.5.1 Ganglioglioma
1.5.2 Desmoplastic infantile ganglioglioma/desmoplastic infantile astrocytoma
1.5.3 Dysembryoplastic neuroepithelial tumour
1.5.4 Diffuse glioneuronal tumour with oligodendroglioma-like features and nuclear clusters
1.5.5 Papillary glioneuronal tumour
1.5.6 Rosette-forming glioneuronal tumour
1.5.7 Myxoid glioneuronal tumour
1.5.8 Diffuse leptomeningeal glioneuronal tumour
1.5.9 Gangliocytoma
1.5.10 Multinodular and vacuolating neuronal tumour
1.5.11 Dysplastic cerebellar gangliocytoma (Lhermitte–Duclos disease)
1.5.12 Central neurocytoma
1.5.13 Extraventricular neurocytoma
1.5.14 Cerebellar liponeurocytoma
1.6 Ependymal tumours
1.6.1 Supratentorial ependymoma
1.6.1.1 Supratentorial ependymoma, ZFTA fusion-positive
1.6.1.2 Supratentorial ependymoma, YAP1 fusion-positive
1.6.2 Posterior fossa ependymoma
1.6.2.1 Posterior fossa ependymoma, group PFA
1.6.2.2 Posterior fossa ependymoma, group PFB
1.6.3 Spinal ependymoma
1.6.3.1 Spinal ependymoma, MYCN-amplified
1.6.4 Myxopapillary ependymoma
1.6.5 Subependymoma
2. Choroid Plexus Tumours
2.1 Choroid plexus papilloma
2.2 Atypical choroid plexus papilloma
2.3 Choroid plexus carcinoma
3. Embryonal Tumours
3.1 Medulloblastoma
3.2 Atypical teratoid/rhabdoid tumour
3.3 Cribiform neuroepithelial tumour
3.4 Embryonal tumour with multilayered rosettes
3.5 CNS neuroblastoma, FOXR2-activated
3.6 CNS tumour with BCOR internal tandem duplication

Table 1. *Cont.*

4. Pineal Tumours
4.1 Pineocytoma 4.2 Pineal parenchymal tumour of intermediate differentiation 4.3 Pineoblastoma 4.4 Papillary tumour of the pineal region 4.5 Desmoplastic myxoid tumour of the pineal region, SMARCB1-mutant
5. Cranial and Paraspinal Nerve Tumours
5.1 Schwannoma 5.2 Neurofibroma 5.3 Perineurioma 5.4 Hybrid nerve sheath tumour 5.5 Malignant melanotic nerve sheath tumour 5.6 Malignant peripheral nerve sheath tumour 5.7 Paraganglioma
6. Meningioma
Subtypes: 6.1 Meningothelial meningioma 6.2 Fibrous meningioma 6.3 Transitional meningioma 6.4 Psammomatous meningioma 6.5 Angiomatous meningioma 6.6 Microcystic meningioma 6.7 Secretory meningioma 6.8 Lymphoplasmacyte-rich meningioma 6.9 Metaplastic meningioma 6.10 Chordoid meningioma 6.11 Clear-cell meningioma 6.12 Atypical meningioma 6.13 Papillary meningioma 6.14 Rhabdoid meningioma 6.15 Anaplastic (malignant) meningioma
7. Mesenchymal, Non-Meningothelial Tumours
7.1 Soft-tissue tumours 7.1.1 Fibroblastic and myofibroblastic tumours 7.1.1.1 Solitary fibrous tumour 7.1.2 Vascular tumours 7.1.2.1 Haemangiomas and vascular malformations 7.1.2.2 Haemangioblastoma 7.1.3 Skeletal muscle tumours 7.1.3.1 Rhabdomyosarcoma 7.1.4 Uncertain differentiation 7.1.4.1 Intracranial mesenchymal tumour, FET-CREB fusion-positive 7.1.4.2 CIC-rearranged sarcoma 7.1.4.3 Primary intracranial sarcoma, DICER1-mutant 7.1.4.4 Ewing sarcoma 7.2 Chondro-osseous tumours 7.2.1 Chondrogenic tumours 7.2.1.1 Mesenchymal chondrosarcoma 7.2.1.2 Chondrosarcoma 7.2.2 Notochordal tumours 7.2.2.1 Chordoma (including poorly differentiated chordoma)
8. Melanocytic Tumours
8.1 Diffuse meningeal melanocytic neoplasms 8.1.1 Meningeal melanocytosis and meningeal melanomatosis 8.2 Circumscribed meningeal melanocytic neoplasms 8.2.1 Meningeal melanocytoma and meningeal melanoma

Table 1. *Cont.*

9. Haematolymphoid Tumours
9.1 Lymphomas
9.1.1 CNS lymphomas
9.1.1.1 Primary diffuse large B-cell lymphoma of the CNS
9.1.1.2 Immunodeficiency-associated CNS lymphoma
9.1.1.3 Lymphomatoid granulomatosis
9.1.1.4 Intravascular large B-cell lymphoma
9.1.2 Miscellaneous rare lymphomas in the CNS
9.1.2.1 MALT lymphoma of the dura
9.1.2.2 Other low-grade B-cell lymphomas of the CNS
9.1.2.3 Anaplastic large cell lymphoma (ALK+/ALK−)
9.1.2.4 T-cell lymphomas and NK/T-cell lymphomas
9.2 Histiocytic tumours
9.2.1 Erdheim–Chester disease
9.2.2 Rosai–Dorfman disease
9.2.3 Juvenile xanthogranuloma
9.2.4 Langerhans cell histiocytosis
9.2.5 Histiocytic sarcoma
10. Germ Cell Tumours
10.1 Mature teratoma
10.2 Immature teratoma
10.3 Teratoma with somatic-type malignancy
10.4 Germinoma
10.5 Embryonal carcinoma
10.6 Yolk sac tumour
10.7 Choriocarcinoma
10.8 Mixed germ cell tumour
11. Tumours of the Sellar Region
11.1 Adamantinomatous craniopharyngioma
11.2 Papillary craniopharyngioma
11.3 Pituicytoma, granular cell tumour of the sellar region, and spindle cell oncocytoma
11.4 Pituitary adenoma/PitNET
11.5 Pituitary blastoma
12. Metastases to the CNS
12.1 Metastases to the brain and spinal cord parenchyma
12.2 Metastases to the meninges

Source: Authors' compilation based on data from WHO Classification of Tumours Editorial Board (2021).

3. Intrinsic Brain Tumours

3.1. Gliomas

3.1.1. Introduction

Glioma susceptibility seems to be hereditary, according to studies of syndromes, linkage, familial aggregation, and mutagen sensitivity in adulthood. Syndromes including medulloblastoma or gliomas, with gene names and chromosome location, are neurofibromatosis 1 (NF1, 17q11) and 2 (NF2 22q12), retinoblastoma (RB1; 13q14), tuberous sclerosis (TSC1 9q34, TSC2 16p13), and Li–Fraumeni (TP53 17p13), as well as Turcot's syndrome and multiple hamartoma (APC 5q21, hMLH1 3p21.3, hMSH2 2p22-21, PMS2 7p22, PTEN 10q23.3) (Bondy et al. 2008). Gliomas are linked to a number of polymorphisms, the most prevalent of which are found in carcinogen metabolism, DNA repair, and immune function genes. Ionizing radiation in certain forms and doses is widely recognized as a cause of brain cancers (Ron 2003). There is yet to be a study that identifies a link between mobile phone use and the risk of having a brain tumour (Newton 2016). Meta-analyses of a large body of research based on multiple case–control and two cohort studies show that self-reported allergies are associated with glioma in a way that is unlikely to be due to chance or methodologic biases alone (Linos et al. 2007).

The WHO Revised 4th edition (2016) classification groups diffusely infiltrating gliomas (oligodendroglial tumours and astrocytic tumours) together and then introduces the category "Other astrocytic tumours" for astrocytomas that are more circumscribed (pleomorphic xanthoastrocytoma, pilocytic astrocytoma, subependymal giant-cell astrocytoma). As a result, the term "low-grade glioma" (LGG) is used to refer to grade 2 gliomas as mentioned by the WHO, including diffuse astrocytomas, oligodendrogliomas, and oligoastrocytomas (Louis et al. 2016).

Supporting glial cells in the brain give rise to high-grade gliomas. The pathological classification is determined by the major cell type. According to the WHO grading system, tumours are rated based on light microscopy appearances (grade 1 to 4). WHO grade 3 (anaplastic astrocytoma and anaplastic oligoastrocytoma) and 4 tumours are classified as HGGs (glioblastoma with oligodendrocyte component, glioblastoma, gliosarcoma). Grade 4 tumours are diffusely infiltrating gliomas with focal or distributed anaplasia and a high proliferative capacity, as evidenced by distinct nuclear atypia, enhanced cellularity, and significant mitotic activity on histological examination. Cellular polymorphism, rapid mitotic activity, nuclear atypia, arterial thrombosis, necrosis, and microvascular proliferation are all seen in grade 4 tumours (Price et al. 2019). The introduction of the WHO Classification of Tumours of the CNS has resulted in broad changes in the categorization of high-grade glioma (Pallud et al. 2014). The definition of molecular subgroups has grossly divided glial-origin tumours into three categories: isocitrate dehydrogenase (IDH) wildtype, IDH mutated, and IDH not specified (i.e., where IDH mutation has not been sought). Within this classification (and with the inclusion of the 1p 19q chromosomal codeletion for oligodendroglioma), diffuse glioma, oligodendroglioma, anaplastic astrocytoma, anaplastic oligodendroglioma, and glioblastoma have now all been defined.

3.1.2. Clinical Considerations

LGGs present with seizures in more than 80% cases. Others present with focal neuro-deficits, altered mentation, or raised intracranial pressure (Pallud et al. 2014). Although "gross neurological deficits" such as dysphasia and hemiparesis are uncommon when LGGs appear, objective neuropsychological examinations generally reveal more subtle cognitive problems at the time of diagnosis. Executive function, attention, focus, working memory, and mood disorders are all common. Before beginning oncological treatment, a thorough evaluation of higher mental functions and health-linked quality of life is now suggested (Klein et al. 2012).

In patients with glioblastoma, the symptoms and indications are relatively uniform but nonspecific. Increased intracranial pressure, which can cause headache, vomiting and nausea, double or blurred vision, and drowsiness, is prevalent in affected people. Extraocular palsies, objective papilloedema, pupil irregularities, and a lower degree of consciousness may be related to these signs and symptoms. They are usually more noticeable in the morning and improve over the day. These tumours are characterized by unrelenting, increasing headache. Seizures affect up to a third of glioblastoma patients (Rincon-Torroella et al. 2017). Bases on the extent and location of tumour invasion, neurological deficits are prevalent. These deficits include changes in personality and altered cognition and might be localized or widespread (Tucha et al. 2000). Although neurological abnormalities from anaplastic astrocytoma and glioblastoma are widespread, they are often subtle and may go unnoticed until the brain tumour is discovered.

3.1.3. Neuroradiological Characteristics

Magnetic resonance imaging (MRI) of LGGs demonstrates tumours that are isointense/hypointense on T1W images, are homogeneously hyperintense on T2W images, and are not enhanced with contrast administration. The extent of the tumour has been shown to best correspond to FLAIR hyperintensity (Figure 1). However, it is important to remember that LGG is a diffuse neoplastic disease and that glioma cells have been shown to be present as far as 2 cm beyond FLAIR signal abnormality (Pallud et al. 2010). Sophisticated MRI techniques, such as MR spectroscopy, have been used to differentiate glioma grades and even to detect key LGG metabolic mutations, such as those of the isocitrate dehydrogenase 1 (IDH1) gene. When tumours were graded with use of proton MR spectroscopy of metabolite ratios (choline/N-acetylaspartate, choline/creatine, and N-acetylaspartate/creatine), this yielded significant differences between LGGs and HGGs ($P < 0.01$). An increased choline-creatinine ratio on MR spectroscopy corresponded to a heightened risk of transformation (Law et al. 2003). MRS of glioma generally shows a choline peak that is significantly increased, a decreased NAA peak, and a creatinine peak with no obvious change. With an increase in glioma malignancy degree, the choline peak increases even more. In some cases, an abnormal increase in the lactate peak or lipid peak could also be detected.

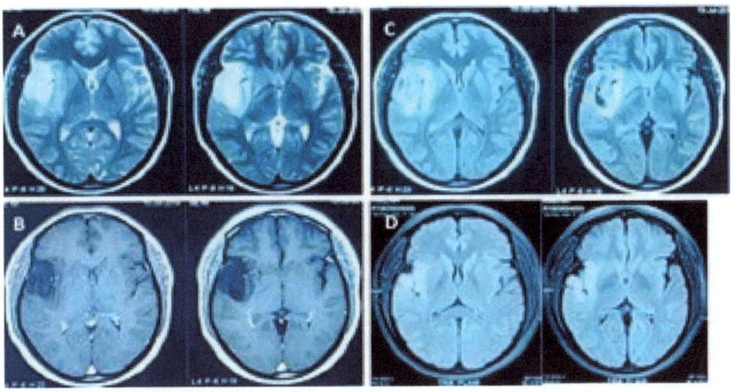

Figure 1. Low-grade gliomas are hyperintense on MRI T2W sequence (**A**), hypointense without contrast enhancement on T1W (**B**), and again hyperintense on FLAIR sequence (**C**). FLAIR sequence is the ideal follow-up sequence and, in this case, shows no tumour recurrence after 1 year (**D**). Source: Figure by authors.

For brain tumours, MRI is now the preferred method of investigation. On T1-weighted MRI, high-grade glioma generally presents as an irregular hypodense lesion with varying degrees of contrast enhancement and oedema (Figure 2).

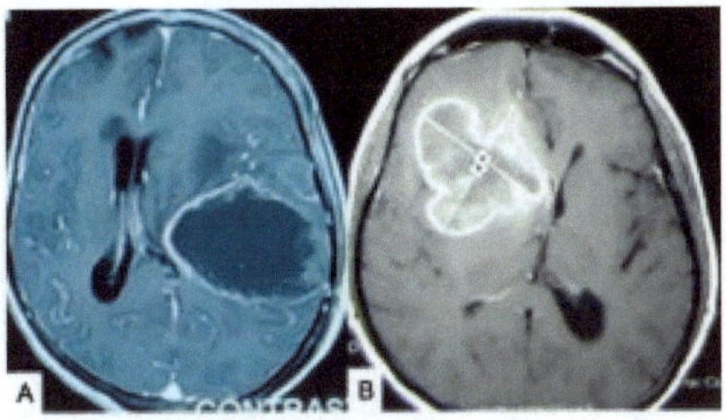

Figure 2. Glioblastomas are typically irregular, peripherally enhancing tumours with central necrosis and mass effect. Contrast MRI axial view: (**A**) parietal GBM and (**B**) frontal GBM. Source: Figure by authors.

Glioblastoma is indicated by the presence of a ring-like enhancement surrounding irregularly shaped regions of putative necrosis. However, non-enhancing tumours such as anaplastic astrocytomas and even glioblastomas might present as non-enhancing lesions at first, especially in elderly patients. Furthermore, low-grade gliomas might sometimes show contrast enhancement. In high-grade malignancies, fluorodeoxyglucose positron emission tomography (FDG-PET) is efficient in revealing hypermetabolism. FDG uptake has long been known to have predictive value. Anaplastic transformation is diagnosed by high FDG uptake in previously known low-grade tumours (Padma et al. 2003). Anatomical imaging is unable to determine tumour margins, which is one of the fundamental drawbacks of using imaging for treatment planning. On both contrast-enhanced T1W MRI and T2W MRI, the tumour expands beyond the margin, according to post-mortem and biopsy studies (Price et al. 2006).

3.1.4. Principles of Glioma Surgery

Glioma surgery aims for the greatest safe resection possible. The surgical removal of these intrinsic brain neoplasms is difficult because they often invade eloquent parts of the brain and lack a distinct border. Preoperative investigations that support anatomical and functional tumour characterization, which aids in defining tumour extent and determining the viability of total resection, are the primary emphasis of this subsection. We also describe intraoperative adjuncts that aid in identifying tumour-infiltrated areas during surgery in order to maximize the extent of resection. Furthermore, the danger of postoperative neurological deficits is reduced while enabling optimal tumour removal with intraoperative functional cortical and subcortical mapping and monitoring. To achieve surgical objectives and guarantee the best possible patient outcomes, it is advised to combine the use of various modalities both before and during surgery (Krivosheya et al. 2016).

Neuronavigation

Neuronavigation (Figure 3) refers to the localizing techniques that indicate the location of an object in relation to the surgical field sans the need for a fixed, rigid coordinate system, such as a frame firmly affixed to the patient's cranium (Willems et al. 2006). The devising of stereotactic systems that do not rely on stereotactic frames was aided by the convergence of three technological achievements: (1) computers that could manipulate large volumes of MRI or CT data at an acceptable cost and efficiency, (2) improved spatial accuracy (nominally within 1 mm) for CT and MRI during the obtaining of data incorporating the patient's head, and (3) low-cost, accurate 3D digitizers to be used as pointing devices in surgery. Frameless stereotactic neuronavigation thus works by acquiring preoperative imaging data (which will serve as a reference map during the surgical approach and tumour resection), using a localizing tool that will be tracked by the neuronavigation system and will serve as a pointer, and a mathematical framework calculating the relationship between the patient's anatomy and preoperative imaging.

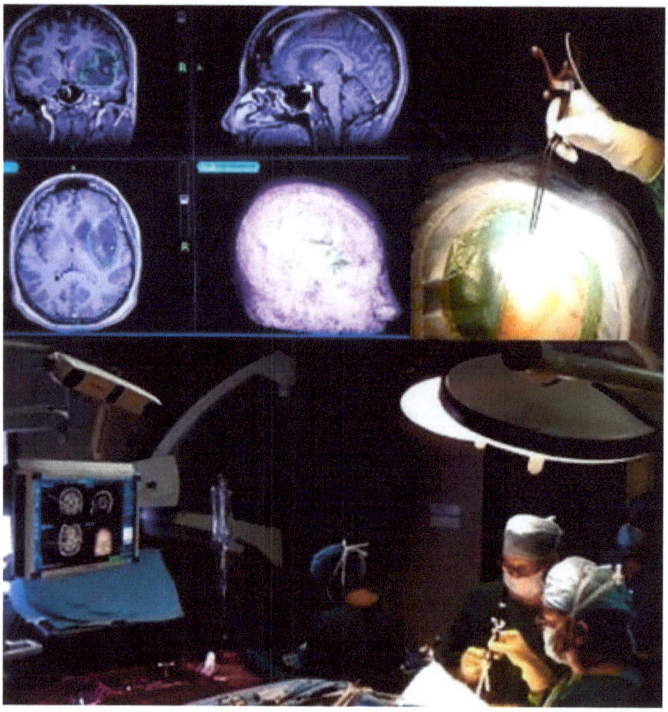

Figure 3. Use of neuronavigation in intrinsic brain tumour surgery (courtesy of Dr. Moududul Haque, Department of Neurosurgery, BSMMU). Source: Figure by authors.

Because there are few, if any, landmarks within the brain's substance, surgical navigation must provide unambiguous guidance to subcortical malignancies. This guidance function is handled in a variety of ways in modern systems. Several research studies have looked at the use of fMRI and DTI for preoperative planning as well as at their intraoperative use as a supplement to surgical navigation for brain tumour removal. It has been found that when fMRI data are paired with DTI data, the accuracy and ability to identify functional structures improves (Kleiser et al. 2010).

Since the 1980s, intraoperative ultrasonography (Figure 4) has been employed for neurosurgery procedures. Intraoperative ultrasonography produces real-time images, has been shown to be helpful in tumour resection, and is faster and considerably cheaper than other intraoperative modalities, such as MRI. Image-guided ultrasonography, which combines the real-time ultrasonographic data with preoperative imaging data, allows for better interpretation of ultrasound images and improved orientation with the use of the ultrasound probe (Miller et al. 2007).

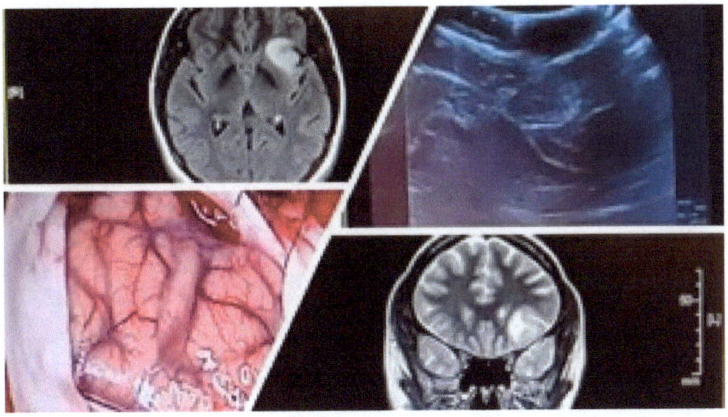

Figure 4. Intraoperative ultrasonography helps in localizing and resecting tumours in real time. Source: Figure authors.

One of the limitations of conventional surgical navigation is decreased accuracy, especially during the final stages of resection, due to tissue deformation and brain shift caused by changes in tumour volume, CSF drainage, intracranial pressure, brain retraction, etc. (Sherman et al. 2011). Intraoperative MRI can be useful in identifying residual tumour, thus allowing for further resection and improved outcomes of gross total resection. Kubben and colleagues concluded that based on available published studies, there was at least level 2 evidence that iMRI-guided surgery was more effective than conventional navigation with respect to their chosen endpoints in patients with glioblastoma (Kubben et al. 2011). But the benefit of iMRI has to be balanced against its significant cost, which remains its main limitation.

Intraoperative Neuromonitoring

Perioperative neuromonitoring (Figure 5) is critical for guiding surgery and perhaps improving neurologic outcomes by minimizing complications. Clinical neurological examination with a co-operative and awake patient is commonly considered the gold standard of neuromonitoring.

According to the International 10–20 electrode placement system, electroencephalography (EEG) can be monitored using electrodes placed on the scalp. During cerebrovascular surgery, EEG is frequently utilized to detect burst suppression. Nonconvulsive seizures can also be diagnosed with intraoperative EEG monitoring. Electrocorticography (ECoG) produces electrical brain signals that have a high signal-to-noise ratio, are less susceptible to artefacts than EEG, and have a high spatial and temporal resolution. Perioperative ECoG is conducted by placing a specific electrode array on the surface or within the material of the brain utilizing strips, depth, or grid electrodes. It is utilized not only to guide the location of the epileptogenic area, but also to examine the extent to which the seizure focus has been resected.

From the point of stimulation along the neural pathway to the response elicited, evoked potentials assess the central nervous system's integrity. Somatosensory evoked potentials (SEPs), brain auditory evoked responses (BAERs), motor evoked potentials (MEPs), and visual evoked potentials (VEPs) are the commonest of these. When the structures that generate the signal are indirectly or directly at risk owing to damage to or disruption in blood supply, SEP monitoring is used. During neurovascular surgery, MEPs are frequently used. The brainstem component of the auditory evoked response is highly resistant to the effects of anaesthetic medicines, and it is used to assess the integrity of cranial nerve VIII following surgery for acoustic schwannoma as well as other cerebellar pontine angle neoplasms. Because VEP monitoring is more technically difficult, it is not routinely used in the operating room. Intraoperative cortical mapping is commonly utilized to locate the motor strip, sensory cortex, or speech centres for surgery in and around these expressive areas. These procedures necessitate an awake patient, with the operation performed under local anaesthetic with sedation.

Patients with intracranial pathology like severe traumatic brain damage, subarachnoid haemorrhage, intracranial tumours, and cerebral oedema may have an elevated ICP. The importance of early detection and treatment of increased ICP cannot be overstated. ICP management has the ability to influence outcomes, especially when care is targeted, personalized, and supported with information from other monitors.

Monitoring cerebral oxygenation with jugular venous oximetry allows for the determination of intraoperative cerebral desaturation and guides anaesthetic interventions like optimizing hyperventilation therapy and managing perfusion pressure, oxygenation, and fluids to optimise cerebral physiology. Transcranial Doppler (TCD) ultrasonography is a non-radioactive, non-invasive, and portable technology that uses a range-gated, pulsed Doppler ultrasound to deliver continuous real-time data about cerebral circulation.

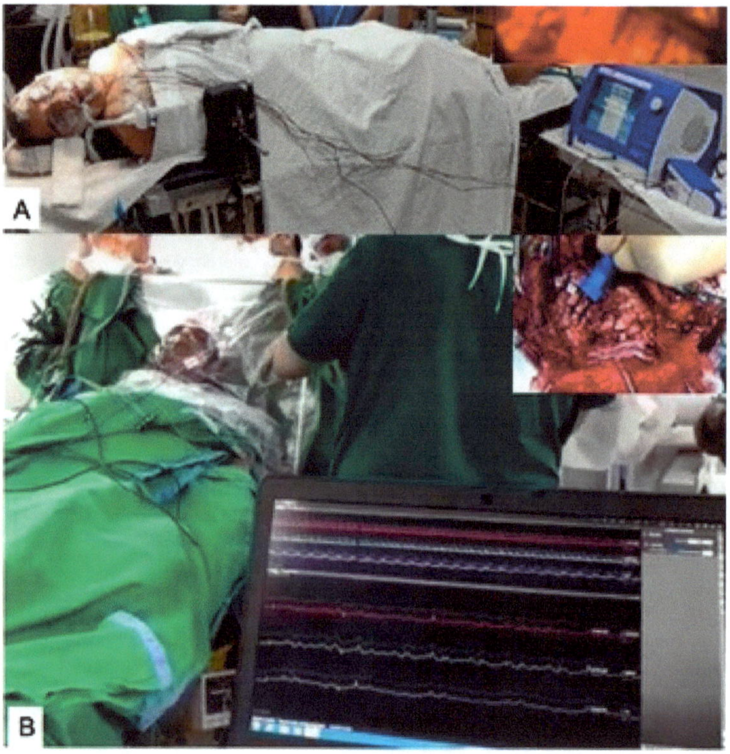

Figure 5. Intraoperative neuromonitoring. (**A**) Facial nerve monitoring in cerebellopontine angle surgery. (**B**) Cortical stimulation in awake patient in glioma surgery. Source: Figure by authors.

Intraoperative Dyes

Intraoperative dyes prove useful in several instances in neurosurgery. They are used in CSF leakage and tumour identification, and also in intraoperative angiography (Raza et al. 2016).

Fluorescein has been used intrathecally to detect CSF leaks; however, it has been linked to seizures in some cases. Fluorescein has also been used intravenously to help identify parts of the brain where the blood–brain barrier (BBB) has been broken, such as in malignancies. During the excision of AVMs, it has also been utilized to perform intraoperative "visible angiograms." Intraoperative angiography is performed using indigocyanine green (ICG). It can be seen in regular light or, in some cases, using near-infrared illumination for a better view. This can only be used on surface vessels. With thick-walled atherosclerotic arteries, or big or wide-neck aneurysms, it may be less reliable (Greenberg 2010).

When tumour cells take up nonfluorescent 5-ALA, it causes the production and accumulation of fluorescent protoporphyrin IX (PpIX). Due to a broken BBB, enhanced neovascularization, and overexpression of membrane transporters in malignant tissues, there is greater ALA absorption in brain tumours. PpIX, which is collected selectively in malignant tissue, generates a red-violet light after being excited with blue light generated from a specific filter attachment on the operational microscope, allowing the surgeon to resect red-violet tumour tissue in a gross total fashion (Belykh et al. 2020).

3.1.5. Treatment Considerations

There are some important prognostic factors which are associated with outcomes in patients with LGGs. Clinically, older age, the existence of neurological impairments or a seizure-free state at the outset, and a low performance status (KPS 70%) are all linked to worse outcomes. There is a negative association between tumour volume and overall survival (OS); also, tumour extension to or location in eloquent areas is associated with shorter OS. Speed of growth, expressed as velocity of diametric expansion (VDE)—a measurement reflecting both initial tumour volume and the increase in volume—has been observed to be an independent prognostic factor for OS and malignant-progression-free survival (PFS) (Pallud et al. 2012). Finally, although overall survival broadly correlates with each histological diagnosis, there is extensive evidence that tumours from individual patients who share the same histological diagnosis do not necessarily share the same biology, and their outcomes may vary widely. The limitations of histological diagnosis prompted the search for more clinically relevant markers for stratifying patients with LGGs. Indeed, a number of glioma-relevant molecular markers have been discovered and seem to be superior to histology in predicting outcomes. These include the presence of mutations of the IDH1 or IDH2, ATRX, and TERT genes and the loss of 1p/19q chromosomal arms. They have been incorporated, for the first time, in the latest WHO classification.

Although the importance of surgery in the management of LGGs was once questionable, in all recent series with objective postoperative evaluation of the extent of resection (EOR) based on the volumetric assessment of FLAIR MRI, a considerable improvement in OS was predicted by the degree of resection. This oncological benefit must be, however, balanced against the risk of functional deficit that may arise from radical surgery (onco-functional balance). Advances in the understanding of the brain, tumours, and brain–tumour interactions, as well as the popularization of awake surgeries and direct electrical brain stimulation (DEBS) techniques, have led to improvements in surgical techniques and to a consequent reduction in permanent neurological deficits to below 5% (Duffau et al. 2008). As a result, the primary therapeutic option to explore in LGGs is maximal and early surgical resection. Needle biopsy is only used in individuals who do not want or are unable to undergo surgery due to medical causes. When subtotal resection is not possible, biopsy may be considered for diffuse tumours such as gliomatoses.

The medical management of the symptoms and signs of malignant glioma accounts for a large part of patient care. When treating these individuals, clinicians should keep in mind that the most prevalent issues are peritumoural oedema, seizures, exhaustion, venous thromboembolisms, and cognitive impairment, all of which should be addressed.

The aims of surgery are to obtain a representative tissue sample of the neoplasm for histological and molecular marker assessment as well as to safely remove the tumour with the aim of improving pressure symptoms, improving the efficacy of adjuvant therapy, delaying deterioration, and improving survival; finally, there is the potential of applying surgically delivered treatments (Figure 6). Although no level 1 data are currently available, modern series that utilize exact volumetric measurements of postoperative neoplasm volume seem to support the benefits of increasing the extent of resection (EOR) on progression-free survival (PFS) as well as on OS. A meta-analysis of 37 retrospective studies covering 41,117 unique patients revealed increased chances of survival after gross total resection (GTR) as an analogy to subtotal resection (STR) (Brown et al. 2016). The difficulty in performing the GTR of these tumours is identifying the limits of resection. As there is a poor margin between the tumour and the normal brain, most studies suggest that a GTR is performed in less than 30% of patients (Albert et al. 1994; Kowalczuk et al. 1997). A variety of tools have been developed to improve this resection rate. Image guidance is essential for planning craniotomies, but unpredictable brain shift restricts its use in identifying tumour limits. Intraoperative ultrasound is a useful method, but it is user-dependent. Intraoperative MRI provides the most accuracy, but it is very expensive and does add time to tumour resection (Mehdorn et al. 2011). 5-aminolevulinic acid (5-ALA) fluorescence guiding is a new surgical adjuvant that uses blue (400 nm) light to locate glioma tissue. In cases of malignant glioma, the administration of 5-ALA permits more thorough removal of contrast-enhancing neoplasms, resulting in greater progression-free survival (Stummer et al. 2006). The oncological neurosurgeon's main task is to resect as much as possible while avoiding any neurological damage. Intraoperative function mapping, employing cortical as well as subcortical mapping, has been shown to decrease the risk of postoperative neurological impairments by half (De Witt Hamer et al. 2012).

Adjuvant therapy for high-grade gliomas has traditionally relied on radiotherapy. The evident tumour is defined as gross tumour volume (GTV) in radiotherapy planning. The clinical target volume (CTV) is then estimated by adding a 2.5 cm margin. To generate the planning target volume (PTV), a 0.5 cm buffer is added to accommodate set-up faults and patient movement. To put it another way, a 3 cm margin is applied around the tumour to protect the normal brain. The dose is thus reduced to decrease the risk of radiation necrosis. In HGGs, two types of radiation are commonly employed. Short-course or palliative radiation delivers a 30-gray dose in six fractions over two weeks, whereas radical radiotherapy delivers a 60-gray dose over thirty daily fractions plus temozolomide during and after radiotherapy (this is known as the Stupp protocol) (Stupp et al. 2005).

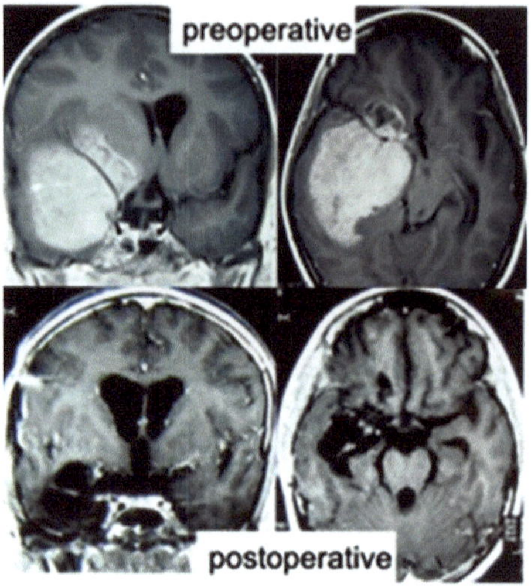

Figure 6. Upper row: preoperative contrast MRI showing right temporal glioma; histology reported GBM. Lower row: contrast MRI six months after the operation and four months after radiotherapy, showing no residual or recurrent tumour. Source: Figure by authors.

The role of chemotherapy as an adjuvant therapy to radiotherapy has been studied in a number of randomized controlled trials. In 2005, a single trial compared the utilization of radiation alone (XRT) to the combination of radiation plus six concurrent cycles of adjuvant temozolomide (XRT/TMZ). Patients who received XRT/TMZ lived an average of two months longer than those who only received XRT. TMZ has a major advantage in that it may be taken orally, and it has quickly become the cornerstone of HGG treatment (Stupp et al. 2005).

In practice, many neurosurgeons use the older classification of gliomas, i.e., low-grade astrocytoma, anaplastic glioma, and glioblastoma multiforme (GBM).

"Low-Grade" Astrocytoma

A total of 5% of all adult primary cerebral tumours are grade 1 or 2 astrocytomas. The average age at which the more common grade 2 tumours arise is 35 years. They consist of well-differentiated astrocytic cells that are further separated into fibrillary, protoplasmic, and gemistocytic types. They are diffuse and grow slowly. The p53 gene is lost in up to 90% of cases. These tumours lack a clear boundary or capsule and extensively invade the surrounding brain, despite being benign.

In children and young adults, pilocytic (grade 1) astrocytomas can develop in the brainstem and cerebellum, in the optic nerve in connection with NF1, and in the hypothalamus. They can frequently stabilize, even regress, and grow extremely slowly.

These may remain asymptomatic for long period. Epilepsy is the most common presentation. Dysphasia, limb weakness, and personality changes can occur over long periods of time. MRI is the investigation of choice and may need to include DTI, tractography, spectroscopy, and fMRI. MRI usually shows a hypointense, non-contrast-enhancing mass in T1W images without or with minimal surrounding oedema.

The excision of low-grade astrocytoma from non-eloquent areas can achieve very good long-term results. However, in eloquent areas, a "safe subtotal/partial resection" of these tumours is performed using awake craniotomy, neuronavigation, brain mapping, or the Duffau concept to avoid neuro-deficits.

About 40% of individuals with grade 2 astrocytomas survive for ten years, and around 50–60% survive for five. Eighty percent of individuals with pilocytic (grade 1) astrocytomas live for twenty years or more (Lindsay et al. 2011).

Glioblastoma Multiforme (GBM)/Anaplastic Astrocytoma

Of all primary cerebral tumours, anaplastic astrocytomas (grade 3) and glioblastoma multiforme (grade 4) account for up to 20%. Anaplastic astrocytoma is four times less prevalent than glioblastoma. The median age upon diagnosis is 45 years old, compared to 64 years old for glioblastoma. These tumours spread widely over the surrounding brain and grow quickly. Histology at autopsy frequently shows dissemination to several distant sites.

Genetic analysis distinguishes between "secondary" glioblastomas, which progress from lower-grade tumours (loss of p53, overexpression of PDGFR, loss of heterozygosity of 10q, abnormalities in the p16 and Rb pathways), and "primary" glioblastomas, which arise de novo (e.g., amplification of EGFR gene, loss of p16, mutation of PTEN, and loss of heterozygosity of 10q).

Clinical presentation includes raised ICP, limb weakness, dysphasia, personality changes, seizures, etc. Clinical features develop gradually, progressing over weeks, months, or years. Sudden deterioration indicates haemorrhage from the tumour. A patient with long-standing epilepsy may experience a quick onset of new symptoms due to a malignant alteration within a "low-grade" lesion. MRI is the investigation modality of choice and may need to include DTI, tractography, spectroscopy and fMRI. MRI usually shows a mixed-intensity (in T1W images) lesion which may be irregularly contrast-enhancing, with surrounding oedema.

Surgery is the mainstay treatment, along with postoperative radiotherapy. Concomitant chemotherapy with radiotherapy is added in GBM patients. The concept of surgical resection is "maximal safe resection". In order to help localize the tumour and assess the extent of tumour removal as the procedure goes on, neuronavigation (frameless stereotaxy), neuromonitoring, or, if possible, real-time CT, MRI, or ultrasound, are frequently used in conjunction with tumour resection. By means of a craniotomy, the physician extracts as much tumour tissue as is safe during an "open" biopsy conducted under direct eyesight. The challenge is that there is no plane of cleavage between the brain and the tumour tissue. The resolution of the imaging limits neuronavigation's ability to identify the boundaries visible on CT or MRI scans. In cases when eloquent regions are nearby, the surgeon may combine tractography or fMRI with the neuronavigation image with or without awake craniotomy to aid in guiding the excision; however, reliability in this regard is still being investigated. An irreparable neurological deficit could be reduced by carrying out the surgery on an awake patient and monitoring the direct effects of electrical stimulation. Large resections in the non-dominant temporal lobe, occipital, or frontal lobes are most securely executed. Most people think that the more cytoreduction—or reduction in tumour bulk—there is, the more effective adjuvant therapy will be.

Although survival has increased due to modern treatments, these tumours still have a poor prognosis. It is impossible to remove everything completely; interhemispheric spread causes even the powerful "hemispherectomy" to fail.

Extensive tumour excision alone increases average survival in surgical patients by only two months; however, when paired with concurrent chemotherapy and radiation therapy, this benefit is increased by an additional twelve months. A total of 25% of patients with this treatment live for two years; more than 40% of patients who have the MGMT gene silenced by promoter methylation survive for more than two years (Lindsay et al. 2011).

3.2. *Ependymomas*

3.2.1. Clinical Considerations

Ependymomas account for 3–5% of all CNS tumours in adults and almost 10% of all CNS tumours in children. Radial glial cells—bipolar progenitor cells that are thought to be a main source of neurons in the developing nervous system—are hypothesized to be the origins of ependymomas. Ependymomas can occur anywhere along the neuro-axis; they are more frequent in the posterior fossa in children, and in adults, they are more common as intramedullary spinal cord tumours. Previously, it was thought that they came from the lining of the central canal of the spinal cord or the cerebral ventricles; however, recent research suggests that radial glial stem cells may be the source (Taylor et al. 2006). Ependymomas are classified as grade 1 (subependymoma or myxopapillary; though some believe that these are different entities than grade 1), grade 2 (ependymoma with definitions of cellular, clear-cell, papillary, or tanycytic), and grade 3 (anaplastic ependymoma).

The clinical appearance of ependymomas varies according to their size, location, and histologic grade. Hydrocephalus, cranial nerve impairments, and cerebellar dysfunctions are all symptoms of infratentorial ependymoma. Supratentorial extraventricular lesions may present with seizures and focal neurological deficits (e.g., hemiparesis, visual field defects, speech difficulty, behavioural changes, memory deficits); lateral ventricular lesions may present with hydrocephalus and focal neurological deficits; and third ventricular lesions with hydrocephalus, focal neurological deficits, or Parinaud's syndrome (Vellimana et al. 2017). There are no conventional staging criteria for ependymomas. The work-up of patients with suspected ependymoma should include a detailed history as well as a physical examination, followed by MRI of the entire neuro-axis.

3.2.2. Investigative Considerations

On computed tomography (CT) scans, ependymomas may be isodense or hyperdense to the brain parenchyma. Nearly half of these tumours show calcifications, which appear as hyperdense regions on CT. On contrast-enhanced CT scans, these tumours usually demonstrate varying degrees of enhancement that may be heterogeneous; they sometimes enhance homogeneously (Yuh et al. 2009). These MRI appearances are not unique to ependymoma (Figure 7), but they are most often iso/hypointense on T1 sequences, high-signal on T2 sequences, and enhance avidly after contrast. FIESTA (fast imaging employing steady-state acquisition) sequences may allow for more accurate resolution of cranial nerves and vascular structures, and both diffusion-weighted imaging (DWI) and apparent diffusion co-efficient (ADC) mapping are now routinely used to identify high-grade tumours. MRS may also be useful with ependymomas showing a low NAA/choline ratio somewhere between that of a PNET and a glioma. A particular imaging feature which is strongly suggestive of ependymoma is when the tumour fills the lateral recesses of the fourth ventricle or even extends out through the foramina of Luschka and Magendie into the cerebellopontine angle (CPA) and spinal canal, respectively (Chandler 2019).

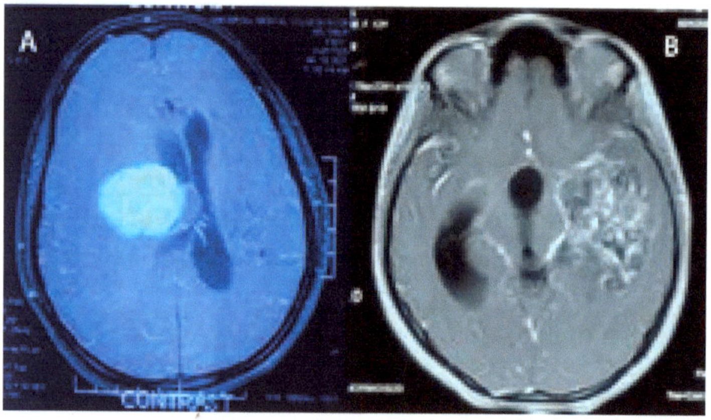

Figure 7. (**A**) Supratentorial extraventricular ependymoma. (**B**) Ependymoma in temporal horn of left lateral ventricle with hydrocephalus. Source: Figure by authors.

3.2.3. Treatment Considerations

The optimal surgical approach for ependymoma is dependent on tumour location (Figure 8).

Infratentorial tumours may be accessed via a standard midline suboccipital craniotomy/ craniectomy and for more lateral tumours, a retromastoid craniotomy/craniectomy may be used. If a pre-resection CSF drainage procedure has not been undertaken, the surgeon might initially create a posterior burr hole and insert an external ventricular drain (EVD) immediately before undertaking the craniotomy. Many neurosurgeons use a telo-velar approach to access fourth ventricular tumours to avoid/minimize damage to the vermis and to try and reduce the risk of posterior fossa mutism/syndrome (Chandler 2019). The aim is always to achieve gross total resection given its paramount importance in prognosis and outcome. Ependymomas are frequently adherent to the brainstem and cranial nerves in the CPA and avoiding damage to these structures can challenge even experienced surgeons. For intraventricular supratentorial ependymomas, an open microsurgical or endoscopic approach can be used. When an open microsurgical approach is chosen, the route commonly includes a trans-sulcal or transcortical or interhemispheric transcallosal corridor for third ventricular lesions (Geffen et al. 1980). For obstructive hydrocephalus caused by posterior fossa, aqueductal, or posterior third ventricular ependymomas, endoscopic third ventriculostomy and biopsy of the intraventricular lesion are a good therapeutic option, provided the interpeduncular cistern is not obliterated by tumour or brainstem displacement (Vellimana et al. 2017).

Craniospinal irradiation (CSI) as an adjuvant therapy has now been replaced by conformal radiotherapy, which uses 3D imaging and software to optimize dose delivery unless metastatic disease is present (Merchant et al. 2009). A range of different radiotherapy paradigms are now available, including hyperfractionated accelerated radiotherapy, IMRT (intensity-modulated radiotherapy), LINAC, SRS (stereotactic radiosurgery), and proton beam radiotherapy.

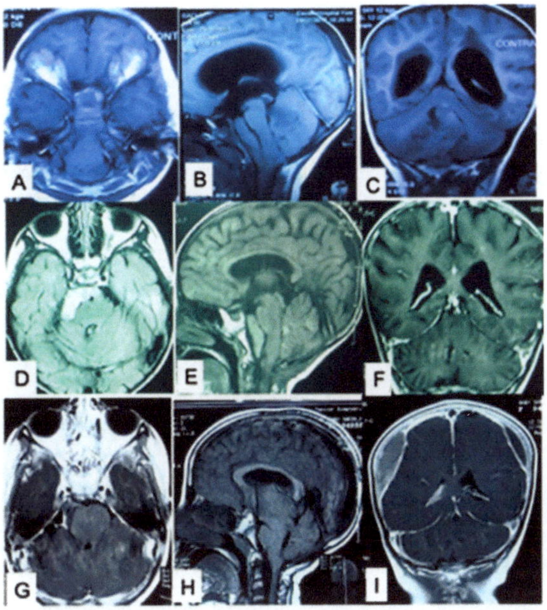

Figure 8. (**A–C**) Preoperative contrast MRI of brain showing posterior fossa extraventricular grade 2 ependymoma (non-contrast-enhancing) in a 4-year-old girl. (**D–F**) Postoperative (subtotally resected and shunted) contrast MRI of brain showing prepontine and premedullary contrast-enhancing residual tumour 3 months after operation. (**G–I**) Postoperative contrast MRI of brain showing no tumour (but there is bilateral parietal asymptomatic subdural effusion) 5 years after operation and adjuvant chemo–radiotherapy. Source: Figure by authors.

3.3. Medulloblastoma

3.3.1. Clinical Considerations

Although medulloblastoma (MB) is a rare disease in adults, accounting for about 1% of all CNS tumours, it is the most prevalent malignant CNS neoplasm in children (Jukich et al. 2001). MB has four different molecular variations, according to the current genomic method. Wingless (WNT), sonic hedgehog (SHH), group 3, and group 4 are the major molecular groupings of MB, with each group having distinct demographics, genetics, recurrence patterns, and outcomes (Northcott et al. 2011). MB is a grade 4 tumour with five variations: classic, desmoplastic nodular, extreme nodular medulloblastoma, anaplastic, and large-cell (Louis et al. 2007). The presenting symptoms and signs depend on the patient's age. Obstructive hydrocephalus and elevated intracranial pressure are common symptoms of a posterior fossa midline tumour. This would result in macrocephaly and a bulging fontanel in infants and toddlers with open sutures. Poor feeding, irritability, regression of milestones, and vomiting usually follow. Older children typically suffer from morning headache and vomiting episodes which relieve the headache. Symptoms due to direct mass effect depend on tumour location. Midline lesions cause truncal ataxia and long tract signs, while more lateral locations—as seen in older children and adolescents—present with cranial nerve palsy, vertigo, and appendicular ataxia. The most common presenting symptoms in adults are headache, ataxia/gait disturbance, and nausea/vomiting, followed by dizziness/vertigo (vestibular symptoms) and diplopia (Ang et al. 2008).

3.3.2. Investigative Considerations

Head ultrasound can be utilized as an initial imaging tool for the diagnosis of hydrocephalus caused by posterior fossa tumour in children with open fontanel. Computed tomography (CT) would show a midline cerebellar lesion with surrounding vasogenic oedema and obstructive hydrocephalus. Medulloblastomas are hypercellular tumours and they present as hyperdense lesions on CT. Calcifications can be seen in 22% of the cases and cystic formation in 59% (Poretti et al. 2012). All patients with a posterior fossa tumour should undergo a detailed examination of the head and spine with MRI. The imaging characteristics of medulloblastomas are variable in adults, perhaps more so than in children. Whereas tumour locations are predominantly midline (vermian) in children (Figure 9), they are more frequently lateral or hemispheric in adults. The intense or homogeneous contrast enhancement pattern that is frequent in children may not be as common in adults. Tumour margins may appear less distinct in adult medulloblastoma as well. Adult medulloblastomas may appear hypointense on T1W MRI but variable on T2W MRI. The hypercellularity of high-grade tumours such as medulloblastomas, with a high nucleus/cytoplasm ratio, results in reduced free water and gives a high signal (restriction) on diffusion-weighted imaging (DWI) (Fruehwald-Pallamar et al. 2011).

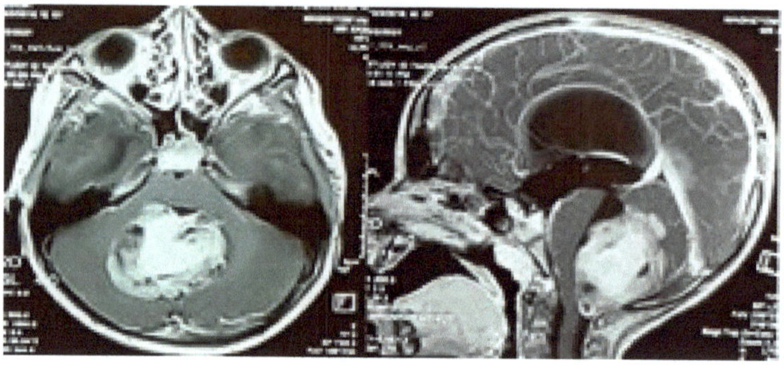

Figure 9. Medulloblastomas are more or less homogenous, highly contrast-enhancing tumours arising from the roof of the fourth ventricle. Source: Figure by authors.

3.3.3. Treatment Considerations

For hydrocephalus due to MB, the routine insertion of ventriculoperitoneal shunts (VPSs) should be avoided because only 10–40% of children will eventually need permanent CSF diversion postoperatively, and these patients will be exposed to a significant risk of VPS complications throughout their lives (Lee et al. 1994). Most surgeons prefer to perform a midline suboccipital craniotomy with the patient in the prone position. Intraoperative neuromonitoring is important. Persistent bleeding usually indicates residual tumour. The endoscope is a useful tool to inspect remnants "around the corners". The target is gross total resection (GTR) under maximum safety. If the tumour invades the floor of the fourth ventricle or is firmly attached to the lower cranial nerves, the surgeon should avoid aggressive resection due to resulting palsies, which significantly decrease the patient's quality of life. According to one study, there is no prognostic dissimilarity between near-total and GTR; hence, there is no need to pursue GTR at the risk of postoperative neurologic morbidity (Thompson et al. 2016).

MB subgroups have various clinical behaviours and may respond favourably to therapies tailored to their particular needs. Norcantharidin, a protein phosphatase inhibitor, has been demonstrated to affect WNT signalling and reduce MB development by promoting nuclear catenin depletion (Cimmino et al. 2011). Smoothened (SMO) inhibitors like vismodegib and sonidegib are the main targets of therapies to modify SHH signalling (Kool et al. 2014). The majority of research on group 3 and group 4 MBs focuses on compounds that block MYC-related pathway activity (Morfouace et al. 2014).

In patients aged under 3 years, even in cases of disseminated disease, current protocols follow radiation-free approaches. In those who are more than 3 years old, adjuvant therapies are stratified into average- and high-risk patients, as per the clinical criteria. Patients in the high-risk group receive 3600 cGy of craniospinal irradiation with a boost at the tumour bed and to focal metastases. Average-risk patients receive reduced craniospinal irradiation (2340 cGy) with a boost to the tumour bed of 5400–5580 cGy (Gottardo et al. 2014).

3.4. *Intracranial Metastasis*

3.4.1. Clinical Considerations

Metastatic brain tumours are the commonest brain tumours in adults (Zigouris et al. 2009). Approximately one-third of patients present with a solitary lesion, one-third with oligometastatic (2–3 lesions), and another third with polymetastatic lesions (Norden et al. 2005). The commonest sources of brain metastases in this patient group are cancers of the lung and breast and melanoma, in descending order. In children, the commonest cause of brain metastases is leukaemia, followed by lymphoma (Takakura et al. 1982). Patients with metastases present with signs and symptoms of increased intracranial pressure, CSF pathway obstruction, neurological mass effect, and, in the untreated situation, coning and death. Irritation of the cortex may lead to focal or generalized seizure presentation in 15–20% of patients, but more so (50%) in those with melanoma (Taillibert and Delattre 2005). Solitary or oligometastatic disease presents with headache (80%), focal neurological deficit (30–40%), and visual disturbance (6%), while polymetastatic disease may present as an encephalopathic or acute confusional state (Gaspar et al. 1997).

3.4.2. Investigative Considerations

The grey/white junction is commonly the site of supratentorial cerebral metastases. Sometimes, they are dural-based. There is typically peripheral or heterogeneous enhancement on contrast CT or MRI examination. Brain metastases are frequently accompanied by severe surrounding oedema that is often out of proportion to the size of the tumour. High-grade glioma, subacute infarct, and brain abscess are among the possible diagnoses for ring-enhancing cerebral lesions. These can be distinguished using advanced MRI.

Magnetic resonance spectroscopy (MRS) analysis of malignancies reveals increased choline (CHO) and decreased creatine (CRE) and n-acetyl aspartate (NAA) (Figure 10). Areas of necrosis with higher lactate are frequent in high-grade gliomas, which typically have lower myoinositol levels (Castillo et al. 2000).

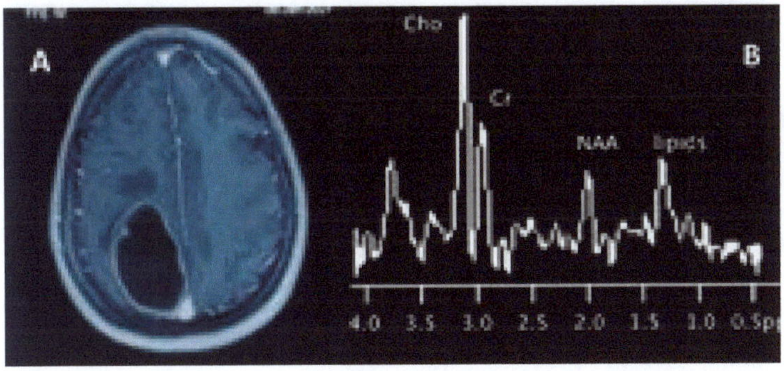

Figure 10. (**A**) Cerebral metastases are usually peripherally enhancing lesions with surrounding oedema which are occasionally dural-based. (**B**) MRS typically shows elevated choline (Cho) and depressed creatine (Cre) and n-acetyl aspartate (NAA). Source: Figure by authors.

3.4.3. Treatment Considerations

High-dose corticosteroids are used in the early stage of the management of patients with symptomatic brain metastases in order to decrease the oedema that classically surrounds these tumours and to help restore neurological function. Individual treatment options can be divided into focal (surgery, stereotactic radio surgery (SRS), interstitial laser therapy, and focused ultrasound treatment) and whole-brain or -body techniques (whole-brain radiotherapy (WBRT), chemotherapy, and targeted or immune therapies). Patient-related factors like age, performance status, the occurrence of extracranial metastases, and the condition of the primary tumour continue to be the key determinants of patient outcome (Gaspar et al. 1997).

The preferred treatment for individuals with a solitary brain metastasis is gross surgical resection, followed by WBRT or SRS to the tumour bed to stop local recurrence and perhaps increase survival. This is especially true for younger patients with stable extracranial illness and a KPS 70. WBRT, along with SRS, offers the best survival benefit in patients with tumours that are inaccessible to surgery, who have several concomitant conditions, have a low KPS, or who choose not to have surgery. However, WBRT may have considerable adverse cognitive effects, and the risk must be balanced with the benefit. Although WBRT remains the standard of care for patients with polymetastatic brain disease, improved planning algorithms have allowed for the use of SRS in these patients. Multiple lesions can be managed with acceptable toxicity due to the sharp dose drop-off and conformity provided by stereotactic systems. According to a recent trial, stereotactic radiosurgery in patients with five to ten brain metastases is not inferior to that in patients with two to four brain metastases when performed without WBRT (Yamamoto et al. 2014). For patients with up to ten brain metastases, stereotactic radiosurgery may be a good alternative because of its low level of invasiveness and favourable side effect profile in comparison to WBRT. In patients with multiple brain metastases (BM), survival following whole-brain radiation therapy (WBRT) is currently predicted using group-based scoring systems that have limited decision-making utility. For the assessment of survival in patients with short life expectancy, however, a more pertinent tailored predictive model can be utilized, such as the Diagnosis-Specific Graded Prognostic Assessment (DS-GPA) or the Radiation Therapy Oncology Group Recursive Partitioning Analysis (RTOG-RPA) (Marchand-Crety et al. 2021).

If surgical intervention is chosen, an en bloc resection technique including dissection just outside or inside the pseudocapsule should be tried. This approach limits the spillage of tumour cells, in addition to meticulously devascularizing the tumour. Piecemeal resection was found to be inferior to this approach (Patel et al. 2009). If the tumour is close to the eloquent cortex, a margin of less than 5 mm is desired but not always possible. As it avoids piecemeal resection, the Cavitron ultrasonic aspirator (CUSA) is frequently useful in achieving this goal.

4. Extrinsic Tumours and Tumour-like Conditions

4.1. *Meningioma*

4.1.1. Clinical Considerations

Meningiomas were first described by Harvey Cushing in 1922 and have since been recognized as the commonest intracranial nonglial tumour (Ostrom et al. 2016). Meningiomas are thought to originate from meningothelial cells (also known as arachnoidal cap cells). Meningothelial cells are most abundant on the surface of arachnoid villi around major venous sinuses, large cerebral veins, crista galli, and over the basilar venous plexus, but are also found in the arachnoid membrane in all its locations and other parts of the CNS (Haines and Frederickson 1991). In descending order of occurrence, the approximate distribution of intracranial meningiomas is as follows: convexity (35%), sphenoid ridge (20%), parasagittal (20%), intraventricular (5%), tuberculum sellae (3%), infratentorial (13%), and others (4%) (Almefty et al. 2017).

Depending on the location (Figures 11 and 12), meningiomas can produce a wide array of symptoms. Symptoms and signs can be related directly to the compression of adjacent neural structures or secondary to the effects of elevated intracranial pressure. For example, if the tumour is located on the medial part of the sphenoid wing, decreased vision and eye movement paralysis may be commonplace, whereas a tumour at the posterior fossa may give rise to a different constellation of symptoms, including hydrocephalus and dysphonia. As a consequence of the irritation of the cerebral cortex, seizures may occur with supratentorial meningiomas (Birk et al. 2019). WHO recognizes three grades of meningioma on the basis of pathologic criteria and the risk of recurrence and aggressive growth. Diagnosis of atypical (grade 2) and anaplastic (grade 3) meningiomas is made primarily based on mitotic count, regions of hypercellularity, nuclear/cytoplasmic ratio, sheet-like growth, prominent nucleoli, and spontaneous necrosis. However, some rare meningioma subtypes, characterized by particular tumour cell phenotypes, are linked to more common recurrence and are automatically (regardless of the presence of the aforementioned histological "features of malignancy") graded as WHO grade 2 (chordoid and clear-cell) or WHO grade 3 (papillary and rhabdoid) meningiomas (Raza et al. 2016).

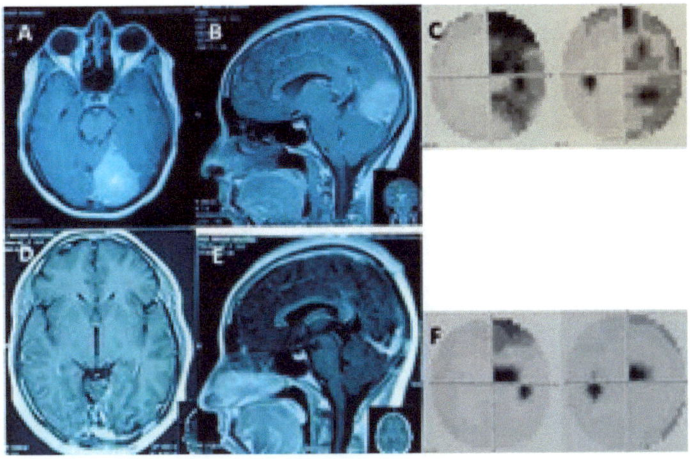

Figure 11. A case of peritorcular meningioma with right homonymous hemianopia (**A–C**). Improvement in visual field after tumour excision (**D–F**). Source: Figure by authors.

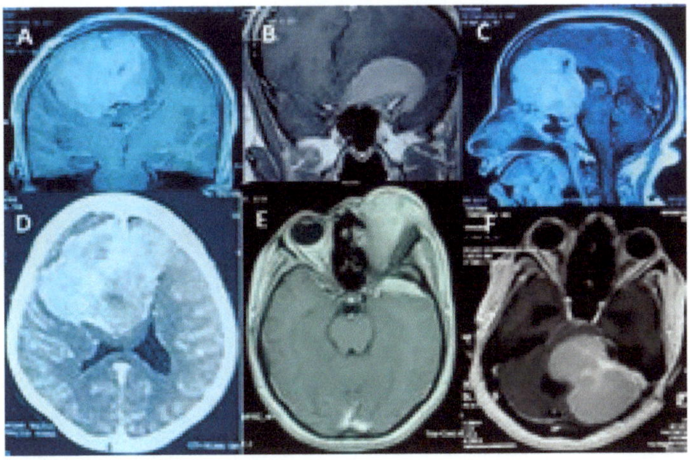

Figure 12. Meningiomas in different locations: (**A**) convexity meningioma; (**B**) clinoidal meningioma; (**C**) olfactory groove meningioma; (**D**) falcine meningioma; (**E**) spheno-orbital meningioma; (**F**) posterior fossa meningioma. Source: Figure by authors.

4.1.2. Investigative Considerations

Patients with meningioma have three distinctive features on plain radiographs: hyperostosis, enhanced vascular patterns, and calcification. Meningiomas often appear isodense to slightly hyperdense on non-contrast-enhanced CT scans in comparison to the contiguous brain parenchyma. There could be calcification. Meningiomas typically grow uniformly and strongly. The tumour usually has a large base and a sharp edge against a bone structure or dural margin. They may appear isointense to the brain on T1W and T2W MRI scans, but gadolinium enhancement is the norm. On T2W images, hyperintensity indicates a meningothelial meningioma, a vascular meningioma, or an aggressive meningioma, all of which have a higher water content. It does, however, point to a tumour that may be removed with ease during surgery. After receiving a contrast agent, the dura mater next to a meningioma's connection may seem enhanced on a CT or MRI scan (Figures 11 and 12). Histological analysis conducted on these alleged dural tails found meningioma cell nests, despite some cases only exhibiting connective tissue and vascular tissue development (Nakau et al. 1997).

DSAs (digital subtraction angiograms) are another tool used in diagnosis. The tumour contrast blush comes early (in the arterial phase), persists late (beyond the venous phase), and is quite thick. Usually, the external carotid artery serves as a feeder for meningiomas. Venograms are only performed to evaluate the dural venous sinuses when treating a parasagittal meningioma, and angiograms are only performed when preoperative embolization would be advantageous (Alalade and Kitchen 2018).

4.1.3. Treatment Considerations

In meningioma surgery, Simpson grading is used to level the extent of excision.

Simpson grading (Simpson 1957) is as follows:

Grade 1—macroscopically complete tumour resection with excision of involved dura and bone.
Grade 2—macroscopically complete tumour removal with coagulation of involved dura only.
Grade 3—macroscopically complete tumour removal without removal of involved dura and bone.
Grade 4—subtotal tumour resection.
Grade 5—decompression with or without biopsy.

Complete surgical resection is the only effective form of management for meningioma (Figures 13–16). Less likelihood of recurrence exists with more thorough excision. Simpson established a five-grade system for categorizing meningioma surgery in 1957. The recurrence rate for grade 1 is about 10%, while it is twice as high for grade 2. It is understandable that the rates of recurrence are higher in the higher Simpson grades. Grade 0 removal is defined as the addition of a 2 cm dural margin.

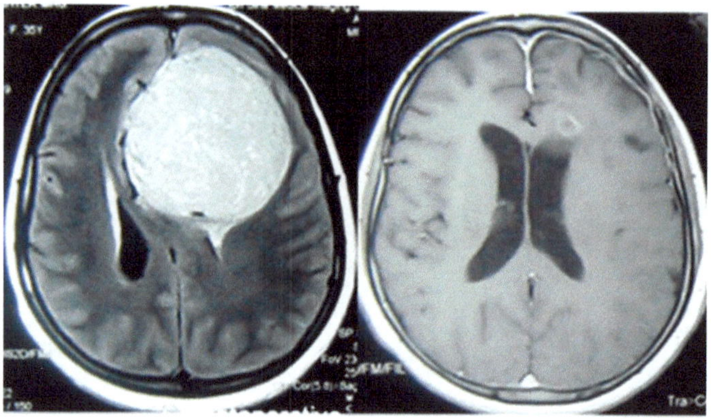

Figure 13. Contrast MRI of brain axial sections; left side shows huge preoperative anterior falcine meningioma and right side shows postoperative complete excision of meningioma. Source: Figure by authors.

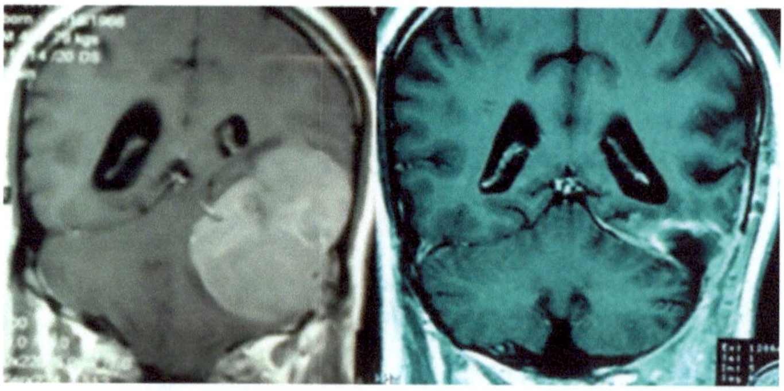

Figure 14. Contrast MRI of brain coronal sections; left side shows huge preoperative tentorial meningioma and right side shows postoperative complete excision of meningioma. Source: Figure by authors.

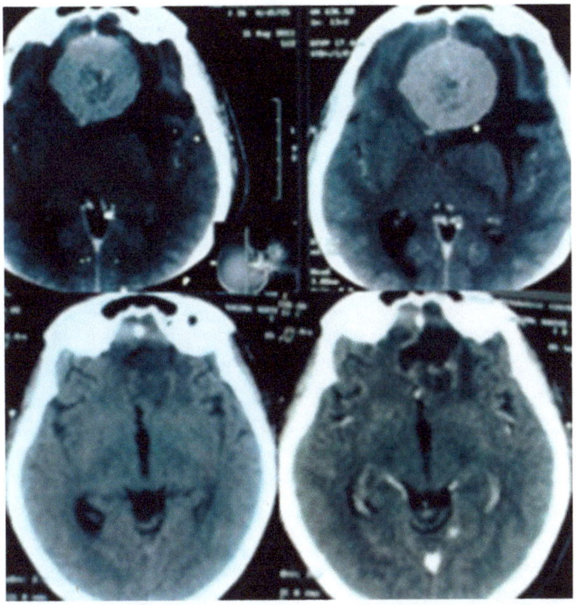

Figure 15. Contrast CT scan of brain axial sections; upper row shows preoperative olfactory groove meningioma, and lower row shows postoperative complete excision of meningioma. Source: Figure by authors.

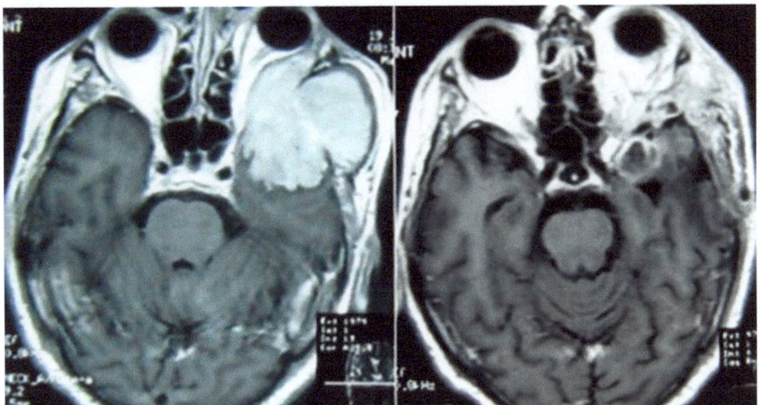

Figure 16. Contrast MRI of brain axial sections; left side shows huge preoperative anaplastic sphenoidal wing meningioma, and right side shows postoperative complete excision of meningioma. Source: Figure by authors.

While surgical resection is the preferred course of treatment, radiation therapy (Figure 16) should be taken into consideration in the following situations: (1) following surgery for a malignant meningioma; (2) after incomplete excision of a meningioma for which the risk of excision of a later recurrence is judged to be excessive; (3) for patients with multiple recurrent neoplasms for whom the surgeon finds that repeat surgery will be very hazardous; and (4) as the only therapy in a patient with progressive symptoms (Guthrie et al. 1991).

Given the relative ease of access, Simpson grade 1 or even grade 0 resection should be conducted in convexity meningiomas. When the bone is involved, removal of the hyperostotic bone with a healthy margin and of the pericranium in an en bloc resection is recommended (Kinjo et al. 1993).

Parasagittal meningioma arises from the dura of the superior sagittal sinus (SSS). The superior sagittal sinus is often not involved in falcine meningioma, which develops from the falx and may be totally hidden by the overlying cortex (Cushing and Eisenhardt 1938).

The most crucial decision in the treatment of parasagittal and falcine meningiomas is selecting the best way to handle the affected sinus. In these situations, a very useful preoperative adjunct may be an MR venogram (Asari et al. 1995). The patient's age and symptoms, patency of the sinus, the site and side of the tumour, and the cerebral venous collateral system should all be taken into account while making decisions about the sinus in each situation (Birk et al. 2019). A sinus that is completely obstructed can be removed at any time. It is crucial for the procedure, and cannot be overstated how important it is, to maintain collateral venous pathways. It is possible to remove the front section of the sinus with or without a graft or replacement. After the tumour has been removed from the sinus, the infiltration of the tumour in one wall can mostly be healed. Early devascularization through interhemispheric exposure along the falx is recommended in falcine tumours when there is a unilateral tumour. To protect the pericallosal arteries in the inferior margin of the dissection and prevent damage to the surrounding cerebral cortex and pial tissue, larger tumours should first undergo central debulking, followed by microsurgical separation of the tumour capsule from the arachnoidal areas (Almefty et al. 2017).

The surgical removal of tentorial meningiomas is based on their specific location. The petrous apex with extension into the perimesencephalic region can be removed utilizing the anterior petrosal approach in malignancies affecting the anterior to midmedial incisural ring. For lesions spreading posteriorly into the lateral pontine region, this method can be used in conjunction with an anterior petrosectomy. The petrosal technique can be used to access lesions that affect the middle-to-posterior portion of the inner ring of the tentorium, as well as the petroclival area and extension into the perimesencephalic cistern (Almefty et al. 2017). A posterior interhemispheric transtentorial technique can be used to access falcotentorial lesions. A supracerebellar infratentorial technique can be used to address tumours at the falcotentorial junction, which are primarily infratentorial (Asari et al. 1995). The supra–infratentorial technique can be used to access larger tentorial leaf tumours with superior extension into the occipital lobe as well as inferior extension into the cerebellum (Sakaki et al. 1987).

For olfactory groove meningioma, a frontal transbasal approach with a supraorbital osteotomy or its modifications allows for the early control of its blood supply, which is predominantly from the anterior ethmoidal artery, and for the placement of a pericranial flap to repair the skull base after cranialization of the frontal sinus and drilling of the hyperostotic bone at its origin (Cusimano and Meier 2019). Tuberculum sellae and planum sphenoidale meningiomas that are small or extend into the sphenoid sinus with an absence of vascular encasement and do not extend laterally to the carotid may be considered for extended endoscopic endonasal approaches (Neil and Couldwell 2019). For others, the pterional approach allows the surgeon to deal with further extensions into the interpeduncular cistern and around the internal carotid artery, but it will likely involve a degree of manipulation of the ipsilateral optic nerve and the area medial to the nerve could be a blind spot. The anterior interhemispheric, rather than subfrontal, approach can preserve olfaction more readily and avoid manipulation of the optic nerves, but a retroclival extension, especially with a prefixed chiasm, is a blind spot (Nimmannitya et al. 2016).

Following extradural drilling of the sphenoid ridge, which also helps to devascularize the tumour, lateral sphenoid wing meningiomas can be removed. After extradural drilling of the sphenoid wing, meningiomas that develop from the middle part of the sphenoid wing are also removed. A cranio-orbital zygomatic craniotomy might be the most effective treatment for malignancies that affect the orbit and superior orbital fissure and progress toward the cavernous sinus (Almefty et al. 2017). The cranio-orbital zygomatic approach can also be used for the resection of clinoidal meningiomas. This offers the surgeon a low-based approach, numerous dissection options, little brain retraction, and, if necessary, the possibility to penetrate the cavernous sinus (Al-Mefty 1991). The larger sphenoid wing, anterior clinoid, superior and lateral orbital walls, and the afflicted dura are all completely removed during surgery for spheno-orbital meningiomas. After carefully repairing the dura with an autologous graft, a cranioplasty is performed for cosmetic purposes (Bikmaz et al. 2007).

According to the description, petroclival meningiomas develop from the top two-thirds of the clivus and from the medial to the trigeminal nerve, at the petroclival junction. Petroclival meningiomas may involve the cavernous sinus through the Meckel cave and cross the middle and posterior cerebral fossae. Sphenopetroclival meningiomas are the most severe ones and invade the sella turcica, sphenoid sinus, and/or cavernous sinus(es) (Alalade and Kitchen 2018). It is debatable which method should be used to remove petroclival meningiomas. Some surgeons like the retrosigmoid approach with the patient in the sitting position, citing its simplicity, while others favour petrosal techniques (Samii and Tatagiba 1992). The transpetrosal partial labyrinthectomy–petrous apicoectomy approach takes a much longer time to accomplish than the retrosigmoid approach. In these two approaches, the temporal lobe and cerebellum, respectively, are retracted. The transpetrosal approach permits a direct view of the tumour, whilst in the retrosigmoid approach, cranial nerve traction is extensive (Al-Mefty et al. 1988). A trans-zygomatic approach may be used when the tumour involves the upper clivus. Tumours involving the lower and mid-clivus are approached by a presigmoid approach, occasionally with division of the non-dominant sinus (Erkmen et al. 2005). Skull base reconstruction is a must in all approaches to prevent CSF leaks.

4.2. *Solitary Fibrous Tumour (Haemangiopericytomas)*

4.2.1. Clinical Considerations

Haemangiopericytomas–solitary fibrous tumours (HPC-SFTs) were once classified as meningiomas and haemangiopericytomas (HPCs). Since the 2013 edition of the WHO Classification of Tumours of Soft Tissue and Bone, HPCs and SFTs are considered one entity. The term HPC has been abandoned and both entities are now called SFTs (Fletcher et al. 2013). This is because they share the same NAB2-STAT6 fusion gene. Molecular studies on HPCs of the dura/meninges have detected similar genetic aberrations, and the most recent WHO Classification of Tumours of the CNS also considers haemangiopericytomas–solitary fibrous tumours as the same entity (Louis et al. 2016). HPCs are generally WHO grade 2 and grade 3. Although the ultimate diagnostic test is identifying the NAB2-STAT6 fusion gene, this is not practical as the first step. Instead, identification of nuclear staining of STAT6 using immunohistochemistry is a good surrogate test (Schweizer et al. 2013).

4.2.2. Investigative Considerations

On imaging tests, meningiomas and HPCs may look similar. A thin- or broad-based meningeal attachment is often visible on CT. On unenhanced CT images, the tumours typically appear hyperdense with focal areas of hypodensity, and after the administration of a contrast agent, they show areas of heterogeneous enhancement (Chiechi et al. 1996). More than 50% of haemangiopericytomas exhibit bone erosion. Hyperostosis is not a characteristic of these tumours (Sibtain et al. 2007). On T1- and T2-weighted MRI, haemangiopericytomas typically show large vascular flow voids and are isointense to grey matter. The most frequent appearance on T1-weighted gadolinium-enhanced images is heterogeneous enhancement (Chiechi et al. 1996). The dural tail sign is present in about half of the malignancies. If the diagnosis is of HPC, body staging is conducted, as the frequency of systemic metastases is high (25–50%) (Damodaran et al. 2014).

4.2.3. Treatment Considerations

The surgical excision of an HPC follows similar concepts as that of a meningioma. The main treatment for HPC is surgery, with a goal of a Simpson grade 1 gross total resection. This requires the removal of bone, dura, and, if necessary, brain or vascular structures, provided that doing so will not result in an unacceptable severe neurological loss. Every effort should be made to accomplish total removal during the initial resection, as surgery for recurrent tumour is usually more challenging and less effective. Due to the high vascularity of many HPCs, significant bleeding during surgery is the biggest potential challenge. After surgery, 60–75% of HPC cases return. At ages 5, 10, and 15, metastatic rates are 13%, 33%, and 64%, respectively, according to Guthrie and colleagues (Guthrie et al. 1989). Studies have shown that stereotactic radiosurgery can effectively cure recurrent or residual disease (Chang and Sakamoto 2003).

4.3. *Dermoids and Epidermoids*

4.3.1. Clinical Considerations

Dermoid and epidermoid cysts, also termed congenital ectodermal inclusion cysts, are commonly derived from retained surface ectoderm trapped by two fusing neuroectodermal surfaces during neural tube closure. Dermoid cysts have a tendency to occur near the midline. The most common intracranial sites are near the anterior fontanelle extradurally and in the sellar, parasellar, and intraventricular regions intradurally. The commonest intraspinal site is near the cauda equina; this localization can be linked to a dermal sinus tract and subsequent increased risk of bacterial infection. Dermoid cysts are composed of epithelial cell debris and keratin and also include elements of the dermis like hair follicles, sebaceous glands, and sweat glands. Epidermoid cysts are mainly intracranial and are found away from the midline. The commonest site is the cerebellopontine angle (40–50%), where they make up the third commonest lesion in adults after vestibular schwannomas and meningiomas. They are also found in the fourth ventricle, the sellar and parasellar regions, the cerebral hemispheres, and the brainstem. Epidermoid cysts are composed of only epithelial cell debris, including cholesterol and keratin, laid down in a lamellar pattern, with no dermal involvement. Compared to patients with epidermoids, patients with dermoid cysts typically present at a younger age. For dermoid cysts, the average age at presentation is 15 years, while it is 35 years for epidermoids, according to Gormley and colleagues (Gormley et al. 1994). In a study by Love and Kernohan, patients with dermoid tumours experienced symptoms for an average of 8.5 years, compared to those with epidermoid tumours, who experienced symptoms for an average of 16 years (Chowdhury et al. 2013; Love and Kernohan 1936). Symptoms and indicators vary depending on the site of the tumour. Extradural lesions often present as local masses with or without headache (Gormley et al. 1994). Due to their frequent parasellar position, intradural tumours are more frequently linked to headache, visual impairment, and, to a lesser extent, changes in the hypothalamus. While tumours near the cerebellopontine angle may result in ataxia, vertigo, or localized impairments in the cranial nerves, those in the middle fossa grow quite slowly and frequently exhibit no symptoms (Akar et al. 2003). Sometimes, a more acute presentation results from a cyst rupture, which causes the contents of the cyst to flow into the subarachnoid space and cause chemical meningitis. This should be distinguished from the septic meningitis seen in intraspinal dermoid cysts, caused by the presence of a dermal sinus tract. Cyst rupture can lead to several neurological sequelae, including headache, seizures, vasospasm, neurological deficit, and death (Chowdhury et al. 2013; Love and Kernohan 1936).

4.3.2. Investigative Considerations

In epidermoids, the subarachnoid space typically contains a homogeneous, non-enhancing, hypodense lesion without surrounding oedema. Arachnoid cysts are the most problematic cystic tumours, with craniopharyngioma, Rathke's cleft cyst, and other cystic tumours also included in the differential diagnosis. The preferred imaging method for identifying these lesions today is MRI (Figure 17a,b and Figure 18). The tumour signal typically exhibits hypointensity on T1W imaging and hyperintensity on T2W images and is heterogeneous (Kumari et al. 2009). On proton density investigations, a rim of strong signal intensity may be seen; some tumours exhibit rim enhancement after gadolinium injection. The previously described cystic entities are part of the differential diagnosis. On standard and spin echo MRI pulse sequences, it is challenging to distinguish between epidermoids and arachnoid cysts; however, DW, FLAIR, constructive interference in steady state, and fast imaging with steady state precession studies can frequently distinguish between epidermoid tumours (Figure 19) and CSF within arachnoid cysts (Hakyemez et al. 2005). On a CT scan, dermoids are often avascular and hypodense, and they do not exhibit contrast enhancement. Dermoid cysts can have a variable appearance on MRI, depending on the balance of their contents, which may include fat, hair, sebum, and teeth. They differ from lipomas in that they do not feature consistent fat densities on all sequences (Osborn and Preece 2006). Dermoid tumours tend to be more localized and exhibit a greater local mass effect than epidermoid tumours because they are often more solid than epidermoid tumours.

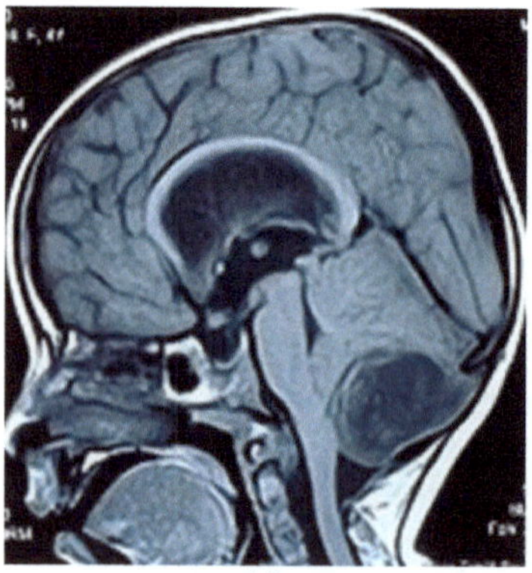

(a)

Figure 17. *Cont.*

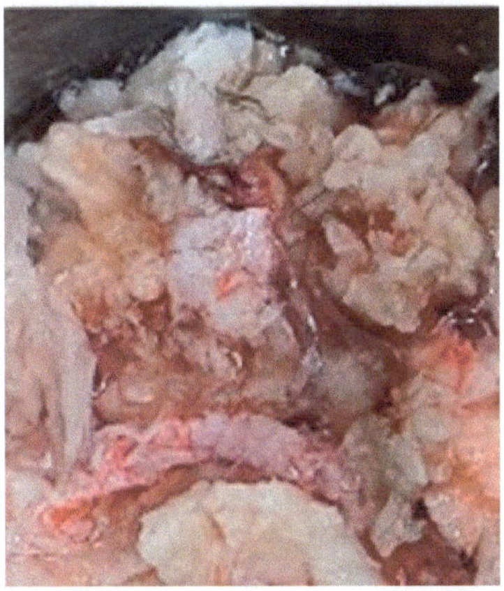

(b)

Figure 17. (**a**) Sagittal section of MRI of a child with a posterior fossa dermoid. (**b**) Typical content of dermoid found perioperatively in the patient in. Source: Figure by authors.

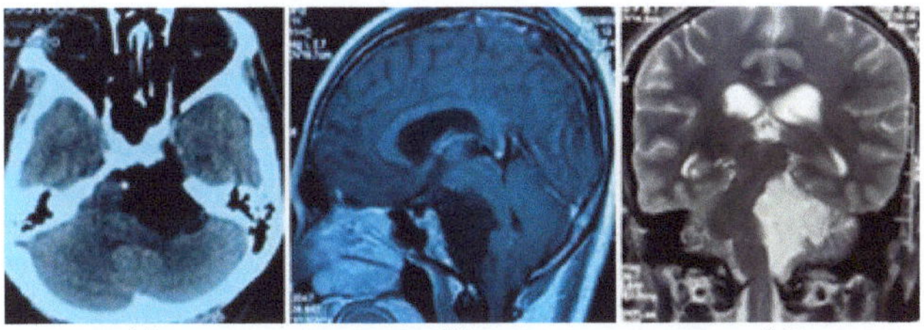

(a) (b) (c)

Figure 18. (**a**) Epidermoids are non-contrast-enhancing irregular isodense lesions along the CSF cisterns in CT images. (**b**,**c**) They also show the same intensity as the CSF in MR images, with DWI being the main differentiating sequence. Source: Figure by authors.

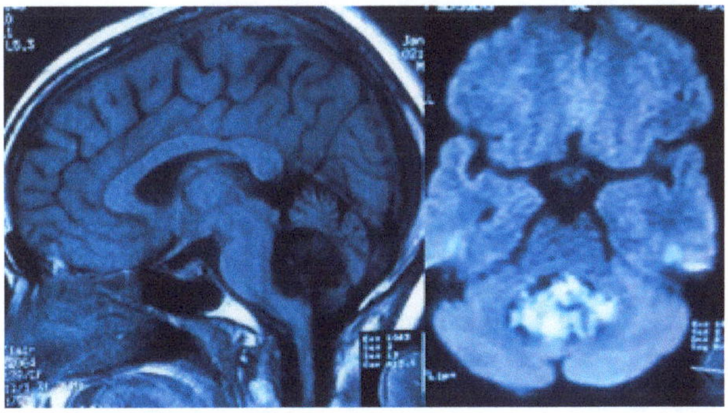

Figure 19. MRI of brain. (**left**) TW1 sagittal image; (**right**) DW axial image showing 4th ventricular epidermoid. Source: Figure by authors.

4.3.3. Treatment Considerations

The main aim of the operation should be the stark removal of the cyst, including the epithelial lining, to provide curative treatment and remove the risk of recurrence. However, surgery can be technically demanding on account of the deep, critical location of the tumours and their relationship to the surrounding neurovascular structures (Gormley et al. 1994). Independent of the surgical approach, resection can be technically demanding for several reasons. Tumour adhesion to adjacent structures on the skull base and also to the surrounding brain parenchyma is common. This is most pronounced with dermoid cysts, which tend to cause a greater granulomatous reaction with the arachnoid mater and occasionally the pia mater. On the other hand, cysts can extend between different anatomical compartments, which is more pronounced in epidermoid cysts (McEvoy 2019). These cysts contain characteristic pearly flakes (Figure 17) (Hassaneen and Sawaya 2017).

5. Sellar, Suprasellar, and Parasellar Tumours

5.1. Pituitary Tumours

5.1.1. Clinical Considerations

The sella turcica, in which the pituitary gland is located, is an intricate assembly of anatomical structures which include neural, endocrine, vascular, osseous, and meningeal tissues and which are in close relation to the cavernous sinus, hypothalamus, and major blood vessels. Lesions of the sella turcica are diverse and include neoplastic and non-neoplastic lesions. Pituitary adenomas are the most common lesions; these are usually benign tumours and comprise 10–12% of all intracranial tumours. Most of these tumours arise from the anterior pituitary, which comprises 80% of the gland's mass. Pituicytomas are tumours of the neurohypophysis. Both sexes are equally affected. Pituitary adenomas in children are about ten times less common than in adults, contributing to 2 to 6% of all intracranial tumours (Keil and Stratakis 2008). The majority of pituitary tumours are sporadic (95%). A small minority are familial (5%) and occur as either isolated lesions or as part of a familial genetic syndrome like multiple endocrine neoplasia (Vandeva et al. 2010; Marques and Korbonits 2017).

Pituitary tumours have a diversity of presentations, including endocrine syndrome, mass effect, incidental finding, pituitary apoplexy, CSF rhinorrhoea, and headache. Prolactin hypersecretion may occur due to prolactinoma or pituitary stalk syndrome. Growth hormone excess may produce acromegaly in adults and gigantism in prepubertal children. Excess corticotropin may produce Cushing's disease or Nelson syndrome in patients who undergo bilateral adrenalectomy. Thyrotropin excess may cause secondary hyperthyroidism, which is very rare, and FSH- and LH-secreting tumours usually do not result in any clinical syndrome.

The hyposecretion of pituitary hormones may cause pituitary cachexia or Simmond's cachexia. Growth hormone deficiency may cause growth delays in children and vague symptoms in adults. Hypogonadism may lead to amenorrhoea, loss of libido, and infertility. Mass effect is usually caused by non-functioning tumours. They may compress the optic nerve and may cause classical bitemporal hemianopia. Other field defects could be superior temporal quadrantonopia, monocular blindness, junctional scotoma, homonymous hemianopia, and central scotoma. Cavernous sinus compression may cause pressure on cranial nerves III, IV, V1, V2, and VI, as well as causing chemosis and proptosis.

Pituitary apoplexy is a condition where neurologic and/or endocrinologic deterioration occurs due to the sudden enlargement of a mass within the sella turcica due to haemorrhage, necrosis, or infarction of a pituitary adenoma. The patient may present with headache, visual disturbance, ophthalmoplegia, ptosis, Horner's syndrome, and alteration of consciousness level. Hypothalamic involvement may also produce hypotension, thermal dysregulation, cardiac dysrhythmia, respiratory pattern disturbance, altered mental state, and diabetes insipidus (DI). CT scan or MRI reveals a haemorrhagic mass. Urgent management includes endocrine evaluation, rapid administration of corticosteroids, and rapid decompression by surgery.

Prolactinoma is the most common tumour among functioning tumours. It may cause amenorrhoea–galactorrhoea syndrome in female patients and impotence and decrease libido in male patients, as well as infertility and bone loss in both sexes. The most common tumours in the posterior pituitary are metastases, and granular cell tumours are the most common tumours of the neurohypophysis.

5.1.2. Investigative Considerations

For the assessment of a pituitary tumour, it is essential to evaluate the levels of all anterior pituitary hormones, like growth hormone, prolactin, ACTH, TSH, LH, and FSH. It is also important to assess morning and evening cortisol levels, insulin-like growth factor 1 and blood sugar levels, and HbA1c and testosterone levels. Formal visual assessment gives details of visual impairment, which are particularly important for macroadenoma. Acromegaly patients may have high growth hormone as well as insulin-like growth factor 1 levels. Cushing's syndrome patients may have hyperglycaemia, loss of diurnal variation in cortisol level, hypokalaemic alkalosis, increased 24-h urine free cortisol, and a positive dexamethasone suppression test.

A plain X-ray of the skull gives little information about pituitary tumours, but is sometimes required for documentation; in acromegaly patients especially, X-ray of the skull, hands, and feet is required. CT scan of the brain with contrast gives information regarding tumour details, contrast enhancement, micro- or macroadenoma, haemorrhage, and calcification. MRI of the brain is the diagnostic investigation of choice and gives the complete picture of tumour details (Figure 20).

On T1WI, the posterior pituitary shows high signal, also referred to as the "bright spot". Tumours are usually hypointense in T1WI and hyperintense in T2 WI. Sometimes, a cerebral angiogram is required to see the carotid encasement. Dynamic MR imaging relies upon the altered contrast enhancement of pituitary microadenomas in relation to the normal gland. Tumours usually enhance at a later time point compared to the normal gland. This timing correlates with tumour size, vascularity, integrity of the blood–brain barrier, and also physical consistency (Kanou et al. 2002). Inferior petrosal sinus sampling (IPSS) is a useful test in determining the site of ACTH overproduction in Cushing's disease (Deipolyi et al. 2011).

Pituitary tumours are graded as microadenoma (diameter less than 1 cm) and macroadenoma (diameter more than 1 cm). Some pituitary adenomas that do not breach the sellar floor are classified as non-invasive and those that breach it are invasive adenomas (Table 2) (Hardy and Vezina 1976).

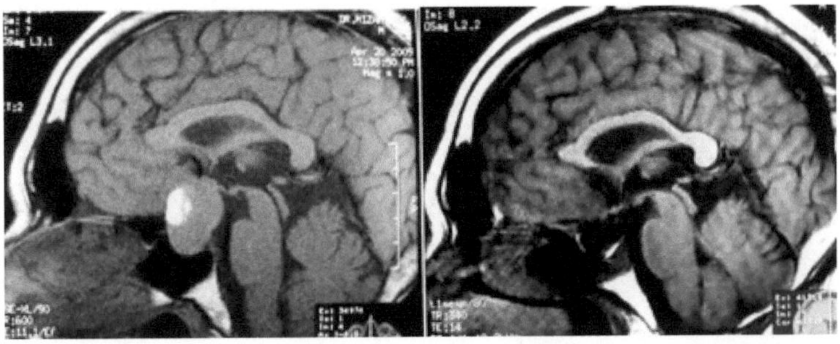

Figure 20. Non-functioning macroadenomas usually present with visual symptoms due to their suprasellar extension. MRI of brain sagittal sections in TW1. (**left**) preoperative image showing pituitary macroadenoma; (**right**) postoperative image showing excision of tumour. Source: Figure by authors.

Table 2. Description of the Hardy and Vezina classification.

Grade/Type	Description
	Hardy classification grade
	Sellar invasion
Grade 0	The enclosed adenoma is described as a tumour that remains within the anatomical confines of the osteoaponeural sheath of the sella turcica. The floor of the sella is always intact.
Grade 1	The sella turcica is within normal limits in size (less than 16×13 mm; 208 mm^2) but shows a lowering of the floor on one side or a bulging of the cortex.
Grade 2	The sella turcica is enlarged to various degrees but the floor remains intact.
Grade 3	The sella is more or less enlarged but there is a local erosion or destruction of the floor.
Grade 4	The entire floor of the sella is diffusely eroded or destroyed, producing a characteristic "phantom sella" with all the boundaries barely visible.
	Suprasellar extension
Type A	The suprasellar expansion bulges into the chiasmatic cistern but does not reach the floor of the anterior third ventricle.
Type B	The tumour reaches the floor of the third ventricle, producing the image of an inverse cupula of the anterior recesses of the third ventricle.
Type C	A voluminous suprasellar expansion bulges largely into the third ventricle up to the foramen of Monro.
Type D	Rare aberrant expansions occur in temporal or frontal fossa.

Source: Authors' compilation based on data from Hardy and Vezina (1976).

One of the most often used methods to assess the risk of pituitary macroadenomas invading the cavernous sinus is the Knosp classification. The Knosp classification primarily assesses the extent of the tumour extending across into the cavernous sinus, with a focus on its relation to the cavernous carotid (Knosp et al. 1993).

Predicting residual tumour after resection and operational planning benefit from the Knosp classification, which stratifies the probability of cavernous sinus invasion. Following resection, low Knosp grades are linked to a noticeably higher likelihood of surgical remission.

Knosp Classification

Three lines (Knosp et al. 1993) are drawn between the supraclinoid internal carotid artery and intracavernous internal carotid artery on coronal MR images (Figure 21).

1. Medial tangent;
2. Intercarotid line;
3. Lateral tangent.

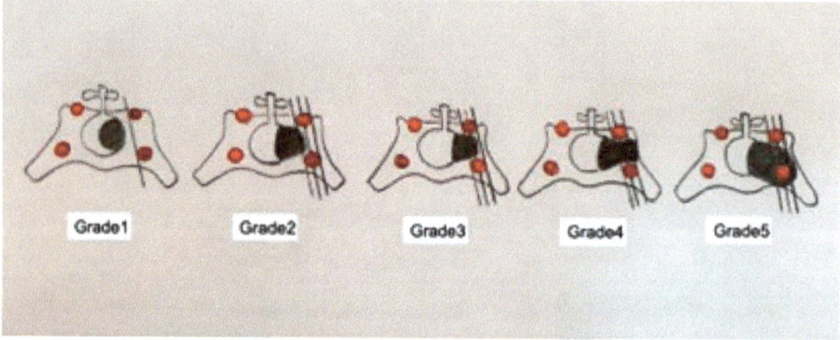

Figure 21. Schematic presentation of Knosp grading of pituitary tumours. Source: Figure by authors; courtesy of Dr. Hafiz Asif Raihan, Neurosurgeon, National Institute of Neurosciences and hospital, Dhaka.

These lines are used to define four grades of tumour invasion:

Grade 0: tumour remains medial to the medial tangent;
Grade 1: tumour extends to between the medial tangent and the intercarotid line;
Grade 2: tumour extends to between the intercarotid line and the lateral tangent;
Grade 3: tumour extends lateral to the lateral tangent;
Grade 3A: tumour extends above the intracavernous internal carotid artery into the superior cavernous sinus compartment.

5.1.3. Treatment Considerations

The principal management of pituitary tumours is both medical and surgical. The only pituitary tumour for which medicinal therapy is the major mode of treatment is prolactinoma. The usual drugs are bromocriptine, cabergoline, and pergolide. Indications for the surgical resection of prolactinoma include drug resistance and intolerance, prolactinoma with cerebrospinal fluid (CSF) leak, acute onset of severe visual or neurological symptoms, or pituitary tumour apoplexy. For acromegaly patients, there are some options for medical treatment with dopamine agonists, somatostatin analogues, and GH antagonists.

The surgical approach could be trans-sphenoidal or transcranial.

The trans-sphenoidal approach could be sublabial or endonasal. Endonasal endoscopy is a versatile approach to deal with pituitary tumours. In endoscopy, there is no external scar and no brain retraction; it is an extra-arachnoid approach and provides a direct landing to the tumour. However, a few complications, like electrolyte imbalance or CSF leak, may occur with this approach.

The transcranial approach still plays an important role in giant and complex pituitary adenomas with wide intracranial extension, brain parenchymal involvement, and the encasement of neurovascular structures. Conventional indications for transcranial approaches include the following:

- Absent pneumatization of the sphenoid sinus;
- Ectatic/kissing internal carotid arteries;

- Reduced dimensions of the sella;
- Lateral involvement of the cavernous sinus lateral to the internal carotid artery;
- Dumbbell-shaped tumours caused by sharp diaphragmatic constriction;
- Calcified/fibrous tumour consistency;
- Wide supra-, para-, and retrosellar extension;
- Arterial encasement;
- Brain invasion;
- Co-existing cerebral aneurysms;
- Separate coexisting pathologies of the sphenoid sinus, especially infections.

Residual/recurrent tumours and postoperative pituitary apoplexy after trans-sphenoidal surgery require individualized considerations (Luzzi et al. 2023).

Radiotherapy is mainly used as an adjuvant therapy to reduce tumour growth in the postsurgical residuum when it cannot be removed safely. Chemotherapy is rarely used in pituitary tumours, except as a salvage treatment for very aggressive pituitary adenomas where other treatment modalities have been exhausted. Oral temozolamide has been used in this regard, with favourable response (Syro et al. 2011).

Acromegaly

Acromegaly is a rare condition brought on by an overabundance of growth hormone (GH), usually as a result of an anterior pituitary adenoma. Insulin-like growth factor 1 (IGF-1) is produced as a result, which leads to the typical proliferation of some tissues. This causes the hands and feet to enlarge, the facial features to coarsen, and it also affects several bodily systems. Acromegaly has three main causes: excess growth hormone-releasing hormone (GHRH), ectopic or iatrogenic GH excess, and primary GH excess (Adigun et al. 2023).

A somatotroph GH-secreting adenoma of the anterior pituitary gland is the most common cause of acromegaly. Additionally, GH excess can be ectopic and generated by cancers other than pancreatic islet cell tumours and lymphomas. Excessive GH administration can potentially lead to iatrogenic GH overload. More rarely, the causes of acromegaly are associated with high GHRH. These can be separated into two categories: core and peripheral causes. Choristomas, ganglioneuromas, and hypothalamic hamartomas are examples of central causes. Adrenal adenoma, small-cell lung carcinoma, and bronchial carcinoid tumours are examples of peripheral causes that release GHRH (Adigun et al. 2023).

The clinical features of acromegaly include joint pain, wrist pain, snoring and sleep apnoea, headaches and visual disturbances, erectile dysfunction or low sex drive, abnormal menses in women, sweaty palms and soles (hyperhidrosis), deepening of the voice, coarse facial features, prominent forehead, prominent brow, prognathism (mandibular enlargement), prominent forehead crease and nasolabial folds, macroglossia and widely spaced dentition, thick eyelids, large nose, acral enlargement (i.e., large hands (with stubby fingers) and feet), proximal myopathy, carpal tunnel syndrome, acromegalic cardiomyopathy, dorsal kyphosis, systemic hypertension, and diabetes mellitus (Adigun et al. 2023).

Serum IGF-1 is employed because, unlike serum GH, it is not affected by changes in sleep patterns, levels of exercise, or the time of day. Elevated IGF-1 levels validate GH excess, and the next step should be imaging to pinpoint the cause. A pituitary MRI is the preferred imaging modality. A CT scan is useful in operative planning. Control of diabetes and hypertension, perioperative airway management, and paying attention to myopathy and cardiomyopathy are very important (Adigun et al. 2023).

Surgery (trans-sphenoidal/transcranial) is the treatment of choice for all microadenomas and macroadenomas. Patients who do not want surgery, are too high risk for surgery, are not candidates for surgery because the tumour might not be resectable, and who have recurrent disease after initial surgical care but are not eligible for repeat surgery are taken into consideration for this. As previously mentioned, neoadjuvant medication therapy may potentially be beneficial prior to surgery. Somatostatin analogues (octreotide, Lanreotide, pasireotide) and GH-receptor antagonists (pegvisomant) are used for medical management. When medical therapy fails to control a patient's disease or there is a recurrence after surgery, radiotherapy (conventional/stereotactic) may be explored as a treatment option. It is imperative to properly follow patients receiving radiation therapy for hypopituitarism (Adigun et al. 2023).

Cushing's Disease

Increased anterior pituitary production of adrenocorticotropic hormone (ACTH) causes the adrenal glands to release too much cortisol, which is the hallmark of Cushing's syndrome, an endocrine disorder. This is frequently brought on by an adenoma of the pituitary gland or by the hypothalamus producing too much corticotropin-releasing hormone (CRH). Pituitary adenomas, which are frequently invisible on imaging tests, are almost always present in Cushing's disease patients. Still, even in the absence of ectopic release of corticotropin-releasing hormone (CRH), rare cases may arise from diffuse corticotroph cell hyperplasia. Microadenomas, which are less than 10 mm in size, make up the majority of these tumours; only 5–10% are macroadenomas (Kairys et al. 2023).

Menstrual irregularities, high blood pressure, diabetes mellitus, widespread weakness, and psychological disorders are among the disease's symptoms. Excess cortisol can be physically manifested as a moon face, buffalo hump, abdominal striae, easy bruising, obesity, facial plethora, and hirsutism. Individuals diagnosed with hypercortisolism typically have a 50% increase in body weight, acne, flushing, poor wound healing, lower limb oedema, fatigue, osteoporosis, myopathy, skin hyperpigmentation, mood and memory abnormalities, decreased sexual drive, or recurrent infections (Kairys et al. 2023).

Biochemical testing includes salivary and serum cortisol testing, 24-h urinary free cortisol testing, serum ACTH assay, and a low-dose overnight dexamethasone suppression test. If an ACTH-secreting tumour is present, a pituitary MRI may reveal it. Nonetheless, in 40% of Cushing's disease patients, MRI is unable to identify a tumour. Tumours visible on MRI have an average size of roughly 6 mm. Implicit petrosal sinus sampling is the most reliable diagnostic test for distinguishing between an adrenal or ectopic Cushing's syndrome and a pituitary tumour. This invasive technique quantifies the variation in ACTH levels between the periphery and the inferior petrosal sinus, which is where the pituitary gland drains (Kairys et al. 2023).

In the event that a primary ACTH-secreting tumour is discovered, trans-sphenoidal surgery is the initial line of treatment for the adenoma. Pituitary radiation therapy is an alternative that may be utilized following a failed trans-sphenoidal surgery. Finally, individuals with Cushing's disease may have an instant decrease in cortisol levels with bilateral adrenalectomy, but after that, they will need to take glucocorticoid and mineralocorticoid replacement medication for the rest of their lives. Nelson's syndrome is one of the main side effects of this treatment (Kairys et al. 2023).

5.2. *Craniopharyngioma*

5.2.1. Clinical Considerations

Craniopharyngioma is a rare tumour which is considered histologically benign but acts in a malignant way because of its close proximity to eloquent brain structures, unexpected biologic behaviour, and high local recurrence rate. It may result in significant endocrine, visual, and neurocognitive morbidity. Across all ages, it constitutes only around 1% of all new CNS tumours found per year, although this rises to 4% in the paediatric group of patients (Dolecek et al. 2012). There is a bimodal age distribution with two peaks, one in middle-to-late adulthood (45–65 years of age) and the other during school age (5–14 years). There is no sex-based preference. While adamantinomatous tumours can be found in both groups, the papillary form of a craniopharyngioma is typically observed in adults.

From an embryological point of view, craniopharyngiomas develop as a result of an improper or incomplete involution of the craniopharyngeal duct and Rathke's pouch, which results in nests of resting epithelial cells that later develop into neoplasms (Prabhu and Brown 2005; Senthilvel et al. 2014). In the mature adult pituitary gland, metaplasia is thought to give rise to papillary tumours.

Craniopharyngiomas and the circle of Willis and its branch are intimately related. The exact anatomical relationship with the optic nerve is very important when planning a surgical approach (Steno et al. 2004), whether normal (above the midpoint of the sella), prefixed (above the tuberculum sella), or postfixed (above the dorsum sella). It can be infradiaphragmatic or supradiaphragmatic (suprasellar extraventricular, intraventricular extraventricular, or purely intraventricular). Intraventricular extraventricular craniopharyngiomas are the most commonly encountered configuration (Steno et al. 2004). These are WHO grade 1 tumours.

According to gross pathologic examination, craniopharyngiomas can be categorized as cystic (50%), mixed cysto-solid (35%), and solid (15%). Secondary changes like fibrosis, calcification, ossification, and cholesterol deposits may occur (Fernandez-Miranda et al. 2012). Cysts are noted to have a brownish-coloured fluid often described as resembling machine oil. Calcification is frequently identified in these tumours.

The symptoms of a craniopharyngioma can be diverse due to the involvement of very important surrounding neurovascular structures. They can be visual (due to injury to or compression of the optic apparatus), endocrine (hypothalamic–pituitary axis), neurocognitive (hypothalamus, mammillary bodies, and associated limbic structures), and of obstructive hydrocephalus. Hydrocephalus and endocrinopathies are commoner in paediatric patients, and impaired vision and neurocognitive changes are commoner in adult patients.

Visual impairment can either be reduced acuity or visual field defects. The different patterns of field defects include bitemporal hemianopia, concentric field defect, homonymous hemianopia, and paracentral or central scotoma. Fundal examination may reveal papilloedema with hydrocephalus or optic atrophy with direct chasmal compression. Children may have stunted development or delayed puberty. Adults may experience amenorrhoea in women or a diminished libido in men due to erectile dysfunction. A thorough neuro-ophthalmologic and endocrine evaluation of the anterior and posterior pituitary gland is necessary at presentation. Obesity and diabetes insipidus resulting from antidiuretic hormone deficiency can also occur with these tumours. Children may have decreased school performance and have the classical triad of hypothyroidism, hypogonadism, and growth retardation (Fernandez-Miranda et al. 2012).

5.2.2. Investigative Considerations

Endocrinopathies can be fatal and significantly reduce a patient's quality of life. Growth hormone is the most often affected hormone in people with hypopituitarism, with 85% of patients affected presentation (Van Effenterre and Boch 2002). A plain X-ray of the skull reveals patchy or rim calcification, erosion of the dorsum sellae, a copper beaten appearance of the skull, and sutural diastasis due to raised intracranial pressure. A CT scan is useful to delineate tumour morphology, hydrocephalus, and calcification.

Craniopharyngiomas are usually lobulated, cystic suprasellar masses. Cyst contents may have increased density compared to the CSF. Calcification is around 85% to 90% in childhood and around 40% to 50% in adult tumours. One of the typical features is eggshell calcification. MRI of the brain gives a detailed view of the tumour, including compression of the optic nerve and of vascular structures, especially the internal carotid artery, and its relationship with delicate neural structures. On MRI, these tumours are usually heterogenous (Figure 22). Sometimes, an angiogram is required to see the vascular relationship before surgical exploration (Fernandez-Miranda et al. 2012).

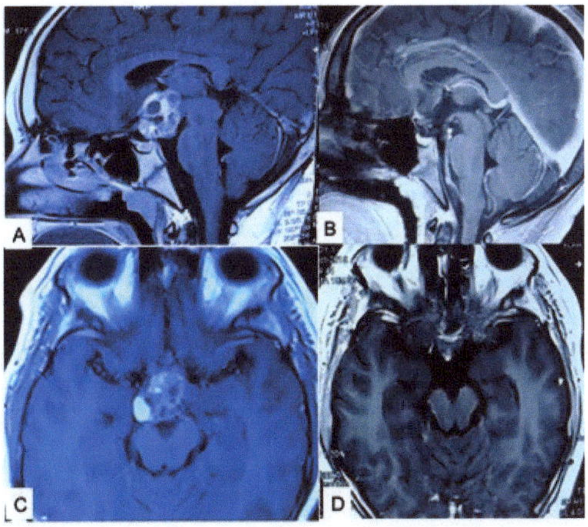

Figure 22. Contrast MRI of brain. (**A,C**) Preoperative craniopharyngiomas typically have both solid and cystic components, associated with calcifications. (**B,D**) Postoperative contrast MRI showing a very small portion of residual tumour adherent to the pituitary stalk. Source: Figure by authors.

5.2.3. Treatment Considerations

Before definitive surgical treatment, it is important to correct the endocrine and biochemical abnormalities. There are different surgical approaches, like transcranial and trans-sphenoidal. The surgical approach will differ based on the site and area of involvement of the tumour. An essential factor in choosing an approach is the stalk and optic chiasm's location with respect to the sella. The location of the chiasm can vary: it might be postfixed above the dorsum sellae, above the diaphragm or the middle of the sellae (normal), or above the tuberculum (prefixed) (Rhoton 2002). Subfrontal and/or trans-sylvian approaches can be employed to deal with these tumours in different craniotomies, like pterional, frontotemporal, or frontotemporal–orbito-zygomatic. The surgical corridors can be interoptic, optico-carotid, carotico-sylvian, or trans-lamina terminalis. The edonasal endoscopic trans-sphenoidal approach is a very good option to deal with infradiaphragmatic tumours. Sometimes, in cystic tumours, endoscopic cyst aspiration with the placement of an Ommaya reservoir can be used in order to aspirate the cyst from time to time in case of raised ICP. Intralesional bleomycin can also be given through this reservoir. Other treatment modalities include conventional radiotherapy, proton beam therapy, and stereotactic radiosurgery (SRS) (Fernandez-Miranda et al. 2012).

The prognosis of these tumours depends upon the maximal safe surgical resection and on the regular endocrine and biochemical assessment of the patients. Because of the critical anatomical location, no tumour should be forcibly pulled away from the optic nerve, vessels, or hypothalamus, and accepting a subtotal resection is often the safest option.

5.3. *Rathke's Cleft Cyst*

5.3.1. Clinical Considerations

Rathke's pouch is the region where the anterior and posterior pituitary glands converge. Normally, this pouch closes quite early in embryonic development. When a remnant enlarges into a cleft, it is known as Rathke's cleft cyst. It is a primary brain tumour that is extremely uncommon and often affects adults. Typically, it is a non-neoplastic lesion that is predominantly intrasellar and rarely suprasellar. A single layer of cuboidal epithelium lines it. This tumour may present as visual impairment and hypopituitarism. It can be asymptomatic or may present with headache and/or variable presentation due to compression of the hypothalamus, pituitary stack, pituitary gland, and optic chiasma (Naik and Thakore 2013).

5.3.2. Investigative Considerations

Thorough neuro-ophthalmic and endocrine evaluation is required. Both CT scan and MRI scan can reveal the cystic lesion. CT scans depict a discrete low-density intrasellar lesion which usually does not calcify. MRI reveals increased intensity on T1 WI in two-thirds of cases; this is variable on T2 WI. This lesion usually does not enhance on contrast but an enhancing rim may sometimes be seen (Naik and Thakore 2013).

5.3.3. Treatment Considerations

The cystic fluid may resemble motor oil. Surgery for this cystic lesion includes draining the fluid from the cyst. Most neurosurgeons now prefer the minimally invasive endoscopic approach, which minimizes complications, hospitalization time, and discomfort.

6. Pineal Tumours

6.1. *Clinical Considerations*

The pineal region is surrounded by the tentorial apex from the back, by the culmen of the cerebellar vermis from below, by the splenium of the corpus callosum from above, and by the third ventricle, quadrigeminal plate, and midbrain tectum from the front. The great cerebral vein of Galen, which is created by the union of the internal cerebral veins above the pineal gland and the basal vein of Rosenthal that emerges laterally from the ambient cisterns, is one of a number of crucially significant venous systems that converge in the pineal area.

The pineal area is prone to both neoplastic and non-neoplastic tumour development. Pineal tumours, 60% of which are germ cell tumours, comprise germinoma, mature teratoma, and immature teratoma with malignant transformation; they also include embryonal carcinoma, yolk sac tumours, and choriocarcinoma. Pineocytoma, pineal parenchymal neoplasms of intermediate differentiation, pineoblastoma, and papillary tumours of the pineal area are tumours originating from glandular tissue. Astrocytoma, ependymoma, glioma, choroid plexus papilloma, meningioma, haemangioma, chemodectoma, and metastases are examples of other tumours (Al-Hussaini et al. 2009). Arachnoid cysts, cysticercoses, arteriovenous malformations, cavernomas, and vein of Galen malformations are non-neoplastic abnormalities of this area. Tumours of the pineal region affect children more frequently than adults. While meningioma and glioma predominate in adults, germinoma or astrocytoma are the commonest tumour types in children.

The symptoms of raised intracranial pressure, cerebellar signs, hydrocephalus, and local compression of the dorsal midbrain are those most frequently associated with pineal region tumours (Konovalov and Pitskhelauri 2003). The typical symptoms of these tumours include headache, nausea, Parinaud syndrome, and double vision. Compression of the posterior commissure and of the rostral interstitial nucleus of the medial longitudinal fasciculus results in Parinaud syndrome (dorsal midbrain syndrome). Upgaze paralysis, convergence–retraction nystagmus induced by a quick upward gaze, pseudo-Argyll Robertson pupils, retraction of the eyelids (Collier's sign), and, occasionally, a conjugate downward look at baseline (i.e., setting sun sign) are the symptoms of this syndrome. The patient may also exhibit extrapyramidal movement disorder, precocious puberty, hypothalamic dysfunction, DI, thalamic pain, and endocrine instability. Pineal cell tumours, ependymoma, and germ cell tumours metastasize quickly in the CSF (drop metastasis).

6.2. *Investigative Considerations*

For germ cell tumours, tumour markers can occasionally be employed as diagnostic as well as prognostic tools. Increased levels of AFP are often linked to yolk sac tumours, but high levels of β-HCG are classically linked to choriocarcinoma (moderate rise in germinoma and embryonal carcinoma; mild elevation in teratoma and embryonal carcinoma). A higher level of placental alkaline phosphatase is also observed in germinoma, yolk sac tumours, and choriocarcinoma. A worse prognosis is linked to higher serum tumour marker levels.

For diagnosis, CT scan and MRI (Figure 23a,b) can delineate the tumour details, hydrocephalus, and compression of surrounding structures. To evaluate drop metastasis, MRI of the cervical, thoracic, and lumbar spine is occasionally performed. The major purpose of tumour markers is to determine the prognosis.

Pure germinomas comprise 55–65% of all intracranial germ cell tumours and are identified synchronously in both the pineal gland and in the suprasellar region in 10% of cases (Matula 2012; Raiyawa et al. 2012). Here, alpha-fetoprotein (AFP) in the CSF as a tumour marker, lumbar puncture, and stereotactic biopsy can be used as diagnostic tools, and radio-chemotherapy is used as the standard of care, as these lesions are very sensitive to both radiation and chemotherapy.

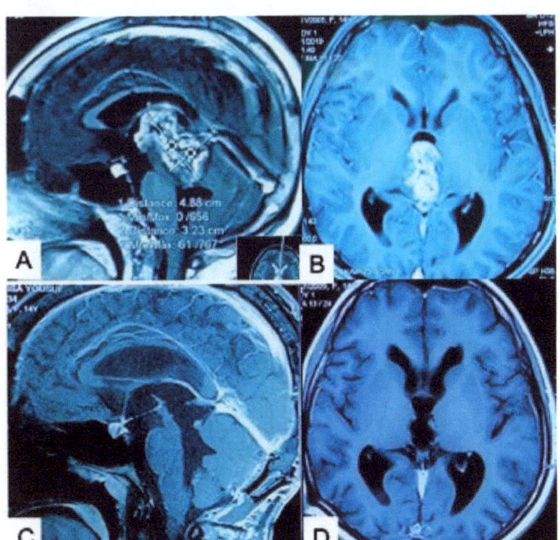

(a)

Figure 23. *Cont.*

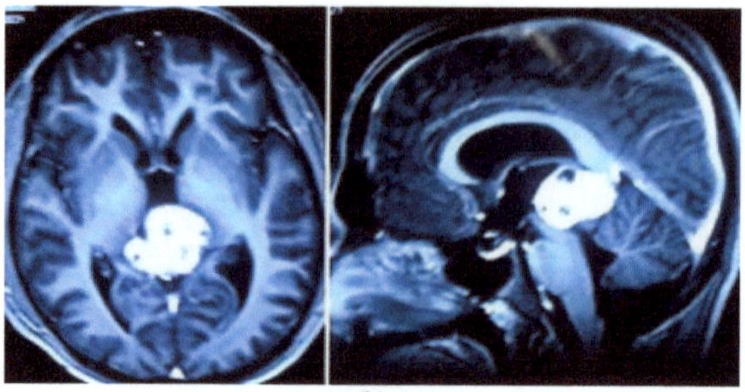

(b)

Figure 23. (**a**) Contrast MRI of brain showing preoperative (**A**,**B**) and postoperative (**C**,**D**) images of pineal and posterior 3rd ventricular grade 2 ependymoma. (**b**) Contrast MRI of brain; axial and sagittal view showing pineal immature teratoma in a 15-year-old boy. Source: Figure by authors.

6.3. Treatment Considerations

The most emergency triage or urgent approach is to place an external ventricular drainage. The standard approach in some institutions is a simultaneous endoscopic pineal tumour biopsy and an endoscopic third ventriculostomy, particularly for radio- and chemosensitive tumours like germinoma. Alternatively, some neurosurgeons insert a preoperative ventriculoperitoneal shunt first and plan for a definitive surgery once the acute condition is resolved. Some surgeons insert a shunt between the third ventricle and the cisterna magna after tumour excision (Figure 24).

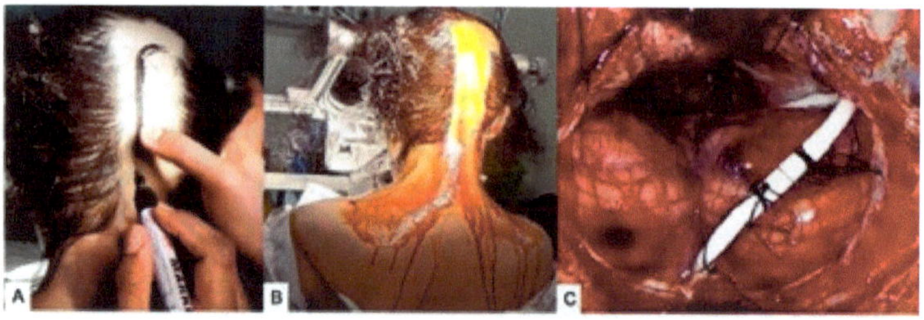

Figure 24. Intraoperative pictures: (**A**,**B**) Sitting position and incision mark for supracerebellar infratentorial approach to pineal tumour. (**C**) Intraoperative insertion of 3rd ventriculo-cisternal (cisterna magna) shunt after tumour removal. Source: Figure by authors.

In 1931, Oppenheim and Krause became the pioneers in the surgical removal of a pineal region tumour via a supracerebellar infratentorial approach (Oppenheim and Krause 1913). Dandy reported the first GTR with the interhemispheric transcallosal approach. Van Wagenen (Van Wagenen 1931) described a transcortical transventricular approach in 1931. Poppen described the occipital transtentorial approach. The anterior transchoroidal approach is preferred when the pineal tumour has spread into the anterior third ventricle.

7. Intraventricular Tumours

7.1. Clinical Considerations

According to the US Central Brain Tumour Registry, about 1.2% of primary brain tumours are intraventricular in location. They represent a diverse group of tumours of variable histopathology, but most are low-grade tumours. They can be confined to one ventricle or can extend into an adjacent ventricle or into an adjacent cistern through the outflow foramina. Large tumours can extend into the parenchyma through the ependymal wall (Ostrom et al. 2013; Louis et al. 2016).

Some of the most common tumours arising from the lateral ventricles are ependymomas, subependymal giant-cell astrocytomas, subependymomas, central neurocytomas, astrocytomas, meningiomas, lymphomas, and choroid plexus tumours. Among third ventricular tumours, colloid cysts, choroid plexus papillomas and carcinomas, meningiomas, craniopharyngiomas, and germ cell tumours are common. Ependymomas and subependymomas are fourth ventricular tumours. Medulloblastomas are usually vermian tumours but frequently present as large tumours within the cerebellar hemispheres. Large, intraparenchymal, high-grade astrocytic tumours can become exophytic into the lateral ventricles and may obliterate the foramen of Monro or cut off the posterior lateral ventricle and cause obstructive hydrocephalus.

Central neurocytomas originate from precursors of neuronal cells that exist within the septum pellucidum. They have a wide attachment on the septum pellucidum and can grow to a significant size within the lateral ventricles and third ventricle through the foramen of Monro. They are well circumscribed, can be lobulated, contain cysts and heterogenous signal and flow voids, and can contain calcification.

Subependymomas are well-circumscribed non-enhancing benign tumours most frequently seen in the ventricle. Surgical resection is indicated if they become symptomatic or progressive on imaging. Subependymal giant-cell astrocytomas are tumours of mixed and neuronal differentiation arising from subependymal nodules and are common in patients with tuberous sclerosis. Ependymomas in adults are more frequent in the fourth ventricle but they can also be seen within the lateral ventricles. They are also the most common intramedullary spinal cord tumours. They are well-circumscribed tumours that enhance and frequently contain calcifications.

Meningiomas are the commonest intraventricular tumours in the trigone of the lateral ventricle. They presumably originate from arachnoid cap cells trapped within the choroid plexus during embryonal life. They may reach a large size and cause symptoms suggestive of high intracranial pressure, but they can be also incidental. Treatment options include surgery, SRS, and surveillance.

Choroid plexus tumours arise from the choroid plexus and are most commonly located in the lateral ventricle in children and the fourth ventricle in adults. Histologically, they can be choroid plexus papillomas (WHO grade 1), atypical choroid plexus papillomas (WHO grade 2), and choroid plexus carcinomas (WHO grade 3). They tend to present with hydrocephalus both due to increased CSF production and due to obstruction.

Colloid cysts are the commonest third ventricular tumours. They are benign lesions consisting of epithelial-lined cysts filled with gel-density material which contains mucin, cholesterol, and hyaloid substances. They can be diagnosed as an incidental finding or present with acute, intermittent, or chronic obstructive hydrocephalus. Sudden death is rare but has been reported. Surgical options include open surgery via a transcortical or transcallosal approach, endoscopic excision, or frameless stereotactic aspiration.

The extension of a sellar mass into the third ventricle may produce visual field disturbances and hormone disturbances on endocrine profile. Suprasellar tumours extending into the ventricles include craniopharyngioma, germinoma, meningioma, and optic pathway and hypothalamic glioma. Common posterior third ventricular tumours include pineal region tumours, meningiomas, arachnoid cysts, and dermoid cysts.

Medulloblastomas originate from the cerebellar vermis and most commonly occur in the paediatric population. They usually present with acute hydrocephalus. The 2016 WHO CNS tumour classification provides a very useful presentation of the usual combinations of the well-established histological subtypes of these tumours (desmoplastic/nodular, medulloblastoma with extensive nodularity, large-cell, and anaplastic) and of the four currently established genetic subtypes (WNT-activated, SHH-activated, group 3 subtype, and group 4 subtype). At the time of presentation, a significant percentage of patients already have secondary deposits in the spine.

The presentation of intraventricular tumours depends on their location, size, and progression rate. Rapid progression can cause acute hydrocephalus that requires CSF diversion before the definite management of the tumour. Slow-growing tumours are asymptomatic for a long time before they become symptomatic and usually present with a chronic, NPH-like clinical picture. Apart from diagnostic imaging, preoperative imaging of the whole craniospinal axis and CSF sampling are indicated for tumours with known potential for CSF dissemination. Head CT and MRI of the head with contrast are needed for diagnosis, evaluation of anatomical details, and surgical planning (Figure 25) (Ostrom et al. 2013; Louis et al. 2016).

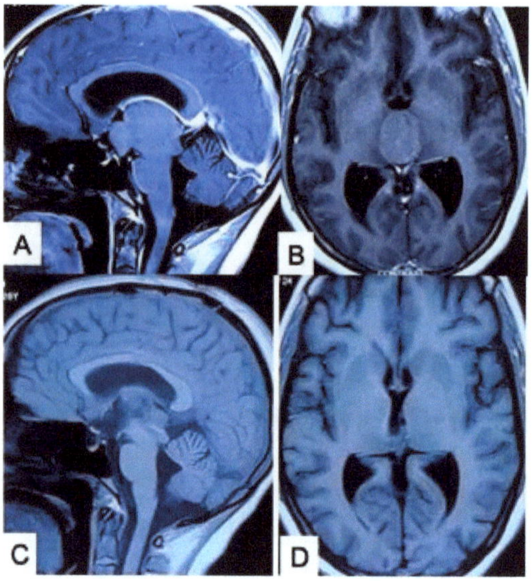

Figure 25. MRI of brain. (**A**,**B**) T1-weighted contrast-enhanced preoperative images showing non-contrast-enhancing 3rd ventricular grade 1 glioma. (**C**,**D**) Postoperative images showing removal of tumour via interhemispheric transcallosal transchoroidal approach. Source: Figure by authors.

7.2. Treatment Considerations

The management of hydrocephalus is the first consideration. For third ventricular tumours, neuro-endoscopy can obtain both CSF diversion (ETV+/- septostomy) and a biopsy. CSF diversion should be carried out first as the biopsy can cause bleeding from the tumour, causing reduced visibility. Conservative management with serial imaging follow-up may be the best option if the patient is asymptomatic, the tumour is not growing, or the patient is not fit for surgery. For older and unfit patients and when the tumour is considered low-grade with an indolent clinical course, CSF diversion alone may be the best alternative. The surgical approach for tumour resection depends on the specific site and extension of the tumour (Ostrom et al. 2013; Louis et al. 2016).

Author Contributions: Conceptualization, methodology, validation, formal analysis, investigation, resources, data curation, M.R.H., R.A.K. and S.I.M.K.N.K.; writing—original draft preparation, M.R.H. and R.A.K.; writing—review and editing, visualization, supervision, F.H.C. All authors have read and agreed to the published version of the manuscript.

Funding: This research received no external funding.

Conflicts of Interest: The authors declare no conflicts of interest.

References

Adigun, Oluwaseun O., Minhthao Nguyen, Tamaryn J. Fox, and Catherine Anastasopoulou. 2023. Acromegaly. In *StatPearls [Internet]*; Treasure Island: StatPearls Publishing. Available online: https://www.ncbi.nlm.nih.gov/books/NBK431086/ (accessed on 2 February 2023).

Akar, Ziya, Necmettin Tanriover, Saffet Tuzgen, Ali M. Kafadar, and Cengiz Kuday. 2003. Surgical treatment of intracranial epidermoid tumors. *Neurologia Medico-Chirurgica* 43: 275–80. [CrossRef] [PubMed]

Alalade, Andrew Folusho, and Neil D. Kitchen. 2018. Convexity and Parasagittal Versus Skull Base Meningiomas. In *Principles of Neurological Surgery*. Edited by R. G. Ellenbogen, L. N. Shekhar and N. D. Kitchen. Philadelphia: Elsevier, pp. 593–601.

Albert, Friedrich K., Michael Forsting, Klaus Sartor, Hans-Peter Adams, and Stefan Kunze. 1994. Early postoperative magnetic resonance imaging after resection of malignant glioma: Objective evaluation of residual tumor and its influence on regrowth and prognosis. *Neurosurgery* 34: 45–60. [CrossRef] [PubMed]

Al-Hussaini, Maysa, Iyad Sultan, Najyah Abuirmileh, Imad Jaradat, and Ibrahim Qaddoumi. 2009. Pineal gland tumours: Experience from the SEER database. *Journal of Neuro-Oncology* 94: 351–58. [CrossRef] [PubMed]

Al-Mefty, Ossama. 1991. Clinoidal meningiomas. In *Meningiomas*. Edited by Ossama Al-Mefty. New York: Raven Press, pp. 427–43.

Al-Mefty, Ossama, John L. Fox, and Robert R. Smith. 1988. Petrosal approach for petroclival meningiomas. *Neurosurgery* 22: 510–17. [CrossRef]

Almefty, R., G. F. Haddad, and O. Al-Mefty. 2017. Meningiomas. In *Youmans & Winn Neurological Surgery*. Edited by H. R. Winn. Philadelphia: Elsevier, pp. 1107–33.

Ang, Celina, David Hauerstock, Marie-Christine Guiot, Goulnar Kasymjanova, David Roberge, Petr Kavan, and Thierry Muanza. 2008. Characteristics and outcomes of medulloblastoma in adults. *Pediatric Blood & Cancer* 51: 603–607. [CrossRef]

Asari, Shoji, Tomohide Maeshiro, Susumu Tomita, Masamitsu Kawauchi, Nobuyoshi Yabuno, Kazushi Kinugasa, and Takashi Ohmoto. 1995. Meningiomas arising from the falcotentorial junction: Clinical features, neuroimaging studies, and surgical treatment. *Journal of Neurosurgery* 82: 726–38. [CrossRef]

Belykh, Evgenii, Kurt V. Shaffer, Chaoqun Lin, Vadim A. Byvaltsev, Mark C. Preul, and Lukui Chen. 2020. Blood-Brain Barrier, Blood-Brain Tumor Barrier, and Fluorescence- Guided Neurosurgical Oncology: Delivering Optical Labels to Brain Tumors. *Frontiers in Oncology* 10: 739. [CrossRef]

Bikmaz, Kerem, Robert Mrak, and Ossama Al-Mefty. 2007. Management of bone-invasive, hyperostotic sphenoid wing meningiomas. *Journal of Neurosurgery* 107: 905–12. [CrossRef]

Birk, Harjus S., Seunggu J. Han, Ramez W. Kirollos, Thomas Santarius, and Michael W. McDermott. 2019. Meningiomas and haemangiopericytoma (HPC). In *Oxford Textbook of Neurological Surgery*. Edited by Ramez Kirollos, Adel Helmy, Simon Thomson and Peter Hutchinson. Oxford: Oxford University Press, pp. 175–89.

Bondy, Melissa L., Michael E. Scheurer, Beatrice Malmer, Jill S. Barnholtz-Sloan, Faith G. Davis, Dora Il'yasova, Carol Kruchko, Bridget J. McCarthy, Preetha Rajaraman, Judith A. Schwartzbaum, and et al. 2008. Brain tumor epidemiology: Consensus from the Brain Tumor Epidemiology Consortium. *Cancer* 113: 1953–68. [CrossRef]

Brown, Timothy J., Matthew C. Brennan, Michael Li, Ephraim W. Church, Nicholas J. Brandmeir, Kevin L. Rakszawski, Akshal S. Patel, Elias B. Rizk, Dima Suki, Raymond Sawaya, and et al. 2016. Association of the extent of resection with survival in glioblastoma: A systematic review and meta-analysis. *JAMA Oncology* 2: 1460–69. [CrossRef]

Castillo, Mauricio, J. Keith Smith, and Lester Kwock. 2000. Correlation of myo-inositollevels and grading of cerebral astrocytomas. *AJNR American Journal of Neuroradiology* 21: 1645–49. [PubMed]

Chandler, C. 2019. Ependymoma. In *Oxford Textbook of Neurological Surgery*. Edited by Ramez Kirollos, Adel Helmy, Simon Thomson and Peter Hutchinson. Oxford: Oxford University Press, pp. 361–66.

Chang, Steven D., and Gordon T. Sakamoto. 2003. The role of radiosurgery for hemangioperi- cytomas. *Neurosurgical Focus* 14: e14. [CrossRef] [PubMed]

Chiechi, Maria V., James G. Smirniotopoulos, and Hernando Mena. 1996. Intracranial hemangiopericytomas: MR and CT features. *AJNR American Journal of Neuroradiology* 17: 1365–71. [PubMed]

Chowdhury, Forhad, Mohammod Haque, and Mainul Sarker. 2013. Intracranial epidermoid tumor; microneurosurgical management: An experience of 23 cases. *Asian Journal of Neurosurgery* 8: 21–28. [CrossRef]

Cimmino, Flora, Maria Nunzia Scoppettuolo, Marianeve Carotenuto, Pasqualino De Antonellis, Valeria Di Dato, Gennaro De Vita, and Massimo Zollo. 2011. Norcantharidin impairs medulloblastoma growth by inhibition of Wnt/catenin signaling. *Journal of Neuro-Oncology* 106: 59–70. [CrossRef]

Cushing, Harvey, and Louise Eisenhardt. 1938. *Meningiomas: Their Classification, Regional Behaviour, Life History, and Surgical End Results*. Springfield: Charles C Thomas.

Cusimano, Michael D., and Michael Patrick Meier. 2019. Surgical management of anterolateral skull base lesions. In *Oxford Textbook of Neurological Surgery*. Edited by Ramez Kirollos, Adel Helmy, Simon Thomson and Peter Hutchinson. Oxford: Oxford University Press, pp. 241–51.

Damodaran, Omprakash, Peter Robbins, Neville Knuckey, Michael Bynevelt, George Wong, and Gabriel Lee. 2014. Primary intracranial haemangiopericytoma: Comparison of survival outcomes and metastatic potential in WHO grade II and III variants. *Journal of Clinical Neuroscience* 21: 1310–14. [CrossRef]

De Witt Hamer, Philip C., Santiago Gil Robles, Aeilko H. Zwinderman, Hugues Duffau, and Mitchel S. Berger. 2012. Impact of intraoperative stimulation brain mapping on glioma surgery outcome: A meta-analysis. *Journal of Clinical Oncology* 30: 2559–65. [CrossRef]

Deipolyi, Amy, Ali Karaosmanoğlu, Cicero Habito, Scott Brannan, Stephan Wicky, Joshua Hirsch, and Rahmi Oklu. 2011. The role of bilateral inferior petrosal sinus sampling in the diagnostic evaluation of Cushing disease. *Diagnostic and Interventional Radiology* 18: 132–38. [CrossRef]

Dolecek, Therese A., Jennifer M. Propp, Nancy E. Stroup, and Carol Kruchko. 2012. CBTRUS Statistical report: Primary Brain and Central Nervous System Tumors Diagnosed in the United States in 2005–2009. *Neuro-Oncology* 14: v1–v49. [CrossRef]

Duffau, Hugues, Peggy Gatignol, Emmanuel Mandonnet, Laurent Capelle, and Luc Taillandier. 2008. Intraoperative subcortical stimulation mapping of language pathways in a consecutive series of 115 patients with grade II glioma in the left dominant hemisphere. *Journal of Neurosurgery* 109: 461–71. [CrossRef]

Erkmen, Kadir, Svetlana Pravdenkova, and Ossama Al-Mefty. 2005. Surgical management of petroclival meningiomas: Factors determining the choice of approach. *Neurosurgical Focus* 19: E7. [CrossRef] [PubMed]

Fernandez-Miranda, Juan C., Paul A. Gardner, Carl H. Snyderman, Kenneth O. Devaney, Primož Strojan, Carlos Suárez, Eric M. Genden, Alessandra Rinaldo, and Alfio Ferlito. 2012. Craniopharyngioma: A pathologic, clinical, and surgical review. *Head & Neck* 34: 1036–44. [CrossRef]

Fletcher, C., K. K. Unni, and F. Mertens. 2013. *World Health Organization Classification of Tumours of Soft Tissue and Bone*, 4th ed. Geneva: WHO.

Fruehwald-Pallamar, Julia, Stefan B. Puchner, Andrea Rossi, Maria L. Garre, Armando Cama, Claus Koelblinger, Anne G. Osborn, and Majda M. Thurnher. 2011. Magnetic resonance imaging spectrum of medulloblastoma. *Neuroradiology* 53: 387–96. [CrossRef] [PubMed]

Gaspar, Laurie, Charles Scott, Marvin Rotman, Sucha Asbell, Theodore Phillips, Todd Wasserman, W. Gillies McKenna, and Roger Byhardt. 1997. Recursive partitioning analysis (RPA) of prognostic factors in three Radiation Therapy Oncology Group (RTOG) brain metastases trials. *International Journal of Radiation Oncology Biology Physics* 37: 745–51. [CrossRef]

Geffen, G., A. Walsh, D. Simpson, and M. Jeeves. 1980. Comparison of the effects of transcortical and transcallosal removal of intraventricular tumours. *Brain* 103: 773–88. [CrossRef] [PubMed]

GLOBOCAN. 2002. *Worldwide Incidence and Mortality of Cancer, 2002 [Computer Program]*. Lyon: IARC.

Gormley, W. B., F. J. Tomecek, N. Qureshi, and G. M. Malik. 1994. Craniocerebral epidermoid and dermoid tumours: A review of 32 cases. *Acta Neurochirurgica* 128: 115–21. [CrossRef] [PubMed]

Gottardo, Nicholas G., Jordan R. Hansford, Jacqueline P. McGlade, Frank Alvaro, David M. Ashley, Simon Bailey, David L. Baker, Franck Bourdeaut, Yoon-Jae Cho, Moira Clay, and et al. 2014. Medulloblastoma Down Under 2013: A report from the third annual meeting of the International Medulloblastoma Working Group. *Acta Neuropathologica* 127: 189–201. [CrossRef]

Greenberg, Mark S. 2010. *Handbook of Neurosurgery*. New York: Thieme.

Gupta, Anshu, and Tanima Dwivedi. 2017. A simplified overview of world health organization classification update of central nervous system tumors 2016. *The Journal of Neurosciences in Rural Practice* 8: 629–41. [CrossRef]

Guthrie, Barton L., Michael J. Ebersold, Bernd W. Scheithauer, and Edward G. Shaw. 1989. Meningeal hemangiopericytoma: Histopathological features, treatment, and long-term follow-up of 44 cases. *Neurosurgery* 25: 514–22. [CrossRef]

Guthrie, B. L., S. C. Carabell, and E. R. Laws, Jr. 1991. Radiation therapy for intracranial meningiomas. In *Meningiomas*. Edited by Ossama Al-Mefty. New York: Raven Press, p. 255.

Haines, D. E., and R. G. Frederickson. 1991. The meninges. In *Meningiomas*. Edited by Ossama Al-Mefty. New York: Raven Press, pp. 9–25.

Hakyemez, Bahattin, Umit Aksoy, Harun Yildiz, and Necdet Ergin. 2005. Intracranial epidermoid cysts: Diffusion-weighted, FLAIR and conventional MR findings. *European Journal of Radiology* 54: 214–20. [CrossRef]

Hardy, J., and J. L. Vezina. 1976. Transsphenoidal neurosurgery of intracranial neoplasm. In *Advances in Neurology*. Edited by R. A. Tompson and J. R. Green. New York: Raven Press, pp. 261–75.

Hassaneen, Wael, and Raymond Sawaya. 2017. Epidermoid, Dermoid, and Neurenteric Cysts. In *Youmans & Winn Neurological Surgery*. Edited by H. Richard Winn. Philadelphia: Elsevier, pp. 1186–91.

Jukich, Patti J., Bridget J. McCarthy, Tanya S. Surawicz, Sally Freels, and Faith G. Davis. 2001. Trends in incidence of primary brain tumors in the United States, 1985–1994. *Neuro-Oncology* 3: 141–51. [CrossRef] [PubMed]

Kairys, N., C. Anastasopoulou, and A. Schwell. 2023. Cushing Disease. In *StatPearls [Internet]*; Treasure Island: StatPearls Publishing. Available online: https://www.ncbi.nlm.nih.gov/books/NBK448184/ (accessed on 23 March 2023).

Kanou, Yukari, Kazunori Arita, Kaoru Kurisu, A. Tomohide, and Kohji Iida. 2002. Clinical implications of dynamic MRI for pituitary adenomas: Clinical and histological analysis. *Journal of Clinical Neuroscience* 9: 659–63. [CrossRef] [PubMed]

Keil, Margaret F., and Constantine A. Stratakis. 2008. Pituitary tumours in childhood: An update in their diagnosis, treatment and molecular genetics. *Expert Review of Neurotherapeutics* 8: 563–74. [CrossRef]

Kinjo, Toshihiko, Ossama Al-Mefty, and Imad Kanaan. 1993. Grade zero removal of supratentorial convexity meningiomas. *Neurosurgery* 33: 394–99. [PubMed]

Klein, Martin, Hugues Duffau, and Philip C. De Witt Hamer. 2012. Cognition and resective surgery for diffuse infiltrative glioma: An overview. *Journal of Neuro-Oncology* 108: 309–18. [CrossRef] [PubMed]

Kleiser, Raimund, Philipp Staempfli, Anton Valavanis, Peter Boesiger, and Spyros Kollias. 2010. Impact of fMRI-guided advanced DTI fiber tracking techniques on their clinical applications in patients with brain tumors. *Neuroradiology* 52: 37–46. [CrossRef] [PubMed]

Knosp, Engelbert, Erich Steiner, Klaus Kitz, and Christian Matula. 1993. Pituitary adenomas with invasion of the cavernous sinus space: A magnetic resonance imaging classification compared with surgical findings. *Neurosurgery* 33: 610–17. [CrossRef]

Konovalov, Alexander N., and David I. Pitskhelauri. 2003. Principles of treatment of the pineal region tumours. *Surgical Neurology* 59: 250–68. [CrossRef]

Kool, Marcel, David T. W. Jones, Natalie Jäger, Paul A. Northcott, Trevor J. Pugh, Volker Hovestadt, Rosario M. Piro, L. Adriana Esparza, Shirley L. Markant, Marc Remke, and et al. 2014. Genome sequencing of SHH medulloblastoma predicts genotype-rdated response to smoothened inhibition. *Cancer Cell* 25: 393–405. [CrossRef]

Kowalczuk, Andrew, R. Loch Macdonald, Chris Amidei, George Dohrmann III, Robert K. Erickson, Javad Hekmatpanah, Stuart Krauss, Swarna Krishnasamy, Gregory Masters, Sean F. Mullan, and et al. 1997. Quantitative imaging study of extent of surgical resection and prognosis of malignant astrocytomas. *Neurosurgery* 41: 1028–36. [CrossRef]

Krivosheya, Daria, Sujit S. Prabhu, Jeffrey S. Weinberg, and Raymond Sawaya. 2016. Technical principles in glioma surgery and preoperative considerations. *Journal of Neuro-Oncology* 130: 243–52. [CrossRef] [PubMed]

Kubben, Pieter L., Karlien J. ter Meulen, Olaf EMG Schijns, Mariël P. ter Laak-Poort, Jacobus J. van Overbeeke, and Henk van Santbrink. 2011. Intraoperative MRIguided resection of glioblastoma multiforme: A systematic review. *The Lancet Oncology* 12: 1062–70. [CrossRef] [PubMed]

Kumari, Rima, Bhuvnesh Guglani, Nitij Gupta, and Sujata Chaturvedi. 2009. Intracranial epidermoid cyst: Magnetic resonance imaging features. *Neurology India* 57: 359–60. [CrossRef] [PubMed]

Law, Meng, Stanley Yang, Hao Wang, James S. Babb, Glyn Johnson, Soonmee Cha, Edmond A. Knopp, and David Zagzag. 2003. Glioma grading: Sensitivity, specificity, and predictive values of perfusion MR imaging and proton MR spectroscopic imaging compared with conventional MR imaging. *AJNR American Journal of Neuroradiology* 24: 1989–98. [PubMed]

Lee, Mark, Jeffrey H. Wisoff, Rick Abbott, Diana Freed, and Fred J. Epstein. 1994. Management of hydrocephalus in children with medulloblastoma: Prognostic factors for shunting. *Pediatric Neurosurgery* 20: 240–47. [CrossRef]

Levin, V., S. Liebel, P. Gutin, V. T. J. DeVita, S. Hellman, and S. A. Rosenberg. 2001. Neoplasms of the Central Nervous System (section 2). In *Cancer: Principles and Practice of Oncology*. Philadelphia: Lipincott, Williams, and Wilkins, pp. 2100–60.

Lindsay, K. W., I. Bone, and G. Fuller. 2011. *Neurology and Neurosurgery Illustrated. General Approach to History and Examination*. London: C L Elsevier.

Linos, Eleni, Tim Raine, Alvaro Alonso, and Dominique Michaud. 2007. Atopy and risk of brain tumors: A meta-analysis. *Journal of the National Cancer Institute* 99: 1544–50. [CrossRef]

Louis, David N., Arie Perry, Guido Reifenberger, Andreas Von Deimling, Dominique Figarella-Branger, Webster K. Cavenee, Hiroko Ohgaki, Otmar D. Wiestler, Paul Kleihues, and David W. Ellison. 2016. The 2016 World Health Organization Classification of Tumors of the Central Nervous System: A summary. *Acta Neuropathologica* 131: 803–20. [CrossRef]

Louis, David N., Arie Perry, Pieter Wesseling, Daniel J. Brat, Ian A. Cree, Dominique Figarella-Branger, Cynthia Hawkins, H. K. Ng, Stefan M. Pfister, Guido Reifenberger, and et al. 2021. The 2021 WHO Classification of Tumors of the Central Nervous System: A summary. *Neuro-Oncology* 23: 1231–51. [CrossRef]

Louis, David N., Hiroko Ohgaki, Otmar D. Wiestler, Webster K. Cavenee, Peter C. Burger, Anne Jouvet, Bernd W. Scheithauer, and Paul Kleihues. 2007. The 2007 WHO classification of tumours of the central nervous system. *Acta Neuropathologica* 114: 97–109. [CrossRef]

Love, J. Grafton, and And James W. Kernohan. 1936. Dermoid and epidermoid tumors (cholesteatomas) of central nervous system. *JAMA* 107: 1876–83. [CrossRef]

Luzzi, Sabino, Alice Giotta Lucifero, Jessica Rabski, Paulo A. S. Kadri, and Ossama Al-Mefty. 2023. The Party Wall: Redefining the Indications of Transcranial Approaches for Giant Pituitary Adenomas in Endoscopic Era. *Cancers* 15: 2235. [CrossRef] [PubMed]

Marchand-Crety, C., J. Riverain, Y. Drouet, F. Felici, C. L. Jeandidier, J. Thariat, and S. Servagi- Vernat. 2021. A new model outperforming RPA and DS-GPA scores for individualized survival prediction of patients following whole brain irradiation for brain metastasis. *Cancer/Radiothérapie* 25: 447–56. [CrossRef] [PubMed]

Marques, Pedro, and Márta Korbonits. 2017. Genetic aspects of pituitary adenoams. *Endocrinology and Metabolism Clinics of North America* 46: 335–74. [CrossRef]

Matula, C. 2012. Tuours of the pineal region. In *Principles of Neurosurgery*. Edited by Richard G. Ellenbogen and Laligam N. Shekhor. Philadelphia: Elsvier, pp. 565–78.

McEvoy, A. 2019. Dermoid and epidermoid cysts. In *Oxford Textbook of Neurological Surgery*. Edited by RRamez Kirollos, Adel Helmy, Simon Thomson and Peter Hutchinson. Oxford: Oxford University Press, pp. 197–203.

Mehdorn, H. Maximilian, Felix Schwartz, Stefan Dawirs, Jürgen Hedderich, Lutz Dörner, and Arya Nabavi. 2011. High-field iMRI in glioblastoma surgery: Improvement of resection radicality and survival for the patient? *Acta Neurochirurgica Supplement* 109: 103–6. [CrossRef] [PubMed]

Merchant, Thomas E., Chenghong Li, Xiaoping Xiong, Larry E. Kun, Frederic A. Boop, and Robert A. Sanford. 2009. Conformal radiotherapy after surgery for paediatric ependymoma: A prospective study. *The Lancet Oncology* 10: 258–66. [CrossRef] [PubMed]

Miller, Dorothea, Stefan Heinze, Wuttipong Tirakotai, Oliver Bozinov, Oguzkan Sürücü, Ludwig Benes, Helmut Bertalanffy, and Ulrich Sure. 2007. Is the image guidance of ultrasonography beneficial for neurosurgical routine? *Surgical Neurology* 67: 579–87. [CrossRef]

Morfouace, Marie, Anang Shelat, Megan Jacus, Burgess B. Freeman, David Turner, Sarah Robinson, Frederique Zindy, Yong-Dong Wang, David Finkelstein, Olivier Ayrault, and et al. 2014. Pemetrexed and gemcitabine as combination therapy for the treatment of Group 3 medulloblastoma. *Cancer Cell* 25: 516–29. [CrossRef]

Naik, Vismay Dinesh, and Nilay Rajendra Thakore. 2013. A case of symptomatic Rathke's cyst. *BMJ Case Reports* 2013: bcr2012006943. [CrossRef]

Nakau, H., T. Miyazawa, S. Tamai, K. Tsuchiya, K. Shima, T. Shirotani, and H. Chigasaki. 1997. Pathologic significance of meningeal enhancement ("flare sign") of meningiomas on MRI. *Surgical Neurology* 48: 584–90. [CrossRef]

Neil, Jayson A., and William T. Couldwell. 2019. Surgical management of sellar and suprasellar tumours. In *Oxford Textbook of Neurological Surgery*. Edited by Ramez Kirollos, Adel Helmy, Simon Thomson and Peter Hutchinson. Oxford: Oxford University Press, pp. 339–49.

Newton, Herbert B. 2016. Overview of brain tumor epidemiology. In *Handbook of Neurooncology Neuroimaging*. Edited by Herbert B. Newton. London: Elsevier.

Nimmannitya, Pree, Takeo Goto, Yuzo Terakawa, Hidetoshi Sato, Toshiyuki Kawashima, Hiroki Morisako, and Kenji Ohata. 2016. Characteristic of optic canal invasion in 31 consecutive cases with tuberculum sellae meningioma. *Neurosurgical Review* 39: 691–7. [CrossRef]

Norden, Andrew D., Patrick Y. Wen, and Santosh Kesari. 2005. Brain metastases. *Current Opinion in Neurology* 18: 654–61. [CrossRef] [PubMed]

Northcott, Paul A., Andrey Korshunov, Hendrik Witt, Thomas Hielscher, Charles G. Eberhart, Stephen Mack, Eric Bouffet, Steven C. Clifford, Cynthia E. Hawkins, Pim French, and et al. 2011. Medulloblastoma comprises four distinct molecular variants. *Journal of Clinical Oncology* 29: 1408–14. [CrossRef] [PubMed]

Oppenheim, H., and F. Krause. 1913. Operative erfolge bei geschwulsten derschuuugel und vierhugelgent. *Berliner Klinische Wochenschrift* 50: 2116–322.

Osborn, Anne G., and Michael T. Preece. 2006. Intracranial cysts: Radiologic-pathologic correlation and imaging approach. *Radiology* 239: 650–64. [CrossRef] [PubMed]

Ostrom, Quinn T., Haley Gittleman, Jordan Xu, Courtney Kromer, Yingli Wolinsky, Carol Kruchko, and Jill S. Barnholtz-Sloan. 2016. CBTRUS statistical report: Primary brain and other central nervous system tumors diagnosed in the United States in 2009–2013. *Neuro-Oncology* 18 S5: v1–v75. [CrossRef]

Ostrom, Quinn T., Haley Gittleman, Paul Farah, Annie Ondracek, Yanwen Chen, Yingli Wolinsky, Nancy E. Stroup, Carol Kruchko, and Jill S. Barnholtz-Sloan. 2013. CBTRUS statistical report: Primary brain and central nervous system tumours diagnosed in the United States in 2006–2010. *Neuro-Oncology* 15: ii1–ii56. [CrossRef]

Padma, M. V., S. Said, M. Jacobs, D. R. Hwang, K. Dunigan, M. Satter, B. Christian, J. Ruppert, T. Bernstein, G. Kraus, and et al. 2003. Prediction of pathology and survival by FDG PET in gliomas. *Journal of Neuro-Oncology* 64: 227–37. [CrossRef]

Pallud, Johan, Etienne Audureau, Marie Blonski, Nader Sanai, Luc Bauchet, Denys Fontaine, Emmanuel Mandonnet, Edouard Dezamis, Dimitri Psimaras, Jacques Guyotat, and et al. 2014. Epileptic seizures in diffuse low-grade gliomas in adults. *Brain* 137, Pt 2: 449–62. [CrossRef]

Pallud, Johan, Luc Taillandier, Laurent Capelle, Denys Fontaine, Matthieu Peyre, François Ducray, Hugues Duffau, and Emmanuel Mandonnet. 2012. Quantitative morphological magnetic resonance imaging follow-up of lowgrade glioma: A plea for systematic measurement of growth rates. *Neurosurgery* 71: 729–39. [CrossRef]

Pallud, J., P. Varlet, B. Devaux, S. Geha, M. Badoual, C. Deroulers, P. Page, E. Dezamis, C. Daumas-Duport, and F. X. Roux. 2010. Diffuse low-grade oligodendrogliomas extend beyond MRI-defined abnormalities. *Neurology* 74: 1724–31. [CrossRef]

Patel, Akash J., Dima Suki, Mustafa Aziz Hatiboglu, Hiba Abouassi, Weiming Shi, David M. Wildrick, Frederick F. Lang, and Raymond Sawaya. 2009. Factors influencing the risk of local recurrence after resection of a single brain metasrasis. *Journal of Neurosurgery* 113: 181–89. [CrossRef] [PubMed]

Poretti, Andrea, Avner Meoded, and Thierry A. G. M. Huisman. 2012. Neuroimaging of pediatric posterior fossa tumors including review of the literature. *Journal of Magnetic Resonance Imaging* 35: 32–47. [CrossRef] [PubMed]

Prabhu, Vikram C., and Henry G. Brown. 2005. The pathogenesis of craniopharyngiomas. *Child's Nervous System* 21: 622–27. [CrossRef] [PubMed]

Price, S. J., H. Bulstrode, and R. Mair. 2019. High-grade gliomas and molecular biology of neurosurgical oncology. In *Oxford Textbook of Neurological Surgery*. Edited by Ramez Kirollos, Adel Helmy, Simon Thomson and Peter Hutchinson. Oxford: Oxford University Press, pp. 89–106.

Price, Stephen J., R. Jena, N. G. Burnet, P. J. Hutchinson, A. F. Dean, A. Pena, J. D. Pickard, T. A. Carpenter, and J. H. Gillard. 2006. Improved delineation of glioma margins and regions of infiltration with the use of diffusion tensor imaging: An image-guided biopsy study. *AJNR American Journal of Neuroradiology* 27: 1969–74. [PubMed]

Raiyawa, Tassapong, Chonlakiet Khorprasert, Chawalit Lertbutsayanukul, Panya Seksarn, Darintr Sosothikul, Jiraphorn Amornfa, and Kanjana Shotelersuk. 2012. Management of intracranial germ cell tumours at the king Chulalongkorn Memorial Hospital. *Journal of the Medical Association of Thailand* 95: 1327–34.

Raza, Shaan M., Matei A. Banu, Angela Donaldson, Kunal S. Patel, Vijay K. Anand, and Theodore H. Schwartz. 2016. Sensitivity and specificity of intrathecal fluorescein and white light excitation for detecting intraoperative cerebrospinal fluid leak in endoscopic skull base surgery: A prospective study. *Journal of Neurosurgery* 124: 621–26. [CrossRef]

Rhoton, A. L., Jr. 2002. The Sellar Region. *Neurosurgery* 51: S335–S374. [CrossRef]

Rincon-Torroella, J., H. Brem, and Alfredo Quiñones-Hinojosa. 2017. Malignant Gliomas. Anaplastic Astrocytoma, Glioblastoma, Gliosarcoma, and Anaplastic Oligodendroglioma. In *Youmans & Winn Neurological Surgery*. Edited by H. R. Winn. Philadelphia: Elsevier, pp. 1006–25.

Ron, Elaine. 2003. Cancer risks from medical radiation. *Health Physics* 85: 47–59. [CrossRef]

Sakaki, Saburo, Sadanori Takeda, Hitoshi Fujita, and Shinsuke Ohta. 1987. An extended middle fossa approach combined with a suboccipital craniectomy to the base of the skull in the posterior fossa. *Surgical Neurology* 28: 245–52. [CrossRef]

Samii, M., and M. Tatagiba. 1992. Experience with 36 surgical cases of petroclival menigiomas. *Acta Neurochirurgica* 118: 27–32. [CrossRef]

Schweizer, Leonille, Christian Koelsche, Felix Sahm, Rosario M. Piro, David Capper, David E. Reuss, Stefan Pusch, Antje Habel, Jochen Meyer, Tanja Göck, and et al. 2013. Meningeal hemangiopericytoma and solitary fibrous tumors carry the NAB2- STAT6 fusion and can be diagnosed by nuclear expression of STAT6 protein. *Acta Neuropathologica* 125: 651–58. [CrossRef] [PubMed]

Senthilvel, Hari Nivas Periyakottai, Shyam Sundar Krishnan, and Madabhushi Chakravarthy Vasudevan. 2014. Extracranial infrasellar craniopharyngioma. *Neurology India* 62: 100–3. [CrossRef] [PubMed]

Sherman, Jonathan H., Kathryn Hoes, Joshua Marcus, Ricardo J. Komotar, Cameron W. Brennan, and Philip H. Gutin. 2011. Neurosurgery for brain tumors: Update on recent technical advances. *Current Neurology and Neuroscience Reports* 11: 313–19. [CrossRef] [PubMed]

Sibtain, N. A., S. Butt, and S. E. Connor. 2007. Imaging features of central nervous system haemangiopericytomas. *European Radiology* 17: 1685–93. [CrossRef]

Simpson, Donald. 1957. The recurrence of intracranial meningiomas after surgical treatment. *Journal of Neurology Neurosurgery and Psychiatry* 20: 22–39. [CrossRef]

Steno, Juraj, Martin Malacek, and Ivan Bizik. 2004. Tumor-third ventricular relationships in supradiaphragmatic craniopharyngiomas: Correlation of morphological, magnetic resonance imaging, and operative findings. *Neurosurgery* 54: 1051–58. [CrossRef]

Stummer, Walter, Uwe Pichlmeier, Thomas Meinel, Otmar Dieter Wiestler, Friedhelm Zanella, and Hans-Jürgen Reulen. 2006. Fluorescence-guided surgery with 5-aminolevulinic acid for resection of malignant glioma: A randomised controlled multicentre phase III trial. *The Lancet Oncology* 7: 392–401. [CrossRef]

Stupp, Roger, Warren P. Mason, Martin J. Van Den Bent, Michael Weller, Barbara Fisher, Martin J. B. Taphoorn, Karl Belanger, Alba A. Brandes, Christine Marosi, Ulrich Bogdahn, and et al. 2005. Radiotherapy plus concomitant and adjuvant temozolomide for glioblastoma. *The New England Journal of Medicine* 352: 987–96. [CrossRef]

Syro, Luis V., Leon D. Ortiz, Bernd W. Scheithauer, Ricardo Lloyd, Queenie Lau, Ricardo Gonzalez, Humberto Uribe, Michael Cusimano, Kalman Kovacs, and Eva Horvath. 2011. Treatment of pituitary neoplasm with temozolamide: A review. *Cancer* 117: 454–62. [CrossRef]

Taillibert, Sophie, and Jean-Yves Delattre. 2005. Palliative care in patients with brain metastases. *Current Opinion in Oncology* 17: 588–92. [CrossRef]

Takakura, Kintomo, K. Sano, S. Hojo, and A. Hirano. 1982. *Metastatic Tumors of the Central Nervous System*. New York: Igaku-Shoin.

Taylor, Michael D., Helen Poppleton, Christine Fuller, Xiaoping Su, Yongxing Liu, Patricia Jensen, Susan Magdaleno, James Dalton, Christopher Calabrese, Julian Board, and et al. 2006. Radial glia cells are candidate stem cells of ependymoma. *Cancer Cell* 9: P70. [CrossRef]

Thompson, Eric M., Thomas Hielscher, Eric Bouffet, Marc Remke, Betty Luu, Sridharan Gururangan, Roger E. McLendon, Darell D. Bigner, Eric S. Lipp, Sebastien Perreault, and et al. 2016. Prognostic value of medulloblastoma extent of resection after accounting for molecular subgroup: A retrospective integrated clinical and molecular analysis. *The Lancet Oncology* 17: 484–95. [CrossRef] [PubMed]

Tucha, Oliver, Christian Smely, Michael Preier, and Klaus W. Lange. 2000. Cognitive deficits before treatment among patients with brain tumors. *Neurosurgery* 47: 324–33. [CrossRef] [PubMed]

van den Bent, Martin J., Michael Weller, Patrick Y. Wen, Johan M. Kros, Ken Aldape, and Susan Chang. 2017. A clinical perspective on the 2016 WHO brain tumor classification and routine molecular diagnostics. *Neuro-Oncology* 19: 614–24. [CrossRef]

Van Effenterre, Rémy, and Anne-Laure Boch. 2002. Craniopharyngima in adult and children: A study of 122 surgical cases. *Journal of Neurosurgery* 97: 3–12. [CrossRef]

Vandeva, S., V. Vasilev, L. Vroonen, L. Naves, M-L. Jaffrain-Rea, A. F. Daly, S. Zacharieva, and A. Beckers. 2010. Familial pituitary adenomas. *Annales Endocrinologie* 71: 479–85. [CrossRef]

Van Wagenen, William P. 1931. A surgical approach for the removal of certain pineal tumours. *Surgery, Gynecology & Obstetrics* 37: 216–20.

Vellimana, A. K., G. P. Dunn, and I. F. Dunn. 2017. Intracranial Ependymomas in Adults. In *Youmans & Winn Neurological Surgery*. Edited by H. R. Winn. Philadelphia: Elsevier, pp. 1069–74.

WHO Classification of Tumours Editorial Board. 2021. *World Health Organization Classification of Tumours of the Central Nervous System*, 5th ed. Lyon: International Agency for Research on Cancer.

Willems, P. W., J. W. van der Sprenkel, C. A. Tulleken, M. A. Viergever, and M. J. Taphoorn. 2006. Neuronavigation and surgery of intracerebral tumours. *Journal of Neurology* 253: 1123–36. [CrossRef]

Yamamoto, Masaaki, Toru Serizawa, Takashi Shuto, Atsuya Akabane, Yoshinori Higuchi, Jun Kawagishi, Kazuhiro Yamanaka, Yasunori Sato, Hidefumi Jokura, Shoji Yomo, and et al. 2014. Stereotactic radiosurgery for patients with multiple brain metastases (JLGK0901): A multi-institutional prospective observational study. *The Lancet Oncology* 15: 387–95. [CrossRef]

Yuh, E. L., A. J. Barkovich, and N. Gupta. 2009. Imaging of ependymomas: MRI and CT. *Child's Nervous System* 25: 1203–13. [CrossRef]

Zigouris, Andreas, Dimitrios Pahatouridis, Evaggelos Mihos, George A. Alexiou, John Nesseris, Anastasia K. Zikou, Maria I. Argyropoulou, Anna Goussia, and Spyridon Voulgaris. 2009. Solitary cystic cerebral metastasis from transitional cell carcinoma of the bladder. *Acta Neurologica Belgica* 109: 322–25. [PubMed]

Skull Base Tumours

Forhad H. Chowdhury, Mohammod Raziul Haque, Robert Ahmed Khan and Khandkar Ali Kawsar

Abstract: Skull base tumours pose a significant challenge to the neurosurgeon. Skull base tumours can be benign or malignant. Primary skull base neoplasms can originate from the meninges, cranial nerves, bones of the cranial vault and skull base, cavernous sinus, or from the orbit and its contents. Tumours of the nose, paranasal sinuses, ears, or the infratemporal fossa can extend to the skull base and cranial cavity. Common skull base tumours are chondrosarcoma, chordoma, schwannoma, adenocarcinoma, and metastatic tumours. They can affect patients at almost any age. The clinical presentation depends on the site, size, and on the age of the patient. The most common presentation includes headache, nasal bleeding, hearing loss, cranial nerve palsy, and focal neuro-deficit/s. Head CT scan and MRI with contrast are enough to diagnose most of the tumours of the skull base. Surgery is the primary modality of management. Surgical approaches differ according to size, site, patient age, nature of neoplasm, and operator experience and expertise as well. Prognosis depends on histological type, extent of resection, and postoperative therapy (where needed) as well. In this chapter, we will briefly discuss the surgical management of all common skull base tumours, along with a short orientation of the surgical approaches used for the removal of skull base tumours.

Abbreviations

CP	cerebellopontine	ICP	intracranial pressure
CPA	cerebellopontine angle	JNA	juvenile nasopharyngeal angiofibroma
CS	cavernous sinus	MRI	magnetic resonance imaging
CSM	cavernous sinus meningioma	SRS	stereotactic radiotherapy
CT	computed tomography	TS	trigeminal schwannoma
IAC	internal acoustic canal	VS	vestibular schwannoma

1. Introduction

Because of their diverse histology, tumours of the base of the skull can be difficult to diagnose and treat before surgery. The precise determination of which tumours are regarded as tumours of the base of the skull is a controversial matter. Any tumour involving or adjacent to the base of the skull would fall under the broadest definition, which would include numerous tumours of the posterior fossa and cavernous sinus as well as pituitary tumours. However, a more specific definition would only include tumours that originate from the connective tissues and bones that make up the base of the skull. Practically speaking, it is occasionally impossible to discern between lesions that originate in the cranial cavity, the upper neck, or the paranasal sinuses and those that subsequently damage bone and cartilage tissues. Common skull base tumours are chondrosarcoma, chordoma, schwannoma, adenocarcinoma, and metastatic tumours. They can affect patients at almost any age. The most common presentation includes headache, aural/nasal bleeding, hearing loss, cranial nerve palsy, and focal neuro-deficit/s. Head CT scan and MRI of the head with contrast are enough to diagnose most tumours of the skull base. Surgery (endoscopic/microscopic) is the primary modality of management. Surgical approaches differ according to size, site, patient age, nature of neoplasm, and operator experience and expertise as well. Prognosis depends on histological type, extent of resection, and postoperative therapy (where needed) as well.

2. Esthesioneuroblastoma

2.1. Clinical Considerations

Esthesioneuroblastoma, also called olfactory neuroblastoma, generally begins as a tumour in the upper part of the nasal cavity and may grow or extend into the sinus, eyes, and brain. It can also spread to the cervical lymph nodes and the parotid glands. In advanced cases, it can also spread to other parts of the brain and body, such as the lungs, liver, bone marrow, bones, and skin. It is believed to originate from sensory neuroepithelial cells, also known as neuroectodermal olfactory cells (Fiani et al. 2019).

It can present at any age in both adult male and female patients. It is considered a relatively rare skull base tumour and constitutes only 3–5% of all tumours in the nasal cavity.

Patients may usually present with anosmia, epistaxis, nasal congestion, sinus infection, nasal obstruction, and difficulty breathing. The lesion may also cause eye pain, proptosis, ophthalmoplegia, diplopia, loss of vision, facial pain, facial numbness, rhinorrhoea, headache, nausea, vomiting, seizure, and, rarely, dental problems. The clinical features depend on the site of the pathology. The most commonly used staging systems are the modified Kadish staging, Dulguerov classification, and Haymes histopathological grading system (Fiani et al. 2019; Kumar 2015).

2.2. *Investigative Considerations*

Any patient with persistent nasal symptoms should undergo a thorough evaluation by an ear, nose, and throat specialist. Flexible endoscopy may reveal a fleshy, reddish-yellow mass filling the nasal cavity covered by the mucosa, with possible ulceration. CT scan of the skull base, paranasal sinus, and neck with and without contrast will reveal a hyperdense mass and heterogenous contrast enhancement. CT can also reveal bony destruction of the lamina papyracea, cribriform plate, and sphenoid sinus wall. MRI is the best neuroimaging modality to detect tumour extension and consistency. A cerebral angiogram is sometimes required to see carotid encasement by the tumour (Fiani et al. 2019; Kumar 2015).

2.3. *Treatment Considerations*

The various treatment modalities include a transcranial approach, endoscopic endonasal surgery, a craniofacial approach, stereotactic radiation therapy, chemotherapy, and palliative therapy. The choice of modality of treatment depends on tumour location and on its extension. It is a slow-growing but malignant tumour with high recurrence rates (Fiani et al. 2019; Kumar 2015).

3. Juvenile Nasopharyngeal Angiofibroma

3.1. *Clinical Considerations*

Juvenile nasopharyngeal angiofibroma (JNA) is a rare, benign tumour of the nasopharynx. It is aggressive locally and causes bone resorption by invading the surrounding tissue (Figure 1). A total of 0.5% of head and neck tumours are caused by it. There is a definite masculine predominance among young people. The Indian subcontinent has a higher tumour prevalence than the West.

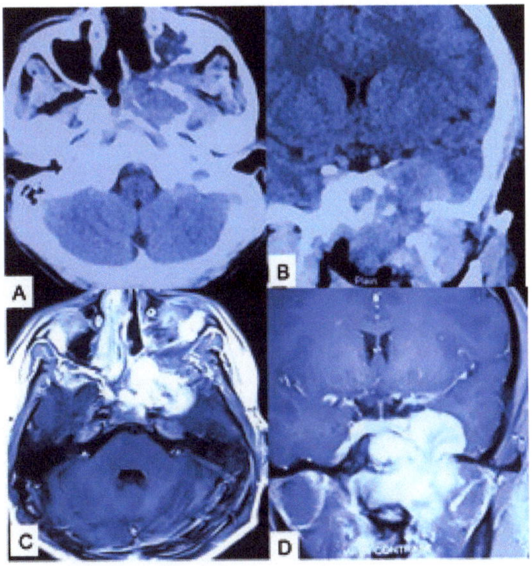

Figure 1. A case of juvenile nasopharyngeal angiofibroma in a 14-year-old boy. Contrast CT, axial and coronal view (**A,B**), and contrast MRI, axial and coronal view (**C,D**), show left-sided juvenile nasopharyngeal angiofibroma. Source: Figure by authors.

The tumour begins in the nasal cavity's lateral wall, near to the superior border of the sphenopalatine foramen. The growth begins in the submucosa of the nasopharynx's floor, progresses to the nasal septum, and grows into the posterior region of the nose, eventually obstructing the airway. Continuous growth involves the sphenoidal sinus, nasal fossa and middle turbinate, and pterygopalatine fossa, as well as the posterior wall of the maxillary sinus. Eventually, the tumour may invade the infratemporal fossa and the middle cranial fossa.

JNA typically manifests as a unilateral, painless nasal blockage that worsens with time. There may also be epistaxis, rhinorrhoea, and face discomfort. There may be facial deformities, proptosis, altered visual acuity, and impaired eustachian tube function. Cranial nerve palsy can result from an invasion of the intracranial space. In the nose and nasopharynx, a hard and friable mass may be found during a clinical examination (Martins et al. 2013; Garça et al. 2010).

3.2. *Investigative Considerations*

The precise location, extent, and relationship of the tumour to nearby structures like blood vessels and nerves can be determined using a CT scan, MRI (Figure 1), and angiography. Pathognomonic for JNA is the antral sign or Holman–Miller sign (forward bowing of the maxillary posterior wall). Nasal endoscopy clearly delineates the lesion and can be used to perform a biopsy for histopathological confirmation.

JNA is categorized into three types based on its radiological and clinical characteristics. Lesions classified as type 1 are primarily localized to the nasopharynx, paranasal sinus, nasal cavity, or pterygopalatine fossa. Type 2 JNAs are those with intact dura mater and little anterior and/or middle cranial fossa expansion that extend into the infratemporal fossa, buccal area, or orbital cavity. Type 3 is a giant, calabash-like tumour lobe in the middle cranial fossa (Martins et al. 2013; Garça et al. 2010).

3.3. *Treatment Considerations*

The preferred treatment is angiography followed by preoperative embolization and surgical resection. The supply of these tumours is usually via the external carotid artery (ascending pharyngeal artery, internal maxillary artery, and palatine artery) and less commonly the internal carotid artery (sphenoidal branch and ophthalmic artery).

Treatment is primarily surgical. The different surgical approach modalities include the transpalatine approach, infratemporal approach, transpalatine plus sublabial approach, middle fossa approach, maxillary swing approach or facial translocation, transmaxillary approach, and extended endonasal endoscopic approach.

These are benign tumours, and metastasis usually does not occur, but they are highly vascular and grow rapidly locally (Martins et al. 2013; Garça et al. 2010).

4. Clival Chordoma

4.1. *Clinical Considerations*

Chordoma is a rare tumour, presumably originating from remnants of the primitive notochord. The sacrococcygeal region accounts for about 50% of chordoma development, the spheno-occipital region for 35%, and the vertebrae for 15%. The upper and middle clivus and the spheno-occipital synchondrosis are all areas where skull base chordomas can be found. They are regarded as low-grade malignancies that grow slowly, but because of local bone infiltration, extension into nearby soft tissue, a high risk of recurrence, and occasional metastasis, they behave more aggressively.

No age group is immune to chordoma, but it is usually seen in adults (30–70 years). Sacrococcygeal is the commonest location, and chordoma is the commonest primary malignant sacral tumour.

The clinical presentation depends on the extension of the tumour. Clival chordomas are classified as upper, middle, lower, or of the craniovertebral junction. Sometimes they are classified as basisphenoidal or basioccipital, depending on whether they arise above or below the spheno-occipital synchondrosis. They may present with diplopia due to abducens palsy, visual loss, pituitary encephalopathy, chiasmal syndrome, cavernous sinus syndrome, nasopharyngeal mass, multiple cranial nerve involvement, brainstem sign, cerebellopontine angle involvement, hydrocephalus, and lower cranial nerve palsy (Chugh et al. 2007; Walcott et al. 2012; Tamura et al. 2015).

4.2. Investigative Considerations

On CT scan, clival chordomas are usually isodense on non-contrast-enhancing. CT also shows bony destruction and areas of calcification. MRI usually shows a lobulated tumour which is hypointense in T1WI and hyperintense in T2 WI, with variable contrast enhancement (Figure 2).

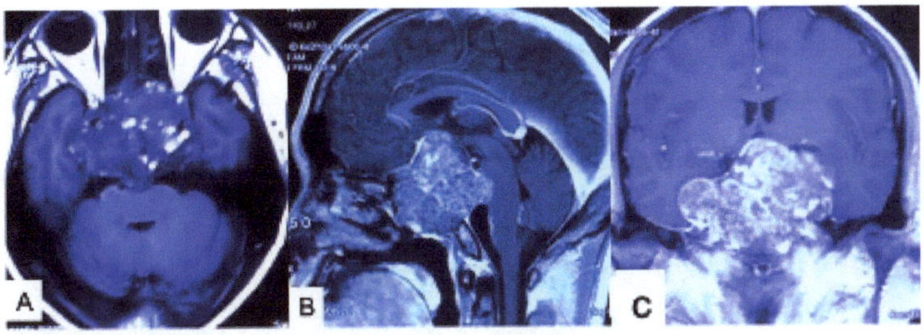

Figure 2. MRI of brain; (**A**) axial, (**B**) sagittal, and (**C**) coronal images showing large clival chordoma. Source: Figure by authors.

4.3. Treatment Considerations

Radical surgical removal is the primary treatment choice. But by the time these tumours are diagnosed, they will have reached a considerable size and invaded many critical structures, which makes surgical access very difficult. There are different anterior and lateral approaches to deal with these lesions depending on their extension. The extended subfrontal, trans-sphenoidal, endoscopic endonasal, transfacial, transoral, and transmandibular circumglossal retropharyngeal are among some of the anterior approaches. The lateral approaches include frontotemporo-zygomatic, preauricular subtemporal and infratemporal, presigmoid combined supratentorial and infratentorial, and also extreme lateral transcondylar.

Radiotherapy, i.e., C12, can be used for residual tumour. There are some restrictions on the utilization of radiation therapy for chordoma treatment because of its close vicinity to the optic nerve, chiasm, brainstem, and pituitary gland (Chugh et al. 2007; Walcott et al. 2012; Tamura et al. 2015).

5. Trigeminal Schwannoma

5.1. Clinical Considerations

Only 0.2–0.4% of all intracranial tumours are trigeminal schwannomas (TSs). The Gasserian ganglion is where they mostly manifest. Compared to acoustic neuroma, they are less common. Patients are usually middle-aged, commonly in their third or fourth decade of life, on first presentation. There is a relationship with neurofibromatosis type 2, just like there is with other schwannomas (Chowdhury et al. 2014; Agarwal 2015).

They can be preganglionic (cisternal), ganglionic (trigeminal ganglion), or postganglionic. Preganglionic TSs are confined to the prepontine cistern and cerebellopontine cistern. Ganglionic TSs are confined to Meckel's cave and they are the commonest. Postganglionic TSs are only found in the cavernous sinus or through the appropriate foramina at the base of the skull. Classically, the ophthalmology division is involved.

Women are somewhat more likely to develop TS. Patients typically have facial pain, most frequently conventional trigeminal neuralgia or atypical facial pain, when they first present with trigeminal nerve dysfunction. Trigeminal neuralgia is a sudden, typically unilateral, intense, fleeting, stabbing, recurrent pain that affects one or more trigeminal nerve branches. Numbness or a burning feeling are additional frequent clinical characteristics. Long-standing lesions can also cause motor symptoms such difficulties chewing, jaw deviation, and masseter and temporalis muscle weakness (Chowdhury et al. 2014; Agarwal 2015).

In 1955, Jefferson created the first classification scheme and divided TS into three categories (Jefferson 1955). Type A tumours arise from the Gasserian ganglion in the middle cranial fossa. Type B tumours develop from the roots of the trigeminal nerve roots in the posterior cranial fossa. The middle and posterior cranial fossa are both occupied by type C tumours, often known as hourglass tumours. Tumours with extracranial extension were introduced as a fourth categorization, type D, by some writers. Six types of TSs were proposed by Yoshida and Kawase (Yoshida and Kawase 1999) in their classification of TSs. Trigeminal nerve tumours of type P come from the root of the trigeminal nerve. Type M tumours arise from the Gasserian ganglion or the peripheral branch at the lateral wall of the cavernous sinus. Extracranial peripheral branches of trigeminal nerves are the source of type E tumours. Combinations of P, M, and E tumours are indicated as types MP, ME, and MPE.

5.2. Investigative Considerations

Conventional X-ray delineates a bony erosion of the petrous apex. The margins are usually smooth without sclerosis. Large tumours may cause erosion of the sella turcica and of the clinoid process as well as the widening of superior orbital fissure. CT scan with bone window reveals all bony changes and iso- to hyperdense lesions with contrast enhancement. These tumours appear as hypointense on T1WI and hyperintense on T2WI MRI, with intense contrast enhancement (Figures 3 and 4). Cerebral angiography sometimes demonstrates an enlarged feeder artery and vessel encasement or displacement.

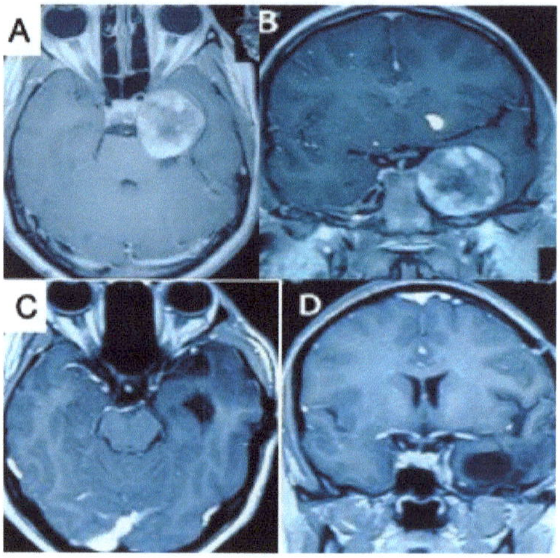

Figure 3. Contrast MRI of brain; pre- (**A**,**B**) and postoperative (**C**,**D**) images of a case of trigeminal schwannoma. Source: Figure by authors.

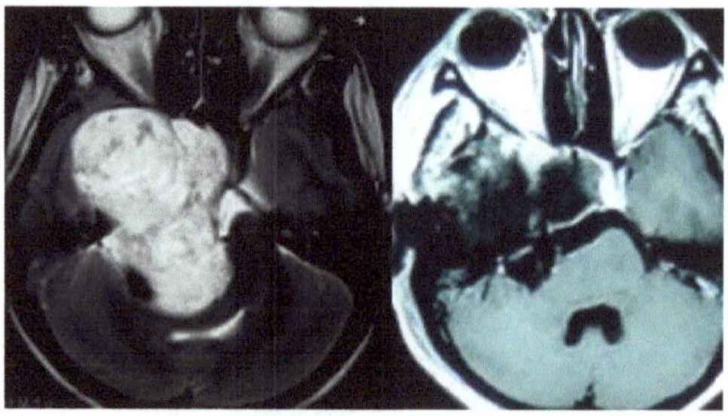

Figure 4. Contrast MRI of brain showing preoperative image of right trigeminal schwannoma occupying both middle and posterior cranial fossa on left-hand side and postoperative image of the same case on right-hand side. Source: Figure by authors.

5.3. Treatment Considerations

The site and size of the tumour determines the appropriate surgical approach (Figures 3 and 4). The commonest approaches are a middle fossa, retrosigmoid, presigmoid, and combined approach. Smaller tumours or residual tumours may be subjected to stereotactic radiosurgery (SRS) (Chowdhury et al. 2014; Agarwal 2015; Jefferson 1955; Yoshida and Kawase 1999).

6. Tumours of the Cerebellopontine Angle (CPA) and Vestibular Schwannoma

6.1. Clinical Considerations

The most frequent location for posterior fossa tumours is the cerebellopontine angle. Acoustic neuromas or vestibular schwannomas (VSs) make up 80% of all intracranial tumours that are found in this area, which in turn represent around 10% of all intracranial tumours. Meningiomas, arachnoid cysts, epidermoids, dermoids, lipomas, various cranial nerve schwannomas, and metastases are further tumours in this area (Carlson and Link 2021).

The petrosal surface of the cerebellum is folded around the lateral side of the pons and around the middle cerebellar peduncle to create the V-shaped CPA or fissure. The middle cerebellar peduncle serves as the floor of this space. The facial, cochlear, superior, and inferior divisions of the vestibular nerve are the four nerves that make up the internal acoustic meatus. Most frequently, VS is caused by the vestibular nerve (80%). In about 65–75% of cases, the inferior branch of the vestibular nerve is the origin of the tumour (Carlson and Link 2021; Komatsuzaki and Tsunoda 2001).

The junctional (Obersteiner–Redlich) zone where central and peripheral myelin converge is where VS originates from, although recent data point to a relationship with the sensory ganglia of the vestibular nerve in the internal auditory canal. The tumour initially grows within the canal and thereafter extrudes into the CPA. Depending on the direction of growth of the tumour, the facial nerve may run in a different direction: anterior to the tumour in about 70% of cases, superior in 10%, posterior in 7%, and inferior in 13% of cases (Carlson and Link 2021; Komatsuzaki and Tsunoda 2001; Xenellis and Linthicum 2003; Roosli et al. 2012; Tryggvason et al. 2012).

VS is the most common of CPA tumours. It is a benign, slow-growing tumour with WHO grade 1. The annual growth rate of VS is 1 to 10 mm. The highest incidence is in patients between their fourth and sixth decade of life. VS developing in patients with neurofibromatosis type 2 tends to present earlier. Most VS cases are unilateral and sporadic in nature. Bilateral VS is a hallmark of NF-II. Iodizing radiation is considered a risk factor.

The signs and symptoms of VS are those due to the involvement of cranial nerve VIII itself, as well as those due to involvement of adjacent cranial nerves (VII, V, IX, and X), the cerebellum, and the brainstem. Compression of the fourth ventricle may also produce features of raised ICP. The commonest symptoms of VS are unilateral progressive sensorineural hearing loss, tinnitus, unsteadiness, headache, facial numbness, and diplopia. Usually, they are slow-growing and present insidiously, but they can have acute presentation when there is haemorrhage within the tumour or due to the rapid expansion of a cyst (Carlson and Link 2021; Komatsuzaki and Tsunoda 2001; Xenellis and Linthicum 2003).

6.2. Investigative Considerations

A neuro-otological work-up is necessary to evaluate these tumours. Clinically, the Rinne test and Waber test are conducted to determine the type of deafness. Other specialized testing includes pure-tone audiometry, impedance audiometry, speech discrimination, and auditory evoked response monitoring.

Plain X-ray of the mastoid (Towne view) is still useful as a first step to see the enlargement and/or erosion of the porus acusticus and the internal acoustic canal (IAC). The transorbital projection (Caldwell view) depicts the canal and the meatus in their actual form and size in one single film without interference from other natural artifacts. CT scan with contrast can easily detect a tumour with bone window to demonstrate the classical widening of the internal acoustic meatus. Brain MRI depicts the tumour details, its consistency, and its relationship with critical neurovascular structures (Figure 5). On T1WI, they are isointense, and on T2WI and heterogenous contrast enhancement, they are slightly hyperintense. Due to their containment in the IAC and growth in the extracanalicular region, they can have a recognizable ice cream cone appearance (Carlson and Link 2021; Tryggvason et al. 2012). The Hannover classification (Table 1) is a dependable grading system for grading the size of vestibular schwannomas (Atchley et al. 2022) and can be used in counselling and in the evaluation of postoperative facial nerve and hearing outcomes.

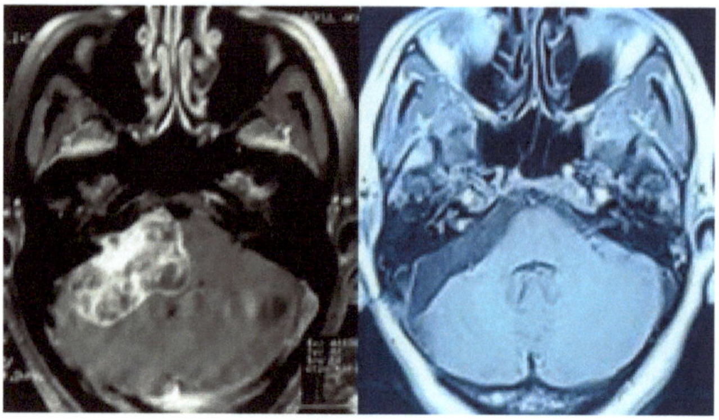

Figure 5. Preoperative and postoperative MRI of a patient with right-sided acoustic schwannoma. Source: Figure by authors.

Table 1. The Hannover classification of vestibular schwannomas.

Grade	Tumour
T1	Purely intracanalicular
T2	Intrameatal or extrameatal
T3A	Filling the cerebellopontine cistern
T3B	Reaching the brainstem
T4A	Compression of brainstem
T4B	Compression of brainstem with dislocation of fourth ventricle

Source: Authors' compilation based on data from Atchley et al. (2022).

6.3. Treatment Considerations

These tumours are very slow-growing. So, if the lesion does not produce significant symptoms, conservative treatment is an option. The therapeutic goals have changed from radical tumour removal to tumour control and to the preservation of neurological function. There are mainly three operative approaches to VS. They are the retromastoid retrosigmoid suboccipital approach, the middle fossa approach, and the translabyrinthine approach. Other special approaches are the transcanal approach, the suboccipital translabyrinthine approach, and the endoscopic approach. Many small tumours (less than 3 cm) are treated by radiosurgery. Gamma Knife surgery has also been used for residual tumour (Carlson and Link 2021; Koos et al. 1993).

Different strategies can be used in resection. The advantage of the retromastoid method is that it preserves hearing, although there is a chance of incomplete resection. This method involves making an incision behind the ear region and mastoid bone. Depending on the size of the tumour, hearing may be preserved using the middle cranial fossa method, which involves making an incision anterior to the ear. Hearing loss is an inevitable outcome of the translabyrinthine method, which passes through the inner ear. This method can be appropriate for individuals who do not have any functional hearing. In general, individuals with large tumours (larger than 4 cm), recurrent tumours following radiation therapy, compression of the brainstem, cranial neuropathy, and hydrocephalus should undergo surgical resection (Carlson and Link 2021).

The retrosigmoid approach is the most versatile as it offers excellent visualization of the CP angle, brainstem, and the IAC (Figure 5). Neuromonitoring for facial nerve and brainstem function and auditory evoked response monitoring for hearing function during the surgery provide tremendous improvement and reduce postoperative morbidity (Carlson and Link 2021).

After exposure, the tumour is debulked with suction and ultrasonic aspiration. The superior and inferior vestibular nerves are exposed and sectioned following meatal drilling to identify the facial nerve. The tumour is dissected away from the facial nerve and cerebellum using neuromonitoring.

Vestibular schwannomas that are surgically removed have a high chance of resection and low risks of recurrence. For the best results, a skilled surgeon and careful patient selection are essential. When 1000 vestibular schwannoma resections were reviewed, the results showed a 98% complete resection rate, a 68% hearing preservation rate, and a 1.1% mortality rate (Samii and Matthies 1997). With total resection, the local recurrence rate is 0–2%. There is around a 30% probability of regrowth if only subtotal resection is feasible (Carlson and Link 2021).

Complications include postoperative CSF leak (9–13%), headache, CN V and VII neuropathies, hearing loss, hydrocephalus, haematoma, aseptic meningitis (2–4%), and hemiparesis (Samii and Matthies 1997).

The management strategy of vestibular schwannoma in NF2 includes microsurgery with or without adjuvant radiation with the aim of preserving hearing and facial function. When choosing a course of treatment, it is critical to consider the needs of the patient, the features of the tumour, and the resources available to the healthcare facility. Treatment options for medium- or small-sized vestibular schwannomas include radiation, surgery, and/or wait-and-scan. There has been a shift in recent years toward the use of planned SRS subsequent to planned subtotal resection. It appears that the late adverse effect of inducing a secondary neoplasm following radiotherapy has very little danger, and novel therapeutic alternatives based on drugs are emerging (Yao et al. 2020).

7. Glomus Tumour

7.1. *Clinical Considerations*

Glomus tumours are also referred to as chemodectomas or paragangliomas. They are benign neuroendocrine tumours that originate from glomus cells and vegetative nervous cells. They can be encountered in many areas of the body. The temporal bone, close to the jugular foramen, is one of the commonest sites. These are the most common tumours that form in the jugular foramen.

Glomus tumours of the cranial base can be broadly categorized into three anatomical descriptions: glomus tympanicum, which is confined to the middle ear (arises from Jacobson's nerve—inferior tympanic branch of cranial nerve IX); glomus jugulare, which is confined to the jugular foramen (arises from the adventitia of the jugular bulb along Arnold's nerve—auricular branch of cranial nerve X or the jugular fossa course of Jacobson's nerve); and glomus jugulotympanicum, which involves both the jugular foramen and the middle ear.

They are slow-growing, abundantly vascular tumours. They are usually benign; however, they may be locally aggressive and extend into the adjacent petrous bone, cerebellopontine angle, and sometimes the neck. They may be asymptomatic when small in size, but large tumours produce pulsatile tinnitus, conductive hearing loss, otalgia, aural fullness, vertigo, dysphagia and/or dysphonia due to lower cranial nerve palsy, facial palsy, Horner's syndrome, and diplopia. Various syndromes, like Vernet's syndrome, Collet–Sicard syndrome, and Villaret's syndrome, are associated with these lesions. Otoscopy classically reveals a red mass (Jayashankar and Sankhla 2015; Kirollos et al. 2019).

7.2. *Investigative Considerations*

Combined CT and MRI are the investigations of choice for the diagnosis and staging of the disease (Figures 6 and 7). CT delineates the bone invasion, which usually has irregular edges. T1WI and T2WI MRI characteristically show mixed signal intensity, described as a salt-and-pepper appearance, reflecting hypervascular signal voids together with focal areas of signal intensity due to intratumoural blood products. Contrast shows avid contrast uptake and demonstrates a smooth tumour contour. Catheter angiography shows a dense, hypervascular tumour blush, often with early venous filling. The two most common staging classifications are the Glasscock–Jackson classification and the Fisch classification (Jayashankar and Sankhla 2015; Kirollos et al. 2019).

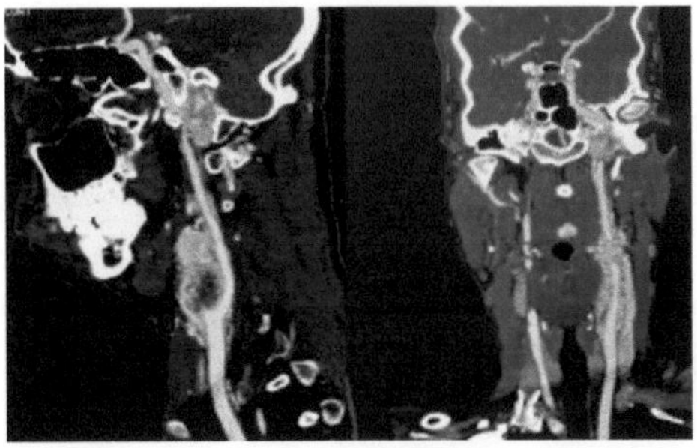

Figure 6. CT and CTA of brain and neck showing left-sided glomus jugulare associated with carotid body tumour. Source: Figure by authhors.

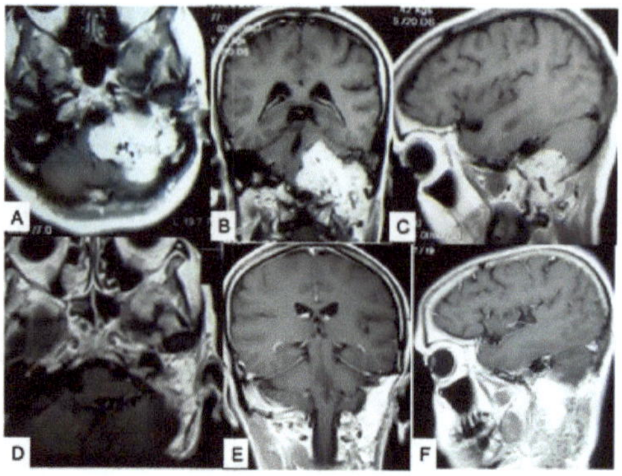

Figure 7. Contrast MRI of head. (**A–C**) Show left-sided large glomus jugulare; (**D–F**) show excision of the tumour. Source: Figure by authors.

7.3. Treatment Considerations

The optimal management of these tumours is challenging and requires a personalized approach administered by an experienced multidisciplinary team. Because of comorbidities, a watch, wait, and rescan policy is often the first line of management. Larger tumours, fast-growing small tumours, and secretory tumours may require treatment with surgery and/or radiotherapy (Jayashankar and Sankhla 2015; Kirollos et al. 2019).

8. Cavernous Sinus Lesion

8.1. Clinical Considerations

The cavernous sinus is a venous plexus located laterally at both sides of the sella turcica which houses important neurovascular structures. For neurosurgeons, the cavernous sinus (CS) region has traditionally presented a difficulty because of its intricate architecture and unique location in the anterolateral skull base. Dolenc's anatomical study and surgical experiences ultimately led to the development of a logical surgical strategy and to the definition of the various relationships between the lesion and the neurovascular structures. Yasargil writes, "There is no doubt that this type of microsurgical anatomical study is a new step in the 100-year history of neurosurgery" in the preface to Dolenc's book (Dolenc and Yasargil 1989). Ali Krisht et al. described the transcavernous microsurgical approach (Krisht et al. 2022).

Pathological findings in the cavernous sinus are diverse and include intrinsic and extrinsic lesions, like vascular, traumatic, inflammatory, congenital, or neoplastic lesions. The primary sites of cavernous sinus metastatic tumours are the breast, prostate, and lung. Primary intracranial tumours include meningioma, haemangioma (Figure 8), neurofibroma, chondroma, and lymphoma. Sometimes, localized tumour spread may occur from nasopharyngeal and pituitary growths.

Cavernous sinus lesions produce symptoms like ophthalmoplegia, chemosis, proptosis, Horner's syndrome, and trigeminal nerve lesions. Depending on the extension of the tumour, it can cause cavernous sinus syndrome or orbital apex syndrome (Chowdhury et al. 2012; Chowdhury and Haque 2017; Al-Mefty and Smith 1988).

8.2. Investigative Considerations

CT scan as well as MRI of the brain delineate the location, extension, and involvement of the cranial nerves and of the internal carotid artery.

8.3. Treatment Considerations

The approach to these tumours is very difficult because of their complex neurovascular structures relationship. The approach can be transcranial or endonasal endoscopic depending on the position of the pathology. In some lesions, SRS is useful (Chowdhury et al. 2012; Chowdhury and Haque 2017; Al-Mefty and Smith 1988).

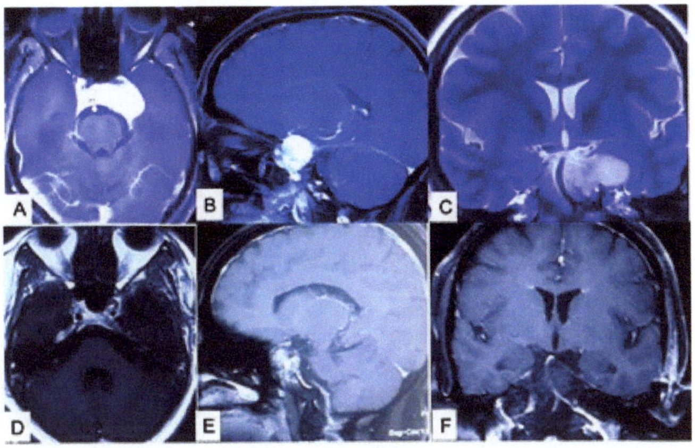

Figure 8. MRI of head. (**A–C**) Preoperative axial, sagittal, and coronal images showing left cavernous haemangioma. (**D–F**) Postoperative images showing excision of tumour. Source: Figure by authors.

8.3.1. Cavernous Sinus Meningioma

Cavernous sinus meningioma (CSM) is the commonest primary cavernous sinus (CS) lesion. The majority of these lesions affect women in their third or fourth decade of life. Any one of the three anatomical presentations of meningiomas can be referred to as a cavernous sinus meningioma. Rarely, a meningioma develops and remains inside the boundaries of the CS proper; other meningiomas mostly originate outside the CS proper and may sporadically penetrate the CS lateral wall; eventually, the majority will spread to encompass both the extracavernous compartments and the CS proper (Raheja and Couldwell 2020).

Clinically, the patient may present with headache, diplopia, visual impairment, (third to sixth) cranial nerve palsy, facial pain, and features of cavernous sinus syndrome. Imaging includes contrast MRI and CT scan of the head and skull base as well as an angiogram.

Today, neurosurgeons face challenges in managing cavernous sinus meningiomas (CSMs) due to inadequate understanding of their natural history, early involvement of critical neurovascular structures, lack of clear tissue planes with normal surrounding structures, and high rate of aggressive surgery-related morbidity. The neurosurgical community's preferred approach has changed over the past few decades from aggressive microsurgical resection to maximal safe resection and the possible application of adjuvant radiotherapy (Raheja and Couldwell 2020). Nowadays, many prefer biopsy and stereotactic radiosurgery (SRS).

8.3.2. Cavernous Sinus Haemangioma

About 3% of benign cavernous sinus masses are cavernous sinus haemangiomas (CSHs), which are more frequent in middle-aged women. Usually slow-growing groups of vascular channels with thin walls, these masses have the ability to affect nearby neurovascular systems mass-wise. These masses can be categorized pathologically into three main categories: mixed, mulberry-like, and sponge-like. The majority of those affected by CSHs are middle-aged women. The symptoms might vary, but headache, altered vision, and cranial nerve palsies, brought on by the mass effect, are common (Noblett et al. 2018).

When it comes to the workup of patients with CSH, MRI is crucial. On T1-weighted imaging, these lesions usually show hypo- or isointensity, and on T2-weighted images, hyperintensity. Resection surgery is the cornerstone of CSH treatment. However, when a tumour is found in the cavernous sinus, up to 40% of tumours show significant intraoperative bleeding; therefore, the decision to perform total surgical excision must be carefully evaluated against the risks of neurovascular injury. Patients who have limited subtotal resection or inoperable lesions may benefit from stereotactic radiosurgery. It has been demonstrated that Gamma Knife radiosurgery (GKS) can considerably reduce tumour size and volume, in addition to relieving some of the neurological symptoms related to CSH (Noblett et al. 2018).

9. Orbital Tumour

There are seven bones that contribute to the bony orbit: 1. pars orbitalis of the frontal bone; 2. lacrimal bone; 3. lamina papyracea of the ethmoid bone; 4. orbital process of the zygomatic bone; 5. orbital surface of the maxillary bone; 6. orbital process of the palatine bone; 7. greater and lesser wings and body of the sphenoid bone. The orbits are bony structures of the skull that house the globe, extraocular muscles, nerves, blood vessels, lacrimal apparatus, and adipose tissue. Common orbital tumours are lymphoma, metastases, lacrimal gland tumours, rhabdomyosarcoma, retinoblastoma, optic nerve glioma, optic nerve sheath meningioma, schwannoma/neurofibroma, choristoma, dermoid, epidermoid, teratoma, haemangioma/cavernoma, lymphangioma, orbital pseudotumour, and orbital sarcoidosis.

9.1. *Clinical Considerations*

Orbital tumours are rare. Tumours may arise from the globe, from the bony orbit, or from any content within the orbit. The commonest malignant orbital tumours in the adult population are metastatic tumours.

Orbital tumours produce symptoms and signs either due to the compression, infiltration, or infarction of orbital structures. Patients with orbital tumours may present with proptosis, diplopia due to external or internal ophthalmoplegia, visual disturbance, eye pain, chemosis, and sensory impairment. Intraconal tumours usually produce axial proptosis; extraconal lesion push the eye out of the lesion. Proptosis may be caused by lesions located outside the orbit, like cavernous sinus lesions. Pulsatile proptosis usually occurs due to a vascular lesion within the orbit or due to a carotid cavernous fistula. Visual impairment may occur in the form of loss of vision—either complete, incomplete, or transient—or visual field defects. Compression of the optic nerve may cause either primary optic atrophy, as in optic nerve glioma and optic nerve sheath meningioma, or optic nerve disc swelling. Usually, inflammatory and malignant lesions produce orbital pain (Chagla 2012; Mercandetti 2019).

9.2. *Investigative Considerations*

The assessment of orbital tumours requires formal visual assessment, which includes visual acuity, visual field analysis, colour vision, and fundoscopy. Plain X-ray of the orbit may reveal bony erosion, sclerosis, or calcification. CT scan of the orbit provides the localization of the tumour, bony changes, calcification, and enhancement of the pathology. Contrast-enhanced MRI is the investigation of choice as it shows soft-tissue structures well (Figure 9). Angiography is sometimes required for vascular lesions like meningioma, haemangiopericytoma, dural AVM, or carotid cavernous fistula. Sometimes, ultrasonography may be helpful in detecting lesions in the anterior segment of retrobulbar tumours (Chagla 2012; Mercandetti 2019).

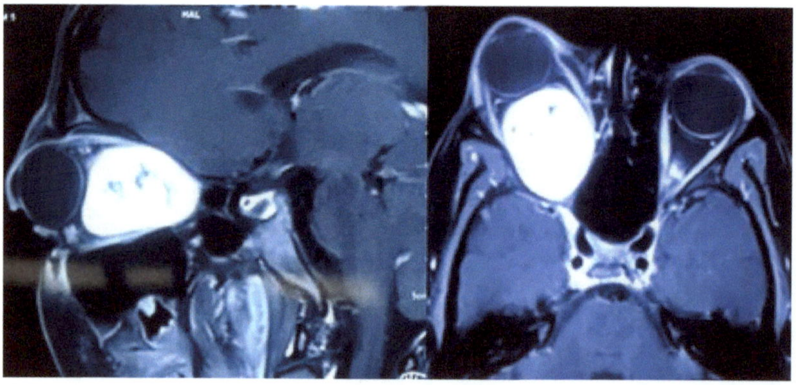

Figure 9. Contrast MRI of brain and orbit showing huge right-sided retrobulbar schwannoma. Source: Figure by authors.

9.3. *Treatment Considerations*

The management of orbital tumours involves clinicians from a variety of surgical disciplines, including neurosurgeons, ophthalmologists, ENT specialists, maxillofacial surgeons, and skull base endoscopic surgeons. The surgical approaches can be transcranial, orbital, and endoscopic. The cranium provides a safe access to the orbit; hence, it is imperative for neurosurgeons to have knowledge on the orbit. There are different ways to approach it transcranially, like a subfrontal approach with superior osteotomy, fronto-orbito-zygomatic craniotomy, fronto-orbito-zygomaticotemporal craniotomy, or lateral orbitotomy. Transcranial approaches are best for lateral, superior, and posteriorly located tumours. The endoscopic approach is best for medially located lesions medial to the optic nerve (Chagla 2012; Mercandetti 2019).

10. Surgical Approaches to the Skull Base

10.1. Pterional Craniotomy

Pterional craniotomy (Figure 10) is a very important daily neurosurgical practice, which is why it requires excellent execution knowledge. Aneurysms of the anterior circulation, basilar apex, the proximal segment of the superior cerebellar and posterior cerebral arteries, arteriovenous malformations and cavernous haemangiomas of the basal forebrain, anterior and middle skull base tumours, gliomas of the frontal, parietal, and temporal opercula, insula, mediobasal temporal region, cerebral peduncles, interpeduncular fossa, and orbital lesions are treated in the pterional trans-sylvian corridor. In order to increase surgical freedom and lower the risk of complications associated with the approach, an overview of the fundamental methods and variations of the pterional approach are described here.

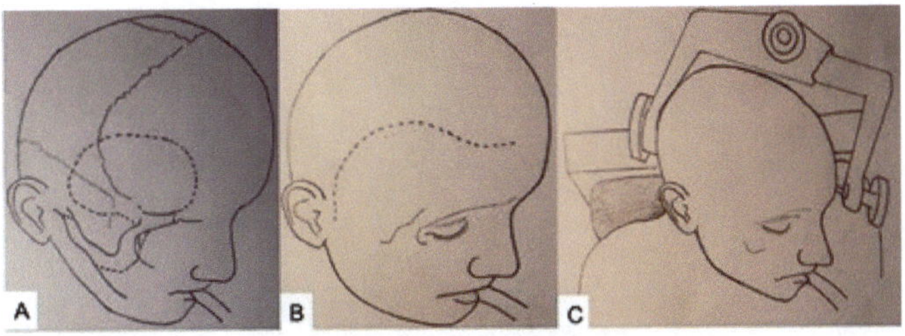

Figure 10. Hand drawings showing (**A**) removal of bone in pterional craniotomy; (**B**) incision mark for pterional craniotomy; (**C**) head positioning and fixation in pterional craniotomy. Source: Figure by authors.

Positioning: To enable the best possible venous outflow, the patient is put supine with their head elevated above the level of the heart by 30° and secured to a Mayfield–Kees or Sugita skull clamp. Yasargil, in 1976, advocated for an extension of about 20° in his classic description. The malar eminence is to be the highest point of the horizon. It is advised to rotate the head contralaterally, with a range of 15°–45° depending on the particular neurovascular target (Yaşargil 1984; Yaşargil et al. 1987).

Incision: Local subcutaneous infiltration of lignocaine and adrenaline diluted in normal saline is useful to reduce pain and enable easier detachment of the skin from the subcutaneous layers. The skin incision starts 1 cm in front of the tragus, anteriorly to the superficial temporal artery and auriculotemporal nerve. The incision curves upward, behind the hairline, to reach the midline. The skin flap is divided by the temporalis muscle and reflected forward. To avoid damaging the frontal branch of the facial nerve, the superficial layer of the temporal fascia and the fat pad within which the nerve courses are separated from the deep layer (interfascial technique).

Two different ways can be followed. In the subfascial technique, an incision into the superficial and deep layers of the superficial temporal fascia is made. In the submuscular technique, an incision into the deep temporal fascia, subperiosteal blunt dissection of the temporalis muscle, and forward reflection of the myocutaneous flap are performed.

The submuscular technique is quicker and poses less risk of intraoperative damage to the frontal branch of the facial nerve, which is why this is mostly practiced. Regardless of the method, the temporalis muscle needs to be cut above the posterior root of the zygoma and subperiosteally detached in a manner that is retrograde, going superior-to-posterior and back-to-front, as described by Oikawa et al. Electrocauterization must be avoided to preserve the anatomical continuity of the deep fascia along with blood supply from the internal maxillary artery. To avoid functional and cosmetic issues as well as atrophy of the temporalis muscle, it is imperative to preserve the deep fascia (Zabramski et al. 1998; Coscarella et al. 2000). Recognizing skull sutures can also be aided by a compulsive subperiosteal dissection of the muscle. The fronto-zygomatic suture and the superior aspect of the posterior root of the zygomatic process of the temporal bone should always be visible.

Craniotomy: The MacCarty keyhole, which is drilled 5 mm behind the point where the fronto-zygomatic, spheno-zygomatic, and frontosphenoidal sutures intersect, allows for access to the dura of the anterior cranial fossa and periorbita (Shimizu et al. 2005). To access the anterior cranial fossa, the first burr hole can be created slightly above the MacCarty keyhole when treating the pathology, which does not require the exposure of the orbit and its contents. The second burr hole is to be made at the level of the temporal squama, above the posterior root of the zygoma.

The extensive drilling of the lateral portion of the larger sphenoid wing until the SOF is a crucial step in the pterional approach. This makes the sphenoidal part of the sylvian fissure, which serves as the entrance to the entire anterior and middle skull base (Figure 11), fully visible. The dural flap can be reflected with the aid of skeletonization and partial expansion of the SOF. It is advised to use a drill to thin the orbital roof in order to create a working corridor and line of sight as close to the anterior cerebral fossa as feasible. This approach is termed the "extended pterional approach". These adjustments allow for unhindered surgical approaches to subfrontal and parasellar targets. Osteotomy along the orbital roof has some of the same advantages as orbito-zygomatic craniotomy, but it is a more effective operation with fewer cosmetic deformities.

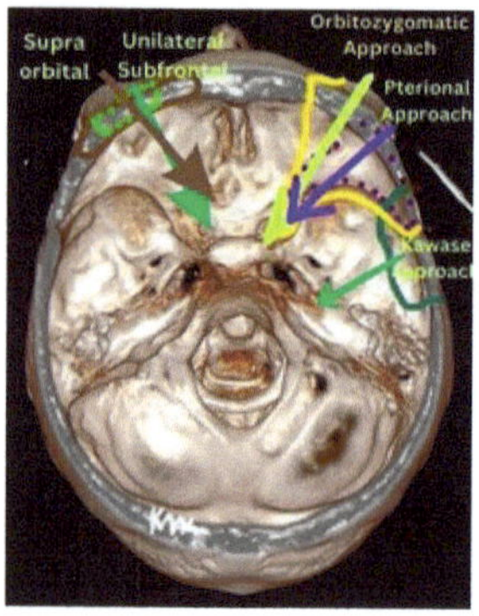

Figure 11. Skull base showing approaches to bony corridor of anterior and middle fossa. Source: Figure by authors.

10.2. Orbito-zygomatic Craniotomy

Skull base approaches were revolutionized in the 1990s, when OZ (Figure 12) began to be the mainstay of the skull base for accessing the sellar and parasellar regions, and complex skull base techniques began to be used. However, there are a few drawbacks and cosmetic concerns to this method. These include diplopia, exophthalmos, enophthalmos, forehead hypaesthesia and dysaesthesia, frontal muscular weakness, and persistent periorbital and eyelid oedema, which can be avoided by deploying the extended pterional approach when possible.

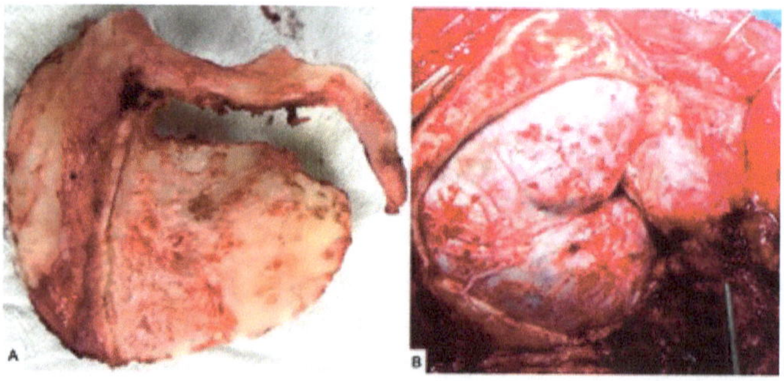

Figure 12. (**A**) Right-sided one-piece OZ craniotomy bone flap; (**B**) right-sided OZ craniotomy after bone flap removal. Source: Figure by authors.

The cranio-orbito-zygomatic (COZ) approach is an extension of the pterional approach, involving the adjunct of orbito-zygomatic (OZ) osteotomy to allow for wider exposure of the anterior and middle skull base and upper retroclival region. It provides advantages when treating giant aneurysms of the anterior communicating artery (ACoA) and distal basilar artery, tuberculum sellae, large anterior clinoidal and spheno-orbital meningiomas, large craniopharyngiomas, giant pituitary adenomas, cavernous haemangiomas of the hypothalamus, and crus cerebri of the midbrain.

Placement and positioning: This is fairly similar to the pterional approach described above. A 30° rotation of the head makes the longer axis of the anterior clinoid process perpendicular to the floor, while at 45°, the surgical view of the subfrontal area is maximized.

Skin incision and soft-tissue dissection: The skin incision is made in a curvilinear fashion behind the hairline and goes from 1 cm anterior to the tragus to the contralateral midpupillary line. The dissection of soft tissue is fairly similar to the pterional approach described above.

Craniotomy: The COZ approach can be executed in a one-piece, two-piece, or three-piece technique.

In the one-piece COZ approach, the MacCarty keyhole is positioned 5 mm behind the junction between the fronto-zygomatic, spheno-zygomatic, and frontosphenoidal sutures. Two further burr holes are placed in the temporal squama, above the posterior root of the zygoma and on the superior temporal line, respectively. The first cut involves the posterior root of the zygoma and is carried out with a reciprocating saw. The second cut connects the keyhole to the inferior orbital fissure (IOF). The third cut starts at the level of the lateral orbital wall and is advanced across the malar eminence. The fourth cut is made at the intraorbital side and crosses the superior orbital rim and the orbital roof until the lateral aspect of the SOF. The keyhole, temporal, and frontal burr holes are interconnected with the craniotome. The COZ bone flap is then fractured by inserting and gently rotating a periosteal elevator into the groove made by the cut of the superior orbital rim. The temporalis muscle and the galea-pericranium flap are reflected downward. The tent stitches of the galea displace the eyeball slightly inferiorly, flattening the exposure of the anterior cranial fossa by a few millimetres. Drilling of the temporal squama can adequately expose the middle fossa, whereas drilling of the lesser sphenoid wing, along with an extra- or intradural anterior clinoidectomy, expands the surgical access to most targets related to this approach.

The two-piece COZ approach can be executed through two different techniques. In the Zabramski technique, after the pterional craniotomy, subtraction of the OZ bar is realized through six cuts. As in the one-piece technique, the first cut is made at the level of the posterior root of the zygoma. The second cut involves the malar eminence, from lateral to medial. The third cut is carried out across the lateral orbital wall, from medial to lateral. The fourth cut is intracranial, involves the orbital roof and the superior orbital rim, and is executed starting from the lateral end of the SOF, taking care to preserve the underlying periorbita. The fifth and sixth cuts connect the SOF and the IOF, thus freeing the lateral orbital wall. The fifth cut starts at the level of the IOF and ends at the level of the anterior part of the middle fossa. The sixth cut moves from the IOF toward the fifth cut. The OZ bar is then detached from the masseter muscle (Zabramski et al. 1998).

In the Al-Mefty technique, the orbitopterional two-piece COZ approach includes two zygomatic cuts involving the anterior and posterior root of the zygoma, respectively. The zygomatic arch is mobilized inferiorly without detachment of the masseter muscle, thus avoiding the risk of postoperative masticatory imbalance. The other steps are those of the one-piece variant of the COZ approach, where all the cuts are carried out extracranially (Al-Mefty 1987).

The three-piece COZ approach consists of a combination of both two-piece variants. It involves zygomatic osteotomy without detachment of the masseter, inferior mobilization of the zygomatic arch, pterional bone flap, and orbital osteotomy as separate pieces entailing the superolateral orbital rim and the orbital roof.

After opening the dura, the COZ approach allows for four different corridors: (1) subfrontal, (2) trans-sylvian, (3) pretemporal, and (4) subtemporal. The trans-sylvian and pretemporal corridors are related to four well-defined deep windows to the infratentorial region through the opening of the Liliequist membrane. The deep windows are as follows: (1) optic–carotid, (2) carotid–oculomotor, (3) supracarotid, and (4) oculomotor–tentorial.

10.3. Subtemporal Approach

A surgical pathway to several lesions located in the middle cerebral fossa was made available via temporal craniotomies. By the 1960s, Drake's groundbreaking work in surgically treating over 1700 posterior circulation and basilar aneurysms had brought the subtemporal technique into a thriving phase. To access the perimesencephalic and midclival regions, various variants of the subtemporal routes were created, including the subtemporal keyhole approach, expanded exposure with zygomatic excision, and removal of the petrous apex (Drake 1965).

Steps of approach: After anaesthesia, lumbar drain should strongly be considered based on the pathology for which surgery is being undertaken. The head is rotated to the contralateral side, aligning the anterior–posterior axis parallel with the floor. The vertex is slightly tilted down toward the floor for efficient intraoperative viewing trajectory as the base of the middle cranial fossa inclines upward steeply. Operating as close to the base of the middle cranial fossa of the skull as possible is the goal of the subtemporal approach. As a result, the skin incision should be made so that the temporal squama is exposed, at the very least, to the zygomatic arch root. An inverted U-shaped skin incision is often performed 1–2 cm anterior to the tragus, starting at the level of the zygomatic arch root. The incision is made around the ear, curving anteriorly, upwards, and finally backward across the pinna. Alternatively, for a minimized temporal bone flap, a linear skin incision can be made from the inferior rim of the zygomatic arch, approximately one finger's width, anterior to the external auditory canal.

The skin flap is then reflected inferiorly, and the temporalis muscle is divided and reflected as well, exposing the zygomatic process of the temporal bone and the root of the zygomatic arch. A 4–5 cm-sized craniotomy at the exposed temporal squama is performed, placing the inferior border of the bone flap as low as possible. If mastoid air cells are inadvertently opened, careful closure by bone waxing or temporal muscle flap should be completed. The inferior overhanging edge of the temporal bone needs to be drilled down flush with the base of the middle cranial fossa (Yasargil et al. 1976; Kawase et al. 1991; Hernesniemi et al. 2005).

10.4. Kawase Approach

The Kawase approach, first described by Kawase et al. in 1985, has added the step of removal of the bones in the petrous apex to the standard subtemporal approach. As the Kawase approach and the extended Kawase approach significantly expanded the exposure range in the upper, middle, and partial inferior regions of the clivus, this approach is used extensively. The approach overcomes the obstructions of the petrosal range and extends the region exposed in the posterior cranial fossa without bringing more retraction of the temporal lobe and Labei's vein, due to which many lesions in the petrosal apex and the upper and middle clivus, including meningioma, chordoma, basilar trunk aneurysm, prepontine epidermoid, trigeminal schwannoma, and pontine cavernoma, could be satisfactorily exposed and safely resected. The gains in the exposure volume and area are more when the manipulation angle is less than 135° (Kawase et al. 1985).

When using the traditional Kawase method, the drilling range of the bone is restricted to the petrosal apex, with a rhomboid shape by the view from the lateral–superior direction. The posterior margin of the trigeminal nerve anteriorly, the petrosal ridge medially, the greater superficial petrosal nerve or petrosal segment of the internal carotid artery laterally, and the arcuate eminence posteriorly define the boundaries of the rhomboid. Restricted is the deep boundary of debone, which is also the boundary between clivus and the petrosal apex. It would be possible to expand the Kawase method by drilling bones outside of the IPS. It could expand the deboning range to the upper and middle clivus and the jugular tubercle (JT).

10.5. Transpetrosal Approaches to the Posterior Fossa

Different degrees of resection of the petrous temporal bone provide for varying degrees of access to posterior fossa lesions. The many variations of transpetrosal techniques can be roughly divided into anterior and posterior groups, despite the nomenclature often being unclear. While the techniques in the anterior group are variations of the fundamental middle fossa approach, the posterior transpetrosal procedures comprise the retrolabyrinthine, translabyrinthine, and transcochlear approaches. The petroclival region and the cerebellopontine angle can potentially be exposed from both the anterior and posterior approaches. The posterior techniques entail varying degrees of petrous bone resection and are based on standard mastoidectomy. This results in progressively increased exposure anteriorly, but in the translabyrinthine approach, hearing is lost, and in the transcochlear approach, hearing and facial strength are lost. On the other hand, the middle fossa techniques entail varying degrees of medial petrous bone excision while sparing the lateral petrous bone. The goal of any middle fossa method is to protect hearing. In order to expose the posterior fossa, extensions of the middle fossa techniques entail the resection of bone within the Kawase rhomboid and division of the tentorium (Tummala et al. 2005).

10.6. Retrosigmoid Approach

In Figure 13 surgical approaches to the bony corridor of the posterior skull base are shown. The retrosigmoid approach (Figure 14) is the workhorse for posterior fossa surgery because of its advantage in providing a versatile corridor to tackle different types of lesions in and around the cerebellopontine angle. Bony anatomical landmarks are helpful in localizing the venous sinuses and planning the craniotomy. Extensions of the approach include, among others, the transmastoid, supracerebellar, far lateral, jugular foramen, and perimeatal approaches. The retrosigmoid approach applies to a broad range of pathologies and, with its extensions, can provide adequate exposure, obviating the need for extensive and complicated approaches.

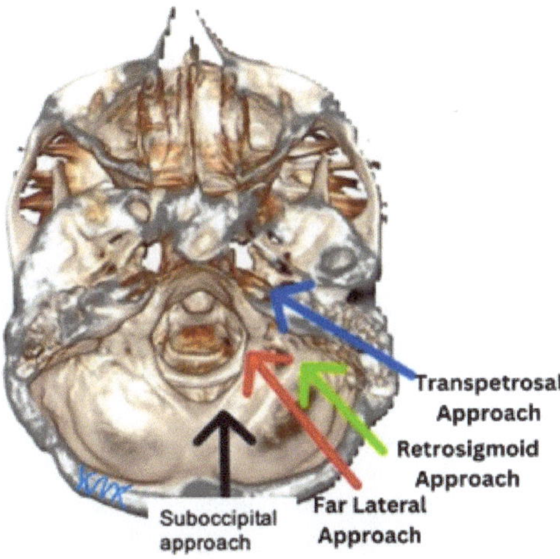

Figure 13. Skull base showing the approaches to the bony corridor of the posterior skull base. Source: Figure by authors.

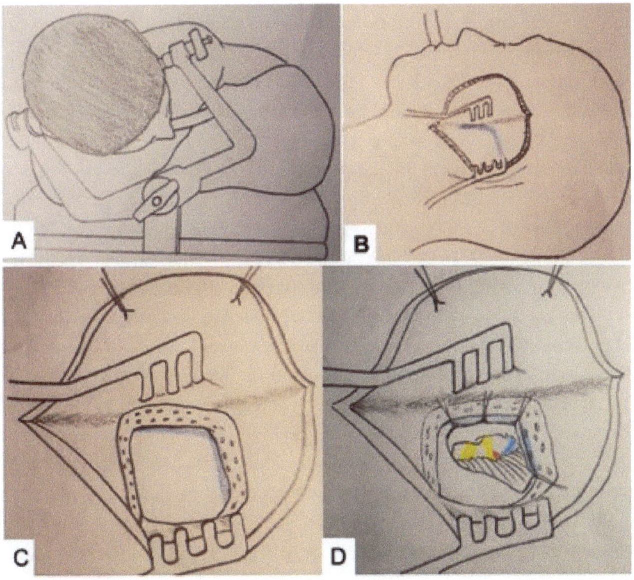

Figure 14. Hand drawings of retrosigmoid craniotomy. (**A**) Positioning and head fixation; (**B**) skin incision and exposure; (**C**) craniotomy; (**D**) after dural opening. Source: Figure by authors.

The retrosigmoid or lateral suboccipital approach was popularized by Woolsey and Krause in the early 1900s. After several modifications, the lateral suboccipital approach evolved into what is now called the retrosigmoid approach. This approach provides optimal access to the cerebellopontine and cerebellomedullary cisterns. The retrosigmoid approach uses a lateral suboccipital craniotomy combined with a partial mastoidectomy to enter the dorsolateral aspect of the posterior fossa. This is the most widely used approach for vestibular schwannoma and other lesions which require the exposure of the brainstem and cranial nerves. It is also used for aneurysms of the anterior inferior cerebellar artery, the posterior inferior cerebellar artery, and basilar trunk. Microvascular decompression of the trigeminal nerve can also be treated through this approach. Small-to-medium-size tumours of the internal auditory canal can be excised with the preservation of hearing (Elhammady et al. 2012).

These patients can be positioned in a sitting, supine, or lateral decubitus position, with lateral decubitus being the most common. Care should be taken to preserve the lesser occipital and greater auricular nerves to reduce postoperative headache and dysaesthesia. Hearing preservation is one of the main advantages of the retrosigmoid approach to resection in vestibular schwannoma treatment, as opposed to the translabyrinthine approach, in which the inner ear structures are sacrificed. Postoperative complications include retraction injury to the cerebellum, venous sinus injury, damage to the cranial nerves and brainstem, as well as postoperative CSF leaks. In particular, the mastoid emissary vein should be located during craniotomy exposure because it can cause substantial bleeding and be the source of an air embolism. Injury to the vertebral artery can also occur during osteotomy of the lower portion of the exposure at the occipital bone.

The RS approach may be carried out with the patient in the supine, lateral, park-bench, sitting, or semi-sitting position. While every surgeon may have different preferences according to the specific case, this section will describe the operation in the semilateral position. The patient is positioned supine on the operating table with the operative side up. The ipsilateral shoulder is bolstered to rotate the patient's torso into a semilateral position, and the patient should be well secured onto the operating table. The head is rotated about 70-80 degrees to the contralateral side, flexed slightly anteriorly and towards the floor to open the angle between the occiput and the neck, and secured in place with a Mayfield clamp pin fixation.

In the RS approach, the single-pin arm is positioned just above the ipsilateral superior temporal line, behind the hairline and anterior to the EAM, avoiding the forehead, and the double-pin arm is positioned just superior and posterior to the contralateral superior nuchal line, avoiding the suboccipital muscles. To widen the angle even more and create more workspace, the ipsilateral shoulder could also be taped down. In the surgical field, the mastoid tip ought to be the highest point. Patients with medium-sized to large tumours may benefit from the placement of a lumbar drain at this time to aid in the draining of cerebrospinal fluid (CSF).

Incision of the skin: The common variations of skin incisions for the RS approach are the linear, lazy S-shaped, C-shaped, and curvilinear inverted U-shaped incisions. After using the zygoma–inion line and mastoid tip–asterion line to approximate the TS, SS, and TSSJ, a C-shaped incision is drawn from 2 cm superior to the middle of the pinna to 1 cm medial to the mastoid tip with the apex of the curve 5 cm posterior to the postauricular crease. The incision may be extended inferiorly depending on the case.

The skin is incised over the region of the temporalis muscle. The incision continues towards the mastoid tip, making sure to cut through subcutaneous adipose tissue, which may decrease the risk of greater auricular nerve and lesser occipital nerve (LON) damage. Special attention needs to be paid to the superior half of the incision to visualize and preserve the LON because it is more superficial and enters the region at the posterior edge of the subcutaneous tissue (approximately at the 4 o'clock position for the left side and at the 8 o'clock position for the right side). The skin flap is then elevated with the fascia of the posterior auricular muscle and the sternocleidomastoid muscle and retracted anteriorly over the mastoid process.

Dissection of the muscles: Traditionally, muscle dissection in the RS approach has been described as following the skin incision. The underlying muscles can be incised in line with the skin to create a single myocutaneous flap and retracted anteriorly in a C-shaped skin incision, divided in line with the skin and retracted anteriorly and posteriorly in a slightly curved skin incision, or a single myocutaneous flap based along the suboccipital muscles can be reflected inferiorly in an inverted U-shaped skin incision.

Craniotomy: Following the retraction of soft tissues, a craniectomy or craniotomy may be performed. The number of burr holes depends on the patient's underlying pathology and on their age. Typically, more burr holes or a craniectomy should be employed for patients over 60 years old because the dura is more attached to the cranial surface. The craniotomy may be limited to just the edge of the TS and SS in the standard RS approach or further extended to expose the sinuses with a limited posterior mastoidectomy in the extended approach.

In the standard RS approach, the most important burr hole, which should expose the junction of posterior fossa dura and the margins of the adjacent transverse sinus and sigmoid sinus, is conventionally placed over the asterion or slightly below it; however, it is also argued that the Teranishi technique (placing the burr hole 6.5mm inferior and 6.5mm anterior to the asterion) or the Ribas technique (10 mm anterior to the asterion with the superior edge of burr hole adjacent to the parietomastoid suture) are the most suitable approaches for the placement of the initial burr hole in the standard and extended RS approach, respectively.

When performing the craniotomy, it is preferable to preserve its shape by starting and completing the cut from the outermost edge of the burr hole to keep the perimeter of the craniotomy as flush as possible. Any exposed mastoid air cells are sealed with bone wax or fibrin glue to prevent postoperative CSF leakage.

10.7. Suboccipital Craniotomy

Suboccipital craniotomy and craniectomy are performed by removing the caudal portion of the occipital bone. Wide exposure to approach the posterior fossa was performed early in the disease course to avoid brainstem compression during surgery and to allow for posterior fossa decompression. Suboccipital craniectomy is the standard treatment for Chiari 1 malformation. The posterior fossa is the deepest of the three cranial fossae, containing a complex anatomy, including the cerebellar hemispheres and vermis, brainstem, cranial nerves, and vasculature. Neurophysiological monitoring is used during risky procedures. Access to the posterior fossa can be gained through the suboccipital approach, allowing for the treatment of the cerebellar hemispheres, cerebellar tonsils and vermis, medulla, and fourth ventricle. In addition, lesions of the craniocervical junction and foramen magnum can be accessed. Patients with Chiari 1 malformation also undergo resection of the C1 posterior arch (Perneczky and Reisch 2008).

Patients can be operated in either the prone, lateral decubitus, or sitting position. The prone position has a lower risk of venous air embolism, but blood may pool within the operative bed, limiting visibility. There is also more pressure placed on the face. The lateral position carries a decreased risk of venous air embolism than the sitting position, but the upper cerebellar hemisphere may fall into the surgical field and interfere with the approach. The sitting position carries a higher risk of cardiopulmonary instability, venous air embolism, and rapid CSF leak, which can result in brain herniation. In cases where opening of the dura is necessary, duraplasty is performed using the nuchal ligament, pericranium from the occipital bone, or a dural substitute. Surgery in the posterior fossa has been reported to carry a complication rate as high as 32%. CSF leaks are the most common surgical complication in the posterior fossa. Cerebellar mutism is a rare complication, occurring in less than 1% of patients and manifesting as slow or frank mutism (Ngwenya et al. 2012). It is transient and thought to be secondary to oedema or ischaemia to the dentate nucleus or pathways of the dentatorubrothalamic tract.

Author Contributions: Conceptualization, F.H.C.; methodology, validation, formal analysis, investigation, resources, data curation, M.R.H., R.A.K. and K.A.K.; writing—original draft preparation, R.A.K. and K.A.K.; writing—review and editing, visualization, supervision, F.H.C. All authors have read and agreed to the published version of the manuscript.

Funding: This research received no external funding.

Acknowledgments: Hafiz Asif Raihan, neurosurgeon, National Institute of Neurosciences and hospital.

Conflicts of Interest: The authors declare no conflict of interest.

References

Agarwal, Ajay. 2015. Intracranial trigeminal schwannoma. *The Neuroradiology Journal* 28: 36–41. [CrossRef] [PubMed]

Al-Mefty, Osama. 1987. Supraorbital-Pterional Approach to Skull Base Lesions. *Neurosurgery* 21: 474–77. [CrossRef] [PubMed]

Al-Mefty, Osama, and Robert R. Smith. 1988. Surgery of tumors invading the cavernous sinus. *Surgical Neurology* 30: 370–81. [CrossRef]

Atchley, Travis J., Nicholas Erickson, Gustavo Chagoya, Matthew Fort, Beverly C. Walters, Benjamin McGrew, and Winfield S. Fisher III. 2022. Hannover Classification of Vestibular Schwannomas: A Reliability Study. *World Neurosurgery* 158: e179–e183. [CrossRef] [PubMed]

Carlson, Matthew L., and Michael J. Link. 2021. Vestibular Schwannomas. *The New England Journal of Medicine* 384: 1335–48. [CrossRef]

Chagla, Aadil S. 2012. Orbital Tumours. In *Textbook of Neurosurgery*. Edited by Prakash Narain Tandon and Ravi Ramamurthi. Joypur: Jaypee Brothers Medical Publishers, pp. 2026–44. [CrossRef]

Chowdhury, Forhad H., and Mohammod Haque. 2017. Microsurgical management of benign lesions interior to the cavernous sinus: A case series. *Asian Journal of Neurosurgery* 12: 398–406. [CrossRef] [PubMed]

Chowdhury, Forhad H., Mohammod R. Haque, Khandkar A. Kawsar, Mainul H. Sarker, M. Hasan, and Atul H. Goel. 2014. Intracranial nonvestibular neurinomas: Young neurosurgeons' experience. *Journal of Neurosciences in Rural Practice* 5: 231–43. [CrossRef]

Chowdhury, Forhad H., Mohammod R. Haque, Khandkar A. Kawsar, Shamim Ara, Quazi D. Mohammod, Mainul H. Sarker, and Atul Goel. 2012. Transcranial Microsurgical and Endoscopic Endonasal Cavernous Sinus (CS) Anatomy: A Cadaveric Study. *Journal of Neurological Surgery Part A* 73: 296–306. [CrossRef]

Chugh, Rashmi, Hussein Tawbi, David R. Lucas, J. Sybil Biermann, Scott M. Schuetze, and Laurence H. Baker. 2007. Chordoma: The nonsarcoma primary bone tumor. *Oncologist* 12: 1344–50. [CrossRef]

Coscarella, Ernesto, A. Giancarlo Vishteh, Robert F. Spetzler, Eduardo Seoane, and Joseph M. Zabramski. 2000. Subfascial and submuscular methods of temporal muscle dissection and their relationship to the frontal branch of the facial nerve. *Journal of Neurosurgery* 92: 877–80. [CrossRef]

Dolenc, Vinko V., and Mahmut G. Yasargil. 1989. *Anatomy and Surgery of the Cavernous Sinus*. Wien: Springer.

Drake, Charles G. 1965. Surgical treatment of ruptured aneurysms of the basilar artery. Experience with 14 cases. *Journal of Neurosurgery* 23: 457–73. [CrossRef]

Elhammady, Mohamed Samy, Fred F. Telischi, and Jacques J. Morcos. 2012. Retrosigmoid approach: Indications, techniques, and results. *Otolaryngologic Clinics of North America* 45: 375–97. [CrossRef]

Fiani, Brian, Syed A. Quadri, Alessandra Cathel, Mudassir Farooqui, Anirudh Ramachandran, Imran Siddiqi, Hammad Ghanchi, Atif Zafar, Blake W. Berman, and Javed Siddiqi. 2019. Esthesioneuroblastoma: A Comprehensive Review of Diagnosis, Management, and Current Treatment Options. *World Neurosurgery* 126: 194–211. [CrossRef] [PubMed]

Garça, Mehmet Fatih, Sevil Ari Yuca, and Koksal Yuca. 2010. Juvenile Nasopharyngeal Angiofibroma. *European Journal of General Medicine* 7: 419–25. [CrossRef]

Hernesniemi, Juha, Keisuke Ishii, Mika Niemelä, Leena Kivipelto, M. Fujiki, and Hu Shen. 2005. Subtemporal approach to basilar bifurcation aneurysms: Advanced technique and clinical experience. *Acta Neurochirurgica Supplement* 94: 31–38. [CrossRef] [PubMed]

Jayashankar, Narayan, and Suresh Sankhla. 2015. Current perspectives in the management of glomus jugulare tumors. *Neurology India* 63: 83–90. [CrossRef]

Jefferson, Geoffrey. 1955. The trigeminal neurinomas with some remarks on malignant invasion of the Gasserian ganglion. *Clinical Neurosurgery* 1: 11–54. [CrossRef] [PubMed]

Kawase, Takeshi, Ryuzo Shiobara, and Shigeo Toya. 1991. Anterior transpetrosal-transtentorial approach for sphenopetroclival meningiomas: Surgical methods and results in 10 patients. *Neurosurgery* 28: 869–76. [CrossRef]

Kawase, Takeshi, Shigeo Toya, Ryuzo Shiobara, and Toru Mine. 1985. Transpetrosal approach for aneurysms of the lower basilar artery. *Journal of Neurosurgery* 63: 857–61. [CrossRef]

Kirollos, Ramez W., Adel Helmy, Simon Thomason, and Peter J. A. Hutchinson. 2019. *Oxford Textbook of Neurological Surgery*. Oxford: Oxford University Press.

Komatsuzaki, Atsushi, and Atsunobu Tsunoda. 2001. Nerve origin of the acoustic neuroma. *The Journal of Laryngology & Otology* 115: 376–79. [CrossRef]

Koos, Wolfgang T., Robert F. Spetzler, and Johannes Lang. 1993. Neurinoma of the statoacoustic nerve. In *Colour Atlas of Microneurosurgery*. Edited by Wolfgang T. Koos and Robert F. Spetzler. Stuttgart: Georg Thieme Verlag, p. 530.

Krisht, Ali F., Jaafar Basma, and Li Cai. 2022. Transcavernous Approach in Vascular Neurosurgery. *Neurosurgery Clinics of North America* 33: e1–e6. [CrossRef] [PubMed]

Kumar, Ritesh. 2015. Esthesioneuroblastoma: Multimodal management and review of literature. *World Journal of Clinical Cases* 3: 774–78. [CrossRef]

Martins, Mariane Barreto Brandão, Francis Vinicius Fontes de Lima, Carlos Alberto Mendonça, Eduardo Passos Fiel de Jesus, Arlete Cristina Granizo Santos, Valéria Maria Prado Barreto, and Ronaldo Carvalho Santos Júnior. 2013. Nasopharyngeal angiofibroma: Our experience and literature review. *International Archives of Otorhinolaryngology* 17: 14–9. [CrossRef] [PubMed]

Mercandetti, Michael. 2019. Orbital Tumors. Available online: https://emedicine.medscape.com/article/1218892-overview?scode=msp&st=fpf&anfErrHint=true&icd=login_error_gg_mismatch_fpf&client=205502&urlCache=aHR0cHM6Ly9lbWVkaWNpbmUubWVkc2NhcGUuY29tL2FydGljbGUvMTIxODg5Mi1vdmVydmlldz9mb3JtPWZwZiZzY29kZT1tc3Amc3Q9ZnBmJnNvY2lhbFNpdGU9Z29vZ2xl&su=jL4upPHuiWTJgj0/YssAXwkUJ/7c7W7HHmGquUjiPzKFke/7ELbJjLhp658Y5czh&form=fpf (accessed on 27 July 2022).

Ngwenya, Laura B., Mirza N. Baig, Manish K. Aghi, and E. Antonio Chiocca. 2012. Cerebellar tumors in adults. In *Schmidek and Sweet Operative Neurosurgical Techniques: Indications, Methods, and Results*, 6th ed. Edited by Alfredo Quiñones-Hinojosa. Philadelphia: Saunders, pp. 169–77.

Noblett, Dylan A., Jennifer Chang, Atrin Toussi, Arthur Dublin, and Kiarash Shahlaie. 2018. Hemangioma of the Cavernous Sinus: A Case Series. *Journal of Neurological Surgery Reports* 79: e26–e30. [CrossRef]

Perneczky, Axel, and Robert Reisch. 2008. Suboccipital approach. In *Keyhole Approaches in Neurosurgery*. Edited by Axel Perneczky and Robert Reisch. Vienna: Springer, pp. 179–204. [CrossRef]

Raheja, Amol, and William T. Couldwell. 2020. Cavernous sinus meningioma. In *Handbook of Clinical Neurology*. Edited by Michael W. McDermott. Amsterdam: Elsevier, vol. 170, pp. 69–85.

Roosli, Christof, Fred H. Linthicum Jr, Sebahattin Cureoglu, and Saumil N. Merchant. 2012. What is the site of origin of cochleovestibular schwannommas? *Audiology and Neurotology* 17: 121–25. [CrossRef]

Samii, Madjid, and Cordula Matthies. 1997. Management of 1000 vestibular schwannomas (acoustic neuromas): Surgical management and results with an emphasis on complications and how to avoid them. *Neurosurgery* 40: 11–21. [PubMed]

Shimizu, Satoru, Necmettin Tanriover, Albert L. Rhoton Jr, Nobutaka Yoshioka, and Kiyotaka Fujii. 2005. MacCarty keyhole and inferior orbital fissure in orbitozygomatic craniotomy. *Neurosurgery* 57: 152–59. [CrossRef] [PubMed]

Tamura, Takamitsu, Taku Sato, Yugo Kishida, Masahiro Ichikawa, Keiko Oda, Eiji Ito, Tadashi Watanabe, Jun Sakuma, and Kiyoshi Saito. 2015. Outcome of clival chordomas after skull base surgeries with mean follow-up of 10 years. *Fukushima Journal of Medical Science* 61: 131–40. [CrossRef]

Tryggvason, Geir, Andrew Barnett, John Kim, Hakan Soken, Joan Maley, and Marlan R. Hansen. 2012. Radiographic association of schwannommas with sensory ganglia. *Otology & Neurotology* 33: 1276–82. [CrossRef]

Tummala, Ramachandra P., Ernesto Coscarella, and Jacques J. Morcos. 2005. Transpetrosal approaches to the posterior fossa. *Neurosurgical Focus* 19: E6. [CrossRef] [PubMed]

Walcott, Brian P., Brian V. Nahed, Ahmed Mohyeldin, Jean-Valery Coumans, Kristopher T. Kahle, and Manuel J. Ferreira. 2012. Chordoma: Current concepts, management, and future directions. *The Lancet Oncology* 13: e69–e76. [CrossRef]

Xenellis, John E., and Fred H. Linthicum, Jr. 2003. On the myth of the glial/Schwann junction (Obersteiner-Redlich zone): Origin of vestibular nerve schwannommaa. *Otology & Neurotology* 24: 1.

Yao, Longping, Mohammed Alahmari, Yasin Temel, and Koos Hovinga. 2020. Therapy of Sporadic and NF2-Related Vestibular Schwannoma. *Cancers* 12: 835. [CrossRef] [PubMed]

Yaşargil, M. G. 1984. *Interfascial Pterional (Frontotemporosphenoidal) Craniotomy*. New York: Georg Thieme Verlag, vol. 1, pp. 217–20.

Yasargil, M. G., J. Antic, R. Laciga, K. K. Jain, R. M. Hodosh, and R. D. Smith. 1976. Microsurgical pterional approach to aneurysms of the basilar bifurcation. *Surgical Neurology* 6: 83–91.

Yaşargil, M. Gazi, Mark V. Reichman, and Stefan Kubik. 1987. Preservation of the frontotemporal branch of the facial nerve using the interfascial temporalis flap for pterional craniotomy. *Journal of Neurosurgery* 67: 463–66. [CrossRef] [PubMed]

Yoshida, Kazunari, and Takeshi Kawase. 1999. Trigeminal neurinomas extending into multiple fossae: Surgical methods and review of the literature. *Journal of Neurosurgery* 91: 202–11. [CrossRef]

Zabramski, Joseph M., Talat Kiriş, Suresh K. Sankhla, Josep Cabiol, and Robert F. Spetzler. 1998. Orbitozygomatic craniotomy. *Journal of Neurosurgery* 89: 336–41. [CrossRef]

Section X: Spinal Neurosurgery

Spinal Anatomy, Mobility, Balance, and Deformity

Khandkar Ali Kawsar and Forhad H. Chowdhury

Abstract: The spinal column is formed of vertebrae and intervertebral discs. The vertebral column contains the spinal cord, nerve roots, dura, and blood vessels within the vertebral canal. In brief, the spine allows for flexion, extension, lateral flexion, and rotatory movement. Human mobility and posture importantly depend on the structural integrity and homeostasis of spinal balances (particularly sagittal and coronal balances). The derangement of structural integrity and the alteration of spinal balance homeostasis lead to spinal deformities like kyphosis, scoliosis, and kyphoscoliosis. This chapter will shortly discuss spinal anatomy, mobility, spinal balance, and spinal deformity. The principles of the management of common spinal deformities such as kyphosis and scoliosis will also be discussed.

Abbreviations

ALV	apical lumbar vertebrae	ASD	adult spinal deformity
CSVL	central sacral vertical line	CT	computed tomography
DDD	degenerative disc disease	FDA	Food and Drug Administration
MRI	magnetic resonance imaging	MT	main thoracic
PT	proximal thoracic	TL/L	thoracolumbar/lumbar
SVA	sagittal vertical axis	TDR	total disc replacement

1. Anatomy of the Spine

1.1. History

Before proceeding to understand the concept of modern spine surgery, knowledge on the anatomy and physiology of the spine needs to be acquired. Herophilus of Chalcedon (300 B.C.), known as the father of anatomy, as well as Galen of Pergamon (130–200 A.D.) were early pioneers who made observations on the nervous system and the spine. Following his 1543 publication of then most up-to-date anatomical textbook *De Humani Corporis Fabrica Libri Septi*, Andreas Vesalius (1514–1564) became regarded as the founder of modern spinal anatomy (Acar et al. 2005).

1.2. Basic Concepts

Vertebrates are an animal subphylum in the phylum Chordata and are defined by their possessing a vertebral column, or spine, which contains vertebrae. In humans, the spine is made up of thirty-three vertebrae, which are divided as follows: seven cervical, twelve thoracic, five lumbar, five sacral, and four coccygeal. The spinal column runs from the occiput to the coccyx. The neurological system and physical structure supported by the vertebral column also make possible correct movement and sensation. Spinal pathology can have a crippling effect on one's quality of life. The axial skeletal system is composed of the vertebrae, the skull, the ribs, and the sternum.

The vertebrae vary in terms of shape and size. This is more applicable to different regions of the spinal column, though they share a similar basic structure.

The vertebral body is the weight-bearing component positioned anteriorly of each vertebra. The superior and the inferior aspects of the vertebral body, lined with hyaline cartilage, are known as superior and inferior endplates. The posterior part is the vertebral arch, with several bony prominences which act as attachment sites for muscles and ligaments. Each vertebra has a single centrally placed spinous process, posteriorly at the point of the arch. On both sides, the transverse processes, which articulate with the ribs, extend laterally and posteriorly. Pedicles are bony structures that connect the vertebral body to the transverse processes. The lamina connects the transverse processes to the spinous processes (Figure 1a,b).

Intervertebral discs are short, cylindrical fibrocartilaginous structures between the vertebrae. They are wedge-shaped in the thoracic and lumbar regions to support the spinal curvature and absorb jolts. Each disc has two parts—a tough fibrous annulus fibrosus and a jelly-like nucleus pulposus, which it surrounds. Disc herniation occurs when the nucleus pulposus herniates in the posterolateral direction, breaking through the annulus fibrosus.

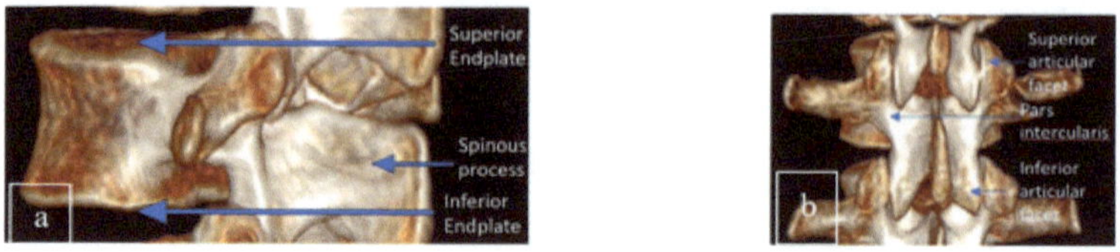

Figure 1. Lateral (**a**) and posterior (**b**) view of lumbar vertebra showing different parts. Source: Figure by authors.

1.2.1. Classification of the Vertebrae

Cervical Vertebrae

There are seven cervical vertebrae. They have three features that distinguish them from other vertebrae (Figure 2a,b):

1. The spinous process is bifid at its distal end, except in the atlas (C1), which has no spinous process, and C7, which has the longest spinous process among the cervical vertebra and may not be bifid.
2. In the first six cervical vertebrae, the vertebral artery and vein run in the transverse foramen. In the seventh, only the vertebral vein occupies the transverse foramen (also known as the foramen transversarium). The vertebral artery is especially significant due to it supplying oxygenated blood to the brain and spinal cord.
3. Cervical vertebrae have a triangular vertebral foramen, except for the atlas (C1) and axis (C2), as those are specialized to allow for the movement of the head.

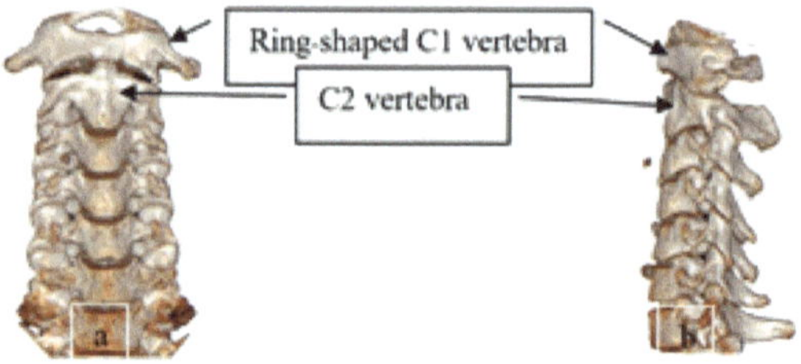

Figure 2. Anterior (**a**) and lateral (**b**) view of cervical spine (3D view). Source: Figure by authors.

Thoracic Vertebrae

The twelve thoracic vertebrae are medium-sized and increase in size as they go down. To produce the bony thorax, there are demifacets in the upper and lower half of each side of the vertebral body. Those demifacets articulate with the heads of two different ribs (Figure 3a,b).

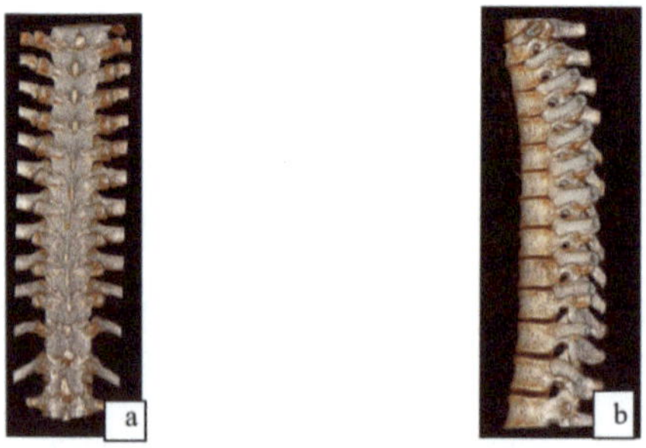

Figure 3. Posterior (**a**) and lateral (**b**) view of the thoracic spine along with the L1 vertebra, showing the position and attachment of the ribs and the anatomy of the facets, joints, and spinous processes of the thoracic vertebra (3D view). Source: Figure by authors.

The spinous processes of the thoracic vertebrae are positioned obliquely inferiorly and posteriorly. The vertebral foramen of the thoracic vertebrae is circular, in contrast to that of the cervical vertebrae.

Lumbar Vertebrae

The largest vertebrae in the spinal column are the lumbar vertebrae, and there are five of them in most individuals (Figure 4a,b). They have a specialized structural design to bear the weight of the torso.

The kidney-shaped vertebral bodies of the lumbar vertebrae are very big. They share a triangular-shaped vertebral foramen with the cervical vertebrae. Compared to the thoracic vertebrae, their spinous processes are shorter and do not reach inferiorly beyond the level of the vertebral body.

Because of their shape and size, needles can enter the spinal cord and spinal canal in this region of the spine, which is not feasible between the thoracic vertebrae. A lumbar puncture and the injection of epidural anaesthesia are two examples of this.

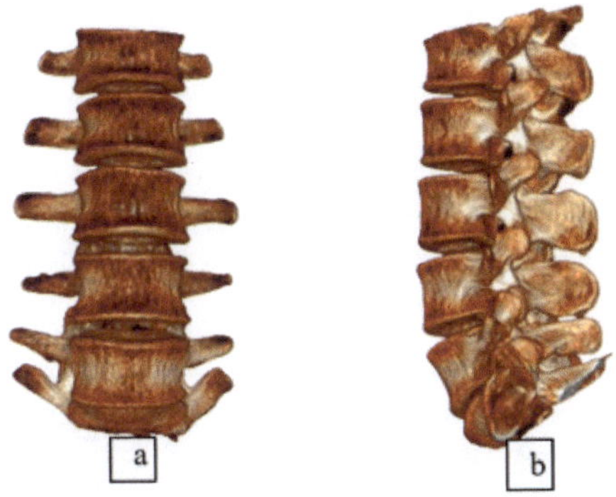

Figure 4. Anterior (**a**) and lateral (**b**) view of lumbar spine (3D view). Source: Figure by authors.

Sacrum and Coccyx

There are five fused vertebrae that make up the sacrum. With the apex pointing downwards, it resembles an inverted triangle. There are facets for articulation with the pelvis at the sacroiliac joints on the lateral sides of the sacrum.

A little bone called the coccyx articulates with the sacrum's apex. It can be identified by the absence of vertebral arches. There is no spinal canal because there are no vertebral arches.

"Sacralization" refers to the fusion of L5 with the sacrum, whereas "lumbarization" describes the separation of S1 from the sacrum. These are developmental in nature.

Ligaments and Joints

The articular facets and joints connecting the bodies of the mobile vertebrae allow them to articulate with one another.

Left and right superior articular facets articulate with the upper vertebrae, while left and right inferior articular facets articulate with the lower vertebrae. Through intervertebral discs, vertebral bodies indirectly articulate with one another. The cartilaginous joints that make up the vertebral body are designed for weight bearing. Intervertebral discs connect the articular surfaces, which are covered by hyaline cartilage.

The anterior and posterior longitudinal ligaments, which extend the whole length of the vertebral column, are two ligaments that support the vertebral body joints. Because of its thickness, the anterior longitudinal ligament keeps the spinal column from overextending. Even though the posterior longitudinal ligament is weaker, it inhibits hyperflexion.

The joints between the articular facets are called facet joints. They allow for some gliding motions between the vertebrae. They are strengthened by several ligaments:

- Ligamentum flavum—extends between the lamina of adjacent vertebrae;
- Interspinous and supraspinous ligaments—join the spinous processes of adjacent vertebrae. Interspinous ligaments attach between processes, and supraspinous ligaments attach to the tips;
- Intertransverse ligaments—extend between transverse processes.

The spinal cord is approximately 45cm long and originates from the medulla. It descends down through the foramen magnum and ends as the conus medullaris, which terminates at S2 in foetuses, L3 in newborns, and at the lower border of L1 in adults. There are two enlargements: cervical C5–T1 for the brachial plexus and lumbosacral L2–S3 for the lumbar and sacral plexuses. The meningeal coverings of the cord are continuous with the brain, and the cord is closely ensheathed by pia mater. The pia continues inferiorly as filum terminale, piercing the distal extremity of the dural sac and attaching to the coccyx. Pia mater forms the denticulate ligaments which secure the cord within the dural sac (Bican et al. 2013). The dura forms a tough sheath and ends distally at S2, anchored to the coccyx by the filum terminale. The space between the arachnoid and pia mater contains CSF. All layers continue along spinal nerve roots. The anterior spinal artery is made up of two branches, one from each vertebral artery (VA). Radicular arteries arise from different levels—C3 (VA), C6 (from the deep cervical artery, with branches from the costocervical trunk and from the left subclavian), C8 (from the costocervical trunk), and D4/D5 (from the intercostal artery). The artery of Adamkiewicz (arteria radicularis anterior magna), which needs special mention, arises between T9 and L2 in 85% and between T5 and T8 in 15% of the population. It is the principal source of blood for the spinal cord from the T8 segment to the conus and comes from the left side in 80% of cases (Frostell et al. 2016). Two paired posterior spinal arteries arise from the posterior inferior cerebellar artery (PICA), which is less prominent than the anterior, and receive additional supply from 10–23 radicular branches. The midthoracic part has poor blood circulation, with a radicular artery from T4/5. This is a "watershed zone" and is more susceptible to vascular insult. There is anatomical variation, as at the conus medullaris, the anterior spinal artery joins the paired posterior spinal arteries. Ascending and descending tracts of spinal cord are shown in Tables 1 and 2, respectively.

Table 1. Ascending tracts.

Tract	Function	Point of Decussation
Dorsal columns Fasciculus gracilis Fasciculus cuneatus	Joint position, vibration, light touch	Brainstem: lower medulla and medial lemniscus
Posterior spinocerebellar	Unconscious proprioception (stretch receptors)	Uncrossed
Anterior spinocerebellar	Unconscious proprioception (whole limb position)	Uncrossed
Lateral spinothalamic	Pain and temperature	Spinal cord: at level of entry across anterior white commissure
Anterior spinothalamic	Light touch	Spinal cord: 2–3 segments above point of entry

Source: Authors' compilation based on data from Diaz and Morales (2016).

Table 2. Anatomy: descending tracts (motor).

Tract	Function	Point of Decussation
Lateral corticospinal	Skilled movement	Medullary pyramids
Anterior corticospinal	Skilled movement	Uncrossed
Rubrospinal	Facilitates flexor muscle tone	Midbrain
Vestibulospinal	Facilitates extensor muscle tone	Uncrossed

Source: Authors' compilation based on data from Diaz and Morales (2016).

2. Concept of Balances

2.1. *Spine Sagittal Balance*

2.1.1. Introduction

Humans stand and move in an environment subject to gravity. Constraints are placed on the spine as a result. Due to the bipedal stance, the pelvis and spine have a close association. The spine and body function inside a cone of equilibrium to maintain sagittal as well as coronal alignment with little energy consumption. This involves lumbar lordosis, dorsal kyphosis, cervical lordosis, and the pelvic anatomy. The primary goal is to retain mechanical equilibrium in both the sagittal and coronal planes, with the centre of cranial load, heads of the femur, and inferior extremities as the focal points. Scoliosis and spinal deformity surgery in the past emphasized coronal plane alignment (Glassman et al. 2005; Schwab et al. 2010).

According to White and Panjabi (White and Panjabi 1990), spinal instability, both acute and chronic, points to substantial spinal displacement that would lead to neuro-deficit, pain. or deformity. Spinal stability is the capability to restrict patterns of deformation under physiologic stresses so as not to harm the spinal cord and nerve roots and, furthermore, to avoid pain or incapacitating deformity resulting from structural alteration.

2.1.2. Aetiology

The aetiologies of sagittal imbalance include congenital, degenerative, traumatic, and iatrogenic. The majority of individuals with spinal sagittal imbalance have a kyphotic or hypolordotic fusion mass, with degenerated segments below and above the fusion (Booth et al. 1999).

Spinal biomechanics can be altered in case of congenital scoliosis, which can involve underdeveloped vertebrae or fixed kyphotic segments (Figure 5). Surgical intervention by fusion of long segments for adolescent idiopathic scoliosis may result in spinal degeneration distally that will affect sagittal balance later on (Wang et al. 2008).

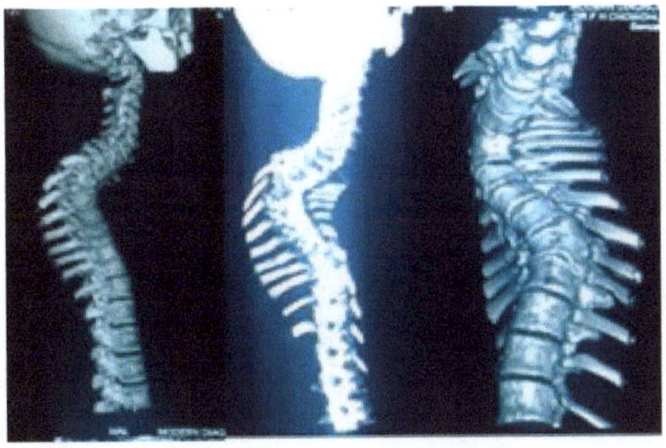

Figure 5. Three-dimensional CT scan of spine showing upper dorsal kyphoscoliosis due to D4 hemivertebra. Source: Figure by authors.

Spinal trauma, regardless of operative or nonoperative treatment, can result in chronic alterations in spinal balance, particularly when the thoracolumbar junction is involved. This phenomenon can be seen in disease conditions which cause degenerative or fixed alterations of the spine, like ankylosis spondylitis or rheumatoid arthritis (Bradford et al. 1987).

Because of the proximal lumbar hyperlordosis caused by thoracolumbar fusion, increased lordosis or kyphosis compensate for the rest of the lumbar and thoracic segments, respectively. The resultant compensating effect wears off over time, resulting in flat back syndrome and thoracic hyperkyphosis (Rose et al. 2009).

2.1.3. Epidemiology

Sagittal imbalance is a complicated problem that can arise from a variety of causes of spinal deformity. Table 3 shows the prevalence of sagittal imbalance based on a large cohort study (Glassman et al. 2005).

Table 3. Distribution of causes of sagittal imbalance (Figures 6–9).

Causes	Percentage (%)
Adolescent idiopathic scoliosis (Figures 6–9)	30.4
Kyphotic angulation	20.7
Iatrogenic imbalance and combined junctional degeneration	14
Congenital, neuromuscular, or scoliosis	25.5

Source: Authors' compilation based on data from Glassman et al. (2005).

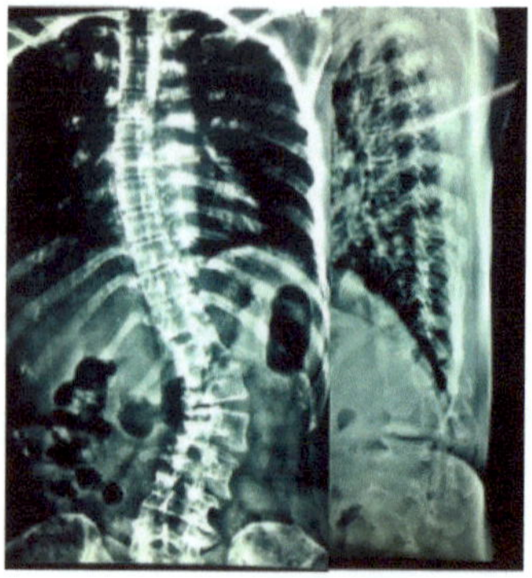

Figure 6. X-ray of dorsolumbar spine, with anterior–posterior and lateral views showing lumbar scoliosis. Source: Figure by authors.

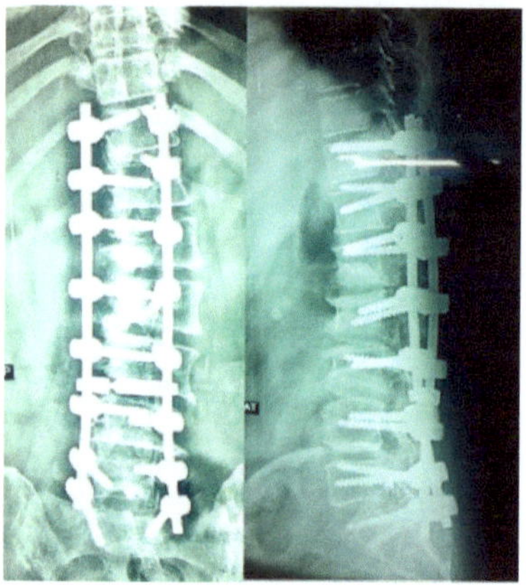

Figure 7. Postoperative X-rays of patient in Figure 6 showing correction of lumbar kyphosis with pedicular screws and rods. Source: Figure by authors.

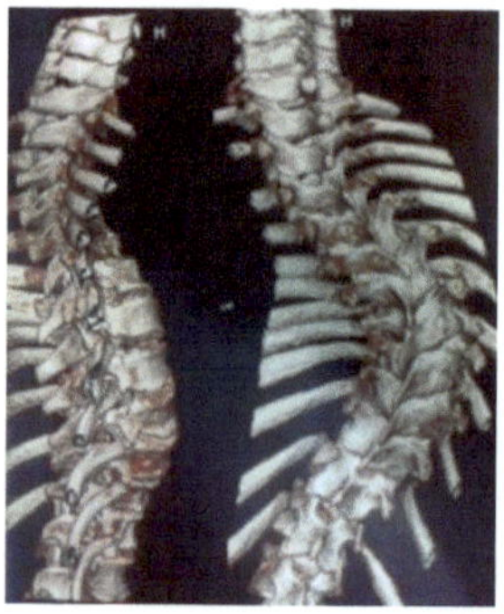

Figure 8. Three-dimensional CT scan of spine showing dorsal kyphosis. Source: Figure by authors.

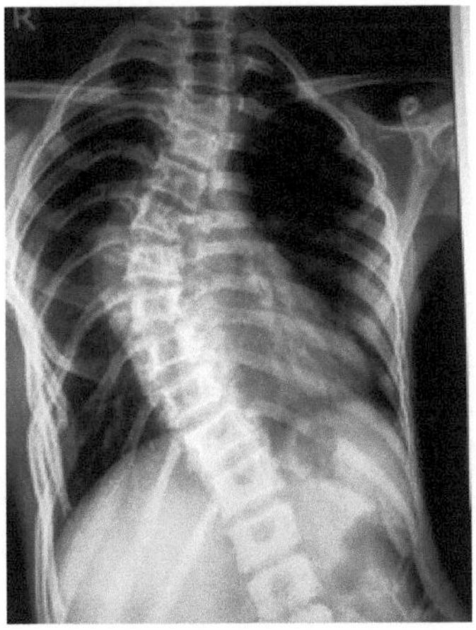

Figure 9. X-ray showing dorsal scoliosis with altered cardiac shadow in a patient with compromised cardiopulmonary function. Source: Figure by authors.

Angular measurement of spinal curves are shown in Table 4.

Table 4. Angular measurement of spinal curves.

Spinal Zone	Normal Curvature
Cervical lordosis	20°–40°
Dorsal kyphosis	20°–50° (can usually range 30° more than lumbar lordosis)
Thoracolumbar junction	D12/L1 junctional area should be neutral, with less than 10° or regional kyphosis
Lumbar lordosis	Mean 60°
Pelvic tilt	<20°
Pelvic incidence	55° ± 10°
Pelvic incidence/lumbar lordosis mismatch	<10°
Sagittal vertical axis	<5 mm

Source: Table by authors.

Sagittal Vertical Axis (SVA) and C7 Plumb Line

The C7 plumb line is the commonest method of determining spinal sagittal balance. An imaginary vertical line is drawn in a caudal direction from the centre of the vertebral C7 body, and it should intersect with or remain within 05 mm of the S1 posterior–superior endplate. For health-related quality of life outcomes, this is regarded to be within the acceptable range. Patients lean forwards and acquire slightly more positive sagittal alignment as they get older.

Preserving the harmonious anatomy of sagittal plane considerations is crucial. To preserve an approximately neutral posture, the cervical spine might compensate with a hyperlordotic presentation. Knee flexion as well as an increased pelvic tilt can help the patient compensate even more. However, this is a physically demanding and tiring position that is not anatomically typical (Schwab et al. 2010).

Pelvic Incidence

Pelvic incidence (PI) (Figure 10) is the angle created by a line drawn 90° to the surface of the sacrum's superior endplate as well as a line from the midpoint of the sacrum's superior endplate to the femoral head's centre. This measurement's usual range is 55° ± 10° (Rose et al. 2009).

PI is a roentgenographic comparison of the biomechanic interaction between the lumbar spine as well as the pelvis in individuals with different pelvic morphologies. An individual's lumbar lordosis (LL) and PI may change. However, to maintain sagittal balance in the lumbopelvic junction as well as SVA in the whole spine, their relationship must be maintained. Changes in pelvic and hip posture often compensate for fixed sagittal abnormalities in the lumbar spine, preserving SVA.

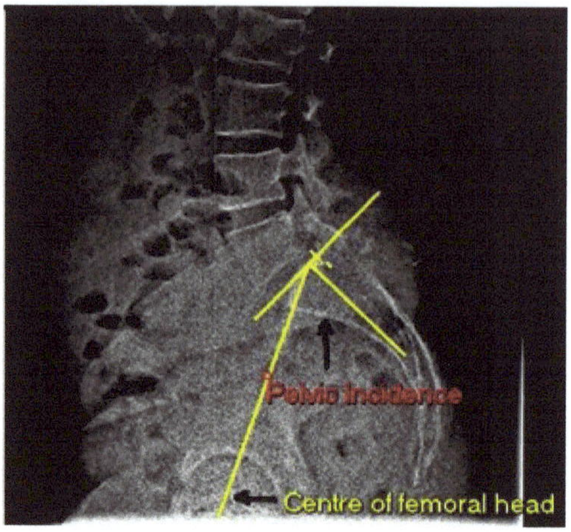

Figure 10. X-ray of lumbosacral spine (lateral view) demonstrating calculation of "pelvic incidence". Source: Figure by authors.

Pelvic Tilt

Pelvic tilt (Figure 11) is the angle between the following two roentgenographic lines:

- A line drawn from the centre of the S1 endplate to the centre of the femoral head;
- A vertical line intersecting the femoral head's centre.

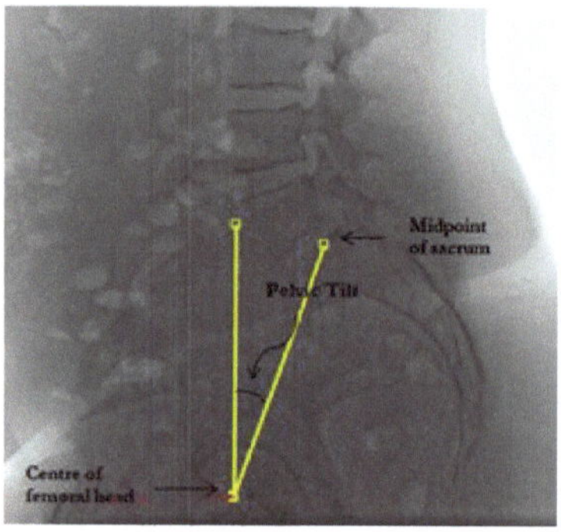

Figure 11. X-ray of lumbosacral spine (lateral view) demonstrating calculation of "pelvic tilt". Source: Figure by authors.

The normal measurement is <20°, but it can vary with differences in position and contracture (Roussouly et al. 2005).

2.1.4. History

A detailed medical history, as well as a history of spinal pathology, must be collected, with special attention paid to any previous spine procedures. Discogenic, mechanical, and neuropathic causes of pain must be distinguished.

A comprehensive musculoskeletal and neurologic examination should be carried out. The patient must be examined in both the standing and supine positions. Gait analysis should be carried out to look for secondary compensatory mechanisms.

The range of motion of the patient's hip and their pain or discomfort should be examined for any probable contractures or dysfunction in addition to the spinal assessment. The cranium must also be considered in terms of the cervical spine's range of motion. Vertical gaze functional constraints, which are fairly frequent consequences of sagittal imbalance, should similarly be evaluated (Kim et al. 2021).

2.1.5. Neurological Examination Related to Spinal Pathologies

Neurological examination (Boyraz et al. 2015; Fuller 2019; Shimizu et al. 1993; Walker 1990; Watson et al. 1997) is a very important tool in diagnosis, especially in the case of spinal pathologies. In this chapter, important examinations relevant to diagnosing the level of spinal pathology will be described.

MOTOR System

Grading of muscle power: Muscle power is conventionally graded using the Medical Research Council (MRC) scale. This is usually amended to divide grade 4 into 4+, 4, and 4−. The scale is as follows:

5 = normal power;
4+ = submaximal movement against resistance;
4 = moderate movement against resistance;
4− = slight movement against resistance;
3 = moves against gravity but not resistance;
2 = moves with gravity eliminated;
1 = flicker;
0 = no movement.

Power should be graded according to the maximum power attained, even it is maintained for a brief period.

Myotomes: Myotomes can be remembered by counting numerically:

"1, 2"—S1 and S2 supply the back of the legs (hip extension, knee flexion, and plantar flexion). This is also the root value of the ankle reflex.

"1, 2"—hip flexion is supplied by L1 and L2.

"3, 4"—L3 and L4 supply the quadriceps and the knee reflex (below the hip).

"5"—foot dorsiflexion is below L3 and L4, so it is supplied by L5.

"5"—the biceps are mainly supplied by C5 and this is the root value of the biceps reflex.

"6"—the brachioradialis is mainly supplied by C6 and this is the root value of the supinator reflex.

"7"—C7 supplies elbow extensors, i.e., the triceps, and extensors of the wrist and fingers; this is the root value of the triceps reflex.

"8"—finger flexion is below C7 and so it is supplied by C8.

"1"—small muscles of the hands are innervated by T1.

Tone: Testing muscle tone is a very important indicator of the presence and site of pathology. It can be surprisingly difficult to evaluate. Patients need to be fully relaxed. Commands to relax usually do not help. Irrelevant conversation or asking the patient to count down may help.

Normal tone is slight resistance through the whole range of motion. When the knee is lifted, the heel will lift minimally off the bed.

Decreased tone means loss of resistance throughout the range of motion. The heel does not lift off the bed when the knee is lifted quickly. Flaccid means marked loss of tone. This happens in lower motor neuron lesions or cerebellar lesions. Rare causes are myopathies, "spinal shock" (e.g., early after a stroke), and chorea. Increased tone means resistance increases suddenly ("a catch"). When the knee is lifted quickly, the heel easily leaves the bed. This is spasticity, which is a consequence of upper motor neuron lesions. Increased tone through the whole range of motion, as if bending a lead pipe, is named lead pipe rigidity. Regular intermittent breaks in tone through the whole range of motion are known as cogwheel rigidity. If the patient seems to oppose your attempts to move their limb, this is called gegenhalten or paratonia, and can happen in bilateral frontal lobe damage. Common causes are cerebrovascular disease and dementia.

Special situations:

- Myotonia: slow relaxation following action. This is demonstrated by asking the patient to make a fist and then release it suddenly. In myotonia, the hand will only unfold slowly.
- Dystonia: patient maintains posture at the extreme end of motion with contractions of agonists and antagonists.
- Percussion myotonia: may be demonstrated when a muscle dimples following percussion with a patella hammer. Most commonly seen in the abductor pollicis brevis and the tongue.

Basic Neurological Screening Examination

Upper limbs: A simple screening procedure can be performed as outlined below. It is to be tested on one side and then compared to the other side.

Shoulder abduction—this can be tested by asking the patient to lift both elbows out to the side. This tests the deltoid muscle, which is innervated by the axillary nerve, C5 root. Elbow flexion—patient's elbow and wrist are held and the hand is pulled towards their face. This tests the biceps brachii, which is innervated by the musculocutaneous nerve, C5 and C6 roots. Elbow extension—the patient is asked to extend the elbow against resistance. This tests the triceps muscle, which is innervated by the radial nerve, (C6), C7, and (C8) roots. Wrist extension—the patient's forearm is supported and the wrist is bent backwards. This tests the flexor carpi ulnaris and radialis muscles, which are innervated by the radial nerve, (C6), C7, and (C8) roots. Finger extension—the patient's hand is supported and extended fingers are to be pressed downward for the test. This tests the extensor digitorum muscle, which is innervated by the posterior interosseous nerve (a branch of the radial nerve), C7 and (C8) roots. Finger flexion—the examiner's fingers are placed on the patient's fingers, palm to palm, so that both sets of fingertips are on the other's metacarpophalangeal joints. The patient is then asked to "flex the fingers" or to "grip your fingers"; the examiner will attempt to "resist the finger flexion" or will try to "open the patient's grip". The flexor digitorum superficialis and profundus, which are innervated by the median and ulnar nerves, C8 root, are tested here. Finger abduction—the patient is asked to spread their fingers out against resistance. This tests the first dorsal interosseous muscle, which is innervated by the ulnar nerve, T1 root. Finger adduction—this can be tested using the card test, i.e., putting a card between the index and middle, middle and ring, or ring and little fingers. This tests the second palmar interosseous muscle, which is innervated by the ulnar nerve, T1 root.

Serratus anterior—the patient is examined from the back while standing in front of a wall. The patient is asked to push against the wall with their arms straight and their hands at shoulder level. If the muscle is weak, the scapula lifts off the chest wall, forming a "winged scapula". The long thoracic nerve, formed from C5, C6, and C7 roots, is tested here.

Brachioradialis—the examiner should hold the patient's semipronated forearm and wrist. The patient is asked to pull their hand towards their face. This tests the brachioradialis muscle, which is innervated by the radial nerve, C6 root.

Flexor digitorum profundus (FDP)— the patient is asked to grip the examiner's fingers while the examiner attempts to extend the distal interphalangeal joint of the little and ring fingers. The medial part of the muscle, which inserts to the fourth and fifth digits, is innervated by the ulnar nerve (C8-T1). The lateral part, which inserts to the second and third digits, is innervated by the median nerve via the anterior interosseous branch (C8-T1).

Lower limbs: The femoral and sciatic nerves are the two major nerves that supply the lower limbs; the former for knee extension and the later for knee flexion. The posterior tibial branch of the sciatic nerve supplies foot plantar flexion and inversion and the small muscles of the foot. The common peroneal branch of the sciatic nerve supplies dorsiflexion and eversion of the ankle.

The examination starts, ideally, by an inspection of the legs for wasting and fasciculation. Wasting is to be checked especially on the quadriceps, the anterior compartment of the shin, the extensor digitorum and brevis, and the peroneal muscles.

A simplified root distribution in the legs can be demonstrated as follows: L1 and L2 for hip flexion, L3 and L4 for knee extension and knee reflex, L5 for dorsiflexion of the foot, inversion and eversion of the ankle, and extension of the big toe, and S1 for hip extension, knee flexion, plantar flexion, and ankle reflex.

Screening Examination for the Lower Limbs

One side is to be compared with the other side. Hip flexion—the patient can be asked to lift their knee towards the chest. When the knee is at a right angle, the patient should be asked to pull it up as hard as they can against resistance applied by the examiner. This tests the iliopsoas muscle, which receives nerve supply from the lumbosacral plexus, L1 and L2 roots. Hip extension—this can be tested while the patient is lying flat with their legs straight. The patient is asked to push down on the examiner's hand, placed under the patient's heel. The gluteus maximus muscle is responsible for the movement and is innervated by the inferior gluteal nerve, (L5) and S1 root. Knee extension—the patient is asked to bend their knee. When it is flexed at 90 degrees, they are asked to straighten the leg against resistance applied at the ankle. This tests the quadriceps femoris muscle, which is innervated by femoral nerve, L3 and L4 roots. Knee flexion—the patient is asked to bend the knee and to bring the heel towards their bottom against resistance applied at the ankle. This tests the hamstring muscles (semitendinosus, semimembranosus, and biceps femoris), which are innervated by the sciatic nerve, (L5) and S1 root. Foot dorsiflexion—the patient is asked to move their ankle back and bring their toes towards their head. When the ankle is past 90 degrees, resistance is applied in the other direction. This tests the tibialis anterior muscle, which is innervated by the deep peroneal nerve, L4 and L5 roots. Plantar flexion of the foot—the patient is asked to point their foot and toes downwards with the leg straight against resistance applied under the foot. This tests the gastrocnemius muscle, which is innervated by the posterior tibial nerve, S1 root.

Big toe extension—the patient is asked to pull their big toe up towards their face against resistance applied by the examiner. This tests the extensor hallucis longus muscle, which is innervated by the deep peroneal nerve, L5 root. Extension of the toes—the patient is asked to bring all toes towards their head against resistance. This tests the extensor digitorum brevis muscle, which is innervated by the deep peroneal nerve, L5 and S1 roots. Foot inversion—the patient is asked to turn their foot inwards while the ankle is at 90 degrees. This tests the tibialis posterior muscle, L4 and L5 roots. Foot eversion—the patient is asked to turn their foot out to the side. This tests the peroneus longus and brevis muscles, which are innervated by the superficial peroneal nerve, L5 and S1 nerve roots.

Tendon Reflexes

Tendon reflexes are increased in upper motor neuron lesions and decreased in lower motor neuron lesions and muscle abnormalities.

Reflexes can be graded as follows (Walker et al.):

0 = absent;
± = present only with reinforcement;
1+ = present but depressed;
2+ = normal;
3+ = increased;
4+ = clonus.

Biceps—the biceps muscle tendon is stretched with a tendon hammer above the elbow. The involved nerve is the musculocutaneous nerve and the root value is C5 (C6). Supinator—the brachioradialis muscle tendon is stretched with a tendon hammer above the wrist with the hand on a semipronated position. The involved nerve is the radial nerve and the root value is C6 (C5). Triceps—the triceps muscle tendon is stretched by stroking the back of the elbow with a tendon hammer. The involved nerve is the radial nerve and the root value is C7. Finger reflex—the examiner holds the patient's hand in a neutral position, places their hand opposite the fingers, and strikes the back of their fingers. The involved muscles are the flexor digitorum profundus and superficialis, the involved nerves are the median and ulnar nerves, and the root value is C8. Scapulohumeral reflex (SHR)—the SHR of Shimizu is elicited by tapping the tip of the spine of the scapula and acromion in a caudal direction. The SHR is classified as hyperactive only when an elevation of the scapula or an abduction of the humerus have been clearly defined after tapping at these points. The major muscles involved are the upper portion of the trapezius, the levator scapulae, and the deltoid. The reflex centre of the SHR is clinically presumed to be located between the posterior arch of C1 and the caudal edge of the C3 body. The implication of a hyperactive SHR provides useful information about dysfunctions of upper motor neuron lesions cranial to the C3 vertebral body level (Shimizu et al. 1993).

Pectoralis reflex—the examiner lightly places the index finger of their left hand on the tendon of the pectoralis major at the deltopectoral groove and strikes the finger with a reflex hammer. The pectoralis major muscle is to be observed. A brisk pectoralis jerk is seen only in patients with spinal cord compression at the C2–3 and/or C3–4 levels. The presence of a hyperactive pectoralis reflex is specific to lesions of the upper cervical spinal cord.

If the pectoralis reflex is brisk, the SHR is be tested to determine the level, as the SHR centre is higher on the spinal cord. If the SHR and jaw jerk are both positive, then the lesion is at the level of the pons or above. If the jaw jerk is negative, the lesion is below the level of the pons.

Lower Limb Reflexes

Knee reflex—the patient's knee on one side is supported by the examiner at 90 degrees. The examiner strikes the knee below the patella and watches the quadriceps. The involved nerve is the femoral nerve and the root value is L3 and L4. Ankle reflex—the examiner holds the patient's foot at 90 degrees, with the medial malleolus facing the ceiling if the patient is lying on a bed. In the sitting position, one leg can be crossed over the other. The Achilles tendon is to be stroked directly. The muscles of the calf are to be watched. The involved nerve is the tibial nerve and the root value is S1 and S2.

Ankle Reflex Alternatives

1. The ankle reflex can also be tested by keeping the patient's legs straight and placing the examiner's hand on the ball of the patient's foot, with the ankles at 90 degrees. The examiner's hand is to be stroked with a tendon hammer and the muscles of the calf are to be watched. If the reflex is absent, reinforcement is needed. 2. Another way to check the ankle reflex is to ask the patient to kneel on a chair so that their ankles are hanging loose over the edge of the chair. The Achilles tendon is to be stroked directly.

Reinforcement of Reflexes

Jendrassik Ernő, a Hungarian physician, described the Jendrassik manoeuvre, where the patient clenches the teeth, flexes both sets of fingers into a hook-like form, and interlocks those sets of fingers together and at the same time, the reflexes are elicited with a tendon hammer. This can be used to reinforce the reflexes of the lower limbs when they cannot be normally elicited.

Clonus

Clonus is a rhythmic oscillating stretch reflex that occurs in upper motor neuron lesions and is generally accompanied by hyper-reflexia. Testing for clonus is performed as part of the neurological exam.

The ankle or Achilles reflex (S1/S2 nerve roots) is the most common site to test for clonus. This is tested while keeping the patient in the supine position. The hip and knee are flexed at a right angle; the knee is supported, the ankle is stretched to a dorsiflex position, then free movement is allowed. A persisted flapping movement of the ankle (plantar flexion) is positive for ankle clonus.

Some other commonly tested clonus reflexes are as follows (Boyraz et al. 2015):

- In the lower limbs, the patella/quadriceps/knee, L2 to L4 (mostly L4), are tested just inferior to the patella (or by pushing the patella distally);
- In the upper limbs:
    - Biceps: C5 to C6, just anterior to the elbow;
    - Triceps: C7 to C8 (mostly C7), just posterior to the elbow;
- For lesions in the brainstem, jaw jerk/masseter (trigeminal nerve) is tested at the chin/mental protuberance.

Interpretation:

- Increased reflex or clonus indicates an upper motor neuron lesion above the root at that level.
- Absent reflexes indicate peripheral neuropathy.
- Reduced reflexes (more difficult to judge) occur in peripheral neuropathy, muscle disease, and cerebellar syndrome. Reflexes can be absent in the early stages of severe upper motor neuron lesion, like "spinal shock".
- Reflex spread indicates an upper motor neuron lesion occurring above the level of innervation of the muscle to which the reflex has spread. The reflex being tested is present but this response goes beyond the muscle normally seen to contract. For example, the fingers are seen to flex when the supinator reflex is tested, or the hip adductors are seen to contract when testing the knee reflex.
- An inverted reflex is a combination of loss of the reflex tested with reflex spread to a muscle at a lower level. The level of the absent reflex indicates the level of the lesion. For example, a biceps reflex is absent but produces a triceps response. This indicates a lower motor neuron lesion at the level of the absent reflex (in this case, C5) with an upper motor neuron lesion below indicating spinal cord involvement at the level of the absent reflex.

Superficial Reflexes

Abdominal reflexes—using the sharp end of a reflex hammer, the examiner lightly scratches the abdominal wall from the abdominal margins toward the umbilicus, observes a quivering motion of the abdominal muscles, and watches the abdominal wall. It should contract on the same side. The afferents are the segmental sensory nerves and the efferents are the segmental motor nerves. The root value above the umbilicus is T8–T9; below the umbilicus, it is T10–T11.

An absent abdominal reflex may occur due to obesity, previous abdominal operations, frequent pregnancy or age, as well as due to pyramidal tract involvement above that level or a peripheral nerve abnormality. Brisk abdominal reflexes are not clinically significant, though they are said to be brisk in cerebral palsy and motor neuron disorders.

Plantar response—the examiner draws the sharp end of the reflex hammer up a lateral border of the foot and across the foot pad. The big toe and the remainder of the foot are observed.

If all toes flex, this is a flexor plantar response. This will be interpreted as negative Babinski's sign, i.e., normal. If the big toe extends (goes up) and the other toes flex or spread, this is extensor plantar response, or positive Babinski's sign. This indicates upper motor neuron lesion. If the big toe extends (goes up), the other toes extend, and the ankle dorsiflexes, this is a withdrawal response. The test needs to be repeated gently or alternative stimuli need to be tried. If there is no movement of the hallux (even if the other toes flex), this indicates no response. A positive test at clinical examination should be reproducible.

Alternative stimuli for plantar response—these alternative stimuli are only useful when the plantar response is present. A stimulus on the lateral aspect of the foot can be tried to elicit a plantar response known as Chaddock's reflex. The same can be elicited by running the thumb and index finger down the medial aspect of the tibia; this is known as Oppenheim's reflex.

An upper motor neuron lesion pattern includes the signs and symptoms of increased tone, brisk reflexes, pyramidal pattern of weakness, and extensor plantar responses. A lower motor neuron lesion pattern includes wasting, fasciculation, decreased tone, decreased or absent reflexes, and flexor plantar responses.

If the reflexes are absent, the diagnosis will go towards polyradiculopathy, peripheral neuropathy, or myopathy. Sensory testing should be normal in myopathy.

In the state of "spinal shock", which occurs after a recent acute and severe upper motor neuron lesion, tone will be reduced and reflexes may be absent, even though this is an upper motor neuron lesion.

Mixed upper motor neuron (in the legs) and lower motor neuron (in the arms) weakness suggests motor neuron disease, which can either be associated with no sensory loss or with mixed cervical myelopathy and radiculopathy, which feature sensory loss.

Weakness in both legs with increased reflexes and extensor plantar responses suggests a lesion in the spinal cord. The lesion must be above the root level of the highest motor abnormality. The level may be ascertained with sensory signs.

Weakness in both legs, along with absent reflexes in the legs, indicates polyradiculopathy, cauda equina lesion, or peripheral neuropathy. Unilateral arm and leg weakness indicates upper motor neuron lesion in the high cervical cord, brainstem, or above.

Laterality of the Lesion

The corticospinal tracts (the pyramidal tracts) cross over in the pyramids in the medulla. Thus, lesions in the brain and brainstem above the medulla result in weakness on the opposite side of the body, and lesions in the spinal cord result in weakness on the same side of the body.

Upper motor neuron signs limited to a single limb can be caused by lesions in the spinal cord, brainstem, or cerebral hemisphere. Motor signs need to be assessed along with cranial nerve or sensory abnormality investigation to reach a diagnosis. If lower motor neuron lesion occurs, the following symptoms are seen.

Upper Limb

Lesion of the C5 root causes weakness of shoulder abduction, external rotation, elbow flexion, impaired sensation in the outer aspect of the upper arm, and loss of biceps reflex. Lesion of the C6 root causes weakness of elbow flexion, pronation, impaired sensation of the lateral aspect of the forearm and thumb, and loss of supinator reflex. Lesion of the C7 root causes weakness of elbow and wrist extension, impaired sensation of the middle finger, and loss of triceps reflex. Lesion of the C8 root causes weakness of finger flexion, impaired sensation of the medial aspect of the forearm, and loss of finger reflex. Lesion of the T1 root causes wasting of all small muscles of the hand and impaired sensation of the medial forearm.

Lesion of the median nerve causes weakness and wasting of the thenar eminence in the abductor pollicis brevis and impaired sensation of the thumb, index, and middle fingers. Lesion of the ulnar nerve causes weakness with or without wasting of all muscles in the hand excepting the LOAF muscles (lateral two lumbricals, opponens pollicis, abductor pollicis brevis, flexor pollicis brevis, and impaired sensation of the little and half ring fingers). Lesion of the radial nerve causes weakness of finger, wrist, and probably triceps and brachioradialis extension, impaired sensory changes at the anatomical snuffbox, and loss of reflex of the supinator and triceps, if the lesion is above the spiral groove.

Bilateral wasting of small muscles can be the presentation of peripheral neuropathy (with distal sensory loss) or motor neuron disease (without sensory loss). Lesion of the axillary nerve causes weakness of shoulder abduction by paralyzing the deltoid and impaired sensation of a small patch on the lateral part of the shoulder.

Lesion of the L4 root will result in weakness of knee extension and foot dorsiflexion; sensation in the medial shin will be impaired and the knee reflex will be affected. Lesion of the L5 root will result in weakness of foot dorsiflexion, inversion, and eversion, extension of the big toe, and hip abduction, and sensation will be impaired in the lateral shin and the dorsum of the foot. Common peroneal palsy results in weakness of foot dorsiflexion and eversion with preserved inversion, and sensation will be impaired in the lateral shin and the dorsum of the foot. Lesion of the S1 root causes weakness of plantar flexion and foot eversion, impaired sensation in the lateral border of the foot and sole of the foot, and ankle reflex loss. If in doubt, re-examine them with these factors in mind.

Sacral Sensation

This is not usually screened. However, it is important to test sacral sensation in any patient with urinary or bowel symptoms, bilateral leg weakness, sensory loss in both legs, and a possible cord conus medullaris or cauda equina lesion.

Patterns of Sensory Loss

Sensory deficits can be classified into eight levels of the nervous system:

1. Single nerve: sensory loss within the distribution of a single nerve may occur. This happens most commonly in the median, ulnar, peroneal, and lateral cutaneous nerves of the thigh.
2. Root or roots: sensory deficit may be confined to a single root or several roots in close proximity. Common roots in the arm are C5, C6, and C7, and in the leg, these are L4, L5, and S1. An important example is cauda equina syndrome, which involves multiple nerve roots in the lumbosacral spine (usually the S1–S5 roots bilaterally). This causes sensory loss in the perianal region and buttocks (saddle anaesthesia) and the back of both thighs.
3. Peripheral nerves can be affected by neuropathy, e.g., in distal glove and stocking deficit.
4. Spinal cord: five patterns of loss can be recognized:
    (a) Complete transverse lesion: hyperaesthesia (increased appreciation of touch/pinprick) at the upper level, with loss of all modalities a few segments below the lesion.
    (b) Hemisection of the cord (Brown-Séquard syndrome): loss of joint position and vibration sensation on the same side as the lesion and pain and of temperature sensation on the opposite side a few levels below the lesion.
    (c) Central cord: loss of pain and temperature sensation at the level of the lesion, where the spinothalamic fibres cross in the cord, with other modalities preserved. This is also known as dissociated sensory loss and is seen in syringomyelia.
    (d) Posterior column loss: loss of joint position and vibration sensation, but pain and temperature sensation are preserved.
    (e) Anterior spinal syndrome: loss of pain and temperature sensation below the level of the lesion, but joint position and vibration sensation are preserved.
5. Brainstem: loss of pain and temperature sensation on the face and on the opposite side of the body. This is found in lateral medullary syndrome.
6. Thalamic sensory loss: hemisensory loss of all modalities.
7. Cortical loss: in parietal lobe damage, the patient is able to recognize all sensations but localizes them poorly and the damage results in the loss of two-point discrimination, astereognosis, and sensory inattention.
8. Functional loss: this diagnosis is suggested by a non-anatomical distribution of sensory deficit, frequently with inconstant findings.

Tinel's Test

Tinel's test is the percussion of a nerve at the putative site of compression (usually using a tendon hammer). It is positive when paraesthesiae are produced in the distribution of the nerve concerned. It is commonly performed to test for median nerve compression at the wrist. Lhermitte's phenomenon is when forward flexion of the neck produces a feeling of electric shock, usually running down the back. The patient may complain of this spontaneously or you can test for it by flexing the neck. Occasionally, patients have the same feeling on extension (reverse Lhermitte's). This indicates cervical pathology, usually demyelination. It occasionally occurs with cervical spondylitic myelopathy, or, rarely, with B12 deficiency or cervical tumours.

Straight leg raising (SLR): this is a test for lumbosacral radicular entrapment. The examiner lifts the leg straight by the heel while patient is lying flat on the bed. The angle and any differences between the two sides are noted. It is regarded as normal when it is >90°, less in older patients. SLR is considered positive when it evokes radiating pain along the course of the sciatic nerve and below the knee between 30° and 70° of hip flexion. Hoover's sign: Hoover's sign demonstrates functional weakness by showing a discrepancy between voluntary hip extension and automatic hip extension. A patient lying on a bed flexing the hip to lift their left leg off the bed will inevitably automatically extend their right hip.

Bladder and Bowel Function

Spinal bladder: initially, the patient presents with urinary retention with or without overflow incontinence. Later, the bladder contracts and automatically voids small volumes of urine and dribbles. This is associated with constipation, but with normal anal tone. The patient may develop reflex penile erections, called priapism (after the Greek god Priapus). This is commonly caused by trauma and multiple sclerosis, rarely by spinal tumours.

Peripheral neurogenic bladder: this is a painless distension of the flaccid bladder with overflow incontinence and large residual volumes. This is associated with faecal incontinence and impotence. Anal tone is reduced. There may be saddle anaesthesia. This occurs in cauda equina lesions. A common cause is central lumbar disc protrusion; rarer causes are spina bifida, ependymomas, cordomas, and metastases. This also occurs in peripheral nerve lesions, where the most common cause is diabetes mellitus and rarer causes are pelvic surgery or malignancy.

2.1.6. Evaluation

Thirty-six-inch erect posture films are the gold standard for imaging spinal alignment. To demonstrate appropriate alignment, symmetry, and compensation, the pelvis, femoral heads, and spinal structure must be evaluated. Certain measures are quite important.

The most recent innovation in X-ray technology enables 2D-to-3D reconstructions using biplanar X-rays, which expose the patient to 800–1000 times lower radiation than a CT scan to produce the same image. MRI and CT can be used as part of a neurosurgical preoperative study or to assess the individual's clinical condition. Plain films, on the other hand, remain the mainstay of diagnosis.

2.1.7. Treatment

The main aim is to arrange the body in a physiological position that allows it to preserve its cone of stability with the lowest possible effort. The effects of sagittal and coronal plane spinal misalignment on pain and impairment in adults are now well recognized. Nonoperative treatment options include bracing for anatomical structural support and physiotherapy for strengthening. When surgical treatment is considered, spinal osteotomies are becoming more common in cases where nonoperative treatment has failed (Menger et al. 2020).

Adult scoliosis, iatrogenic fixed sagittal imbalance, flat back syndrome, kyphotic decompensation syndrome, as well as flat buttocks are all common disorders that necessitate surgical treatment. Smith-Petersen osteotomy, pedicle subtraction osteotomy, Ponte osteotomy, total/partial corpectomies, as well as spinal column resections are some of the main realignment procedures mentioned in the literature for these pathologies (Boachie-Adjei et al. 2006; Bridwell et al. 2004; Smith-Petersen et al. 1969; Thomasen 1985).

Schwab et al. described a complete classification of spinal osteotomies based on anatomy and established the inter- and intra-rater reliability of this classification system (Schwab et al. 2014) (Table 5).

Prevalence of Adult Spinal Deformity (ASD) and Role of Surgery Depending on the Magnitude of the Disease

Schwab and colleagues (Schwab et al. 2003) utilized the Short Form (SF)-36 questionnaire in the US to assess the illness burden in cases with adult scoliosis, comparing the findings to data from the general US population and those with other medical comorbidities. In all eight SF-36 domains, adults with scoliosis performed worse than the general population. For the US population with symptomatic spinal deformity, Bess and colleagues (Bess et al. 2016) gathered summary values of the SF-36 physical and mental components and observed comparable findings with a faster generational decline than the average (Roussouly et al. 2005).

ASD is a matter of discussion in healthcare due to its frequency among people over the age of 65, a population that is growing due to a variety of circumstances. Nonoperative care of ASD has been shown to be ineffective, with individuals with smaller abnormalities and people who are already happy with their spine-related health benefiting the most. Surgical treatment is favoured by patients hoping to improve their quality of life, according to publications, but complications are common (Diebo et al. 2019).

Table 5. Spinal osteotomy classification.

Grade	Description of Osteotomy
1	Partial facet joint excision—resection of the joint capsule and inferior facet at a particular spinal level.
2	Total facet joint resection—both inferior and superior facets at a specific spinal segment are excised with whole ligamentum flavum excision; other posterior parts of the vertebra incorporating the spinous processes and the lamina may also be excised.
3	Partial body/pedicle resection—partial wedge excision of a segment of the posterior vertebral body and of a part of the posterior vertebral elements, including the pedicle.
4	Partial body/pedicle/disc—wider wedge excision through the vertebral body, including a substantial part of the posterior vertebral body, posterior elements with pedicles, as well as excision of at least a portion of 1 endplate with the nearby intervertebral disc.
5	Discs and total vertebra—total excision of a vertebra and of both nearby discs (rib excision in the dorsal region).
6	Discs and multiple vertebrae—excision of more than one total vertebra and of nearby discs. Grade 5 excision as well as additional nearby vertebral excision.

Source: Authors' compilation based on data from Schwab et al. (2014).

Degenerative Spine Disease Without Instability

Without overt instability, whether a degenerative spine needs fusion or not is a matter of debate. There are no class I data to prove the efficacy of fusion. With the fact that the fusion reduces the range of movement, novel surgical plans are required to substitute surgical fusion.

Dynamic Stabilization

Two techniques are being studied: disc arthroplasty and posterior dynamic stabilization devices. The US Food and Drug Administration (FDA) has approved some artificial disc brands to manage symptomatic degenerative lumbar disc disease. Disc arthroplasty and lumbar fusion yielded similar results in short-term studies (Lin and Wang 2006).

A prospective, randomized, controlled multicentre trial aimed at demonstrating the "noninferiority" of cervical total disc replacement (TDR) in terms of outcome at 24 months found that this technique was at least similar in terms of outcome to anterior cervical discectomy and fusion (Murrey et al. 2009). Though most key outcome criteria (like pain scores and neurologic success) were comparable across both arms at 24 months, the disc replacement arm required fewer analgesics and had a lesser number of reoperations than the fusion arm.

Despite the fact that these findings are encouraging for total disc replacement, they should not be applied to the group of cases with multilevel disc herniations, spondylolisthesis, spondylosis, or degenerative disc disease (DDD), as this research was applicable to patients with radiculopathy and single-level disc disease. Long-term follow-up studies are essential to see whether these advantages are long-lasting, whether motion preservation using artificial discs is maintained over time, and whether the frequency of adjacent segment disease is reduced.

There are various types of posterior dynamic stabilization devices. Pedicle screw-based systems, in which the screws are joined by flexible elements rather than rigid rods, are the most promising. Theoretically, their purpose is to restrict movement to an area where spine loading is near-neutral or neutral or to avoid movement into a zone where excessive loading happens. Again, the studies undertaken thus far have generated clinical outcomes that are comparable to fusion (Schwarzenbach et al. 2005).

Contrary to conventional spinal instruments, which are sheltered from biomechanical stress as soon as the bony fusion is established, artificial discs and posterior dynamic stabilization devices should have better outcomes than fusion surgery and must function for the lifetime of the patient. Biologic management strategies aimed at repairing and preserving deteriorated spine elements, rather than mechanical treatment strategies, are more likely to give an acceptable remedy to degenerative spine disease in the future. Until then, lumbar TDR may be a preferable way of treatment over lumbar fusion for young patients with degenerative disc disease (DDD) who do not have severe facet joint degeneration, deformity, instability, or osteopenia/osteoporosis (Salzmann et al. 2017).

3. Kyphosis

When the dorsal spine curve is outside of the usual limit on the sagittal plane, it is called kyphosis. The Cobb angle is taken to determine the angle of the thoracic curve. Angle calculations between the superior endplate of D5 and the inferior endplate of D12 were reported by the Scoliosis Research Society (SRS) to range from 10 to 40 degrees (O'Brien et al. 2004). Thoracic kyphosis develops more commonly in men than in women (9.6%) (Yaman and Dalbayrak 2014).

3.1. Aetiology of Kyphosis

- Congenital kyphosis (Figure 12);
- Scheuermann kyphosis;
- Degenerative disc disease;
- Tumour-related kyphosis;
- Post-traumatic kyphosis;
- Postlaminectomy iatrogenic kyphosis;
- Infection-related kyphosis (Pott);
- Kyphosis developing due to neuromuscular diseases;
- Muscular dystrophy;
- Myelomeningocele;
- Spinal muscular atrophy;
- Paget's disease;
- Neurofibromatosis;
- Skeletal dysplasia (Yaman and Dalbayrak 2014).

The most important aetiologies of kyphosis will be discussed here.

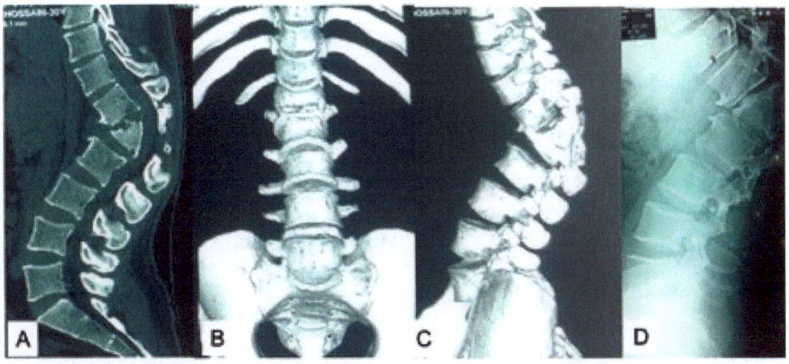

Figure 12. (**A**) Sagittal view; (**B**,**C**) three-dimensional reconstruction of CT scan of lumbodorsal spine and (**D**) X-ray lumbodorsal spine lateral view showing congenital kyphosis due to anomalous L1 vertebra. Source: Figure by authors.

3.2. *Scheuermann Kyphosis*

The Danish radiologist Holger Werfel Scheuermann was the first to define Scheuermann disease, also called "osteochondritis deformans juvenilis dorsi". The osteochondritis of secondary ossification centres causes rigid kyphosis which is commonest in young adults (Scheuermann 1920). It most frequently affects the lower dorsal and upper lumbar regions. It mostly affects adolescents between the ages of 13 and 16. The majority of patients are taller than their peers (Fotiadis et al. 2008).

Sorenson proposed the first diagnostic criteria for Scheuermann disease (Sörensen 1964):

1. Angulation of wedging of at least three adjacent vertebrae greater than 5°.
2. Kyphosis in the sagittal plane of more than 40°.
3. Irregularities of vertebral endplate.
4. Though Scheuermann's disease generally affects the dorsal spine (classic type), Edgren et al. also published an atypical type affecting the lumbar spine (Edgren and Vainio 1957).

3.2.1. Clinical Findings

1. Pain: after being seated for a long time, pain develops in the apical area. This pain diminishes once growth stops. Type 2 Scheuermann kyphosis causes greater pain than type 1 kyphosis.
2. Deformity: it is most commonly found during school age. To counteract kyphosis, lordosis of the lumbar and cervical spine may increase (Yaman and Dalbayrak 2014).

3.2.2. Treatment

When kyphosis can be minimized, rehabilitation is indicated to relieve discomfort and enhance sagittal balance. Postural control, trunk stretching and strengthening, and musculotendinous stretching, notably of tense pectoral and hamstring muscles, are all examples of rehabilitation treatments. In the event of restrictive pulmonary disease, respiratory rehabilitation can be beneficial (Zaina et al. 2009). For uncomfortable Scheuermann's disease with mild kyphosis or for mild kyphosis itself, bracing is recommended (Bradford et al. 1974).

When kyphosis between 55° and 80° is diagnosed before skeletal maturity, brace treatment is almost always successful, according to Lowe (Lowe 2007; Lowe and Line 2007). Until the patient achieves skeletal maturity, the brace should be put on for 21 h every day (Zaina et al. 2009; Gutowski and Renshaw 1988). Due to both the psychological and aesthetic influence of a neck ring, compliance may be lower with the Milwaukee brace than with other braces.

Scheuermann's disease rarely needs surgery. Surgery is suggested for stiff and symptomatic kyphosis (neurological impairment) with considerable and increasing curvature (>70°) when conservative measures fail (Lowe and Line 2007; Papagelopoulos et al. 2008; Palazzo et al. 2014). In skeletally mature patients, it must be performed by qualified surgeons. The first surgical procedure for treating Scheuermann's kyphosis was the posterior operative technique (Papagelopoulos et al. 2008). Various approaches have been developed. They all have the following steps: spinal structures are released, kyphosis is corrected (at least 50% of the curve is corrected), and instrumentation with arthrodesis is performed.

A number of authors paired an anterior release with a posterior correction to make the curve easier to adjust. The benefits of the additional anterior technique, on the other hand, are uncertain, and side effects may be more common (Lee et al. 2006; Lonner et al. 2007). Electrophysiologic monitoring is increasingly used to control neurological problems that may develop after surgery, especially during kyphosis reduction. Neurological (paraplegia), infectious, and respiratory problems are the most common (Lowe and Line 2007). The degeneration of the segment above or below the arthrodesis is known as junctional syndrome (Kim et al. 2012).

3.3. *Postlaminectomy Kyphosis*

Following extensive laminectomy, the likelihood of developing kyphosis increases. The facets of the posterior column in the neck area carry 65% of the load, while the rest is transmitted to the forearm. It is important to remember that when the posterior tension band (the ligamentum flavum, interspinous ligaments, and the ligamentum nuchae) is destroyed, stability is compromised (Yaman and Dalbayrak 2014).

The removal of more than a third of the cervical facets has been linked to instabilities (Epstein 1988). In certain studies, the rate of postlaminectomy kyphosis development in the paediatric age group was reported to be 100% (Dickson et al. 1978). To preclude the development of postlaminectomy kyphosis, cases should be carefully opted for laminectomy. The likelihood of developing postlaminectomy kyphosis is reduced if there is preoperative lordosis (10 degrees or more), no instability findings on extension and flexion radiographs, and the facets are preserved perioperatively. In patients without cervical lordosis, the likelihood of postlaminectomy kyphosis is twice as high. In patients in whom the facets could not be protected, posterior fusion after decompression is indicated (Rao et al. 2011; Scioscia et al. 2011). When 30%–50% of the facets are eliminated, McAllister et al. recommend fusion (McAllister et al. 2012). In one study, anterior corpectomy with instrumentation, posterior fusion plus instrumentation and combined anterior corpectomy and posterior fusion with instrumentation were offered as surgical options for postlaminectomy kyphosis. During follow-up, none of the patients managed with cervical laminectomy and fused with lateral mass screws developed kyphosis, according to Kumar et al. (Kumar et al. 1999).

Post-traumatic kyphosis is a type of kyphosis that develops at the thoracolumbar junction after a trauma or surgery (Vaccaro and Jacoby 2002). The loads posed on the thoracic spinal segment during compression and flexion may create segmental kyphosis by causing a height decrease in the anterior column. Progressive kyphosis can occur as a result of pseudoarthrosis that occurs following surgery to cure the patient's spinal fracture and lack of fusion. Progressive neurological deficit and discomfort are the specific surgical signs of post-traumatic kyphosis (Yaman and Dalbayrak 2014; Vaccaro and Jacoby 2002).

4. Scoliosis

4.1. Introduction and Classification

Scoliosis is a broad term that describes a range of disorders characterized by alterations in the shape and the position of the spine, trunk, and thorax. Hippocrates used the term "spina luxate" to refer to all spinal abnormalities. Galen is credited with coining the term "scoliosis" (from the Greek skolios, which means "crooked or curved") (Vasiliadis et al. 2009) to describe an abnormal lateral spinal curvature.

"Structural scoliosis," or simply scoliosis, must be distinguished from "functional scoliosis," which is a curvature of the spine caused by extraspinal factors (e.g., paraspinal muscle tone asymmetry or shortening of a lower limb). When the underlying cause is removed, it usually reduces or disappears completely (e.g., in a recumbent position) (Negrini et al. 2018).

Kleinberg (Kleinberg 1922) coined the phrase "idiopathic scoliosis," which refers to all cases in which a specific disease is unable to be identified as the reason of the deformity; in reality, it can arise in otherwise healthy children and it progresses in response to a variety of stimuli throughout the fast interval of growth. Idiopathic scoliosis, by definition, has no known aetiology and is most likely caused by a combination of factors.

Idiopathic scoliosis is an aetiopathogenetically characterized spinal deformity that is an indication of a syndrome with a complex aetiology (Xiong et al. 1994; Burwell et al. 1983; Brooks et al. 1975). Scoliosis almost often appears as a single deformity, but careful examination may uncover several significant subclinical signs (Grivas et al. 2002; Weinstein 1999).

An "upper-end vertebra" and a "lower-end vertebra," both used as a control level to determine the Cobb angle, limit the curvature in the frontal plane (AP X-ray in upright posture) (Figure 13). The diagnosis is verified, according to the Scoliosis Research Society (SRS), when the Cobb angle is 10 degrees or above and axial rotation is visible. At the apical vertebra, the maximum axial rotation is measured. A Cobb angle of less than 10° (Xiong et al. 1994), however, can indicate structural scoliosis with the possibility of progression.

Progression is more prevalent in female children during the puberty growth spurt, and it is known as progressive idiopathic scoliosis then. If left untreated, it can progress to significant trunk abnormalities, limiting chest capacity as well as functional biomechanics, exercise capability, work abilities, and overall fitness, all of which are linked to a decrease in the quality of life (Negrini et al. 2018).

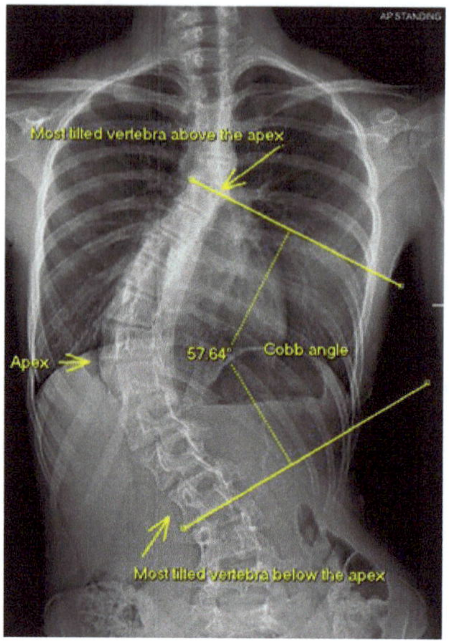

Figure 13. X-ray showing dorsolumbar scoliosis and demonstration of calculation of Cobb angle. Source: Figure by authors.

The three-step Lenke (Lenke et al. 2001) classification for adolescent idiopathic scoliosis has gained acceptance.

1. Label primary curve as type 1 to 6.

- Calculate regional curves:
  - Proximal thoracic (PT);
  - Main thoracic (MT);
  - Thoracolumbar/lumbar (TL/L).
- Define major curve (biggest curve): always either MT (type 1–4) or MT/L (type 4*, 5, 6).
- Detect whether minor curve is structural or not:

  Definition of structural: >25 degrees in the coronal plane on standing AP and not bending out to <25 degrees on bending films OR >20 degrees in the sagittal plane.

Assign type 1 to 6 based on the chart from Table 6.

Table 6. Assignment of types 1 to 6 based on chart below.

Curve Type	Curve Name	Comment on PT **, MT, TL/L
1	Main thoracic	Structural (major*) for MT, none for PT, TL/L
2	Double thoracic (DT)	Structural for PT and structural (major*) for MT, none for TL/L
3	Double major (DM)	None for PT, structural (major*) for MT, structural for TL/L
4	Triple major (TM)	Structural for PT, structural (major*) for MT and TL/L
5	TL/L	None for PT and MT, structural (major*) for TL/L
6	TL/L-MT	None for PT, structural for MT, structural (major*) for TL/L

Structural (major*)—has the largest Cobb angle and is always structural. In type 4, it can be either MT or FL/L based on which Cobb angle is greater. ** If PT is the largest curve, then by default assign major curve to MT. Source: Authors' compilation based on data from Lenke et al. (2001).

2. Assign lumbar modifier (A, B, C).

- Identify apical lumbar vertebrae (ALV): is it the lower lumbar body which falls outside of the curve?
- Draw the central sacral vertical line (CSVL) and determine its relationship to the pedicles of the ALV.
- Modifier:

- A if CSVL runs between pedicles of apical lumbar vertebrae (ALV);
  CSVL falls between pedicles of the lumbar spine up to stable vertebra.
- B modifier if CSVL touches pedicle of apical lumbar vertebrae (ALV);
- C modifier if CSVL does not touch apical lumbar vertebrae (ALV);
  Apex of lumbar curve falls completely off the midline, showing a curve with complete apical translation off the CSVL.

3. Assign sagittal modifier (-,N,+).

- Measure the sagittal Cobb angle from D5 to D12.
- Modifier:

  (a) hypokyphotic (−) if <10°;
  (b) normal if 10°–40°;
  (c) hyperkyphotic (+) if >40°.

4.2. Management

Scoliosis is a difficult condition to treat medically. Observation, bracing, and surgery are the traditional alternatives, in order. Spinal deformities are surgically corrected or improved to maintain sagittal balance, improve or preserve lung function, limit pain or morbidity, maximise postoperative function, and elevate or at least not affect lumbar spine function (Canale and Beaty 2008).

Developed curvature in a growing paediatric patient, severe deformity C > 50 with asymmetry of the trunk in teens, discomfort that is not contained by nonsurgical management, dorsal lordosis, and considerable physical deformity are all indications for the surgical treatment of AIS. Fusion surgery approaching from the anterior, posterior, or a combination of both are among the surgical options. Anterior procedures for idiopathic scoliosis include anterior instrumentation and fusion, which is now considered a standard procedure for certain dorsolumbar and lumbar curves (Canale and Beaty 2008; Muschik et al. 2006). Without using the anterior method, posterior instrumented fusion with pedicle screws or hooks is used. There are two stages in the combined technique:

(1) Anterior release plus fusion.
(2) Posterior fusion plus instrumentation with multi-hook segments (Canale and Beaty 2008; Muschik et al. 2006).

In more serious cases, a combination of these two steps is used.

In skeletally immature patients, the anterior technique has long been recommended because it can effectively prevent the crankshaft phenomenon (Dwyer 1973; Giehl et al. 1992) and it has historically been recorded to achieve better curve and rib hump correction as well as save fusion levels caudally. Another benefit derived from anterior spinal instrumentation is that it can treat thoracic hypokyphosis, which is common in AIS patients (Betz et al. 1999).

The results of thoracoscopic anterior instrumented spinal fusion are likewise excellent. Many surgeons, on the other hand, are unfamiliar with thoracoscopic surgery (Geck et al. 2009). When compared to anterior open or posterior methods, the learning curve remains steep, and operating times appear to be much longer (Lonner et al. 2006; Newton et al. 2009). All of these factors have limited its widespread adoption among orthopaedic surgeons. For the same duration of time, posterior pedicle screw instrumentation with posterior Ponte osteotomies (Geck et al. 2009) for both dorsal and dorsolumbar idiopathic scoliosis have gained popularity due to less morbidity, better respiratory function outcomes, and similar roentgenographic outcomes compared to anterior surgery (Lonner et al. 2006; Newton et al. 2009).

Although anterior thoracoscopic instrumentation can produce significant scoliosis correction (average 55–65%) with favourable cosmetic results, the danger of instrumentation problems (proximal screw pull-out) and of pseudoarthrosis is considerable (Reddi et al. 2008).

In the literature, there are several studies that compare anterior releasing and posterior fusing procedures for the treatment of scoliosis (Muschik et al. 2006). SA-phased treatment for extreme inflexible scoliosis with a Cobb angle > 80° at the coronal plane was described in a retrospective study by Yamin et al. (Yamin et al. 2008). The first stage involved anterior release and halopelvic tension, while the second stage involved posterior instrumentation plus spinal fusion. They came to the conclusion that staged surgery is a reliable method for managing serious stiff scoliosis (Yamin et al. 2008). Min et al. (Min et al. 2007) investigated the radiological and clinical results of patients who had selective short anterior fusion of the main thoracolumbar/lumbar (TL/L) curve for the management of idiopathic AIS. They came to the conclusion that a balanced and satisfactorily repaired spine is produced by selected short anterior fusion of the TL/L curve scoliosis with a dorsal curve of less than 25 degrees. Short fusions allow for global spinal equilibrium by leaving enough movable lumbar segments (Min et al. 2007).

An anterior approach is, therefore, unnecessary with thoracic pedicle screw instrumentation. When compared to segmental hook instrumentation, posterior pedicle screw instrumentation results in much superior major and minor curvature correction frequencies sans any neurological problems and enhanced lung function (Sanders et al. 2003). According to Betz et al., both the anterior and posterior groups had equal coronal correction and balancing (Betz et al. 1999). In both the axial and coronal planes, thoracic pedicle screws enhanced correction. When compared to posterior segmental hook instrumentation, lumbar lordosis can be adequately managed to allow for more dorsal hypokyphosis (Pourfeizi et al. 2014).

Due to an increased risk of wound- or anaesthesia-related issues, two-stage surgery to repair scoliosis may give rise to some difficulties. Other potential hazards include thoracotomy complications (haemothorax, pneumothorax, etc.). Because of the unique challenges of ICU admissions, statistically significant differences are a critical aspect to consider when making an ICU admission decision. Another element to consider is the total length of stay in the hospital. Long-term hospitalization can raise hospitalization risks (medical errors, nosocomial infections, psychological impacts, and so on) (Weiss and Goodall 2008).

Scoliosis can cause soft-tissue inflammation or deep inflammatory processes as well as respiratory difficulties, haemorrhage, and nerve injury. Approximately 5% of individuals require reoperation as little as five years after surgery (Hawes and O'Brien 2008). The physical consequences of surgery are not always predictable (Kouwenhoven and Castelein 2008). In severe scoliosis, posterior segmental pedicle screw fixation without anterior release resulted in plausible deformity correction with minimal loss of curvature correction (Pourfeizi et al. 2014).

Growth modulation procedures, like the Shilla operation, growing rods, stapling of vertebral body, and, recently, vertebral body tethering (VBT), all rely on the Hueter–Volkmann principle to control growth and to rectify the curvature in adolescent idiopathic scoliosis (Aronsson and Stokes 2011; McCarthy et al. 2014; Betz et al. 2010; Hueter 1863). These approaches are expected to help maintain the underlying structure of the spine, which can result in a variety of advantages (Hoernschemeyer et al. 2020).

Author Contributions: Conceptualization, methodology, validation, formal analysis, investigation, resources, data curation, writing—original draft preparation, K.A.K.; writing—review and editing, visualization, supervision, F.H.C. All authors have read and agreed to the published version of the manuscript.

Funding: This research received no external funding.

Conflicts of Interest: The authors declare no conflicts of interest.

References

Acar, Feridun, Sait Naderi, Mustafa Guvencer, Ugur Türe, and Mahmut N. Arda. 2005. Herophilus of Chalcedon: A Pioneer in Neuroscience. *Neurosurgery* 56: 861–67. [CrossRef]

Aronsson, David D., and Ian A. F. Stokes. 2011. Nonfusion treatment of adolescent idiopathic scoliosis by growth modulation and remodeling. *Journal of Pediatric Orthopaedics 31 S* 1: S99–S106. [CrossRef]

Bess, Shay, Breton Line, Kai-Ming Fu, Ian McCarthy, Virgine Lafage, Frank Schwab, Christopher Shaffrey, Christopher Ames, Behrooz Akbarnia, Han Kim Jo, and et al. 2016. The health impact of symptomatic adult spinal deformity: Comparison of deformity types to United States population norms and chronic diseases. *Spine (Phila Pa 1976)* 41: 224–33. [CrossRef]

Betz, Randal R., Ashish Ranade, Amer F. Samdani, Ross Chafetz, Linda P. D'Andrea, John P. Gaughan, Jahangir Asghar, Harsh Grewal, and Mary Jane Mulcahey. 2010. Vertebral body stapling: A fusionless treatment option for a growing child with moderate idiopathic scoliosis. *Spine (Phila Pa 1976)* 35: 169–76. [CrossRef]

Betz, Randal R., Jürgen Harms, David H. Clements, III, Lawrence G. Lenke, Thomas G. Lowe, Harry L. Shufflebarger, Dezsö Jeszenszky, and Bruno Beele. 1999. Comparison of anterior and posterior instrumentation for correction of adolescent thoracic idiopathic scoliosis. *Spine (Phila Pa 1976)* 24: 225–39. [CrossRef]

Bican, Orhan, Alireza Minagar, and Amy A. Pruitt. 2013. The spinal cord: A review of functional neuroanatomy. *Neurologic Clinics* 31: 1–18. [CrossRef]

Boachie-Adjei, Oheneba, John AI Ferguson, Richard G. Pigeon, and Melissa R. Peskin. 2006. Transpedicular lumbar wedge resection osteotomy for fixed sagittal imbalance: Surgical technique and early results. *Spine (Phila Pa 1976)* 31: 485–92. [CrossRef]

Booth, Kevin C., Keith H. Bridwell, Lawrence G. Lenke, Christy R. Baldus, and Kathy M. Blanke. 1999. Complications and predictive factors for the successful treatment of flatback deformity (fixed sagittal imbalance). *Spine* 24: 1712–20. [CrossRef]

Boyraz, Ismail, Hilmi Uysal, Bunyamin Koc, and Hakan Sarman. 2015. Clonus: Definition, mechanism, treatment. *Medicinski Glasnik* 12: 19–26.

Bradford, David S., John H. Moe, Francisco J. Montalvo, and Robert B. Winter. 1974. Scheuermann's kyphosis and round-back deformity. Results of Milwaukee brace treatment. *The Journal of Bone and Joint Surgery* 56: 740–58.

Bradford, David S., Walter L. Schumacher, John E. Lonstein, and Robert B. Winter. 1987. Ankylosing spondylitis: Experience in surgical management of 21 patients. *Spine* 12: 238–43. [CrossRef] [PubMed]

Bridwell, Keith H., Stephen J. Lewis, Anthony Rinella, Lawrence G. Lenke, Christy Baldus, and Kathy Blanke. 2004. Pedicle subtraction osteotomy for the treatment of fixed sagittal imbalance. Surgical technique. *The Journal of Bone and Joint Surgery* 86 S1: 44–50. [PubMed]

Brooks, H. L., S. P. Azen, E. Gerberg, R. Brooks, and L. Chan. 1975. Scoliosis: A prospective epidemiological study. *The Journal of Bone and Joint Surgery* 57: 968–72. [CrossRef] [PubMed]

Burwell, R. G., N. J. James, F. Johnson, J. K. Webb, and Y. G. Wilson. 1983. Standardised trunk asymmetry scores. A study of back contour in healthy school children. *The Journal of Bone & Joint Surgery British* 65: 452–63.

Canale, S. Terry, and James H. Beaty. 2008. *Campbell's Operative Orthopaedics*. Philadelphia: Mosby.

Diaz, Eric, and Humberto Morales. 2016. Spinal Cord Anatomy and Clinical Syndromes. *Seminars in Ultrasound, CT and MRI* 37: 360–71. [CrossRef]

Dickson, Jesse H., P. R. Harrington, and W. D. Erwin. 1978. Results of reduction and stabilization of the severely fractured thoracic and lumbar spine. *The Journal of Bone and Joint Surgery* 60: 799–805. [CrossRef]

Diebo, Bassel G., Neil V. Shah, Oheneba Boachie-Adjei, Feng Zhu, Dominique A. Rothenfluh, Carl B. Paulino, Frank J. Schwab, and Virginie Lafage. 2019. Adult spinal deformity. *Lancet* 394: 160–72. [CrossRef]

Dwyer, A. F. 1973. Experience of anterior correction of scoliosis. *Clinical Orthopaedics and Related Research* 93: 191–214. [CrossRef]

Edgren, Walter, and Sakari Vainio. 1957. Osteochondrosis juvenilis lumbalis. *Acta Chirurgica Scandinavica Supplementum* 227: 3–47.

Epstein, Joseph A. 1988. The surgical management of cervical spinal stenosis, spondylosis and myeloradiculopathy by means of the posterior approach. *Spine* 13: 864–69. [CrossRef]

Fotiadis, E., E. Kenanidis, E. Samoladas, A. Christodoulou, P. Akritopoulos, and K. Akritopoulou. 2008. Scheuermann's disease: Focus on weight and height role. *European Spine Journal* 17: 673–78. [CrossRef]

Frostell, Arvid, Ramil Hakim, Eric Peter Thelin, Per Mattsson, and Mikael Svensson. 2016. A Review of the Segmental Diameter of the Healthy Human Spinal Cord. *Frontiers in Neurology* 7: 238. [CrossRef]

Fuller, Geraint. 2019. *Neurological Examination Made Easy E-Book*. Amsterdam: Elsevier Health Sciences.

Geck, Matthew J., Anthony Rinella, Dana Hawthorne, Angel Macagno, Linda Koester, Brenda Sides, Keith Bridwell, Lawrence Lenke, and Harry Shufflebarger. 2009. Comparison of surgical treatment in Lenke 5C adolescent idiopathic scoliosis:anterior dual rod versus posterior pedicle fixation surgery. A comparison of two practices. *Spine* 34: 1942–51. [CrossRef]

Giehl, J. P., J. Volpel, and E. Heindrich. 1992. Correction of the sagittal plane in idiopathic scoliosis undergoing the Zielke procedure (VDS). *International Orthopaedics* 16: 213–18. [CrossRef]

Glassman, Steven D., Keith Bridwell, John R. Dimar, William Horton, Sigurd Berven, and Frank Schwab. 2005. The impact of positive sagittal balance in adult spinal deformity. *Spine* 30: 2024–29. [CrossRef]

Grivas, Theodoros B., Panagiotis Samelis, Theodoros Chadziargiropoulos, and Basilios Polyzois. 2002. Study of the rib cage deformity in children with 10°-20° of Cobb angle Late Onset Idiopathic Scoliosis, using Rib-Vertebra Angles. *Studies in Health Technology and Informatics* 91: 20–24. [CrossRef]

Gutowski, W. Thomas, and Thomas S. Renshaw. 1988. Orthotic results in adolescent kyphosis. *Spine (PhilaPa 1976)* 13: 485–89. [CrossRef]

Hawes, Martha C., and Joseph P. O'Brien. 2008. A century of spine surgery: What can patients expect? *Disability and Rehabilitation* 30: 808–17. [CrossRef]

Hoernschemeyer, Daniel G., Melanie E. Boeyer, Madeline E. Robertson, Christopher M. Loftis, John R. Worley, Nicole M. Tweedy, Sumit U. Gupta, Dana L. Duren, Christina M. Holzhauser, and Venkataraman M. Ramachandran. 2020. Anterior Vertebral Body Tethering for Adolescent Scoliosis with Growth Remaining A Retrospective Review of 2 to 5-Year Postoperative Results. *The Journal of Bone & Joint Surgery* 102: 1169–76. [CrossRef]

Hueter, C. 1863. Anatomic studies on the joints of the extremities in newborns and adults. *Archiv für Pathologische Anatomie und Physiologie und für klinische Medicin* 26: 484–519.

Kim, Daniel, Donald D. Davis, and Richard P. Menger. 2021. Spine Sagittal Balance. In *StatPearls [Internet]*. Treasure Island: StatPearls Publishing.

Kim, Han Jo, Lawrence G. Lenke, Christopher I. Shaffrey, Ellen M. Van Alstyne, and Andrea C. Skelly. 2012. Proximal junctional kyphosis as a dis-tinct form of adjacent segment pathology after spinal deformity surgery: Asystematic review. *Spine (Phila Pa 1976)* 37: S144–S164. [CrossRef]

Kleinberg, Samuel. 1922. The operative treatment of scoliosis. *Archives of Surgery* 5: 631–45. [CrossRef]

Kouwenhoven, Jan-Willem M., and René M. Castelein. 2008. The pathogenesis of adolescent idiopathic scoliosis: Review of the literature. *Spine (Phila Pa 1976)* 33: 2898–908. [CrossRef]

Kumar, Vijay G. R., Gary L. Rea, Lawrence J. Mervis, and John M. McGregor. 1999. Cervical spondylotic myelopathy: Functional and radiographic longterm outcome after laminectomy and posterior fusion. *Neurosurgery* 44: 771–77. [CrossRef]

Lee, Stanley S., Lawrence G. Lenke, Timothy R. Kuklo, Luis Valenté, Keith H. Bridwell, Brenda Sides, and Kathy M. Blanke. 2006. Comparison of Scheuermann kypho-sis correction by posterior-only thoracic pedicle screw fixation ver-sus combined anterior/posterior fusion. *Spine (Phila Pa 1976)* 31: 2316–21. [CrossRef]

Lenke, Lawrence G., Randal R. Betz, Jürgen Harms, Keith H. Bridwell, David H. Clements, Thomas G. Lowe, and Kathy Blanke. 2001. Adolescent idiopathic scoliosis: A new classification to determine extent of spinal arthrodesis. *The Journal of Bone and Joint Surgery* 83: 1169–81. [CrossRef]

Lin, Eric L., and Jeffrey C. Wang. 2006. Total disk arthroplasty. *Journal of the American Academy of Orthopaedic* 14: 705–14. [CrossRef]

Lonner, Baron S., Dimitriy Kondrashov, Farhan Siddiqi, Victor Hayes, and Carrie Scharf. 2006. Thoracoscopic spinal fusion compared with posterior spinal fusion for the treatment of thoracic adolescent idiopathic scoliosis. *The Journal of Bone and Joint Surgery* 88: 1022–34. [CrossRef]

Lonner, Baron S., Peter Newton, Randy Betz, Carrie Scharf, Michael O'Brien, Paul Sponseller, Lawrence Lenke, Alvin Crawford, Tom Lowe, Lynn Letko, and et al. 2007. Operative management of Scheuermann'skyphosis in 78 patients: Radiographic outcomes, complications, and technique. *Spine (Phila Pa 1976)* 32: 2644–52. [CrossRef]

Lowe, Thomas G. 2007. Scheuermann's kyphosis. *Neurosurgery Clinics of North America* 18: 305–15. [CrossRef]

Lowe, Thomas G., and Breton G. Line. 2007. Evidence based medicine: Analysis of Scheuermann kyphosis. *Spine* 32: S115–S119. [CrossRef]

McAllister, Beck D., Brandon J. Rebholz, and Jeffery C. Wang. 2012. Is posterior fusion necessary with laminectomy in the cervical spine? *Surgical Neurology International* 3: S225–S231. [CrossRef]

McCarthy, Richard E., Scott Luhmann, Lawrence Lenke, and Frances L. McCullough. 2014. The Shilla growth guidance technique for early-onset spinal deformities at 2-year follow-up: A preliminary report. *Journal of Pediatric Orthopaedics* 34: 1–7. [CrossRef]

Menger, Richard P., Donald D. Davis, and Joe H. Bryant. 2020. Spinal Osteotomy. In *StatPearls [Internet]*. Treasure Island: StatPearls Publishing.

Min, Kan, Frederik Hahn, and Kai Ziebarth. 2007. Short anterior correction of the thoracolumbar/lumbar curve in King 1 idiopathic scoliosis: The behaviour of the instrumented and non-instrumented curves and the trunk balance. *European Spine Journal* 16: 65–72. [CrossRef]

Murrey, Daniel, Michael Janssen, Rick Delamarter, Jeffrey Goldstein, Jack Zigler, Bobby Tay, and Bruce Darden. 2009. Results of the prospective, randomized, controlled multicenter Food and Drug Administration investigational device exemption study of the ProDisc-C total disc replacement versus anterior discectomy and fusion for the treatment of 1-level symptomatic cervical disc disease. *The Spine Journal* 9: 275–86. [CrossRef]

Muschik, Michael Thomas, Holger Kimmich, and Thomas Demmel. 2006. Comparison of anterior and posterior double-rod instrumentation for thoracic idiopathic scoliosis: Results of 141 patients. *European Spine Journal* 15: 1128–38. [CrossRef]

Negrini, Stefano, Sabrina Donzelli, Angelo Gabriele Aulisa, Dariusz Czaprowski, Sanja Schreiber, Jean Claude de Mauroy, Helmut Diers, Theodoros B. Grivas, Patrick Knott, Tomasz Kotwicki, and et al. 2018. SOSORT guidelines: Orthopaedic and rehabilitation treatment of idiopathic scoliosis during growth. *Scoliosis and Spinal Disorders* 13: 3. [CrossRef]

Newton, Peter O., Vidyadhar V. Upasani, Juliano Lhamby, Valerie L. Ugrinow, Jeff B. Pawelek, and Tracey P. Bastrom. 2009. Surgical treatment of main thoracic scoliosis with thoracoscopic anterior instrumentation. Surgical technique. *The Journal of Bone and Joint Surgery* 91 S2: 233–48. [CrossRef]

O'Brien, M. F., T. R. Kuklo, K. M. Blanke, and L. G. Lenke. 2004. *Radiographic Measurement Manual*. Memphis: Medtronic Sofamor Danek, pp. 1–110.

Palazzo, Clémence, Frédéric Sailhan, and Michel Revel. 2014. Scheuermann's disease: An update. *Joint Bone Spine* 81: 209–14. [CrossRef]

Papagelopoulos, Panayiotis J., Andreas F. Mavrogenis, Olga D. Savvidou, Evanthia A. Mitsiokapa, George G. Themistocleous, and Panayotis N. Soucacos. 2008. Current concepts in Scheuermann's kyphosis. *Orthopedics* 31: 52–58, quiz 9–60.

Pourfeizi, Hossein Hojjat, Jafar Ganjpour Sales, Ali Tabrizi, Ghanbar Borran, and Sahar Alavi. 2014. Comparison of the Combined Anterior-Posterior Approach versus Posterior-Only Approach in Scoliosis Treatment. *Asian Spine Journal* 8: 8–12. [CrossRef]

Rao, R. D., I. A. Madom, and J. C. Wang. 2011. Cervical laminectomy and fusion. In *Advanced Reconstruction Spine*. Rosemont: American Academy of Orthopedic Surgeons, pp. 97–104.

Reddi, Vasantha, Douglas Vinton Clarke Jr, and Vincent Arlet. 2008. Anterior thoracoscopic instrumentation in adolescent idiopathic scoliosis. A systematic review. *Spine* 33: 1986–94. [CrossRef]

Rose, Peter S., Keith H. Bridwell, Lawrence G. Lenke, Geoffrey A. Cronen, Daniel S. Mulconrey, Jacob M. Buchowski, and Youngjung J. Kim. 2009. Role of pelvic incidence, thoracic kyphosis, and patient factors on sagittal plane correction following pedicle subtraction osteotomy. *Spine* 34: 785–91. [CrossRef]

Roussouly, Pierre, Sohrab Gollogly, Eric Berthonnaud, and Johanes Dimnet. 2005. Classification of the normal variation in the sagittal alignment of the human lumbar spine and pelvis in the standing position. *Spine* 30: 346–53. [CrossRef]

Salzmann, Stephan N., Nicolas Plais, Jennifer Shue, and Federico P. Girardi. 2017. Lumbar disc replacement surgery—Successes and obstacles to widespread adoption. *Current Reviews in Musculoskeletal Medicine* 10: 153–59. [CrossRef]

Sanders, Albert E., Richard Baumann, Hugh Brown, Charles E. Johnston, Lawrence G. Lenke, and Ernest Sink. 2003. Selective anterior fusion of thoracolumbar/lumbar curves in adolescents: When can the associated thoracic curve be left unfused? *Spine (Phila Pa 1976)* 28: 706–13. [CrossRef]

Scheuermann, H. W. 1920. Kyphosis dorsalis juvenilis. *Ugeskrift for Laeger* 82: 385–93.

Schwab, Frank, Ashish Patel, Benjamin Ungar, Jean-Pierre Farcy, and Virginie Lafage. 2010. Adult spinal deformity-postoperative standing imbalance: How much can you tolerate? An overview of key parameters in assessing alignment and planning corrective surgery. *Spine* 35: 2224–31. [CrossRef]

Schwab, Frank, Ashok Dubey, Murali Pagala, Lorenzo Gamez, and Jean P. Farcy. 2003. Adult scoliosis: A health assessment analysis by SF-36. *Spine (Phila Pa 1976)* 28: 602–6. [CrossRef]

Schwab, Frank, Benjamin Blondel, Edward Chay, Jason Demakakos, Lawrence Lenke, Patrick Tropiano, Christopher Ames, Justin S. Smith, Christopher I. Shaffrey, Steven Glassman, and et al. 2014. The comprehensive anatomical spinal osteotomy classification. *Neurosurgery* 74: 112–20. [CrossRef]

Schwarzenbach, Othmar, Ulrich Berlemann, Thomas M. Stoll, and Gilles Dubois. 2005. Posterior dynamic stabilization systems: DYNESYS. *Orthopedic Clinics of North America* 36: 363–72. [CrossRef]

Scioscia, T., A. C. Crowl, and Jeffrey C. Wang. 2011. Posterior subaxial cervical fusion. In *Advanced Reconstruction Spine*. Edited by Jeffrey C. Wang. Rosemont: American Academy of Orthopedic Surgeons, pp. 89–95.

Shimizu, Takachika, Haruhiko Shimada, and Kenji Shirakura. 1993. Scapulohumeral reflex (Shimizu). Its clinical significance and testing maneuver. *Spine (Phila Pa 1976)* 18: 2182–90. [CrossRef]

Smith-Petersen, M. N., Carroll B. Larson, and Otto E. Aufranc. 1969. Osteotomy of the spine for correction of flexion deformity in rheumatoid arthritis. *Clinical Orthopaedics and Related Research* 66: 6–9. [CrossRef]

Sörensen, K. Harry. 1964. *Scheuermann's Juvenile Kyphosis*. Copenhagen: Munksgaard.

Thomasen, E. 1985. Vertebral osteotomy for correction of kyphosis in ankylosing spondylitis. *Clinical Orthopaedics and Related Research* 194: 142–52. [CrossRef]

Vaccaro, A. R., and S. M. Jacoby. 2002. Thoracolomber fractures. In *Orthopaedic Knowledge Update Spine*, 2nd ed. Edited by David F. Fardon and Steven R. Garfin. Illinois: American Academy of Orthopedic Surgeons, pp. 263–78.

Vasiliadis, Elias S., Theodoros B. Grivas, and Angelos Kaspiris. 2009. Historical overview of spinal deformities in ancient Greece. *Scoliosis* 4: 6. [CrossRef]

Walker, H. Kenneth. 1990. Deep Tendon Reflexes. In *Clinical Methods: The History, Physical, and Laboratory Examinations*, 3rd ed. Edited by H. Kenneth Walker, W. Dallas Hall and J. Willis Hurst. Boston: Butterworths.

Wang, Yan, Yonggang Zhang, Xuesong Zhang, Peng Huang, Songhua Xiao, Zheng Wang, Zhengsheng Liu, Baowei Liu, Ning Lu, and Keya Mao. 2008. A single posterior approach for multilevel modified vertebral column resection in adults with severe rigid congenital kyphoscoliosis: A retrospective study of 13 cases. *European Spine Journal* 17: 361–72. [CrossRef]

Watson, Joseph C., William C. Broaddus, Maurice M. Smith, and Wayne S. Kubal. 1997. Hyperactive pectoralis reflex as an indicator of upper cervical spinal cord compression: Report of 15 cases. *Journal of Neurosurgery* 86: 159–61. [CrossRef]

Weinstein, Stuart L. 1999. Natural history. *Spine* 24: 2592–600. [CrossRef]

Weiss, Hans-Rudolf, and Deborah Goodall. 2008. Rate of complications in scoliosis surgery: A systematic review of the Pub Med literature. *Scoliosis* 3: 9. [CrossRef]

White, A. A., and M. M. Panjabi. 1990. *Clinical Biomechanics of the Spine*. Philadelphia: Lippincott, pp. 30–342.

Xiong, Bo, John A. Sevastik, Rune Hedlund, and Bo Sevastik. 1994. Radiographic changes at the coronal plane in early scoliosis. *Spine* 19: 159–64. [CrossRef]

Yaman, Onur, and Sedat Dalbayrak. 2014. Kyphosis: Diagnosis, Classification and Treatment Methods. *Turkish Neurosurgery* 24 S1: 62–74.

Yamin, Shi, Li Li, Wei Xing, Gao Tianjun, and Zhang Yupeng. 2008. Staged surgical treatment for severe and rigid scoliosis. *Journal of Orthopaedic Surgery and Research* 3: 26. [CrossRef]

Zaina, F., S. Atanasio, Claudio Ferraro, C. Fusco, A. Negrini, M. Romano, and Stefano Negrini. 2009. Review of rehabilitation and orthopedic conservative approach to sagittal plane diseases during growth: Hyperkyphosis, junctional kyphosis, and Scheuermann disease. *European Journal of Physical and Rehabilitation Medicine* 45: 595–603.

Spinal Injuries

Md Moshiur Rahman, Nazmin Ahmed and Forhad H. Chowdhury

Abstract: Spinal injury can be devastating for the patient and their family. It can be a big economic burden for families and society. Most spinal injury patients are young and injuries are usually caused by road traffic accidents, falls from heights, or by acts of violence. Injury can occur in any part of the spine. Spinal injury can be with or without neuro-deficit and with or without instability; for this reason, in these patients, clinical and radiological evaluations are very important. Management ranges from simple immobilization to complex decompression and stabilization. The early part of this chapter will discuss the history and epidemiology of spinal injury, the three-column theory of spinal stability, the clinical and radiological evaluation of spinal injury patients, and the classification of spinal injury. The later part of this chapter will briefly demonstrate the principles of management of specific types of spinal injury, as well as their complications and outcome prediction.

Abbreviations

AD	autonomic dysreflexia	AIS	ASIA Impairment Scale
CNS	central nervous system	CV	Cardiovascular
CVJ	craniovertebral junction dislocation	DBH	dopamine-S-hydroxylase
DVT	deep vein thrombosis	GW	Gardner–Wells
ICU	intensive care unit	MAO	monamine oxidase
MRI	magnetic resonance imaging	NLI	neurological level of injury
PE	pulmonary embolism	SCI	spinal cord injury

1. Introduction

Spinal injury can cause an overwhelming debilitation in the patient's life. Adjusting to the new condition is a test for all who are included, as it is particularly costly from the monetary perspective, both for the patient and their family and for healthcare administrations, as improving the patient's quality of life requires a wide range of assorted costs. Furthermore, most patients who experience the ill effects of spinal injury are of working age; therefore, they lose their source of revenue and become absolutely contingent upon their family, both monetarily and in terms of their basic needs, for example, eating, getting dressed, bathing, and so on, requiring in-home, personalized medical care. As indicated by different epidemiological examinations, spinal cord injury affects somewhere in the range of 236–1298 people per million worldwide (Guttman 1973). Spinal cord injury (SCI) can result from acute trauma, compression, and from hemisection. These three causes are reflected in the clinical scores for the study of SCI. Each of the three results in various levels of essential tissue damage. Despite noteworthy advancements in the recovery of SCI patients, the following areas have not been satisfactorily researched: (1) the overall fundamental pathophysiologic issues that happen in severely affected subjects, such as osteoporosis, periarticular bone alterations, hypertensive emergencies, etc.; (2) moderation of serious injury: anti-inflammatories or careful intervention to protect as much sensory and motor function as possible; and (3) the potential recovery of lost motor function. Acute injury to the spinal cord results in an immediate loss of motor function. The capacity to walk requires the support of a number of long tracts of the spinal cord. Moreover, pathophysiologic changes happen following SCI. If we are mindful of the specific pathophysiologic condition of the patient, it is conceivable to diminish the pace of progressive loss of function after acute spinal cord injury and to preserve some level of motor and sensory function by proper intervention. The morphologic changes that result from fall-related spinal cord injuries in exploratory animal models are like those that happen in most human spinal cord injuries. The cell layers of neurons, glia, and veins go through irreversible pathologic changes that lead to the degeneration of the spinal cord and incorporate mechanical and vascular disruption and the influx of free radicals. In spinal cord injury models, blood flow to the affected fragment is especially diminished, indicating that ischaemia might be a significant pathogenic component (DeVivo 2002). The reduced blood flow might lead to vasospasm or microvascular dysfunction, or both. The spinal cord and the remainder of the central nervous system (CNS) have high requirements to function correctly, more so than other vital organs. The blood–CNS barrier maintains a special climate for the CNS by barring certain substances and improving the transport of others, for example, ascorbic acid. Accordingly, lipid and protein membranes must be physicochemically flawless to maintain the functioning of the sensitive films engaged in their transport. Minor disruptions in the arrangement of key atoms in the membranes of the lipids that help keep up the dynamic state of key catalysts, for example, Na+, K+-ATPase, adenylate cyclase, and prostaglandin synthetase, can have adverse outcomes. Modifying lipid transmission will influence synaptosome arrangement and the coupling of transmitter receptors. Biogenic amines delivered inside the spinal cord after injury have been studied.

2. Epidemiology and History

SCI was first mentioned as "an illness not to be cured" by a mysterious physician from Egypt in the supposed Edwin Smith Papyrus over 5000 years ago (Guttman 1973). The prognosis for people with SCI has only recently improved. Before World War II, an individual with SCI had a future that was rarely longer than two years; the majority succumbed to renal failure, septic infections, and pressure ulcers. With the appearance of anti-microbials and improved restorative strategies, noteworthy advancement has been made toward viably alleviating and dealing with the various unexpected problems stemming from SCI. People with SCI have improved their capability for self-care and mobility, which typically enables them to reintegrate into their social networks. This has been made possible by improved intensive care strategies as well as early and comprehensive rehabilitation. The prevalence of SCI has slowly increased, and the relevance of this problem as a medical issue for society has increased, despite the fact that the annual frequency of SCI in the USA has remained stable and that the chances of death every year after injury have decreased. Even though the general incidence has stayed consistent in recent decades, the most prevalent causes of SCI have changed. Car accidents are the main cause of SCI, followed by falls and violence-related reasons (National Spinal Cord Injury Statistical Center 2005). Over time, the severity of injuries associated with sports has decreased while the severity of injuries from falls has increased. Before 1980, 13% of SCI cases were attributed to acts of violence. This percentage peaked at 25% between 1990 and 1999, then started to decline to 14% starting in 2000. Despite the fact that most injuries happen in people between the ages of 16 and 30, the mean age at acute SCI has increased to 37.6 years.The percentage of affected people over 60 years old increased from 5% prior to1980 to 11% after 2000. The origin of the injury differs between age groups, with sports-related and violence-related injuries commoner in the younger population and falling-related injuries commoner in the elderly population. There is a more prominent occurrence of SCI in the hotter months and on weekends. There has been an ongoing pattern toward a higher number of incomplete injuries, perhaps because of differing aetiology (e.g., falls cause an incomplete injury and violent trauma a complete injury), improved therapy at the site of injury by emergency services, and the availability of immediate medical attention. At the time of injury, over half of the individuals with SCI are secondary school graduates and of working age. Less than 33% of people are married at the time of spinal cord injury, with the majority (30%) being single (Go et al. 1995). Cervical injuries make up about 13% of all acute SCIs, whereas thoracic injuries make up the remaining 33%. The most common level of injury resulting in paraplegia is T12, and the most common injury resulting in neurological sequelae is C5, followed by C4 and C6, in the cervical region.

3. Three-Column Concept of the Spine

Francis Denis, in 1983, published a novel classification of spinal fractures as well as their management among stakeholder medical professionals (Zhang and Chauvin 2021; Denis 1983). In place of Sir Frank Holdsworth's earlier two-column theory, he devised a three-column theory (Holdsworth 1970). This newly developed three-column hypothesis later served as the cornerstone of a system for categorizing spinal injuries.

In the Denis classification system, the spinal architecture is divided into three columns including the following components (Figure 1) (Zhang and Chauvin 2021; Denis 1983; Holdsworth 1970):

Anterior column:

- ALL (anterior longitudinal ligament);
- Anterior two-thirds of the vertebral body and the annulus.

Middle column:

- Posterior one-third of the vertebral body and the annulus;
- Posterior vertebral wall;
- PLL (posterior longitudinal ligament).

Posterior column:

- Everything that is behind the PLL plus the posterior ligamentous complex as well as the posterior bony arch (supraspinous ligament, capsule of facet joint, interspinous ligament, and ligamentum flavum).

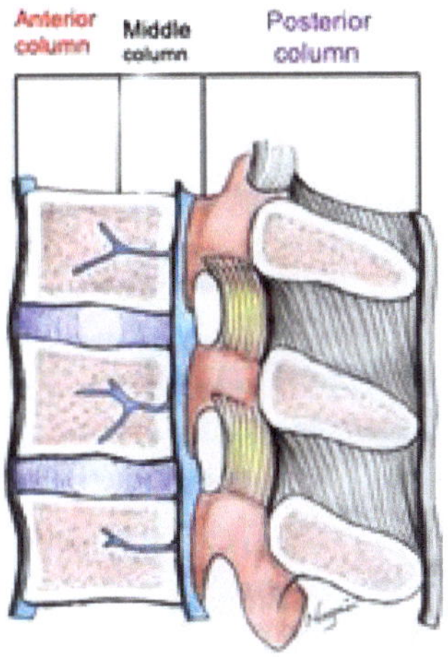

Figure 1. Three-column model of the spine. Source: Figure by authors.

To explain the innate instability of the middle column, the third column was created (Denis 1983; Denis 1984). When the posterior longitudinal ligament is injured in conjunction to the posterior annulus fibrosis, middle column fractures are deemed unstable, but an isolated total breakdown of the posterior ligamentous complex is not enough to cause complete instability (Zhang and Chauvin 2021).

4. Clinical Evaluation of SCI

The International Standards for Neurological Classification of Spinal Cord Injury, more commonly referred to as the American Spinal Injury Association (ASIA) guidelines, are the most precise method for evaluating SCI (Figure 2) (Sapru 2002; American Spinal Injury Association and International Spinal Cord Society 2006). This enables the clinician to determine the motor, physical, and neurological consequences of the injury, the level of the injury, and the ASIA Impairment Scale (AIS) score. The sensory and motor components, along with certain mandatory and optional components, make up the two main segments of the neurologic evaluation of a person with SCI. The necessary components include the assessment of neurological, motor, and sensory function levels, motor and sensory scores, and an assessment of the injury level. An anal examination that checks for voluntary anal contraction and deep anal pressure sensation is also necessary. A standardized neurological scale should be used to capture this information so that it may be retained in clinical records. The optional components are those portions of the neurological evaluation that do not contribute to the mathematical scoring but may reflect a more accurate scenario of the patient's clinical status. These include tests of additional muscles, proprioception, as well as reflexes. An instruction handbook and videotapes on the international regulations in this regard are available via the ASIA office in Atlanta, Georgia. These recommendations provide the definitions for the most often used terminology that doctors use to assess neurological function and evaluate SCI. The Model System Spinal Cord Injury information network uses the international recommendations since they are the most comprehensive and reliable system for evaluating SCI. This information network, which is maintained by designated SCI Model System centres in the USA, keeps track of information about spinal cord injury, provides rehabilitation services, and conduct research on SCI from the onset of injury to its progression over the long term.

For sensory functioning in incomplete spinal cord injury, a mathematical scale is utilized, which is as follows:

0—lack of sensation;
1—weakened sensation, characterized as fractional or modified sensation, encompassing hyperaesthesia;
2—typical sensation, with the face being the ordinary reference point.

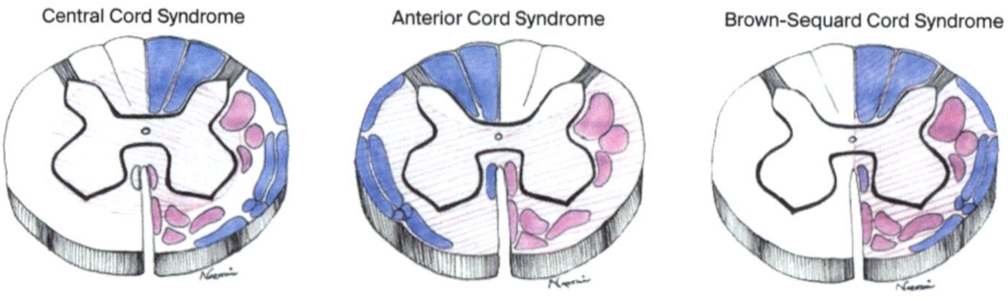

Figure 2. Illustrations of different types of incomplete spinal cord injury. Source: Figure by authors.

The patient must be capable of differentiating between a safety pin's sharp and dull edges in a pinprick test. The failure to distinguish between the two results in a score of 0. When a patient can differentiate between the sharp and dull end but the pin is not felt as sharply as it would be on the face, the patient receives a score of 1 for a weaker response to the pinprick test. If the pain the same as on the face, a score of 2 (normal) is assigned. A cotton swab is utilized to assess light touch, with a normal score of 2 representing a touch sensation equivalent to that on the face and a weakened score of 1 representing less sensation than on the face. The tactile level is described as having a characteristic sensation for both the pinprick and light touch on both sides of the body. This is also assessed on the caudal dermatome. For each dermatome, the scores for pinprick and light touch are added separately to produce a possible absolute score of 112 for tactile record scoring (56 on each side). A digital examination is conducted to evaluate deep anal sensation. The clinician approaches the patient and firmly presses a digit on the inside of the anus to feel for any tactile awareness, whether related to touch or pressure. One or the other must be present in order for deep anal sensation to be recorded. Proprioception, which refers to the ability to sense joint position and movement, temperature, and force, is an optional component of the sensory function assessment. In the unlikely event that precise tactile examination of any dermatome cannot be carried out, "not tried" should be noted, or another site within the dermatome can be examined, with proof that a different site was used. Ten important muscles on each side of the body—five in the upper appendages and five in the lower appendages—are tested as part of the motor assessment. Beginning with the elbow flexors (i.e., C5 innervated muscles) and ending with the plantar flexors, muscles should be tested in a cranial-to-caudal pattern. Although the majority of muscles are supplied by more than one nerve root, these muscles have been chosen for examination as they are consistently essentially innervated by the relevant segment and because they are straightforward to test while lying in a reclined position. A muscle is regarded to have complete innervation by at least one of its innervating segments in SCI if it receives a rating of 3/5. A muscle is regarded as important for useful activities if it has a grading of over 3 and if it can generate resistance against gravity (Welch et al. 1986). Different major muscles (such as the deltoids, abdominal muscles, and hip adductors) may be used; however, they are not utilized to detect the connection of specific regions of the spinal cord or to determine a motor level. In addition to the major muscles, the external anal sphincter should be tested by digital examination to identify voluntary contraction. To avoid confusing reflex contraction of the anal sphincter with voluntary contraction, care must be exercised. The most caudal key muscle group that is rated three or higher on the ASIA scale, with the portions cephalad to it retaining normal function, is known as the motor level (American Spinal Injury Association and International Spinal Cord Society 2006). The motor level is calculated when the motor scores for each muscle are recorded during a standard examination. The highest absolute motor score is 100, or 50 on each side. In many cases, the patient's clinical state may prevent the completion of an accurate assessment, like when a patient is unconscious owing to traumatic brain injury, has a lumbosacral or brachial plexus injury, or has an immobilized limb due to a broken bone. The clinician should enter NT, for "not tried", rather than a numerical score, when the patient is not entirely tested in any way at all. The NLI (neurological level of injury) is the most caudal level above which the body's motor and sensory modalities on the two sides are both normal. For instance, the NLI is C7 if the motor level is C7 and the sensory level is C8. It is advised to note each side separately, as this may provide a clearer picture of the individual's status because the motor or sensory level may differ from side to side (i.e., right C6 motor, C7 sensory, left C7 motor, C6 sensory). Compared to the overall NLI, the motor level in the upper extremities is a good reflection of the level of function and of the severity of injury and disability after tetraplegia (total loss of motor function) (Marino et al. 1995).

5. Neurological Evaluation

Stabilizing spine protections, such as immobilization, should be continued until thorough clinical and radiological evaluations are completed. The underlying examination should include an itemized neurological examination that is completed as early as is practical and includes a time and date stamp. It is crucial that all motor and sensory function be assessed in an awake patient. The American Spine Injury Association (ASIA) framework should be used to assess muscle strength and pinprick and light touch sensation. In unconscious patients, muscular tone, deep tendon reflexes, long tract signs, and priapism in the male patient should all be noted at first. The evaluation should include an anal examination to check sphincter tone, types of contraction, the absence or presence of the bulbocavernosus response, the anal wink, and perineal sensation. The use of a feeding tube and of a Foley urinary catheter can occur as treatment progresses. This is because it is normal for these patients to develop paralytic ileus, which puts them at risk of malnutrition. Not only is the Foley urinary catheter useful for recording urinary production, but it can also prevent bladder overdistention, which frequently accompanies the urinary retention experienced by these individuals.

6. Radiographic Evaluation

A lateral cervical spine series is the first thing that the radiographs of patients with spinal injury are evaluated for. About 70–83% of the time, this view accurately detects significant deviations from the norm. This view has to be examined for arrangement, abnormalities in the bone and intervertebral disc spaces, and soft-tissue injuries. At the C3 level, prevertebral tissues often measure close to 4 mm in thickness. Prevertebral soft-tissue swelling should be taken into account just as much as vertebral facture. In 30–40% of patients, prevertebral soft-tissue swelling could be the primary radiological evidence of traumatic spinal cord injury (Harris 1986). Imaging should include each of the seven cervical vertebrae and the C7-D1 junction (Nichols et al. 1987). Consider using a "swimmer's perspective", offsetting the humeral heads, to visualize the cervical spine. Atlantoaxial, atlanto-occipital, or other instabilities identified in the initial examination are contraindications to using this view. An AP view, together with an odontoid view (also called open mouth), is typically all that is required to sufficiently view the cervical spine. Limitations of plain X-rays include the difficulty in identifying tendon injuries, over- and underexposure, and decreased perception of the cervicothoracic, occipitocervical, and thoracolumbar areas. CT scanning should also be used to investigate any areas or junctions that ordinary views are unable to adequately visualize. Bone dislocation is also better viewed with CT, and CT filters are more sensitive to vertebral fractures (Blackmore et al. 1999). The limitations of this method encompass missing fractures that correlate falsely to the imaging plane. This is no longer a major worry thanks to the use of transforms. However, CT is the imaging modality of choice for viewing neurological components because X-ray has limited sensitivity in diagnosing fractures. CT can be used in patients who have unexplained neurological damage, an additional neurological conditions, or who have inconsistent assessment results between the skeletal and neurological systems. This occurs in cases of traumatic spinal fracture. Spinal cord compression, intramedullary oedema and discharge, plate disruption, ligament injury, and vascular obstruction can all be identified with an X-ray. MRI also provides a better image of recurring injuries such myelomalacia and syrinx arrangement. The great majority of these cases can be assessed using sagittal T2W images. Cases with altered mental states and fractures that involve decussation always be suspected of this (Golueke et al. 1987). When MRI cannot be performed or when there is an MRI contraindication, like a pacemaker, emergency myelography is performed.

7. Types of Spinal Cord Injury

7.1. General Types of Spinal Cord Injury

To link the various types of SCI with their sequelae, clinicians have attempted to classify them depending on clinical symptoms. The Frankel classification is broadly considered to be useful and objective. Cases are evaluated as (A) complete neurological injury; (B) preserved sensation only; (C) preserved motor, nonfunctional; (D) preserved motor, functional; and (E) normal motor function. According to this classification, complete neurological injury has no preservation of motor or sensory function in at least three segments underneath the level of injury. As indicated by the guidelines published by the American Spinal Injury Association in 1992, for a spinal cord injury to be classified as incomplete, motor or sensory function or both should be preserved in the S4–S5 sacral segments (American Spinal Injury Association 1992). Otherwise, the patient is regarded to have a complete spinal injury. These definitions are significant in that, as far as prognosis goes, patients with incomplete

SCI have greater likelihood of achieving some functional recovery, while in those with complete SCI, avoiding spinal shock is the best-case scenario. In large cohort studies of patients with spinal cord injury, the majority are classified as incomplete SCI cases.

7.2. Specific Types of Spinal Cord Injuries

7.2.1. Injury to the Cervical Spine

Different pattern and classification of cervical spinal injuries are shown in Figures 3–11 and Table 1.

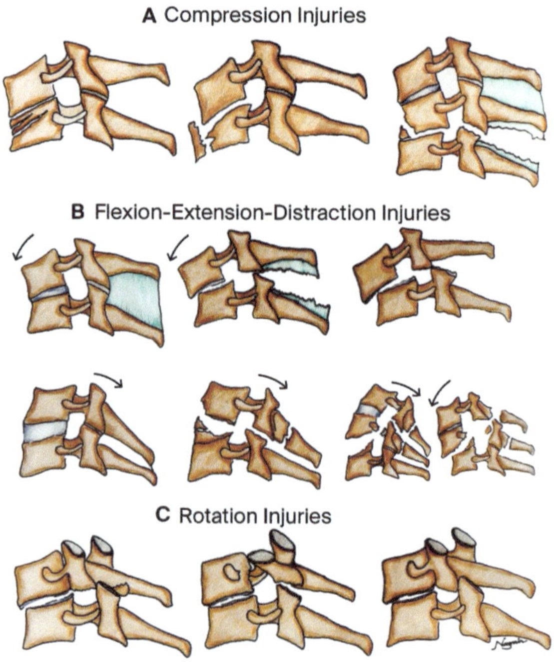

Figure 3. Illustration showing a schema for the classification of lower cervical spine injuries (Argenson et al. 1997). Source: Figure by authors.

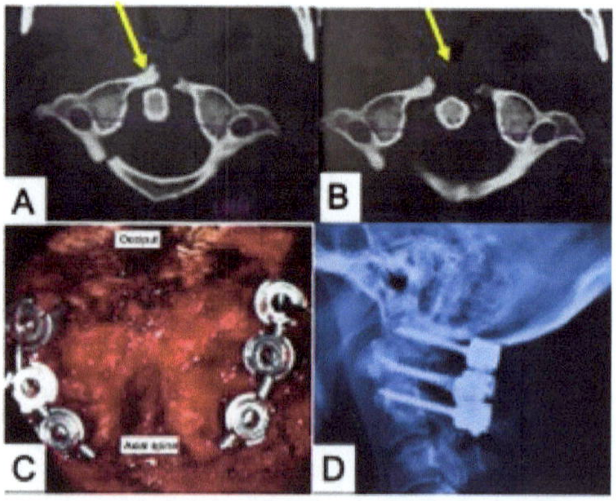

Figure 4. (**A**) CT scan of CVJ showing Jefferson fracture; (**B**) CT scan after 6 weeks showing unstable fracture; (**C**) perioperative picture of fixation of the occipital condyles (Co), C1 lateral mass, and C2 lateral mass with fusion for unstable Jefferson fracture; (**D**) postoperative X-ray showing fixation of Co-C1-C2. Source: Figure by authors.

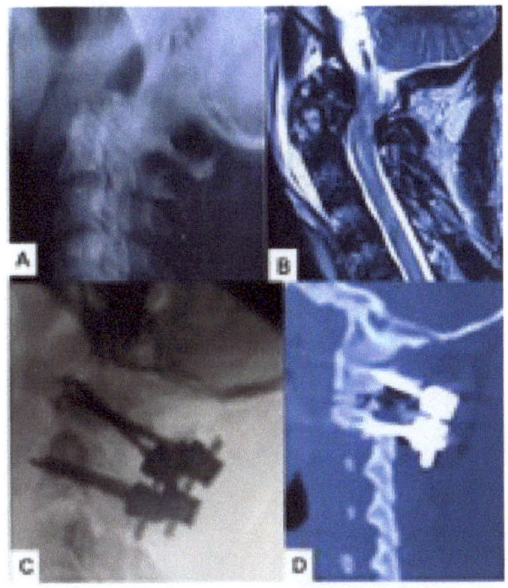

Figure 5. (**A**,**B**) X-ray of cervical spine and MRI of CVJ showing traumatic AAD. (**C**,**D**) X-ray of CVJ showing fixation of C1 and C2 by lateral mass screws and rods, respectively. Source: Figure by authors.

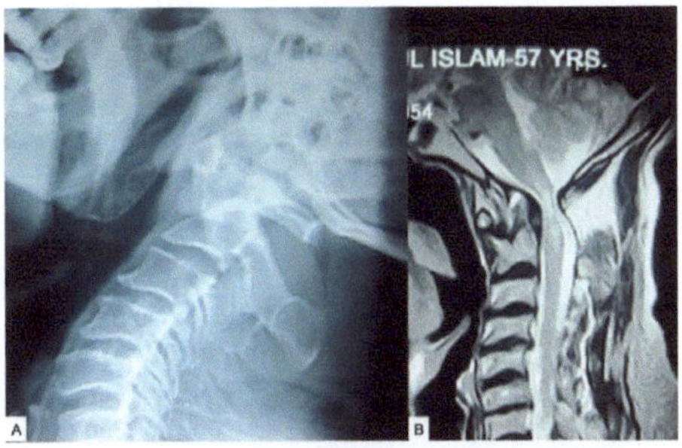

Figure 6. (**A**) X-ray of cervical spine showing AAD (traumatic); (**B**) MRI of CVJ showing AAD with spinal cord compression. Source: Figure by authors.

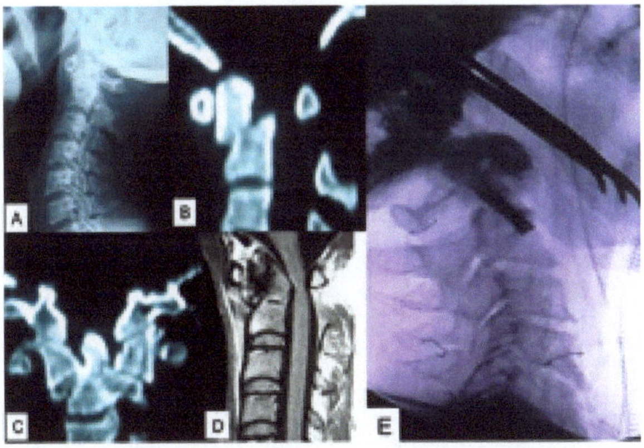

Figure 7. (**A**) X-ray of CVJ showing odontoid fracture with AAD; (**B**,**C**) CT scan of CVJ showing type 2 unstable odontoid fracture. (**D**) MRI of CVJ showing cord compression with instability. (**E**) Intraoperative X-ray showing reduction of odontoid fracture with fixation. Source: Figure by authors.

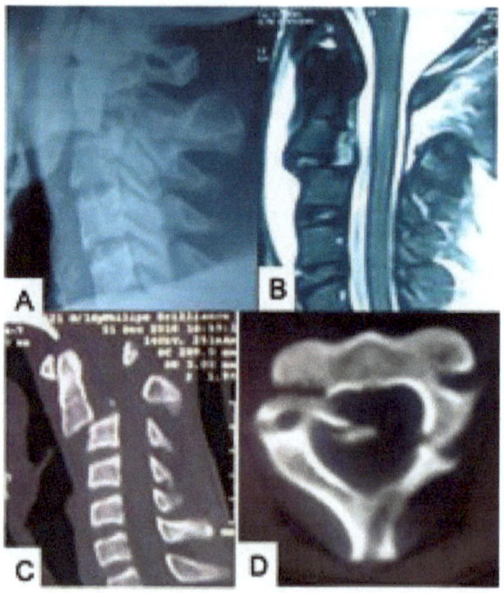

Figure 8. (**A**) X-ray, (**B**) MRI, and (**C,D**) CT scan of cervical spine showing hangman's fracture. Source: Figure by authors.

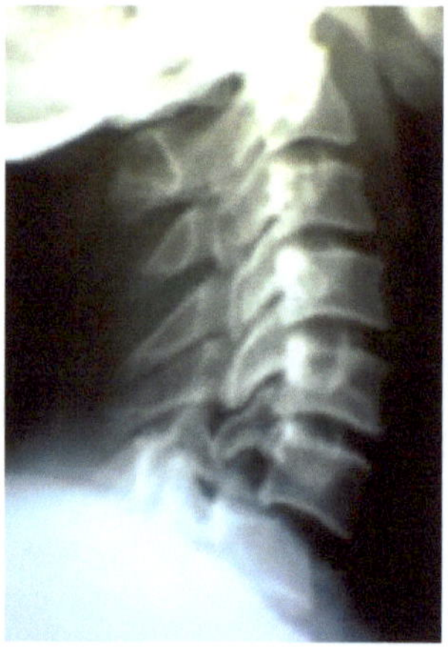

Figure 9. X-ray of cervical spine (lateral view) showing fracture and dislocation of C7 with locked facet. Source: Figure by authors.

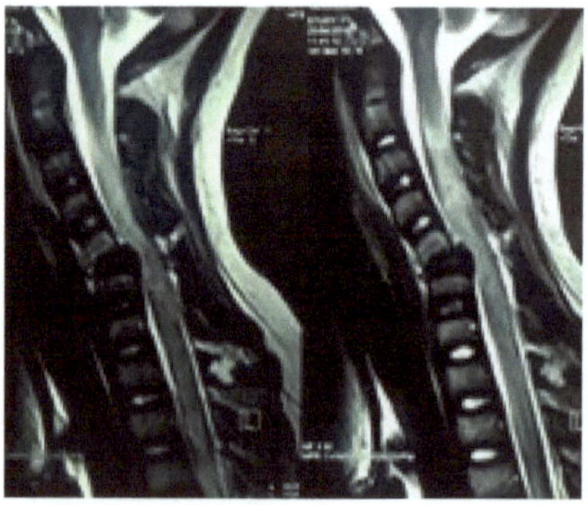

Figure 10. MRI of cervical spine (sagittal view) showing traumatic fracture and subluxation at C5/6 with spinal cord injury. Source: Figure by authors.

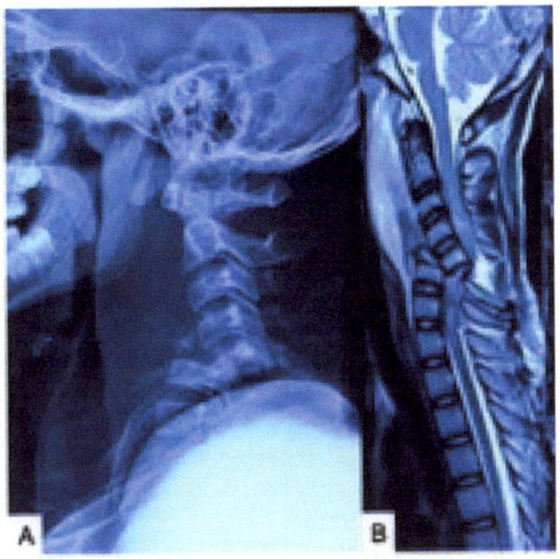

Figure 11. (**A**) X-ray of cervical spine (lateral view) showing complete fracture and dislocation at C5/6. (**B**) MRI of cervical spine showing complete transection of cervical spinal cord. Source: Figure by authors.

Table 1. Classification of cervical spinal injury.

A. Cervicocranial Injuries—Anatomical Types		
Occiput	Atlanto-occipital dislocation (AOD)	Severe combined distractive force; often fatal
Atlas (C1)	Jefferson burst fractures	Axial compression
Odontoid process (Figure 7)	Type 1 Type 2 Type 3	Tip of dens (stable) Through base of dens (unstable) Through C2 vertebral body (stable)
Axis (C2)	Hangman's fracture	Pars fracture ("traumatic spondylolisthesis"')
B. Lower Cervical Spinal Injuries—Classified by Mechanism of Injuries (bones fail in compression and ligaments fail in distraction)		
Distractive flexion	Posterior ligament tear Hyperflexion sprain Bilateral "perched facets" Bilateral facet dislocation Unilateral facet dislocation (with rotational component)	
Compressive flexion	Anterior vertebral body fracture Wedge compression fracture Flexion teardrop	
Distractive extension	Anterior ligament tear Hyperextension sprain Hyperextension teardrop Hyperextension dislocation	
Compressive extension	Posterior element fractures Unilateral or bilateral laminar, lateral mass or spinous process fracture	
Axial compression	Vertebral body burst fracture	
Lateral bending	Uncinate process fracture Unilateral vertebral body Posterior element fracture	
Clay shoveler's fracture	Isolated spinous process fracture of C7 (C6 or T1)	

Source: Authors' compilation based on data from Schwartz (2008).

Most spine injuries happen at the cervical spine, which is the most flexible section of the vertebral column. Car accidents represent a large portion of these wounds. Tears and fractures are the most widely recognized types of injury, and subluxations and spinal cord injury without radiographic abnormality (SCIWORA), although generally rare, happen more habitually in younger patients (Hamilton and Mylks 1992).

According to estimates, 15% of people with spine injuries experience neurological and physical problems (Hagen 2015). The cervical spine is the most frequently involved segment, and it is calculated that 40–60% of all cervical spine injuries result in neurological morbidity and mortality (Hagen 2015). After clinical and radiographic evaluations are completed, unstable or severe injury should be treated immediately with cervical traction using Gardner–Wells (GW) pins (Hagen 2015).

Following careful cleansing of the skin in the area and administration of a local anaesthetic, pins are placed 1 cm cephalad to the pinna by the external acoustic meatus (Labronici et al. 2015). The pins are tightened until the spring-loaded indicator protrudes 1 mm above the surface (Labronici et al. 2015). Keeping the patient compliant and awake enough to comply with subsequent neurological examinations is crucial. Complications such pin dislodging, site contamination, and skull penetration are connected to cervical traction (Patel et al. 2009). Distracting injuries, skull fractures, and unstable upper cervical spine injuries are among the indications against using this technique (Iida et al. 1999).

Recommendations of the WFNS Spine Committee 2019 for Cervical Spine Trauma

Guidelines for preventing spine damage include the following (World Federation of Neurosurgical Societies Spine Committee 2019):

- The following are the most effective measures for preventing spinal cord injuries linked to auto accidents:
  - The implementation of measures such as enacting and upholding laws against drunk driving, which mandate a 0.05 g/dL blood alcohol limit for all drivers;
  - The use of head restraints;
  - The use of seatbelts and kid passenger restraints;
  - The setting and enforcement of speed limits.
- The best interventions for the prevention of spinal cord injury associated with road traffic motorcycle accidents comprise the following:
  - Motorcycle helmets;
  - Motorcycle daytime running lights;
  - Designs of roads that keep autos and larger vehicles apart from people and two-wheelers. comprehensive traffic-calming strategies;
  - Graduated driver licensing laws.
- The following interventions are included in the prevention of SCI caused by falls:
  - Clear floors free of debris and loose carpets; Adequate lighting; Handrails and furniture at the right height; Window guards in high-rise buildings; Roof barriers;
  - Safe harvesting equipment. When appropriate, wheelbarrows.

Guidelines for the transportation and immobilization of patients with cervical spine trauma include:

- In the prehospital context, immobilization of patients over 12 years old who are at high risk of spinal cord injury (SCI) should involve the use of a hard cervical collar and a spinal backboard with straps or tape to immobilize the patient completely.
- Alert individuals with mild blunt trauma without penetrating damage and any spinal discomfort can be carried without being immobilized in the event of a human resource shortage.
- As soon as possible, patients with acute traumatic spinal cord injuries should be sent to the primary hospital facility for SCI treatment.
- For alert, asymptomatic individuals, collar immobilization may be stopped after arrival at the hospital.
- Following a negative high-quality C-spine CT scan, an alert, symptomatic patient may no longer require in-hospital collar immobilization.

Guidelines for closed reduction of cervical spine fractures:

- Awake patients with partial injuries are better candidates for a closed reduction if one is attempted.
- There is no evidence that closed reduction of cervical locked facets is more beneficial than open reduction.
- Pre-reduction MRI and open reduction should be chosen when attempting a reduction in patients who have lost consciousness.
- Surgical reduction and prompt anterior decompression are preferable options in the event that a closed reduction attempt is unsuccessful.

- Although most publications recommend it should be done as soon as feasible, the ideal period for a closed reduction is not well established.
- Following closed reduction, all patients ought to undergo surgery to achieve stabilization and fusion. An anterior, posterior, or mixed anterior and posterior route may be used for this procedure.

Guidelines for radiologic evaluation of upper cervical trauma include the following:

- Cervical CT is the first study to be performed for cervical spine screening in patients whose history and physical examination results raise suspicions of cervical spinal trauma. It is crucial for diagnosis and surgical planning.
- Transverse atlantal ligament disruption and instability in C1–C2 may be indicated by an anterior atlanto-dental interval (AADI) > 3 mm or a posterior atlanto-dental interval (PADI) < 13 mm.
- In patients with cervical injuries, preoperative 3D CT scanning should be carried out to rule out anatomical bone abnormalities before to the implantation of screws at the upper cervical spine.

Suggesations for occipital condyle fractures:

- For the treatment of occipital condyle fractures (OCF), Mueller et al. (2012)'s classification scheme would be better.
- For OCF diagnosis and treatment, CT imaging is the best option.
- To evaluate the stability of OCFs and determine the integrity of the craniocervical ligaments, MRI is advised in addition to CT scan.
- For OCFs without atlanto-occipital dislocation (AOD), conservative care should be given priority over surgical care.

Guidelines for atlanto-occipital dislocation injuries:

- In patients suspected of having atlanto-occipital dislocation (AOD), CT may be sufficient to define the condylo-C1 interval (CCI).
- An atlanto-occipital dislocation may be suspected in cases of severe traumatic brain injury (TBI), lower cranial nerve impairments, and/or spinal cord injury.
- Patients with AOD should have occipitocervical fixation surgery if their overall status is stable.
- Cervical traction is not advised for AOD.

Guidelines for atlas fractures:

- In order to determine the type of fracture and the integrity of the transverse atlantal ligament (TAL), treatment for isolated atlas fractures should be based on CT and MRI criteria.
- Most atlas fractures are stable and respond well to conservative management.
- Any "unstable" atlas fracture as well as atlanto-occipital instability and an intraligamentous TAL rupture are indications for surgery for atlas fractures.

Guidelines for odontoid fractures:

- An anterior atlanto-dental interval (AADI) > 3 mm in adult patients with odontoid fractures suggests disruption of the transverse atlantal ligament (TAL) and instability in C1–C2, whereas an AADI $\geq$ 5 mm suggests rupture of the transverse ligament and accessory stabilizing ligaments.
- If type 2 odontoid fractures are fixed with a posterior C1 lateral screw in conjunction with a C2 pedicle/laminar screw, the following factors increase the risk of fracture nonunion: advanced age, prolonged duration, and preoperative separation of the odontoid fracture > 4 mm.
- The "gap" in the fracture and the time between injury and operation are important predictors of fusion failure in anterior odontoid screw fixation.

Guidelines for Hangman Fractures:

- In addition to a CT scan, an upright X-ray taken under physician supervision may be helpful for hangman's fractures.
- Surgery is advised for hangman's fractures of Levine type 2A.
- Due to its complexities, conservative therapy for hangman's fracture should be done with a rigid collar rather than with Halovest.
- Levine type 3 hangman's fractures may require both anterior and posterior surgery.

Treatment recommendations for combined atlas and axis fractures are as follows:

- No superior evidence exists for combination atlas–axis fractures.
- In the majority of C1–C2 combination fracture cases, external immobilization is employed.
- The following are suggestions for the classification of subaxial cervical spine injuries:

- The Subaxial Injury Classification (SLIC) system is a safe and useful tool for directing subaxial cervical spine injury therapy. The SLIC score (morphology, neurology, and disco-ligamentous complex—DLC) and the selected course of treatment have a high degree of agreement (>90%).
- We also recommend the use of MRI to obtain a more accurate categorization of subaxial fractures.

Strategies for managing injuries to the subaxial cervical spine include:

- Treating C1 hangman's fractures with C2–C3 angulation of $\geq$11 degrees and C1 type 2 odontoid combination fractures with an atlanto-dental interval of $\geq$5 mm with surgery.
- For injuries with a SLIC score of less than 3, nonsurgical treatment with a rigid collar for 6–12 weeks is advised.
- Early surgery is advised for injuries with a SLIC score greater than 4.
- Anterior operations are advised for major anterior column injuries.
- Surgery is indicated for stable incomplete impairments with significant spinal canal disruption or for growing neurological deficits.
- Patients with significant dislocation (complex) injuries and those in need of multilevel corpectomy should be evaluated for additional posterior procedures.
- There is disagreement over the recommendation to do posterior procedures on patients who have ankylosing spondylitis and osteoporosis.

Recommendations for traumatic locked facets:

- Preoperative MRI is advised in the management of locked facets if a posterior approach is being investigated.
- Traction aids in immobilizing the shaky section and could facilitate reduction.
- Anterior surgical procedures are sufficient for effective therapy of most acute ($\leq$3 days) locked aspects.
- When an anterior approach is impractical, a posterior technique is recommended for lower cervical locked facets with no or minimal disc prolapse, as well as chronic locked aspects lasting more than two weeks.

The following are recommendations for paediatric cervical spine injuries:

- MRI is required for children without abnormal X-ray or CT scan results who have neurological spinal cord symptoms.
- For irreducible rotatory atlanto-occipital dislocation, surgery is recommended.
- If a child under five years old has a cervical spine fracture or dislocation and there is no surgical rationale, a Minerva cast may be utilized in place of a halo.

Guidelines for cervical trauma-related vertebral artery damage include the following:

- Computed tomographic angiography (CTA) should be used as a screening method in certain individuals who have experienced blunt cervical trauma and have fractures close to the vertebral artery course.
- Conventional catheter angiography is advised if CTA is abnormal for vertebral artery injury (VAI) and endovascular therapy is a possible course of treatment.
- The choice of therapy—anticoagulation therapy versus antiplatelet therapy versus no treatment—for patients in whom endovascular treatment for VAI is not advised should be tailored to the patient's specific characteristics of the vertebral artery injury, the accompanying injuries, and the risk of bleeding.
- Since the function of endovascular therapy in VAI is yet unclear, no advice can be given regarding its application in treating VAI.

7.2.2. Craniocervical Fracture and Dislocation

Occipital Condylar Fractures

Classifications of occipital condylar fractures are shown in Table 2.

Jefferson Fracture

This fracture (Figure 4) was first described by Sir Geoffrey Jefferson (Jefferson 1920). Typically, it is a four-point (burst) fracture of the C1 ring, yet the term is presently regularly utilized to incorporate the more frequent three- or two-point fractures of the arches of C1 (the most delicate of the vertebra) (Papadopoulos 1993; Alker et al. 1975). The most common cause of Jefferson fractures are diving accidents. There is a 41% possibility of a related C2 break. In children, it is essential to separate a C1 fracture from the standard synchondroses. A fracture may additionally happen through the unfused synchondrosis.

Table 2. Classifications for evaluating occipital condylar fractures.

Classification	Type	Description	Stability	Treatment
Anderson and Montesano (1988)	I	Comminuted: minimal/no displacement	Stable	Collar
	II	Direct trauma with basilar skull fracture	Stable	
	III	Avulsion fracture involving the alar ligament	Unstable	Surgical or halo fixation
Tuli et al. (1997)	1	Nondisplaced	Stable	Collar
	2A	Displaced, ligaments intact	Stable	
	2B	Displaced plus craniocervical instability	Unstable	Surgical or halo fixation

Source: Authors' compilation based on data from Anderson and Montesano (1988); Tuli et al. (1997).

Hangman's Fractures

- Vertical or angled fractures (Figure 8) of the C2 pars interarticularis, disengaging the posterior arch from the vertebral body.
- Usually brought about by hyperextension (MVA or diving accident); the posterior C1 arch as well as C2–C3 disc should likewise be assessed for injury.
- Most isolated fractures can be managed with a collar; displaced, unstable fractures can be dealt with halo immobilization.
- Surgery might be indicated if there is C2–C3 facet dislocation or if the patient has another significant unstable spinal injury.

Classification of hangman fracture is shown in Table 3.

Table 3. Levine and Edwards classification of hangman fractures.

Type	Description	Notes
I	<3 mm anterolisthesis, no angulation	Axial load and hyperextension
II	>3 mm anterolisthesis, angulation and disruption of posterior longitudinal ligament	Hyperextension and axial loading force linked to severe flexion
IIa	Horizontal fracture line and angulation without anterolithesis	Flexion, distraction; no or mild displacement but very severe angulation
III	Type I plus bilateral facet joint dislocation	Flexion, compression

Source: Authors' compilation based on data from Levine and Edwards (1985).

The commonest subluxation of the axis on C3 occurs regularly. Schneider et al. (1965) coined the term "Hangman's fracture" (HF), despite the fact that the most common causes of HFs nowadays are hyperextension and secondary flexion from MVAs or diving accidents. Nonetheless, modern-day HFs share some similarities with those seen in judicial hangings (where the submental position of the noose brings about hyperextension as well as distraction) (Wood-Jones 1913).

Craniovertebral Junction Dislocations

CVJ dislocations are uncommon and are categorized as atlantoaxial subluxation without fracture, vertical atlanto-axial dislocation (vertical AAD), and joint vertical dislocations (vertical AOD and vertical AAD). Typically occurring in children and adolescents, traumatic posterior atlantoaxial subluxation can be accompanied by odontoid fracture (Fielding et al. 1978). It is a rare occurrence in elderly patients and adults and has only been described in eight case reports (Fox and Jerez 1977; Haralson and Boyd 1969; Jamshidi et al. 1983; Sassard et al. 1974; Sud et al. 2002; Wong et al. 1991; Yoon et al. 2003). The C2 odontoid process/dens is physically joined with the C1's anterior arch and the TAL's synovial joint, and thanks to its special anatomical configuration, it can act as a pivot for the rotation of C1 above C2. As a result, it is extremely difficult to achieve the dislocation of the

C2 odontoid process from the C1 arch, meaning that this traumatic lesion is associated with extensive ligament damage. This unusual injury's nature can be confirmed by radiological analysis using an X-ray, CT scan, and 3D MRI. In the acute stage, neuroimaging is helpful to accurately define the ligament damage and to prevent the presence of a traumatic haematoma in the spinal canal. Spinal cord injury was not severe in any of the cases discussed in the text. Three patients had no neurological deficits (Yoon et al. 2003; Haralson and Boyd 1969), and the remaining five displayed mild or temporary motor weakness (Sud et al. 2002; Wong et al. 1991; Yoon et al. 2003). This illustrates that before spinal cord compression occurs at the C1-2 junction, there is a significant amount of free space. The vast extent of the spinal canal suggests that there can be a lot of instability in this area. Amir Jamshidi et al. (Jamshidi et al. 1983), in 2009, hypothesized that severe rotating hyperextension of the neck is the basis of these uncommon and traumatic events. The pathophysiology of the injury is still under debate. Rotating subluxation is caused by general damage and injury to the C1-2 lateral facet joints. Currently, clinical treatment is debatable and is being discussed. It is clear that the reduction of dislocation is difficult when the patient is alert (Jamshidi et al. 1983). This is because of extent of ligament damage.

Atlanto-Occipital Dislocation (AOD)

Until recently, treating this kind of injury was unusual because most patients would either die at the site of the accident or right away after reaching at the hospital due to traumatic brain stem injury (Consortium for Spinal Cord Medicine 1997). Strong resuscitative measures taken on the scene have transformed AOD into a physical problem that may be treatable (Consortium for Spinal Cord Medicine 1997). Untreated AOD is associated with extreme morbidity and mortality (Hagen 2015). Clinically, individuals may exhibit complete tetraplegia, respiratory distress, or neurological normalcy (Hagen 2015). When a patient is conscious, it is occasionally possible to hear them complain of occipital pain, and lower cranial nerve paralysis can be seen (Schneider et al. 1965). Brown–Sequard syndrome, focal neurological deficits, or Bell's palsy have been described with this injury (Schneider et al. 1965). Increased signal intensity in and around the tendons on MRI may indicate tendon injury. Numerous symptoms, ranging from mild neurological issues to bulbar–cervical separation leading to respiratory arrest and death, may be present.

Atlantoaxial Dislocation (AAD)

This term indicates a loss of continuity between atlas and axis (C1 and C2) (Figures 5 and 6). The expected distance between the anterior arch of C1 and the dens is <2–3 mm in adults and <5 mm in children. The causes of AAD can be traumatic or secondary to specific infections. Following a comminuted C1 fracture, the cross over tendon is currently attached to a bone segment. The spine is weak, and the C1 lateral mass has been dislodged. Rheumatoid arthritis, Down syndrome, and Morquio syndrome are related disorders (Consortium for Spinal Cord Medicine 1997). Patients with the aforementioned diseases should be carefully assessed, and these conditions should be excluded in individuals with deficits limited to the upper cervical spinal cord. A traumatic atlanto-axial dislocation alone, without further displacement, is uncommon (Consortium for Spinal Cord Medicine 1997). Treatments include posterior fixation and fusion.

7.2.3. Subaxial Cervical Spine Injuries

These will, in general, happen in young patients because of a car accident or some sports injury (Figures 3 and 9–11). In this age group, if cervical immobilization is used, one-level arthrodesis be employed to avoid further injury and preserve the range of motion. Similarly, a posterior approach may be used depending on the number of levels involved.

- The most regularly affected levels are C5 and C6.
- The three categories of injury are compression fractures, burst/distraction fractures, or translational injuries.
- These injuries may affect either bony tissue or soft tissue.

A schematic drawing from Argenson et al.'s classification of lower cervical spine injuries is shown in Figure 3 (Argenson et al. 1997).

7.2.4. Dorsolumbar Fracture and Sacral Fracture

Injuries to the Dorsal, Dorsal–Lumbar, and Lumbar Spine

Illustrations in Figure 12 show the AO/Magerl classification of dorsolumbar spinal injuries.

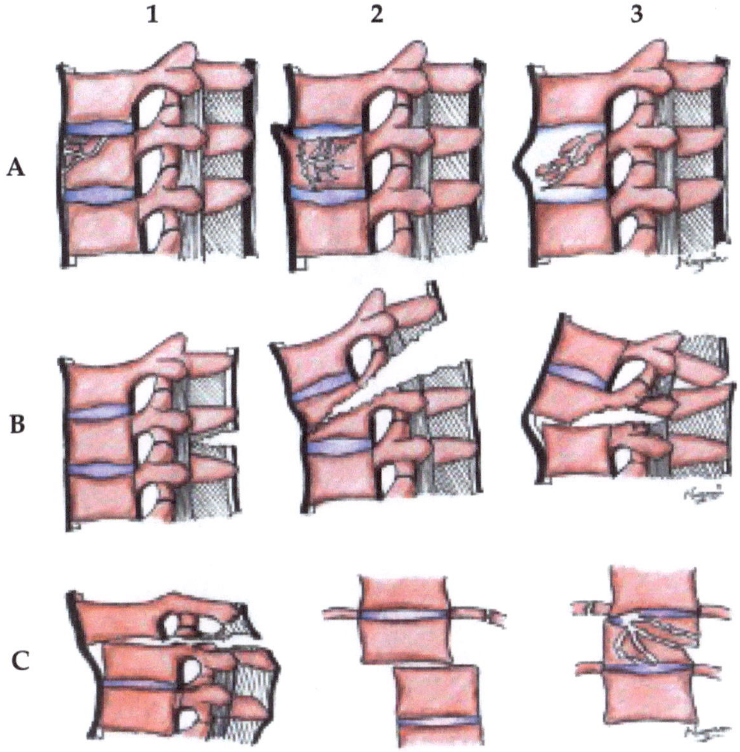

Figure 12. Illustrations showing AO/Magerl classification of dorsolumbar spinal injuries showing three main types ((**A**) compression, (**B**) distraction, (**C**) torsional injury) and their subtypes (**1**, **2** and **3**). Source: Figure by authors.

Injuries to the dorsal (D2 to D10), dorsolumbar (D11 to L2), and lumbar (L3 to L5) spine (Figures 12–18) are managed separately, as the bone arrangement, biomechanics, and neurological functions of each of these segments are unique. Even though the fracture mechanisms that happen in these segments are similar, the clinical interpretation and, thus, the treatment and prognosis shifts as indicated by the degree of the injury.

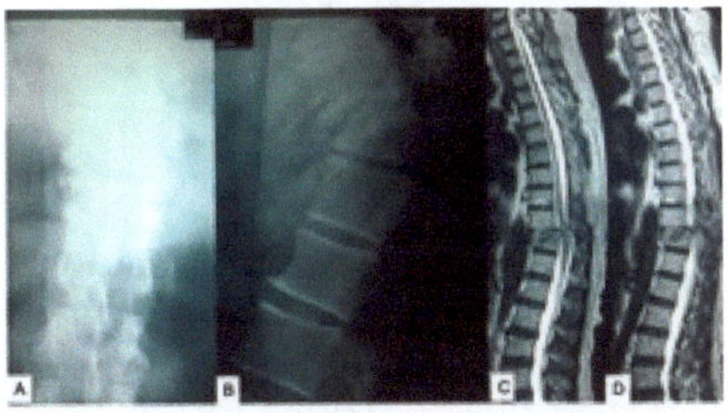

Figure 13. (**A**,**B**) X-ray and (**C**,**D**) MRI of dorsal spine showing unstable fracture and posterior dislocation of D11 with cord compression. Source: Figure by authors.

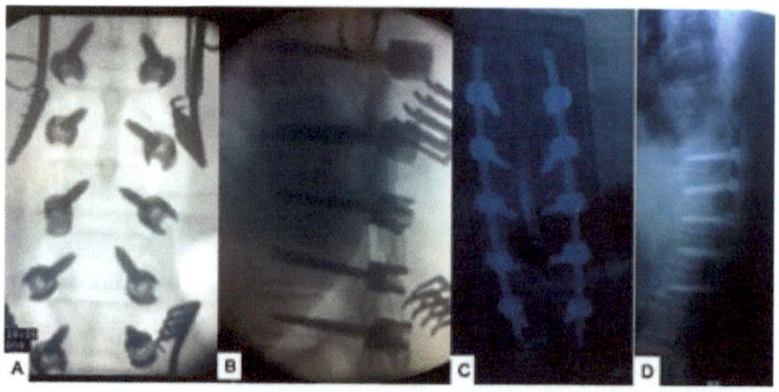

Figure 14. (**A**,**B**) Intraoperative X-ray of fracture reduction, stabilization (with pedicular screws and rods), and fusion of D11 fracture and dislocation in patient in Figure 13. (**C**,**D**) Postoperative X-ray of patient in Figure 13. Source: Figure by authors.

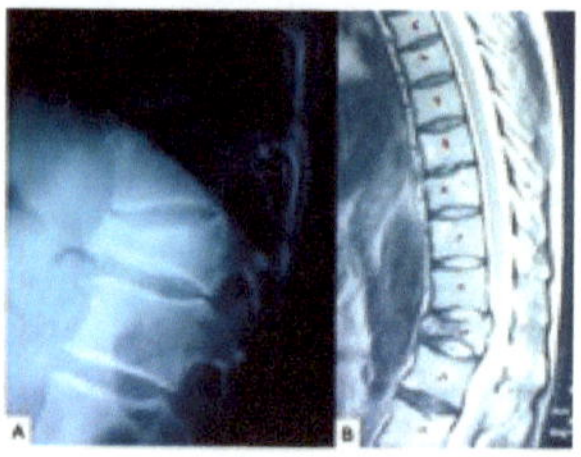

Figure 15. (**A**) X-ray and (**B**) MRI of dorsal spine showing relatively stable D12 compression fracture which was managed conservatively. Source: Figure by authors.

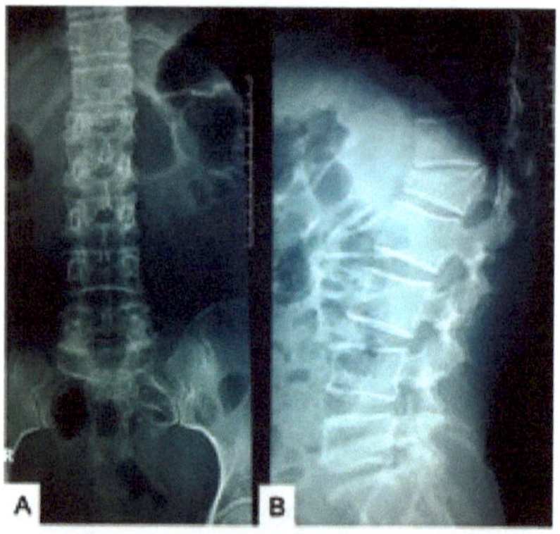

Figure 16. (**A**,**B**) X-ray of dorsolumbar spine showing L1 wedge fracture. Source: Figure by authors.

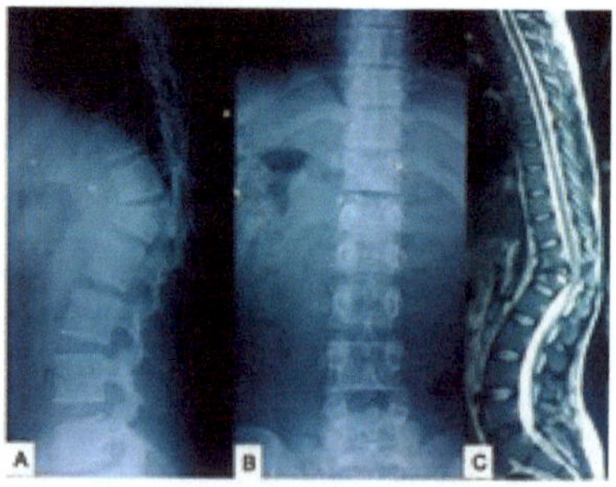

Figure 17. (**A**,**B**) X-ray and (**C**) MRI of dorsolumbar spine showing unstable L1 wedge fracture with compression of conus medullaris. Source: Figure by authors.

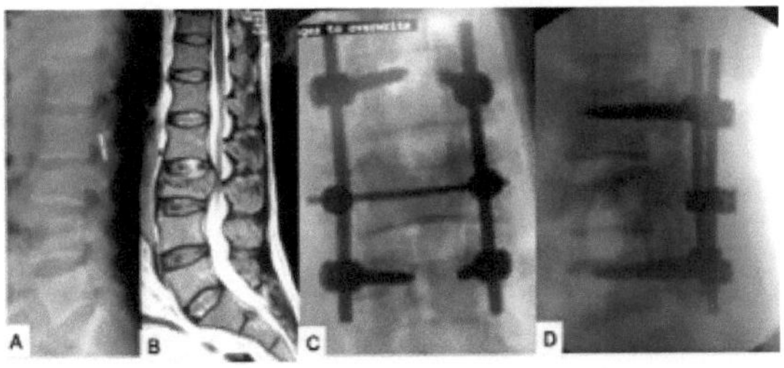

Figure 18. (**A**) X-ray lumbar spine showing L3 compression fracture and (**B**) MRI of lumbar spine showing L3 compression fracture with cauda equina compression. (**C,D**) Postoperative X-ray after decompression, fusion, and stabilization of L3 fracture. Source: Figure by authors.

Thoracic Spine Injuries

Thoracic spinal injuries are shown in Figures 12–15. Fifteen percent of all spinal cord injuries are to the thoracic spine (Tator 1994). Even though the the thoracic spine is difficult to damage, the spinal canal is extremely vulnerable to injury and has the worst chance of recovering in a way that will be useful. Solely 10% of dorsal vertebral body injuries are caused by spinal cord injuries. In contrast, the cervical spine comprises 39% of this total. The degree of the neurological deficits commonly associated with injuries to this area is represented by a weak spinal-canal-to-spinal-cord ratio and weak CSF flow. The sternum, the back, the costovertebral tendons, the ribs, the chest enclosure and divider muscles, and this region's musculature all serve to stabilize the spinal column here. In addition to strengthening the thoracic region, they also limit the amount of physiological growth that is permitted. For instance, the ribcage restricts expansion movement by around 70% (White and Panjabi 1979). The fact that a healthy ribcage is associated with a fourfold rise in the compression resistance of the adjacent vertebral segment confirms that the ribcage also gives stiffness to the spine (White and Panjabi 1979). The upper thoracic region's flexion and expansion are also constrained by the ribs, and the back structures mostly prevent expansion (White and Panjabi 1979).

Injury to the Lower Spinal Cord and the Cauda Equina: The Role of Surgical Decompression

Individuals with lesions to the lower spinal cord and the cauda equina may sustain total or partial injury (Germon et al. 2015). Decompressive surgery typically does not produce positive results in patients who have complete injuries for longer than 48 h (Germon et al. 2015). Both early and late decompression have been shown to improve function, which suggests that the role of time is yet unknown.

Injury to the T11–L1 Segment

Anterior and posterohorizontal methods of decompression are used for this part of the spine (Figures 16 and 17). The main ways to deal with T11 lesions include a thoracotomy cut, while the involvement of T12 and L1 requires a thoracoabdominal surgical approach (Germon et al. 2015). This methodology might be used in incomplete SCI or compressive cauda equina lesions (Germon et al. 2015). Where there is evidence of posterior neural compression, this system is contraindicated. Postero-lateral surgeries incorporate the extracavitary and costotransversectomy technique (Gokaslan et al. 1998). These procedures also necessitate the excision of at least one rib and the use of cross-over cycles to gain access to the lateral vertebral body. Posterior instrumentation can be refined with the two procedures, even though the extracavitary approach considers the perception of the level inverse to the pedicle base (Gokaslan et al. 1998). With this form, it is difficult to excise of large midline bone pieces. These methodologies are related to the danger of inadequate decompression because of the presentation, and there is a high risk of deformation without anterior bone joining (Germon et al. 2015).

Injury to the L2–L4 Segment

In injuries to L2-L4 segment (Figure 18) functional recovery is varied because these lesions cause damage to the cauda equina. If there is neurological compression, a laminectomy with transpedicular decompression might offer sufficient exposure (Gokaslan et al. 1998). With an S-shaped incision from the tip of the 12th rib into the lower abdomen, a retroperitoneal surgery enables the viewing of the peritoneum and the contents of the abdominal cavity (Zindrick et al. 1986). The lumbar segmental vessels are then linked, and the psoas muscle is subsequently mobilized to give caudal access from L2 to the anterolateral region of the lumbar spine (Zindrick et al. 1986). After instrumentation, a vertebrectomy plus grafting is accomplished (Gokaslan et al. 1998). Maintaining physiological lordosis in this area is important since losing it can result in postural abnormalities and a flat back.

Injury to the L5 Segment

At L5, neural decompression with a transpedicular approach can be successfully accomplished following a laminectomy. In cases of extreme neural compression, a paramedian abdominal incision can be used to conduct anterior decompression. Through a retroperitoneal or transperitoneal approach, the lower lumbar spine may then be revealed. More extensive exposure is provided by the transperitoneal method, but it also involves mobilizing the large vessels and the plexus of the hypogastric nerve. An increased probability of impotence is correlated with the mobilization of the above structure. For L5 fractures, sacral fixation is required. Excellent fixation is provided by the utilization of posterior instrumentation with the positioning of pedicle screws laterally at 45° in the sacrum ala or medially in the first pedicle (Zindrick et al. 1986). To improve the build, sacral sublaminar wiring is often used. Patients are put in a lumbosacral orthotic system postoperatively.

Thoracolumbar Spine Trauma: WFNS Spine Committee Recommendations

Epidemiology and incidence (World Federation of Neurosurgical Societies Spine Committee 2020):

- The most frequent causes of thoracolumbar fractures are falls and traffic accidents.
- Including osteoporotic fractures, the annual incidence of TL fractures is around 30 per 100,000 people.
- Little is known about the true prevalence and epidemiology in poor nations.
- Low-velocity falls are becoming more common, particularly among the elderly.
- In industrialized nations, the mortality rate following a spinal injury is declining. This is particularly true for spinal injuries sustained in auto accidents because of advancements in traffic laws and vehicle safety.
- Many vertebral fractures occur in youngsters;
- The death rate from thoracolumbar trauma is relatively high in male older patients.

Radiological diagnosis and classification:

- In clinical practice, the revised AO classification and TLICS should be utilized as trustworthy classifications of traumatic thoracolumbar fractures.
- Recent research indicates that the new AO classification may be more beneficial in the treatment of thoracolumbar fractures even if it is more complicated.
- In the event that an MRI or CT scan are not accessible, AP and lateral standard radiographs may be taken.
- Although MRI should be taken into consideration, CT still plays a significant role in the assessment of trauma because it is unable to accurately show the disco-ligamentous complex.
- The most popular advanced imaging technique is magnetic resonance imaging (MR imaging), which is the preferred tool for disco-ligamentous abnormalities, spinal cord abnormalities, and other disorders related to spinal trauma.

Indications for nonsurgical and surgical treatment:

- It is preferable not to treat AO type B and C fractures conservatively.
- There is no clinical evidence that bracing for the conservative treatment of TL fractures will improve the outcome.
- AO type A2, A3, and A4 fractures can be treated conservatively if there is no significant kyphotic angulation, significant vertebral body collapse, or canal compromise with neurological impairment.
- It is preferable to operate on fracture dislocations and instances with substantial instability (TLISS classification score > 5).
- Although there is insufficient data to support it, surgical decompression and stabilization may be considered for burst fractures resulting in neurological impairments.
- Conservative or surgical methods can be used to treat burst fractures in the absence of neurological impairments.

Surgical approaches for thoracolumbar fractures:

- Short-segment posterolateral pedicle screw fixation is usually enough for burst fractures.
- In order to strengthen the construct in cases of burst fractures of the thoracolumbar junction, a fracture-level screw should be used. If it is not possible to incorporate a fracture-level screw, long-segment fixation ought to be used.

- There is no proof that fusion is necessary when utilizing long-segment screws because the results are the same with or without fusion.
- The clinical results for TL burst fractures are insensitive to the choice of anterior or posterior approach.
- There is insufficient data to conclude that nonoperative treatment for burst fractures of the lumbar and thoracic spine is superior in terms of clinical results.
- Since the data points to comparable clinical results, minimally invasive methods of treating thoracolumbar burst fractures may be taken into consideration.
- Non-fusion surgery for thoracolumbar burst fractures has the following benefits over fusion surgery: less donor site problems, shorter recovery times, and less bleeding.
- There is no statistical evidence that suggests regional kyphosis will worsen following non-fusion surgery.

Factors influencing surgical results:

- After thoracolumbar burst fracture surgery, obesity may exacerbate segmental kyphosis.
- Bad things seem to happen to those who are older.
- Poor results are predicted by smoking, comorbidities, and long-term high-dose steroid use.
- It is not recommended to rule out early surgery due to polytrauma or high injury severity scores.
- Kyphotic deformity may worsen if there is a greater than 50% loss of anterior vertebral body height.
- Since it greatly affects the result, it is crucial to identify injuries to the posterior longitudinal ligament complex.
- Burst fractures with sagittal–transverse canal diameter ratio <0.40 are substantially related with brain damage and outcomes.
- After surgery, Cobb's angle greater than 10.5° may indicate unfavorable results.

Post-traumatic kyphosis following thoracolumbar fractures:

- Untreated, unstable burst fractures are the most frequent cause of post-traumatic kyphosis.
- There is no specific kyphosis angle that would require surgery in the treatment of post-traumatic kyphosis. Instead, one must evaluate the global sagittal equilibrium.
- Remarkable kyphosis correction can be obtained with posterior surgery, with minimal blood loss and complications.

Sacral Fractures

These are uncommon and are regularly brought about by shear forces (Jefferson 1920). They can harm sacral roots and plexus and influence pelvic and spinopelvic stability. Injuries beneath S2 ought not to influence ambulation; however, they might be unstable and lead to trauma that improves after careful intervention (Bellabarba and Bransford 2015).

8. Medical Complications of Spinal Injuries

8.1. Cardiovascular Complications

Direct cardiovascular (CV) issues after SCI are caused by the disruption of the autonomic nervous system and the loss of interaction between receptor organs and brainstem regions (Hagen 2015). SCI-related CV problems encompass pulmonary embolism, deep vein thrombosis (DVT), autonomic dysreflexia (AD), orthostasis, cardiac arrhythmia, abnormalities of the thermoregulatory system, and orthostasis (PE) (Hagen 2015). The most common CV abnormalities in acute SCI are bradycardia and hypotension, both of which are brought on by a lack of sympathetic tone (Tator 1994).

8.2. Orthostatic Hypotension

Orthostatic hypotension is a reduction in circulatory effort caused by an alteration in body posture toward the upright. There are several warning signs, including drowsiness, unsteadiness, syncope, and pallor. People with a complete injury above the T6 level are prone to orthostasis. The orthostatic hypotension component includes preganglionic sympathetics in the spinal cord and interferes with the sensory CV contribution to the brainstem. Aortic and carotid baroreceptors sense a decrease in blood pressure when the patient stands up. This can often result in an increase in sympathetic tone, causing vasoconstriction and tachycardia. But the efferent route is blocked in SCI, preventing an increase in sympathetic outflow (i.e., norepinephrine and epinephrine). Due to these factors, the pulse only slightly increases as a result, which is insufficient to counteract the decline in blood pressure. Additionally, venous pooling occurs, which reduces venous return to the right atrium and, as a result, decreases cardiovascular output. Orthostasis's adverse effects depend more on cerebral blood flow than on high blood pressure (Gonzalez et al. 1991). As spinal postural reflexes that generate vasoconstriction develop and cerebrovascular autoregulation of dissemination improves in response to low perfusion pressures, this condition gradually worsens (Corbett et al. 1971).

8.3. Thermoregulation

Body temperature is usually under hypothalamic control (i.e., thermoregulation). When the core temperature needs to be raised, the hypothalamus may utilize shivering and vasoconstriction, which increase heat production and decrease heat loss. Similar to sweating, vasodilation reduces temperature by boosting heat loss. SCI reduces the peripheral nervous system's capacity to direct the hypothalamus. Individuals with lesions above T5 frequently exhibit poikilothermy, or difficulties in responding to local temperature. For instance, a person with a high level of SCI may have a high core temperature while in a hot environment or outdoors, which could be misconstrued for an infectious source-induced fever. Therefore, it is critical to teach patients self-protection strategies against both hypothermia and hyperthermia.

8.4. Autonomic Dysreflexia

Autonomic dysreflexia, also called autonomic hyper-reflexia, is a syndrome that occurs in cases with SCI above the T6 level and leads to an uncoordinated sympathetic response. It is is a medical emergency that needs prompt detection and care. The rate ranges from 48% to 85% in SCI patients, and it is caused by an exaggerated sympathetic response below the level of injury that the patient is unaware of as they lack feeling (Lindan et al. 1980; Erickson 1980). Overdistention, frequently of the bladder, is the primary cause of these dangerous hypertensive episodes. They may also result from inappropriate catheterization or a clogged indwelling Foley catheter. Any injury, regardless of the cause, such as constipation, a pressure ulcer, tight clothing, an ingrown toenail, or a fracture, may worsen the disease, as these causes and trigger an episode of dysreflexia. A lack of compensatory descending parasympathetic stimulation and intrinsic post-traumatic hypersensitivity cause the sympathetic response to be exaggerated. The outcome is local vasoconstriction despite maximum parasympathetic vasodilatory efforts and a steep rise in blood pressure. Reflex bradycardia might be caused by this increased blood pressure; however, it is not sufficient to decrease it altogether. When it comes to older adult patients, who may naturally be hypertensive, monitoring hypertension is especially important. AD can cause headaches, excessive sweating, and piloerections due to intentional stimulation of hair follicles. Flushing may occur above the level of injury. The patient typically complains of nasal congestion and discomfort. Retinal discharge, myocardial localized necrosis, subarachnoid or intracerebral drain, seizures, and potentially death are all expected complications of AD. AD may occur soon after injury and exists in many patients within six months of injury. Within one year of injury, 92% of patients are affected by AD (Lindan et al. 1980).

8.5. Deep Vein Thrombosis

The most well-recognized CV-related risk after SCI is deep vein thrombosis (DVT). Its occurrence fluctuates somewhere in the range of 8% and 100% depending on the analytic tests used (Green et al. 1992, 2005). Recent information shows that the rate of DVT might be decreasing, maybe because of prophylaxis (Green et al. 2005; Ragnarsson et al. 1995). Virchow's triad, namely venous stasis, vascular injury, and hypercoagulability, comprises the risk factors for the development of DVT in SCI. A lower appendage fracture, obesity, older age, diabetes, a history of past thrombosis, and vascular disease are additional risk factors. Individuals with tetraplegia and those who have neurologically recovered from SCI have DVT more frequently. The onset often occurs within fourteen days, and after two months, the frequency starts to decline. One of the leading aetiologies of death in patients during the intensive phase of SCI is PE, which occurs in 1–7% of those with the condition (Green et al. 2005). Most incidences occur in the lower appendages' deep veins. The degree or severity of SCI has no bearing on PE. After SCI, DVT prevention is crucial. Clinical testing is important but less effective in SCI patients due to the absence of some of the common signs and symptoms, like sensitivity to palpation. The degree of apoplexy is inversely correlated with the perimeter of the legs; in any event, a 1 cm difference between perimeter of the two lower limbs at the calf or thigh should arouse suspicion. Clinical recommendations for the prevention and management of DVT in SCI have been made available by the Consortium for Spinal Cord Injury (Consortium for Spinal Cord Medicine 1997). A plan for anticoagulant prophylaxis and mechanical prophylaxis—i.e., pneumatic pressure devices—is suggested. Usually, it is advised to employ mechanical prophylaxis when the patient is sleeping, 24 h a day. If there is no evidence of brain injury, or coagulopathy, anticoagulant prophylaxis with either unfractionated or low-molecular-weight heparin should begin within 72 h of the initial injury. The duration of DVT prevention depends on the kind and severity of SCI as well as any concurrent clinical conditions that are present (Consortium for Spinal Cord Medicine 1997). Patients in whom anticoagulant prophylaxis has failed or who are contraindicated to anticoagulation may be eligible for the placement of retrievable vena cava filters; nonetheless, this is by no means a replacement for pharmacological thromboprophylaxis. When using mechanical coagulation, lower appendage preparation and exercise are typically continued for 48–72 h following the implementation of the appropriate therapeutic treatment.

8.6. Respiratory Complications

Following SCI, respiratory complications such as atelectasis, pneumonia, and aspiration are very common (Jackson and Groomes 1994). All things considered, the older the patient, the higher the neurological level, and the more severe the neurological injury, the more likely these conditions are to arise. Patients with SCI are more vulnerable to the development of respiratory complications due to prior respiratory problems (e.g., having a history of smoking, ongoing bronchial asthma, chronic obstructive pulmonary disease, and excess weight). Several factors may contribute to inadequate respiratory function during severe SCI. Severe SCI causes the respiratory muscles to lose all or some of their mobility. Patients who have an injury at or above the C3 level are typically unable to breathe on their own at first and need artificial ventilation. Mechanical ventilation may be necessary for a while for injuries below the C3 vertebra. These individuals may not be able to empty their lungs of secretions because their abdominal muscles are losing mobility to varying degrees, which affects their ability to cough. Thoracic SCI is typically associated with chest injuries, such as rib fractures, hemopneumothorax, and lung injuries, which can result in acute respiratory failure. To prevent any potential respiratory complications following severe SCI, careful respiratory management is essential. Following SCI, a preventative respiratory treatment program should start as soon as possible. For those with severe SCI, breathing medications with saline solutions or bronchodilators should be available. Significant components of respiratory management include dynamic chest stretches and exercises, incorporating percussion, clearing lung secretions as needed, and assisted coughing techniques. Regularly placing the patient in the Trendelenburg and reverse Trendelenburg positions, and side-lying positions, if possible, should help with perfusion. Due to the weakness of the cough in people with high-level SCI, assisted coughing is provided by different manual techniques (such as the quad cough) or by using mechanical insufflation–exsufflation equipment. When treating a patient with a freshly implanted inferior vena cava filter, caution should be taken when using the quad coughing method. In contrast to suctioning, people with SCI prefer mechanical insufflation–exsufflation for the treatment of their secretions. Strengthening the abdominals as well as other innervated accessory muscles of respiration should begin as soon as possible after injury (Jackson and Groomes 1994; Garstang et al. 2000). During mechanical ventilation, the abdominal muscles may weaken quickly, and if mechanical ventilation stops, they will not be able to provide enough aspiratory work.

9. Prognosis for Recovery and Prediction of Outcome

The primary factor in determining how well the injured brain will recover neurologically is the actual assessment. Once the patient's physical condition has been identified, it will be possible to predict when the injury will be resolved. The use of radiographic and electrodiagnostic testing, as well as neurological assessment, are just a few clinical techniques that can be used to predict neurological recovery after SCI (Kirshblum and O'Connor 2000). The neurological assessment's determination of whether a person has a neurologically complete or incomplete injury is the primary predictor of recovery (Kirshblum and O'Connor 2000). The degree of the underlying injury, the underlying muscular strength, and the subject's age are other significant assessment factors (Theisen et al. 2014). Recovery from spinal injuries below the cervical spine that cause paraplegia is been the same as recovery from injuries causing quadriplegia, although some predictions regarding future recovery are comparable (Theisen et al. 2014). Numerous studies have linked MRI observations to neurological status and recovery following SCI and discovered that the kind and degree of MRI change correlate with the severity and prognosis of the injury (Ditunno et al. 2002). In the immediate aftermath of an SCI, numerous electrophysiological tests are used to assess the severity and level of the SCI and predict neurological and functional outcomes (Ditunno et al. 2002). Techniques for improving clinical and neuroradiological tests include nerve conduction studies, late responses (H-reflex and F-wave), motor evoked potentials, somatosensory evoked potentials, and sympathetic skin responses (Theisen et al. 2014).

10. Pharmacological and Surgical Procedures to Increase Recovery and Regeneration

After the underlying injury, various changes happen inside the spinal cord that prevent the return of function. In recent decades, various pharmacological techniques for the treatment of SCI to improve recuperation have emerged. No significant differences in neurological or functional results were found between the two regimens at 6 months or 1 year; notwithstanding this, the maximum tolerated dose was below the therapeutic threshold. Patients with cauda equina injuries and injuries to the cervical spine were not included in the study. A month and a half, half a year, and a year later, the study revealed that methyl prednisolone (MP) given within 8 h of injury increased neurological recovery, even though practical recovery was not explicitly taken into account. Patients treated after 8 h exhibited no beneficial effects. Enhancing blood flow to the spinal cord, preventing lipid peroxidation, being a free radical scavenger, and having a moderating capacity are all aspects of MP activity. Tirilizad is a potent steroid that has no glucocorticoid effect, providing the positive effects of MP (such as lipid peroxidation and the movement of cancer prevention agents) without the negative effects. According to the study, patients who are treated within three hours of injury should receive steroids for 24 h, and those who are treated between three and eight hours after the accident should have them for 48 h. There are several recent reports that call into doubt the current normal use of steroids, and this more recent practice using 48 h of therapy has not been widely accepted. In the central nervous system (CNS), GM-1 ganglioside (Sygen) is present in high concentration and is involved in the structures of a large portion of cell membranes. It is hypothesized that GM-1 ganglioside can stimulate and protect protein kinases, inhibit glutamate-induced neuronal excitotoxicity, increase neurite outgrowth, and reduce CNS tissue damage. An unpublished small study that treated individuals within 48 h of injury for an average of 26 days found greater mean recovery after 1 year, with somewhat better recovery for muscles that were weak at the time of the study (Geisler et al. 1991). At the primary endpoint of 26 weeks, no significant effects were seen in the entire group of patients being evaluated (Bracken 2001). In a pharmacological trial, fampridine-SR, a long-acting version of 4-aminopyridine (4-AP), was used on people with chronic incomplete spinal cord injury. The potassium (K+) channel blocker 4-AP binds to internodal axonal K+, improving nerve conduction. Phase 2 research on SCI showed trends toward improvement in pain and stiffness (Gokaslan et al. 1998; Davis et al. 1990; Segal and Brunnemann 1997). A phase 1 clinical trial of electrical stimulation was carried out on 10 participants with neurologically complete SCI. Their injuries ranged between C5 and T10 in severity, and MRI did not reveal any evidence of other lesions. Pain scores assessed using a visual analogue scale indicated a reduction in their level of pain at one year, and improvements in light touch and pinprick sensitivity as well as in the strength of some muscles were found (Shapiro et al. 2005). The Food and Drug Administration approved the enrolment of 10 more severe SCI patients after it was determined that the use of this therapy in patients with severe SCI was safe and could be useful. Additional results and preliminary clinical reports have shown similar outcomes.

11. Conclusions

The progressive degradation of both vascular and brain tissue, which undermines the anatomical substrate required for neurological recovery, is linked to all cellular and molecular alterations and events. These neurodegenerative mechanisms increase the need for various therapeutic approaches to lessen the harm brought on by secondary injury. These approaches are frequently based on knowledge of the pathophysiology of spinal cord injury, which aids in the development of systematic and multivariable therapies that facilitate functional recovery, prevent secondary injury, and promote regeneration. Spine injuries can be neurologically damaging. To avoid neurological worsening, prompt identification in the setting of multiple injury is important. Initial evaluation includes a thorough history and physical examination, which includes a thorough neurological assessment, in addition to airway safety and haemodynamic stability. The radiographic evaluation of life-threatening injuries starts in the emergency room. A high index of scepticism should always be maintained in order to recognize and treat such injuries, like atlanto-occipital dislocation. The most frequently injured area of the spinal cord is the cervical spine. The identification and treatment of injuries in this region are crucial due to the high morbidity and mortality rates associated with them. For certain types of injuries that, if effective, can be repaired without surgery, closed reduction can be explored.

Author Contributions: Conceptualization, methodology, validation, formal analysis, investigation, resources, data curation, M.M.R. and F.H.C.; writing—original draft preparation, M.M.R. and N.A.; writing—review and editing, visualization, supervision, F.H.C. All authors have read and agreed to the published version of the manuscript.

Funding: This research received no external funding.

Conflicts of Interest: The authors declare no conflicts of interest.

References

Alker, George, Jr., Young S. Oh, Eugene V. Leslie, Judith Lehotay, Victor A. Panaro, and Edward G. Eschner. 1975. Postmortem radiology of head neck injuries in fatal traffic accidents. *Radiology* 114: 611–17. [CrossRef] [PubMed]

American Spinal Injury Association. 1992. *Standards for Neurological and Functional Classification of Spinal Cord Injury*. revised. Chicago: American Spinal Injury Association.

American Spinal Injury Association and International Spinal Cord Society. 2006. *International Standards for Neurological Classification of Spinal Cord Injury*, 6th ed. Chicago: ASIA and ISCS.

Anderson, Paul A., and Pasquale X. Montesano. 1988. Morphology and treatment of occipital condyle fractures. *Spine (Phila Pa 1976)* 13: 731–36. [CrossRef] [PubMed]

Argenson, Claude, F. de Peretti, A. Ghabris, P. Eude, J. Lovet, and I. Hovorka. 1997. Classification of lower cervical spine injuries. *European Journal of Orthopaedic Surgery & Traumatology* 7: 215–29. [CrossRef]

Bellabarba, Carlo, and Richard J. Bransford. 2015. Spinopelvic fixation. In *AOSpine Masters Series, Volume 6: Thoracolumbar Spine Trauma*. New York: Thieme.

Blackmore, C. Craig, Scott S. Emerson, Frederick A. Mann, and Thomas D. Koepsell. 1999. Cervical spine imaging in patients with trauma: Determination of fracture risk to optimize use. *Radiology* 211: 759–65. [CrossRef] [PubMed]

Bracken, Michael B. 2001. Summary statement: The Sygen (GM-1 ganglioside) clinical trial in acute spinal cord injury. *Spine* 26: S99–S100. [CrossRef]

Consortium for Spinal Cord Medicine. 1997. *Prevention of Thromboembolism in Spinal Cord Injury: Clinical Practice Guidelines*. Washington: Paralyzed Veterans of America.

Corbett, J. L., H. L. Frankel, and P. J. Harris. 1971. Cardiovascular reflex responses to cutaneous and visceral stimuli in spinal man. *The Journal of Physiology* 215: 395–409. [CrossRef]

Davis, Floyd A., Dusan Stefoski, and Jean Rush. 1990. Orally administered 4-aminopyridine improves clinical signs in multiple sclerosis. *Annals of Neurology* 27: 186–92. [CrossRef]

Denis, Francis. 1983. The three column spine and its significance in the classification of acute thoracolumbar spinal injuries. *Spine (Phila Pa 1976)* 8: 817–31. [CrossRef]

Denis, Francis. 1984. Spinal instability as defined by the three-column spine concept in acute spinal trauma. *Clinical Orthopaedics and Related Research* 189: 65–76. [CrossRef]

DeVivo, Michael J. 2002. Epidemiology of traumatic spinal cord injury. In *Spinal Cord Medicine*. Edited by Steven Kirshblum, Denise I. Campagnolo and Joel A. DeLisa. Philadelphia: Lippincott Williams & Wilkins, pp. 69–81.

Ditunno, J. F., A. E. Flanders, S. Kirshblum, V. Graziani, and A. Tessler. 2002. Predicting outcomes in traumatic spinal cord injury. In *Spinal Cord Medicine*. Edited by Steven Kirshblum, Denise I. Campagnolo and Joel A. DeLisa. Philadelphia: Lippincott Williams & Wilkins, pp. 108–22.

Erickson, R. P. 1980. Autonomic hyperreflexia: Pathophysiology and medical management. *Archives of Physical Medicine and Rehabilitation* 61: 431–40.

Fielding, J. William, Richard J. Hawkins, Robert N. Hensinger, and William R. Francis. 1978. Atlantoaxial rotary deformities. *Orthopedic Clinics of North America* 9: 955–67. [CrossRef] [PubMed]

Fox, John L., and Alvaro Jerez. 1977. An unsual atlantoaxial dislocation: Case report. *Journal of Neurosurgery* 47: 115–18. [CrossRef]

Garstang, Susan V., Steven C. Kirshblum, and Kenneth E. Wood. 2000. Patient preference for inexsufflation for secretion management in spinal cord injury. *The Journal of Spinal Cord Medicine* 23: 80–85. [CrossRef] [PubMed]

Geisler, Fred H., Frank C. Dorsey, and William P. Coleman. 1991. Recovery of motor function after spinal-cord injury: A randomized, placebo-controlled trial with GM-1 ganglioside. *The New England Journal of Medicine* 324: 1829–38. [CrossRef] [PubMed]

Germon, Timothy, Sashin Ahuja, Adrian TH Casey, Nicholas V. Todd, and Am Rai. 2015. British Association of Spine Surgeons standards of care for cauda equina syndrome. *The Spine Journal* 15 S3: S2–S4. [CrossRef] [PubMed]

Go, B. K., M. J. DeVivo, and J. S. Richards. 1995. The epidemiology of spinal cord injury. In *Spinal Cord Injury: Clinical Outcomes from the Model Systems*. Edited by Samuel L. Stover, Joel A. DeLisa and Gale G. Whiteneck. Gaithersburg: Aspen Publishers.

Gokaslan, Ziya L., Julie E. York, Garrett L. Walsh, Ian E. McCutcheon, Frederick F. Lang, Joe B. Putnam, David M. Wildrick, Stephen G. Swisher, Dima Abi-Said, and Raymond Sawaya. 1998. Transthoracic vertebrectomy for metastatic spinal tumors. *Journal of Neurosurgery* 89: 599–609. [CrossRef]

Golueke, P., S. Sclafani, T. Phillips, A. Goldstein, T. Scalea, and A. Duncan. 1987. Vertebral artery injury: Diagnosis and management. *Journal of Trauma and Acute Care Surgery* 27: 856–65. [CrossRef]

Gonzalez, F., J. Y. Chang, K. Banovac, D. Messina, A. Martinez-Arizala, and R. E. Kelley. 1991. Autoregulation of cerebral blood flow in patients with orthostatic hypotension after spinal cord injury. *Paraplegia* 29: 1–7. [CrossRef]

Green, David, Russell D. Hull, Eberhard F. Mammen, Geno J. Merli, Saul I. Weingarden, and James S. T. Yao. 1992. Deep vein thrombosis in spinal cord injury summary and recommendations. *Chest* 102: 633S–635S. [CrossRef]

Green, David, Susan Sullivan, Janet Simpson, Robert C. Soltysik, and Paul R. Yarnold. 2005. Evolving risk for thromboembolism in spinal cord injury (SPIRATE Study). *American Journal of Physical Medicine & Rehabilitation* 84: 420–22. [CrossRef]

Guttman, Ludwig. 1973. *Spinal Cord Injuries: Comprehensive Management and Research*. Oxford: Blackwell Scientific Publications.

Hagen, Ellen Merete. 2015. Acute complications of spinal cord injuries. *World Journal of Orthopedics* 6: 17–23. [CrossRef] [PubMed]

Hamilton, Mark G., and S. Terence Mylks. 1992. Pediatric spinal injury: Review of 174 hospital admissions. *Journal of Neurosurgery* 77: 700–4. [CrossRef] [PubMed]

Haralson, Robert H., III, and Harold B. Boyd. 1969. Posterior dislocation of the atlas without fracture. Report of a case. *The Journal of Bone and Joint Surgery* 51: 561–66. [PubMed]

Harris, John H., Jr. 1986. Radiographic evaluation of spinal trauma. *Orthopedic Clinics of North America* 17: 75–86. [CrossRef] [PubMed]

Holdsworth, Frank. 1970. Fractures, dislocations, and fracture-dislocations of the spine. *The Journal of Bone & Joint Surgery* 52: 1534–51.

Iida, Hideo, Shigekuni Tachibana, Takao Kitahara, Shigeharu Horiike, Takashi Ohwada, and Kiyotaka Fujii. 1999. Association of head trauma with cervical spine injury, spinal cord injury, or both. *The Journal of Trauma and Acute Care Surgery* 46: 450–52. [CrossRef]

Jackson, Amie B., and Thomas E. Groomes. 1994. Incidence of respiratory complications following spinal cord injury. *Archives of Physical Medicine and Rehabilitation* 75: 270–75. [CrossRef]

Jamshidi, Saied, Michael W. Dennis, Charles Azzam, and Najmaldin Karim. 1983. Traumatic posterior atlantoaxial dislocation without neurological deficit. Case report. *Neurosurgery* 12: 211–13. [CrossRef]

Jefferson, Geoffrey. 1920. Fractures of the atlas vertebra: Report of four cases, and a review of those previously recorded. *British Journal of Surgery* 7: 407–22. [CrossRef]

Kirshblum, Steven C., and Kevin C. O'Connor. 2000. Levels of spinal cord injury and predictors of neurologic recovery. *Physical Medicine and Rehabilitation Clinics of North America* 11: 1–27. [CrossRef]

Labronici, Pedro José, Diogo do Nascimento Pereira, Pedro Henrique Vargas Moreira Pilar, José Sergio Franco, Marcos Donato Serra, José Carlos Cohen, and Rogério Carneiro Bitar. 2015. Safe localization for placement of percutaneous pins in the calcaneus. *Revista Brasileira de Ortopedia* 47: 455–59. [CrossRef] [PubMed]

Levine, Alan M., and C. C. Edwards. 1985. The management of traumatic spondylolisthesis of the axis. *The Journal of Bone and Joint Surgery* 67: 217–26. [CrossRef] [PubMed]

Lindan, R., E. Joiner, A. A. Freehafer, and C. Hazel. 1980. Incidence and clinical features of autonomic dysreflexia in patients with spinal cord injury. *Paraplegia* 18: 285–92. [CrossRef] [PubMed]

Marino, R. J., D. Rider-Foster, G. Maissel, and J. F. Ditunno. 1995. Superiority of motor level over single neurological level in categorizing tetraplegia. *Paraplegia* 33: 510–13. [CrossRef] [PubMed]

Mueller, Franz Josef, Bernd Fuechtmeier, Bernd Kinner, Michael Rosskopf, Carsten Neumann, Michael Nerlich, and Carsten Englert. 2012. Occipital condyle fractures. Prospective follow-up of 31 cases within 5 years at a level 1 trauma centre. *European Spine Journal* 21: 289–94. [CrossRef]

National Spinal Cord Injury Statistical Center. 2005. Spinal cord injury: Facts and figures at a glance. *The Journal of Spinal Cord Medicine* 28: 379–80.
Nichols, Constance G., David H. Young, and William R. Schiller. 1987. Evaluation of cervicothoracic junction injury. *Annals of Emergency Medicine* 16: 640–42. [CrossRef]
Papadopoulos, Stephen M. 1993. Biomechanics of Occipito-Atlanto-Axial Trauma. In *Spinal Trauma: Current Evaluation and Management*. Edited by AANS Publications Committee, Gary L. Rea and Carole A. Miller. Hoboken: WileyBlackwell, pp. 17–23.
Patel, Shanon, Shalini Kanagasingam, and Thomas Pitt Ford. 2009. External cervical resorption: A review. *Journal of Endodontics* 35: 616–25. [CrossRef]
Ragnarsson, Kristjan T., Karyl M. Hall, Conal B. Wilmot, and R. Edward Carter. 1995. Management of pulmonary, cardiovascular and metabolic conditions after spinal cord injury. In *Spinal Cord Injury: Clinical Outcomes from the Model Systems*. Edited by Samuel L. Stover, Joel A. DeLisa and Gale G. Whiteneck. Gaithersburg: Aspen Publishers.
Sapru, Hreday N. 2002. Spinal cord: Anatomy, physiology and pathophysiology. In *Spinal Cord Medicine*. Edited by Steven Kirshblum, Denise I. Campagnolo and Joel A. DeLisa. Philadelphia: Lippincott Williams & Wilkins.
Sassard, Walter R., Charles F. Heining, and William R. Pitts. 1974. Posterior atlantoaxial dislocation without fracture. Case report with successful conservative treatment. *The Journal of Bone & Joint Surgery* 56: 625–28.
Schneider, Richard C., Kenneth E. Livingston, A. J. E. Cave, and Gilbert Hamilton. 1965. 'Hangman's Fracture' of the Cervical Spine. *Journal of Neurosurgery* 22: 141–54. [CrossRef]
Schwartz, David T. 2008. Section 5. Cervical Spine. In *Emergency Radiology: Case Studies*. Edited by David T. Schwartz. New York: McGraw-Hill. Available online: https://accessemergencymedicine.mhmedical.com/ (accessed on 31 May 2023).
Segal, Jack L., and Sherry R. Brunnemann. 1997. 4-Aminopyridine improves pulmonary function in quadriplegic humans with longstanding spinal cord injury. *Pharmacotherapy* 17: 415–23. [CrossRef] [PubMed]
Segal, Jack L., and Sherry R. Brunnemann. 1998. 4-Aminopyridine alters gait characteristics and enhances locomotion in spinal cord injured humans. *The Journal of Spinal Cord Medicine* 21: 200–4. [CrossRef] [PubMed]
Shapiro, Scott, Richard Borgens, Robert Pascuzzi, Karen Roos, Michael Groff, Scott Purvines, Richard Ben Rodgers, Shannon Hagy, and Paul Nelson. 2005. Oscillating field stimulation for complete spinal cord injury in humans: A phase 1 trial. *Journal of Neurosurgery: Spine* 2: 3–10. [CrossRef] [PubMed]
Sud, S., S. Chaturvedi, T. B. S. Buxi, and S. Singh. 2002. Posterior atlantoaxial dislocation without associated fracture. *Skeletal Radiology* 31: 529–31. [CrossRef] [PubMed]
Tator, Charles H. 1994. Epidemiology and general characteristics of the spinal cord injured patient. In *Contemporary Management of Spinal Cord Injury*. Edited by Edward C. Benzel and Charles H. Tator. Park Ridge: American Association of Neurological Surgeons.
Theisen, D., L. Malisoux, R. Seil, and A. Urhausen. 2014. Injuries in youth sports: Epidemiology, risk factors and prevention. *Deutsche Zeitschrift für Sportmedizin* 65: 248–52. [CrossRef]
Tuli, Sagun, Charles H. Tator, Michael G. Fehlings, and Margot Mackay. 1997. Occipital condyle fractures. *Neurosurgery* 41: 368–76. [CrossRef]
Welch, Robert D., Susanne J. Lobley, Susan B. O'Sullivan, and Murray M. Freed. 1986. Functional independence in quadraplegia: Critical levels. *Archives of Physical Medicine and Rehabilitation* 67: 235–40.
White, Augustus A., and Manohar M. Panjabi. 1979. The basic kinematics of the human spine: A review of past and current knowledge. *Spine* 3: 12. [CrossRef]
White, Augustus A., and Manohar M. Panjabi. 1990. *Clinical Biomechanics of the Spine*. Philadelphia: JB Lippincott.
Wong, David A., Robert P. Mack, and Thomas K. Craigmile. 1991. Traumatic atlantoaxial dislocation without fracture of the odontoid. *Spine* 16: 587–89. [CrossRef]
Wood-Jones, Frederic. 1913. The Ideal Lesion Produced by Judicial Hanging. *Lancet* 181: 53. [CrossRef]
World Federation of Neurosurgical Societies Spine Committee. 2019. Cervical Spine Trauma Recommendations. Available online: https://wfns-spine.org/cervical-spine-trauma-recommendations (accessed on 5 March 2024).
World Federation of Neurosurgical Societies Spine Committee. 2020. Thoracolumbar Spine Trauma: WFNS Spine Committee Recommendations. Available online: https://wfns-spine.org/pdf/Thoracolumbar%20Spine%20Trauma%20Recommendations.pdf (accessed on 5 March 2024).
Yoon, Do Heum, Kook Hee Yang, Keung Nyun Kim, and Sung Han Oh. 2003. Posterior atlantoaxial dislocation without fracture: Case report. *Journal of Neurosurgery: Spine* 98: 73–76. [CrossRef] [PubMed]

Zhang, Andrew, and Brad J. Chauvin. 2021. Denis Classification. In *StatPearls [Internet]*; Treasure Island: StatPearls Publishing. Available online: https://www.ncbi.nlm.nih.gov/books/NBK544310/ (accessed on 23 July 2022).

Zindrick, Michael R., Leon L. Wiltse, Eric H. Widell, James C. Thomas, W. Russell Holland, B. Ted Field, and Curtis W. Spencer. 1986. A biomechanical study of intrapeduncular screw fixation in the lumbosacral spine. *Clinical Orthopaedics and Related Research* 203: 99–111. [CrossRef]

Degenerative Spinal Disease

Mohammod Zahed Hossain and Forhad H. Chowdhury

Abstract: Degenerative spinal disease is the commonest spinal problem dealt with by a neurosurgeon. Degenerative spine disease takes up significant working hours for neurosurgeons throughout the world. It is a progressive deterioration of the elements of the spinal cord and includes disc abnormality, facet joint abnormality, osteophytes spondylolisthesis, spondylolysis, ligamentum flavum hypertrophy, etc. All the aforementioned conditions can result in spinal canal stenosis, which can lead to neural compression and can produce compression on the cord or root and lead to myelopathy, radiculopathy, myeloradiculopathy, and cauda equina syndrome. Most of the time, MRI, CT, and X-ray of the spine are enough for diagnosing these conditions. Surgical intervention is needed when there is myelopathy, radiculopathy, or instability. This chapter will briefly discuss the management of disc prolapses (lumbar, cervical, and dorsal); degenerative spinal canal stenosis (spondylosis with myelopathy and radiculopathy); spondylolisthesis; ossified posterior longitudinal ligaments; and ligamentum flavum hypertrophy. It will also discuss degenerative diseases of the craniovertebral junction with instability and myelopathy (atlantoaxial dislocation and atlanto-occipital dislocation).

Abbreviations

AAD	atlantoaxial dislocation	ADI	atlanto-dental interval
AOD	atlanto-occipital dislocation	AF	annulus fibrosis
ALL	anterior longitudinal ligament	AP	anterior–posterior
CCJ	craniocervical junction	CES	cauda equina syndrome
CT	computed tomography	CTA	CT angiogram
CSF	cerebrospinal fluid	CSM	cervical spondylotic myelopathy
CVJ	craniovertebral junction		
DISH	diffuse idiopathic skeletal hyperostosis	DVT	deep vein thrombosis
ECM	extracellular matrix	EP	endplate
HRQOL	health-related quality of life	ITF	intertransverse fusion
IV	Intravenous	IVD	intervertebral disc
LBP	low back pain	LDD	lumbar disc disease
LDH	lumbar disc herniation	LFH	ligamentum flavum hypertrophy
MDCT	multidetector CT	mJOAS	modified Japanese Orthopedic Association Score
MMP	matrix metalloproteinase		
MRI	magnetic resonance imaging	NP	nucleus pulposus
ODI	Oswestry disability index	OALL	ossified anterior longitudinal ligament
OPLL	ossified posterior longitudinal ligament	PEEK	poly ether ether ketone
PLIF	posterolateral interbody fusion	PLL	posterior longitudinal ligament
SLR	straight leg raising	UTI	urinary tract infection
VB	vertebral body		

1. Introduction

The human spine is made up of highly specialized structures and tissues that are designed to provide a wide range of movement and significant load-transmitting capacity for daily physical activity (Ferguson and Steffen 2003). The human spinal column is the body's main support structure. Along with the intervertebral discs and ligaments, it is supported by paraspinal muscles. The spine consists of 33 separate bones, called the vertebrae. With age, five sacral vertebrae become fused and give rise to one sacrum, and four coccygeal vertebrae become fused and become one coccyx. So, in adults, there are 26 vertebral bones. The flexibility of the discs between the vertebrae allows for a cushioning effect. The spine, which must be both stable and flexible, is particularly vulnerable to damage and can degenerate over time. The spinal column is composed of (1) the vertebral column, composed of vertebrae, intervertebral discs, and ligaments, and (2) the spinal cord, including nerve roots and the cauda equina, covered by the meninges.

In men, the spine is typically 60–65 cm long, while it is 45–50 cm long in women. Of this length, 1/4th–1/5th is contributed by discs. The diameter of the canal varies in different regions of spine. It is widest in the cervical region (anterior–posterior AP diameter 17–18 mm), followed by the lumbar region (AP diameter average 11.5 mm) (Karantanas et al. 1998). It is narrowest in the thoracic region. The functions of the spine are weight transmission, acting as a shock absorber, like a cushion, and giving flexibility to the spine for movement. Bony structures protect the neural structures. The vertebral column is composed of vertebral bodies (VBs), pedicles, intervertebral discs, synovial facet joints, ligaments, and transverse and spinous processes. All these components can show signs of normal ageing as well as degenerative or regenerative changes (Pytel et al. 2006).

Spondylosis is an "umbrella" term to describe some type of degeneration in the spine. In the spine, the degenerative process involves the bony components (i.e., VBs), intervertebral discs, joints, and ligaments.

Degenerative spine disease is a progressive deterioration of the elements of the spinal cord and includes the following (Greenberg 2010):

1. Disc abnormality;
2. Facet joint abnormality;
3. Osteophytes;
4. Spondylolisthesis;
5. Spondylolysis;
6. Ligamentum flavum hypertrophy.

All the above conditions can cause spinal canal stenosis, which can lead to neural compression and can produce compression over the cord or root and lead to myelopathy, radiculopathy, myeloradiculopathy, and cauda equina syndrome.

2. Degenerative Disc Disease

2.1. *Anatomy and Physiology of the Disc*

The seven cervical, twelve thoracic, and five lumbar discs (twenty-three in all) are basically similar in structure, but they differ in size and shape according to the vertebrae in between which they are interposed (Easwaran 2012a). The nucleus pulposus (NP), a gelatinous inner core, the annulus fibrosus (AF), an outer rim, and cartilage endplates on both the upper and lower sides make up an intervertebral disc (Choi 2009; Easwaran 2012a). The outer AF, which is rich in type 1 collagen, is a circular layer that resists tensile tension because the collagen fibres run alternately between the lamellae of the annulus in an oblique fashion. The proteoglycan and water gel that make up the NP are connected by a loose network of type 2 collagen and elastin fibres (Karantanas et al. 1998). Aggrecan-1, the NP's most important proteoglycan, offers essential osmotic characteristics to resist compression, contributing to the shock-absorbing mechanism. One of the major avascular parts of the body is the intervertebral disc. Nutrients for the disc tissues are delivered by vessels in the subchondral bone close to the hyaline cartilage of the endplate. Small molecules like glucose and oxygen are carried over the endplate by passive diffusion. Proteoglycan and collagen, which make up a disc's basic skeletal framework, are produced by chondrocytes. The annulus fibrosus fibres, as well as the neighbouring dura and PLL, are innervated by the recurrent sinuvertebral nerve of Luschka, a meningeal branch of the spinal nerve that develops from the posterior ramus of each nerve root. Innervation is present in the outer annular regions, but not in the inner annular regions or the nucleus pulposus (Panigrahi and Reddy 2012).

2.2. *Biomechanics of the Spine*

The water content of the nucleus pulposus is vital for its biomechanical properties. On applying a compression force, water is expelled from the disc and it is reabsorbed into the disc once the force is removed. At low loads, the disc does not resist deformation but, beyond a certain load, the stiffness increases abruptly. This property allows the disc to remain flexible on minimal loading, while it contributes to stability as the loading increases. When the load limits are exceeded, the endplates fail first before the annulus fibrosus. This happens with compression loads of about 14,000 N in lumbar disc and 3000 N in the cervical disc (Kaiser et al. 2000). Water loss in the disc, associated with ageing, reduces the viscoelastic adaptability of the disc, making it prone to failure. The dehydrated disc behaves as a fibrous solid rather than a watery gel in terms of its biomechanical properties. Apart from compression loads, the other loads that the disc withstands are tension, shear, and torsion loads. During day-to-day activities, the loads acting on the disc are a combination of these pure loads (Easwaran 2012a).

2.3. *Changes Caused by Ageing*

With ageing, the water content in the nucleus pulposus (NP) becomes reduced. This dehydration is caused by a decrease in the proteoglycan content of the matrix in the NP. There is a reduction in collagen content with the replacement of type 2 collagen by type 1 collagen in the inner part of annulus (Singh et al. 2009). Type 1 collagen fibres become coarser and more cross-linked, thus increasing their stiffness. The collagen becomes non-enzymatically glycated, which further increases cross-linking. These biochemical changes are accompanied by histological changes such as the appearance of microstructural clefts, which have been observed as early as at the age of 15 years. There is fissuring and clumping of parts of the NP. The endplate (EP) undergoes changes like thinning, formation of fissures, and alteration of cell density, and there is subchondral bone sclerosis (Roberts et al. 2006). The changing microstructure and biochemistry alter the biomechanical characters of the ageing disc. As the NP becomes desiccated, the annulus fibrosus (AF) has to bear more of the compression load. The AF becomes stiffer but structurally weakened (Easwaran 2012a).

3. Lumbar Disc Herniation

3.1. *Introduction*

The term "lumbar degenerative disc disease" includes a spectrum of disorders like disc bulge, disc protrusion—which can be (i) central, (ii) paracentral, (iii) intraforaminal, or (iv) far lateral—disc extrusion (with or without a mitigated fragment), and internal disc disruption. Patients suffering from this condition present with low back pain (LBP) and/or radiculopathy of long duration or, acutely, with cauda equina syndrome (Panigrahi and Reddy 2012). Over 80% of the general public will experience LBP at some point in their lives, and it is responsible for about 15% of all sick days used at work. LBP is mostly brought on by lumbar disc disorders (LDDs), which include lumbar disc degeneration, including lumbar disc herniation. Studies have been conducted to identify the origins of LDDs. Genetic and environmental factors have been used to classify the causes (Kawaguchi 2018). Physical activity, sports, driving, and smoking can be classified as environmental risk factors (Kawaguchi 2018). Throughout the last century, mechanical load injury was proposed as the most important cause of disc prolapses (Luoma et al. 1998). Recent studies have revealed that genetic factors are a key factor in LDDs (Kawaguchi 2018).

The integrity and structure of both the nucleus and annulus in conjunction determine the mechanical characteristics of a disc. A change in each of these characteristics can have an impact on the disc's overall qualities. The disc gap is further strengthened by the anterior and posterior longitudinal ligaments (ALLs and PLLs). The ALL functions as a tension band to counteract pressures applied in extension because its attachment to the vertebral body margins is stronger than its attachment to the annulus. Even though it is weaker than the ALL, the PLL firmly adheres to the annulus fibrosus and functions as a tension band to fend against flexion stresses. In cases of free fragment disc herniation, it is usually ripped. The endplate's purpose is more biological than biomechanical in that it is crucial for the passage of nutrients into the disc (Easwaran 2012a).

3.2. *Causes*

The most frequent cause of disc herniation is disc degeneration, which is a slow, ageing-related wear-and-tear process. Discs lose flexibility as they age, making them more likely to rupture or rip at the slightest twist or strain. Most people struggle to identify the reason behind their ruptured disc. Twisting and turning when lifting can sometimes result in a herniated disc, as can using your back muscles rather than your leg and thigh muscles to raise heavy objects. Rarely is the cause a traumatic incident like a fall or a knock to the back.

3.3. *Risk Factors*

Factors that may increase the danger of a herniated intervertebral disc include the following:

- Weight. Weight is one factor that can make a herniated disc more likely to occur. Discs are put under additional strain due to excess body weight.
- Occupation. Those who have physically demanding occupations are more likely to experience back issues. Herniated discs are also more likely to occur if someone repeatedly lift, pull, push, bend laterally, or twist.
- Genetics. Herniated disc development is predisposed by genetics in some people.
- Smoking. Smoking is believed to reduce oxygen flow to the disc, hastening its degeneration.

3.4. Pathophysiology

Mechanical and metabolic disturbances both contribute to the complex processes of lumbar disc degeneration and herniation (Panigrahi and Reddy 2012). Twin studies have shown a genetic propensity to disc degeneration (Choi 2009). Disc herniation reaches a peak in the fourth decade of life, despite the fact that disc degeneration worsens with age (Panigrahi and Reddy 2012). The elastic modulus, which distributes stress to the most important areas of the disc, is aberrant and non-uniform in degenerated discs. They also have abnormal vascularity, collagen distribution, and collagen cross-linking. Repetitive or continuous axial overloading is the key determinant in the pathogenesis of lumbar degenerative disease. Obese individuals, manual labourers, truck drivers, and those involved in athletic activities like weightlifting and gymnastics are at risk of repetitive axial overloading of the spine (Panigrahi and Reddy 2012). Degenerated discs can no longer support a load hydrostatically. The endplate and annulus are where the load's stress is most concentrated (Choi 2009).

LDH is hypothesized to be caused by a number of alterations in the biology of the intervertebral disc:

1. Degradation of collagen and extracellular matrix (ECM) materials;
2. Upregulation of degradation systems like apoptosis and matrix metalloproteinase (MMP) expression;
3. Inflammation pathways;
4. Decreased water retention in the NP, increased type 1 collagen percentage in the NP and inner AF;
5. Degradation of collagen and extracellular matrix (ECM) materials (Amin et al. 2017; Kalb et al. 2012; Brayda-Bruno et al. 2014; Mayer et al. 2013).

The majority of disc herniations occur in a posterolateral direction, i.e., corresponding to the area of the spinal canal between the midline and the neural foramen, because the nucleus pulposus is situated somewhat posteriorly within the annulus and the PLL reinforces the annulus fibrosus in the midline posteriorly.

LDH symptoms are generated by several mechanisms. Among these are the presence and effects of *Propionibacterium acnes*, contributions from an acidic environment, microstructural alterations to the nerve root, and, most critically, the stretching effect of herniated disc material on the nerve root (Amin et al. 2017).

The types of disc herniation are as follows: (1) disc bulge; (2) protruded; (3) contained/entrapped; (4) extruded; (5) migrated,

The zones of lumbar disc herniation are as follows: (1) central canal zone— paramedian, midline, and subarticular zone; (2) foraminal zone; (3) extraforaminal zone (Greenberg 2010).

The most common spaces involved, according to frequency, are L4/5, L5/S1, L3/4, and others.

3.5. Clinical Features

3.5.1. Symptoms

An individual with a herniated lumbar disc can present with radiculopathy, neurogenic claudication, or cauda equina syndrome. The initial symptom in an individual with a disc herniation is pain, which may be in the back, buttock, thigh, leg, or foot and which may be present either in all or a few of these areas. Radicular pain is aggravated by bending, coughing, sneezing, and lifting a grounded object. The pain is usually relieved by lying down in a hip-and-knee-flexed posture.

The symptoms of lumbar disc herniation can be summarized as follows:

- Back pain that comes and goes. Moving about, coughing, sneezing, or standing for extended amounts of time may make it worse.
- Muscle spasms in the back.
- Sciatica, which causes pain to radiate from the back or buttock down the leg and into the calf or the foot.
- Leg muscles that are weakened.
- Numbness in the foot or the leg.
- Diminished knee- or ankle-level reflexes.
- Modifications in bowel or bladder function.

The level of disc herniation can be determined according to the motor and sensory functions of the respective nerve root. These are summarized in Table 1.

Patients who have large central disc herniation and resultant spinal canal stenosis present with neurogenic claudication which is asymptomatic at rest. They experience bilateral lower extremity pain after a variable duration of exertion, associated with numbness which is relieved with a brief period of rest. A central lumbar disc herniation may result in cauda equina syndrome with perineal numbness, loss of bladder and bowel control, and some degree of motor weakness in the legs (Panigrahi and Reddy 2012). It is important to look for spasms of the paraspinal muscles and the range of movement of the spine and perform a rectal examination when cauda equina syndrome is suspected. It is important to interpret the straight leg raising test (Lasegue test)—a positive test implies a reproduction of radicular pain and not back pain.

Table 1. Common neurologic changes in herniated lumbar discs according to root level.

Root-Level	Motor Weakness	Sensory Loss	Reflex Depression	Muscle Wasting
L2	Hip flexion and abduction	Lat thigh	Nil	Thigh
L3	Knee extension	Patellar region	Knee	Thigh
L4	Knee extension, ankle dorsiflexion	Medial shin below knee	Knee	Thigh
L5	Extensor hallucis longus	Dorsum of foot, lateral calf		Calf
S1	Plantar flexion at ankle	Lateral border of foot, posterior calf	Ankle	Calf

Source: Authors' compilation based on data from Panigrahi and Reddy (2012).

3.5.2. Physical Findings in Radiculopathy

Nerve root impingement produces a set of symptoms and signs that help to identify the level of disc herniation. These include motor weakness, sensory changes, and reflex changes as described in Table 1. Nerve root tension signs also help to determine the level. These include the following:

1. Lasegue sign, also known as straight leg raising test (SLR): roots involved are L5 and S1 and, to small extent, L4.
2. Crossed SLR: more specific for the same roots than SLR.
3. Femoral stretch test, also known as reverse SLR: roots involved are L2, L3, and L4.

Some other tests, not practiced much, are the bowstring sign, cram test, sitting knee extension, the FABER test, etc. (Greenberg 2010).

3.6. Differential Diagnosis

Although back pain is the commonest symptom of a herniated lumbar disc, in making the diagnosis, it is also the least useful symptom. The following conditions also present with symptoms similar to those of a herniated lumbar disc:

1. Tumours involving the nerves (neurofibroma, Schwannoma, ependymoma) or metastatic deposits in the pedicle;
2. Peripheral neuropathy in diabetes mellitus and entrapment neuropathies involving the sciatic nerve in the pelvis;
3. Osteoarthritis of the hip;
4. Fractures involving the vertebra caused by trauma, osteoporosis, or metastatic deposits;
5. Arachnoid cyst and Tarlov's cysts of the spinal region;
6. Vascular claudication.

Some serious conditions involving low back pain should be excluded by the "red flag signs" depicted in the Table 2.

3.7. Investigations

3.7.1. Plain Radiograph

Plain X-rays are the first-line imaging tools utilized in low back pain. A diagnosis of lumbar disc herniation cannot be made from a plain radiograph, but it can help by providing indirect evidence, like features of degenerative changes including narrowing of intervertebral disc space, disc calcification, marginal osteophytes, and sclerosis of the nearby vertebral body endplate. Standard anteroposterior and lateral radiographs exclude other aetiologies of back pain. Dynamic extension and flexion views are needed to rule out associated spondylolisthesis.

Table 2. Red flag signs for individuals with low back problems.

Condition	Red Flags
Infection or cancer	1. Age > 50 or <20 years 2. History of malignancy 3. Immunosuppression 4. Unexplained wt. loss 5. IV drug abuse, UTI, fever, or chills 6. Back pain not relieved with rest
Spinal fracture	1. History of significant trauma 2. Prolong utilization of steroids 3. Age > 70 years
Severe neurologic compromise or cauda equina syndrome	1. Acute onset of overflow incontinence or urinary retention 2. Loss of sphincter tone or faecal incontinence 3. Progressive or global weakness in lower extremities

Source: Authors' compilation based on data from Greenberg (2010).

3.7.2. Magnetic Resonance Imaging (MRI)

MRI (Figure 1) is the preferred initial study for the assessment of lumbar degenerative diseases including disc herniations and lateral recess, central canal, and neural foraminal stenoses. It is the gold standard of neuroimaging in diagnosing suspected lumbar disc herniation, with an accuracy of about 97% (Roberts et al. 2006).

MR imaging findings consistent with a degenerated disc are as follows (Panigrahi and Reddy 2012):

- Decreased signal intensity on T2W scans of the nucleus pulposus, compared with a normal disc, because of a desiccation of the degenerated disc and resultant diminished water content in the nucleus pulposus.
- Irregularity of the outline of the nucleus pulposus.
- Decrease in disc height.
- An intense dot-like high-intensity signal in the posterior annulus signifying an annulus tear.

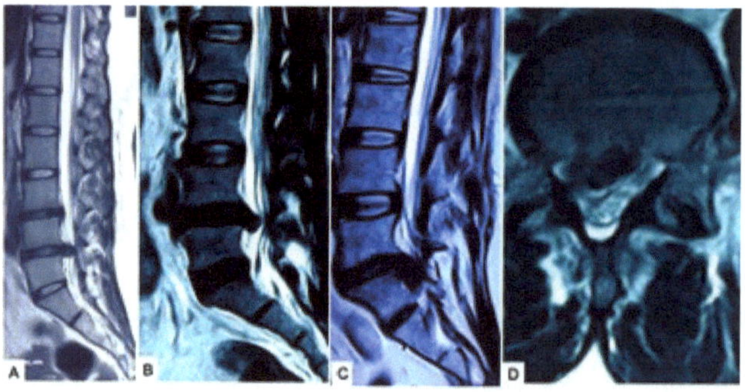

Figure 1. (**A**,**B**) MRI of lumbosacral spine (T2W sagittal images) showing PLID at L4 and 5. (**C**,**D**) MRI of lumbosacral spine (T2W sagittal and axial images) showing, respectively, PLID at L5 and S1 (left). Source: Figure by authors.

A disc herniation is best detected on axial images (either computed tomography or MR imaging) because in this plane, the focal, usually eccentric posterior extension of the disc material is readily visualized. The protruding disc obliterates epidural fat and displaces the nerve root sleeve, or both. Sagittal T1W and T2W MR images often demonstrate posterior bulging of the IVD. Sagittal T1W and moderately and heavily T2W images provide information regarding the level of herniation and the presence of extruded or sequestrated fragments, if any.

There are some contraindications to MRI. These include the following (Greenberg 2010):

(a) Cardiac pacemaker;
(b) Ferromagnetic aneurysmal clip;
(c) Metallic implants inside the body;
(d) Metallic FB within the eye;
(e) H/O of placement of coil, vascular stent, or filter in last 6 months;
(f) H/O of bullet of pellet within the body;
(g) Claustrophobia is a relative contraindication.

In these situations, CT scan and myelography are the solution.

3.7.3. Myelography

It is possible to delineate the dural sac, spinal cord, and exiting nerve roots on myelography. The myelographic signs of disc herniation include the following:

- Compression of the root of the nerve and thecal sac with an angular indentation on the anterolateral surface of the thecal tube.
- Compression of the nerve root with fusiform widening of the more distal end of the involved root.
- Central compression of the thecal tube by a centrally located herniated nucleus pulposus.

Myelographic findings are more appropriate for L4/5 than for L5/S1 because of the wider diameter of the epidural space at this level. Myelography cannot detect lateral or foraminal discs.

The disadvantages of myelography include the fact that it is an invasive procedure, occasionally needs overnight hospitalization, and cannot give information about lateral or foraminal disc herniation, as well as the issue of iodine allergy (Panigrahi and Reddy 2012; Greenberg 2010).

3.7.4. Computed Tomography

With multidetector CT (MDCT) substantially improving computed tomography (CT), which was previously regarded to be clinically inferior to MRI in LDH detection, the diagnostic level of CT is now almost on par with that of MRI. There are a number of scenarios where CT or myelography might be preferred over MRI, such as when MRI is unavailable or impractical (such as with pacemakers or cochlear implants) or when patients would feel too uncomfortable (intractable back pain or claustrophobia) (Amin et al. 2017).

3.7.5. Nerve Conduction Study and Electromyography

This study is sometimes required to exclude peripheral neuropathy and some conditions of the nerves.

3.8. Management

Successful management of LDH depends on the correct diagnosis of the problem and the selection of the appropriate mode of treatment. It is to be ensured that the symptoms are due to LDH. There are lot of causes of low back pain. For this purpose, careful history-taking is very important. The patient should be thoroughly examined, and scans, films, and reports should be carefully interpreted.

The management options for a patient with degenerative disc disease are as follows:

(1) Nonoperative;
(2) Operative.

3.8.1. Nonoperative Management

Initial nonsurgical treatment is warranted except in cases of absolute indications for surgery (discussed later on). It includes the following:

(a) Bed rest: for severe radicular discomfort, a brief (4-day) duration of bed rest is advised. Many patients find respite from their problems by lying flat, which is one justification for bed rest. Using the supine position to reduce intradiscal pressure is another justification.
(b) Nevertheless, a Cochrane review of nine trials with 1435 patients that compared bed rest with other therapies or different lengths of bed rest came to the conclusion that bed rest in comparison to staying active has, at best, no effect on low-back pain and, at worst, may have slightly harmful effects (Hagen et al. 2000). In patients with low back pain of varying durations, both with and without radiating pain, there was no discernible difference between the effects of bed rest compared to exercises, or between 7 days and 2–3 days of bed rest, in the management of acute low back pain.
(c) Activity modification: patients should temporarily restrict heavy weightlifting, prolonged sitting, and bending and twisting of the back.
(d) Physiotherapy: in the acute phase, this includes the use of hot packs, short-wave diathermy, and microwave therapy. After the acute phase, a graduated regime of back exercises is instituted.
(e) Analgesics.
(f) Muscle relaxants.

(g) Spinal manipulation therapy.
(h) Epidural injection.
(i) Patient education: the condition should be explained to the patient, and the patient should be reassured. The correct posture during work and sleep should be explained (Greenberg 2010; Panigrahi and Reddy 2012).

3.8.2. Operative Management

(a) Open techniques,
(b) Microdiscectomy,
(c) Minimally invasive surgery, including endoscopic techniques,
(d) Minimally invasive techniques:

- Chemonucleolysis;
- Automated percutaneous lumbar discectomy;
- Laser assisted percutaneous discectomy;
- Arthroscopic microdiscectomy;
- Intradiscal electrothermal therapy;
- Percutaneous nucleoplasty.

Operative therapy of LDH has previously been linked to increased short-term benefits and inconsistent value in the medium- to long-term range (Amin et al. 2017; Weinstein et al. 2006; Atlas et al. 1996) in a number of sizable investigations. A recent randomized Finnish study comparing nonoperative care with microdiscectomy in LDH (Amin et al. 2017; Österman et al. 2006) supported this conclusion. A subgroup analysis which revealed that microdiscectomy of L4-5 LDH produced better patient-reported outcomes than nonoperative therapy, including subjective job ability, ODI (Oswestry disability index), and HRQOL (Health-Related Quality of Life) scores, was the study's most innovative discovery (Amin et al. 2017; Österman et al. 2006).

Indications for Surgery

(1) Failure of nonsurgical measure to control pain for 5–8 weeks.
(2) Emergency surgery—(a) cauda equine syndrome (CES) (b); progressive motor deficit; (c) intolerable pain despite adequate narcotic analgesics.
(3) Patients who do not want to wait or try out nonsurgical treatment (Greenberg 2010).

Surgery is recommended if symptoms persist after 6 weeks of supervised conservative management, although the optimal timing of surgery is still being debated. Quick pain alleviation is the primary benefit of early surgery, although similar clinical outcomes one year later allow for prolonged conservative treatment in some patients (Panigrahi and Reddy 2012).

Microdiscectomy

The microsurgical approach in lumbar discectomy is currently the gold standard in the management of herniated lumbar disc disease. The success frequency of microdiscectomy ranges from 88 to 98.5%, while the complication rate is around 1.5%. The biggest advantage is the shorter incision and hence reduced postoperative pain, which reduces the length of hospital stay.

The complication rate following microdiscectomy is 15–30%. Intraoperative complications include the following:

- Exploration of the wrong site or level;
- Dural tears resulting in postoperative CSF leak or pseudomeningocoele;
- Injury to the nerve root;
- Retroperitoneal injury to great vessels and bowel;
- Facet joint fracture;
- Haemorrhage.

Wrong-level exploration can be minimized by using perioperative C-Arm X-ray. Postoperative complications include the following:

- Discitis (septic or aseptic);
- Arachnoiditis;
- Soft-tissue infection;

- Failure of pain relief;
- Recurrence of pain due to failed back surgery.

Minimally Invasive Surgery

Over the past 15–20 years, minimally invasive techniques for spine surgery have been developed and are being used more frequently. These methods are linked to lesser soft-tissue and skeletal trauma, cheaper acute care costs, and shorter hospital stays. Interlaminar, posterolateral, transforaminal, and transiliac are a few acknowledged percutaneous endoscopic methods for treating LDHs (Amin et al. 2017; Bai et al. 2017; Tonosu et al. 2016). When compared to open discectomy, endoscopic discectomy is often associated with shorter operating times, less blood loss, and lower reoperation rates, with no rise in overall complications or wound infections (Amin et al. 2017; Phan et al. 2017). However, a double-blind randomized control trial with 325 patients was unable to distinguish between open and endoscopic surgery in terms of long-term patient-centred results (Amin et al. 2017; Overdevest et al. 2017).

3.8.3. Complications of Lumbar Disc Surgery

The most common complications of lumbar disc surgery are as follows:

(a) Discitis;
(b) Recurrent disc herniation;
(c) Failed back syndrome (failure to relieve symptoms);
(d) Wrong site of operation;
(e) Unintended durotomy: CSF fistula, pseudomeningocele;
(f) Nerve root injury;
(g) Postop urinary retention: usually transient.

Some rare complications are CES, DVT, great vessel injury (aorta, vena cava), compression neuropathy due to positioning, and postoperative visual loss.

Discitis

The nucleus pulposus is infected. Disc and vertebral body (VB) damage could begin in the cartilaginous endplate and progress from there. Postop discitis can develop following a variety of surgeries, but lumbar discectomy is the most prevalent one.

Failed Back Syndrome

This occurs when, after having back surgery, the low back pain or radiculopathy symptoms do not improve in a satisfactory manner. These individuals frequently need analgesics and cannot go back to work. Factors that may contribute to or cause failed back syndrome include the following (Greenberg 2010):

(a) Wrong initial diagnosis due to inadequate clinical or radiological (imaging) preop work-up.
(b) Continued cauda equina or nerve root compression due to residual or recurrent disc herniation, wrong site operation, adjacent-level pathology, adhesive scar formation, pseudomeningocele, or segmental instability.
(c) Deafferentation pain, which is typically continuous and scorching or ice cold, is a symptom of permanent nerve root injury brought on by the initial disc herniation or following surgery.
(d) Discitis.
(e) Adhesive arachnoiditis.
(f) Postoperative reflex sympathetic dystrophy.

These patients should be thoroughly evaluated, including a detailed history, clinical examination, and re-checking all investigation documentation prior to the operation. Then, total blood count, lumbar spine X-ray, MRI with contrast, and CT scan with contrast and with bone window view should be repeated to identify any infection, residual disc herniation, and spinal instability, as well as to ascertain whether surgery was performed at the correct site and to assess the condition of the previous lesion for which surgery was performed.

Treatment is mostly symptomatic if there is no radiculopathy and includes bed rest, analgesics, and physical therapy. Sometimes, a short course of steroids can be given. Patients who have radiculopathy for residual/recurrent disc herniation and spinal instability need reoperation. For instability, fusion and fixation is needed.

3.9. Cauda Equina Syndrome

The cauda equina, a group of nerves near the end of the spinal cord, is so named because it resembles a horse's tail. These nerve roots continue in the lumbar and sacral region as the cauda equina. The clinical condition CES is caused by the malfunctioning of several lumbar and sacral nerve roots within the lumbar spinal canal, typically as a result of cauda equina compression. The lumbar region's most severe herniated disc is the most frequent cause of CES. Cauda equina syndrome requires immediate surgical treatment because it is a neurosurgical emergency.

The causes of CES include the following (Greenberg 2010):

1. Compression of the cauda equina:
    - (a) massive herniated lumbar disc;
    - (b) neoplasm;
    - (c) free fat graft after discectomy;
    - (d) spinal epidural haematoma;
    - (e) trauma: fracture fragments compressing the cauda equina.
2. Infection—epidural abscess;
3. Neuropathy—ischaemic or inflammatory;
4. Ankylosing spondylitis.

Patients with CES may have some or all of the following "red flag" symptoms:

- Urinary retention: the commonest symptom.
- Urinary and/or faecal incontinence.
- "Saddle anaesthesia"—sensory impairment that can involve the genitals, anus, and the buttock region.
- Paralysis or weakness of more than one nerve root that leads to weakness of both lower extremities.
- Back pain and/or leg pain (also known as sciatica).
- Numbness and altered sensation in the back and/or legs.
- Bilateral absence of Achilles reflex.
- Sexual dysfunction.

Symptoms of cauda equina syndrome can be of (a) acute onset, developing suddenly within 24 h, or of (b) gradual onset, developing within several weeks.

Surgical decompression is frequently required as soon as possible in cases of cauda equina syndrome to lessen or remove pressure on the damaged nerves. Although there are conflicting findings in the literature about the best time to start treatment, it is widely accepted that having surgery within 24–48 h has the highest chance of improving sensory and motor impairments.

Although lumbar laminectomy is the preferred method of treating cauda equina syndrome, lumbar microdiscectomy may be performed in some specific circumstances. The degree of nerve injury present at the time of surgery and the speed with which the nerve is decompressed are two variables that affect the prognosis for cauda equina syndrome. Physical therapy is needed for rehabilitation.

Depending on the cause of CES, antibiotics or a high dose of corticosteroids may also be needed. Radiotherapy and chemotherapy may be needed after surgery in case of a tumour, but radiotherapy may delay the recovery of nerve function.

4. Spondylolisthesis

4.1. Introduction

One vertebra being displaced over the following lower vertebra in the sagittal plane is known as spondylolisthesis. Since the superior vertebra is usually displaced anteriorly and since this most frequently occurs in the lumbar region, it is also referred to as the forward slipping of lumbar vertebra (Easwaran 2012b).

Spine instability, or spondylolisthesis, causes the vertebrae to move more than they should. L5 over S1 is the most frequent pairing, followed by L4 over L5 (Greenberg 2010).

At the level of the listhesis, lumbar disc herniation is uncommon; but, once the disc is exposed, it may "roll" out and produce MRI abnormalities that may mimic a herniated disc (Greenberg 2010). If the listhesis causes nerve root compression, it involves the root that exits below the pedicle of the slipped upper vertebra and causes low back pain with radiculopathy.

4.2. Classification and Aetiology

An aetiological classification that is widely accepted was proposed in 1976 by Wiltse, Newman, and MacNab (Table 3).

Table 3. Wiltse–Newman–MacNab classification of spondylolisthesis.

Type	Aetiology
Isthmic	Pars interarticularis (isthmus) defect
Subtype A	Bilateral chronic spondylolytic defect in the isthmus
Subtype B	Healed spondylolysis with elongated isthmus
Subtype C	Acute bilateral fracture of isthmus
Degenerative	Abnormal motion due to disc and facet joint degeneration
Dysplastic	Congenital abnormality of neural arch such as malformed L5 inferior or superior S1 facet, abnormal sacral surface, no pars defect
Traumatic	Acute fracture of the neural arch at a site other than the isthmus
Pathological	A. Generalized bone disease B. Localized bone disease disrupting the integrity of the neural arch

Source: Authors' compilation based on data from Wiltse et al. (1976).

Nowadays, this classification system has been rearranged into six types (with the inclusion of a new type).

Type 1: Dysplastic—the congenital arch of L5 or the upper sacrum permits spondylolisthesis. No pars defect. A total of 94% are associated with spina bifida occulta.
Type 2: Isthmic—a failure of the neural arch due to a defect in the pars interarticularis. There are three sub types: (a) lytic: fatigue fracture or insufficiency fracture of the pars; (b) elongated but intact pars; (c) acute fracture of the pars.
Type 3: Degenerative—as a result of long-standing intersegmental instability.
Type 4: Traumatic—as a result of fractures usually in areas other than the pars.
Type 5: Pathological—local or generalized bone disease.
Type 6: Postsurgical—caused by complications after surgery, e.g., laminectomy and discectomy.

Classification by the severity of slippage, calculated as the percentage of the width of the vertebral body (Massachusetts General Hospital 2016):

- Grade 1: 0–25%;
- Grade 2: 25–50%;
- Grade 3: 50–75%;
- Grade 4: 75–100%;
- Grade 5: >100%.

4.3. Presentation

Spondylolysis and spondylolisthesis may be entirely asymptomatic. Common presentations are as follows (Easwaran 2012b; Greenberg 2010):

(1) Low back pain: poorly localized, central, sometimes referred to the sacral and perineal region.
(2) Sciatica.
(3) Neurogenic claudication.
(4) Radiculopathy: commonly L4, L5, and S1.
(5) Postural abnormality: sagittal imbalance and scoliosis.

4.4. Investigations

Xray, MRI and CT scan are important in the management of spodylilisthesis (Figures 2–4).

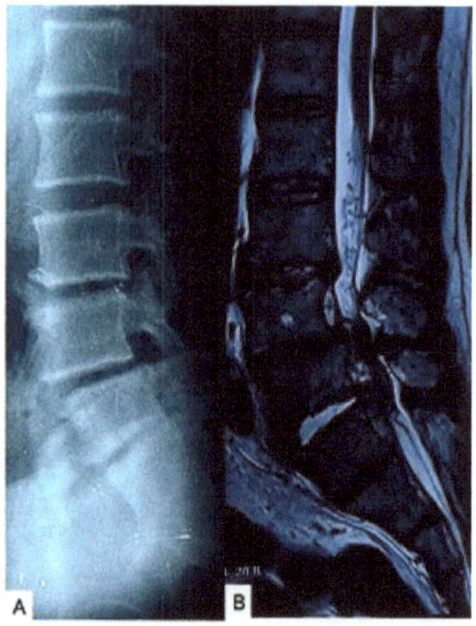

Figure 2. (**A**) X-ray of lumbosacral spine (lateral view) and (**B**) MRI of lumbosacral spine (T2W sagittal image) showing grade 1 spondylolisthesis at L4 and 5. Source: igure by authors.

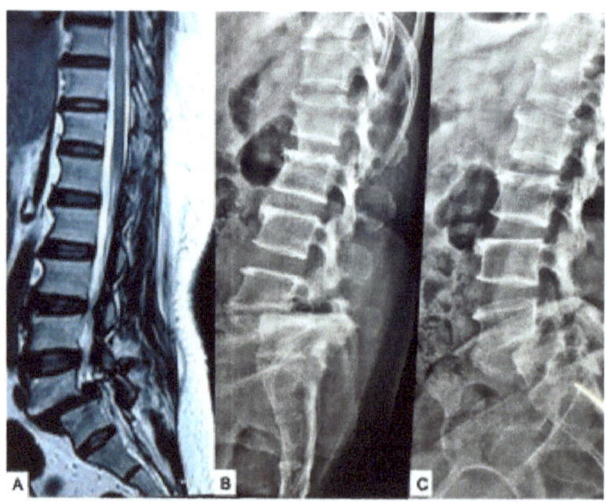

Figure 3. (**A**) MRI of lumbosacral spine (T2W sagittal image) and (**B**,**C**) dynamic X-ray of lumbosacral spine (lateral view) showing unstable grade 2 spondylolisthesis at L4 and 5 and fractured pars interarticularis with L5 sacralization. Source: Figure by authors.

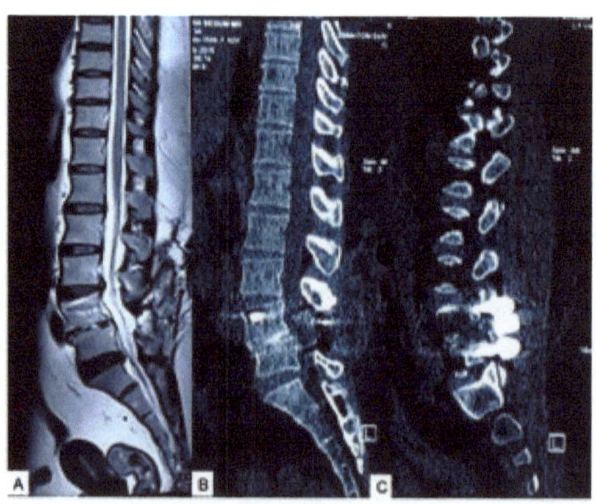

Figure 4. (**A**) MRI of lumbosacral spine (T2W sagittal image); (**B**,**C**) CT scan of lumbosacral spine (sagittal images) showing reduction, stabilization, and fusion of L4 and 5 in a case of spondylolisthesis. Source: Figure by authors.

4.4.1. Plain Radiographs

Plain X-rays are the best way to diagnose spondylolisthesis. The standard projections used are as follows: (1) The anteroposterior view, which also covers the sacroiliac joints and both hip joints and demonstrates scoliosis and sagittal balance; (2) The lateral view in the standing posture in a neutral position, flexion, and extension. The lateral neutral position shows the degree of slipping and the canal diameter. The flexion–extension dynamic film shows sagittal spinal instability. A forward movement of up to 2 mm in flexion is acceptable in healthy patients (Hayes et al. 1989). (3) The oblique view may demonstrate pars defects with the "Scottie dog collar" sign.

4.4.2. MRI

MRI provides details on soft tissues such ligaments, nerve roots, the synovium, and intervertebral discs (Easwaran 2012b). Loss of CSF signal on T2WI may be attributable to juxtafacet cysts, increased fluid in the facet joint, and vacuum discs, as well as lateral recess stenosis, central canal stenosis, and foraminal stenosis (Greenberg 2010).

4.4.3. Computed Tomography (CT)

A conventional CT scan or one conducted after water-soluble myelography typically reveals a "trefoil" channel (cloverleaf shaped, with three leaflets). Additionally, hypertrophied ligaments, AP canal diameter, facet arthropathy, and pars fractures, as well as, rarely, bulging annuli or herniated discs, are all visible on a CT scan (Greenberg 2010). CT scan is a *sine qua non* in preoperative planning (Easwaran 2012b).

4.5. Management

4.5.1. Conservative Management

Conservative management is warranted in individuals with no or minimal symptoms. This is offered to young patients with low-grade spondylolisthesis or spondylolysis and to older patients with non-disabling degenerative spondylolisthesis.

The modalities consist of 3–5 days of rest till the acute episode of back pain resolves. Longer periods of bed rest are counterproductive. Oral analgesics, bracing, various physical therapies, epidural/facetal steroid injections, and spinal flexion exercises are also prescribed (Easwaran 2012b).

4.5.2. Surgical Management

Indications for Surgery

Surgical management is warranted in (1) patients with disabling symptoms that are unrelieved by conservative management; (2) asymptomatic spondylolisthetic patients with a possible high risk of progression. The aims of surgery are halting the progression of neuro-deficit, pain relief, and, possibly, improving some presenting neurologic deficit (Greenberg 2010; Easwaran 2012b).

Surgical Options

These include (1) decompression by laminectomy, facetectomy, and foraminotomy; excision of thickened ligamentum flavum or hypertrophic synovium, drainage of synovial cysts, discectomy, and epidural scar release are the soft-tissue manoeuvres to relieve root compression; (2) reduction is seldom necessary to achieve the twin aims. Reduction is easier to achieve and becomes neurologically safer when it is attempted after decompression is completed. Distraction force applied to pedicle screws can help achieve reduction; (3) fusion: (a) interbody (PLIF); (b) interfacetal and (c) interspinous process; (d) intertransverse fusion (ITF); and (4) stabilization by instrumentation using a (a) transpedicular screw or a (b) transfacetal screw.

5. Dorsal Disc Prolapses

5.1. Introduction

Clinically symptomatic thoracic herniated discs are rare. Both sexes are affected equally. Most thoracic herniations usually happen centrally or posterolaterally, and less than 10% can be herniated laterally (McInerney and Ball 2000).

5.2. Clinical Features

Thoracic disc herniations are mostly asymptomatic. There is no typical pattern of clinical features that differentiates a herniated thoracic disc from other dorsal lesions. The usual signs and symptoms are pain (localized, axial, or radicular), motor impairment (myelopathy), hyper-reflexia and spasticity, and bowel and bladder dysfunction. Herniated thoracic disc myelopathy is usually progressive and often associated with sensory impairment down to the level of compression. Lateral thoracic disc prolapse is often associated with radicular pain in the dermatome of the root with or without paraesthesia or dysaesthesia. This radicular neuralgia is usually positional and nocturnal. Thoracic disc herniation is usually static or reduces in actual size in most cases (McInerney and Ball 2000; Shirzadi et al. 2013).

5.3. Neuroimaging

MRI of the thoracic spine is the primary imaging modality of choice for diagnosis, evaluation, and surgical planning. Plain CT is needed to evaluate the degree of calcification as thoracic herniated discs are often calcified (Figures 5 and 6).

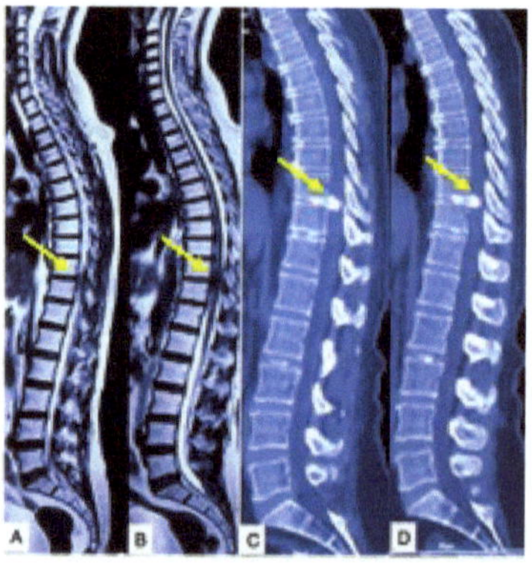

Figure 5. (**A**,**B**) MRI of spine (T2W sagittal images) showing thoracic disc prolapse at D10 and 11 with compressive myelopathy (marked with an arrow). (**C**,**D**) CT scan of spine (sagittal views) in the same patient showing the prolapsed disc was calcified (marked with an arrow). Source: Figure by authors.

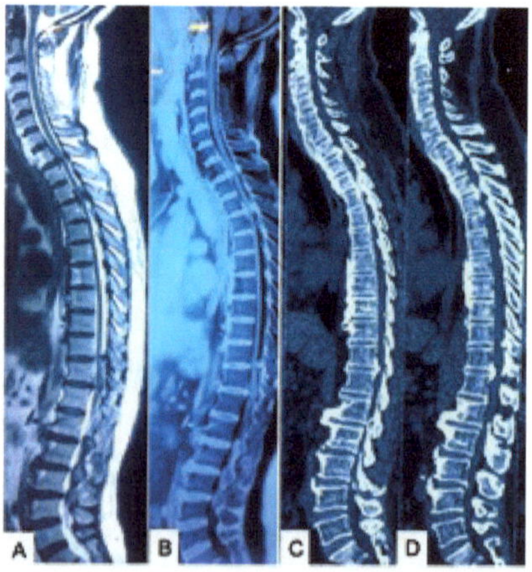

Figure 6. (**A**,**B**) MRI of the spine (T2W sagittal images) showing thoracic disc prolapse at D1 and 2 and D3 and 4 as well as ligamentum flavum hypertrophy (LFH) at the same levels with LFH at D10 and 11. (**C**,**D**) CT scan of the spine (sagittal views) in the same patient showing the prolapsed discs were calcified and LFH was also calcified. This patient also had an ossified anterior longitudinal ligament (OALL) and OPLL, indicating a case of diffuse idiopathic skeletal hyperostosis (DISH). Source: Figure by authors.

5.4. *Treatment*

5.4.1. Conservative

Conservative treatment is the first therapeutic option in most cases and usually consists of rest, analgesics, muscle relaxation, and movement restriction.

5.4.2. Surgical

Surgical indications are as follows:

(i) Severe myelopathy;
(ii) Progressive myelopathy;
(iii) Severe radiculopathy.

Surgical approaches include posterolateral (costotransversectomy, transpedicular, lateral extracavitary approach, lateral parascapular extrapleural approach) and anterolateral approaches (thoracotomy/thoracoscopic). The surgical treatment of herniated thoracic disc prolapses is associated with significant complications, such as neurological deterioration, wrong-level surgery, incomplete disc resection, postoperative instability, cerebrospinal fluid leaks, pulmonary complications, infection, intercostal neuralgia, etc. (McInerney and Ball 2000; Shirzadi et al. 2013).

6. Cervical Spondylosis and Myeloradiculopathy

The term "cervical spondylosis," which is occasionally used interchangeably with "cervical spinal stenosis," is typically used to describe cervical degenerative disc degeneration (Greenberg 2010). Age-related wear and tear in the cervical spine (neck), known as cervical spondylosis, can cause neck discomfort, stiffness, and other symptoms. Spondylosis usually implies more widespread age-related degenerative pathologies of the cervical spine, including intervertebral disc herniation, hypertrophy of the lamina, articular facets, and ligaments (lig. flavum, PLL), and subluxation of the spine. Common symptoms include neck pain or stiffness, nagging soreness in the neck, muscle spasms, dizziness, and headaches (Greenberg 2010). There are three main presentations linked to cervical spondylosis: (1) neck pain and brachialgia; (2) radiculopathy; (3) myelopathy (Deopujari and Kumar 2012).

6.1. *Cervical Disc Herniation*

6.1.1. Introduction

The nucleus pulposus is displaced as a result of cervical disc herniation, which may impinge on these crossing neurons as they leave the neural foramen or directly compress the spinal cord inside the spinal canal. When the nucleus pulposus partially or completely protrudes through the annulus fibrosus, disc herniation occurs. Acute or chronic occurrences of this mechanism are also possible. Chronic herniations are caused by the intervertebral disc degenerating and drying out as a result of normal ageing; these symptoms typically appear slowly or gradually and are usually less severe. Contrarily, acute herniations are typically brought on by trauma, with the nucleus pulposus protruding via a tear in the annulus fibrosus as a result (Caridi et al. 2011; Sharrak and Al Khalili 2021).

Cervical disc herniation is more common in women than in men as they age, and it is most commonly diagnosed in people between the ages of 51 and 60 (Sharrak and Al Khalili 2021).

6.1.2. Pathophysiology

A bulging nucleus pulposus is hypothesized to mechanically compress the nerve, contributing to the pathophysiology of herniated discs and to a localized rise in inflammatory cytokines (interleukin (IL)-1 and IL-6, substance P, bradykinin, TNF-alpha, and prostaglandins). Microvascular injury caused by compression forces can range in severity from a minor restriction of venous flow that produces congestion and oedema to a severe obstruction that can lead to arterial ischaemia (Sharrak and Al Khalili 2021; Rhee et al. 2007; Doughty and Bowley 2019). Posterolaterally, where the annulus fibrosus is thin and lacking the structural support of the posterior longitudinal ligament, herniations are more likely to happen (Dydyk et al. 2020).

The most commonly affected roots are C5 and C6. This can be explained by Sunderland's (Sunderland 1974) observation that the C4, C5, and C6 roots have a strong attachment to the vertebral column, while the others are relatively free (Deopujari and Kumar 2012). Patients under 55 are much more likely to present with herniated nucleus pulposus-related radiculopathy, whereas patients over 55 are more likely to develop canal or foraminal stenosis as a result of osteophyte formation (Deopujari and Kumar 2012).

6.1.3. Clinical Features

The C5–C6 and C6–C7 vertebral bodies are the ones where cervical disc herniations most frequently happen. Symptoms will then develop at C6 and C7, respectively, as a result of this (Table 4). Axial neck ache or ipsilateral arm pain or paraesthesia in the concomitant dermatomal distribution are the most frequent subjective symptoms (Sharrak and Al Khalili 2021).

Table 4. Features of nerve root involvement as a result of compression by a herniated intervertebral disc in the cervical spine (radiculopathy).

Root Involved	Distribution of Pain	Distribution of Paraesthesia	Weak Muscles	Reflex Change
C2	Ear or eye pain, headache			
C3, C4	Ill-defined neck pain		Neck muscle spasm	
C5	Lateral arm, shoulder, neck	Lateral arm	Deltoid, supraspinatus, infraspinatus	Biceps reflex
C6	Lateral arm, forearm, thumb	Lateral arm and forearm, thumb and index finger	Biceps, brachioradialis, wrist extensors	Biceps, brachioradialis
C7	Dorsal arm and forearm, interscapular area	Middle and index finger	Triceps and wrist extensors	Diminished triceps
C8	Medial forearm and hand, 5th digit	Medial forearm and hand, 5th digit	Intrinsic muscles of hand	Finger flexor

Source: Authors' compilation based on data from Deopujari and Kumar (2012); Sharrak and Al Khalili (2021).

Cervical myelopathy occurs from the compression of the cervical spinal cord. This compression may be discogenic or spondylotic. When a herniated disc (large central disc), also called a soft disc, causes compression over the cord, this is called discogenic myelopathy. When the bony spur of an osteophyte also called a hard disc or an ossified posterior longitudinal ligament, causes a narrowing of the cervical spinal canal and results in the compression of the spinal cord, this is called spondylotic myelopathy.

The symptoms of cervical myelopathy may include the following:

- Neck pain;
- Reduced motion range;
- Stiffness;
- Weakness in the arms and hands;
- Difficulty handling small objects, such as coins or pens;
- Tingling or numbness in the arms and hands;
- Poor coordination and clumsiness of the hands;
- Balance issues.

The Spurling test, Lhermitte sign, and Hoffman test are examples of provocative tests. Acute radiculopathy can be diagnosed with the Spurling test. To detect spinal cord compression and myelopathy, the Hoffman test and the Lhermitte sign can be employed (Sharrak and Al Khalili 2021). The clinical pattern of myelopathy is characterized by the existence of long tract signs, which include hyporeflexia of deep tendon reflexes at the level of affection and hyper-reflexia below the level of affection in the upper and lower limbs, increased muscle tone or clonus, and the presence of pathological reflexes, including Hoffman's sign or Babinski's sign (UMNL below the level of the lesion and LMNL at the level of lesion) (Deopujari and Kumar 2012).

6.1.4. Classification of Cervical Myelopathy

Nurick Classification, founded on ambulatory function and gait (Derek 2021; Nurick 1972; Lasanianos et al. 2015):

Grade 0: Normal or root symptoms only;
Grade 1: Signs of spinal cord compression; normal gait;
Grade 2: Gait difficulties; however, fully employed;
Grade 3: Gait difficulties deter employment, walks unassisted;
Grade 4: Unable to walk without assistance;
Grade 5: Bed- or wheelchair-bound.

6.1.5. Investigation

Radiologic Evaluation

The diagnostic workup includes dynamic and static cervical spine X-ray, CT scan, and MRI. Cervical X-rays should be taken in the anteroposterior, lateral neutral, flexion, and extension, and oblique views, and may show loss of disc space height, foraminal osteophyte, spondylotic bars, kyphosis, posterior compression from facet arthropathy, subluxations, or late auto fusion of adjacent cervical segments. Flexion–extension lateral X-ray films may be helpful to evaluate significant instability. Oblique views can also demonstrate foraminal osteophytes.

MRI

MRI (Figure 7) is the preferred diagnostic modality for cervical disc herniation and spondylosis. MRI is helpful in assessing the spinal cord, spinal canal diameter, and various components responsible for stenosis and compression, viz., intervertebral discs, ligamentum flavum hypertrophy, and vertebral ligaments. Individuals with cervical spondylotic myelopathy frequently have greater increases in signal intensity changes on T2W MRI images at the level of spinal compression. This could be a sign of gliosis, myelomalacia, ischaemia, inflammation, or oedema (Deopujari and Kumar 2012; McCormick et al. 2003).

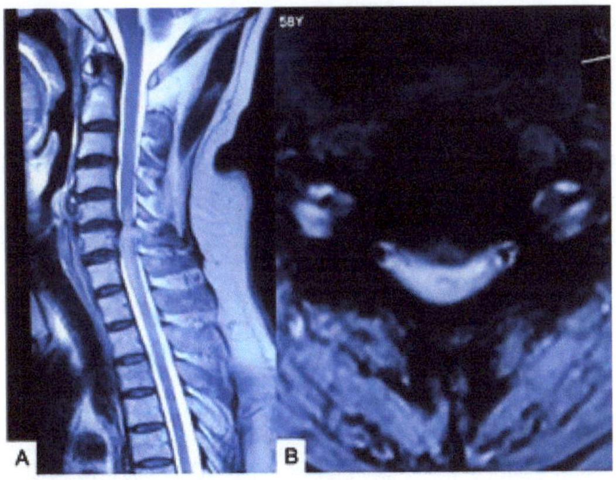

Figure 7. MRI T2W images of the cervical spine ((**A**) sagittal and (**B**) axial) showing prolapsed cervical intervertebral disc at C5 and 6 causing compression of the spinal cord with changes in signal intensity. Source: Figure by authors.

CT Scan

CT is required for better delineation of bone anatomy and OPLL. CT is also helpful in assessing the transverse foramina, facets, and the size, shape, and diameter of the spinal canal, as well as uncovertebral joints. Dynamic CT scans are the most helpful in the assessment of instability. CT myelography provides excellent visualization of radicular or cord compression in patients in whom MRI cannot be done for some reasons (Deopujari and Kumar 2012).

Neurophysiology

Patients with ambiguous symptoms or imaging results may benefit from nerve conduction and electromyography tests, which can also be used to rule out peripheral neuropathy. Brachial plexitis, carpal tunnel syndrome, and thoracic inlet syndromes can be accurately diagnosed with the help of neurophysiological studies (Deopujari and Kumar 2012; McCormick et al. 2003).

6.1.6. Treatment

A frequent degenerative condition known as cervical disc disease or spondylosis is characterized by the intervertebral disc's progressive degradation and ensuing alterations to the bones and soft tissues. Medical therapy and surgery are the two potential therapeutic treatments for cervical spondylosis and disc herniation.

(i) Medical or nonsurgical treatment: The majority of patients (75–90%) will recover from acute cervical radiculopathies brought on by a herniated disc; therefore, nonsurgical procedures are commonly used to treat them. The modalities that can be utilized include the following:

- Collar immobilization.
- Traction: intermittent cervical traction.
- Pharmacotherapy: NSAIDs and short courses of steroids, anti-neuralgic drugs, and muscle relaxants can help.
- Physical therapy: includes range-of-motion exercises, ice, strengthening exercises, heat, electrical stimulation, and ultrasound therapy.
- Cervical spine manipulation.

(ii) Interventional treatment: Injections of spinal steroids are a typical nonsurgical option. With pathological confirmation by MRI, perineural injections (translaminar and transforaminal epidurals, selective nerve root blocks) are an alternative. These procedures ought to be carried out with radiologic supervision (Sharrak and Al Khalili 2021; Eubanks 2010; Childress Marc A. 2016).

Surgical

Surgical intervention is indicated for patients with spondylosis and cervical disc herniation with the following presentations:

- disabling pain intractable to conservative therapy;
- acute spinal cord compression;
- progressive neuro-deficit and progressive muscular weakness or sensory disturbance.

Decompression of the nerve root and spinal cord and the removal of anteroposterior flattening and cervical cord distortion are the three main objectives of surgical care of patients with radiculopathy or myelopathy (Deopujari et al. 2012).

Surgical Options:

1. Anterior approach:

    - Anterior cervical discectomy without fusion (it is rarely performed nowadays).
    - Anterior cervical discectomy with fusion.

The anterior cervical discectomy with fusion procedure continues to be the gold standard because it enables the pathology to be removed and prevents recurring neural compression by conducting a fusion. Fusion can be performed by bone grafts taken from the iliac crest or cadaveric irradiated bone or using artificial devices like cages made of PEEK or titanium filled with osteogenic material. These bone grafts or devices may need stabilization with plates and screws. The disadvantage of anterior approaches is that immobility at fused level may elevate stress on adjacent disc spaces, leading to disc herniation at those levels.

Without performing fusion, mobility can be restored by artificial disc placement. This is called dynamic fusion. Normal biomechanics are restored when motion is maintained at the damaged disc level, and this has a number of benefits, including the prevention of adjacent segment degeneration and donor site morbidity and achieving early postoperative mobilization. Instability, prior fusion at an adjacent level, elderly patients (>60 years old), and severe facet arthrosis at the afflicted level are among the exclusion criteria for artificial discs (Deopujari et al. 2012).

The purposes of spinal internal fixation techniques are to establish anatomical alignment, safeguard neuronal components, and mechanically stabilize the spine while making an effort to maintain the motion of healthy spinal segments (Deopujari et al. 2012).

Hoarseness, paralysis of the tongue, difficulty swallowing, Horner's syndrome, oesophageal perforation and fistula, spinal cord/root injury, and vertebral artery injury are only a few of the potential side effects of anterior cervical surgery. A postoperative infection or haemorrhage may also result (Deopujari et al. 2012).

Graft-related complications are infection, collapse, extrusion, and donor site complications like pain and infection followed by failure of fusion (Deopujari et al. 2012; Hafez and Crockard 1997).

2. Posterior approach:

- Cervical laminectomy with or without lat. mass fixation.
- Keyhole laminotomy and foraminotomy.
- Laminoplasty.

The advantages of posterior surgical techniques are numerous. They commonly do not need stabilization, fusion, or instrumentation, and they typically take less operative time. Under direct observation, the nerve roots are decompressed with minimum risk to significant arteries and tissues. Disadvantages include postoperative neck pain, spinal instability stimulating further bone spur formation, and an inability to evaluate ventral canal osteophytes (Deopujari et al. 2012).

Foraminotomy

Root compression by extreme lateral disc herniation in the absence of cord compression is best managed by foraminotomy. It can sometimes be performed along with laminotomy.

Recommendations of the WFNS Spine Committee 2019 for Cervical Spondylotic Myelopathy

Guidelines for cervical spondylotic myelopathy (CSM) clinical presentation (WFNS Spine Committee 2019):

- Clonus, Hoffmann sign, Babinski's sign, inverted brachioradialis reflex, hyper-reflexia, and other myelopathic symptoms are essential to the clinical diagnosis of cervical myelopathy. They may, however, be absent in 20% of myelopathic individuals and are not highly sensitive.
- While not all patients may exhibit every myelopathic sign, a severe myelopathy will exhibit at least one of these.
- A patient's history and physical examination, together with other indicators, play a major role in the clinical diagnosis of CSM. These indicators and symptoms then trigger additional research using cervical spine imaging.
- In severe myelopathy patients, after laminoplasty, major recovery and improvement in myelopathic signs occur during the first 6 months and thereafter plateau.
- Treatment recommendations for individuals exhibiting myelopathic signs must be based on a mix of imaging examinations and clinical complaints, provided that no other plausible causes exist. Myelopathic indications do not always indicate CSM, and their successful surgical treatment is not impeded by their absence.

Suggestions for the natural course of cervical stenosis:

- Patients exhibiting indications of myelopathy and cervical stenosis may have a wide range of natural outcomes.
- Although it's conceivable for the disease to advance, the prognosis for those patients is unknown. Some people with severe disabilities may progress on their own without treatment, while others may remain stagnant for extended periods of time.
- The annual chance of developing myelopathy with cervical stenosis is about 3% for patients with substantial stenosis but no symptoms (pre-myelopathic).

Recommendations for electrophysiology:

- The following electrophysiological tests, in order of benefit, should be used on patients with CSM: electromyography (EMG), motor evoked potential (MEP), spinal cord evoked potential (SCEP), and somatosensory evoked potential (SEP).
- Regular electrophysiological studies help distinguish CSM from other neurological disorders in the differential diagnosis process. However, differential diagnosis is exceedingly challenging, particularly

in the early stages of the disease; specific testing are required, and it may be difficult to distinguish between moderate types of polyneuropathy and ALS.

- While it has been determined that MEP and SEP are useful tests for predicting the results of CSM surgery, there is no proof that they are more useful than clinical indicators.
- MR alterations may not be as good in predicting results as electrophysiological testing.
- Monitoring lower extremity power with electrophysiological tests is not very useful, and its usefulness during ACDF surgery is debatable.
- During CSM surgery, it has been discovered that EMG and MEP monitoring are helpful in reducing C5 root palsy.
- Clinical deterioration is not always evident in instances with intraoperative MEP/SEP worsening, and it is not specific. Modifications to the MEP/SEP during surgery may not always prevent brain damage and enhance results.

Recommendations for canal diameters on CT and MRI:

- Despite contradictory data, the preoperative workup should incorporate magnetic resonance imaging (MRI) morphometric examination of the spine, as it plays a major role in the assessment and prognostication of CSM.
- Compression ratio (CR), maximal canal compromise (MCC), and transverse area (TA) are the three factors measured by MRI that have the strongest correlations with the functional outcomes of patients with CSM after surgery. Since each parameter has advantages and disadvantages of its own, an evaluation of the MR parameters as a whole yields a more accurate prediction.

Suggestions for MRI signal intensity variations:

- A poorer prognosis in CSM may be associated with intense spinal cord T2 hyperintensity on cervical MRI.
- Patients should not be denied surgical treatment for cervical stem cell disease (CSM) if their cervical MRI shows less T2 signal abnormalities.
- More research is required to establish new grading schemes or to validate the ones that have been suggested.
- T1 hyposignal should be interpreted as an indication of a more severe illness with less hope for recovery.
- Additional research is required to determine how variations in the sagittal and axial extensions of the T1 signal affect the result.

Guiedlines for recent imaging techniques for CSM:

- Other than conventional MRI, diffusion MRI, MR spectroscopy, and dynamic MRI (dMRI) may be a part of MR examinations in a CSM imaging protocol. We recommend using them in outcome research. We will be better able to prognosticate and identify patients before the alterations and lasting harm set in with data gathered from clinical and imaging findings.

The following are recommendations for CSM, both surgical and nonsurgical:

- The WFNS Spine Committee supports Fehlings and colleagues' guidelines. Following consensus, the revised and modified WFNS Spine Committee Recommendations are outlined below.
- Surgical surgery is advised for people with moderate to severe CSM. To categorize CSM as severe, moderate, or mild, we advise utilizing the modified Japanese Orthopedic Association (mJOA) scale or its regional variants.
- For patients with mild CSM (mJOA score of 15–17), we advise providing surgical surgery or rehabilitation. If nonoperative therapy was used initially, we advise operative intervention when symptoms start to worsen quickly. For an illness that progresses slowly, nonoperative treatment may be taken into consideration.
- Prophylactic surgery should not be recommended for non-myelopathic individuals who have radiologic evidence of cord compression but do not exhibit radiculopathy symptoms. These individuals ought to receive clinical follow-up on a regular basis, counseling regarding the possibility of deterioration, and education regarding the indications and symptoms of advancement. Patients should be made aware of the possibility of neurological impairments following minor injuries.
- Non-myelopathic patients who exhibit clinical signs of radiculopathy and radiologic evidence of cord compression are high-risk candidates who should receive counseling since they may worsen. It is advised that these people have surgery, or if they decline, be under close observation and get rehabilitation. If they start exhibiting myelopathic symptoms, they should get surgery as soon as possible. Patients should be informed about neurological deficits that may follow trivial injury.

- The literature consistently shows a deficiency of data regarding the effectiveness of nonoperative treatment for cervical myelopathy. Therefore, in most circumstances, nonoperative treatment may not be the best option.
- Circumferential cord compression on axial MRI, decreased CSF space diameter, hypermobility of spinal segments, angular edged deformity, instability, greater angle of vertebral slip, lower segmental lordotic angle, and presence of OPLL are predictive factors that suggest a potential deterioration during nonoperative management. Prolonged MEPs and SEPs, symptomatic radiculopathy, and EMG indications of anterior horn cell lesions are significant predictors of the development of myelopathy (poor evidence).
- The duration of symptoms has the greatest impact on outcomes. Subpar results are the result of significant delays in surgical care. Put another way, patients who experience less symptoms for a shorter period of time following surgery are more likely to have better outcomes (poor evidence).
- The WFNS Spine Committee strongly recommends randomized controlled trials comparing surgical versus nonsurgical therapies in mild CSM, as there is still clinical equipoise between surgery and conservative treatment.
- There is also a need to analyse the cost-effectiveness and standardized methodology of long-term follow-up in mild CSM.

The following are recommendations for surgical indications for the treatment of CSM:

- Patients with CSM who have progressive neurological deficit, recurrent or persistent radiculopathy that is not responding to conservative treatment (after three years), static neurological deficit with severe radicular pain when accompanied by confirmatory imaging (CT, MRI), and clinical–radiological correlation are candidates for surgery.
- Patients with CSM who have anterior surgery indications include a straightened spine or kyphotic spine with a compression level below three.

Suggesations for comparison of anterior surgical techniques for CSM:

- There are numerous alternatives for anterior decompression, including anterior cervical discectomy and fusion (ACDF), anterior cervical corpectomy and fusion (ACCF), oblique corpectomy, skip corpectomy, and hybrid surgery.
- A corpectomy is a good option for a ventral compression of fewer than three vertebral segments in patients with CSM in whom a single-level disc and osteophyte excision are insufficient to decompress the cord. A corpectomy can correct a cervical spine kyphotic deformity and return the lordotic curvature alignment to normal.
- Alternate-segment discectomy/osteophyte removal with preservation of the intervening vertebra's body is biomechanically more stable than a total corpectomy with contiguous segment discectomy in situations of multi-segment illness with contiguous multi-segment thecal compression.

Recommendations for endoscopic as well as partial corpectomy interventions:

- The sagittal canal diameter can be significantly increased with an oblique partial corpectomy. However, in cases of bilateral radiculopathy, this surgery could be challenging to carry out. It is not advisable to choose an oblique corpectomy if there is a lot of instability.
- Some surgical method adjustments have reduced the incidence of Horner's syndrome (caused by unilateral disruption of the sympathetic chain) to less than 5%.

The following are recommendations for CSM in the elderly:

- In patients with osteophytes at C5-6-7 causing bony ankylosis, CSM may appear at lower levels, like the C7-T1 level, or at higher levels where mobility segments are intact, such as the C3-4 level.

Suggestions regarding complications from anterior procedures for CSM:

- There is a wide range of reported complications from anterior surgeries for CSM. Compared to neurologic and implant-related consequences, approach-related issues (dysphagia, dysphonia, oesophageal damage, respiratory distress, etc.) are more frequent. Surgical issues should be extremely infrequent when using careful surgical techniques and the right implants.

Suggestions for improving the success rate of anterior surgeries for CSM include:

- Improvements in 70% to 80% of patients have been documented following anterior surgery for CSM.
- Recoveries from JOA typically range from 60% to 70%.
- The success rates for ACDF, ACCF, and oblique corpectomy are not significantly different.

- Compared to ACCF, ACDF is typically linked with less intraoperative blood loss and fewer surgical complications. Functional outcomes are found to be the same when use the Neck Disability Index (NDI), JOA, and Odom's criteria.

Recommendations for choosing a surgical method:

- Patients with CSM should take into account a variety of factors when choosing a surgical strategy, including patient comorbidities, the number of levels implicated, the location of the compressive pathology, and the sagittal curvature.

Suggestions for posterior surgical techniques for CSM include:

- Posterior surgical decompression is a useful method for enhancing patients' neurological function.
- For CSM, the three posterior surgical approaches are laminectomy, laminectomy with fusion, and laminoplasty. If there are three or more levels of anterior compression, these methods are frequently applied. However, posterior decompressive procedures are required in cases when there is considerable posterior compression at one or both levels.
- It is unclear how beneficial each posterior decompression technique is in comparison to the others. When a patient has kyphosis, laminectomy and posterior fixation with fusion are the best options, particularly if the kyphosis is flexible. On the other hand, anterior surgery in conjunction with posterior decompression is the optimum treatment for rigid kyphosis. Laminotorosis preservation can benefit from laminoplasty. Laminoplasty cases with severe axial neck pain should not be considered. Nonetheless, there are always cases that fall into the gray area, such patients with a straightened cervical spine, where it's difficult to determine which course of action is preferable.
- When treating patients with substantial dorsal and ventral osteophytic compression, which cannot be addressed comprehensively with a single anterior or posterior operation, a combination approach should be used.
- Selecting the right procedure for a given patient requires consideration of a number of factors. Surgeons should customize their preoperative counseling to make patients aware of these details.

Recommendations for complications of posterior surgeries for CSM:

- Complications resulting from posterior surgeries for CSM include injury to the spinal cord and nerve roots, implant-related complications, C5 palsy, spring-back closure of the lamina after laminoplasty, and postlaminectomy kyphosis.

Recommendations for the success rate of posterior procedures for CSM include:

- A tendency indicates that laminoplasty is superior to standard laminectomy but about equal to the more recent, minimally invasive skip laminectomies.

Suggestions for the future of surgical approaches:

- The current body of knowledge is inadequate, particularly when it comes to weighing the costs and benefits of different surgical approaches, comparing the effectiveness of different surgical approaches using different techniques, and conducting long-term follow-up to ascertain results. Therefore, ongoing study on the results of cervical spine surgery is crucial.
- Prospective registries with long-term follow-up will be crucial for our future decisions, as doing randomized controlled studies in spine surgery is exceedingly challenging.

Suggestions for CSM outcome measures include the following:

- There are numerous outcome measures available. We suggest Nurick's grade, the Myelopathy Disability Index (MDI), and the modified Japanese Orthopedic Association (mJOA) scale as functional measures.
- Walking tests are useful for quantitative assessments, and the Short Form 36 (SF-36) is a useful tool for assessing functional quality of life.

Suggestions for clinical factors influencing results:

- Age, length of symptoms, and severity of myelopathy upon presentation are the three clinical factors most frequently associated with CSM. More unfavorable outcomes can be anticipated following surgery the older the patient is, the longer the symptoms have persisted, and the more severe the symptoms were at presentation.

- Nevertheless, further research is needed to confirm the impact of examination results on surgical outcomes. The following predictive characteristics have been researched and appear to influence the results in CSM: clonus, leg spasticity, hand atrophy, and Babinski's sign.

The following are recommendations for radiological characteristics that impact outcomes:

- There is a correlation between the severity of myelopathy and overall health scores and cervical alignment metrics. One of the most crucial factors has been determined to be the cervical spine's curvature.
- Worse results are predicted by cervical spine kyphosis. Notably, those with normal cervical lordosis experience significant neurological improvement.
- Results are predicted by cervical spine instability. Longer symptom duration, a worse preoperative JOA score, and more preoperative physical indicators are substantially predictive of a poor surgical outcome in patients with single-segmental CSM with instability.
- An important consideration in the prognosis of CSM is the spinal cord compression ratio. The spinal canal's AP diameter, however, is not clinically significant.
- The results of spinal cord atrophy cannot be predicted.
- On T2-weighted MR images, high signal intensity is a poor prognostic indicator.

Suggestions for surgical factors influencing results:

- If the disease is localized (affecting one or two levels), surgery should be done from the anterior or posterior.
- Posterior decompression need to be selected if the anterior compression is diffuse-narrowing or consists of more than two levels.
- When making decisions in cases involving many levels (more than two) CSM, the cervical sagittal vertical axis is the most crucial consideration.

7. Ossification of the Posterior Longitudinal Ligament (OPLL)

7.1. Introduction

Although OPLL (Figure 8a,b and Figure 9) occurs in many ethnic groups, patients of Asian heritage frequently experience it. Patients with OPLL are between the ages of 32 to 81 (mean: 53), with a small male predominance. With age, the prevalence rises (Greenberg 2010). OPLL's precise pathophysiology is not entirely established (Saetia et al. 2011). The posterior longitudinal ligament first undergoes fibrosis, then calcifies, and finally ossifies (Greenberg 2010).

Location:

- Cervical: 75%.
- Thoracic: 15%.
- Lumbar: 10%.

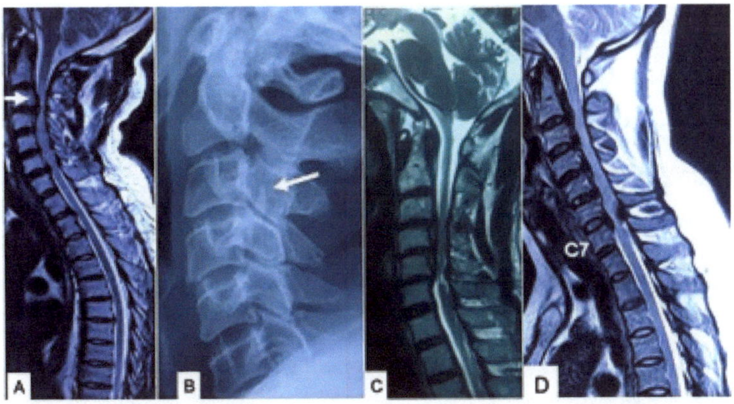

(a)

Figure 8. *Cont.*

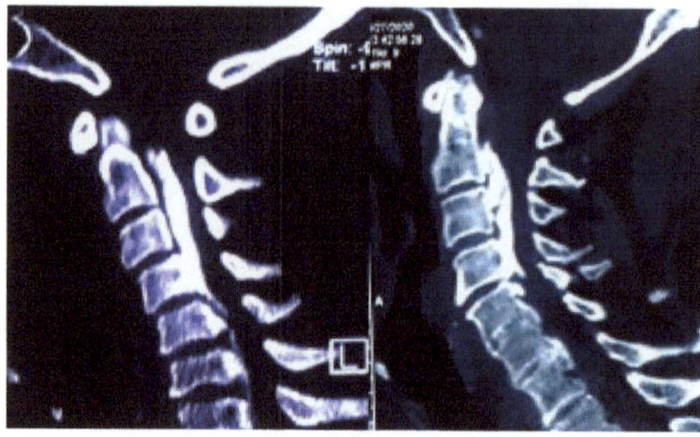

(b)

Figure 8. (**a**) MRI of cervical spine (T2W sagittal images) showing OPLL at C3-6, with cord compression mostly at C3 and 4 (**A**). X-ray of cervical spine of patient in Figure 8A (lateral view) showing calcification of OPLL at C3 and 4 (marked with an arrow) (**B**). MRI of cervical spine (T2W sagittal images) showing OPLL with cord compression at C4 & 5 and C6 & 7, respectively (**C**,**D**). (**b**) CT scan of cervical spine showing C2-4 level OPLL in two different patients. Source: Figure by authors.

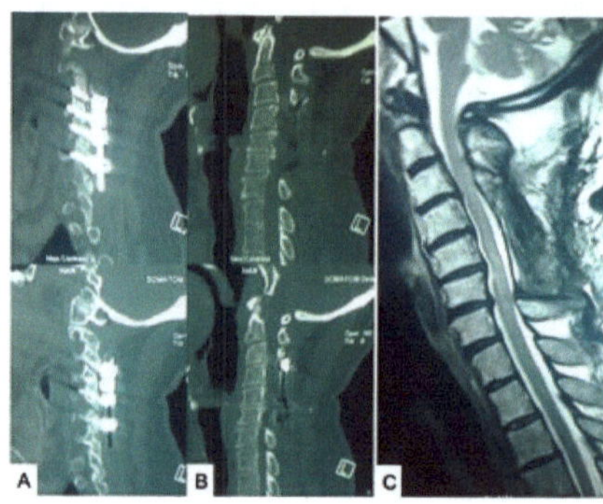

Figure 9. (**A**,**B**) CT scan of cervical spine (sagittal views) and (**C**) MRI of cervical spine (T2W sagittal view) in the same patient showing cord decompression by laminectomy at C3-6 with bilateral lateral mass fixation in a patient with OPLL. Source: Figure by authors.

7.2. Stages of Spinal Cord Damage Due to OPLL

- Stage 0: normal or mild compression of the anterior horn, no neuronal loss.
- Stage 1: mild compression of the anterior horn plus partial neuronal loss.
- Stage 2: marked deformity of anterior horn with severe neuronal loss.
- Stage 3: serious spinal cord damage.

Due to the spinal cord's ossification and aberrant signal intensity, T2W sequences are thought to be the most useful in evaluating spinal cord compression (Hirai et al. 2001).

7.3. Pathologic Classification

1. Segmental: limited to the region beneath the vertebral bodies, avoids disc gaps.
2. Continuous: spans the disc space from VB to VB(s).
3. Mixed: incorporates components of the first two while skipping areas.
4. Other variations: one of these is a rare form of OPLL that is restricted to the disc space and is continuous with the endplates and features focal PLL hypertrophy with punctate calcification (Greenberg 2010).

The majority of patients exhibit no symptoms or only minor subjective complaints (Greenberg 2010). The majority of OPLL patients who do have symptoms have them due to neurological impairments such radiculopathy, myelopathy, and/or bowel and bladder complaints (Saetia et al. 2011). The evaluation of OPLL can be achieved via plain X-ray and via CT scan of the spine. MRI of the spine will demonstrate the degree of spinal cord involvement.

7.4. Treatment Decisions Based on Clinical Grade

1. Class I: radiological proof devoid of clinical symptoms or indications. The majority of OPLL patients have no symptoms. Unless severe, conservative management is recommended.
2. Patients in Class II have myelopathy or radiculopathy. Expectantly, a minimal or stable neuro-deficit may follow. Surgical intervention is necessary when there is a significant deficiency or when progression is seen.
3. Class IIIA myelopathy ranges from moderate to severe. Surgery is typically necessary.
4. Class IIIB involves severe to total quadriplegia. For partially quadriplegic patients who are slowly getting worse, surgery is a possibility. A worse prognosis is linked to rapid worsening or total quadriplegia, old age, or poor health (Greenberg 2010).

Approaches to OPLL may be either anterior or posterior. When the OPLL involves one or two segments, an anterior approach is best; this may involve corpectomy and removal of the ossified posterior longitudinal ligament followed by fusion of the spine using a bone graft or cage. If more than two vertebrae are involved, a posterior approach is used. Laminectomy or laminoplasty with or without lateral mass fixation with rods and screws are the choices. The "K-line", which is a virtual line between the midpoints of the anteroposterior canal diameter at C2 and C7, is a useful prognostic indicator for sufficient decompression by laminoplasty for OPLL with kyphosis and/or thick ossification foci. The K-line can reflect both the alignment and the thickness of the OPLL, which determine the surgical outcomes (Fujiyoshi et al. 2008).

8. Degenerative and Inflammatory Craniovertebral Junction (CVJ) Instability: Atlantoaxial Dislocation (AAD)

8.1. Introduction

If not treated promptly and effectively, atlantoaxial dislocation (AAD), a relatively uncommon and potentially catastrophic disturbance of the normal occipital–cervical anatomy, may lead to permanent deficits or sagittal deformity (Yang et al. 2014).

Traumatic, inflammatory (including infectious), idiopathic, or congenital diseases can cause the atlantoaxial joints to become unstable (Subin et al. 1995; Chowdhury et al. 2011).

8.2. Craniocervical Junction: Anatomy

Ligaments (Figure 10) attaching the axis and atlas to the clivus, occipital bone, and occipital condyle secure the connection of the skull and cervical spine. Numerous motions of the craniocervical junction (CCJ) necessitate the stabilization of numerous ligaments. The atlas' superior articular facet and the occipital condyle combine to form the atlanto-occipital joint, which is stabilized by the articular capsule.

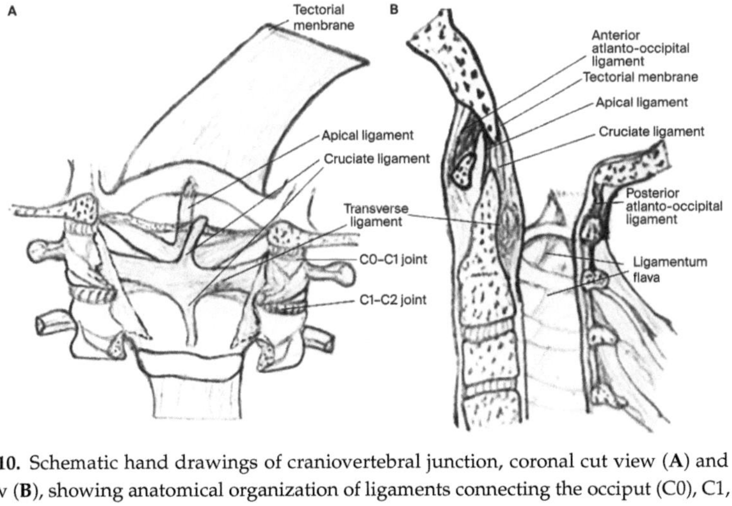

Figure 10. Schematic hand drawings of craniovertebral junction, coronal cut view (**A**) and sagittal cut view (**B**), showing anatomical organization of ligaments connecting the occiput (C0), C1, and C2. Source: Figure by authors.

This joint allows for 5° of axial rotation and 25° of flexion and extension (Hall et al. 2015; Tubbs et al. 2011). The three joints that make up the atlantoaxial segment allow for 30° of axial rotation and 15° of axial flexion. These include an atlanto-dental joint and two lateral mass articulations. The latter limits excessive extension and allows for only 10° of extension in an average individual. From the anterior arch of the C1 to the anterior side of the clivus, the anterior atlanto-occipital membrane attaches. It prevents excessive neck extension by extending the anterior longitudinal ligament. The medial occipital condyle is connected to the lateral aspect of the odontoid process via the alar ligaments. Each side has an atlanto-occipital displacement. At the atlanto-occipital joint, these ligaments prevent flexion and axial rotation on the opposite side. The apical ligament connects the tip of the odontoid process to the occipital bone, the anterior-to-superior band of the cruciate ligament, and behind to the alar ligaments. In 20% of cases, this ligament may be congenitally missing. It is frequently a rudimentary structure that contributes nothing to the mechanical stability of the CCJ. The Barkow ligament, which runs anterior to and parallel to the alar ligaments, joins the tip of the dens to the occipital condyle. This ligament might help stop overly extended neck postures. The medial occipital condyles are where the transverse occipital ligament attaches and spans the foramen magnum. This ligament may help to limit excessive lateral bending, flexion, and axial rotation because it occasionally links with the alar ligaments (Chowdhury et al. 2017; Hall et al. 2015; Tubbs et al. 2011). The superior, transverse, and inferior bands that make up the cruciform or cruciate ligament are positioned directly behind the odontoid in the middle. The odontoid to the basion is stabilized by the superior band. The cruciform ligament's transverse band, which is its strongest component, stabilizes the odontoid to the lateral masses of the C1. It avoids posterior displacement of the dens and restricts C1's lateral mobility in relation to the dens, keeping anterior C1-2 subluxation to 3 to 5 mm. The superior band is carried over into the inferior band, further solidifying the connection between the body of axis and the bason. Immediately behind the cruciate ligament is where the tectorial membrane is located. It joins the clivus laterally to the hypoglossal canals and continues as the posterior longitudinal ligament via the spinal canal. Extra flexion and extension are prevented by this ligament. The lateral masses of C1, which are located anterior to the tectorial membrane, are connected to the auxiliary atlantoaxial ligament by the posterior portion of the C2's body. This ligament's function is unknown. The occipital bone and the posterior atlas arch are connected by the posterior atlanto-occipital membrane. It carries the ligamentum flavum further. The ligamentum nuchae connects the external occipital protuberance to the spinous process of C7 and is a continuation of the supraspinous ligament. The purpose of this ligament is to limit excessive neck flexion (Chowdhury et al. 2017; Hall et al. 2015; Tubbs et al. 2010; Tubbs et al. 2011).

8.3. Aetiology

The aetiology of AAD can be grossly divided into congenital, traumatic, or inflammatory, though the cause is usually multifactorial (Yang et al. 2014).

8.3.1. Traumatic Causes

A purely traumatic AAD in the absence of a background risk factor is extremely uncommon (Venkatesan et al. 2012). It is discussed in the Chapter of spinal trauma.

8.3.2. Congenital Causes

Certain congenital diseases are linked to anomalies in the craniocervical region, which puts these populations at risk for atlantoaxial dislocation (Yang et al. 2014; Menezes et al. 1980). These are as follows:

- Down syndrome (trisomy 21) (Figure 11).
- Skeletal dysplasias (spondyloepiphyseal dysplasia, Goldenhar syndrome, and Morquio syndrome) (Figure 12) (Song and Maher 2007).
- Spondyloepiphyseal dysplasia (Miyoshi et al. 2004).
- Congenital osseous abnormalities (Wang et al. 2013) [failures in segmentation, like os odontorium (Figure 13), C2–C3 fusion, occipitalized atlas, basilar invagination (Figure 14), and asymmetrical occiput–C3 facet joints]

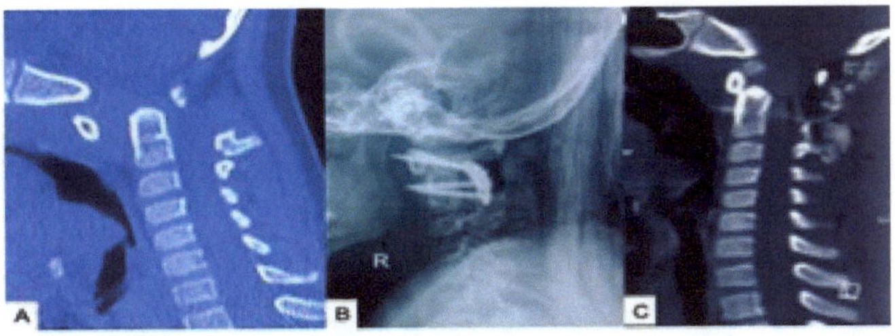

Figure 11. (**A**) CT scan of CVJ (sagittal view) showing AAD in 8-year-old boy with Down syndrome. (**B**) Postoperative plain X-ray of CVJ (lateral view) and (**C**) postoperative CT of CVJ (sagittal view) showing reduction, fixation, and fusion of AAD with lateral mass screws and plates and with facet joint fusion. Source: Figure by authors.

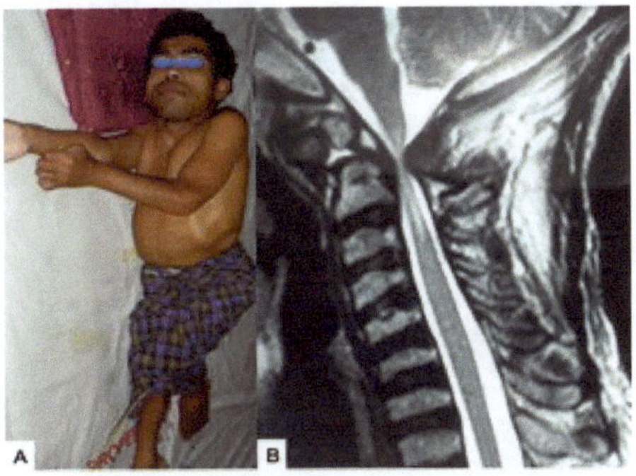

Figure 12. (**A**) A patient with skeletal dysplasia with quadriparesis. (**B**) MRI of the patient's cervical spine showing high cervical "pencil tip" compressed cord due to AAD. Source: Figure by authors.

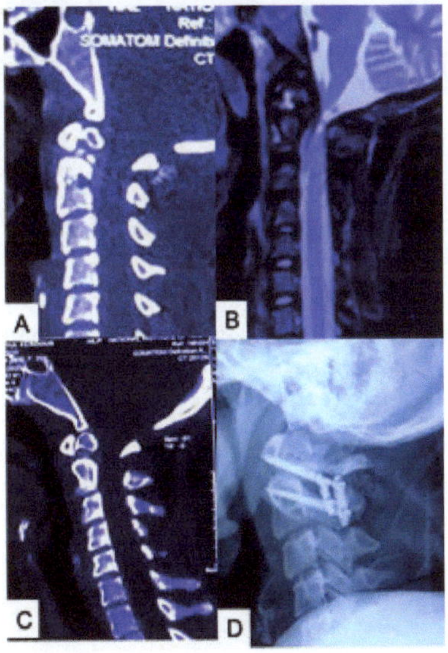

Figure 13. (**A**) CT scan of CVJ (sagittal view) showing "os odontorium" with anterior AAD. (**B**) MRI of CVJ (T2W sagittal view) showing severe cord compression. (**C**) Postoperative CT scan of CVJ in the same patient showing reduced AAD. (**D**) Postoperative X-ray (lateral view) of CVJ in the same patient showing reduction and stabilization with lateral mass screws and plates. Source: Figure by authors.

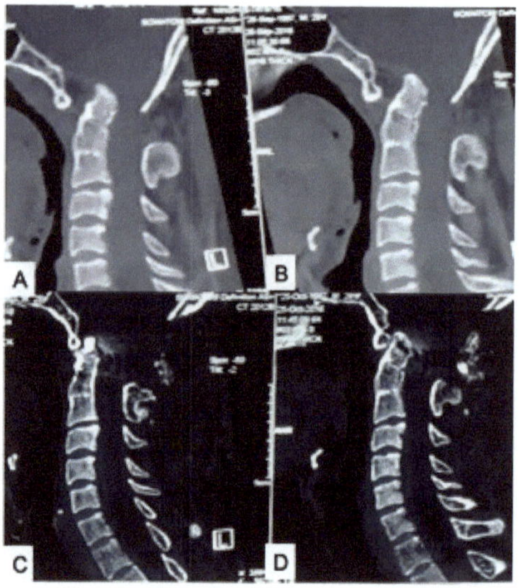

Figure 14. CT scan of CVJ (sagittal images). (**A**,**B**) Preoperative images showing AAD with basilar invagination (BI). (**C**,**D**) Postoperative images showing vertical and horizontal reduction, stabilization, and fusion. Source: Figure by authors.

8.3.3. Inflammatory Causes

Chronic inflammation in rheumatoid arthritis causes chronic synovitis, which results in bone degradation and ligament elasticity, which can cause instability and atlantoaxial dislocation (Figure 15) (Yang et al. 2014).

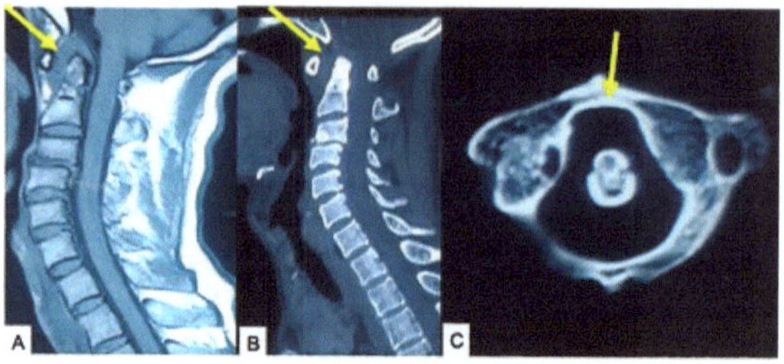

Figure 15. (**A**) MRI of CVJ in a rheumatoid arthritis patient showing atlantoaxial instability with cord compression and soft tissue mass due to pannus formation (marked with an arrow). (**B**,**C**) CT scan of CVJ (sagittal and axial views, respectively) showing AAD in the same patient. Source: Figure by authors.

8.3.4. Degenerative Causes

Osteoarthritis of C1C2 joints.

8.3.5. Infective Causes

Tuberculosis and hydatidosis.

8.3.6. Neoplastic Causes

Metastasis, lymphoma, myeloma, etc.

8.4. Clinical Presentation

Neck pain and restriction of neck movement (50%), weakness and numbness (70%), pyramidal signs (90%) (Passias et al. 2013; Yin et al. 2013), sphincter disturbances, respiratory distress. lower cranial nerve palsy, myelopathy, respiratory failure, neurologic compromise, vertebral artery dissection, and, rarely, quadriplegia or death if left untreated (Yang et al. 2014; Panda et al. 2010).

8.5. Differential Diagnosis

Torticollis (Figure 16), atlantoaxial rotatory fixation, odontoid fractures without atlantoaxial dislocation (Yang et al. 2014).

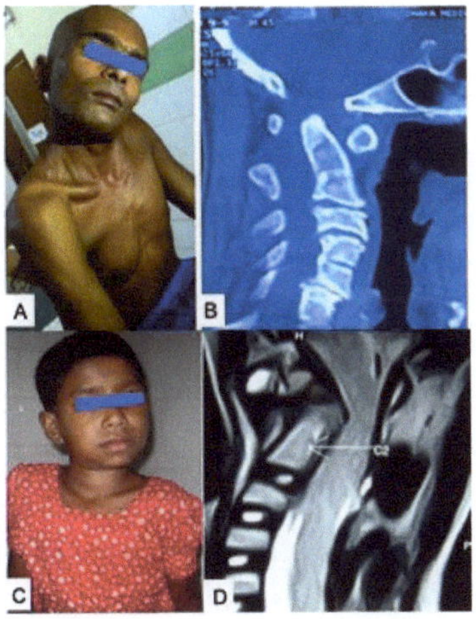

Figure 16. Adult patient with torticollis (**A**) and AAD (**B**). Paediatric patient with torticollis (**C**) and AAD (**D**). Source: Figure by authors.

8.6. Investigations and Diagnosis

8.6.1. X-Ray

Utilizing the atlanto-dental interval, X-ray radiographic measurements of the atlantoaxial joint articulation determine atlantoaxial dislocation (ADI is a small, slit-like space between the posterior aspect of the anterior atlas ring and the anterior aspect of the odontoid process). Radiographs of the neck's dynamic flexion and extension allow for the measurement of the ADI and the definition of joint reducibility (Yang et al. 2014). When the head moves, the ADI typically remains static and does not exceed 3 mm in adults and 5 mm in children (Yang et al. 2014; Passias et al. 2013).

Anterior dislocations are the primary cause of the majority (70%) of symptomatic AAD cases. The space for the spinal cord is limited as a result of anterior dislocation increasing the ADI (Yeom et al. 2013). Less than 14 mm of spinal cord space predicts the beginning of paralysis and has been linked to the severity of neurological deficiency (Yang et al. 2014; Yurube et al. 2012). Neutral and dynamic X-rays have a low diagnostic sensitivity.

8.6.2. Magnetic Resonance Imaging (MRI)

With high sensitivity and specificity, MRI is highly helpful for learning about joints, soft tissues, and the spinal cord. It can also occasionally reveal early warning signals of instability (Yeom et al. 2013).

8.6.3. Computed Tomography (CT)

Computed tomography (CT) has higher specificity for the diagnosis of CVJ instability (Yang et al. 2014). It provides skeletal details and provides essential information for surgical planning. Dynamic CT scan of the CVJ with 3D reconstruction and CTA of the vertebral arteries are warranted.

8.7. Classification of Atlantoaxial Dislocations

AAD was classified early into two subcategories by Greenberg (Yang et al. 2014):

1. Reducible;
2. Irreducible.

Hawkins and Fielding's classification system according to the direction of dislocation is as follows:

1. Posterior;
2. Anterior;
3. Lateral;
4. Rotational (Fielding and Hawkins 1977).

The Wang classification is as follows:

Type 1: instability;
Type 2: reducible dislocation;
Type 3: irreducible dislocation;
Type 4: bony dislocation (Wang et al. 2013).

The Wang classification is used for the classification and treatment strategy of AAD (Wang and Wang 2012; Wang et al. 2013). Here, preoperative assessment is conducted using dynamic X-ray, reconstructive CT, and a skeletal traction test.

8.8. Treatment

The aims of AAD treatment are as follows:

(i) Sagittal alignment correction of the upper cervical spine;
(ii) Fixation close to the anatomical alignment (Ferguson and Steffen 2003).

8.8.1. Surgical Treatment

Indications for surgery:

- Symptomatic atlantoaxial dislocation (to prevent possible respiratory failure, progressive neurological deficit, and death) (Finn et al. 2008).
- Asymptomatic AAD (to avoid myelopathy from persistent instability). In this case, though, there are some controversies (Yang et al. 2014; Panda et al. 2010).

Surgical approaches:

A. Posterior

The main surgical procedures are posterior. Posterior surgical procedures include the following:

(i) C1–C2 reduction, fusion (including facets joint), and stabilization by Goel's/Harm's technique;
(ii) Reduction and transarticular screw fixation;
(iii) Occipitocervical/C1–C2 fusion (periodontoid tissue release or/after transoral odontoidectomy).

The main complications of posterior approaches are vertebral artery injury and mobility reduction (Yeom et al. 2013). The overall complication rate in transoral surgery is 9.4% and includes CSF leakage, wound infection, wound dehiscence, pneumonia, and death (Yang et al. 2014).

B. Anterior

Anterior surgical approaches include the following:

(i) Transoral or endonasal odontoidectomy (posterior fixation is needed with it);
(ii) Anterior C1-C2 transarticular screw fixation or screw and plate fixation (retropharyngeal) (Padua et al. 2013).

A C1 lateral mass screw approach combined with a C2 pedicle screw fixation connected by rods is utilized in C1 lateral mass screw and C2 pedicle screw fixation to stabilize the atlantoaxial joint; screws and plates can also be employed (Harms and Melcher 2001; Goel and Laheri 1994; Abumi et al. 1994). When called upon, the approach permits extension to the occiput or subaxially (De Iure et al. 2009; Deen et al. 2003). Additionally, it encourages intraoperative reduction following screw fixation (Harms and Melcher 2001).

As an alternative, a crossing screw method through the C2 lamina was reported for the C1 lateral mass screw and C2 laminar screw fixation technique in 2004. But it cannot prevent lateral bending (Finn et al. 2008; Wang 2007; Lapsiwala et al. 2006) and it has a high frequency of hardware failure (Yeom et al. 2013).

8.8.2. Nonoperative Treatment

In adults who are symptomatic and there are no surgical contraindications, conservative treatment is typically not advised. Even in cases of asymptomatic AAD, stabilization by posterior arthrodesis is necessary because chronic instability frequently results in myelopathy (Healey et al. 2002).

Prior to ambulatory orthotic immobilization with active range-of-motion exercises until free motion is restored, cervical halter traction in the supine position for 24 to 48 h is recommended (Koval and Zuckerman 2006); this is the case in paediatric transverse ligament disruption and in patients with Grisel syndrome (Yang et al. 2014).

9. Atlanto-Occipital Dislocation (AOD)

The main cause of AOD is injury to the ligaments connecting the occiput to the upper cervical spine, which is frequently without comorbid fractures. As a result, it is more likely to go unnoticed than traumatic cervical spine fractures. A better comprehension of the anatomy of the craniocervical junction (CCJ) is necessary for the accurate diagnosis and management of this injury (Chowdhury et al. 2017). Different traumatic processes can cause AOD, but they are all characterized by the transmission of too much force to the craniovertebral junction (CVJ), which causes widespread ligamentous disruption. These processes can be a combination of lateral flexion, hyperextension, or hyperflexion (Hall et al. 2015; Montane et al. 1991; Yüksel et al. 2008). In the presence of relatively moderate trauma, certain predisposing factors, including neoplastic, inflammatory, neoplastic, and congenital illnesses, may enhance the risk of AOD. The CVJ may be affected by rheumatoid arthritis, which can also weaken the transverse ligament, increasing the chance of C1 subluxation. Up to 30% of the time, Down syndrome is accompanied by laxity of the craniocervical ligaments. By producing a fulcrum-like action, congenital cervical vertebral fusion disorders may also predispose people to AOD (Chowdhury et al. 2017; Montane et al. 1991; Tubbs et al. 2011).

Numerous reports have shown that trauma-related atlanto-occipital instability frequently results in death, while patients who suffer from less severe injuries may live (Papadopoulos et al. 1991; Guigui et al. 1995; Hosalkar et al. 2005). Atlanto-occipital instability caused by non-trauma is uncommon. Non-traumatic AOD (Figure 17) may present with clinical features like those of AAD (Chowdhury et al. 2017). Investigations including dynamic X-ray/fluoroscopy of the CVJ, CT scan with VA-CTA, and MRI of the CVJ are needed for detailed assessment and surgical planning.

Surgical techniques for AOD (Chowdhury et al. 2017) include the following:

- Co–C1 wiring and fusion: a midline lower-occipital burr hole is made and then occipito-atlantal fixation is performed using an epidural wire followed by fusion.
- C0–C1 transarticular fixation: here, condylar joint transarticular screw fixation is performed under fluoroscopic guidance.
- Occipital condyle C1 lateral mass screw–rod fixation and fusion (C0-C1 fixation): condylar joint fixation with screws and rods with fusion.

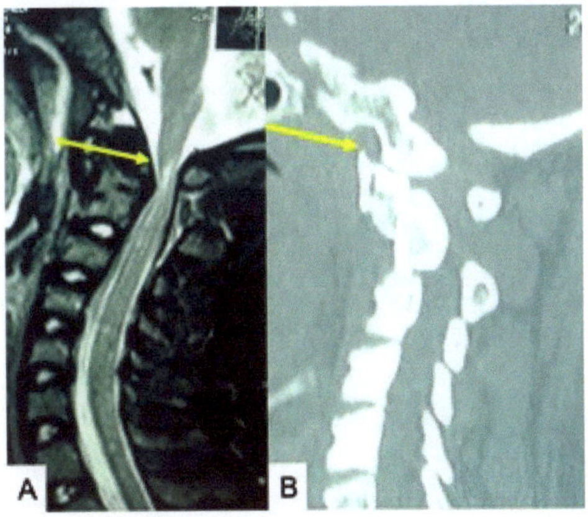

Figure 17. (**A**) MRI of CVJ showing high cervical spinal cord compression due to craniovertebral junction instability. (**B**) CT scan of CVJ in the same patient showing condylar joint or atlanto-occipital dislocation (AOD) (marked with an arrow). Source: Figure by authors.

10. Ligamentum Flavum Hypertrophy (LFH)

Ligamentum flavum hypertrophy (LFH) is a rare cause of compressive myeloradiculopathy. The anterior surfaces of the laminae of an adjacent neural arch are joined by a sequence of paired ligaments called the ligamentum flavum. The main cause of LFH is fibrosis, which develops as a result of the accumulation of mechanical stress due to trauma and age (Safak et al. 2010). Although the prevalence of LFH is unclear, several authors have put out numerous theories to explain the pathophysiology of the disease (Sairyo et al. 2007; Sairyo et al. 2005; Park et al. 2009).

The ligamentum flavum can enlarge due to degeneration, which can result in spinal canal stenosis and root discomfort (Liu et al. 2003). The two main causes of ligamentum flavum hypertrophy— injury and scar tissue—can both be widespread and occasionally unilateral. A portion of the elastic fibres is ruptured during trauma (whether slight or severe), which causes the ligamentum flavum to expand to some extent.

After repair, further hypertrophy occurs due to reparative scar formation. The disease progresses slowly, with repeated cycles of hypertrophy with calcification by repeated trauma resulting in myeloradiculopathy (Ambulgekar and Kulkarni 2021). It can occur in any part of the spinal column. The patient may present with clinical features of slowly progressing myeloradiculopathy. MRI demonstrates a hypertrophied ligamentum flavum with extension and a degree of myeloradicular compression. CT scan shows calcification of LFH (Figure 18).

Surgical decompression by laminectomy and excision of LFH is the treatment of choice in symptomatic cases. During the removal of calcified LFH, careful drilling under a microscope is needed.

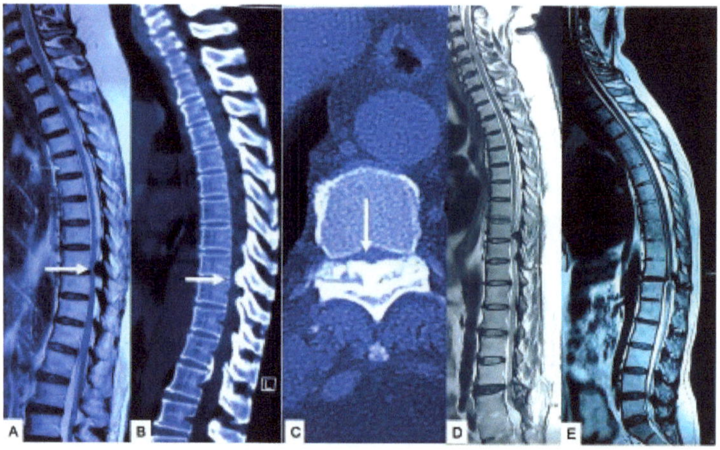

Figure 18. (**A**) MRI of spine (T2W sagittal image) showing ligamentum flavum hypertrophy (LFH), most prominent at D9 and 10. (**B**,**C**) CT scan of spine (sagittal view and axial view, respectively) showing calcification of LFH in the patient in Figure 18A. (**D**,**E**) MRI of spine (T2W sagittal images) showing dorsal LFH with dorsal spinal cord compression in two different patients. Source: Figure by authors.

Author Contributions: Conceptualization, methodology, validation, formal analysis, investigation, resources, data curation, M.Z.H.; writing—original draft preparation, M.Z.H.; writing—review and editing, visualization, supervision, F.H.C. All authors have read and agreed to the published version of the manuscript.

Funding: This research received no external funding.

Conflicts of Interest: The authors declare no conflicts of interest.

References

Abumi, Kuniyoshi, Hajime Itoh, Hiroshi Taneichi, and Kiyoshi Kaneda. 1994. Transpedicular screw fixation for traumatic lesions of the middle and lower cervical spine: Description of the techniques and preliminary report. *Journal of Spinal Disorders* 7: 19–28. [CrossRef]

Ambulgekar, Rajesh K., and Pratik G Kulkarni. 2021. Compressive myelopathy due to Ligamentum flavum hypertrophy leading to spastic paraplegia: A care report. *International Journal of Orthopaedics Sciences* 7: 568–71. [CrossRef]

Amin, Raj M., Nicholas S. Andrade, and Brian J. Neuman. 2017. Lumbar Disc Herniation. *Current Reviews in Musculoskeletal Medicine* 10: 507–16. [CrossRef] [PubMed]

Atlas, Steven J., Richard A. Deyo, Robert B. Keller, Alice M. Chapin, Donald L. Patrick, John M. Long, and Daniel E. Singer. 1996. The Maine lumbar spine study part II: 1-year outcomes of surgical and non-surgical management of sciatica. *Spine* 21: 1777–86. [CrossRef]

Bai, Jiayue, Wei Zhang, Yapeng Wang, Jilong An, Jian Zhang, Yapeng Sun, Wenyuan Ding, and Yong Shen. 2017. Application of transiliac approach to intervertebral endoscopic discectomy in L5/S1 intervertebral disc herniation. *European Journal of Medical Research* 22: 4–13. [CrossRef]

Brayda-Bruno, Marco, Marta Tibiletti, Keita Ito, Jeremy Fairbank, Fabio Galbusera, Alberto Zerbi, Sally Roberts, Ellen Wachtel, Yulia Merkher, and Sarit Sara Sivan. 2014. Advances in the diagnosis of degenerated lumbar discs and their possible clinical application. *European Spine Journal* 23: 315–23. [CrossRef]

Caridi, John M., Matthias Pumberger, and Alexander P. Hughes. 2011. Cervical radiculopathy: A review. *HSS Journal* 7: 265–72. [CrossRef]

Childress Marc A., Blair A. Becker. 2016. Nonoperative Management of Cervical Radiculopathy. *American Family Physician* 93: 746–54.

Choi, Yong-Soo. 2009. Pathophysiology of Degenerative Disc Disease. *Asian Spine Journal* 3: 39–44. [CrossRef]

Chowdhury, Forhad H., Mohammod Raziul Haque, Sarwar Murshed Alam, S.M. Noman Khaled Chowdhury, Shamsul Islam Khan, and Atul Goel. 2017. Condylar Joint Fusion and Stabilization (by Screws and Plates) in Nontraumatic Atlanto-Occipital Dislocation: Technical Report of 2 Cases. *World Neurosurgery* 107: 54–62. [CrossRef]

Chowdhury, Forhad Hossain, Md. Raziul Haque, S. M. Noman Khaled Chowdhury Chowdhury, Md. Shafiqul Islam, Zahid Raihan, and Mainul Haque Sarkar. 2011. Surgery at Cranio-vertebral (CV) Junction: Our Experience of 32 Cases. *Journal of Bangladesh College of Physicians and Surgeons* 29: 78–84. [CrossRef]

De Iure, Federico, R. Donthineni, and Stafeno Boriani. 2009. Outcomes of C1 and C2 posterior screw fixation for upper cervical spine fusion. *European Spine Journal* 18: 2–6. [CrossRef] [PubMed]

Deen, H. Gordon, Barry D. Birch, Robert E. Wharen, and Ronald Reimer. 2003. Lateral mass screw-rod fixation of the cervical spine: A prospective clinical series with 1-year follow-up. *Spine Journal* 3: 489–95. [CrossRef]

Deopujari, C. E., and Rajiv Kumar. 2012. Cervical Disc Disease and Spondylosis—Clinical Features and Diagnosis. In *Ramamurthi and Tandon's Textbook of Neurosurgery*. Edited by Prakash Narain Tandon and Ravi Ramamurthi. New Delhi: Jaypee Brothers Medical Publication, pp. 1248–51.

Deopujari, C. E., Rajiv Kumar, and Rajan Shah. 2012. Cervical Disc Disease and Spondylosis Management. In *Ramamurthi and Tandon's Textbook of Neurosurgery*. Edited by Prakash Narain Tandon and Ravi Ramamurthi. New Delhi: Jaypee Brothers Medical Publication, pp. 1252–61.

Derek, W. Moore. 2021. Cervical Myelopathy. Available online: https://www.orthobullets.com/spine/2031/cervical-myelopathy (accessed on 14 November 2022).

Doughty, Christopher T., and Michael P. Bowley. 2019. Entrapment Neuropathies of the Upper Extremity. *Medical Clinics of North America* 103: 357–70. [CrossRef]

Dydyk, Alexander M., Ruben Ngnitewe Massa, and Fassil B. Mesfin. 2020. Disc Herniation. In *StatPearls [Internet]*. Treasure Island: StatPearls Publishing.

Easwaran, Ramakrishna. 2012a. Pathophysiology of Disc Degeneration. In *Ramamurthi and Tandon's Textbook of Neurosurgery*. Edited by Prakash Narain Tandon and Ravi Ramamurthi. New Delhi: Jaypee Brothers Medical Publication, pp. 1239–47.

Easwaran, Ramakrishna. 2012b. Spondylolisthesis. In *Ramamurthi and Tandon's Textbook of Neurosurgery*. Edited by Prakash Narain Tandon and Ravi Ramamurthi. New Delhi: Jaypee Brothers Medical Publication, pp. 1297–311.

Eubanks, Jason David. 2010. Cervical radiculopathy: Nonoperative management of neck pain and radicular symptoms. *American Family Physician* 81: 33–40. [PubMed]

Ferguson, Stephen J., and Thomas Steffen. 2003. Biomechanics of the aging spine. *European Spine Journal* 12: S97–S103. [CrossRef]

Fielding, J. William, and R. J. Hawkins. 1977. Atlanto-axial rotatory fixation. (Fixed rotatory subluxation of the atlanto-axial joint). *Journal of Bone and Joint Surgery American* 59: 37–44. [CrossRef]

Finn, Michael A., Daniel R. Fassett, Todd D. Mccall, Randy Clark, Andrew T. Dailey, and Darrel S. Brodke. 2008. The cervical end of an occipitocervical fusion: A biomechanical evaluation of 3 constructs. Laboratory investigation. *Journal of Neurosurgery: Spine* 9: 296–300. [CrossRef]

Fujiyoshi, Takayuki, Masashi Yamazaki, Junko Kawabe, Tomonori Endo, Takeo Furuya, Masao Koda, Akihiko Okawa, Kazuhisa Takahashi, and Hiroaki Konishi. 2008. A new concept for making decisions regarding the surgical approach for cervical ossification of the posterior longitudinal ligament: The K-line. *Spine* 33: E990–E993. [CrossRef]

Goel, Ajay, and Vishal Laheri. 1994. Plate and screw fixation for atlanto-axial subluxation. *Acta Neurochirurgica* 129: 47–53. [CrossRef]

Greenberg, Mark S. 2010. *Handbook of Neurosurgery*. New York: Thieme.

Guigui, P., M. Milaire, G. Morvan, B. Lassale, and A. Deburge. 1995. Traumatic atlanto-occipital dislocation with survival: Case report and review of the literature. *European Spine Journal* 4: 242–47. [CrossRef] [PubMed]

Hafez, R. F., and H. A. Crockard. 1997. Failure of osseous conduction with interbody B.O.P. graft. *British Journal of Neurosurgery* 11: 57–59. [CrossRef] [PubMed]

Hagen, Kåre B., Gunvor Hilde, Gro Jamtvedt, and Michael F. Winnem. 2000. The Cochrane review of bed rest for acute low back pain and sciatica. *Spine* 25: 2932–39. [CrossRef] [PubMed]

Hall, Graham C., Michael J. Kinsman, Ryan G. Nazar, Rob T. Hruska, Kevin J. Mansfield, Maxwell Boakye, and Ralph Rahme. 2015. Atlanto-occipital dislocation. *World Journal of Orthopedics* 6: 236–43. [CrossRef]

Harms, Jürgen, and Robert P. Melcher. 2001. Posterior C1-C2 fusion with polyaxial screw and rod fixation. *Spine* 26: 2467–71. [CrossRef] [PubMed]

Hayes, Mark A., Thomas C. Howard, Curtis R. Gruel, and Joseph A. Kopta. 1989. Roentgenographic evaluation of lumbar spine flexion- extension in asymptomatic individuals. *Spine* 14: 327–31. [CrossRef]

Healey, David, Merv Letts, and James G. Jarvis. 2002. Cervical spine instability in children with Goldenhar's syndrome. *Canadian Journal of Surgery* 45: 341–4.

Hirai, Toshinori, Yukunori Korogi, Mutsumasa Takahashi, and Osamu Shimomura. 2001. Ossification of the posterior longitudinal ligament and ligamentum flavum: Imaging features. *Seminars in Musculoskeletal Radiology* 5: 83–8. [CrossRef]

Hosalkar, Harish S., Eric L. Cain, David Horn, Kingsley R. Chin, John P. Dormans, and Denis S. Drummond. 2005. Traumatic atlanto-occipital dislocation in children. *Journal of Bone & Joint Surgery American* 87: 2480–88. [CrossRef]

Kaiser, M. G., A. T. Parsa, B. D. Birch, and P. C. McCormick. 2000. The Intervertebral Disc. In *Neurosurgery. The Scientific Basis of Clinical Practice*. Edited by Alan Crockard, Richard Hayward and Julian T. Hoff. London: Blackwell Science, pp. 1061–72.

Kalb, Samuel, Nikolay L. Martirosyan, M. Yashar S. Kalani, Guy G. Broc, and Nicholas Theodore. 2012. Genetics of the degenerated intervertebral disc. *World Neurosurgery* 77: 491–501. [CrossRef]

Karantanas, A. H., A. H. Zibis, M. Papaliaga, E. Georgiou, and S. Rousogiannis. 1998. Dimensions of the lumbar spinal canal: Variations and correlations with somatometric parameters using CT. *European Radiology* 8: 1581–5. [CrossRef] [PubMed]

Kawaguchi, Yoshiharu. 2018. Genetic background of degenerative disc disease in the lumbar spine. *Spine Surgery and Related Research* 2: 98–112. [CrossRef]

Koval, Keneth J., and Joseph D. Zuckerman. 2006. *Handbook of Fractures*. Philadelphia: Lippincott Williams & Wilkins.

Lapsiwala, Samir B., Paul A. Anderson, Ashish Oza, and Daniel K. Resnick. 2006. Biomechanical comparison of four C1 to C2 rigid fixative techniques: Anterior transarticular, posterior transarticular, C1 to C2 pedicle, and C1 to C2 intralaminar screws. *Neurosurgery* 58: 516–21. [CrossRef]

Lasanianos, Nick G., George K. Triantafyllopoulos, and Spiros G. Pneumaticos. 2015. Myelopathy: Nurick Grading System. In *Trauma and Orthopaedic Classifications*. Edited by Nick G. Lasanianos, Nikolaos K. Kanakaris and Peter V. Giannoudis. Berlin and Heidelberg: Springer, pp. 255–56.

Liu, L. M., Y. M. Song, and Quan Gong. 2003. Treatment of lumbarstenosis and root pain resulting from simple hypertrophy of lumbar Ligamenta flava. *ZhongguoXiu Fu ChongJianWai Ke Za Zhi* 17: 50–51.

Luoma, Katariina, Hilkka Riihimäki, Raili Raininko, Ritva Luukkonen, Antti Lamminen, and Eira Viikari-Juntura. 1998. Lumbar disc degeneration in relation to occupation. *Scandinavian Journal of Work, Environment & Health* 24: 358–66.

Massachusetts General Hospital. 2016. *Spondylolysis and Spondylolisthesis of the Lumbar Spine*. Boston: Massachusetts General Hospital.

Mayer, Jillian E., James C. Iatridis, Danny Chan, Sheeraz A. Qureshi, Omri Gottesman, and Andrew C. Hecht. 2013. Genetic polymorphisms associated with intervertebral disc degeneration. *Spine Journal* 13: 299–317. [CrossRef] [PubMed]

McCormick, William E., Michael P. Steinmetz, and Edward C. Benzel. 2003. Cervical spondylotic myelopathy: Make the difficult diagnosis, then refer for surgery. *Cleveland Clinic Journal of Medicine* 70: 899–904. [CrossRef] [PubMed]

McInerney, James, and Perry A. Ball. 2000. The pathophysiology of thoracic disc disease. *Neurosurgical Focus* 9: E1. [CrossRef]

Menezes, Arnold H., John C. VanGilder, Carl J. Graf, and Dennis E. McDonnell. 1980. Craniocervical abnormalities. A comprehensive surgical approach. *Journal of Neurosurgery* 53: 444–55. [CrossRef]

Miyoshi, Kota, Kozo Nakamura, Nobuhiko Haga, and Yoji Mikami. 2004. Surgical treatment for atlantoaxial subluxation with myelopathy in spondyloepiphyseal dysplasia congenita. *Spine* 29: E488–E491. [CrossRef]

Montane, Ismael, Frank J. Eismont, and Barth A. Green. 1991. Traumatic occipitoatlantal dislocation. *Spine* 16: 112–6. [CrossRef] [PubMed]

Nurick, S. 1972. The pathogenesis of the spinal cord disorder associated with cervical spondylosis. *Brain* 95: 87–100. [CrossRef] [PubMed]

Österman, Heikki, Seppo Seitsalo, Jaro Karppinen, and Antti Malmivaara. 2006. Effectiveness of microdiscectomy for lumbar disc herniation. *Spine* 31: 2409–14. [CrossRef] [PubMed]

Overdevest, Gijsbert M., Wilco C. Peul, Ronald Brand, Bart W. Koes, Ronald H. M. A. Bartels, Wee F. Tan, and Mark P. Arts. 2017. Tubular discectomy versus conventional microdiscectomy for the treatment of lumbar disc herniation: Long-term results of a randomised controlled trial. *Journal of Neurology, Neurosurgery and Psychiatry* 88: 1008–16. [CrossRef] [PubMed]

Padua, Mary R. A., Jin S. Yeom, So Y. Lee, So M. Lee, Ho-Joong Kim, Bong-Soon Chang, Choon-Ki Lee, and K. Daniel Riew. 2013. Fluoroscopically guided anterior atlantoaxial transarticular screws: A feasibility and trajectory study using CT-based simulation software. *The Spine Journal* 13: 1455–63. [CrossRef]

Panda, Samhita, S. Ravishankar, and D. Nagaraja. 2010. Bilateral vertebral artery dissection caused by atlantoaxial dislocation. *Journal of the Association of Physicians of India* 58: 187–89.

Panigrahi, M. K., and S. R. Reddy. 2012. Lumber disc disease. In *Ramamurthi and Tandon's Textbook of Neurosurgery*. Edited by Prakash Narain Tandon and Ravi Ramamurthi. New Delhi: Jaypee Brothers Medical Publication, pp. 1280–89.

Papadopoulos, Stephen M., Curtis A. Dickman, Volker K. H. Sonntag, Harold L. Rekate, and Robert F. Spetzler. 1991. Traumatic atlantooccipital dislocation with survival. *Neurosurgery* 28: 574–79. [CrossRef]

Park, Jong-Beom, Chae-Gwan Kong, Kyung-Hwan Suhl, Eun-Deok Chang, and K. Daniel Riew. 2009. The increased expression of matrix metalloproteinases associated with elastin degradation and fibrosis of the Ligamentum flavum in patients with lumbar spinal stenosis. *Clinics in Orthopedic Surgery* 1: 81–89. [CrossRef]

Passias, Peter G., Shenglin Wang, Michal Kozanek, Shaobai Wang, and Chao Wang. 2013. Relationship between the alignment of the occipitoaxial and subaxial cervical spine in patients with congenital atlantoxial dislocations. *Journal of Spinal Disorders and Techniques* 26: 15–21. [CrossRef]

Phan, Kevin, Joshua Xu, Konrad Schultz, Mohammed Ali Alvi, Victor M. Lu, Panagiotis Kerezoudis, Patrick R. Maloney, Meghan E. Murphy, Ralph J. Mobbs, and Mohamad Bydon. 2017. Full-endoscopic versus micro-endoscopic and open discectomy: A systematic review and meta-analysis of outcomes and complications. *Clinical Neurology and Neurosurgery* 154: 1–12. [CrossRef]

Pytel, Peter, Robert L. Wollmann, Richard G. Fessler, Thomas N. Krausz, and Anthony G. Montag. 2006. Degenerative Spine Disease Pathologic Findings in 985 Surgical Specimens. *American Journal of Clinical Pathology* 125: 193–202. [CrossRef]

Rhee, John M., Tim Yoon, and K. Daniel Riew. 2007. Cervical radiculopathy. *Journal of the American Academy of Orthopaedic Surgeons* 15: 486–94. [CrossRef]

Roberts, Sally, Helena Evans, Jayesh Trivedi, and Janis Menage. 2006. Histology and pathology of the human intervertebral disc. *Journal of Bone and Joint Surgery American* 88: 10–14.

Saetia, Kriangsak, Dosang Cho, Sangkook Lee, Daniel H. Kim, and Sang Don Kim. 2011. Ossification of the posterior longitudinal ligament: A review. *Neurosurgical Focus* 30: E1. [CrossRef]

Safak, Alp Alper, Merih Is, Ozdemir Sevinc, Cagatay Barut, Nesrin Eryoruk, Besir Erdogmus, and Murat Dosoglu. 2010. The thickness of the Ligamenta flava in relation to age and gender. *Clinical Anatomy* 23: 79–83. [CrossRef]

Sairyo, Koichi, Ashok Biyani, Vijay Goel, Douglas Leaman, Robert Booth Jr, Jean Thomas, Daniel Gehling, Lakshmi Vishnubhotla, Rebecca Long, and Nabil Ebraheim. 2005. Pathomechanism of Ligamentum flavum hypertrophy: A multidisciplinary investigation based on clinical, biomechanical, histologic, and biologic assessments. *Spine* 30: 2649–56. [CrossRef]

Sairyo, Koichi, Ashok Biyani, Vijay K. Goel, Douglas W. Leaman, Robert Booth Jr, Jean Thomas, Nabil A. Ebraheim, Ian A. Cowgill, and Suneeth E. Mohan. 2007. Lumbar Ligamentum flavum hypertrophy is due to accumulation of inflammation related scar tissue. *Spine* 32: E340–E347. [CrossRef]

Sharrak, Samir, and Yasir Al Khalili. 2021. Cervical Disc Herniation. In *StatPearls [Internet]*; Treasure Island: StatPearls Publishing. Available online: https://www.ncbi.nlm.nih.gov/books/NBK546618/ (accessed on 15 November 2022).

Shirzadi, Ali, Doniel Drazin, Sunil Jeswani, Leah Lovely, and John Liu. 2013. A typical presentation of thoracic disc herniation: Case series and review of literature. *Case Report in Orthopedics* 2013: 621476. [CrossRef]

Singh, Kern, Koichi Masuda, Eugene J-M. A. Thonar, Howard S. An, and Gabriella Cs-Szabo. 2009. Age-related changes in the extracellular matrix of nucleus pulposus and anulus fibrosus of human intervertebral disc. *Spine* 34: 10–6. [CrossRef]

Song, Debbie, and Cormac O. Maher. 2007. Spinal disorders associated with skeletal dysplasias and syndromes. *Neurosurgery Clinics of North America* 18: 499–514. [CrossRef]

Subin, Bill, Jin-Fa Liu, G. June Marshall, Hua-Yang Huang, Jin-Hua Ou, and Gue-Zou Xu. 1995. Transoral anterior decompression and fusion of chronic irreducible atlantoaxial dislocation with spinal cord compression. *Spine* 20: 1233–40. [CrossRef]

Sunderland, Sydney. 1974. Meningo neural relations in the intervertebral foramen. *Journal of Neurosurgery* 40: 756–63. [CrossRef]

Tonosu, Juichi, Yasushi Oshima, Ryutaro Shiboi, Akihiko Hayashi, Yuichi Takano, Hirohiko Inanami, and Hisashi Koga. 2016. Consideration of proper operative route for interlaminar approach for percutaneous endoscopic lumbar discectomy. *Journal of Spine Surgery* 2: 281–88. [CrossRef]

Tubbs, R. Shane, Joshua Dixon, Marios Loukas, Mohammadali M. Shoja, and Aaron A. Cohen-Gadol. 2010. Ligament of Barkow of the craniocervical junction: Its anatomy and potential clinical and functional significance. *Journal of Neurosurgery: Spine* 12: 619–22. [CrossRef]

Tubbs, R. Shane, Justin D. Hallock, Virginia Radcliff, Robert P. Naftel, Martin Mortazavi, Mohammadali M. Shoja, Marios Loukas, and Aaron A. Cohen-Gadol. 2011. Ligaments of the craniocervical junction. *Journal of Neurosurgery: Spine* 14: 697–709. [CrossRef]

Venkatesan, Muralidharan, Raj Bhatt, and Martyn L. Newey. 2012. Traumatic atlantoaxial rotatory subluxation (TAARS) in adults: A report of two cases and literature review. *Injury* 43: 1212–15. [CrossRef]

Wang, Michael Y. 2007. Cervical crossing laminar screws: Early clinical results and complications. *Operative Neurosurgery* 61: 311–15. [CrossRef]

Wang, Shenglin, and C. Wang. 2012. A novel surgical classification and treatment strategy for atlantoaxial dislocations based on 1106 cases over 14 years. Paper presented at Cervical Spine Research Society, Chicago, IL, USA, December 7.

Wang, Shenglin, Chao Wang, Ming Yan, Haitao Zhou, and Gengting Dang. 2013. Novel surgical classification and treatment strategy for atlantoaxial dislocations. *Spine* 38: E1348–E1356. [CrossRef]

Weinstein, James N., Tor D. Tosteson, Jon D. Lurie, Anna N. A. Tosteson, Brett Hanscom, Jonathan S. Skinner, William A. Abdu, Alan S. Hilibrand, Scott D. Boden, and Richard A. Deyo. 2006. Surgical vs nonoperative treatment for lumbardisk herniation. *JAMA* 296: 2441. [CrossRef]

WFNS Spine Committee. 2019. Cervical Spondylotic Myelopathy. Available online: https://wfns-spine.org/pdf/Recommendations-of-WFNS-Spine-Committee.pdf (accessed on 12 March 2024).

Wiltse, Leon L., P. H. Newman, and Ian Macnab. 1976. Classification of spon-dylolisis and spondylolisthesis. *Clinical Orthopaedics and Related Research* 117: 23–9.

Yang, Sun Y., Anthony J. Boniello, Caroline E. Poorman, Andy L. Chang, Shenglin Wang, and Peter G. Passias. 2014. A review of the diagnosis and treatment of atlantoaxial dislocations. *Global Spine Journal* 4: 197–210. [CrossRef]

Yeom, Jin S., Jacob M. Buchowski, Ho-Joong Kim, Bong-Soon Chang, Choon-Ki Lee, and K. Daniel Riew. 2013. Risk of vertebral artery injury: Comparison between C1-C2 transarticular and C2 pedicle screws. *Spine Journal* 13: 775–85. [CrossRef]

Yin, Yi-Heng, Guang-Yu Qiao, Xin-Guang Yu, Huai-Yu Tong, and Yuan-Zheng Zhang. 2013. Posterior realignment of irreducible atlantoaxial dislocation with C1-C2 screw and rod system: A technique of direct reduction and fixation. *Spine Journal* 13: 1864–71. [CrossRef]

Yüksel, K. Zafer, Murvet Yüksel, L. Fernando Gonzalez, Seungwon Baek, Joseph E. Heiserman, Volker KH Sonntag, and Neil R. Crawford. 2008. Occipitocervical vertical distractioninjuries: Anatomical biomechanical, and 3-tesla magnetic resonance imaging investigation. *Spine* 33: 2066–73. [CrossRef]

Yurube, Takashi, Masatoshi Sumi, Kotaro Nishida, Hiroshi Miyamoto, Kozo Kohyama, Tsukasa Matsubara, Yasushi Miura, Daisuke Sugiyama, and Minoru Doita. 2012. Incidence and aggravation of cervical spine instabilities in rheumatoid arthritis: A prospective minimum 5-year follow-up study of patients initially without cervical involvement. *Spine* 37: 2136–44. [CrossRef]

Spinal Tumours

Md Moshiur Rahman and Forhad H. Chowdhury

Abstract: Spinal tumours arise from a wide spectrum of different tissues. Primary spinal tumours originate from the spinal cord or the vertebral segment. Metastatic tumours of the spine are secondary tumours of the spine that metastasise to or reach these spinal regions from a distant area. Intramedullary neoplasms arise from glial and support cells in the spinal cord; extramedullary neoplasms originate from peripheral nerve roots. Between 4% and 16% of all adult central nervous system (CNS) tumours are primary neoplasms of the spinal cord. Dumbbell tumours are tumours that may be located in various compartments. Intradural–intramedullary neoplasms and dumbbell neoplasms make up 18% and 22%, respectively, of all primary spinal cord neoplasms; intradural–extramedullary tumours account for 54% of all such neoplasms. Meningioma and schwannoma are the most common intradural–extramedullary spinal tumours. Glioma, ependymoma, cavernoma, and haemangioblastoma are frequent intramedullary tumours. Clinical features include pain, weakness (paresis/paralysis), and sphincter dysfunction. Contrast MRI and CT scan of the spine are the right imaging modalities in most cases. Microsurgical treatment is the definitive treatment. This chapter briefly discusses the management of common and rare spinal tumours, including meningioma, schwannoma, astrocytoma, ependymoma, dumbbell tumours, and metastatic tumours.

Abbreviations

ABC	aneurysmal bone cyst	CNS	central nervous system
CT	computed tomography	CSF	cerebrospinal fluid
DWI	dissemination-weighted imaging	EG	eosinophilic granuloma
GCT	giant-cell tumour	IDEM	intradural–extramedullary
IM	intradural–intramedullary	IMSCT	intramedullary spinal cord tumour
MPNST	malignant peripheral nerve sheath tumour	NF	neurofibromatosis type 1
NST	nerve sheath tumour	NF2	neurofibromatosis type 2
NOMS	neurological, oncological, mechanical, systemic	PCNSL	primary CNS lymphoma
SEC	spinal extraosseous chordoma	STIR	short TI inversion recovery

1. Epidemiology of Spinal Tumours

Spinal and spinal cord tumours arise from a wide spectrum of different tissues, like bone, nerves, soft tissues, and blood vessels. These tumours should be assessed with very different preoperative treatment strategies according to the benign or malignant behaviour of the tumour. Primary spinal tumours are a group of tumours which originate from the spinal cord or the vertebral segment. In opposite, metastatic tumours in these areas are secondary tumours of the spine that metastasise to or reach these spinal regions from an area that is significantly far away via a haematogenous route or from nearby organs. The primary tumour group incorporates a wide variety of tumours which can occur all through the spine. These tumours of the spine usually originate from neural, osseous, cartilaginous, and perineural structures. However, these tumours contrast from one another in terms of location and origin. An inappropriate utilization of the terminology related to spinal tumour origin and subtypes can be seen in the literature. To correct it, and for the sake of simplicity, an explanation of this nomenclature is greatly needed. Logical inconsistency is often seen in the use of the expressions "spinal tumour" and "spinal cord tumour." These two terms are sometimes utilized interchangeably. Even when it does not originate from the spinal cord, any pathology influencing the spinal cord, regardless of whether it is a primary tumour of a vertebral segment or a metastatic (extradural) tumour, can be named a spinal cord tumour, regardless of its root. The expression "spinal tumour" is a general term and incorporates both extradural and intradural lesions. Spinal tumours are comprehensively ordered by their cause and comprise both "spinal cord tumours" and "vertebral segment tumours." Vertebral segment tumours can be primary or metastatic and originate from osseous and cartilaginous components. Intradural–intramedullary tumours are the term used to describe spinal cord neoplasms that essentially develop from the spinal cord's cell components. However, complete intradural–extramedullary pathologies, such as meningiomas, can be considered primary spinal cord tumours even though they do not arise from the spinal cord. Extramedullary, intramedullary, or both types of intradural tumours are possible. While intramedullary neoplasms arise from glial and support cells of the spinal cord, extramedullary neoplasms originate from peripheral nerve roots, which are not a fundamental component of the spinal cord. The nomenclature "spinal cord tumour" will be utilized to refer to all intradural diseases in this section. Between 4 and 16% of all adult central nervous system (CNS) tumours are primary neoplasms of the spinal cord. The overall age-dependent incidence rate ranges from 0.74 to 2.5 per 100,000 individuals (Elia-Pasquet et al. 2004; Kurland 1958; Liigant et al. 2000; Materljan et al. 2000). Despite sharing a comparable histopathology with their cranial counterparts, primary spinal cord neoplasms are less typical. Dumbbell tumours are tumours that may be located in various locations. Intradural–intramedullary neoplasms and dumbbell neoplasms make up 18% and 22%, respectively, of all primary spinal cord neoplasms; intradural–extramedullary tumours account for 54% of all such neoplasms (Conti et al. 2004) (Table 1).

No specific neurological sign or symptom may be used to diagnose these tumours. The compression of neural tissues is a characteristic of spinal cord tumours. These tumours' clinical manifestations can cover a wide variety of adverse effects, from minor sensory complaints to serious motor impairments.

Table 1. Classification of spinal tumours.

Extradural	Intradural
Primary (malignant tumours)	**Primary (intramedullary tumours)**
Chordoma	Astrocytoma
Chondrosarcoma	Ependymoma
Fibrosarcoma	Dermoid tumour
Ewing's sarcoma	Epidermoid tumour
Lymphoma	Teratoma
Osteosarcoma	Lipoma
	Haemangioblastoma
	Ganglioglioma
Benign tumours	**Extramedullary tumours**
Osteoid osteoma	Meningioma
Osteoblastoma	Neurofibroma
Osteochondroma	Schwannoma
Chondroblastoma	
Fibroma	
Giant-cell tumour	
Haemangioma	
Aneurysmal bone cyst	
Secondary	**Secondary**
Metastatic tumours	Metastatic tumours

Source: Authors' compilation based on data from Conti et al. (2004).

2. Classification of Spinal Tumours

2.1. Intradural–Extramedullary Tumours

Intradural–extramedullary (IDEM) tumours mostly consist of nerve sheath tumours (neurofibromas and schwannomas), meningiomas, and myxopapillary ependymomas at the filum terminale. Spinal meningiomas are the most continuous intradural tumours and typically occur in the dorsal region. The psammomatous subtype, which mimics the intracranial subtypes in which numerous psammoma bodies can be seen, is the most well-known histologic subtype (Gottfried et al. 2003; Schaller 2005). Meningiomas tend to affect older people aged 50–70 and are more frequent in women, with a female-to-male ratio of 3 to 1 (Preston-Martin 1990). Both genders are affected by nerve sheath tumours in a similar way, and their occurrence peaks in the fourth and fifth decades of life. The far more prevalent subtype in this group, schwannomas, typically occurs sporadically but can also be detected in neurofibromatosis (Seppälä et al. 1995). The dorsal nerve rootlet gradually becomes normal as spinal nerve sheath tumours (NSTs) develop from either the ventral or dorsal nerve rootlets. These neoplasms can be intradural only, particularly in the cervical regions, or extradural; they can also have both extra- and intradural segments and manifest as dumbbell-like patterns. Schwannomas are thought to form in the area where oligodendrocytes transition into Schwann cells, where they provide myelin. As they swell up, these all-around-capsulated neoplasms can put pressure on nearby functioning fascicles (Kim et al. 1989). Depending on the kind, schwannomas can have a reduced cell structure with palisading Verocay bodies (Antoni A) or have fewer cells (Antoni B) (Requena and Sangüeza 1995). Neurofibromas are most frequently encountered in people with neurofibromatosis type 2, but they can also occur randomly. In these tumours, which differ significantly from schwannomas in that they can involve different nerve fascicles and grow along the entire nerve, it can occasionally be challenging to completely excise the neoplasm without the deliberate cutting of the nerve root. Damage from schwannomas can be distinguished thanks to the close proximity of axons in net pathology. The most common age for the incidence of filum terminale ependymomas, which are all-around-capsulated tumours, is 36 years old (Sonneland et al. 1985). Histologic smears show myxopapillary-appearing vascularized myxoid cores surrounded by well-differentiated cuboidal or columnar cells that are radially oriented.

IDEM tumours (Figure 1) are often benign, slow-growing neoplasms, and there may be a long lag interval between the onset of clinical features and discovery. The main side effect, axial back discomfort, may not be discovered for quite some time. Another negative effect, particularly in NST patients, is radicular pain. Cauda equina syndrome or myelopathy may result from spinal cord compression. Affected patients may become aware of adverse effects at a younger age if a functional or neurological deficit progresses quickly over time.

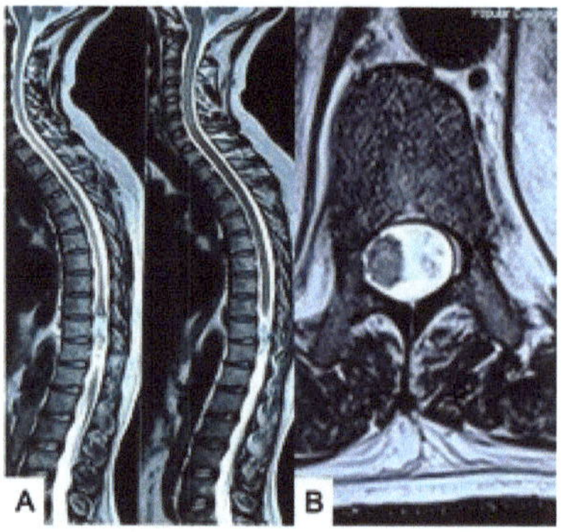

Figure 1. (**A**,**B**) MRI dorsal spine (T2W sagittal and axial images) showing intradural–extramedullary tumour (schwannoma). Source: Figure by authors.

Surgery should be performed on all individuals with dynamic neural or practical impedance as well as those whose sequential MR tests show rapid tumour progression. Surgery is not required (on symptomatic grounds only) in asymptomatic patients; the main exception would be in the case of myxopapillary ependymoma, where asymptomatic cases would be asked to undergo cautious excision to prevent CSF leaks (Mridha et al. 2007; Fassett et al. 2005). Due to the difficulties and limitations of the transthoracic approach published by Bohlman, which necessitates the resection of significant portions of the lung and may result in severe vascular injury, thoracic IDEM tumours are typically treated using traditional methods (Bohlman and Zdeblick 1988). Various techniques for removing ventral thoracic lesions have been published; these include the conventional extracavitary procedure described by Larson, which is appropriate for both ventrally located neoplasms and neoplasms with large extraforaminal parts, and the costotransversectomy strategy, which is also appropriate for lateral and ventrolateral injuries, but not for anteriorly located neoplasms due to limited view of the opposite side of the lung (McCormick 1996).

2.1.1. Nerve Sheath Tumours (Schwannoma and Neurofibroma)

About 25% of neoplasms that appear in the intradural–extramedullary region are nerve sheath tumours (Figures 1–4) (Levy et al. 1986).

Nerve sheath tumours occasionally extend to the spinal cord or extramedullary compartment, although the most of the intradural–extramedullary spinal tumours are constrained to the intradural–extramedullary region. Schwannomas make up about 65% of intradural nerve sheath tumours, and neurofibromas make up the majority of the remainder. Malignant NSTs are rare, making up only 5% of these tumours. Both schwannomas and neurofibromas are rare diseases that most frequently present as solitary neoplasms and have no underlying hereditary disease. One of three genetic diseases, namely neurofibromatosis type 1 (NF1), neurofibromatosis type 2 (NF2), or schwannomatosis, will be responsible for a small percentage of isolated lesions and nearly all occurrences of metastases. Neurofibromas can develop at any age, although schwannomas seldom affect children and peak in incidence in the fourth to sixth decades of life.

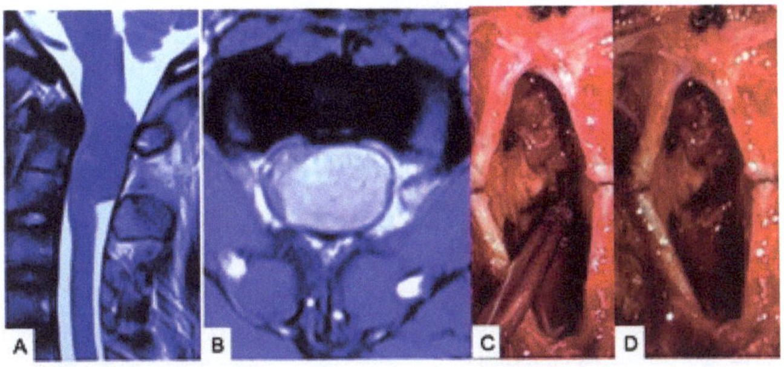

Figure 2. (**A**,**B**) MRI of craniovertebral junction (CVJ) (sagittal and axial T2W images) showing intradural C2 schwannoma. (**C**,**D**) Intraoperative images after removal of tumour. Source: Figure by authors.

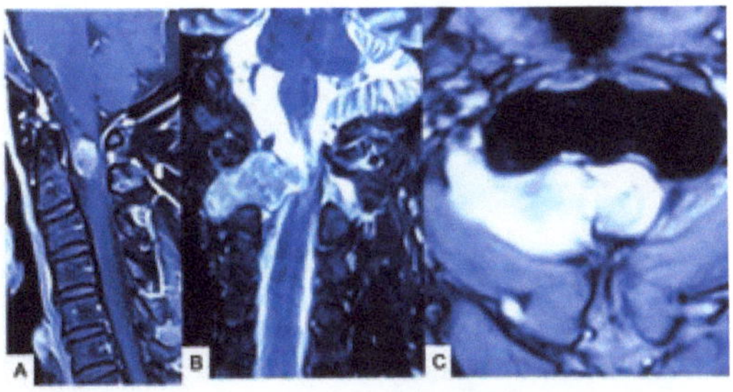

Figure 3. MRI of craniovertebral junction (**A**) contrast sagittal view; (**B**,**C**) T2W coronal view) showing C2 schwannoma with both extra- and intradural (extra-arachnoidal) extension on right side. Source: Figure by authors.

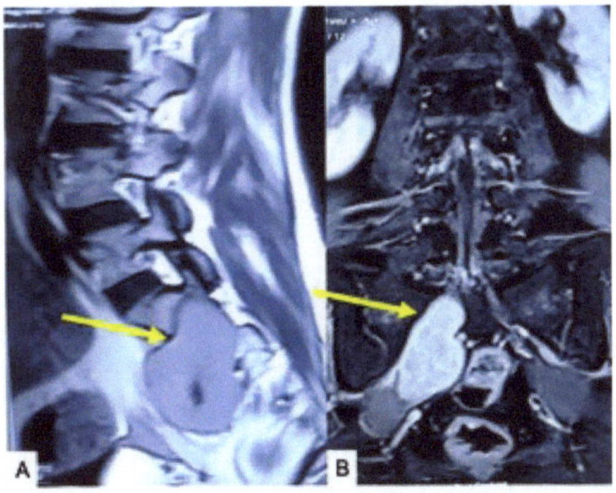

Figure 4. MRI of lumbosacral spine (**A**) T1W sagittal image and (**B**) contrast coronal image showing right S2 schwannoma (arrow marked) extending into pelvis (posterior to rectum). Source: Figure by authors.

According to histology, conventional schwannomas have two distinct morphologies and are made of neoplastic Schwann cells (Figure 1). Schwann cells that are constantly spindled to a minimum are organized in fascicles that run in diverse directions in the Antoni A pattern. Spinal schwannomas have a strong propensity for tactile nerve roots and much less frequently affect the autonomic or motor nerves. The majority of schwannomas are relatively slow-growing neoplasms that do not recur and sporadically undergo detrimental alteration. Recurrences occur in 32–40% of cases of plexiform schwannomas and spinal cell schwannomas, which are fairly common.

The majority of irregular neurofibromas manifest as cutaneous lesions, and occasionally, the spinal roots are also involved. However, spinal inclusion is common in NF1 patients, and many neoplasms can be connected to scoliosis and the risk of detrimental alteration (Khalid et al. 2018). Atypical and plexiform neurofibromas are two different types of neurofibromas. High cellularity, scattered mitotic figures, cytological atypia, monomorphic cytology, as well as/or fascicular development characterizes atypical neurofibromas, which can be challenging to distinguish from low-grade peripheral nerve sheath tumours.

2.1.2. Malignant Peripheral Nerve Sheath Tumours (MPNSTs)

Even though there have been a few rare cases of spinal MPNSTs, these tumours usually develop in the retroperitoneum, appendages, head, and neck and make up 3–10% of all soft-tissue sarcomas. If the tumour is resectable, careful excision is the preferred course of treatment because MPNSTs have a high risk of metastasizing (Ducatman et al. 1986); nevertheless, there is currently no effective primary therapy available. The visualization of metastatic or unresectable MPNSTs is incredibly poor, especially in the spinal region, where the mortality rates can reach 80%; larger lesions are therefore inevitably associated with more morbidity (Lang et al. 2012; Endo et al. 2011). The extremely rare condition known as spinal extraosseous chordoma (SEC) typically affects the cervical and epidural regions. SECs are more accurate, less malignant, and recur and metastasize at a slower rate than those originating from the bone. An unusual, dangerous tumour that develops from bone or soft tissues is called mesenchymal chondrosarcoma. Tumours may contain calcification, which could influence or reflect the progression of the disease.

2.1.3. Spinal Meningiomas

Spinal meningioma (Figure 5) develops in the membranes that surround the spinal cord (Duong et al. 2012). Compared to men, women experience these much more frequently (Hoa and Slattery 2012). Meningiomas are intradural–extramedullary in 90–95% of cases (Conti et al. 2004), and the shape of an intradural tumour, also known as a dumbbell tumour, is particularly characteristic. Spinal meningiomas comprices nearly 1.2–12.7% of all meningiomas as well as 25% of all spinal cord tumors. The thoracic region is where these tumours are most frequently encountered, followed by the cervical and lumbar regions. The peak incidence of meningiomas occurs in the sixth and seventh decades of life and they are often only diagnosed after the age of 50.

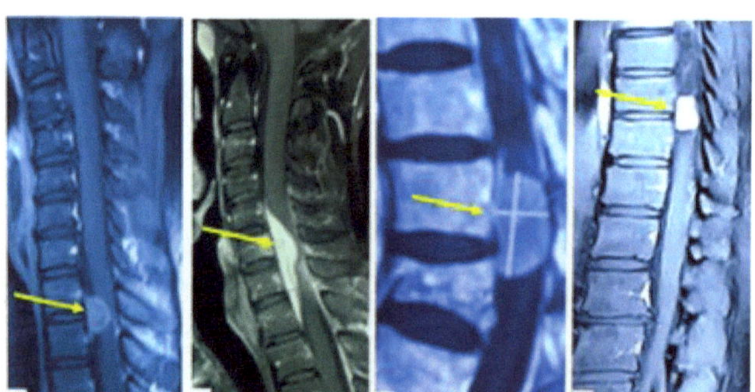

Figure 5. Contrast MRI of spine (sagittal view) showing (**A**) upper dorsal meningioma, (**B**) cervical en plaque meningioma, and (**C**,**D**) lower dorsal meningiomas (arrow marked). Source: Figure by authors.

Spinal meningiomas have a low risk of tumor recurrence and a generally good oncological and surgical prognosis. Slowly expanding and occasionally engulfing the nearby arachnoid, but infrequently the pia, spinal meningiomas grow laterally into the subarachnoid region. Surgery is the usual course of treatment, with the goals being full excision of the tumor and the restoration and improvement of neurologic function. Although radiotherapy is usually used as an adjuvant therapy for spinal meningioma, it may be explored in cases of tumor recurrence, for difficult surgical cases, and for individuals with higher-grade lesions. Novel molecular and genetic profiling contributes to our understanding of spinal meningioma and could lead to the discovery of new therapeutic avenues (Hohenberger et al. 2023).

2.2. *Intradural–Intramedullary Tumours*

Intradural–intramedullary tumours (Figures 6 and 7) can be of the following varieties.

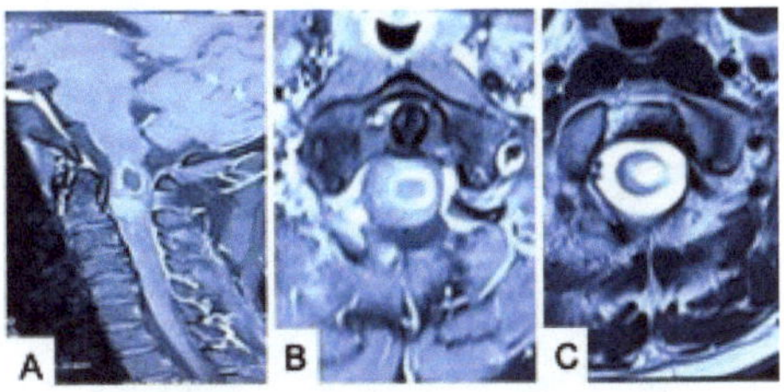

Figure 6. Contrast-enhanced MRI of cervical spine (**A**) contrast sagittal, (**B**) contrast axial, and (**C**) T2W axial images) revealing cystic and solid lesions to the upper cervical spine (astrocytoma grade 2). Source: Figure by authors.

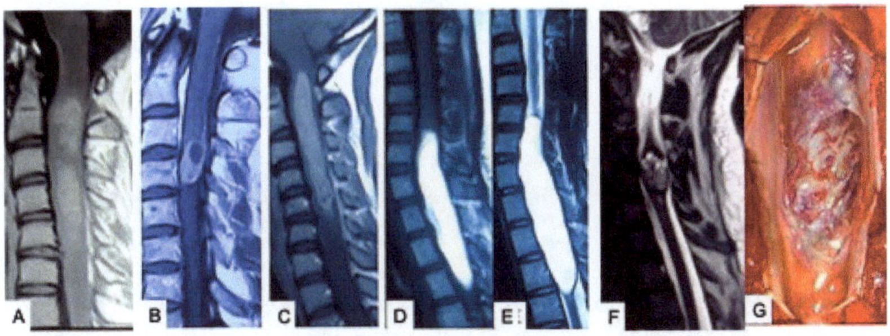

Figure 7. MRI of spine (sagittal sections) showing intramedullary spinal tumours: (**A**) long-segment cervical ependymoma; (**B**) cervical haemangioblastoma; (**C**) cervical astrocytoma; (**D**,**E**) cervicodorsal lipoma; and (**F**) cervical cavernoma. (**G**) Intraoperative picture of cervical cavernoma after durotomy in patient in (**F**). Source: Figure by authors.

2.2.1. Astrocytoma

This tumour (Figures 6 and 7C) has a low rate of one-year survival. Incidence is most common between the third and fifth decades of life. The female-to-male = 1:1.5. The proportion of low-grade to high-grade tumours is 3:1 in all age groups. It can occur at all possible levels.

A total of 38% of cases are cystic; the cystic fluid, as a rule, has a high protein content (Greenberg 2010).

2.2.2. Ependymoma

The most widely occurring tumours of the lower spinal cord, conus, and filum are ependymomas (Figures 7A and 8), and they are slow to develop. There is a slight male predominance, and they are commoner in the third to the sixth decades of life. The majority occur in the filum, and the cervical region comes in second. Histologically speaking, myxopapillary ependymoma (Figure 8) is the most frequent. Other histological types include papillary, cell, epithelial, and mixed. A total of 46% of affected people have cystic degeneration, which may extend into the spinal canal. In the filum, it is typically barely vascular (Greenberg 2010).

2.2.3. Haemangioblastoma

Haemangioblastoma (Figure 7B) is generally non-invasive, sharply demarcated, and may include peripheral cysts. Some 33% of cases of spinal haemangioblastoma are linked to von Hippel–Lindau disease. It requires a microsurgical approach like AVM, and may be associated with intraoperative hypotension (Greenberg 2010).

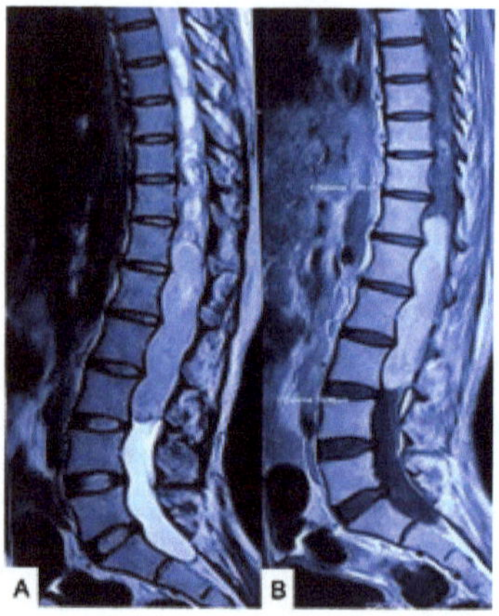

Figure 8. (**A**,**B**) MRI of lumbosacral spine showing myxopapillary ependymoma at D12 to L3. Source: Figure by authors.

2.2.4. Dermoid and Epidermoid

Epidermoids are uncommon before the late teens/young adulthood. There is a slight female predominance. Upper thoracic and cervical localizations are uncommon; incidence in the conus is frequent. Generally, these are IDEM neoplasms, yet in the conus/cauda equina they may have an IM (intramedullary) part.

2.2.5. Lipoma

Lipoma (Figure 7D,E) may develop related to spinal dysraphism. Below, we consider lipomas that happen without spinal dysraphism. Onset peaks in the second, third, and fifth decades of life. There is no sex prevalence. Typically, they are IDEM (there is a sub-type that is exclusively IM, in the spinal cord); the cervicothoracic level is the most well-known area of occurrence. Faecal incontinence is common with low tumours. Nearby subcutaneous dimples or masses are visible. Malis suggests early subtotal resection at around 1 year from onset in symptomless patients (Malis 1978). Superficial extrasacral resection is insufficient, as it results in thick intraspinal scarring which may prompt acute serious neurological damage with poor salvageability.

3. Extradural Tumours

3.1. Chordoma

The primary sacral spine tumour that is most commonly diagnosed today is chordoma. These tumours rarely develop in persons under the age of 40 and are twice as frequent in men than in women. The sacral spine, the notochord's embryologic endpoint, is where it typically develops from remaining notochord cells. Chordomas develop gradually but are malignant. Patients commonly present with bladder and bowel incontinence, sexual dysfunction, dull pain, or neurological repercussions. Huge sacral chordomas in patients might press on the internal organs, resulting in bowel blockages, urine incontinence, and abdominal pain. CT scans of the sacrum might be insufficient for visualizing these tumours. Magnetic resonance imaging is the favoured imaging methodology, permitting the clinician to assess the size of the tumour, explicit tumour segments, and the degree of soft-tissue involvement. On separate T1W imaging and T2W imaging scans, chordomas are frequently isointense and hyperintense. With gadolinium, they improve heterogeneously. The sacral cortex can be reconstructed in computed tomography (CT), and neuroforaminal widening can be shown. Additionally, some chordomas may have calcifications. A thorough biopsy is frequently recommended for tissue analysis and to manage additional treatment. Endoscopy and biopsy of disputed lesions should be completed if it is proven that the lesion originated primarily from the rectum. Transrectal biopsy should be avoided to prevent the spread of tumour cells to unaffected regions. The remaining tumours should be analyzed via CT-guided biopsy, and the biopsy tract is confined within the confines of the concomitant excision. Several histologic subtypes exist. Conventional chordomas contain a bottomless myxoid framework and the cell cytoplasm has a "bubble-like" physaliferous design. Other types of chordomas incorporate chondroids and de-differentiated chordomas. For the most part, chordomas affect soft tissues, and are typically avascular (Arnautovic and Gokaslan 2019).

3.2. Epidural Tumours

This section on extradural spinal cord tumours must make a distinction between two categories: bone and soft-tissue tumours. It is possible to further classify the latter into primary and secondary neoplasms. These neoplasms differ in a number of crucial ways: although soft-tissue tumours are typically benign and do not directly affect the biomechanical qualities of the spinal column, bony tumours interfere with spinal cohesion and are predominately caused by malignant agents. In the past two years, there have been notable advancements in the surgical management of bone tumours, including a better perception of the spinal cord's biomechanics and improved repair and reconstruction techniques (Klekamp and Samii 2007).

3.2.1. Sign and Symptoms

Pain, motor weakness, gait ataxia, sensory deficits, dysaesthesias, sphincter issues, localized swelling, etc., are the earliest symptoms of epidural spinal tumours (including soft-tissue and bone tumours). Most patients with epidural tumours have a characteristic clinical presentation, which includes systemic pain, spastic para- or tetraparesis, and radicular symptoms. Local discomfort is the primary symptom in most individuals with epidural neoplasms (65% with soft-tissue and 79% with bone tumours). At first, only a small number of patients are seen to have motor or gait issues (Klekamp and Samii 2007).

Soft-tissue tumours that originate from the epidural region push epidural veins and fat aside before compressing the dura. They frequently advance into the paraspinal spaces in the direction of the intervertebral foramina as they grow along and around the dural sac. The foramina may then become enlarged as a result of bone erosion. The vertebral bodies may become twisted or dysplastic if this phenomenon starts in early childhood.

Depending on whether they are benign or malignant, bone tumours tend to damage or alter the bony anatomy but otherwise have similar clinical characteristics. Local pain, which is the primary initial symptom in 79% of patients and is brought on by periosteum and bone infiltration, is present. Before the tumour affects the spinal cord, radicular symptoms may appear after it compresses the intervertebral foramina or bursts into the soft tissue. In a paper on spinal metastases, for instance, it was demonstrated that 80% of patients progressed from local discomfort to neurological features within 2 months (Helweg-Larsen and Sørensen 1994).

However, due to the risk that malignant tumours, in particular, pose to the integrity of the spine, quick clinical diagnoses following vertebral collapse and spinal instability are not unheard of.

Patients with bone tumours (Figure 9) typically experience gait issues and localized pain. Analogously to patients with extra- and intramedullary tumours, people with epidural tumours have noticeably higher levels discomfort (McCormick et al. 1990; Solero et al. 1989). People with epidural neoplasms had the highest percentage of progressive spinal cord damage, in contrast (i.e., they are incapable of walking or experience bowel and bladder incontinence). This is mostly caused by bony tumours that suddenly compress the cord following pathological fractures and by a high rate of malignant tumours. In other words, because indications of spinal dysfunction may obscure those of tumour progression as in intra- or extramedullary tumours, the clinical course is not always straightforward.

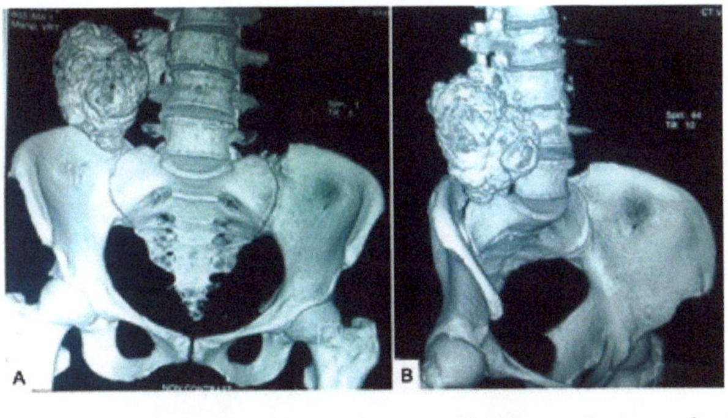

Figure 9. (**A**,**B**) Three-dimensional reconstruction CT scan of lumbosacral spine and pelvis showing L3 right transverse process-originating osteochondroma. Source: Figure by authors.

3.2.2. Neuroradiology

While MRI is currently almost exclusively used to make a neuroradiological diagnosis of extra- and intramedullary tumours (Figures 1–8 and 10–12), this is not the case with extradural tumours, notably bone tumours. CT and straightforward X-rays are absolutely necessary for spine bone tumours and are also advised for extradural soft-tissue tumours, despite the fact that contemporary MRI affords excellent visualization of soft-tissue and bone structures.

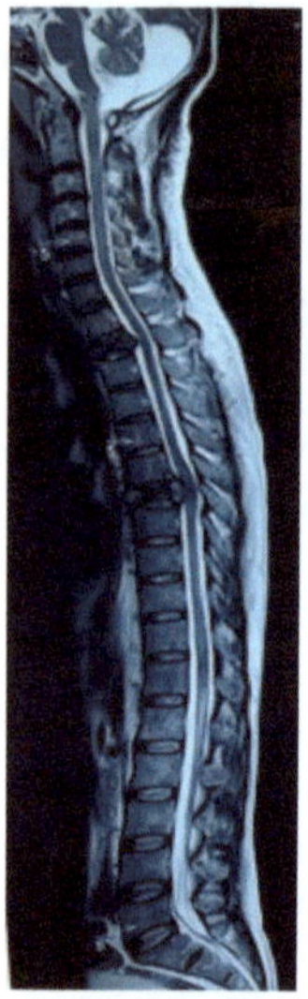

Figure 10. MRI of spine (sagittal view) showing D2 and D7 vertebral body collapse due to metastatic tumours (with compression of thecal sac). Source: Figure by authors.

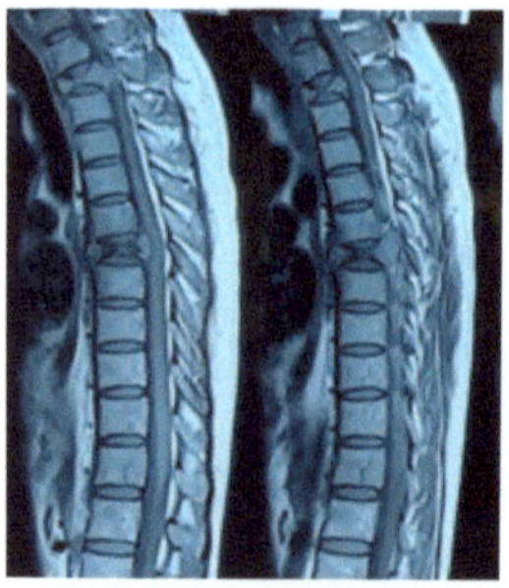

Figure 11. MRI of dorsal spine (sagittal views) showing multiple vertebral involvement of tumours (multiple myeloma) with collapse of multiple vertebral bodies. Source: Figure by authors.

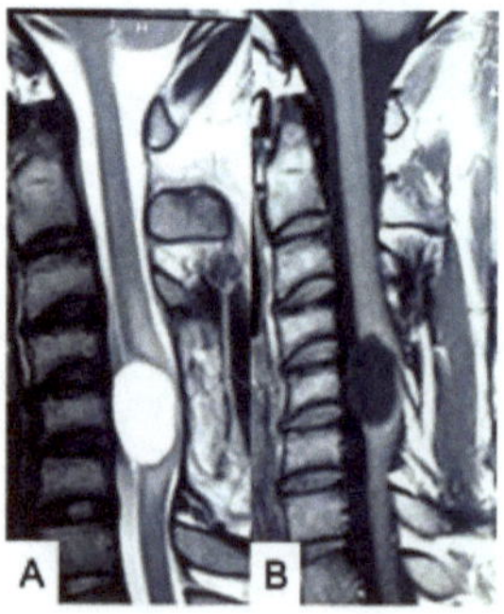

Figure 12. (**A**,**B**) MRI of cervical spine (sagittal views) showing cervical neuro-enteric cyst. Source: Figure by authors.

An extradural tumour's neuroradiological evaluation must reveal the following information:

1. The tumour's location and size, to start.
2. Distinction between bone tumours and soft-tissue tumours.
3. Distinction between a metastatic and a malignant tumour.
4. The reaction of the surrounding tissues.
5. Major vessel involvement.
6. Spinal stability.

Oblique X-ray imaging can show the intervertebral foramina. Although schwannomas account for the majority of cases, widening of the foramina can also be seen in a range of other histologies, including osteoblastomas, chondrosarcomas, and meningoceles (Zibis et al. 2000). Some epidural tumours can grow to huge sizes within the paraspinal spaces. Epidural schwannomas with bright contrast enhancement can be solid or cystic. They are generally laterally placed, compress the dura, and develop in the extraspinal space along the sheath of the nerve via the neuroforamen. The neuroforamen is widened. The extraspinal part is in most cases larger than the intraspinal part. Sometimes, minor intradural tumour extensions cannot be ruled out on MRI; in these cases, the dura needs to be extended along the nerve root for intradural examination. Epidural cavernomas show a varied signal pattern on MRI based on the quantity and chemical condition of haemoglobin derivatives linked to smaller haemorrhages. They may relate to significant haemorrhagic cysts. Synovial cysts have fatty liquid in them. The signal pattern on MRI is inhomogeneous and can look like a cavernoma. Computed tomography shows the linkage to the intervertebral joint and facilitates the differential diagnosis.

Epidural arachnoid cysts are very simple to spot. The degree of spinal compression exerted by those cysts is complicated to ascertain. Some behave as slit-like dura dissections, while others only slightly or severely pinch the dura and spinal cord. The diagnostic difficulty is to show a dura shortage and, consequently, the communication location between the cyst and the subarachnoid space. The surgical plan is determined by this location. When there has been a history of trauma, dura deficiencies along a nerve root sleeve are more commonly linked to epidural arachnoid cysts. To show this communication, myelography and post-myelographic CT may be necessary. The spinal cord may occasionally herniate into this dura defect. On T1W images, lymphomas and other infiltrating neoplasms like soft-tissue sarcomas are iso- or hypointense, but on T2W images, they exhibit high signal intensity. They develop in the epidural region around the dural sac and homogenously accumulate contrast without breaking down the bone (Boukobza et al. 1996).

Epidural diseases that may be mistaken for neoplasms include spinal lipomatosis, disc prolapses, abscesses, and chronic epidural haematomas. MRI signal intensities for chronic extradural haematomas vary according to the age of the haemorrhage. In patients with haemorrhagic diatheses, they may spread throughout numerous spinal segments or be localized. No trauma history is required. Sequential exams may be used to prove spontaneous resorption. Spinal epidural abscesses can be brought on by haematologic conditions or local spread from a nearby vertebral abscess or spondylodiscitis. Spinal lipomatosis, which is correlated with total body fat, can be seen in patients who are very overweight. It might also be connected to steroid therapy. Severe compression of fat tissue by the dural sac is the distinguishing feature.

3.3. Metastasis

The most prevalent spinal tumours are spinal metastases (Figures 10 and 11), which account for around 90% of the masses seen on spinal imaging. Although not restricted to bone metastases, spinal metastases are more frequently detected as bone metastases and about 20% of patients also have invasion of the spinal canal and cord compression. The dorsal region of the spinal column is where metastasis is most frequently discovered, followed by the lumbar region. The cervical region is where metastasis is least likely to be discovered (Mundy 2002).

The sparing of intervertebral disc space is a distinguishing characteristic of these lesions when analysing spinal metastases on MRI images. This disc area is almost always involved during an infection. The pathways by which metastatic spine disorders spread include direct tumour growth, venous haematogenic dissemination as opposed to arterial spread, and, eventually, lymphatic spread. The most frequent route for tumour embolization and spinal invasion among these is haematogenous dissemination through Batson's plexus system. The following tumours, listed in descending order, are the most prevalent primary malignancies that largely spread to the spine: thyroid (2.5%), renal (5%), gastrointestinal (4.5%), lung (19%), prostate (7.5%), and breast (21%). All tumours have the potential to spread to the spine; however, the cancers indicated above metastasize into the spinal cord at an early stage of the disease (Ziu et al. 2022).

3.3.1. Epidemiology

When treating cancer patients, doctors frequently run into the situation of spinal metastases. The morbidity associated with spinal metastasis includes spinal cord compression brought on by the invasion of epidural space, pathological bone fractures needing large dosages of narcotic drugs for therapy, and hypercalcemia. Rarely will spinal metastasis with no apparent involvement of the bone seed within the spinal cord itself. In such cases, the diagnosis of metastatic lesions is complicated because there is no known history of the primary tumour, so the proper diagnosis is only determined after testing identifies the type of tumour.

3.3.2. Clinical Symptoms and Physical Examination

Pain is the primary symptom experienced by people with spinal metastases. Any oncologic patient who experiences back or neck pain should be given a high level of clinical suspicion. Pain is the most common starting symptom that needs to be evaluated by the doctor in therapy, despite the fact that it is not the most dreadful or deadly symptom of spinal metastases. In addition to being an early symptom, metastasized neck and back pain frequently requires additional diagnostic imaging in patients who cannot undergo imaging of the full spine. Patients sometimes awaken from sleep due to the severe and excruciating pain. Additionally, if nerve injury has occurred, the pain is intense and firing in a particular dermatomal range, which may signal a greater tumour enlargement. In the event that the tumour has spread into the spinal canal, sensory and motor impairment could be permanent and even more concerning. The degree to which the deficit is weak and extends is a key concept for treating spinal metastases. The larger the deficit at presentation, the worse the odds of recovery. Furthermore, the amount of time between the onset of the deficiency and the doctor discovering the cause affects the possibility and probability of regeneration.

3.3.3. Diagnosis

The simplest and most frequently accessible diagnostic for evaluating an oncologic patient with neck or back discomfort is an X-ray of the spine. Simple anterior, posterior, and lateral pictures are frequently insensitive or complicated and need at least 50% bone disintegration before an issue may be noticed. MRI of the spine is the gold standard for assessing these abnormalities (Figures 10 and 11). Expansion, invasion rates, spinal canal obstruction, and metastatic aetiology are all revealed by MRI. However, it is not always available, for example if a patient has an internal or external pacemaker. Myelography should be utilized with or without CT imaging for patients who are not suitable for MRI. Myelography has the advantage of sending CSF for pathological investigation; however, its utility is severely limited when the canal is entirely blocked by a lesion. In these cases, multiple contrast injections into the spinal cord could be required to overcome the obstruction stage.

3.3.4. Treatment

Spinal Instability Neoplastic Score (SINS) (Fisher et al. 2010). Scoring is as follows:

- Location:
    - Junctional (occiput–C2, C7-T1, T11-L1, L5-S1)—3 points;
    - Mobile spine (C3-6, L2-4)—2 points;
    - Semirigid (t3-T10)—1 point; rigid (s2-5)—0 points.
- Pain:
    - Yes—3 points;
    - Occasional but not mechanical pain—2 points;
    - Pain-free lesion—0 points.
- Bone lesion:
    - Lytic—2 points;
    - Mixed (lytic/blastic)—1 point;
    - Blastic—0 points.
- Spinal alignment:
    - Subluxation/translation present—4 points;
    - De novo deformity (kyphosis/scoliosis)—2 points;
    - Normal alignment—0 points.

- Vertebral body collapse:
    - >50% collapse—3 points;
    - <50% collapse—2 points;
    - No collapse with >50% body involved—1 point;
    - None of the above—0 points.
- Posterolateral involvement of the spinal elements:
    - Bilateral—3 points;
    - Unilateral—1 point;
    - None of the above—0 points.

A score of 0–6 indicates stability, a score of 7 to 12 defines intermediate (possibly impending) instability, and a score of 13–18 indicates instability. A score of more than 7 warrants a surgical consultation.

Patients can be managed without surgery if metastasis affects many bony structures without compromising the cord or causing a bone fracture. However, consulting a spine surgeon is crucial if you want guidance on spinal instability caused by several spine metastases. However, radiation therapy and chemotherapy may be the main treatment options for the majority of patients with multiple spinal metastases and normal neurological examinations. An image-guided bone lesion biopsy may be beneficial if tissue is required for pathological diagnosis and there are no primary metastases or metastases that are easily accessible using any other approach. Rarely is an open diagnosis necessary after numerous unsuccessful efforts with a needle biopsy (Aielli et al. 2019; Kam et al. 2019; Yang et al. 2018).

When a spinal cord tumour is present, the approach to treatment must change considerably, and immediate surgical consultation is necessary because these patients may proceed to bed-bound status within days. Research has demonstrated that paralysis brought on by metastatic spine disease considerably reduces the life expectancy of malignant patients. Contrarily, surgical intervention will greatly lower the mortality and morbidity linked to acute paralysis in patients with acute paralysis brought on by metastatic disease compression of the spinal cord (Patchell et al. 2005; van den Bent 2005).

3.3.5. Role of Steroids

Depending on the speed and severity of neurological deterioration, treatment may require the administration of steroids. In clinical trials, dexamethasone has been found to reduce pain and ameliorate symptoms. The precise dose that would help the patient the most is unknown, though. No discernible therapeutic advantage was seen with the larger dose in research comparing a 100 mg dexamethasone bolus dose with a 10 mg initial injection of dexamethasone bolus. A 10 mg IV bolus dosage followed by a 4 mg maintenance dose given every 6 h, tapered over the course of 2 weeks, as permitted by the clinical scenario, could serve as a successful starting dose. Immediate scans to assess growth and possible surgical involvement should be made available.

Surgical intervention is acceptable when there is little reason to suspect the presence of an extremely radiosensitive tumour, when total paralysis has been present for longer than 24 h, or when the patient's projected survival is shorter than 3 or;4 months. Following surgery, further care should include chemotherapy and targeted radiation using a multidisciplinary approach. Radiation therapy typically involves 30–40 Gy in ten treatments. After radiation and chemotherapy, wound closure becomes a worry; thus, the patient needs to be continuously watched to spot and treat the wound as soon as possible (Le et al. 2018; Osborn et al. 2018).

The NOMS (neurological, oncological, mechanical, systemic) paradigm is the foundation of the current therapeutic strategy for spinal metastases. This framework's neurological component evaluates the patient's neurological status and the grade of epidural spinal cord compression as determined by MRI; the oncological and mechanical components describe the radiosensitivity of the primary tumour and the mechanical stability of the spine as determined by the neoplastic spinal instability score, respectively. These parameters determine the broad management categories for these patients, which may include decompression and surgical stabilization, spinal stereotactic radiation therapy, conventional external beam radiation therapy alone or with stabilization, or a combination of these following separation surgery (Table 2).

Table 2. Augmentation and radiosurgery in spinal metastases.

Surgery	Vertebral Augmentation	Radiosurgery
Manifested spinal cord compression by a tumour that is not highly radiosensitive, mechanical instability, uncertain diagnosis.	Vertebral body fracture with pain without significant epidural spinal cord compression.	Failure of radiotherapy to control disease.

Patients without any of the above are generally candidates for radiation therapy. Source: Authors' compilation based on data from Patchell et al. (2005); van den Bent (2005); Bilsky et al. (1999).

3.3.6. Indications for Surgery

Primary surgery (Bilsky et al. 1999):

- Radioresistant tumour (sarcoma, renal cell carcinoma);
- Spinal instability;
- Pathological fracture with bone in the spinal canal;
- Occult primary tumour;
- Circumferential epidural tumour; moderate to highly radioresistant tumour (colon, lung).
- Secondary surgery after chemo/radiotherapy.
- Progressive neurologic symptoms.

4. Sacral Spinal Tumours

Up to 7% of all spinal tumours are sacral spine tumours, which are extremely unusual (Feldenzer et al. 1989). They can be categorized thoroughly into primary or metastatic groups. In addition, primary sacral neoplasms may be divided into three categories based on their origin: congenital, osseous, or neurogenic. Chordoma is the most well-known primary sacral neoplasm. Metastasis-related sacral tumour is the most well-known type. It is worth identifying the differences between primary and metastatic sacral tumours since they may have a big impact on future treatment paradigms and interdisciplinary debates. For example, a primary sacral neoplasm should be given cautious consideration for biopsy, with detailed technique considerations and follow-up treatment plans. On the other hand, biopsy is probably unsuitable for patients who have complete spinal injury and a metastatic tumour with sacral linkage. In these patients, carefully removing tumour tissue or plans for palliative care that include chemotherapy or radiation might be more appropriate. Sacral tumours present noteworthy management difficulties and require careful treament because of a wide range of accompanying side effects, tumour types, and complex accessory bone structures. The bone structure of the sacral spine is one of a kind as it is close to neighbouring neurovascular structures, bony components, joints, and retroperitoneal organs, which requires an interdisciplinary approach before starting treatment.

4.1. Lymphoma

The CNS may be afflicted by lymphoma, a deadly lymphocytic tumour, either as the primary or secondary manifestation of another systemic illness. "Primary CNS lymphoma" (PCNSL) is lymphoma of the spinal cord or brain that excludes all other regions (apart from the visual structures). Over the past 20 years, CNS lymphoma has increased in frequency across all age groups.

4.2. PCNSL

PCNSL has also been referred to in the literature as microgliomatosis, immunoblastic sarcoma, malignant reticulosis, and perivascular sarcoma. When present, it most frequently manifests as single or multiple central brain damage in middle-aged adults. The patient's immunologic capacity affects how the neurologic involvement presents. Nearly 4% of intracranial tumours are primary CNS lymphomas. For up to two decades, critical CNS lymphoma rates have been steadily rising (Grommes and DeAngelis 2017).

An isodense or tolerably hyperdense lesion that improves firmly and uniformly with differentiation is seen by a CT scan. Oedema that is mild to moderate is usual. Particularly in immunocompromised patients, tumours may exhibit an upgraded ring structure. A typical region is the periventricular zone, where most tumours border the ependyma. On T1W MR images, primary CNS lymphomas are often isointense or mildly hypointense, and on T2W MR images, they are isointense or mildly hyperintense. Benign tumours have been seen; however, they are uncommon. Treatment modalities for PCNSL have advanced significantly in the last decade. Chemotherapy and radiotherapy, separately or in combination, have altogether expanded the prognosis of numerous immunocompetent patients with PCNSL.

5. Rare Spinal Cord Tumours

5.1. Epidemiology

Although the most recent classification of intramedullary spinal cord tumours (IMSCTs) states they only comprise 2–4% of all CNS tumours, spinal cord neoplasms actually make up about 15% of all primary central nervous system (CNS) tumours (Kopelson et al. 1980). Astrocytoma and ependymoma, two of the more prevalent intramedullary lesions, are described in detail elsewhere in this book. Astrocytomas and ependymomas are the commonest IMSCTs and usually occur in children, although ependymomas have also been seen in adults. Haemangioblastomas and spinal cord metastases, which are far commoner in the adult population, are less common IMSCTs.

5.2. Diagnostics

Assessment should initially start with a careful physical test with an emphasis on distinguishing upper motor neuron signs to identify the neurologic level of injury. When the physical test has been finished, the highest-quality imaging modality is magnetic resonance imaging (i.e., MRI). Gadolinium is commonly used as the contrast material. Histologic conclusions can sometimes be reached by surveying the MRI qualities of the lesion, as every subtype has a particular imaging appearance. T2W imaging is the modality of choice to detect spinal canal widening as lesions are traditionally hyperintense (Arima et al. 2014). Thus, primary intramedullary spinal cord lymphoma appears hyperintense on T2W MRI. These neoplasms are frequently multicentral and ineffectively described without syrinx evidence (Nakamizo et al. 2002). Homogenous enhancement and solid qualities are visible on gadolinium-enhanced images and an isointense signal on T1 (Flanagan et al. 2011). On T1 and T2W imaging, intramedullary lipomas are hyperintense and follow fat signal on all sequences (Shen et al. 2001). Cord lipomas are usually singular; however, some patients have multiple lipomas (Patwardhan et al. 2000). Tumours are generally situated along the ventral segment of the spinal cord in the intradural–extramedullary area, yet they can invade the intramedullary space in rare cases (Menezes and Traynelis 2006).

6. Dumbbell Tumours of the Spine

Heuer first used the phrase "dumbbell tumour" in 1929 to refer to spinal tumours that develop an hourglass shape as they grow inside an anatomical barrier, like a nerve root foramen, the dura mater, or other bone components (Heuer 1929; Eden 1941; Love and Dodge 1952). Based on the site of the tumour, spinal tumours with significant intraspinal or/and paravertebral involvement are categorized into four groups: intramedullary, intradural–extramedullary, epidural, and dumbbell (McCormick 1996). Dumbbell tumours can be divided into different groups as indicated by the constricting structure and details of tumour location (Asazuma et al. 2004).

Today, the phrase "dumbbell tumour" refers to a specific type of tumour that involves at least two distinct places and is associated with them, like the intradural or epidural space or regions external to the spinal canal, rather than the hourglass shape (Ozawa et al. 2007).

The location and size of spinal dumbbell tumours influence their presentation. The majority of individuals with spinal dumbbell neoplasms present with similar clinical features, regardless of the underlying pathology. Non-radicular pain is a typical side effect, followed by sensory deficits, gait difficulties, radiculopathy, motor impairments, ataxia, and bowel and bladder dysfunction (Safaee et al. 2015; Sowash et al. 2017). Non-radicular pain can continue as the disease progresses, while radiculopathy will in general settle following surgery (Sowash et al. 2017). Dumbbell tumours are more likely to be malignant among paediatric patients than among adult patients.

7. Spinal Arachnoid Cysts

Arachnoid cysts may compress the spinal cord and nerve roots, or simply obstruct the flow of the CSF, depending on their size and position, which could be the cause of a syrinx (Clifton et al. 1987; Inoue et al. 2001; Mallucci et al. 1997; Wang et al. 2003). They might be brought about by injury or another condition that causes arachnoid scarring, for example, meningitis, subarachnoid drain, or surgery, to name but a few (Andrews et al. 1988; Bassiouni et al. 2004; Buczek and Jagodziński 1994; Fobe et al. 1998; Kang et al. 2000; Osenbach et al. 1992). Patients with ankylosing spondylitis have been shown to experience multiple lumbar arachnoid cysts (Rosenkranz

1971; Shaw et al. 1990). Congenital cysts and cysts related to various of mutations have also been described (Baysefer et al. 2001; Jamjoom et al. 1991; Wakai and Chiu 1984). Some of them may be a benign mutation (Fortuna and Mercuri 1983; Perret et al. 1962). Arachnoid cysts can communicate with or be separated from the subarachnoid area. The weight of the cyst and, thus, the clinical side effects, may change during the course of the patient's treatment depending on how well they correspond with the subarachnoid space. Rarely, spinal cord herniation and dura abnormalities are linked to intradural arachnoid cysts. Arachnoid cysts may be detected posteriorly in the midline or may only affect one side of posterior back subarachnoid space if they are limited to either side of the posterior median arachnoid septum (Perret et al. 1962). Anterior cysts are usually a consequence of a surgical procedure, such as a lumbar puncture or an injection, or a sequela of trauma or meningitis.

8. Cysts and Tumour-like Lesions

Throughout the CNS, there are a few locations where cysts with cuboidal to columnar mucin-delivering epithelium are seen. These refer to Rathke's cleft cysts in the sella, colloid lesions in the third ventricle, and neurenteric (neuroepithelial, neuroglial, enterogenous, or bronchogenic) lesions (Figure 12) when they develop in the anterior spinal canal or intracranially. These cysts are thought to be benign rather than malignant. Radiographic presentation is comparable among these benign lesions, including Rathke's cleft cysts, colloid lesions, enterogenous lesions, neuroglial growths, and epidermoid and dermoid cysts (Berger and Wilson 1985).

9. Diagnostics and Differential Diagnostics of Spinal Cord Tumours

Spinal cord tumours are uncommon tumours with vague clinical indications; they are usually diagnosed late. Radicular symptoms, for example, back pain, progressive neurologic deficiencies, or skeletal deformities, are ordinarily seen in children. Approximately 20–30% of primary intradural spinal tumours are spinal cord tumours. The intradural–extramedullary compartment is where the remaining approximately 70–80% of primary intradural neoplasms are located (Duong et al. 2012). Spinal cord tumour detection and evaluation are performed via magnetic resonance imaging. T1W and T2W sagittal and axial views should be used in the imaging protocol. In the sagittal, axial, and coronal planes, those configurations should include contrast-enhanced T1W series. Similar to when abnormal bone is found, short-TI inversion recovery (STIR) must be used to detect spinal cord tumours. As of late, some CT procedures, for example, dissemination-weighted imaging (DWI) and diffusion tensor imaging (DTI), have been described in the assessment spinal lesions (Landi et al. 2016).

10. Benign Tumours of the Spinal Column

Benign tumours of the axial skeleton are usually found in children and young people. When they happen in adults, they are commonly found in people somewhere in the range of 20 and 30 years old, in a posterior area. Osteochondroma, osteoid osteoma, and osteoblastoma are the more common types of benign lesions that are less likely to recur if a thorough resection can be performed. The removal of the primary tumour itself is typically therapeutic, unlike in malignant tumours, which call for the removal of a large portion of healthy tissue surrounding the lesion. Other "benign" tumours, such as eosinophilic granulomas, giant-cell tumours, aneurysmal bone cysts, and haemangiomas can be linked to underlying infection, occur in many locations, or be locally aggressive, respectively. Osteochondroma (Figure 9) is a ligament-topped, hard projection that may develop from a cartilaginous remnant of the physis or from a nearby physis. Of all benign bone tumours, osteochondromas are the most well-known. Osteochondromatosis, one of the commonest skeletal dysplasias, can manifest as a consequence of hereditary osteochondromas. Clinical features range from dull spinal pain (smaller tumours) to decreased mobility or deformity (bigger tumours). Although they have similar pathogenic origins, osteoblastoma and osteoid osteoma differ in size and frequency of spinal contribution. These lesions are thought to represent chronic inflammatory responses rather than actual neoplasms. Neurological disorders are rare, but the most well-known cause of painful scoliosis is osteoid osteoma. It can be seen radiographically as a radiolucent area with a focal nidus and an appropriate degree of surrounding sclerosis. Treatment is through extraction. Even though small deformities will be resolved with resection alone, severe scoliosis may necessitate combination treatment. Aneurysmal bone cysts (ABCs) are benign, non-neoplastic, proliferative lesion. ABCs affect the axial skeleton in 12–25% of all documented cases, although they account for just about 1–2% of all primary bone tumours. Although the pathophysiology is unclear, theories include a concealed tumour or traumatic arteriovenous malformation, which would lead to the formation of a cyst. ABCs have fluid-filled chambers that are partitioned by fibrous septa. ABCs most frequently occur in the thoracolumbar region (Moore and Newell 2006).

Benign bony tumours are usually found in the posterior region, with the posterior segments accounting for 60% of spinal aneurysmal bone cysts. ABCs typically manifest in younger patients, in their second decade of life. A multiloculated, expansile, deeply vascular osteolytic lesion with an eggshell-like cortical edge can be seen on radiographic imaging with CT and MRI. In up to 40% of cases, different degrees of vertebral inclusion can occur. Preoperative embolization, complete resection, or embolization alone for regions of the spine that are challenging to access are all forms of treatment. If not enough edges are resected, postoperative radiotherapy may be necessary (Park et al. 2016).

11. Spinal Osteosarcoma

Osteosarcoma, which makes up 0.5% of all malignant tumours, is the most prevalent type of bone sarcoma. Relatively uncommon, spinal osteosarcoma makes for 3–5% of all spine cancers. The sacral region is the primary affected area, with the lumbar and thoracic segments following suit. Clinical treatment of spinal osteosarcoma has always been difficult due to the disease's diverse anatomic locations and significant neurological abnormalities (Wang et al. 2023).

Pain is the most common symptom of osteosarcoma and affects nearly all patients; over 70% of patients also have neurologic impairment. Research indicates that in 80% of cases of osteolysis, CT shows matrix mineralization; in terms of illustrating cortical damage, CT is more accurate than both plain radiography and MR imaging. MRI findings are nonspecific (Katonis et al. 2013).

The current standard of care for osteosarcoma consists of postoperative adjuvant chemotherapy, surgical removal of all clinically relevant metastases, and surgical resection of the main tumour following neoadjuvant chemotherapy. Although there has been significant progress in treating limb osteosarcoma, treating spinal osteosarcoma still presents significant difficulties because of the disease's high recurrence, susceptibility to metastases, and mortality rate (Wang et al. 2023).

The ideal resection depends on the location and extent of the tumour in the spinal column, even though wide en block resection is the procedure with the best outcomes. When the tumour does not impact at least one pedicle and there is no indication that the disease has spread, wide en block excision should be taken into consideration. En block excision is nearly impossible when tumours that affect both pedicles extend into the lamina, the vertebral artery foramen, or the tip of the odontoid. When this occurs, intralesional surgical resection ought to be taken into account. The prognosis is much poorer than that of limb osteosarcoma (Katonis et al. 2013).

Author Contributions: Conceptualization, methodology, validation, formal analysis, investigation, resources, data curationwriting—original draft preparation, M.M.R.; writing—review and editing, visualization, supervision, F.H.C. All authors have read and agreed to the published version of the manuscript.

Funding: This research received no external funding.

Conflicts of Interest: The authors declare no conflicts of interest.

References

Aielli, Federica, Marco Ponzetti, and Nadia Rucci. 2019. Bone Metastasis Pain, from the Bench to the Bedside. *International Journal of Molecular Sciences* 20: 280. [CrossRef] [PubMed]

Andrews, Brian T., Philip R. Weinstein, Mark L. Rosenblum, and Nicholas M. Barbaro. 1988. Intradural arachnoid cysts of the spinal canal associated with intramedullary cysts. *Journal of Neurosurgery* 68: 544–49. [CrossRef] [PubMed]

Arima, H., T. Hasegawa, D. Togawa, Y. Yamato, S. Kobayashi, T. Yasuda, and Y. Matsuyama. 2014. Feasibility of a novel diagnostic chart of intramedullary spinal cord tumours in magnetic resonance imaging. *Spinal Cord* 52: 769–73. [CrossRef] [PubMed]

Arnautovic, Kenan I., and Ziya L. Gokaslan. 2019. *Spinal Cord Tumors*. Cham: Springer.

Asazuma, Takashi, Yoshiaki Toyama, Hirofumi Maruiwa, Yoshikazu Fujimura, and Kiyoshi Hirabayashi. 2004. Surgical strategy for cervical dumbbell tumours based on a three-dimensional classification. *Spine* 29: E10–E14. [CrossRef]

Bassiouni, Hischam, Anja Hunold, Siamak Asgari, Uwe Hübschen, Hermann-Josef König, and Dietmar Stolke. 2004. Spinal intradural juxtamedullary cysts in the adult: Surgical management and outcome. *Neurosurgery* 55: 1352–60. [CrossRef]

Baysefer, Alper, Yusuf Izci, and Ersin Erdoğan. 2001. Lateral intrathoracic meningocele associated with a spinal intradural arachnoid cyst. *Pediatric Neurosurgery* 35: 107–10. [CrossRef]

Berger, Mitchel S., and Charles B. Wilson. 1985. Epidermoid cysts of the posterior fossa. *Journal of neurosurgery* 62: 214–19. [CrossRef]

Bilsky, Mark H., Eric Lis, Jeffrey Raizer, Henry Lee, and Patrick Boland. 1999. The diagnosis and treatment of metastatic spinal tumor. *The Oncologist* 4: 459–69. [CrossRef]

Bohlman, H. H., and T. A. Zdeblick. 1988. Anterior excision of herniated thoracic discs. *The Journal of Bone and Joint Surgery. American* 20: 1038–47. [CrossRef]

Boukobza, M., C. Mazel, and E. Touboul. 1996. Primary vertebral and spinal epidural non-Hodgkin's lymphoma with spinal cord compression. *Neuroradiology* 38: 333–37. [CrossRef]

Buczek, M., and Z. Jagodziński. 1994. Diagnosis and treatment of central nervous system arachnoid cyst. *Neurologia i Neurochirurgia Polska* 28: 211–20. [PubMed]

Clifton, A. G., L. Ginsberg, W. J. S. Webb, and A. R. Valentine. 1987. Idiopathic spinal arachnoid cyst, and syringomyelia. *The British Journal of Radiology* 60: 1023–25. [CrossRef] [PubMed]

Conti, Piero, Gastone Pansini, Homere Mouchaty, Christian Capuano, and Renato Conti. 2004. Spinal neurinomas: Retrospective analysis and long-term outcome of 179 consecutively operated cases and review of the literature. *Surgical Neurology* 61: 34–43. [CrossRef] [PubMed]

Ducatman, Barbara S., Bernd W. Scheithauer, David G. Piepgras, Herbert M. Reiman, and Duane M. Ilstrup. 1986. Malignant peripheral nerve sheath tumours. A clinicopathologic study of 120 cases. *Cancer* 57: 2006–21. [CrossRef]

Duong, Linh M., Bridget J. McCarthy, Roger E. McLendon, Therese A. Dolecek, Carol Kruchko, Lynda L. Douglas, and Umed A. Ajani. 2012. Descriptive epidemiology of malignant and nonmalignant primary spinal cord, spinal meninges, and cauda equina tumours, United States, 2004–2007. *Cancer* 118: 4220–27. [CrossRef]

Eden, Kenneth. 1941. The dumb-bell tumours of the spine. *British Journal of Surgery* 28: 549–70. [CrossRef]

Elia-Pasquet, Sandrine, Dorothée Provost, Anne Jaffré, Hugues Loiseau, Anne Vital, Guy Kantor, Jean-Philippe Maire, Michel Dautheribes, Vincent Darrouzet, Jean-François Dartigues, and et al. 2004. Incidence of central nervous system tumours in Gironde, France. *Neuroepidemiology* 23: 110–17. [CrossRef]

Endo, Makoto, Chikashi Kobayashi, Nokitaka Setsu, Yusuke Takahashi, Kenichi Kohashi, Hidetaka Yamamoto, Sadafumi Tamiya, Shuichi Matsuda, Yukihide Iwamoto, Masazumi Tsuneyoshi, and et al. 2011. Prognostic significance of p14ARF, p15INK4b, and p16INK4a inactivation in malignant peripheral nerve sheath tumours. *Clinical Cancer Research* 17: 3771–82. [CrossRef]

Fassett, Daniel R., James Pingree, and John RW Kestle. 2005. The high incidence of tumour dissemination in myxopapillary ependymoma in pediatric patients. Report of five cases and review of the literature. *Journal of Neurosurgery* 102: 59–64. [CrossRef]

Feldenzer, John A., James L. McGauley, and John E. McGillicuddy. 1989. Sacral and presacral tumours: Problems in diagnosis and management. *Neurosurgery* 25: 884–91. [CrossRef]

Fisher, Charles G., Christian P. DiPaola, Timothy C. Ryken, Mark H. Bilsky, Christopher I. Shaffrey, Sigurd H. Berven, James S. Harrop, Michael G. Fehlings, Stefano Boriani, Dean Chou, and et al. 2010. A novel classification system for spinal instability in neoplastic disease: An evidence-based approach and expert consensus from the Spine Oncology Study Group. *Spine* 35: E1221–E1229. [CrossRef] [PubMed]

Flanagan, E. P., B. P. O'neill, A. B. Porter, G. Lanzino, T. M. Haberman, and B. M. Keegan. 2011. Primary intramedullary spinal cord lymphoma. *Neurology* 77: 784–91. [CrossRef] [PubMed]

Fobe, J. L., K. Nishikuni, and M. A. Gianni. 1998. Evolving magnetic resonance spinal cord trauma in child: From hemorrhage to intradural arachnoid cyst. *Spinal Cord* 36: 864–66. [CrossRef] [PubMed]

Fortuna, A., and S. Mercuri. 1983. Intradural spinal cysts. *Acta Neurochirurgica* 68: 289–314. [CrossRef] [PubMed]

Gottfried, Oren N., Wayne Gluf, Alfredo Quinones-Hinojosa, Peter Kan, and Meic H. Schmidt. 2003. Spinal meningiomas: Surgical management and outcome. *Neurosurgical Focus* 14: e2. [CrossRef]

Greenberg, Mark S. 2010. *Handbook of Neurosurgery*. New York: Thieme.

Grommes, Christian, and Lisa M. DeAngelis. 2017. Primary CNS Lymphoma. *Journal of Clinical Oncology* 35: 2410–18. [CrossRef]

Helweg-Larsen, Susanne, and Per Soelberg Sørensen. 1994. Symptoms and signs in metastatic spinal cord compression: A study of progression from first symptom until diagnosis in 153 patients. *European Journal of Cancer* 30A: 396–98. [CrossRef]

Heuer, George J. 1929. The so-called hour-glass tumours of the spine. *Archives of Surgery* 18: 935–81. [CrossRef]

Hoa, Michael, and William H. Slattery, III. 2012. Neurofibromatosis 2. *Otolaryngologic Clinics of North America* 45: 315–32. [CrossRef]

Hohenberger, Christoph, Peter Hau, Karl-Michael Schebesch, Oliver Kölbl, Markus J. Riemenschneider, Fabian Pohl, Martin Proeschold, and Nils Ole Schmidt. 2023. Spinal meningiomas. *Neuro-Oncology Advances* 5: i112–i121. [CrossRef]

Inoue, Y., Y. Nemoto, K. Ohata, H. Daikokuya, A. Hakuba, T. Tashiro, M. Shakudo, K. Nagai, K. Nakayama, and R. Yamada. 2001. Syringomyelia associated with adhesive spinal arachnoiditis: MRI. *Neuroradiology* 43: 325–30. [CrossRef]

Jamjoom, Abdulhakim B., Bruce G. Mathew, and Hugh B. Coakham. 1991. A variant of the syndrome of spinal arachnoid cysts with multiple congenital defects. *British journal of neurosurgery* 5: 77–82. [CrossRef] [PubMed]

Kam, Tsz Yeung, Oscar Siu Hong Chan, Albert Wai Man Hung, and Rebecca Mei Wan Yeung. 2019. Utilization of stereotactic ablative radiotherapy in oligometastatic & oligoprogressive skeletal metastases: Results and pattern of failure. *Asia-Pacific Journal of Clinical Oncology* 15: 14–19. [CrossRef] [PubMed]

Kang, H. S., C. K. Chung, and H. J. Kim. 2000. Spontaneous spinal subdural hematoma with spontaneous resolution. *Spinal Cord* 38: 192–96. [CrossRef] [PubMed]

Katonis, P., G. Datsis, A. Karantanas, A. Kampouroglou, S. Lianoudakis, S. Licoudis, E. Papoutsopoulou, and K. Alpantaki. 2013. Spinal Osteosarcoma. *Clinical Medicine Insights: Oncology* 7: S10099. [CrossRef] [PubMed]

Khalid, Syed I., Owoicho Adogwa, Ryan Kelly, Ankit Metha, Carlos Bagley, Joseph Cheng, and John O'Toole. 2018. Adult spinal Ependymomas: An epidemiologic study. *World Neurosurgery* 111: e53–61. [CrossRef]

Kim, Phyo, Michael J. Ebersold, Burton M. Onofrio, and Lynn M. Quast. 1989. Surgery of spinal nerve schwannoma. Risk of neurological deficit after resection of involved root. *Journal of Neurosurgery* 71: 810–14. [CrossRef]

Klekamp, Jörg, and Madjid Samii. 2007. Epidural Tumors. In *Surgery of Spinal Tumors*. Berlin and Heidelberg: Springer. [CrossRef]

Kopelson, Gene, Rita M. Linggood, George M. Kleinman, Joanne Doucette, and C. C. Wang. 1980. Management of intramedullary spinal cord tumours. *Radiology* 135: 473–79. [CrossRef]

Kurland, Leonard T. 1958. The frequency of intracranial and intraspinal neoplasms in the resident population of Rochester, Minnesota. *Journal of Neurosurgery* 15: 627–41. [CrossRef]

Landi, Alessandro, Valeria Palmarini, Alessandro D'Elia, Nicola Marotta, Maurizio Salvati, Antonio Santoro, and Roberto Delfini. 2016. Magnetic resonance diffusion tensor imaging and fiber-tracking diffusion tensor tractography in the management of spinal astrocytomas. *World Journal of Clinical Cases* 4: 1–4. [CrossRef]

Lang, Ning, Xiao-Guang Liu, and Hui-Shu Yuan. 2012. Malignant peripheral nerve sheath tumour in spine: Imaging manifestations. *Clinical Imaging* 36: 209–15. [CrossRef]

Le, Robert, Jeremy D. Tran, Mel Lizaso, Ramin Beheshti, and Austin Moats. 2018. Surgical Intervention vs. Radiation Therapy: The Shifting Paradigm in Treating Metastatic Spinal Disease. *Cureus* 10: e3406. [CrossRef]

Levy, Walter J., John Latchaw, Joseph F. Hahn, Buphinda Sawhny, Janet Bay, and Donald F. Dohn. 1986. Spinal neurofibromas: A report of 66 cases and a comparison with meningiomas. *Neurosurgery* 18: 331–34. [CrossRef] [PubMed]

Liigant, Aive, Toomas Asser, Andres Kulla, and Ain-Elmar Kaasik. 2000. Epidemiology of primary central nervous system tumours in Estonia. *Neuroepidemiology* 19: 300–11. [CrossRef] [PubMed]

Love, J. Grafton, and H. W. Dodge. 1952. Dumbbell (hourglass) neurofibromas affecting the spinal cord. *Surgery, Gynecology & Obstetrics* 94: 161–72.

Malis, Leonard I. 1978. Intramedullary Spinal Cord Tumours. *Clinical Neurosurgery* 25: 512–39. [CrossRef] [PubMed]

Mallucci, C. L., R. J. Stacey, J. B. Miles, and B. Williams. 1997. Idiopathic syringomyelia and the importance of occult arachnoid webs, pouches, and cysts. *British Journal of Neurosurgery* 11: 306–9. [CrossRef]

Materljan, Eris, Branka Materljan, J. Sepcic, Lidija Tuskan-Mohar, Gordana Zamolo, and Irene Erman-Baldini. 2000. Epidemiology of central nervous system tumours in Labin area, Croatia, 1974–2001. *Croatian Medical Journal* 45: 206–12.

McCormick, Paul C. 1996. Surgical management of dumbbell and paraspinal tumours of the thoracic and lumbar spine. *Neurosurgery* 38: 67–74. [CrossRef]

McCormick, Paul C., Kalmon D. Post, and Bennett M. Stein. 1990. Intradural extramedullary tumours in adults. *Neurosurgery Clinics of North America* 1: 591–608. [CrossRef]

Menezes, Arnold H., and Vincent C. Traynelis. 2006. Spinal neurenteric cysts in the magnetic resonance imaging era. *Neurosurgery* 58: 97–105. [CrossRef]

Moore, Anne J., and David W. Newell. 2006. *Tumour Neurosurgery*. London: Spinger.

Mridha, A. R., M. C. Sharma, C. Sarkar, V. Suri, A. Rishi, A. Garg, and A. Suri. 2007. Myxopapillary ependymoma of lumbosacral region with metastasis to both cerebellopontine angles: Report of a rare case. *Child's Nervous System* 24: 1209–13. [CrossRef] [PubMed]

Mundy, Gregory R. 2002. Metastasis to bone: Causes, consequences and therapeutic opportunities. *Nature Reviews Cancer* 2: 584–93. [CrossRef] [PubMed]

Nakamizo, Tomoki, Haruhisa Inoue, Fukashi Udaka, Masaya Oda, Makoto Kawai, Kengo Uemura, Makio Takahashi, Kazuto Nishinaka, Hideyuki Sawada, Masakuni Kameyama, and et al. 2002. Magnetic resonance imaging of primary spinal intramedullary lymphoma. *Journal of Neuroimaging* 12: 183–86. [CrossRef] [PubMed]

Osborn, Virginia W., Anna Lee, and Yoshiya Yamada. 2018. Stereotactic Body Radiation Therapy for Spinal Malignancies. *Technology in Cancer Research & Treatment* 17. [CrossRef]

Osenbach, Richard K., John C. Godersky, Vincent C. Traynelis, and Robert D. Schelper. 1992. Intradural extramedullary cysts of the spinal canal: Clinical presentation, radiographic diagnosis, and surgical management. *Neurosurgery* 30: 35–42. [CrossRef]

Ozawa, Hiroshi, Shoichi Kokubun, Toshimi Aizawa, Takeshi Hoshikawa, and Chikashi Kawahara. 2007. Spinal dumbbell tumours: An analysis of a series of 118 cases. *Journal of Neurosurgery: Spine* 7: 587–93. [CrossRef]

Park, Howard Y., Sara K. Yang, William L. Sheppard, Vishal Hegde, Stephen D. Zoller, Scott D. Nelson, Noah Federman, and Nicholas M. Bernthal. 2016. Current management of aneurysmal bone cysts. *Current Reviews in Musculoskeletal Medicine* 9: 435–44. [CrossRef]

Patchell, Roy A., Phillip A. Tibbs, William F. Regine, Richard Payne, Stephen Saris, Richard J. Kryscio, Mohammed Mohiuddin, and Byron Young. 2005. Direct decompressive surgical resection in the treatment of spinal cord compression caused by metastatic cancer: A randomised trial. *Lancet* 366: 643–48. [CrossRef]

Patwardhan, Vasudha, Tufail Patanakar, Diane Armao, and Suresh K. Mukherji. 2000. MR imaging findings of intramedullary lipomas. *American Journal of Roentgenology* 174: 1792–93. [CrossRef]

Perret, George, David Green, and John Keller. 1962. Diagnosis and treatment of intradural arachnoid cysts of the thoracic spine. *Radiology* 79: 425–29. [CrossRef]

Preston-Martin, Susan. 1990. Descriptive epidemiology of primary tumours of the spinal cord and spinal meninges in Los Angeles County, 1972–1985. *Neuroepidemiology* 9: 106–11. [CrossRef] [PubMed]

Requena, Luis, and Omar P. Sangüeza. 1995. Benign neoplasms with neural differentiation: A review. *The American Journal of Dermatopathology* 17: 75–96. [CrossRef] [PubMed]

Rosenkranz, Wolf. 1971. Ankylosing spondylitis: Cauda equina syndrome with multiple spinal arachnoid cysts. Case report. *Journal of Neurosurgery* 34: 241–43. [CrossRef] [PubMed]

Safaee, Michael, Andrew T. Parsa, Nicholas M. Barbaro, Dean Chou, Praveen V. Mummaneni, Philip R. Weinstein, Tarik Tihan, and Christopher P. Ames. 2015. Association of tumour location, extent of resection, and neurofibromatosis status with clinical outcomes for 221 spinal nerve sheath tumours. *Neurosurgical Focus* 39: E5. [CrossRef] [PubMed]

Schaller, Bernhard. 2005. Spinal meningioma: Relationship between histological subtypes and surgical outcome? *Journal of Neuro-Oncology* 75: 157–61. [CrossRef]

Seppälä, Matti T., Matti JJ Haltia, Risto J. Sankila, Juha E. Jääskeläinen, and Olli Heiskanen. 1995. Long-term outcome after removal of spinal schwannoma: A clinicopathological study of 187 cases. *Journal of Neurosurgery* 83: 621–26. [CrossRef]

Shaw, Pamela J., David A. Allcutt, David Bates, and PeterJ Crawford. 1990. Cauda equina syndrome associated with multiple lumbar arachnoid cysts in ankylosing spondylitis: Improvement following surgical therapy. *Journal of Neurology, Neurosurgery & Psychiatry* 53: 1076–79. [CrossRef]

Shen, Shu-Huei, Jiing-Feng Lirng, Feng-Chi Chang, Jing-Ying Lee, Chao-Bao Luo, Shing-Su Chen, and Cheng-Yen Chang. 2001. Magnetic resonance imaging appearance of intradural spinal lipoma. *Chinese Medical Journal (Taipei)* 64: 364–68.

Solero, Carlo L., Maurizio Fornari, Sergio Giombini, Giovanni Lasio, Giuseppe Oliveri, Carlo Cimino, and Franco Pluchino. 1989. Spinal meningiomas: Review of 174 operated cases. *Neurosurgery* 25: 153–60. [CrossRef]

Sonneland, Paula R. L., Bernd W. Scheithauer, and Burton M. Onofrio. 1985. Myxopapillary ependymoma. A clinicopathologic and immunocytochemical study of 77 cases. *Cancer* 56: 883–93. [CrossRef]

Sowash, Madeleine, Ori Barzilai, Sweena Kahn, Lily McLaughlin, Patrick Boland, Mark H. Bilsky, and Ilya Laufer. 2017. Clinical outcomes following resection of giant spinal schwannomas: A case series of 32 patients. *Journal of Neurosurgery: Spine* 26: 494–500. [CrossRef] [PubMed]

van den Bent, Martin J. 2005. Surgical resection improves outcome in metastatic epidural spinal cord compression. *Lancet* 366: 609–10. [CrossRef] [PubMed]

Wakai, Susumu, and Chin-Wen Chiu. 1984. Rare combination of spinal lesions and spina bifida occulta: Case report. *Developmental Medicine & Child Neurology* 26: 117–21. [CrossRef]

Wang, Jing, Xiang-zhi Ni, Ming-lei Yang, Xing Huang, Shu-ming Hou, Cheng Peng, Jia-shi Cao, and Tie-Long Liu. 2023. Prognostic factors and treatment outcomes of spinal osteosarcoma: Surveillance, epidemiology, and end results database analysis. *Frontiers in Oncology* 13: 1083776. [CrossRef]

Wang, Michael Y., Allan DO Levi, and Barth A. Green. 2003. Intradural spinal arachnoid cysts in adults. *Surgical Neurology* 60: 49–55. [CrossRef]

Yang, Xiong-gang, Deng-xing Lun, Yong-cheng Hu, Yong-heng Liu, Feng Wang, Jiang-tao Feng, Kun-chi Hua, Li Yang, Hao Zhang, Ming-you Xu, and et al. 2018. Prognostic effect of factors involved in revised Tokuhashi score system for patients with spinal metastases: A systematic review and Meta-analysis. *BMC Cancer* 18: 1248. [CrossRef]

Zibis, A. H., A. Markonis, and A. H. Karantanas. 2000. Unusual causes of spinal foraminal widening. *European Radiology* 10: 144–48. [CrossRef]

Ziu, Endrit, Vibhu Krishnan Viswanathan, and Fassil B. Mesfin. 2022. Spinal Metastasis. In *StatPearls [Internet]*; Treasure Island: StatPearls Publishing. Available online: https://www.ncbi.nlm.nih.gov/books/NBK441950/?cv=1&msclkid=b63e0727cbd611e (accessed on 23 May 2023).

Spinal Infections and Parasitic Infestation

Mohammod Raziul Haque, Esma Azam Zico and Forhad H. Chowdhury

Abstract: Spinal infection is not uncommon. It can affect both the bone and soft tissue of the spine and it may be spontaneous or iatrogenic following surgery or spinal tap. It usually presents with pain and fever, with or without neurological deficit/spinal deformity, and its causes can be pyogenic, tubercular, viral, fungal, or, very rarely, parasitic. Spinal infection can be treated both conservatively and/or with surgery. Conservative management includes antibiotic and/or antitubercular therapy; surgical intervention ranges from ultrasound-guided aspiration of pus to deformity correction by instrumentation. Neurological outcomes are excellent if there is a neuro-deficit due to tubercular infection; the worst outcomes are following pyogenic infection. This chapter will briefly discuss pyogenic, tubercular, and fungal spinal infections and spinal parasitic infestations, including their neurosurgical management.

Abbreviations

AFB	acid-fast bacilli	ATD	antitubercular therapy
CBC	complete blood count	CRP	C-Reactive Protein
ESBL	extended-spectrum Beta-lactamase	SEA	spinal epidural abscess
CES	cauda equina syndrome	CT	computed tomography
ESR	erythrocyte sediment rate	FDG	5 Fluoro-deoxy Glucose
MRSA	methicillin-resistant *Staphylococcus aureus*	TC	total count
IGRA	interferon-gamma release assay	IV	intravenous
MRI	magnetic resonance imaging	SOL	space-occupying lesion
HIV	human immunodeficiency virus	HSV	Herpes simplex virus

1. Introduction

Spinal infection means infection and inflammation of the spinal and/or paraspinal tissue. It leads to considerable acute and chronic morbidity in the patient and causes significant financial loss to the patient and the healthcare system. Due to the relatively high incidence and difficulty in diagnosis, there must be a thorough understanding of the diagnostic and management principles in order to successfully treat these patients.

2. Incidence

The prevalence of spinal infections ranges from 2% to 7%, with a mortality rate of 2%–15%. Spinal infection has a bimodal occurrence, affecting primarily juvenile patients under the age of 20 and adult patients aged 50–70 years. The frequency of spinal infections has not decreased as antibiotic therapy has advanced, particularly among the elderly, owing to a rise in patients with risk characteristics (Tayles and Buckley 2004; Frangen et al. 2006).

3. Types of Spinal Infection

3.1. According to Anatomical Site

(i) Vertebral osteomyelitis/spondylitis: Infection of the vertebral body without involving the disc is called spondylitis; it most commonly involves the lumbar segment of the spine.
(ii) Spondylodiscitis/discitis: This is an infection of the disc and bone and it can occur spontaneously or postoperatively. Symptoms include severe pain during spine movement and radiating pain in different body regions with fever and chills.
(iii) Spinal epidural abscess: This is a neurosurgical emergency. These infections can cause weakness, back pain, spinal tenderness, and bowel and bladder disturbance.
(iv) Spinal subdural empyema: This infection is rarer and usually spreads from an infection in another anatomical area.
(v) Meningitis/arachnoiditis: This is an infection and inflammation of the meninges of the spine. This infection can spread swiftly and can lead to severe life-threatening complications if not managed properly.
(vi) Spinal cord abscess: This usually presents as an intramedullary SOL. It is caused by both pyogenic and tubercular organisms.

3.2. According to Aetiology

(i) Pyogenic: Most common organisms are *Staphylococcus aureus*, *Streptococcus*, and *E coli*.
(ii) Granulomatous: Most commonly caused by M. Tubercular (Figures 1 and 2); other rare granulomatous infections are caused by M. Brucellar, syphilis, and fungi (aspergillus).
(iii) Viral: Human immunodeficiency virus (HIV), Herpes zoster, Epstein–Barr virus (EBV), Cytomegalo virus, herpes simplex virus (HSV), West Nile virus, human T-cell lymphotropic virus type 1 (HTLV-1), polio virus.
(iv) Parasitic: Parasitic infections of the spine are very rare. Infectious myelopathy is caused by Schistosoma infections, which are one of the most frequent parasites. Africa, South America, and Eastern Asia are the most common places to find these. *Echinococcus granulosus* cysts in dogs can compress the spinal cord (Frangen et al. 2006; Sobottke et al. 2008; Duarte and Vaccaro 2013).

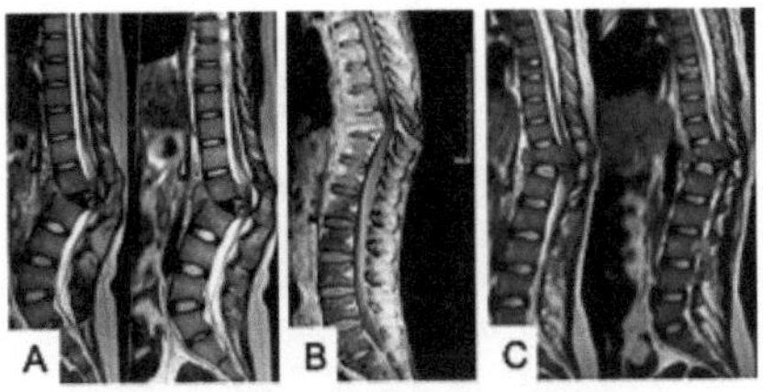

Figure 1. (**A–C**) Tubercular spondylodiscitis with loss of vertebral body with instability. Source: Figure by authors.

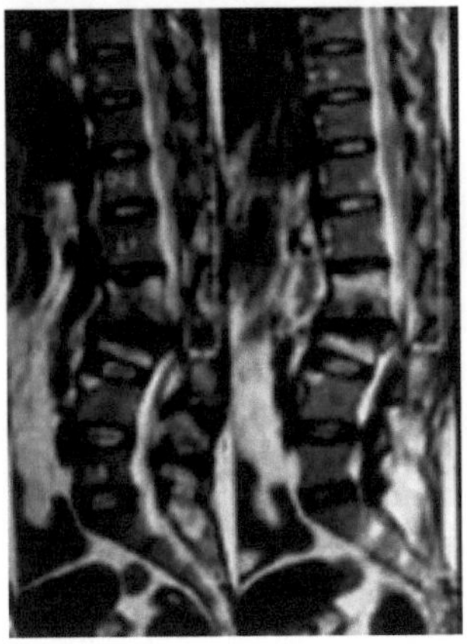

Figure 2. Lumbar tubercular spondylodiscitis. Source: Figure by authors.

4. Predisposing Factors

1. Elderly age;
2. Diabetes mellitus;
3. IV drug abuse;
4. Haemodialysis/kidney or hepatic failure;
5. Oncological history and chemotherapy;
6. Previous spinal surgery;
7. Septicaemia;
8. Infectious endocarditis;
9. Immunosuppressive conditions, including alcohol abuse, HIV infection, chronic steroid use, rheumatologic disease, and Dengue fever (Figure 3) (Sobottke et al. 2008; Duarte and Vaccaro 2013).

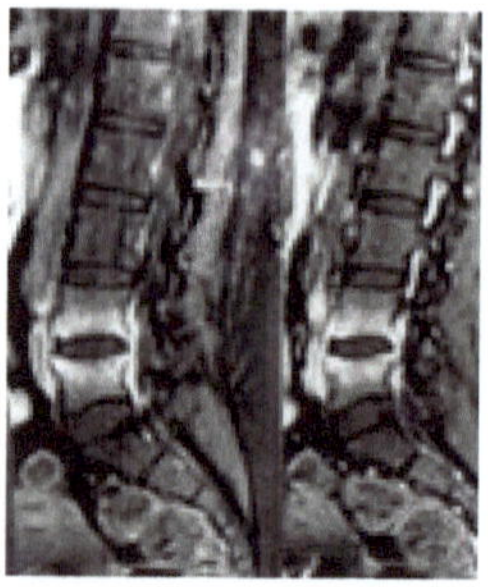

Figure 3. Spontaneous spondylodiscitis after Dengue fever. Source: Figure by authors.

4.1. Post-Procedure Spinal Infection

Spinal infection can follow any intervention, even a single spinal tap (Figure 4).

Post-procedure spinal infection can be superficial or deep and can be early or late. Classification is depending on the grade of infection and likelihood of host response. The severity of infection is divided into three groups: (1) superficial or deep infection with a single organism, (2) deep infection with multiple organisms, and (3) deep infection and myonecrosis with multiple or resistant organisms (Rasouli et al. 2012).

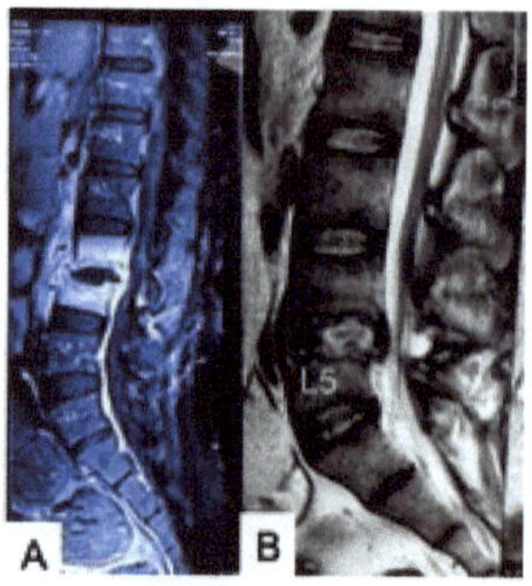

Figure 4. (**A**,**B**) Contrast-enhanced MRI showing spondylodiscitis after spinal anaesthesia at L2/3 and L4/5. Source: Figure by authors.

5. Aetiopathogenesis

Spinal infection can start from three sources; the most common source is haematogenous, then spread from a contiguous site, and, lastly, from the direct entry of an organism due to iatrogenic or penetrating trauma.

Haematogenous spread can be through the arterial or venous system. The Batson plexus is a potential route of infection. Pelvic infections can spread to the lumbar vertebrae; pulmonary infection can spread to the thoracic vertebrae and beyond. The urinary tract also a frequent source of infection. Adjacent structures, such as a retropharyngeal abscess, oesophageal perforation, or aortic implants, can transfer an infection to the spine in a contiguous manner. An iatrogenic aetiology is common, and infection can occur after epidural treatments. In the paediatric group, the spine has extensive arterial anastomosis, so arterial spread is more common and spontaneous disc infection is not rare. However, this extensive blood supply combats infection, resulting in rapid healing and little bone destruction. Discs have blood supply until the age of 15; then, they become avascular (Duarte and Vaccaro 2013; Rasouli et al. 2012; Tyrrell et al. 1999; Butler et al. 2006; Fantoni et al. 2012; Maslen et al. 1993).

6. Clinical Presentation

Spinal infection usually presents with back pain or neck pain which is constant, aggravated by even mild spinal movement, and worse at night. There may be some constitutional symptoms, like fever with chills and rigor if the infection is pyogenic or low-grade evening fever with weight loss and/or loss of appetite if the infection is caused by TB. Clinical features depend on the extent of the involvement of the spine; epidural abscesses usually present with profound neurological deficits and paraplegia/quadriplegia in low-income countries and may present with radiculopathy. Mechanical compression and vascular impairment are prone to cause neurologic abnormalities (most prominently with epidural abscesses) (Frangen et al. 2006; Tyrrell et al. 1999; Fantoni et al. 2012; Broner et al. 1996; Gouliouris et al. 2010).

Localized spinal discomfort, muscular spasms, and a markedly reduced range of motion are all possible symptoms. Neck stiffness is the most common symptom of cervical spinal infections. They can also produce a retropharyngeal abscess, which can lead to dysphagia, dysphonia, and torticollis (Broner et al. 1996; Carragee 1997; Schimmer et al. 2002).

Irritability, refusal to sit, crawl, or walk, and bowel and bladder incontinence are all symptoms that can be seen in children. Lumbar lordosis is also visible. Fever and neurologic impairments, on the other hand, are uncommon in paediatric patients.

Infection may spread to adjacent tissue and may present with psoas abscesses. It may cause bone destruction and spinal instability, leading to spinal deformity like kyphosis or gibbus (Schimmer et al. 2002; Brown et al. 2001; Mylona et al. 2009).

7. Diagnosis

Initially, some haematological tests, like ESR, TC, DC, and CRP, are essential. A high ESR is more sensitive, and 90% of individuals with spondylodiscitis have an elevated CRP. Both can be utilized to track a patient's reaction to therapy. A 25% decrease in ESR at 1 month is a great indicator of a positive treatment response, but CRP is more precise and returns to normal sooner. If patient presents with high-grade fever, blood culture is essential before starting antibiotics (Sobottke et al. 2008; Carragee 1997; Lillie et al. 2008).

At the time of the initial assessment, plain radiography should be taken. The absence of definition and irregularities of vertebral endplates is the first evidence of spinal infection that may be noticed on plain X-rays. This normally happens 2–8 weeks after the first symptom appears. This causes endplate fragmentation and a decrease in the height of the intervertebral disc. X-rays are also useful in determining whether or not there is any global malalignment as a result of illness or bone damage (coronal or sagittal).

The gold standard for diagnosing a spinal infection is MRI. For the imaging of spinal infections, MRI has the highest specificity and sensitivity. It possesses a 96% sensitivity and a 94% specificity. Furthermore, it shows more epidural space with soft-tissue detail. Discs and vertebral bodies show a hypointense signal on T1W and a hyperintense signal on T2W, attributable to oedema in spinal infections. Gadolinium-enhanced MRI improves MRI accuracy by helping to distinguish infection from degenerative and tumour-associated pathology. Endplate alterations cause a hypointense signal on T2W imaging in degenerative disease, although there is no oedema. In comparison to normal bone marrow, tumour lesions show a relatively hypointense signal on T1W image. However, no one imaging feature can tell the difference between a tumour and an infection. Extensive bone deterioration with conservation of the intervertebral disc, heterogeneous augmentation of the body of vertebra, and the development of a paravertebral abscess are among the MRI findings in tuberculous spondylitis (Broner et al. 1996; Krogsgaard et al. 1998; Diehn 2012; Sharif 1992).

CT scan is the modality of choice to see bony details both for diagnostic and surgical planning. Also, where MR imaging is contraindicated, CT myelography can be helpful. Early abnormalities in vertebral endplates can be identified this way (Broner et al. 1996; Jevtic 2004).

Bone scan has an improved specificity over MRI, of 91%–100%, to identify spinal infection. PET scan with FDG shows increased specificity. FDG uptake is highest in sites of inflammation containing macrophages and neutrophils, enabling high-resolution imaging of acute and chronic infections. Degenerative disease, including fractures, has no FDG uptake (Gemmel et al. 2006, 2010).

Tissue diagnosis is essential to differentiate malignancy from infection and to guide antibiotic selection in adults, but empirical antibiotics can be started prior to tissue diagnosis in paediatric patients. Tissue diagnosis is important if a fungal or tubercular infection is suspected and if empirical therapy failed in that group.

Obtaining sufficient and accurate tissue for diagnosis is the key factor. CT-guided FNAC is least invasive, but it has an accuracy of 70% and has some limitations, like inadequate tissue, radiation, and complications. So, core biopsy is preferred to FNAC if the abscess cavity can be accessed easily. Core biopsy can be taken in different ways, like percutaneous fluoroscopic guidance or endoscope assistant (Ratcliffe 1985; Kornblum et al. 1998; Gasbarrini et al. 2012).

Open biopsy is sometimes essential if closed biopsy fails to detect an organism or if the infection site is inaccessible or if the patients needs surgery for a neurological deficit or for a spinal deformity.

The biopsy specimen should be delivered for Gram stain, AFB stain, fungal stain, and anaerobic bacteria, aerobic bacteria, fungal, and tubercular cultures. Gene X-pert for M. tuberculosis with rifampicin sensitivity should also be used. An interferon-gamma release assay (IGRA) from whole-blood plasma, as well as an acid-fast bacilli (AFB) smear including culture, can be employed, with a sensitivity rate of up to 88% if there is a high index of expectation for tuberculosis. Biopsy specimens should be handed over for histopathologic investigation if there is any suspicion of a tumour or fungal illness (Ratcliffe 1985; Cheng et al. 2004; Kumar et al. 2010; de Lucas et al. 2009; Rankine et al. 2004; Michel et al. 2006).

8. Management

The management of spinal infections includes both nonsurgical and surgical techniques.

8.1. Nonsurgical Management

Nonsurgical management includes antibiotics, improvement in nutritional status, immobilization with a thoracolumbar brace or cervical collar, treatment of comorbidities, and close monitoring for any neurological deterioration.

8.1.1. Indications for Nonsurgical Management

Nonsurgical management is indicated for spinal infection that does not cause any neurological deficit or spinal instability, for patients unfit for surgery, or for patients who have been completely paralyzed for more than 36 h. However, recent observations suggest that those who have been completely paralyzed due to compression of the spinal cord by a non-malignant mass for 2–3 months without any vascular compromise can benefit from surgical intervention.

8.1.2. Choice of Antibiotic

Broad-spectrum antibiotics covering *Staphylococcus aureus*, MRSA, ESBL, and *Escherichia coli* should be administered. Intravenous antibiotics should be given for 6–8 weeks, followed by oral antibiotics, depending on clinical and laboratory proof of resolution of infection. Before starting antibiotics, specimens must be collected and/or blood must be drawn for culture if fever is present (Sobottke et al. 2008; Broner et al. 1996; Ratcliffe 1985; Khanna et al. 1996; Del Curling et al. 1990; Danner and Hartman 1987).

8.1.3. Minimally Invasive Nonsurgical Treatment

This is indicated for psoas abscess or other paravertebral abscesses and for pyogenic spondylodiscitis. Here, abscesses can be drained as guided by USG/CT.

8.2. Surgical Management

8.2.1. Aims of Surgical Management

These include the decompression of the neural elements and the debridement of infective necrotic tissue.

8.2.2. Indications

(1) Neurological deficit from compression by phlegmon or any other elements resulting from a destructive consequence of infection. (2) Spinal instability. (3) Failure of conservative management.

8.2.3. Relative Indications

Epidural abscess; sepsis in the cervical and dorsal region with or without neurological deficit; uncontrollable pain.

The threshold for surgery for infections in the cervical and dorsal spine is low, as mild compression may have disastrous consequences.

8.2.4. Surgical Approach

The surgical approach to spine infections depends on the site of the lesion, extent of bony damage, and neurological deficit.

9. Follow-Up

To see the response to treatment, CRP and ESR can be assessed weekly. CRP is a good early measure of how well a treatment is working because it starts to normalize within the first week. Imaging can be performed to see fusion and radiological improvements in the infection.

10. Outcome

Mortality rates are very low, less than 5%; this is because of advancements in radio-imaging have resulted in early diagnosis and prompt treatment. Morbidity is due to neurological deficit; complete paralysis for more than 12 h due to pyogenic infection is very unlikely to improve, but complete paralysis due to Pott's disease without neurovascular compromise has very favourable outcomes (Tyrrell et al. 1999; Schimmer et al. 2002; Del Curling et al. 1990; Delafuente 1991).

11. Recurrence

In the paediatric population, relapses of spinal infections are uncommon. Adults have a recurrence risk of up to 14%, with 75% of recurrences occurring in the first year in patients with medical conditions. Recurrent infection is linked to paravertebral abscesses, recurrent bacteraemia, and chronic draining sinuses, among other things.

12. Spinal Tuberculosis/Pott's Disease

12.1. Introduction

Sir Percival Pott reported tuberculous spondylitis and its clinical manifestation of paraplegia in European patients with kyphotic deformities in 1779 (Sobottke et al. 2008). Spine tuberculosis (STB) is a particularly deadly type of skeletal tuberculosis because it can cause neurological deficits as a result of the compression of nearby nerve tissues and considerable spinal deformity. So, early detection and treatment of spinal tuberculosis is critical for precluding catastrophic consequences (Dobson 1972).

12.2. Incidence

Extrapulmonary tuberculosis (EPTB) has a low incidence of 3%, yet there has been no substantial decrease in the frequency of EPTB as there has been with pulmonary tuberculosis. Skeletal tuberculosis (STB) accounts for about 10% of EPTB cases, and spinal TB is the most prevalent site of STB, accounting for roughly 50% of skeletal EPTB cases. The most frequently impacted part of the spinal column is still the thoracolumbar junction, followed by the cervical and lumbar spine. The spinal column is implicated in less than 1% of all tuberculosis (TB) cases (Luk 1999; Pertuiset et al. 1999; Kulchavenya 2014).

12.3. Pathophysiology of Spinal TB

The mycobacterium tuberculosis complex, which comprises roughly 60 species, causes tuberculosis. Humans are only known to be affected by Mycobacterium TB (the commonest), Mycobacterium bovis, Mycobacterium africanum, and Mycobacterium microti (Jain and Dhammi 2007).

It is a fastidious, slow-growing aerobic bacillus. Infections can start in the lungs, mediastinal lymph nodes, gastrointestinal tract, mesentery, genitourinary system, or any other viscera. When aerobic circumstances are good, the bacilli tend to stay latent for long periods of time and multiply every 20–30 h. Haematogenous diffusion of the bacillus from a primary focus causes spinal infection, which is always secondary (Schirmer et al. 2010; Tuli 1993).

The paradiscal arteries separate on both sides of the disc and then reach the subchondral zone of the top and lower endplates of each disc, making the intervertebral disc an avascular anatomical structure. The fact that the vertebra has an artery supply promotes subchondral bone inclusion on both sides of the disc, known as "paradiscal," which is the most prevalent kind (Rasouli et al. 2012). "Central" involvement results in vertebral body loss; "posterior" involvement involves neural arch structures; and "nonosseous" involvement promotes abscess creation. TB causes granulomatous inflammation, classically characterized by epithelioid cells and lymphocytic infiltration, which may unite to create the characteristic Langhans-type giant cells, resulting in caseating necrosis of the afflicted tissues and the formation of a cold abscess. Kyphosis is a deformity of the spine caused by a gradual destruction of the body of the vertebra, leading to a deformation of the spine (Rajasekaran et al. 2014; Jain 2010).

12.4. Clinical Presentation of Spinal TB

The intensity and length of the disease, as well as the location of the disease and the existence of comorbidities, all influence how spinal TB manifests (Su et al. 2010). There are two types of spinal tuberculosis: complex and simple. Patients with complex tuberculosis have abscesses, sinus formation, deformity, instability, and neurological deficits. Simple spinal tuberculosis is one in which the diagnosis is made before the onset of problems. Backache is by far the most prevalent symptom. It is mostly related to bone inflammation during the active period, and it can be radicular in character on rare occasions. The intensity of rest pain at the affected level is proportional to the extent of bone loss and instability. PTB is more commonly related to constitutional symptoms like weight loss, loss of appetite, malaise, and fever than to spinal TB (Hayes et al. 1996).

12.5. Diagnosis

The diagnosis of spinal tuberculosis is made utilizing clinical and classic MRI findings, and it is proved by either culture with sensitivity, the Gene Xpert PCR test, or histological evidence.

12.6. Management

12.6.1. Conservative

There are some controversies about the duration of ATD therapy, but the authors recommend 18 (3 + 15) months (Figure 5).

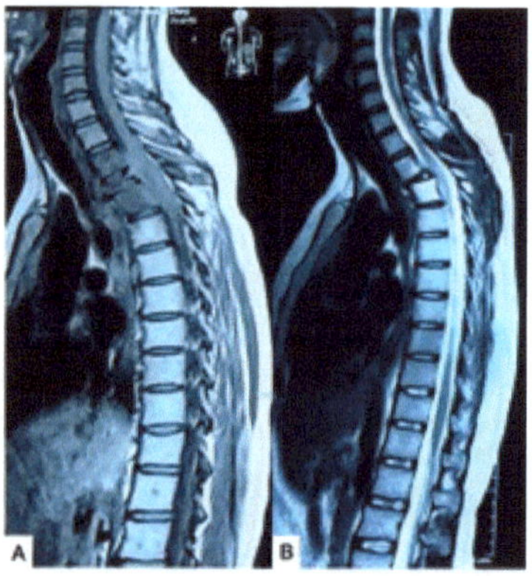

Figure 5. (**A**) MRI of spine showing D1, D2, and D3 tubercular spondylodiscitis with complete collapse of D2, epidural abscess, and cord compression. (**B**) MRI of spine 18 months after surgery and anti-TB therapy. Source: Figure by authors.

Drug Resistance (MDR, XDR)

MDR-TB (Figure 6) is resistant to both INH and rifampicin. It usually happens as a result of poor treatment; however, resistant strains can also spread. Resistance to INH and rifampicin, as well as any fluoroquinolone and at least one injectable second-line anti-TB treatment, is known as extensively drug-resistant TB (XDR-TB) (Jain 2010; Su et al. 2010). Velayati et al. suggested the term "totally drug-resistant tuberculosis" (TDR-TB) in 2009 to describe TB strains that demonstrated in vitro resistance to all first- and second-line medications tested (Pawar et al. 2009).

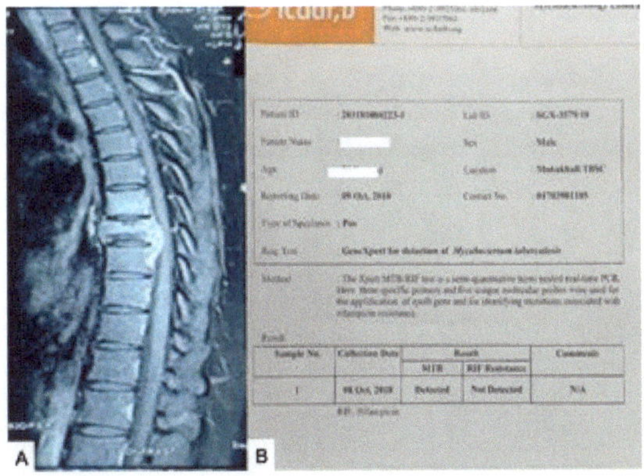

Figure 6. Dorsal Pott's (**A**) with positive gene X-pert and rifampicin sensitivity (**B**). Source: Figure by authors.

12.6.2. Surgical Management

Indications for surgical therapy:

(1) Chemotherapy failure or recurrence;
(2) Significant weakness at presentation;
(3) Instability;
(4) Static or growing neurological impairment even after starting chemotherapy;
(5) Incapacitating pain;
(6) Deformities.

Fundamentals of surgical management:

- Optimum decompression and debridement;
- Maintenance and augmentation of stability;
- Correction or slowing of deformity progression.

Surgical objectives (Figure 7):

- Drainage of abscess;
- Infected material debridement;
- Debridement and fusion +/− stabilization (Velayati et al. 2009).

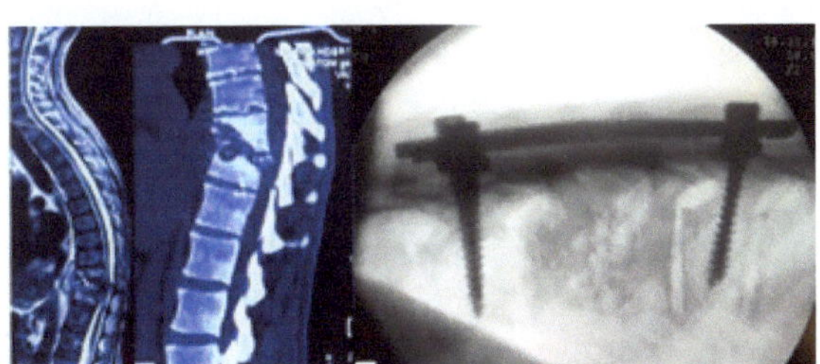

Figure 7. (**A**) MRI of spine and (**B**) CT scan of dorsal spine showing dorsal spinal tuberculosis with cord compression. (**C**) Intraoperative X-ray of after decompression, fusion, and stabilization. Source: Figure by authors.

12.7. Cold Abscess

Chemotherapy alone heals the majority of cold abscesses, with draining being necessary in rare cases, like respiratory discomfort or dysphagia caused by a big cervical paravertebral abscess or pseudo-hip flexion deformity as a result of a huge psoas abscess (Mallick et al. 2004; Oniankitan et al. 2014).

12.7.1. Surgical Approach

The surgical approach to spine infections is based on the site of lesion, the extent of bone loss, and neurological deficit. Anterior and posterior approaches, global reconstruction by posterior approach, or mixed procedures are used to accomplish debridement plus fusion with or without instrumentation.

(i) Anterior approach: usually performed in the cervical region.
(ii) Posterior approach: most commonly performed due to familiarity of route, ease of access, and the easy learning curve.

In the cervical spine, for ventral locations, an anterior approach is recommended, including the debridement of the infected disc and bone followed by normal saline wash, then by the placement of an iliac crest graft/allograft or artificial cage and stabilization with plates and screws. For posterior lesions, a posterior approach and stabilization with lateral mass screws and cervical pedicle screws should be used. In the thoracic spine if the lesion is an epidural abscess only with/without neurological deficit, laminectomy, hemi-laminotomy, or laminoplasty is recommended; if the lesion is associated with bone loss or instability, then stabilization with pedicle screws is recommended. For ventral thoracic lesions, several approaches exist. The ventral approach helps to debride infected ventral bone and tissue and should be followed by ventral or dorsal stabilization; the posterolateral approach (costo-transversectomy) involves decompression and stabilization. In the thoracolumbar junction and lumbar region, decompression and debridement by TLIF followed by stabilization is recommended. TLIF on one or two levels can be accomplished by both MISS and an open technique. Fusion can be performed with a tricortical iliac crest bone graft or with irradiated bone with bone morphogenic protein/autologous small bone chips (Al Sebai et al. 2004; Hodgson et al. 1960; Tuli 2007; Govender and Parbhoo 1999; Benli et al. 2007; Christodoulou et al. 2006; Chen et al. 2003; Lee et al. 2006; Mizuno 1967; Shang et al. 2010).

12.7.2. Outcome

Over 90% of cases of Pott's paraplegia have very good recovery. If the patient develops thromboangiitis obliterans, the outcome is unsatisfactory.

13. Spinal Epidural Abscess

13.1. Introduction

A spinal epidural abscess (SEA) is an emergency subtype of spinal infection which demands prompt diagnosis and treatment; otherwise, disastrous results can be seen.

Incidence: SEAs are a very uncommon ailment. Pyogenic SEAs occur in 0.2–1.2 instances per 10,000 hospital admissions, with the number of cases probably rising. With a male-to-female ratio of roughly 2:1, there is a masculine predominance (Khanna et al. 1996; Del Curling et al. 1990).

13.2. Aetiopathogenesis

Pyogenic and nonpyogenic organisms can cause a spinal epidural abscess. Although the causative pathogen varies by geographical region, *Staphylococcus aureus* is the commonest pathogen (70%), followed by Streptococcus species (7%). But the frequency of SEAs is rising, in part as a result of an increase in the number of elderly people, IV drug abusers, invasive spinal interventions, and HIV cases, as well as due to advancements in radiologic imaging techniques. SEAs caused by Gram-negative bacilli (more frequently seen in IV drug abusers), fungal species, mycobacterium tuberculosis, and parasitic pathogens have been documented, despite their rarity. Around 35% of persons who develop a SEA have used IV drugs in the past; 50%–60% are immunocompromised as a result of a chronic disease; and 10%–20% have had spine surgery (Michel et al. 2006; Khanna et al. 1996; Del Curling et al. 1990).

13.3. Clinical Features and Diagnosis

Systemic features include fever, malaise, and local features according to the site of infection. These are as follows:

- In cervical SEA: neck stiffness, retropharyngeal abscess, quadriparesis.
- In thoracic SEA: back pain, local tenderness, paraparesis.
- In lumber SEA: lower back pain, local tenderness, CES.

Diagnosis: CBC with ESR, CRP, and contrast MRI (Figure 8) are the recommended diagnostic tools. For the detection of organisms, CT-guided aspiration of large ventral abscesses is recommended, but for localized abscesses within the spinal canal, surgical decompression and collection of pus and abscess wall should be performed. The latter should be sent for Gram stain, AFB stain, and culture in blood agar media and Lowenstein–Jensen media; fungal stain should also be sought.

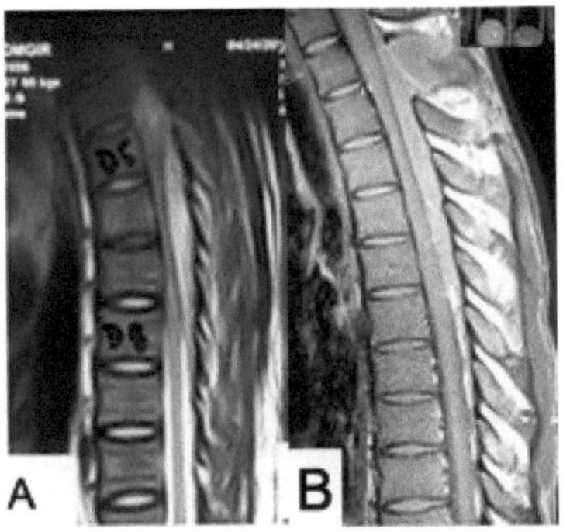

Figure 8. (**A**,**B**) Dorsal spinal epidural abscess. Source: Figure by authors.

13.4. Treatment

Early identification, CT scan-guided aspiration/drainage, and empirical antibiotic therapy followed by cultures with sensitivities are the mainstays of treatment. If the patient has acute neurological deficits, more than minor sensory disturbances, or is neurologically deteriorating, surgical decompression and debridement plus/minus spinal stabilization should be performed; postoperative complications, like arachnoiditis, may permanently worsen the patient's neurological status. As a result, the risks and advantages of a surgical procedure must be carefully weighed (Michel et al. 2006; Khanna et al. 1996; Del Curling et al. 1990).

13.5. Outcome

SEAs are fatal in 4–31% of cases (Tuli 2007). Patients with severe neurologic deficits rarely improve, even with surgical intervention within 6–12 h of the start of paralysis. Pott's disease has a 75% recurrence rate.

14. Pyogenic Spondylodiscitis

14.1. Introduction and Aetiopathogenesis

Pyogenic spondylodiscitis is a potentially fatal infection of the intervertebral disc(s) and/or neighbouring vertebrae (Skaf et al. 2010). It can happen as a result of haematogenous implantation during bacteraemia, direct dissemination from a nearby infection, or implantation during spinal surgery (Skaf et al. 2010). Spondylodiscitis is becoming more common, despite the fact that it is still a rare condition (Govender 2005). Abscess development in the epidural space and neighbouring soft tissues and muscle is common with spondylodiscitis. Localized inflammation and abscess formation can lead to spinal cord compression plus/minus vertebral column instability, resulting in long-term neurological impairment (Skaf et al. 2010).

In paediatric patients, an isolated intervertebral disc infection occurs first, followed by the involvement of the neighbouring endplates. By the age of 15, the anastomoses between the equatorial and circumferential superficial metaphyseal arteries shrink to the point of atrophy. In adults, nutrient end arteries supply the subchondral spongy bone, where a small septic embolus may lodge in the presence of bacteraemia and proceed to grow, resulting in a bone infarct and subsequent osteomyelitis. Infection spreads to neighbouring vertebral bodies by bridging anastomotic vessels from one metaphysis to the next (Skaf et al. 2010). After settling in the subchondral space, the infection usually progresses into the disc, resulting in osteomyelitis and discitis. The infection can then spread across the disc and into neighbouring endplates (Wong-Chung et al. 1999). Unlike spontaneous spondylodiscitis in adults, which begins in the body of the vertebra and then spreads to the disc space, iatrogenic or postoperative spondylodiscitis is characterized by direct disc space involvement. It is important to mention that its incidence, predisposing factors, causative organisms, and management strategies vary throughout the world.

14.2. *Clinical Presentation*

Patient may have symptoms long before the diagnosis. Patients commonly experience pain (up to 90%) and fever (only 52%). The commonest symptom is pain, which is usually confined to the spine, is aggravated by movement, and can radiate (Wong-Chung et al. 1999). The commonest symptoms of spondylodiscitis include paravertebral muscle soreness and spasm, as well as limitations in spine movement. In some situations, neurologic problems like spinal cord or nerve root compression, as well as meningitis, may occur (12%). The development of an epidural abscess is indicated by the evolution of spinal discomfort to radicular symptoms, followed by weakening and paralysis (Sapico and Montgomerie 1990), or by the infected level's kyphotic collapse. Because of mostly anterior cord compression, sensory impairment is uncommon, although motor and long-tract symptoms are more typical (Eismont et al. 1983).

14.3. *Investigations*

14.3.1. Imaging

X-ray of the spine may show reduced disc space, fracture, and deformity. CT scan of the spine shows bone involvement and deformity. MRI of the spine shows soft-tissue involvement, abscess, and cord compression (Figures 9–11).

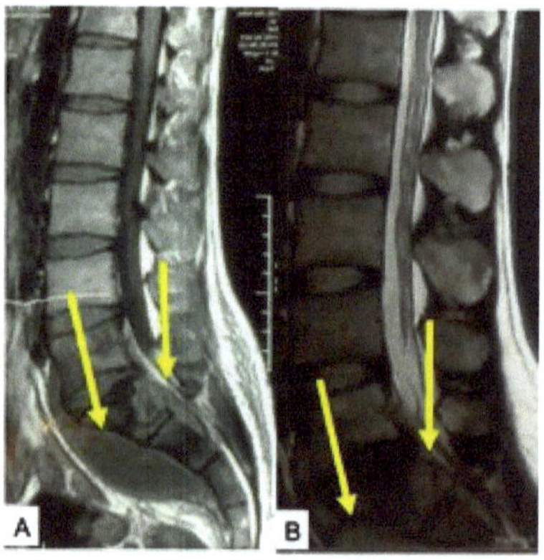

Figure 9. (**A**,**B**) MRI of lumbosacral spine showing lumbosacral spondylodiscitis (pyogenic) with epidural and presacral abscess (arrow marked). Source: Figure by authors.

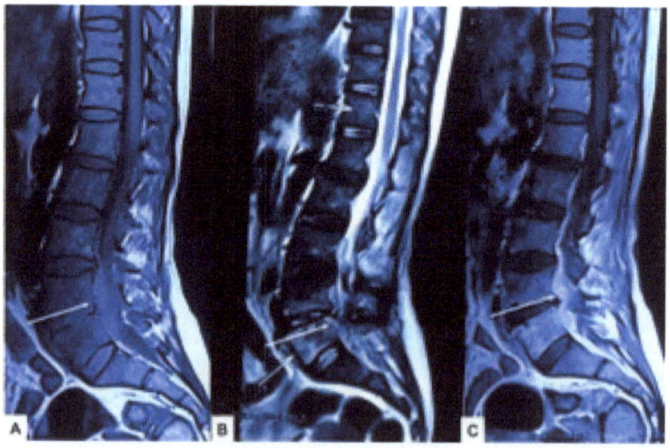

Figure 10. (**A–C**) MRI of lumbosacral spine showing L5 and S1 spondylodiscitis (pyogenic) with epidural abscess. Source: Figure by authors.

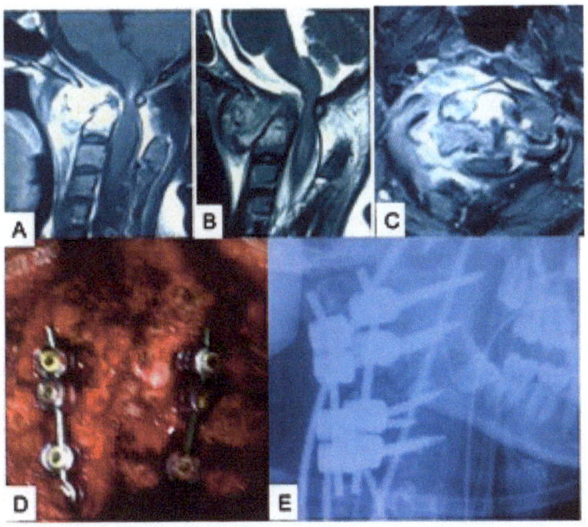

Figure 11. (**A–C**) MRI of craniovertebral junction (CVJ) showing pyogenic spondylodiscitis resulting in CVJ instability and spinal cord compression. (**D**) Intraoperative picture of fixation of CVJ (C1, C2, and C3). (**E**) Intraoperative X-ray of fixation. Source: Figure by authors.

14.3.2. Laboratory Investigations

The WBC could be abnormally high. In almost all situations, an increase in ESR is noted, even if it is nonspecific. A steady decline in ESR is frequently observed with appropriate medical treatment. Although nonspecific, C-reactive protein (CRP) may be a more clinically relevant marker than ESR and should be utilized to track the progression of the disease (Rath et al. 1996). Culture specimens should be taken from the blood, urine, and focused suppurative processes. Blood cultures can be positive in around 50% of patients, and they can help with antimicrobial medication selection.

14.3.3. Image-Guided Needle Biopsy

If an organism cannot be detected using less intrusive culture procedures, direct cultures from the involved vertebral body or/+ disc space are used. Percutaneous needle biopsy guided by CT or fluoroscopy (accuracy rate ranges from 70% to 100%, while open biopsies are accurate in more than 80% of cases) can be performed (An et al. 2006).

14.3.4. Open Biopsy

Open biopsy techniques have an accuracy of 93.3% (Razak et al. 2000) but are associated with morbidity (Lestini and Bell 1990).

14.3.5. PCR

Non-culture amplification-based DNA analysis (PCR) is also highly specific and sensitive; it commonly identifies the Mycobacterium.

Biopsy material should be sent for pyogenic, bacterial, tubercular, and fungal cultures with histological examination, staining (Gram and AFB), and PCR. The bacteria responsible for spontaneous pyogenic spondylo discitis arelisted in Table 1.

14.3.6. Differential Diagnosis

Inflammatory, granulomatous, neoplastic, or degenerative processes are all possible causes of pyogenic spondylodiscitis (Sapico and Montgomerie 1990). Inflammatory disorders such appendicitis, pyelonephritis, abdominal abscesses, and intestinal infarction might mimic spondylodiscitis in terms of clinical presentation.

14.3.7. Complications

Cervical spine infections can cause a retropharyngeal abscess, and dorsal spine infections can be complicated by life-threatening mediastinitis. Spondylodiscitis at any level can cause complications like epidural abscess, meningitis, subdural abscess, absence of lordosis, vertebral collapse with consequent spinal instability, and progressive neurological deterioration. A terrible consequence is epidural abscess. The prognosis of epidural abscesses is worse than that of epidural granulation tissue. Vertebral osteomyelitis can cause long-term spinal impairment. Neurological impairments, a diagnosis delay of at least 8 weeks, and chronic debilitating disorders were all found to be predictors of a poor prognosis. Some SEA patients may still experience irreversible paralysis. Long-term rehabilitation is frequently required. The mortality rate for vertebral osteomyelitis has been published to be between 2 and 20%; it is around 5% for SEA (Kourbeti et al. 2008).

Table 1. Bacterial aetiological organisms in pyogenic spontaneous spondylodiscitis.

Gram-Positive Aerobic Cocci	Percentages
Staphylococcus aureus	57
Streptococcus pyogene	4.1
Coagulase-negative staphylococci	3.4
Other streptococci	2
Enterococcus spp.	0.7
Gram-Negative Aerobic Bacilli	
Escherichia coli	10.5
Proteus spp.	6.7
Pseudomonas aeruginosa	5.7
Klebsiella pneumoniae	1.8
Enterobacter spp.	1.8
Salmonella spp.	1.8
Serratia marcescens	0.5
Anaerobic Bacteria	
Propionibacterium spp.	2
Bacteroides fragilis	0.5
Peptostreptococcus spp.	0.5

Source: Authors' compilation based on data from Sapico and Montgomerie (1990).

14.3.8. Early Diagnosis

Spondylodiscitis is generally recognized at a later stage. Early detection is predicated on a significant index of suspicion, with a focus on the following factors: (1) presence of an infectious focus; (2) presence of predisposing risk factors like increased age, rheumatoid arthritis, diabetes mellitus, immunosuppression, steroid utilization, ethanol abuse, history of recent invasive diagnostic or surgical spinal procedure, and infectious endocarditis (Eismont et al. 1983; Lestini and Bell 1990); (3) localized spinal pain along with paravertebral muscle spasm, fever, restriction of movement, and presence of neurological deficit.

14.3.9. Management and Outcome

Management should attempt to alleviate pain, avoid or aid in recovery from neurologic impairments, eliminate infection, avoid relapse, and restore spinal stability.

Conservative Treatment

Conservative management principles include (a) establishing a correct microbiological diagnosis; (b) treating with proper antibiotics; (c) immobilization of the spine; and (d) monitoring for clinical and radiological sign/s of instability of the spine, infection progression, or neurological impairment.

- Spinal column immobilization.
- Specimens for microbiological tests should be obtained at admission, and blood for blood cultures should be collected three times.
- A percutaneous biopsy of the afflicted disc is required if these tests are negative. Following surgery, blood cultures should be acquired on a regular basis (Cherasse et al. 2003).
- Unless clinical circumstances dictate differently, such as in patients with neutropenia or severe sepsis, antimicrobial therapy should not be started until the organism has been isolated and identified (Grados et al. 2007). Depending on the clinician's best judgement of the likely organism/s (Ozuna and Delamarter 1996) and the patient's risk factors, the patient should be started on empiric wide-spectrum antibiotic therapy.

Direct antibiotics should be given intravenously once an organism has been detected. Treatment failure was found to be more common when parenteral antibiotic therapy was given for fewer than four weeks, according to studies (Eismont et al. 1983). Most guidelines recommend 6–12 weeks of intravenous antibiotic treatment for pyogenic spondylodiscitis. When debridement is adequately accomplished, theoretically, further intravenous antibiotic treatment duration can be shorter than that of conservative therapy alone (Li et al. 2018).

Surgical Treatment

Indications for neurosurgical management in pyogenic spontaneous spondylodiscitis:

1. Failure of conservative therapy to work.
2. Neurologic impairments that are severe or worsening.
3. Septic embolization or big paraspinal abscess causing local mass impact.
4. Substantial osseous disease affecting two nearby vertebral bodies or a single vertebral body with more than 50% loss.
5. Spinal malformation that worsens over time with or without intractable spinal pain.

Principles of neurosurgical treatment (Figure 11):

- Complete debridement and elimination of diseased tissue.
- Decompression of nerve components.
- Spinal alignment restoration.
- Adjustment of spinal instability.
- Infection usually affects just the anterior vertebral components. Intact posterior components normally preserve some degree of rigidity, preventing major subluxation. As a result, decompression laminectomy alone may destabilize the spine even more, leading to a greater neurological deficit (Eismont et al. 1983).
- In situations of dorsally located epidural abscesses, only laminectomy is recommended. A limited disc space infection can be managed with posterolateral debridement in some patients. However, for thoracic and lumbar lesions, anterior procedures are generally recommended for thorough debridement of the intervertebral disc and vertebral bodies to return to healthy bone, followed by autologous bone grafting utilizing either an anterolateral (Gasbarrini et al. 2005) or a posterolateral (Eismont et al. 1983; McGuire and Eismont 1994) route that preserves the facets, pedicles, and laminae. Several studies have recommended the utilization of autologous grafts after appropriate debridement (Schuster et al. 2000). Recent research has backed the usage of titanium mesh cages to avoid the morbidity of autografts and the slow rate of assimilation of structural allografts (Fayazi et al. 2004).
- Moreover, despite surgery, there is a substantial number of studies urging prolonged bed rest du e to a worry of reinfecting the patient with foreign implants.
- Depending on the number of segments affected, bone quality, and the existence of pre-existing kyphotic deformity, a few recent papers have advocated further posterior fixation following anterior decompression and fusion (Rea et al. 1992).
- Patients who have already had posterior fixation or titanium cages have a lower risk of postoperative problems (Hee et al. 2002).
- Recently, Rath et al. revealed that a posterolateral technique can be used to successfully perform debridement, autologous interbody bone grafting, and internal fixation, allowing for early patient mobilization (Rath et al. 1996).
- Recent research has shown that in cases of acute spinal infection, primary arthrodesis and stabilization can be accomplished (Faraj and Webb 2000).
- Spinal instrumentation, when utilized in the case of kyphotic deformity or subluxation, is a very important adjunct that can be used successfully if a careful debridement of contaminated tissue is performed along with antibiotics.

15. Postoperative and Iatrogenic Spondylodiscitis

15.1. Introduction

The only way an adult with an avascular intervertebral disc space can contract genuine discitis is through direct inoculation of the pathogen. After an ordinary lumbar discectomy, postoperative discitis has been documented to occur in between 0.7 and 2.8% of patients (Kraemer et al. 2003). When a fusion is added to the operation, the frequency rates jump from 0.9% to 6%. The rate of infection following spinal instrumentation is, on average, 7% with a range of 1.3–12% (Gepstein and Eismont 1990). Infection can occur after laminectomy, lumbar puncture, myelogram, lumbar sympathectomy, chemonucleolysis, and discography, as well as other spinal operations.

15.2. Predisposing Factors and Aetiology

Age, uncontrolled diabetes, malnutrition, steroid medication, radiated area, pre-existing malignancy, long preoperative hospital stays, insufficient sterile practices, longer procedures, and more operating room traffic are all predisposing factors. Patients with postoperative spondylodiscitis have been shown to be younger, to have fewer underlying disorders, and to have a longer time between the beginning of symptoms and diagnosis than those with spontaneous spondylodiscitis (Dufour et al. 2005).

The most typical symptom of a postoperative infection is a brief respite from symptoms after surgery, preceded by a recurrence of back pain 2–6 weeks later, aggravated by almost any spinal motion and occasionally radiating to the hip, groin, leg, abdomen, scrotum, or perineum. Fever, increased perspiration, and chills are common constitutional complaints. In 33% of the instances, local tenderness is present (Natale et al. 1992). In most cases, the surgical site looks to be benign. Neurologic deficits are uncommon, but if they do occur, an epidural abscess or cauda equina syndrome due to recurrent disc prolapse should be suspected (Heller 1992). ESR is frequently raised despite the lack of leukocytosis, although the trend of alterations on periodic ESR testing might be very informative. Plain radiographs are initially normal in postoperative spondylodiscitis, but later (on average, after 3 months) demonstrate reduced disc space height and a blurring of the affected endplates.

The preferred test is MR imaging, which yields results that are akin to those found in spontaneous pyogenic spondylodiscitis. In postoperative spodylodiscitis, *Staphylococcus epidermidis* is the most prevalent pathogen, followed by *Staphylococcus aureus* bacteria. Gram-negative bacteria such as *Escherichia coli* and Pseudomonas aeruginosa can also be blamed (Jimenez-Mejias et al. 1999).

15.3. Treatment

Analgesics, muscle relaxants, antibiotics, immobilization in a halo vest or brace, and bed rest should be used to treat postoperative and iatrogenic spondylodiscitis. Any suspected postoperative infection should be subject to a CT-guided needle aspirate with culture. If pyogenic infection is confirmed or highly suspected, a minimum of 6 weeks of culture-specific injectable antibiotics is suggested (or until ESR drops sufficiently), starting with an anti-staphylococcal antibiotic (e.g., vancomycin +/− rifampin) and a broad-spectrum anti-Gram-negative antibiotic, pending the identification of the organism, and then modifying the regimen depending on the sensitivity data. When the organism detected is MRSA, and because vancomycin monotherapy has been linked to low success rates, combined therapy or a newer anti-staphylococcal medication should be considered. Epidural abscess formation, sepsis, and increasing neurological impairments all require surgery. The surgical route is mostly determined by the severity of the condition. Patients who are diagnosed earlier in the course of the disease can be managed by re-exploration later on. An anterior approach is recommended in more extensive or chronic situations (Skaf et al. 2010).

16. Fungal Spinal Infection

Fungal infections of the spine are rather infrequent. Fungi like Coccidioides immitis as well as Blastomyces dermatitidis are only found in some parts of the world, although cryptococcus, aspergillus, and candida can be found wherever. Candida and Aspergillus are natural body commensals that cause disease in those who are susceptible (patients with uncontrolled diabetes, immunosuppressed and immunocompromised individuals, patients with HIV infection, etc.) when they enter the circulatory system through intravenous lines, prosthetic device implantation, or surgically. For other fungi, spinal infection is frequently the result of the fungus spreading through the blood or directly from a pulmonary source of infection. Vertebral compression fractures and severe deformities of the spine can occur when the vertebral bodies are involved. Psoas or paravertebral abscesses can develop if an infection spreads along the anterior longitudinal ligament. Early detection of the disease necessitates a surgeon's experience, a high index of suspicion, a thorough travel history, and a thorough physical examination, especially in patients with weakened immune systems. Treatment is mainly founded on the rapid administration of suitable medication (typically injectable at first, then long-term oral medicine) and ongoing clinical monitoring. Indications for surgery (debridement and stabilization plus spinal fusion) include resistance to medicinal therapy, spinal instability, and neurologic impairments. The patient's premorbid status, the variety of the fungal pathogen, and the time of treatment commencement all influence the prognosis (Kim et al. 2006).

17. Parasitic Spinal Infestation

In poorer countries with insufficient sanitation, parasitic illnesses are more common. The spine can be affected by a variety of different parasite infections that impact the CNS. Patients may present with common symptoms like back pain, weakness, numbness, or autonomic incontinence, prompting the clinician to conduct appropriate spine imaging. These lesions can readily be misidentified for other commoner medically curable lesions in cases of parasite infection (Majmundar et al. 2019).

17.1. Neurocysticercosis

Taenia solium is the causal parasite of cysticercosis, the commonest parasitic infestation of the CNS. The disease is brought on by the consumption of embryonated parasite eggs. The parasite enters the bloodstream through the small intestine and travels to a range of locations, including the eyes, skeletal muscles, and neurological systems. This condition is more likely to cause intracranial involvement; spinal cysticercosis accounts for just 1.5 to 3% of all cysticercosis cases (Figure 12).

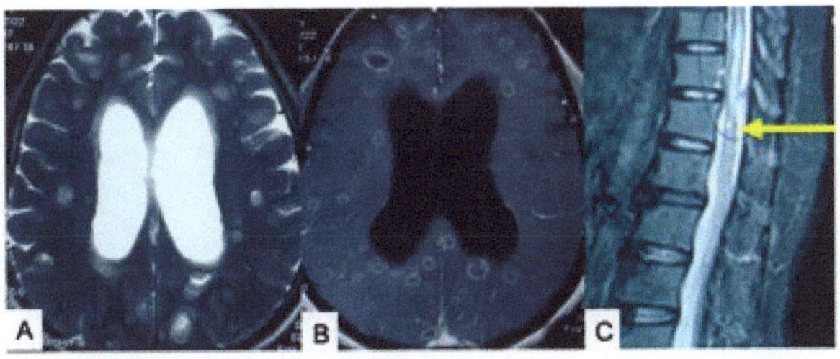

Figure 12. (**A**,**B**) MRI of the brain showing extensive neurocystocercosis. (**C**) MRI of the spine of the same patient showing neurocystocercosis in the spinal cord. Source: Figure by authors.

Spinal neurocysticercosis affecting the spinal cord is exceedingly rare, and it is present in about 1–6% of persons diagnosed with neurocysticercosis (Torabi et al. 2004). The intramedullary type is less prevalent than leptomeningeal involvement (Majmundar et al. 2019; do Amaral et al. 2015). Neurocysticercosis can affect the body of the vertebra, the epidural/subdural/subarachnoid spaces, and the spinal cord itself, similar to (intramedullary) neoplasms. Neurological deficiencies arise as a result of the cysts' mass effect and as an inflammatory response to treatment. The best imaging modality is MRI with contrast, which shows oedema, the mass effect, and enhancement, as well as cystic fluid intensity. Furthermore, the cyst and scolex can be seen using high-resolution T2W images (3D constructive interference in steady state [3D- CISS]). In asymptomatic cases, an antiparasitic drug, frequently albendazole, is administered alongside an anti-inflammatory drug, usually corticosteroids, to minimize inflammation caused by larval death. Surgery is only used in patients who have mass lesions that are causing neurological impairments. The presence of intramedullary lesions is a rare indication for surgery (Majmundar et al. 2019).

17.2. Neuroschistosomiasis

Schistosomiasis is a blood-borne infection caused by platyhelminths (flatworms) of the genus Schistosoma, which is found in Africa, Asia, and the Americas (Carod Artal 2012; Shih and Koeller 2015). Schistosoma japonicum, S. mansoni, and S. hematobium are the three primary species that can infect humans (Shih and Koeller 2015). The dispersion of eggs through venous shunts or retrograde passage of mature worms from the abdominal veins to the vertebral venous plexus are thought to be the mechanisms of CNS infection (Carod Artal 2012; Shih and Koeller 2015; do Amaral et al. 2015). When eggs are deposited into the spinal cord, the host responds with inflammation, resulting in many of the neurological issues related to advanced schistosomiasis. Inflammatory processes can result in space-occupying granulomatous masses in severe situations. Acute or subacute clinical presentation most commonly affects the lower spinal cord (Ferrari and Moreira 2011). Low back discomfort radiating down the legs, lower limb weakness and paraesthesias, deep tendon reflex abnormalities, bladder dysfunction, sexual impotence, and constipation are all clinical characteristics. Conus medullaris syndrome, acute myelopathy, or acute/subacute lower extremity myeloradiculopathy are all possible symptoms. Due to intramedullary granuloma formation, MRI may show swelling of the spinal cord, particularly in the lower part of the spinal cord and in the conus medullaris (Ferrari and Moreira 2011). Thickened cauda equina roots with uneven contrast enhancement are another common result (Ferrari and Moreira 2011; Adeel 2015). The enzyme-linked immunosorbent assay (ELISA) is the most dependable immunological approach for diagnosis, with a sensitivity of 50% and a specificity of 95%. The sensitivity of the indirect haemagglutination assay (IHA) testing ranges from 70% to 90%, and the integration of both immunological tests has a specificity of 93% and a sensitivity of 90%. However, tissue biopsy by surgery is the most conclusive form of diagnosis. A granuloma tissue sample would reveal schistosome ova encircled by necrosis, inflammation, and demyelination Carod Carod Artal (2012).

Schistosomicidal medicines, like praziquantel, and steroids are among the treatment possibilities Carod Carod Artal (2012). However, in cases of significant spinal cord compression and tissue diagnosis, surgical granuloma excision and decompressive laminectomy may be necessary for symptomatic relief (Majmundar et al. 2019).

17.3. *Toxoplasmosis*

Toxoplasmosis is the commonest type of opportunistic CNS infection among AIDS patients. Toxoplasma gondii, which produces the disease, is an obligate intracellular protozoan parasite (Ashraf et al. 2013).

Spinal cord involvement is not common. Furthermore, spinal cord infection is rarely found alone and is frequently coupled with intracranial involvement. Clinical signs include limb weakness, loss of sensation, and incontinence. A typical MRI finding is localized intramedullary ring-enhancing lesions (Garcia-Gubern et al. 2010). Immunological antibody testing and CSF cytology are also very useful. A summation of pyrimethamine, sulfadiazine, and folinic acid is the preferred therapeutic therapy. Trimethoprim–sulfamethoxazole is another option for treatment. Steroids have also been successfully utilized to relieve symptoms (García-García et al. 2015). In many circumstances, surgical intervention has no clearly defined purpose (Majmundar et al. 2019).

17.4. *Echinococcal (Hydatid) Disease*

Echinococcus granulosus and Echinococcus multilocularis are the two most frequent echinococcal pathogens. Although echinococcal disease of the CNS is uncommon, the dorsal spine is the most frequently afflicted area of the CNS (Neumayr et al. 2013). The symptoms of spinal involvement are nonspecific and are caused by spinal cord compression, which leads to myelopathy or radiculopathy (Majmundar et al. 2019). Cystic lesions in adjacent vertebral bodies, spondylitis, and bone lysis can all be seen on plain X-rays. Ultrasonography may aid in the detection of abdominal involvement. Osteolytic lesions of the vertebral bodies can be seen with a CT scan (Czermak et al. 2001). Intravenous contrast does not enhance the lesion (Prabhakar et al. 2005). The most sensitive neuroimaging modality for detecting spinal hydatid disease is MRI (Prabhakar et al. 2005). T1W scans typically show a cystic wall that is hypointense or isointense, but T2W images show a hypointense cystic wall with a hyperintense cyst (Pamir et al. 2002). Spinal tuberculosis, abscess, malignancy, and cystic lesions like spinal arachnoid cysts, epidermoids, or aneurysmal bone cysts are among the differential diagnoses (do Amaral et al. 2015). A definitive diagnosis can only be made through surgical exploration and histological testing. Tests for serodiagnosis are specific but not sensitive. The therapy of choice is surgery (Pamir et al. 2002). Though the necessity for spinal fusion should always be evaluated based on the amount of the lesion, the most commonly performed treatment is simple decompressive laminectomy (Figure 13a,b and Figure 14).

The majority of surgical operations are performed using the posterior approach (Pamir et al. 2002). In most cases, radical surgical excision is preferred. The use of scolicidal drugs intraoperatively to limit parasite dispersion during the operation has been recorded in cases of hydatid cyst excision in the abdomen and pelvis (Majmundar et al. 2019; Besim et al. 1998), but it might theoretically give a comparable protective advantage in cases of hydatid cyst removal in the spine.

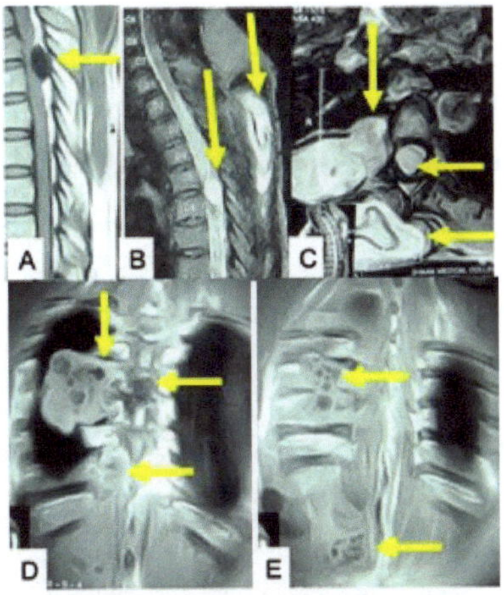

(a)

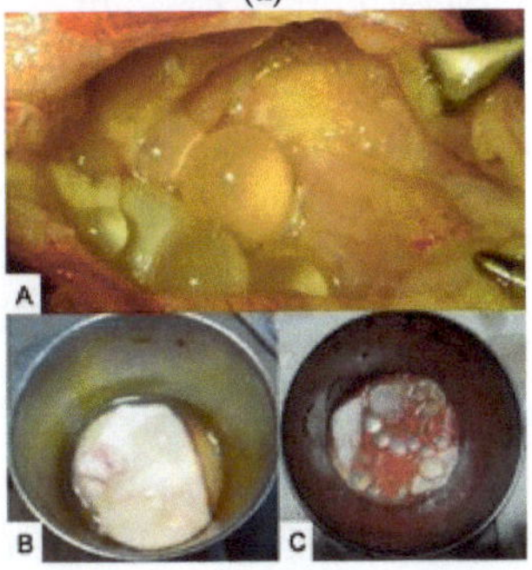

(b)

Figure 13. (a) MRI of dorsal spine (sagittal sections) showing spinal hydatid cyst causing cord compression (**A**,**B**); MRI of dorsal spine (axial section) showing spinal, mediastinal, and intramuscular hydatid cyst (marked with an arrow) (**C**); MRI of chest and upper abdomen (coronal section) showing hydatid cysts in mediastinum and liver (**D**,**E**). (**b**) Intraoperative pictures of patient in (**a**). Daughter cysts in intramuscular hydatid cyst (**A**); hydatid cysts after removal (**B**,**C**). Source: Figure by authors.

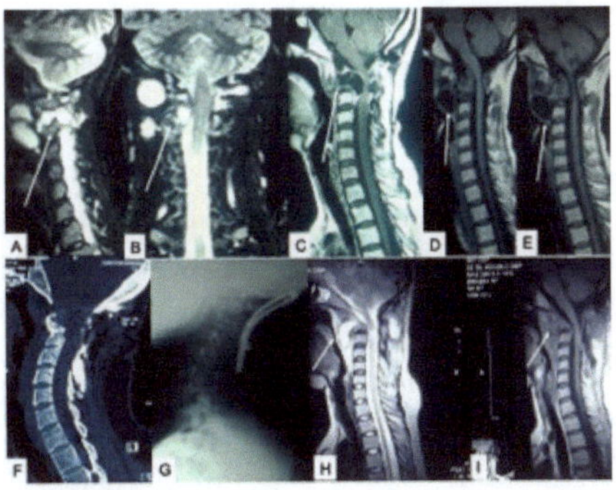

Figure 14. (**A–I**) MRI of CVJ showing hydatidosis (Echinococcosis) with instability and cord compression. Source: Figure by authors.

18. Conclusions

Spinal infections are not common, and presentation is usually nonspecific, so early diagnosis is difficult. Nevertheless, appropriate imaging modalities, like MRI with Gad enhancement, blood tests (ESR, CRP), biopsy, and histopathology can aid in making the diagnosis and can guide the proper management, either surgical or nonsurgical, to preserve neurological function and spinal stability. Assessment of the remission of clinical features and of the normalization of ESR and CRP are part of the long-term follow-up. Recurrent infections frequently necessitate surgical intervention and long-term antibiotic therapy.

Author Contributions: Conceptualization, methodology, validation, formal analysis, investigation, resources, data curation, M.R.H. and F.H.C.; writing—original draft preparation, E.A.Z.; writing—review and editing, visualization, supervision, F.H.C. All authors have read and agreed to the published version of the manuscript.

Funding: This research received no external funding.

Conflicts of Interest: The authors declare no conflicts of interest.

References

Adeel, Ahmed Awad. 2015. Spinal cord schistosomiasis. *Sudanese Journal of Paediatrics* 15: 23–28.

Al Sebai, M. Wasef, M. Monir Madkour, and K. R. Al Moutaery. 2004. Surgical Management of Spinal Tuberculosis. In *Tuberculosis*. Edited by M. Monir Madkour. Berlin: Springer, pp. 493–534.

An, Howard S., Koichi Masuda, and Nozomu Inoue. 2006. Intervertebral disc degeneration: Biological and biomechanical factors. *Journal of Orthopaedic Science* 11: 541–52. [CrossRef]

Ashraf, Aabid, Altaf Kirmani, Abdul Bhat, and Arif Sarmast. 2013. A rare case of recurrent primary spinal echinococcosis. *Asian Journal of Neurosurgery* 8: 206–8. [CrossRef]

Benli, I. Teoman, Alper Kaya, and Emre Acaroglu. 2007. Anterior instrumentation in tuber- culous spondylitis: Is it effective and safe? *Clinical Orthopaedics and Related Research* 460: 108–16. [CrossRef]

Besim, H., K. Karayalçin, O. Hamamci, Ç. Güngör, and A. Korkmaz. 1998. Scolicidal agents in hydatid cyst surgery. *HPB Surgery* 10: 347–51. [CrossRef]

Broner, Frank A., Douglas E. Garland, and Jack E. Zigler. 1996. Spinal infections in the immunocompromised host. *Orthopedic Clinics of North America* 27: 37–46. [CrossRef]

Brown, R., K. McHugh, M. Hussain, V. Novelli, and D. Jones. 2001. Discitis in young children. *Bone & Joint Surgery British Volume* 83: 106–11. [CrossRef]

Butler, Joseph S., Martin J. Shelly, Marcus Timlin, William G. Powderly, and John M. O'Byrne. 2006. Nontuberculous pyogenic spinal infection inadults: A 12-year experience from a tertiary referral center. *Spine* 31: 2695–700. [CrossRef]

Carod Artal, Francisco Javier. 2012. Cerebral and spinal schistosomiasis. *Current Neurology and Neuroscience Reports* 12: 666–74. [CrossRef]

Carragee, Eugene J. 1997. Pyogenic vertebral osteomyelitis. *Journal of Bone and Joint Surgery American* 79: 874–80. [CrossRef]

Chen, Yi-Cheng, Ming-Chau Chang, Shih-Tein Wang, Wing-Kuang Yu, Chien-Lin Liu, and Tain-Hsiung Chen. 2003. One-stage posterior surgery for treatment of advanced spinal tuberculosis. *Journal of the Chinese Medical Association: JCMA* 66: 411–17.

Cheng, V. C., W. C. Yam, I. F. Hung, P. C. Woo, S. K. Lau, B. S. Tang, and K. Y. Yuen. 2004. Clinical evaluation of the polymerase chain reaction for the rapid diagnosis of tuberculosis. *Journal of Clinical Pathology* 57: 281–85. [CrossRef]

Cherasse, A., D. Martin, C. Tavernier, and J. F. Maillefert. 2003. Are blood cultures performed after disco-vertebral biopsy useful in patients with pyogenic infective spondylitis? *Rheumatology (Oxford)* 42: 913. [CrossRef]

Christodoulou, Anastasios G., Panagiotis Givissis, Dimitrios Karataglis, Panagiotis D. Symeonidis, and John Pournaras. 2006. Treatment of Tuberculous Spondylitis with Anterior Stabilization and Titanium Cage. *Clinical Orthopaedics and Related Research* 444: 60–65. [CrossRef]

Czermak, Benedikt V., Karin M. Unsinn, Thaddeus Gotwald, Andreas A. Niehoff, Martin C. Freund, Peter Waldenberger, Wolfgang Vogel, and Werner R. Jaschke. 2001. *Echinococcus granulosus* Revisited: Radiologic Patterns Seen in Pediatric and Adult Patients. *American Journal of Roentgenology* 177: 1051–56. [CrossRef]

Danner, Robert L., and Barry J. Hartman. 1987. Update on spinal epidural abscess: 35 cases and review of the literature. *Reviews of Infectious Diseases* 9: 265–74. [CrossRef]

de Lucas, Enrique Marco, Andrés González Mandly, Agustín Gutiérrez, Raúl Pellón, Laura Martín-Cuesta, Javier Izquierdo, Elena Sánchez, Eva Ruiz, and Fernando Quintana. 2009. CT-guided fine-needle aspiration in vertebral osteomyelitis: True usefulness of a common practice. *Clinical Rheumatology* 28: 315–20. [CrossRef]

Del Curling, O., Jr., David J. Gower, and Joe M. McWhorter. 1990. Changing concepts in spinal epidural abscess: A report of 29 cases. *Neurosurgery* 27: 185–92. [CrossRef]

Delafuente, Jeffrey C. 1991. Nutrients and immune responses. *Rheumatic Diseases Clinics of North America* 17: 203–12. [CrossRef]

Diehn, Felix E. 2012. Imaging of spine infection. *Radiologic Clinics* 50: 777–98. [CrossRef]

do Amaral, Lázaro Luís Faria, Renato Hoffmann Nunes, and Antonio Jose da Rocha. 2015. Parasitic and rare spinal infections. *Neuroimaging Clinics* 25: 259–79. [CrossRef] [PubMed]

Dobson, Jessie. 1972. Percivall Pott. *Annals of The Royal College of Surgeons of England* 50: 54–65. [PubMed]

Duarte, Rui M., and Alexander R. Vaccaro. 2013. Spinal infection: State of the art and management algorithm. *European Spine Journal* 22: 2787–99. [CrossRef]

Dufour, Véronique, Antoine Feydy, Ludovic Rillardon, Aimée Redondo, Laurence Le Page, Frédéric Bert, Nadia Belmatoug, and Bruno Fantin. 2005. Comparative study of postoperative and spontaneous pyogenic spondylodiscitis. *Seminars in Arthritis and Rheumatism* 34: 766–71. [CrossRef]

Eismont, Frank J., H. H. Bohlman, P. L. Soni, V. M. Goldberg, and A. A. Freehafer. 1983. Pyogenic and fungal vertebral osteomyelitis with paralysis. *Journal of Bone and Joint Surgery America* 65: 19–29. [CrossRef]

Fantoni, Massimo, Enrico Maria Trecarichi, Barbara Rossi, Valentina Mazzotta, G. Di Giacomo, L. A. Nasto, E. Di Meco, and E. Pola. 2012. Epidemiological and clinical features of pyogenic spondylodiscitis. *European Review for Medical & Pharmacological Sciences* 16: 2–7.

Faraj, A. A., and J. K. Webb. 2000. Spinal instrumentation for primary pyogenic infection report of 31 patients. *Acta Orthopaedica Belgica* 66: 242–47.

Fayazi, Amir H., Steven C. Ludwig, Michael Dabbah, R. Bryan Butler, and Daniel E. Gelb. 2004. Preliminary results of staged anterior debridement and reconstruction using titanium mesh cages in the treatment of thoracolumbar vertebral osteomyelitis. *The Spine Journal* 4: 388–95. [CrossRef]

Ferrari, Teresa Cristina A., and Paulo Roberto R. Moreira. 2011. Neuroschistosomiasis: Clinical symptoms and pathogenesis. *The Lancet Neurology* 10: 853–64. [CrossRef]

Frangen, T. M., T. Kälicke, M. Gottwald, S. Andereya, H.-J. Andress, O. J. Russe, E. J. Müller, G. Muhr, and C. Schinkel. 2006. Surgical management of spondylodiscitis: An analysis of 78 cases. *Der Unfallchirurg* 109: 743–53. [CrossRef]

García-García, Concepción, Federico Castillo-Álvarez, José M. Azcona-Gutiérrez, María J. Herraiz, Valvanera Ibarra, and José A. Oteo. 2015. Spinal cord toxoplasmosis in human immunodeficiency virus infection/acquired immunodeficiency syndrome. *Infectious Diseases* 47: 277–82. [CrossRef] [PubMed]

Garcia-Gubern, Carlos, Carmen R. Fuentes, Lissandra Colon-Rolon, and Daniel Masvidal. 2010. Spinal cord toxoplasmosis as an unusual presentation of AIDS: Case report and review of the literature. *International Journal of Emergency Medicine* 3: 439–42. [CrossRef] [PubMed]

Gasbarrini, A. L., E. Bertoldi, M. Mazzetti, L. Fini, S. Terzi, F. Gonella, L. Mirabile, G. Barbanti Bròdano, A. Furno, A. Gasbarrini, and et al. 2005. Clinical features, diagnostic and therapeutic approaches to haematogenous vertebral osteomyelitis. *European Review for Medical and Pharmacological Sciences* 9: 53–66. [PubMed]

Gasbarrini, A., Luca Boriani, Caterina Salvadori, S. Mobarec, J. Kreshak, C. Nanni, E. Zamparini, M. Alberghini, Pierluigi Viale, and U. Albisinni. 2012. Biopsy for suspected spondylodiscitis. *European Review for Medical & Pharmacological Sciences* 16: 26–34.

Gemmel, Filip, Nicolas Dumarey, and Christopher J. Palestro. 2006. Radionuclide imaging of spinal infections. *European Journal of Nuclear Medicine and Molecular Imaging* 33: 1226–37. [CrossRef]

Gemmel, Filip, Paul C. Rijk, James MP Collins, Thierry Parlevliet, Katrin D. Stumpe, and Christopher J. Palestro. 2010. Expanding role of 18F-fluoro-D- deoxyglucose PET and PET/CT in spinal infections. *European Spine Journal* 19: 540–51. [CrossRef]

Gepstein, R., and F. I. Eismont. 1990. Post-Operative Spine Infections. In *The Lumbar Spine*. Edited by James N. Weinstein and Sam W. Wiesel. Philadelphia: W.B. Saunders.

Gouliouris, Theodore, Sani H. Aliyu, and Nicholas M. Brown. 2010. Spondylodiscitis: Update on diagnosis and management. *Journal of Antimicrobial Chemotherapy* 65: iii11–iii24. [CrossRef]

Govender, S. 2005. Spinal infections. *The Journal of Bone & Joint Surgery British* 87: 1454–58. [CrossRef]

Govender, S., and A. H. Parbhoo. 1999. Support of the anterior column with allografts in tuberculosis of the spine. *The Journal of Bone & Joint Surgery British* 81: 106–9. [CrossRef]

Grados, Franck, François Xavier Lescure, Eric Senneville, René Marc Flipo, Jean Luc Schmit, and Patrice Fardellone. 2007. Suggestions for managing pyogenic(non-tuberculous) discitis in adults. *Joint Bone Spine* 74: 133–39. [CrossRef]

Hayes, A. J., M. Choksey, N. Barnes, and O. C. Sparrow. 1996. Spinal tuberculosis in developed countries: Difficulties in diagnosis. *Journal of the Royal College of Surgeons of Edinburgh* 41: 192–96. [PubMed]

Hee, Hwan T., Mohammad E. Majd, Richard T. Holt, and David Pienkowski. 2002. Bettertreatment of vertebral osteomyelitis using posterior stabilization and titanium mesh cages. *Clinical Spine Surgery* 15: 149–56.
Heller, J. G. 1992. Postoperative infections of the spine. In *The Spine*. Edited by Richard H. Rothman and Frederick A. Simeone. Philadelphia: W.B. Saunders.
Hodgson, A. R., F. E. Stock, H. S. Y. Fang, and G. B. Ong. 1960. Anterior spinal fusion: The operative approach and pathological findings in 412 patients with Pott's disease of the spine. *Journal of British Surgery* 48: 172–78. [CrossRef] [PubMed]
Jain, A. K. 2010. Tuberculosis of the spine: A fresh look at an old disease. *The Journal of Bone & Joint Surgery British Volume* 92: 905–13. [CrossRef]
Jain, Anil K., and Ish Kumar Dhammi. 2007. Tuberculosis of the spine: A review. *Clinical Orthopaedics and Related Research* 460: 39–49. [CrossRef]
Jevtic, Vladimir. 2004. Vertebral infection. *European Radiology* 14: E43–E52. [CrossRef]
Jimenez-Mejias, Manuel E., Juan de Dios Colmenero, Fernando J. Sánchez-Lora, Julián Palomino-Nicás, José M. Reguera, Joaquín García de la Heras, María A. García-Ordoñez, and Jerónimo Pachón. 1999. Postoperative spondylodiskitis: Etiology, clinical findings, prognosis, and comparison with nonoperative pyo-genic spondylodiskitis. *Clinical Infectious Diseases* 29: 339–45. [CrossRef]
Khanna, Rohit K., Ghaus M. Malik, Jack P. Rock, and Mark L. Rosenblum. 1996. Spinal epidural abscess: Evaluation of factors influencing outcome. *Neurosurgery* 39: 958–64.
Kim, Choll W., Andrew Perry, Brad Currier, Michael Yaszemski, and Steven R. Garfin. 2006. fungal infection of the spine. *Clinical Orthopedics and Related Research* 444: 92–99. [CrossRef]
Kornblum, Martin B., David P. Wesolowski, Jeffrey S. Fischgrund, and Harry N. Herkowitz. 1998. Computed tomography-guided biopsy of the spine: A review of 103 patients. *Spine* 23: 81–85. [CrossRef]
Kourbeti, Irene S., Sotirios Tsiodras, and Dimitrios T. Boumpas. 2008. Spinal infections: Evolving concepts. *Current Opinion in Rheumatology* 20: 471–79. [CrossRef] [PubMed]
Kraemer, Robert, Alexander Wild, Holger Haak, Jörg Herdmann, Rüdiger Krauspe, and Jürgen Kraemer. 2003. Classification and management of early complications in open lumbar microdiscectomy. *European Spine Journal* 12: 239–46. [CrossRef] [PubMed]
Krogsgaard, Michael R., Peter Wagn, and Jörgen Bengtsson. 1998. Epidemiology of acute vertebral osteomyelitis in Denmark: 137 cases in Denmark 1978–1982, compared to cases reported to the National Patient Register 1991–1993. *Acta Orthopaedica Scandinavica* 69: 513–17. [CrossRef] [PubMed]
Kulchavenya, Ekaterina. 2014. Extrapulmonary tuberculosis: Are statistical reports accurate? *Therapeutic Advances in Infectious Disease* 2: 61–70. [CrossRef]
Kumar, Raj, Rupant K. Das, and Ashok Kumar Mahapatra. 2010. Role of interferon gamma release assay in the diagnosis of Pott disease. *Journal of Neurosurgery: Spine* 12: 462–66. [CrossRef]
Lee, Sun-Ho, Joo-Kyung Sung, and Yeun-Mook Park. 2006. Single-stage transpedicular decompression and posterior instrumentation in treatment of thoracic and thoracolumbar spinal tuberculosis: A retrospective case series. *Journal of Spinal Disorders & Techniques* 19: 595–602. [CrossRef]
Lestini, William F., and Gordon R. Bell. 1990. Spinal infections: Patient evaluation. *Journal of Neurosurgery: Spine* 2: 244–56.
Li, Yun-Da, Chak-Bor Wong, Tsung-Ting Tsai, Po-Liang Lai, Chi-Chien Niu, Lih-Huei Chen, and Tsai-Sheng Fu. 2018. Appropriate duration of post-surgical intravenous antibiotic therapy for pyogenic spondylodiscitis. *BMC Infectious Diseases* 18: 468. [CrossRef]
Lillie, Patrick, Hiten Thaker, Peter Moss, Joy Baruah, Lorraine Cullen, Damien Taylor, and Gavin Barlow. 2008. Healthcare associated discitis in the era of antimicrobial resistance. *JCR: Journal of Clinical Rheumatology* 14: 234–37. [CrossRef]
Luk, K. D. K. 1999. Tuberculosis of the spine in the new millennium. *European Spine Journal* 8: 338–45. [CrossRef]
Majmundar, Neil, Purvee D. Patel, Vincent Dodson, Ashley Tran, Ira Goldstein, and Rachid Assina. 2019. Parasitic infections of the spine: Case series and review of the literature. *Neurosurgical focus FOC* 46: E12. [CrossRef] [PubMed]
Mallick, I. H., M. H. Thoufeeq, and T. P. Rajendran. 2004. Iliopsoas abscesses. *Postgraduate Medical Journal* 80: 459–62. [CrossRef] [PubMed]
Maslen, David R., Stephen R. Jones, Mark A. Crislip, Raymond Bracis, Ronald J. Dworkin, and Jeffrey E. Flemming. 1993. Spinal epidural abscess: Optimizing patient care. *Archives of Internal Medicine* 153: 1713–21. [CrossRef] [PubMed]

McGuire, Robert A., and Frank J. Eismont. 1994. The fate of autogenous bone graftin surgically treated pyogenic vertebral osteomyelitis. *Clinical Spine Surgery* 7: 206–15.

Michel, Sven C. A., Christian W. A. Pfirrmann, Norbert Boos, and Juerg Hodler. 2006. CT-guided core biopsy of subchondral bone and intervertebral space in suspected spondylodiskitis. *American Journal of Roentgenology* 186: 977–80. [CrossRef]

Mizuno, S. 1967. Posterior approaches in spondylotomy for spinal tuberculosis. *Seikei Geka* 18: 876–82. (In Japanese).

Mylona, Eleni, Michael Samarkos, Eleni Kakalou, Panagiotis Fanourgiakis, and Athanasios Skoutelis. 2009. Pyogenic vertebral osteomyelitis: A systematic review of clinical characteristics. *Seminars in Arthritis and Rheumatism* 39: 10–17. [CrossRef]

Natale, Massimo, M. Lama, Raffaele D'Avanzo, D. Squillante, and F. A. Cioffi. 1992. Postoperative lumbar discitis. *Minerva Anestesiologica* 58: 209–15.

Neumayr, Andreas, Francesca Tamarozzi, Sam Goblirsch, Johannes Blum, and Enrico Brunetti. 2013. Spinal cystic echinococcosis—A systematic analysis and review of the literature: Part 1. Epidemiology and anatomy. *PLoS Neglected Tropical Diseases* 7: e2450. [CrossRef]

Oniankitan, Owonayo, Eyram Fianyo, Kodjovi Kakpovi, Lama K. Agoda-Koussema, and Moustafa Mijiyawa. 2014. Sacrum Pott's disease: A rare location of spine tuberculosis. *The Egyptian Rheumatologist* 36: 209–11. [CrossRef]

Ozuna, Richard M., and Rick B. Delamarter. 1996. Pyogenic vertebral osteomyelitisand postsurgical disc space infections. *The Orthopedic Clinics of North America* 27: 87–94. [CrossRef] [PubMed]

Pamir, M. Necmettin, Koray Ozduman, and Ilhan Elmaci. 2002. Spinal hydatid disease. *Spinal Cord* 40: 153–60. [CrossRef] [PubMed]

Pawar, Uday M., Vishal Kundnani, Vikas Agashe, Amita Nene, and Abhay Nene. 2009. Multidrug-resistant tuberculosis of the spine—Is it the beginning of the end? A study of twenty-five culture proven multidrug-resistant tuberculosis spine patients. *Spine* 34: E806–E810. [CrossRef]

Pertuiset, Edouard, Johann Beaudreuil, Frédéric Lioté, Anne Horusitzky, Farid Kemiche, Pascal Richette, Dominique Clerc-Wyel, Isabelle Cerf-Payrastre, Henri Dorfmann, Jacques Glowinski, and et al. 1999. Spinal tuberculosis in adults: A study of 103 cases in a developed country, 1980–1994. *Medicine (Baltimore)* 78: 309–20. [CrossRef] [PubMed]

Prabhakar, Mukund, Apurv J. Acharya, Dhaval R. Modi, and Bhavin Jadav. 2005. Spinal hydatid disease: A case series. *The Journal of Spinal Cord Medicine* 28: 426–31. [CrossRef]

Rajasekaran, S., Rishi Mugesh Kanna, and Ajoy Prasad Shetty. 2014. Pathophysiology and treatment of spinal tuberculosis. *JBJS Reviews* 2: e4. [CrossRef]

Rankine, J. J., D. A. Barron, P. Robinson, P. A. Millner, and R. A. Dickson. 2004. Therapeutic impact of percutaneous spinal biopsy in spinal infection. *Postgraduate Medical Journal* 80: 607–9. [CrossRef]

Rasouli, Mohammad R., Maryam Mirkoohi, Alexander R. Vaccaro, Kourosh Karimi Yarandi, and Vafa Rahimi-Movaghar. 2012. Spinal tuberculosis: Diagnosis and management. *Asian Spine Journal* 6: 294–308. [CrossRef]

Ratcliffe, J. F. 1985. Anatomic basis for the pathogenesis and radiologic features of vertebral osteomyelitis and its differentiation from childhood discitis: A microarteriographic investigation. *Acta Radiologica Diagnosis* 26: 137–43. [CrossRef]

Rath, Stefan A., Ulrich Neff, Ortwin Schneider, and Hans-Peter Richter. 1996. Neurosurgical management of thoracic and lumbar vertebralosteomyelitis and discitis in adults: A review of 43consecutive surgically treated patients. *Neurosurgery* 38: 926–33. [CrossRef]

Razak, M. M., Z. H. Kamari, and S. Roohi. 2000. Spinal infection—An overview and the results of treatment. *The Medical Journal of Malaysia* 55: 18–28. [PubMed]

Rea, Gary L., John M. McGregor, Carole A. Miller, and Michael E. Miner. 1992. Surgical treatment of the spontaneous spinal epidural abscess. *Surgical Neurology* 37: 274–79. [CrossRef] [PubMed]

Sapico, Francisco L., and John Z. Montgomerie. 1990. Vertebral osteomyelitis. *Infectious Disease Clinics of North America* 4: 539–50. [CrossRef] [PubMed]

Schimmer, Ralph C., Christina Jeanneret, Pierce D. Nunley, and Bernard Jeanneret. 2002. Osteomyelitis of the cervical spine: A potentially dramatic disease. *Journal of Spinal Disorders & Techniques* 15: 110–17.

Schirmer, Patricia, Cybèle A. Renault, and Mark Holodniy. 2010. Is spinal tuberculosis contagious? *International Journal of Infectious Diseases* 14: e659–E666. [CrossRef]

Schuster, James M., Anthony M. Avellino, Frederick A. Mann, Allain A. Girouard, M. Sean Grady, David W. Newell, H. Richard Winn, Jens R. Chapman, and Sohail K. Mirza. 2000. Use of structural allografts in spinalosteomyelitis: A review of 47 cases. *Journal of Neurosurgery: Spine* 93: 8–14. [CrossRef]

Shang, H., D. Y. Wang, and G. H. Wen. 2010. I-Stage surgical treatment for thoracolumbar spinal tuberculosis with kyphosis. *Chinese General Practice* 32: 42.

Sharif, Hassan S. 1992. Role of MR imaging in the management of spinal infections. *AJR. American Journal of Roentgenology* 158: 1333–45. [CrossRef]

Shih, Robert Y., and Kelly K. Koeller. 2015. Bacterial, fungal, and parasitic infections of the central nervous system: Radiologic-pathologic correlation and historical perspectives. *Radiographics* 35: 1141–69. [CrossRef]

Skaf, Ghassan S., Nathalie T. Domloj, Michael G. Fehlings, Carmel H. Bouclaous, Amira S. Sabbagh, Zeina A. Kanafani, and Souha S. Kanj. 2010. Pyogenic spondylodiscitis: An overview. *Journal of Infection and Public Health* 3: 5–16. [CrossRef]

Sobottke, Rolf, Harald Seifert, Gerd Fätkenheuer, Matthias Schmidt, Axel Goßmann, and Peer Eysel. 2008. Current diagnosis and treatment of spondylodiscitis. *Deutsches Ärzteblatt International* 105: 181–87. [CrossRef] [PubMed]

Su, Shou-Hsin, Wen-Cheng Tsai, Chun-Yu Lin, Wei-Ru Lin, Tun-Chieh Chen, Po-Liang Lu, Pei-Ming Huang, Jong-Rung Tsai, Ya-Ling Wang, Ming-Chu Feng, and et al. 2010. Clinical features and outcomes of spinal tuberculosis in southern Taiwan. *Journal of Microbiology, Immunology and Infection* 43: 291–300. [CrossRef] [PubMed]

Tayles, Nancy, and Hallie R. Buckley. 2004. Leprosy and tuberculosis in Iron Age Southeast Asia? *American Journal of Physical Anthropology* 125: 239–56. [CrossRef]

Torabi, Amir M., Mary Quiceno, Dianne B. Mendelsohn, and Craig M. Powell. 2004. Multilevel intramedullary spinal neurocysticercosis with eosinophilic meningitis. *Archives of Neurology* 61: 770–72. [CrossRef] [PubMed]

Tuli, Surendra Mohan. 1993. *Tuberculosis of the Skeletal System*. New Delhi: JayPee Brothers Medical, pp. 144–53.

Tuli, Surendra Mohan. 2007. Tuberculosis of the spine: A historical review. *Clinical Orthopaedics and Related Research* 460: 29–38. [CrossRef]

Tyrrell, P. N. M., V. N. Cassar-Pullicino, and I. W. McCall. 1999. Spinal infection. *European Radiology* 9: 1066–77. [CrossRef]

Velayati, Ali Akbar, Mohammad Reza Masjedi, Parissa Farnia, Payam Tabarsi, Jalladein Ghanavi, Abol Hassan ZiaZarifi, and Sven Eric Hoffner. 2009. Emergence of new forms of totally drug-resistant tuberculosis bacilli: Super extensively drug-resistant tuberculosis or totally drug-resistant strains in Iran. *Chest* 136: 420–25. [CrossRef]

Wong-Chung, John K., Shaheed A. Naseeb, Sangam G. Kaneker, and Ali J. Aradi. 1999. Anterior disc protrusion as a cause for abdominal symptoms in childhood discitis. A case report. *Spine* 24: 918–20. [CrossRef]

Spinal Vascular Lesions

Forhad H. Chowdhury, Nausher Alam and Mohammod Raziul Haque

Abstract: Spinal vascular lesions are relatively rare. For the the detection and treatment of such lesions, understanding their anatomical and pathophysiological basis is essential. Spinal ischaemic infarctions are probably extremely rare. Spinal dural AV fistulas are the commonest. These lesions may present acutely or chronically. MRI, MRA, CT scan, CTA of the spine, and spinal DSA are necessary investigation modalities for diagnosis and evaluation. Microsurgery is the mainstay of treatments; however, endovascular treatment options are sometimes very useful. In this chapter, spinal vascular malformations (including spinal AVM and AVF), spinal cord infarctions, spinal cord cavernomas and haemangiomas will be discussed briefly encompassing their management options.

Abbreviations

ASA	anterior spinal artery	AVM	arteriovenous malformation
AVF	arteriovenous fistula	CM	cavernous malformation
CT	computed tomography	CTA	computed tomographic angiography
dAVF	dural AVF	dAVM	dural AVM
DSA	digital subtraction angiogram	MRI	magnetic resonance imaging
MRA	magnetic resonance angiography	PSA	posterior spinal artery
SVM	spinal vascular malformation	ST	soft tissue
VB	vertebral body	VH	vertebral haemangioma

1. Spinal Vascular Anatomy

The posterior and anterior spinal arteries are the main blood vessels that perfuse the spinal cord's intricate blood supply system. To appreciate the pathophysiology of spinal vascular pathologies, one must have a comprehensive understanding of the usual spinal blood supply. The posterior and the anterior artery systems supply the spinal cord. The anterior arterial system is created by the anterior spinal artery (ASA), which remains in the anterior median fissure. The anterior horn's grey matter and the corticospinal tracts, including the spinothalamic tracts, are all supplied by sulcal arteries that emerge from the anterior spinal artery. Between the two posterior spinal arteries (PSAs), the posterior artery system creates a plexiform network of collaterals. It nourishes the posterior third of the spinal cord (Singh et al. 2016; Greenberg 2010).

The posterior and anterior spinal arteries typically receive a feeding from 6 to 10 medullary arteries. The vertebral arteries, including branches of the thyrocervical trunk, give rise to the medullary arteries in the cervical region. These medullary arteries arise from the intercostal and lumbar arteries, which in turn develop from the aorta and the iliac arteries in the dorsal and lumbar regions. The biggest of these medullary arteries, the artery of Adamkiewicz, normally arises on the left side to supply the spinal cord from D8 to L2 (Singh et al. 2016; Greenberg 2010; Lindsay et al. 2011).

2. Spinal Cord Ischaemic Conditions

2.1. Anterior Spinal Artery (ASA) Syndrome

2.1.1. Introduction

Ischaemia of the ASA, which results in functional abnormalities of the anterior two-thirds of the spinal cord, is the cause of ASA syndrome. The corticospinal tract, reticulospinal tract (autonomic fibres), spinothalamic tract, and grey matter are among the spinal structures that are impacted. Motor deficit, loss of pain, loss of warmth, and hypotension are signs that are found in this syndrome. The most typical type of spinal cord infarction is ASA syndrome. The anterior spinal cord is more susceptible to ischaemia due to the single anterior spinal artery's limited collaterals (as opposed to the posterior spinal cord, which is perfused by two PSAs) (Schneider 2010).

2.1.2. Aetiology

- Aortic insufficiencies: aortic dissections, aneurysms, direct aortic trauma, surgeries, and atherosclerosis.

- Pathology of the spinal column: acute intervertebral disc herniation, kyphoscoliosis, cervical spondylosis, compromised spinal column, and neoplasms.
- Other aetiologies: vasculitis, sickle cell disease, polycythaemia, decompression sickness, and collagen and elastin diseases (Schneider 2010).
- Any thrombus or embolus in the artery of Adamkiewicz can result in ASA syndrome (Yoon et al. 2002).

2.1.3. Clinical Features

- Total motor paralysis caudal to the level of the infarction.
- Loss of temperature and pain sensation at and caudal to the level of the infarction (Greenberg 2010).
- Intact sense of proprioception (Foo and Rossier 1983.)
- Autonomic dysfunctions: hypotension (either frank or orthostatic), sexual dysfunction, and/or bladder and bowel dysfunction (Cheshire et al. 1996; Cheung et al. 2002).
- Areflexia, flaccid external and internal sphincter tone leading to anal and urinary incontinence, and intestinal obstruction can also be found (Schneider 2010).

Symptoms generally occur very rapidly and are frequently experienced within 1 h of the initial damage.

2.1.4. Investigations

Ten to fifteen hours after the onset of symptoms, MRI can determine the extent and site of the damage. It is possible to employ diffusion-weighted imaging since it can detect impairment within a few minutes after the onset of symptoms (Schneider 2010). MRA, CTA, and DSA can be performed but have little value. Investigations for the identification of causes are needed.

2.1.5. Treatment

The root cause and symptoms will determine the course of treatment. The prognosis is bad when the diagnosis is hidden. The mortality rate is about 20%, and 50% of people die. Typically, there are only minor or no changes in symptoms (Schneider 2010).

2.2. Posterior Spinal Artery Syndrome (PSAS)

PSAS is very rare, as the white matter in the spinal cord is more resistant to ischaemia.
Clinical features:

- Absence of tendon reflexes/motor weakness.
- Absence of joint position sense.

Investigation: MRI T2W and DW images will easily diagnose the condition.
Treatment: Treatment is symptomatic and directed toward the aetiology (Greenberg 2010).

2.3. Venous Infarction (Total Cord Syndrome)

This is a swift "total" cord syndrome with poor outcomes, frequently linked to pelvic sepsis (Greenberg 2010).

3. Spinal Vascular Malformations (SVMs)

SVMs, also commonly termed spinal AVMs, are spinal vascular malformations. Approximately 4% of primary intraspinal masses are SVMs and they mostly occur in middle age (Youmans 1982).

3.1. Classification

The American/English/French Connection Working Formulation Classification (Greenberg 2010; Lindsay et al. 2011; Youmans 1982; Gueguen et al. 1987; Mourier et al. 1993).

3.1.1. Dural AVM (Low Flow)

Type 1: dAVM or dAV–fistula (AVF); 80% of SVMs in adults are type 1 (Strugar and Chyatte 1992). They take their vascular supply from the radicular artery, which creates a fistula (AV shunt) at the dural root sleeve (in the intervertebral foramen); then, it drains into a distended vein on the posterior spinal cord. Generally, it affects the lower thoracic or lumbar spine. These SVMs have a sluggish flow. Congestion of the cord's veins may result from high pressure in the draining vein. Cord involvement could be far from the fistula. Back pain, cauda equina syndrome, progressive myeloradiculopathy, and urine retention are common symptoms in middle-aged individuals. Ninety percent of affected patients are men. Up to 35% of patients report experiencing pain. About 15–20% are connected to other AVMs (cutaneous or other). Rarely does a type 1 SVM bleed. A type 1B SVM contains two or more arterial feeders, whereas type 1A SVM has a single artery feeder.

3.1.2. Intradural AVMs (High Flow)

About 20% of spinal SVMs are intradural. Nearly 75% of intradural AVMs present clinically with sudden onset of symptoms, generally from haemorrhage (intramedullary or SAH).

Type 2 (spinal glomus AVM): These are intramedullary AVMs and the real AVM of the cord. Fifteen to twenty percent of all SVMs are glomus AVMs. A compact nidus supplied by medullary arteries with the AV shunt occupies at least partly the pia or the cord. They may be accompanied by supplying artery aneurysms. They have worse outcomes than dural AVMs. Usually one or at most two to three feeders occur in 80% of cases.

Type 3 (juvenile spinal AVM): It is an enormously engorged glomus AVM that occupies the whole cross-section of the spinal cord and extends down the vertebral body. It may lead to spinal deformity.

Type 4 (intradural perimedullary AVM): Arteriovenous fistulae (AVF) is another name for these. They are direct fistulae between the veins which drain the cord and the ASA, which typically supplies the spinal cord. Varices frequently occur in the vein immediately distal to the fistula. They are usually lethal, with bleeding into the subarachnoid space, and occur in younger individuals than type 1 (Bederson and Spetzler 1996). Based on the size and intricacy of the nidus, Merland and colleagues divided these lesions into three groups (Merland et al. 1980; Singh et al. 2016).

Subtype 1 pathologies are low-flow arteriovenous shunts in the conus or filum terminale composed of a small fistula fed by a solitary small ASA.

Subtype 2 perimedullary AVF are high- or moderate-flow fistulas. Their nidus is medium- or small-size and composed of multiple discrete shunts which are fed by several enlarged ASA sor PSAs.

Subtype 3 are multiple high-flow shunts composed of multiple dilated arteries feeding into a solitary large fistula.

3.1.3. Miscellaneous Vascular Lesions of the Spine

(i) Cavernomas of the spinal cord.
(ii) Venous angiomas of the spinal cord: very rare. Difficult to see in angiography.
(iii) Vertebral body haemangiomas.

Spetzler et al's classification of spinal vascular lesions are shown in Table 1.

3.2. Presentation

Depending on the form of AVM, the clinical characteristics of spinal AVMs can vary. The majority of spinal AV anomalies are seen in the lower dorsal and dorsolumbar spine, and the dural type is the most prevalent variety.

Table 1. Spetzler, et al.'s classification (this system of classification reincorporates vascular spinal tumours).

1. Neoplastic Vascular Lesions	2. Spinal Aneurysms (Rare)	3. Arteriovenous Lesions	
		AVF	AVMs
- Haemangioblastoma - Cavernoma	----- (very rare)	- Intradural: dorsal ventral - Extradural	- extradural–intradural - intradural - intramedullary - intramedullary–extramedullary - conus medullaris

Source: Authors' compilation based on data from Greenberg (2010); Spetzler et al. (2002).

Patients with the dural type typically complain of a myelopathy that is slowly progressing, and many of them have a history of recurrent myelopathy. The engorging vein's direct mechanical compression or a blood flow disturbance (steal/venous hypertension) that results in cord ischaemia are the two causes of the myelopathy.

The most frequent symptom on clinical presentation is motor weakness, which is preceded by paraesthesia plus sphincter abnormalities.

This type of spinal AV malformation is quite uncommonly associated with pain and acute myelopathy onset. Back pain with recent onset and myelopathy are common acute symptoms of the perimedullary and intramedullary types. Here, a burst nidus can result in intramedullary haemorrhage or subarachnoid haemorrhage. The clinical presentation may include indications of meningeal inflammation. However, a low-flow malformation or fistula might manifest symptoms gradually and can mirror the dural type's aetiology and clinical presentation (July and Wahjoepramono 2019; Dumont and Oldfield 2011; Jellema et al. 2003).

Eighty-five percent or so of patients have a growing neurodeficiency (back pain plus quadriparesis or paraparesis over months to years). Less than 5% of SVMs are present, comparable to spinal cord "tumours". About 10–20% of SVMs cause abrupt onset of myelopathy, which typically occurs in individuals under 30 years old (Greenberg 2010; Tobin and Layton 1976) and is brought on by bleeding (SAH, SDH, epidural haematoma, haematomyelia, or watershed infarction). In 2–3% of cases, a bruit is heard during auscultation above the spine. Some 3–25% of people have a lesion across their back; the Valsalva technique may make the angioma redder (Greenberg 2010; Barnwell et al. 1990; Tobin and Layton 1976).

3.3. Evaluation

3.3.1. Magnetic Resonance Imaging (MRI)

While MRI can identify some SVMs more reliably and safely than spinal DSA, it is insufficient for treatment planning. Extramedullary flow voids are present in 82% of lesions. Additionally, several levels of cord contrast enhancement are visible (from venous infarction or venous congestion). The diagnosis is not ruled out by a negative MRI. On T2WI MRI, the core region of the spinal cord may exhibit a diffuse hyperintense signal indicative of spinal cord oedema (Figure 1).

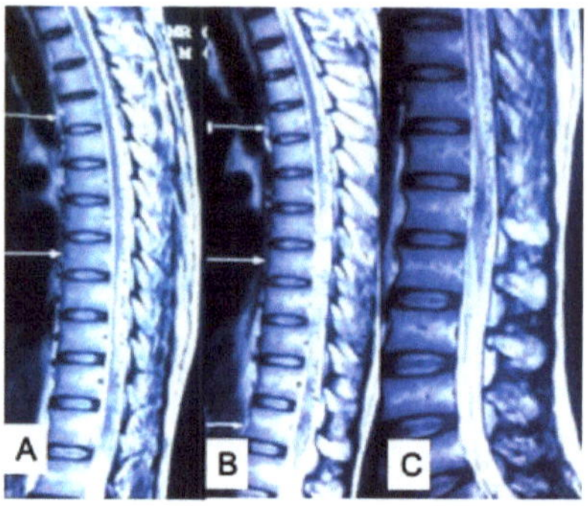

Figure 1. MRI of dorsal (**A**,**B**) and dorsolumbar spine (**C**) (T2W images, sagittal views) showing intradural vascular flow voids suggestive of spinal AVM. Source: Figure by authors.

A hypointense signal, which is more likely to be present at the cord's dorsal surface, may be present in conjunction with this lesion. An obstructed perimedullary venous plexus is represented by these hypointense signals (vascular voids). The spinal cord is frequently seen to be hypointense and enlarged on T1W imaging. When the contrast agent is infused, diffuse enhancement that corresponds to chronically obstructed veins may be visible along with a breach in the blood–spinal cord barrier.

3.3.2. Digital Subtraction Angiography (DSA)

Because DSA may be used to analyse the angiographic architecture of the vessels within or around the lesion, it becomes the preferred course of action. Additionally, DSA provides insightful data regarding the flow dynamics of the lesions, making it a significant tool for choosing treatment approaches (Figures 2 and 3).

For type 1dural AVMs, DSA must include all dural supplying arteries of the neuro-axis, including the following:

1. ICAs: the arteries of Bernasconi and Cassinari;
2. Every radicular artery, including the artery of Adamkiewicz;

3. Internal iliac arteries in search of sacral feeders.

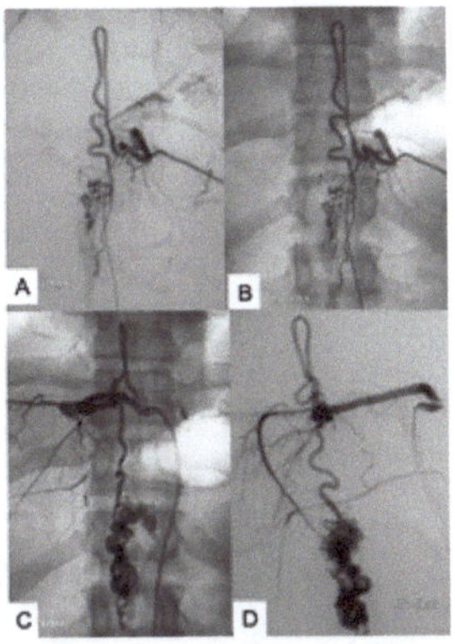

Figure 2. (A–D) Spinal DSA showing spinal AVM at dorsolumbar junction. Source: Figure by authors.

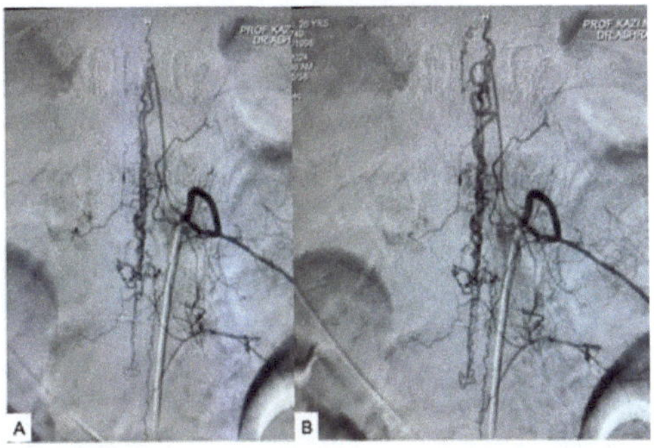

Figure 3. (A,B) Spinal DSA showing lower dorsal spinal AVM with feeding artery. Source: Figure by authors.

3.3.3. MRA

Spinal MRA might be useful if it can identify the fistula at a level that is suspiciously close to a vertebral level (Figure 4), as this information would speed up investigation via DSA. MRA is very important where DSA or CTA contraindicated.

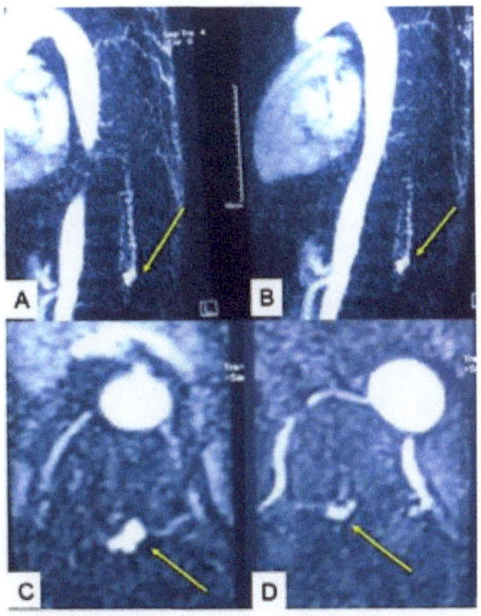

Figure 4. (A–D) Spinal MRA of the patient in Figures 1 and 3, showing the feeder and nidus of the AVM (arrow marked). Source: Figure by authors.

3.3.4. CTA

Spinal CTA can also define spinal AVMs with feeding arteries in the intervertebral foramen (Figures 5 and 6). Three-dimensional CTA is an attractive option for planning microsurgical excision (Singh et al. 2016; Greenberg 2010; Lindsay et al. 2011; July and Wahjoepramono 2019; Dumont and Oldfield 2011; Barnwell et al. 1990).

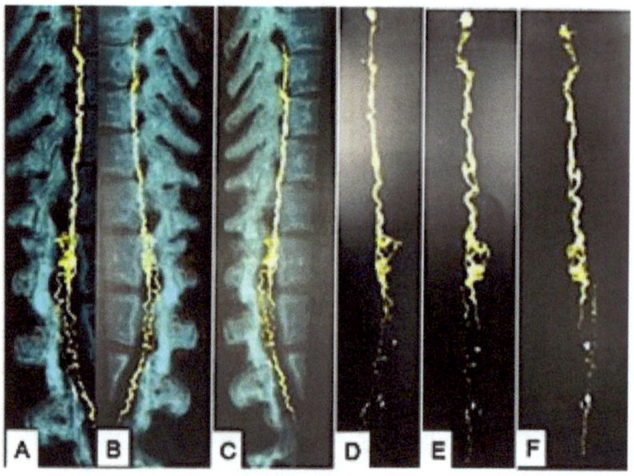

Figure 5. (**A–F**) CTA of dorsolumbar spine showing lower dorsal spinal SVM. Source: Figure by authors.

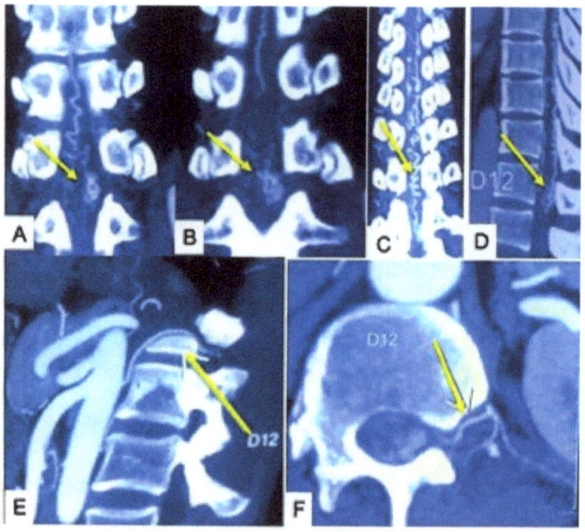

Figure 6. (**A–F**) Spinal CTA of the patient in Figures 1 and 4, showing the feeder and nidus of the AVM (marked with an arrow). Source: Figure by authors.

3.4. *Treatment*

There are two streams of treatments: (1) microsurgery and (2) endovascular therapy.

3.4.1. Microsurgery

Microsurgery (Figure 7) can safely deal with almost all spinal SVMs. The recurrence rate following microsurgery is very low in comparison to endovascular neurosurgery. While spinal AVM microsurgery is comparable to that for cerebral AVMs, the parenchyma cannot be retracted and haemorrhages are seldom life-threatening. Moreover, arteries of passage must be protected to prevent permanent impairments. A preoperative ICG angiography is frequently beneficial. The nidus is small, and the hemosiderin ring surrounding it on MRI frequently serves as a plane that can be used for imaging.

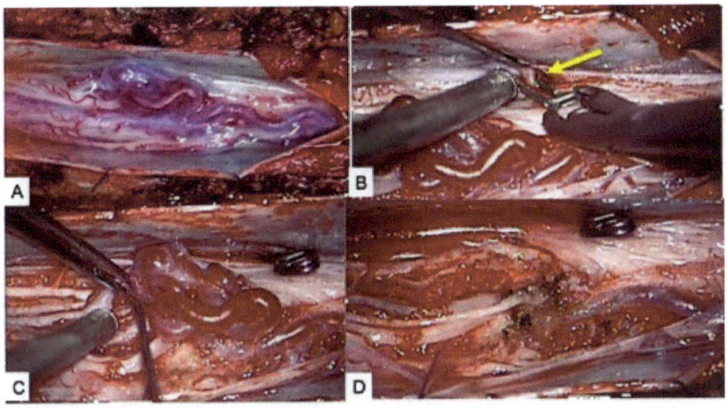

Figure 7. Intraoperative pictures of the patient in Figures 1, 4 and 6. (**A**) After laminotomy and dural exposure; (**B**) feeder occlusion with mini aneurysm clip (marked with an arrow), (**C**) excision of AVM; (**D**) after excision of AVM. Source: Figure by authors.

3.4.2. Endovascular Neurosurgery

It can be used in many cases of spinal AVMs, specially when the feeder vessel is limited with no mechanical compression. Type 1 (dural AVMs) is possibly receptive to glue-based endovascular therapy, in which case the proximal vein also needs to be sealed off. If a dural fistula is not entirely removed by the surgeon, it will return. Some type 2 (spinal glomus AVMs) SVMs, particularly type 2A SVMs (single-feeder), may be treatable with interventional neuroradiologic techniques like embolization. Surgery is frequently used for type 2B (>2 feeders) because recurrence may be more common with endovascular management than with surgical intervention.

3.4.3. Summary of Spinal AVM Treatment

All type 1 SVMs can be safely treated microsurgically. Endovascular therapy may also be effective but recurrence is higher. In type 2 A and B, microsurgery is preferable over endovascular therapy. In type 3 (juvenile type of spinal AVMs), the natural course is possibly better than the outcome with any type of management. But when intervention is inevitable, microsurgery is preferable. Type 4:

- Subtype 1: Microsurgery is recommended as endovascular therapy is difficult; treatment is easy on the filum terminale but challenging on the conus medullaris.
- Subtype 2: Microsurgery if preferable (especially with posterolateral AVF) as endovascular occlusion is incomplete.
- Subtype 3: Endovascular therapy is preferred as microsurgery is difficult (Singh et al. 2016; Greenberg 2010; Lindsay et al. 2011; July and Wahjoepramono 2019; Dumont and Oldfield 2011; Endo et al. 2016).

4. Spinal Cavernous Malformation

These lesions are frequently tiny, have little blood flow, and are fed by sinusoidal vessels with thin walls. Cavernous malformations (CMs) frequently have a gliosis and hemosiderin rim around them. MRI can quickly identify them (Figure 8). Despite being more frequent in the brain than in the spinal cord (See-Sebastian and Marks 2013), CMs nonetheless account for up to 12% of spinal vascular pathologies (Killeen et al. 2014). Cases often exhibit myelopathy symptoms between the third and sixth decades of life, while the disease's progression can vary in both intensity and severity (Scherman et al. 2016).

For individuals with asymptomatic CM or patients with modest, static symptoms, nonsurgical treatment with sequential surveillance imaging is a viable choice (Kivelev et al. 2012). Patients who experience a progressive neurological decline require surgical intervention (Liang et al. 2011) (Figure 9). Complete resection or obliteration of the lesion should be the aim of microsurgery because recurring myelopathic symptoms could result from remaining CM bleeding (Singh et al. 2016; Wang et al. 2016) (Figure 10).

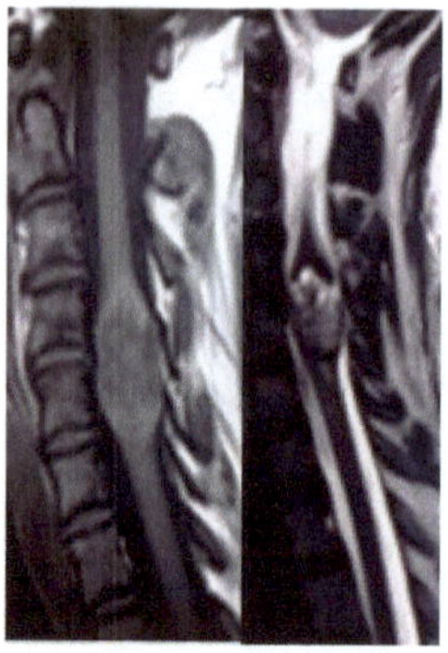

Figure 8. MRI of cervical spine (sagittal views, T1W and T2W images—right and left, respectively) showing intramedullary cavernoma. Source: Figure by authors.

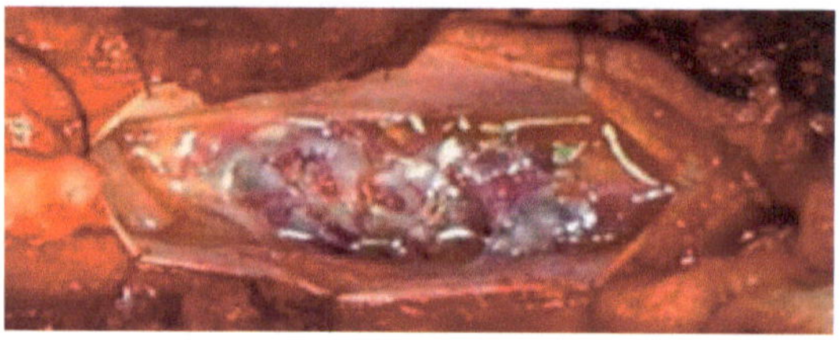

Figure 9. Perioperative picture of cavernoma of patient in Figure 8 after laminectomy, durotomy, and myelotomy. Source: Figure by authors.

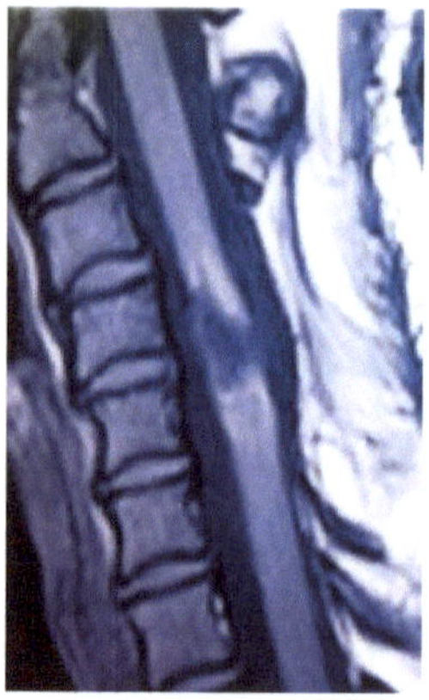

Figure 10. Postoperative MRI of cervical spine of patient in Figures 8 and 9 showing removal of tumour. Source: Figure by authors.

5. Spinal Epidural and Subdural Haematomas

These could exhibit a sudden onset of paraplegia. When a spinal AVM ruptures, an epidural or less frequently a subdural haematoma may develop. This can also happen after lumbar puncture or minor trauma, or it might develop on its own in patients who have a bleeding condition, liver disease, or are using anticoagulant medication. MRI (or myelography) shows the lesion in detail (Figure 11). Without waiting for spinal DSA, spinal decompression is necessary immediately after addressing any coagulation shortage (rapid CTA or MRA can be done on emergency basis). Angiomatous tissue may be seen during a pathological investigation of the haematoma; in many cases, there is no clear cause (Greenberg 2010; Lindsay et al. 2011; Dumont and Oldfield 2011; Jellema et al. 2003).

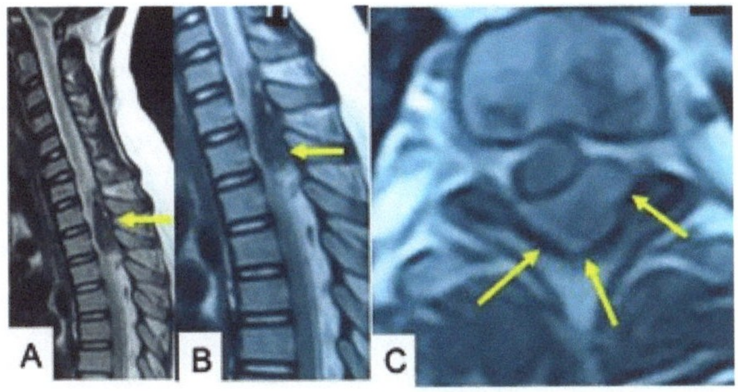

Figure 11. (**A**,**B**) MRI of spine (T2W images, sagittal sections) showing upper dorsal spinal epidural haematoma (marked with an arrow) causing acute paraplegia. (**C**) MRI of spine (T1W axial images) showing epidural haematoma (marked with an arrow). Source: Figure by authors.

6. Vertebral Haemangioma (VH)

6.1. Introduction

VH is also known as spinal haemangioma, cavernous haemangioma, or haemangiomatous angioma. VH classically occurs in post-pubertal female patients. VH is the most common primary spinal bone tumour (10–12% of all primary spinal bone neoplasms). Among these tumours, 70% are solitary and 30% are multiple (Greenberg 2010; Lindsay et al. 2011; Wang et al. 2018; Fox and Onofrio 1993; Healy et al. 1983). The most frequent site for these lesions is the dorsolumbar junction; the cervical and sacral spine are uncommon sites. In 25% of cases, VH only affects the corpus vertebrae; in 25% of cases, it affects the neural arch; and in 50% of cases, it affects both portions. Pure extradural lesions might happen very infrequently (Figure 12). The rarest lesions are intramedullary lesions. These are benign in origin and infrequently (1.2%) present with symptoms; they typically result from compression fractures, disc herniations, and, less frequently, neural compression from bone expansion by tumours. While reported, malignant degeneration is extremely rare (Lindsay et al. 2011; Fox and Onofrio 1993; Healy et al. 1983).

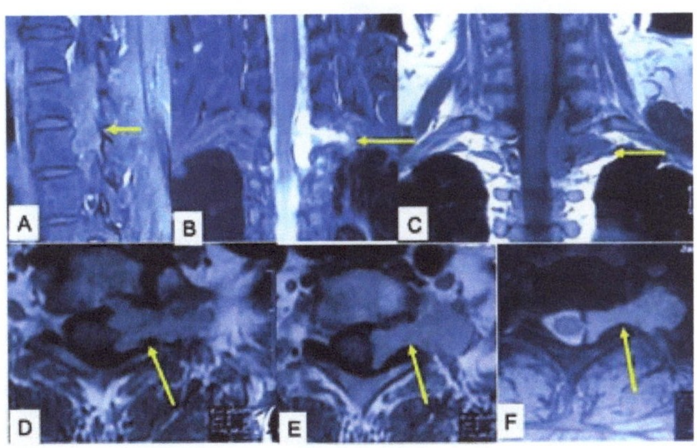

Figure 12. MRI of cervicodorsal spine. (**A**) Contrast sagittal image; (**B**) T2W coronal image; (**C**) T1W coronal image; (**D**,**E**) axial contrast image; and (**F**) T2W axial image showing pure spinal extradural (dumbbell-shaped) haemangioma (marked with an arrow). Source: Figure by authors.

6.2. Clinical Presentation

Most VH cases are asymptomatic and identified incidentally. Only 0.9% to 1.2% of people experience symptoms. The reason why symptoms hardly ever manifest before adolescence may be due to an unproven hormonal effect that causes symptoms to worsen with pregnancy or fluctuate with the menstrual cycle. VH can occasionally result in localized discomfort without radiculopathy at the affected level. However, rather than due to the VH itself, pain is more frequently present in these lesions due to associated pathologies (such as compression fracture, herniated disc, and spinal stenosis). Rarely, progressive neurodeficiency may develop (in the form of myelopathy, generally dorsal). Possible mechanisms of myelopathy include tumour growth into the spinal canal through the epidural space, bone growth (cortical "blistering") with widening of the pedicles including lamina, and formation of a "bony" spinal stenosis. Pressure by feeding and draining vessels, spontaneous epidural haematoma, compression fracture, and cord ischaemia due to a "steal phenomenon" are the other rare causes of myelopathy in VH (Greenberg 2010; Wang et al. 2018; Fox and Onofrio 1993).

6.3. Evaluation

6.3.1. Plain X-Rays

VH typically shows coarse, vertically depicted striations (corduroy pattern) or a "honeycomb" picture. At least >30% of the vertebral body will have been involve before these findings appear on plain X-ray.

6.3.2. CT Scan

Spinal CT scan is the investigation of choice. The "polka-dot sign", i.e., multiple high-density dots, represents cross-sections through thickened trabeculae.

6.3.3. MRI of the Spine

It demonstrates that tiny haemangiomas are hyperintense, spherical, and focal on T1WI and T2WI. Lesions that are more widespread may be hypointense. On T1WI and T2WI, lesions with a propensity to develop exhibit a mottled enhanced signal. They are also isointense on T1WI and hyperintense on T2WI, and they tend to be symptomatic.

6.3.4. Spinal DSA

DSA may be used to differentiate between symptomatic (normal or slightly enhanced vascularity in contrast to neighbouring bone) and non-evolving (moderate to high hypervascularity) VH. If the supplying artery does not also feed the ASA, therapeutic spinal DSA may be performed. If not, the feeding artery may be embolized beforehand or sacrificed during operation (Greenberg 2010; Wang et al. 2018).

6.4. Treatment

6.4.1. Asymptomatic/Incidental VH

It does not warrant routine follow-up or evaluation.

6.4.2. Symptomatic VH (With Pain or Neurologic Deficit)

Treatment options are as follows:

(i) Radiotherapy: It can be used postoperatively after partial resection, preoperatively as a surgical adjuvant, or alone for symptomatic VH. The sclerotic obliteration of VH makes it radiosensitive. Pain relief may take months or years, and there may be no radiological signs of a response.
(ii) Embolization: Endovascular embolization can provide alleviation of pain more quickly in comparison to radiotherapy. It can also be utilized as a neurosurgical adjunct before surgery. If the major radicular artery (the artery of Adamkiewicz) is embolized, there is a danger of spinal cord infarction.
(iii) Vertebroplasty: It is a better option than kyphoplasty as kyphoplasty destroys the trabecular bone.
(iv) Biopsy: Biopsy is needed in cases where diagnosis is not certain (e.g., when metastases are highly probable).
(v) Surgery: Surgery is utilized for painful lesions that do not respond to the aforementioned treatments or for lesions that result in a growing neurological disability.

Surgical treatment options for symptomatic VH:

- Only neural arch involvement, with or without soft tissue (ST) in canal: radical excision.
- Vertebral body (VB) involvement with anterior canal compression: anterior corpectomy and strut graft.
- VB is affected but no bony expansion, ST in lateral canal: laminectomy with excision of soft tissue.
- Significant involvement of the anterior and posterior vertebral segments along with circumferential bone expansion without ST compression: laminectomy combined with radiation or laminectomy with close monitoring.
- Extensive involvement of anterior and posterior vertebral segments with ST in anterior canal: anterior corpectomy and strut graft plus radiotherapy or anterior corpectomy and strut graft and close follow-up.

- Risk of surgery: major surgical risks include blood loss, destabilization, neurological deficit, or postoperative extradural haematoma. In 20–30% cases, the disease recurs after subtotal resection; recurrence is common within 2 years. Patients with subtotal excision should have radiotherapy (Greenberg 2010; Lindsay et al. 2011; Wang et al. 2018; Fox and Onofrio 1993; Healy et al. 1983).

Author Contributions: Conceptualization, methodology, validation, formal analysis, investigation, resources, data curation, F.H.C. and M.R.H.; writing—original draft preparation, writing—review and editing, F.H.C., visualization, supervision, F.H.C. and N.A. All authors have read and agreed to the published version of the manuscript.

Funding: This research received no external funding.

Conflicts of Interest: The authors declare no conflicts of interest.

References

Barnwell, Stanley L., Christopher F. Dowd, Richard L. Davis, Michael S. B. Edwards, Philip H. Gutin, and Charles B. Wilson. 1990. Cryyptic vascular malfonnations of the spinal cord: Diagnosis by magnetic resonance imaging and outcome of surgery. *Journal of Neurosurgery* 72: 403–7. [CrossRef] [PubMed]

Bederson, Joshua B., and Robert F. Spetzler. 1996. Pathophysiology of type I spinal dural arteriovenous malformations. *BNI Quarterly* 12: 23–32.

Cheshire, William P., Cesar C. Santos, E. Wayn Massey, and James F. Howard, Jr. 1996. Spinal cord infarction: Etiology and outcome. *Neurology* 47: 321–30. [CrossRef] [PubMed]

Cheung, Albert T., Stuart J. Weiss, Michael L. McGarvey, Mark M. Stecker, Michael S. Hogan, Alison Escherich, and Joseph E. Bavaria. 2002. Interventions for reversing delayed-onset postoperative paraplegia after thoracic aortic reconstruction. *The Annals of Thoracic Surgery* 74: 413–19. [CrossRef] [PubMed]

Dumont, A. S., and E. H. Oldfield. 2011. Spinal vascular malformations. In *Youmans Neurological Surgery*. Edited by H. Richard Winn. Philadelphia: Elsevier, pp. 4167–202.

Endo, Toshiki, Hidenori Endo, Kenichi Sato, Yasushi Matsumoto, and Teiji Tominaga. 2016. Surgical and Endovascular Treatment for Spinal Arteriovenous Malformations. *Neurologia Medico-Chirurgica* 56: 457–64. [CrossRef]

Foo, Dominic, and Alain B. Rossier. 1983. Anterior spinal artery syndrome and its natural history. *Paraplegia* 21: 1–10. [CrossRef]

Fox, Mark W., and Burton M. Onofrio. 1993. The natural history and management of symptomatic and asymptomatic vertebral hemangiomas. *Journal of Neurosurgery* 78: 36–45. [CrossRef]

Greenberg, Mark S. 2010. *Handbook of Neurosurgery*. New York: Thieme.

Gueguen, B., J. J. Merland, M. C. Riche, and A. Rey. 1987. Vascular malformations of the spinal cord: Intrathecal perimedullary arteriovanous fistulas fed by medullary arteries. *Neurology* 37: 969–79. [CrossRef]

Healy, Michael, David A. Herz, and Lorraine Pearl. 1983. Spinal hemangiomas. *Neurosurgery* 13: 689–91. [CrossRef]

Jellema, Korné, L. R. Canta, C. C. Tijssen, W. J. Van Rooij, P. J. Koudstaal, and Jan van Gijn. 2003. Spinal dural arteriovenous fistulas: Clinical features in 80 patients. *Journal of Neurology, Neurosurgery & Psychiatry* 74: 1438–40. [CrossRef]

July, Julius, and Eka J. Wahjoepramono. 2019. *Neurovascular Surgery*. Singapore: Springer. [CrossRef]

Killeen, Tim, Adam Czaplinski, and Evaldas Cesnulis. 2014. Extradural spinal cavernous malformation: A rare but important mimic. *British Journal of Neurosurgery* 28: 340–46. [CrossRef]

Kivelev, Juri, Mika Niemelä, and Juha Hernesniemi. 2012. Treatment strategies in cavernomas of the brain and spine. *Journal of Clinical Neuroscience* 19: 491–97. [CrossRef] [PubMed]

Liang, Jian-Tao, Yu-Hai Bao, Hong-Qi Zhang, Li-Rong Huo, Zhen-Yu Wang, and Feng Ling. 2011. Management and prognosis of symptomatic patients with intramedullary spinal cord cavernoma: Clinical article. *Journal of Neurosurgery: Spine* 15: 447–56. [CrossRef] [PubMed]

Lindsay, Kenneth W., Ian Bone, and Geraint Fuller. 2011. *Neurology and Neurosurgery Illustrated. General Approach to History and Examination*. London: C. L. Elsevier.

Merland, J. J., M. C. Riche, and J. Chiras. 1980. Intraspinal extramedullary arteriovenous fistulae draining into the medullary veins. *The Neuroradiology Journal* 7: 271–320.

Mourier, K. L., Y. P. Gobin, B. George, G. Lot, and J. J. Merland. 1993. Intradural perimedullary arteriovenous fistulae: Results of surgical and endovascular treatment in a series of 35 cases. *Neurosurgery* 32: 885–91. [CrossRef] [PubMed]

Scherman, Daniel Brian, Prashanth J. Rao, Winny Varikatt, and Gordon Dandie. 2016. Clinical presentation and surgical outcomes of an intramedullary C2 spinal cord cavernoma: A case report and review of the relevant literature. *Journal of Spine Surgery* 2: 139–42. [CrossRef]

Schneider, Gregory S. 2010. Anterior spinal cord syndrome after initiation of treatment with atenolol. *The Journal of Emergency Medicine* 38: e49–e52. [CrossRef]

See-Sebastian, Ester H., and E. Robert Marks. 2013. Spinal cord intramedullary cavernoma: A case report. *West Virginia Medical Journal* 109: 28–30.

Singh, Rahul, Brandon Lucke-Wold, Kymberly Gyure, and Sohyun Boo. 2016. A Review of Vascular Abnormalities of the Spine. *Annals of Vascular Medicine and Research* 3: 1045.

Spetzler, Robert F., Paul W. Detwiler, Howard A. Riina, and Randall W. Porter. 2002. Modified classification of spinal cord vascular lesions. *Journal of neurosurgery* 96: 145–56. [CrossRef]

Strugar, John, and Douglas Chyatte. 1992. *In situ* photocoagulation of spinal dural arteriovenous malformations using the Nd:Yag laser. *Journal of Neurosurgery* 77: 571–74. [CrossRef] [PubMed]

Tobin, W. D., and D. D. Layton. 1976. The diagnosis and natural history of spinal cord arteriovenous malformations. *Mayo Clinic Proceedings* 51: 637–46. [PubMed]

Wang, Ben, Na Meng, Hongqing Zhuang, Songbo Han, Shaomin Yang, Liang Jiang, Feng Wei, Xiaoguang Liu, and Zhongjun Liu. 2018. The Role of Radiotherapy and Surgery in the Management of Aggressive Vertebral Hemangioma: A Retrospective Study of 20 Patients. *Medical Science Monitor: International Medical Journal of Experimental and Clinical Research* 24: 6840–50. [CrossRef] [PubMed]

Wang, Chen, Chien-Min Chen, Fang Shen, Xiao-Dong Fang, Guang-Yu Ying, Yu-Cheng Ren, Dan-Feng Yu, Liang-Liang Zhu, Yong-Jian Zhu, and Jian-Min Zhang. 2016. Microscope-assisted endoscopic interlaminar ligation of spinal arteriovenous fistulas: Technical note. *Journal of Neurosurgery: Spine* 25: 394–97. [CrossRef]

Yoon, Woong, Jae Kyu Kim, Yun Hyun Kim, Tae Woong Chung, and Heoung Keun Kang. 2002. Bronchial and Nonbronchial Systemic Artery Embolization for Life-threatening Hemoptysis: A Comprehensive Review. *Radiographics* 22: 1395–409. [CrossRef]

Youmans, Julian R. 1982. *Neurological Surgery*. Philadelphia: W.B. Saunders.

Section XI: Endoscopic Neurosurgery

Endoscopy and MIS in Neurosurgery

Khandkar Ali Kawsar, Atul H. Goel and Forhad H. Chowdhury

Abstract: The utilization of neuroendoscopes in neurosurgery is a remarkable advancement. It limits neural injury and maximizes the view of operative areas in the brain, spine, and peripheral nerves, which may be remote. The entrance and approaches to ventricles and cisterns have become attractive and easier. Devising optic endoscopic lenses—long and angled instruments—changed endoscopic neurosurgery into a very versatile super-specialty. In this chapter, we will first discuss the history of neuroendoscopy; later, its utility in hydrocephalus, skull base surgery, neuro-oncological surgery, aneurysm surgery, craniosynostosis, and transcranial cystic lesion treatment will be discussed. Some important endoscopic operations will be discussed with relevant anatomical landmarks. In the later part of the chapter, we will address spinal endoscopy and peripheral nerve endoscopy.

Abbreviations

AC	arachnoid cyst	AICA	anterior inferior cerebellar artery
AP	anterior–posterior	CNS	central nervous system
CSF	cerebrospinal fluid	CT	computed tomography
EACS	endoscopy-assisted craniosynostosis surgery	ECTR	endoscopic carpal tunnel release
EEA	endoscopic endonasal approach	EES	endoscopic endonasal surgery
ETV	endoscopic third ventriculostomy	HFS	hemifacial spasm
HH	hypothalamic hamartoma	HPA	hypothalamic–pituitary axis
ICA	internal carotid artery	ICH	intracranial hematoma
ID	internal diameter	MIS	minimally invasive surgery
MRI	magnetic resonance imaging	MVD	microvascular decompression
PECD	percutaneous endoscopic cervical discectomy	PETD	percutaneous endoscopic thoracic discectomy
REZ	root entry zone	SCA	superior cerebellar artery
SIADH	secretion of inappropriate antidiuretic hormone	TELD	transforaminal endoscopic lumbar discectomy
TCL	transverse carpal ligament	TDH	thoracic disc herniation
UN	ulnar nerve	VP	Ventriculoperitoneal

1. Introduction

Using an endoscope, neuroendoscopy treats diseases of the CNS. Two newborns with hydrocephalus underwent the first neurosurgery endoscopic operation with a cystoscope in 1910, and one of them experienced a successful recovery (Li et al. 2005; Sgouros 2013; Walker 2001). In 1922, after more than a decade had passed, Walter Dandy attempted a choroid plexectomy but failed (de Divitiis et al. 2002). Mixter accomplished the first endoscopic third ventriculostomy (ETV) in 1923, on a 9-month-old infant with obstructive hydrocephalus by utilizing a urethroscope (Mixter 1923). After employing a new endoscope with an electrocautery, an irrigation system to preclude ventricular collapse, and a movable operative tip to penetrate the third ventricular floor, Scarff first presented his findings in 1935 (Li et al. 2005; Walker 2001).

Early in the 1970s, developments in optics and electronics led to the creation of high-resolution rigid and flexible endoscopes, which were effectively employed for ventricular surgery. The use of ETV for the management of hydrocephalus with endoscope-assisted, minimally invasive surgical techniques, which started in the 1980s to 1990s and are still used today, has advanced to the current stage of neuroendoscopy (Teo and Mobbs 2004).

Initially, only the ventricles could be used for endoscopic treatments because they are filled with a crystal-clear fluid, the ideal medium. At present, the neuroendoscopic field has expanded beyond ventricular operations and is utilized for all varieties of neurosurgically manageable conditions, including craniosynostosis, rare subtypes of hydrocephalus, intraventricular tumors, intracranial cysts, hypothalamic hamartomas (HH), and skull base tumors (Shim et al. 2017).

Similar to other endoscopic operations, minimum tissue damage, improved visualization, improved cosmetic outcomes, shorter hospital stays, and lower surgical morbidity are the benefits of minimally invasive endoscopic procedures. The utilization of neuroendoscopy approaches may help to reduce this risk. In neurosurgery, the surgeon works to reduce operative trauma by limiting the exposure size and avoiding unintended brain retraction, which can occur via rising local cerebral tissue pressure as well as reduced regional cerebral blood flow and may ultimately affect the neurologic result after micro-neurosurgical operation. The endoscope is a great teaching tool since it improves the surgeon's perspective by enhancing illumination as well as magnification (Perneczky and Fries 1998; Teo 2000). A survey of neurosurgeons comparing the endoscope and the microscope revealed that the endoscope is superior for gazing around corners (30°, 70°, and 110°) and the microscope is preferable only for reduced hand fatigue and 3D vision, advantaged that are now provided by endoscopic holders (Teo and Mobbs 2004).

2. Neuroendoscopic Instruments

Surgeons must own a specific neuroendoscopy kit (Figure 1). The control units of the camera, video camera, light source, monitor, video recorder, and computerized system for storing video clips or single-picture capture should all be included in the endoscopy tower. Endoscope positioning as well as fixation arms that can be secured to the headrest or the operating table assist the surgeon in preventing arm fatigue, which can otherwise impair eye–hand coordination and limit flexibility (Siomin and Constantini 2004).

A pair of scissors and grasping forceps (Figure 2), a coagulation tool (either bipolar or monopolar), a straight scope, an irrigation, and one or more angled telescopes are among the endoscopic tools used by surgeons (Figure 3).

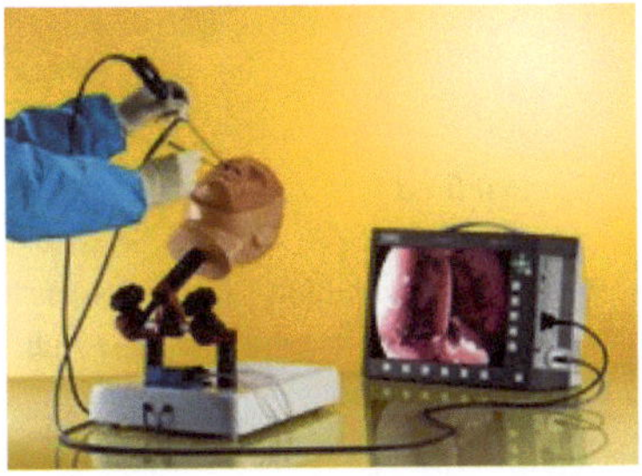

Figure 1. Endoscopic instruments. Source: Figure by authors.

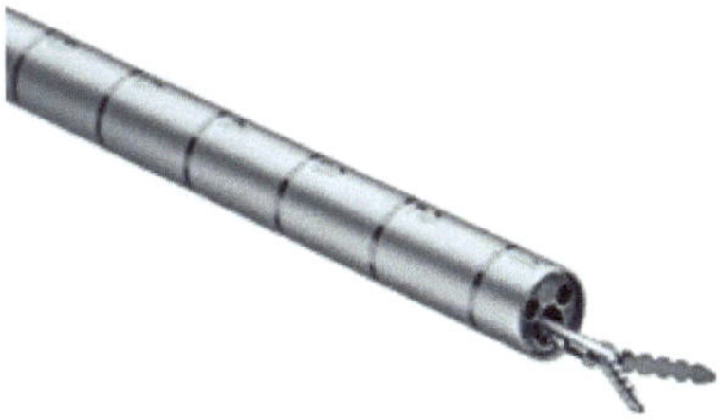

Figure 2. Endoscopic grasping forceps. Source: Figure by authors.

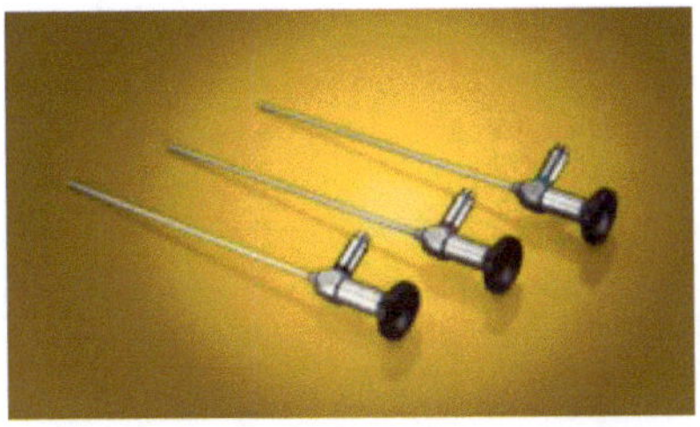

Figure 3. Straight and angled scopes. Source: Figure by authors.

A skilled assistant can show the surgeon the challenging areas and can enable two-handed operation. It is crucial to have recording units that can record images for later analysis in digital or video format (Alberti et al. 2001). Thanks to flexible neuroendoscopes, the range of neuroendoscopy has expanded (Figure 4).

In order to boost the accuracy of the endoscopic approach, frameless computerized navigation is being employed more and more in cranial endoscopic procedures. It was tested to be accurate, dependable, and beneficial in several intracranial neuroendoscopic procedures. Excellent red distinction and remarkable color depth are provided by modern three-chip technology. Even with quick camera movements, the most recent full HD technology produces images without latency. The goals and requirements for endoscopic interventions will evolve as we learn more about various CNS disorders. Future indications for minimally invasive or even ultra-microsurgical access will require the use of supervisory-controlled robotic systems, telemanipulated neurosurgery, shared control systems, or perhaps totally robotic telesurgery (Grotenhuis 2014).

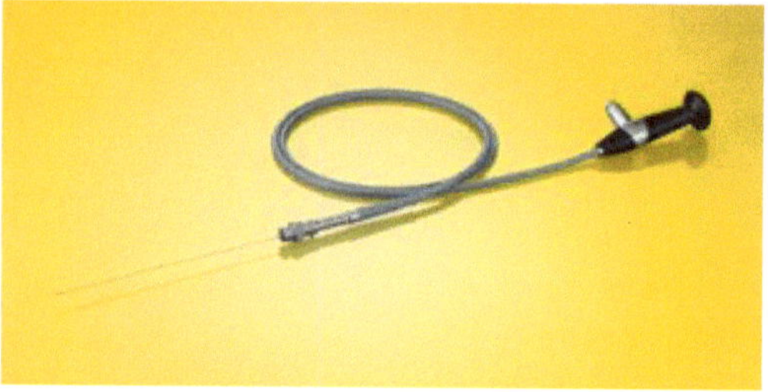

Figure 4. Flexible endoscope. Source: Figure by authors.

3. Endoscopic Third Ventriculostomy (ETV)

3.1. History and Background

The history of ventricular cerebrospinal fluid (CSF) diverting began in 1951 (Nulsen and Spitz 1951). With the enhanced neuroimaging capabilities of endoscopes, intrigue in ETV for the management of obstructive hydrocephalus was revived in the 1970s, after a brief hiatus in the use of this operation. Vries wrote about his experiences treating five hydrocephalus patients in 1978, where he used a fiberoptic endoscope to show that ETVs were theoretically possible (Vries 1978). Jones and colleagues first reported a 50% shunt-free chance of success for ETV in 24 cases with different types of hydrocephalus in 1990 (Jones et al. 1990). In a set of 103 patients, the same researchers reported an elevated rate of success of 61% four years later (Jones et al. 1994). ETV is now utilized to treat obstructive hydrocephalus brought on by compressive periaqueductal tumor lesions or benign aqueductal stenosis. Shunt-free success rates in the modern era range from 80% to 95% (Sgouros 2013).

As knowledge in this area increases, the indications for ETV are being extended to include cases with meningomyelocele, Chiari malformation, hydrocephalus associated with Dandy–Walker syndrome, and even noncommunicating kinds of hydrocephalus. Due to avoiding shunt reliance and associated difficulties, ETV is increasingly preferred to ventriculoperitoneal (VP) shunt implantation in some circumstances (Sufianov et al. 2008).

3.2. Important Operative Landmarks

It is crucial to recognize significant ventricular features and structures for good ETV. Here, we go through a few significant features that surgeons should be familiar with in order to complete the process properly. Figure 5 depicts the equipment needed for ETV as well as an endoscopic view with some significant landmarks.

The choroid plexus is a significant anatomical landmark because it persists at the choroidal fissure despite severe abnormalities in the ventricular architecture, providing the surgeon with an essential navigational tool. The third ventricle is reached after the foramen of Monro by the anterior section of the choroid plexus.

The fornix, which makes up the upper and anterior edge of the Monro's foramen, is another significant anatomical feature. When the endoscope is passed from the lateral to the third ventricle, the fornix is vulnerable to harm because of its placement; the chance of injury and subsequent memory loss increases with more passages. When detected, the thalamostriate vein, which dives into the foramen of Monro along with the choroid plexus, provides another significant landmark. The third ventricle's lateral walls are created by the hypothalamus. The structures most vulnerable to damage during an ETV are the supraoptic and paraventricular arcuate nuclei because of their location in the lateral wall and closeness to the trajectory, which may result in endocrinologic disruption (Unal and Aydoseli 2018).

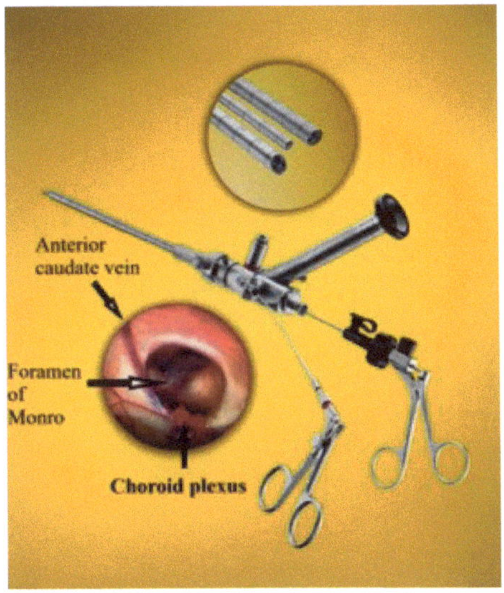

Figure 5. ETV instrument with a working channel and view of the foramen. Source: Figure by authors.

In front of the coupled mamillary bodies, the third ventricle's floor must be carefully fenestrated (Figure 6). The Liliequist membrane needs to be fenestrated and the ETV endoscope has to be advanced in order to boost rates of success. This stage will reveal the basilar artery.

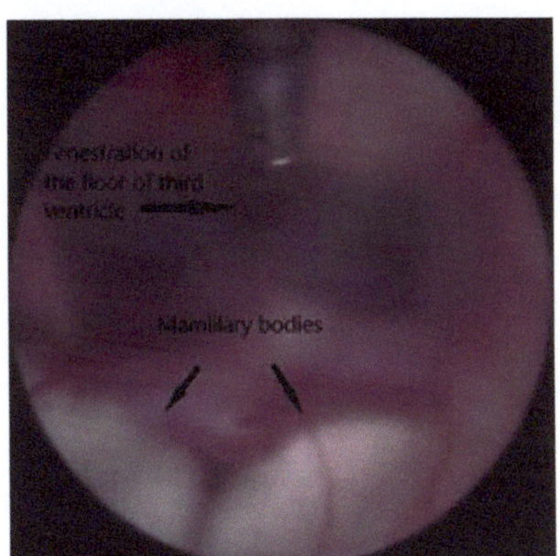

Figure 6. Fenestration of the floor of the ventricle. Source: Figure by authors.

3.3. Precautions

When there is a history of prior tumors, shunt surgery, or a thicker third ventricle floor, there are a number of precautions to be taken when performing an ETV. Tumors, like a brainstem glioma, can change the anatomy. The third ventricle's floor may become distorted as a result, and the basilar artery may move forward, reducing the safe area for floor penetration. When a tumor blocks the third ventricle, hydrocephalus may develop rather quickly, with the third ventricle's floor appearing opaque and unattenuated. Without being able to see the underlying neurovascular systems, perforation will be challenging and inevitably demand sharper technique, increasing the danger.

3.4. Success Rate of ETV

Since they have less pronounced ventricular enlargement, a thicker third ventricle floor, and a frequently aberrant architecture, cases who have previously been shunted are technically more challenging. If the third ventricle's floor is excessively thick, blood obscures the endoscopic vision, or if the basilar artery is situated beneath or dangerously near to the desired point of fenestration, ETV treatment may need to be abandoned in some individuals. Nevertheless, after three years, ETV has an average success rate of about 75%, although this varies depending on the case, including the surgeon's skill. Particularly in individuals with posterior fossa neoplasms, the outcomes of ETV are favorably comparable to those achieved after shunting (Sainte-Rose et al. 2001). Additionally, ETV seems to have a financial benefit over shunting (Barlow and Ching 1997).

ETV failure might happen early or late. Bleeding at the fenestration zone, undiscovered extra arachnoid membranes obstructing the CSF flow, an insufficient fenestration size, and other variables can all lead to early failure. Later sealing of the opening by gliotic tissue or an arachnoid layer causes late failure. This issue may be quite significant. There are now a number of accounts in the literature about deaths that followed late failure of ETV (Hader et al. 2002), and this continues to be a management challenge since this failure can happen suddenly and may be unforeseen. Early or delayed failure may be caused by tumor development and insufficient CSF absorption at the site of the arachnoid villi. Why a patient population with open fenestrations shows deterioration after several months of good health is unknown (Tisell et al. 2000). The literature lists hypothalamic dysfunction, bradycardia, and bleeding from injury to ependymal veins, arteries, or the choroid plexus as procedure-related problems. Short-term problems, which are mostly peroperative and technique-related, and long-term problems, which happen at a significantly lower rate, are the two main categories of complications (Brockmeyer et al. 1998).

4. Complex Hydrocephalus Simplifications and Intracranial Cysts

4.1. Multiloculated Hydrocephalus

Even when a patient has a working VP shunt, multiloculated hydrocephalus is characterized by discrete CSF compartments that tend to expand inside the ventricular system. Meningitis, post-shunt infection, intraventricular hemorrhage, head trauma, ependymal injury during shunt placement, and other inflammatory processes frequently result in multiloculation (Andresen and Juhler 2012). More than 30% of newborns who survive a neonatal meningitis attack will eventually develop hydrocephalus; the majority of these neonates run the risk of having multiloculated hydrocephalus (Reinprecht et al. 2001). The ventricular catheter or typical locations of CSF absorption cannot absorb accumulated CSF because the compartments are divided by septa (Spennato et al. 2004). Several shunts are not recommended since they have a high failure rate and can lead to infections.

By fenestrating the membrane, endoscopy provides a straightforward method of navigating separated CSF compartments and ventricles. Carefully studying the preoperative MRI is essential for effective surgical planning. Entry locations are chosen so that the fewest possible burr holes can be used to fenestrate the greatest number of cysts (El-Tantawy 2018). The burr hole used to insert a ventricular catheter can also be used for this. In most patients with loculated ventricles, septum pellucidum fenestration to join the two lateral ventricles will prevent the need for two shunts (Unal and Aydoseli 2018).

Chronic ependymal inflammation and the emergence of new septa, according to Spennato et al., are explanations for the increased prevalence of shunt blockage in multiloculation. Multiloculated hydrocephalus was viewed as a progressive illness (Spennato et al. 2007). After initial surgery, 38.5% of people with multiloculated hydrocephalus needed extra neuroendoscopic fenestrations, according to Akbari et al., while 33% of patients, according to El-Ghandour, required repeat endoscopic fenestration during the follow-up period (El-Ghandour 2008; Akbari et al. 2015).

It was recently discovered that aqueductoplasty could be used to treat trapped fourth ventricle conditions. Techniques of applied neuroendoscopy have been expanded to include endoscopic fourth ventriculostomy as well as Monro and Magendie foraminoplasty (Li et al. 2005; Oi and Abbott 2004; Sgouros 2013).

4.2. Intracranial Cysts

The ventricular system is capable of harboring a wide variety of cysts. Arachnoid cysts, which are often extra-axial; choroid plexus cysts; neoplastic cysts; and parasitic cysts (e.g., cysticercotic and hydatid cysts) can appear within the ventricles. Arachnoid cysts can often be successfully removed endoscopically or via fenestration in patients.

Approximately 1% of all cerebral mass lesions are intracranial arachnoid cysts (ACs) (Robinson 1971). Due to the improved accessibility of CT and MRI, its incidence appears to have grown recently (Hanieh et al. 1988; Fernández Molina 2013). Different surgical procedures are advised. Pure endoscopic AC fenestration has grown in popularity and is actually favored by many neurosurgeons as a result of the advancement of neuroendoscopy, particularly in situations with suprasellar or quadrigeminal cistern cysts and cysts in the posterior fossa (Oertel et al. 2020; Gangemi et al. 2011; Karabagli and Etus 2012; Wang et al. 2013).

Nine out of fourteen children (64%) with arachnoid cysts in an initial series were managed successfully via neuroendoscopic fenestration through a burr hole, obviating the need for craniotomy (Guiot 1973). Endoscopic transsphenoidal surgery is especially suited for cysts that are restricted to the pituitary fossa. Without the use of shunting, ventriculo-cysto-cisternostomy allows for long-term decompression of suprasellar arachnoid cysts. The majority of patients who have intraventricular cysts or tumors also have hydrocephalus. Given that CSF diversion and tumor therapy may be performed simultaneously, this renders endoscopic surgery especially useful (Di Rocco et al. 2005; Fukushima et al. 1973). Arachnoid cysts, cavum velum interpositum cysts, ventricular neuroepithelial cysts, colloid cysts, and large pineal cysts were all successfully fenestrated by Teo et al. Frameless stereotactic assistance has been helpful in directing the burr hole toward these cysts in circumstances where the ventricles are very small. Arachnoid cyst surgery aims to alleviate symptoms. This is especially important for endoscopic fenestration since, despite significant clinical improvement, the cyst's appearance may only minimally shrink on postoperative imaging (Teo and Mobbs 2004).

5. Endoscopic Applications in Neuro-Oncology

The field of neuro-oncology offers the best setting for endoscopic use. Traditional tumor care can benefit greatly from the advantages of enhanced intraventricular pathology visibility, improved hydrocephalus management of tumors, safer biopsies, and minimally invasive excision of intraventricular tumors (Teo and Mobbs 2004).

A surgeon might utilize an endoscope to gauge the extent of resection after removing a tumor. With an endoscope, the very same neurosurgery can frequently be performed using a smaller craniotomy, according to the idea of minimally invasive but highly successful surgery (Perneczky et al. 1999). Endoscopy may increase the survival chances for people with benign tumors by enabling a more thorough excision (Wallner et al. 1988; Garcia and Fulling 1985). Third ventriculostomy and septostomy are examples of adjunctive treatments that can be carried out via the same access to treat related issues like secondary hydrocephalus without the need for shunt insertion (Teo and Mobbs 2004).

The first description of endoscopic stereotactic imaging and excision of intra-axial brain tumors was published in 1980 (Jacques et al. 1980; Shelden et al. 1980). The excision of tumors using stereotactic endoscopy through a conduit made of a dilator in the shape of a bullet was also reported in 1990 (Otsuki et al. 1990). Through the use of a dilatable conduit, Kassam et al. documented the creation of an entirely endoscopic method for intra-axial tumor removal. In an effort to provide a parafascicular route to the tumor, a channel is constructed through the dilated white matter. The endoscope works parallel to the conduit (port), which generates an air medium that enables bimanual dissection. The procedure carefully abides by established microsurgical principles (Kassam et al. 2009).

For the microscopic removal of deep cerebral tumors, Dr. Kelly invented a stereotactic tubular retraction device with a 20 mm diameter. His work served as the foundation for the initial development of endoscopic resection (Kelly et al. 1986, 1988; Russell and Kelly 2002). Because a cone of light is delivered by a microscope, which tapers from the light source until it lands on the target, the conduit needs to offer microscopic visualization that is greater than an endoscopic conduit. The endoscope, in comparison, uses an inverted light cone to produce illumination and magnification. In order to deliver the endoscope millimeters away from the destination, a considerably smaller port or conduit (11.5 mm) can be employed, producing a "flashlight" effect that illuminates the tumor. Utilizing this benefit of the neuroendoscope, intra-axial tumor resections can be carried out (Kassam et al. 2009).

Despite the endoscope's lack of binocular vision, this was not a serious drawback. Proprioceptive input made possible by bimanual dissection makes up for lost binocular vision with ease. This is comparable to an observer's perspective being used when performing microscopic neurosurgery. After gaining sufficient expertise, a surgeon acquires 3D perception based on movement and touch (tactile feedback). According to Kassam et al., endoscopic visualization for subcortical tumors may be more effective than microscopic visualization as the endoscope enables close-up vision of the pathology to be treated and unfettered "flashlight" lighting in deep areas (Kassam et al. 2009). The benefit of using a microscope is evident and makes it preferable for cortical lesions as well as dissections, but this straight endoscopic view also offers important advantages for deep-seated brain tumors. In fact, once the microscope has been removed from the region, endoscopic vision has been utilized to certify adequate excision for intraparenchymal neoplasms (Teo and Nakaji 2005).

With this method, selected primary and secondary brain neoplasms may be safely excised. Tumors far larger than the tube itself can be efficiently eliminated via dynamic port retraction and piecemeal extirpation. The long-term outcome will ultimately depend on the biology of the neoplasm. The port, however, may present a viable option (in carefully chosen patients) to achieve the objectives of surgery, namely, cytoreduction or total tumor excision with a manageable degree of morbidity, reducing both the volume of the corticectomy and the amount of white-matter dissection necessary for the excision of the neoplasm (Kassam et al. 2009).

The burr hole is positioned to allow the scope to enter the ventricle as far away from the lesion as feasible and to allow the scope to observe the tumor directly, rather than peeping around a corner. Before coming across the problematic anatomy, the surgeon might situate themself by recognizing normal anatomical structures when using the distal technique. The surgeon can move the scope more freely and without risking harm to the surrounding healthy brain because the majority of the remote part of the scope is inside the ventricle (Teo and Mobbs 2004).

Not all intraventricular tumors require endoscopic treatment. The ideal tumor should be histologically low-grade, with accompanying secondary hydrocephalus, moderate to low vascularity, and soft consistency (Teo and Mobbs 2004). It might never be feasible to confirm these characteristics before surgery.

A few rules should be followed when dealing with intraventricular tumors. The surgeon must select a trajectory that avoids ornate structures while providing a clear view of the tumor. To make the tumor removal process easier, the exterior of the lesion is coagulated using either unipolar cautery or a laser. In order to remove blood and debris and to stop the ventricle from becoming too hot, there is extensive irrigation. Cysts must be opened, drained, and their contents extracted piecemeal or by suction, including piecemeal coagulation and removal of the remaining wall. After the procedure is finished, the scope is removed as the tract is checked for intraparenchymal hemorrhage (Teo and Mobbs 2004). Irrigation is used extensively to achieve hemostasis. During intraventricular hemostasis, a cut-end Foley catheter can be utilized to remove blood clots (Kawsar et al. 2015).

A tried-and-true treatment option for intraventricular brain tumors is endoscopic tumor biopsy. Both the diagnostic yield and risk are high (>90% and 3.5%). Endoscopic biopsy can treat Langerhans cell histiocytosis, infiltrative optic/hypothalamic pathway glioma, and germ cell tumors (Sgouros 2013). Tumors or colloid cysts that are pedunculated at the ependymal wall can be removed endoscopically. Except for when the cyst is exceptionally large, which raises the danger of venous damage at the Monro's foramen, endoscopic removal of a colloid cyst is technically feasible through the lateral ventricle in the majority of cases (Sgouros 2013; Yamini et al. 2004). Obstructive hydrocephalus or vision loss may be temporarily or permanently relieved by transventricular endoscopic neoplasm cyst decompression (Shim et al. 2017).

Rare congenital anomalies known as hypothalamic hamartomas that arise from the inferior hypothalamus are linked to epileptic fits, early puberty, and cognitive issues. All patients, with the exception of those who have premature puberty, need surgery. The HH type (as determined by Delalande and Fohlen (2003) or Choi et al. (2004)) should determine whether a single treatment or combination of treatments is utilized. Small HHs have been attempted to be surgically removed using endoscopic excision assisted by stereotactic guidance, although some of the tumors persisted. Surgery for the excision of HHs is frequently carried out in stages. However, according to recent research, endoscopic disconnection of HHs appears to be both safer and more efficient than other methods (Choi et al. 2004; Rekate et al. 2006). Most of the time, navigation assistance is advised due to the clear need for precision in lateral and third ventricles of a normal size (Shim et al. 2017).

6. Endoscope-Assisted Microsurgery

The next step after standard microsurgery is endoscopy, which enables the neurosurgeon to see tumor remains, including those concealed under a cranial nerve, eloquent cerebral tissue, or the tentorial margin.

The field of endoscopic neurosurgery that is expanding the fastest is this one. The goal of microsurgery has been to reduce retraction and increase visibility. Endoscopy enables the neurosurgeon to take these objectives one step closer. In order to remove tumors and clip aneurysms, surgeons often need to view "around corners", which is made possible by acutely angled, rigid, and flexible scopes. The extra-axial components of the skull base can be approached in a number of ways to enhance visibility without risking conventional microsurgical methods. The endoscope is placed down the same surgical field, which is the approach that is most frequently used. While this does not add to the morbidity, it tends to clog the already small operative field. The scope can be placed through a contralateral burr hole to avoid cramming more devices down a small craniotomy. A very small supraorbital incision can be utilized to gain entry to the subarachnoid area, and routine microsurgical dissection is then carried out to determine the lesion. When the pathology is visible, the scope is locked in position and the ipsilateral side is the object of attention. For instance, this method provides superb imaging of the aneurysm clip points or the oblique extent of a neoplasm. Endoscopy is being utilized more frequently to examine aneurysms, tumor resection beds, and other pathologies. The benefits of endoscopy for these uses have been explored by a number of authors (Brockmeyer et al. 1998; Lewis et al. 1994; Gamea et al. 1994).

The endoscope provides an improved and frequently innovative perspective of the anatomy, which can help residents comprehend a surgical strategy. Additionally, the student and the operating surgeon have the same perspective, which is not always the case with an operating microscope. The possibility of striking structures while inserting the endoscope is the most hazardous part of utilizing the endoscope. Instead of focusing on the image on the screen, it is important to direct the endoscope by looking down the length of its barrel. It is crucial to keep an eye on the shaft after inserting the endoscope into the working zone because, if it is not fixed, slight, hardly perceptible movements at the tip may lead to a big excursion at the backside of the scope, that could have devastating results. The surgeon may be able to work with both hands if they are using a fixed endoscope holder. By doing so, the surgeon will be able to employ more sophisticated tools and avoid having the endoscope brush up against important structures in the operational corridor (Teo and Mobbs 2004).

7. Endoscopy for Base of the Skull Lesions

Carrau and colleagues (Carrau et al. 1996), who described their initial experience with endonasal transsphenoidal hypophysectomy at the University of Pittsburgh, are credited with pioneering the use of neuroendoscopy to treat skull base tumors. Other pathologies of the sellar and parasellar areas were included in the scope of this method by de Divitiis and colleagues (de Divitiis et al. 2002). The anterior skull base tumors can now be seen up to the crista galli as well as down to the level of the axis using the bilateral endonasal endoscopic technique. The lesions in (a) the crista galli to tuberculum sellae, (b) the sellae and suprasellar area, (c) the upper clival zone, and (d) the lower clival zone up to the level of the axis are shown in Figure 7.

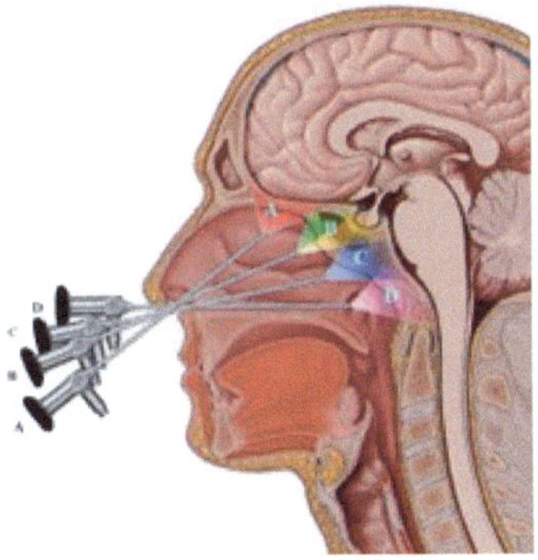

Figure 7. Angulation of endoscope and access to the broad area of the skull base. Source: Figure by author.

With positive outcomes and minimal morbidity, the endoscopic endonasal approach was used for the surgical excision of pituitary tumors and craniopharyngioma (Shim et al. 2017). Based on the size of the mass, the endoscopic approach for sellar and suprasellar neoplasms should be chosen. Endoscopic removal of supradiaphragmatic lesions and transtuberculum–transplanum sphenoidale removal of suprasellar prechiasmatic preinfundibular lesions are both options (Sgouros 2013).

Endoscopic endonasal surgery is particularly challenging when dealing with tumors in the tuberculum sellae region. It is a small anatomical area with delicate but significant microvasculature and probable circle of Willis involvement. The most popular vascularized flap to be used to treat high-flow leaks is the nasal septal flap (Hadad et al. 2006; El-Sayed et al. 2008). Excision of the planum and cribriform anteriorly along the base of the skull is a logical extension of the endoscopic endonasal approach (Roxbury et al. 2016).

The pathologies of the petroclival region, clivus, and intradural posterior fossa (immediately next to the clivus), can now be effectively treated by endoscopic endonasal surgery (EES). The clival and paraclival areas have historically been challenging to access, particularly pathologies that have considerable bilateral extension or significant sagittal plain extension. The typical split of the clivus into thirds, each requiring a different method, shows that for such tumors a mix of open procedures is frequently necessary (Sekhar et al. 1993).

The anterior surgical corridor offers access to pathologies that reach right and left across the midline, whereas EEAs are particularly adaptable to the sagittal plain. This means that a single endonasal conduit can be used to access even larger neoplasms that cover the total clival region. Midline access to the interpeduncular fossa, basilar top, mammillary bodies, and third ventricle floor is made possible using an endoscopic superior transclival approach. The dorsum sellae and the posterior clinoid processes, which must be accessible and excised during this approach, make up the upper clivus, also called the "sellar clivus". The basilar artery, anterior inferior cerebellar artery, ventral pons, prepontine cistern, and cisternal section of the abducens nerve are all accessible via a middle transclival approach. The paraclival ICAs as well as the petroclival fissure obstruct the sphenoidal clivus laterally. The interdural portion of cranial nerve VI restricts the middle transclival exposure laterally (Zwagerman et al. 2016).

A number of experts have written papers on methods for treating Meckel's cave lesions that expand inferiorly as well as laterally to the cavernous sinus (Wang et al. 2016; Raza et al. 2014; Jouanneau et al. 2014). The vertebro-basilar junction, vertebral arteries, posterior inferior cerebellar arteries, IX–XII cranial nerves, premedullary cistern, and ventral medullary surface are all exposed during the lower transclival approach through the lower clival segment, which is located beneath the roof of the choana (Zwagerman et al. 2016). An endoscopic image of the cerebellopontine angle is depicted in Figures 8 and 9 (Chowdhury et al. 2012).

CSF rhinorrhea, which frequently results from trauma and iatrogenic deformation of the base of the skull and is secondary to neoplastic inflammatory and pseudotumor syndromes, has been treated using endoscopic procedures. Endoscopic restructuring of tissue planes and total disconnection of the cranial space from sinonasal cavities can be used to correct faults in the skull base and accomplish a multi-layered reconstruction. A single layer of fascia or fat, followed by tissue glue, can be used to heal small bone defects. Multi-layered closure is necessary for larger skull base lesions with significant intraoperative CSF leakage. A homologous fat graft in the bone deficiency, followed by the fascia lata, an osseous buttress, and tissue glue, can be used to achieve this. A gasket seal repair can be added to these larger skull base abnormalities (Sgouros 2013; Hadad et al. 2006). Kawsar et al. reported positive results in their series, and Fortes et al. demonstrated endoscopic correction of CSF leakage via transpterygoid transposition of a temporoparietal fascia flap (Fortes et al. 2007). Figure 10 illustrates the flap's course through the endoscopic method (Kawsar et al. 2020).

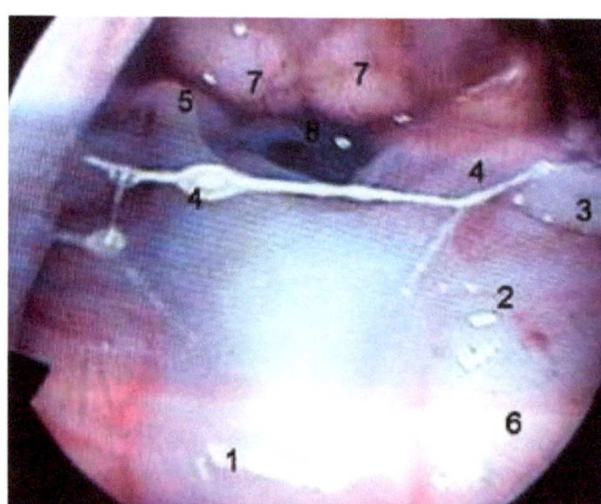

Figure 8. Endoscopic view of the interpeduncular fossa. 1—basilar artery, 2—superior cerebellar artery, 3—3rd nerve, 4—posterior cerebellar artery, 5—posterior communicating artery, 6—basilar pons, 7—mamillary body, and 8—thalamoperforator. Source: Figure by authors.

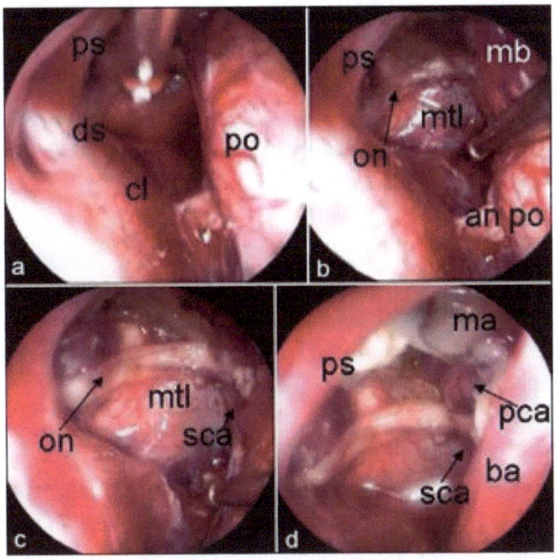

Figure 9. (**a–d**) Intraoperative sequential endoscopic exploration of CP angle. ps—pituitary stalk, ds—dorsum sellae, cl—clivus, po—pons, on—oculomotor nerve, mb—midbrain, mtl—medial temporal lobe, an—abducent nerve, sca—superior cerebellar artery, pca—posterior cerebral artery, ba—basilar artery, and ma—mamillary body. Source: Figure by authors.

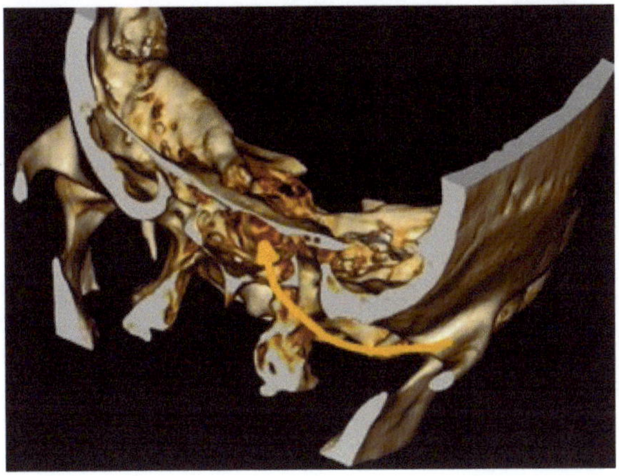

Figure 10. Route of endoscopic transposition of vascularized transpterygoid temporal muscle flap (TPTMF flap). Source: Figure by authors.

8. Endoscopic Transsphenoidal Surgery

8.1. Introduction

Although Gerard Guiot is credited with being the first neurosurgeon to employ the endoscope in the transsphenoidal procedure, he eventually gave up due to poor visibility (Guiot et al. 1963; Liu et al. 2001). Many surgeons (Apuzzo et al. (1977) along with Bushe and Halves (1978); Halves and Bushe (1979)) did not record the utilization of the endoscope as a technical accessory in the microscopic excision of extrasellar pituitary pathologies until the late 1970s. In the beginning, endoscopy was used to supplement microsurgery so that other surgeons could observe things that were out of their line of sight using tilted mirrors (Liu et al. 2001; Hardy 1967). Axel Perneczky, who pioneered the use of the endoscope in cerebral neurosurgery, stressed the importance of an endoscopic understanding of micro-anatomy, which may not be fully understood with a microscope, and developed the idea of minimally invasive neurosurgery (Fries and Perneczky 1998; Perneczky and Fries 1998).

As a consequence of the collaboration between neurosurgical and ENT surgeons, the pure endoscopic transsphenoidal procedure (i.e., utilization of the neuroendoscope as the only viewing instrument) was established in the early 1990s. At the Central Hospital of the University of Nancy, Jankowski and colleagues published their experiences of three instances in which they applied a solely endoscopic transsphenoidal procedure to the sellae turcica in 1992 (Jankowski et al. 1992).

More recently, the idea of extending techniques to the base of the skull has been introduced. Other technical accessories like microvascular Doppler, neuronavigation, and endoscopic endonasal transsphenoidal surgery have been used to treat lesions outside the sellae turcica (Kaptain et al. 2001; Locatelli et al. 2000).

8.2. Operative Procedural Techniques

Under general anesthesia, the patient is in supine position with the trunk raised 10° and the head turned 10° in the direction of the surgeon. The patient's head is fixed with three pins or tape in a horseshoe headrest, but not rigidly. The nasal cavities are crammed with pledgets drenched in dilute adrenaline just before the endoscope is inserted. The following three phases can be used to divide the operation.

8.2.1. Nasal Phase

The major anatomical landmarks, like the nasal septum medially and inferior turbinate laterally, can be recognized after entry with the endoscope. The choana can be seen by moving in that direction and following the inferior turbinate's tail. Medially, the vomer (a midline pointer) and, superiorly, the sphenoid sinus floor limit the choana (Figure 11).

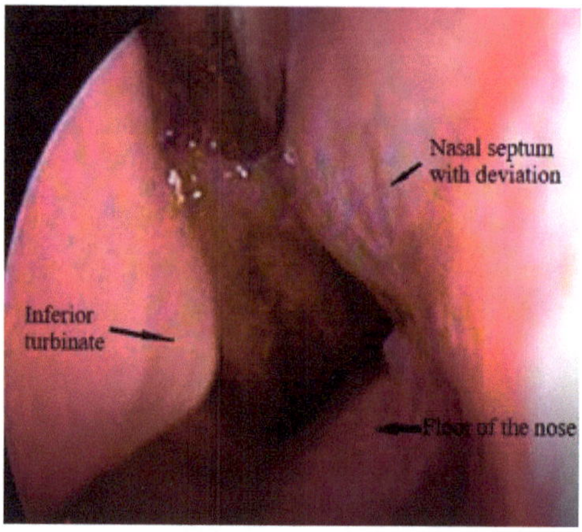

Figure 11. Nasal stage of endoscopic pituitary. Source: Figure by authors.

To increase the surgical passage between the nasal septum and the middle turbinate, the middle turbinate is softly moved laterally. The sphenoid ostium can be seen while looking up with an endoscope; it is typically 1.5 cm superior of the choana's roof. The superior or supreme turbinate, if they cover the sphenoid ostium, can be gently lateralized or eliminated while still preserving the cribriform plate's lateral lamella.

To avoid damaging the ethmoidal plate and causing a CSF leak, great care should be taken when removing or laterally luxating these turbinates.

8.2.2. Sphenoid Phase

In order to prevent arterial hemorrhage from the septal arterial branches of the sphenopalatine artery, this step of the treatment begins with the cauterization of the spheno-ethmoid recess as well as the region surrounding the sphenoid ostium. The septum of the nose is separated from the sphenoid rostrum using a microdrill. With care taken not to over extend the incision in the inferolateral side, at which the sphenopalatine artery and its major branches lie, the ventral wall of the sphenoidal sinus is then extensively opened with a microdrill and rongeur, working circumferentially.

To achieve the correct working direction for the complete instrument when within the sphenoid, with its distal end in the sellae, it is essential to extensively expose and uncover the anterior wall of the sphenoid. The sellar floor, spheno-ethmoid planum, tuberculum sellae, and clival indentation of the sphenoid sinus are all evident after the excision of all sphenoid septa, as well as its posterior and lateral walls. The bony protuberances of the intracavernous internal carotid artery, the second cranial nerve, and the opto-carotid recess can be seen laterally to the sellar floor (Figure 12). The intracavernous carotid artery's bony protuberances should be identified to mark the sellar floor limits, even though it may not always be possible to identify each anatomical feature.

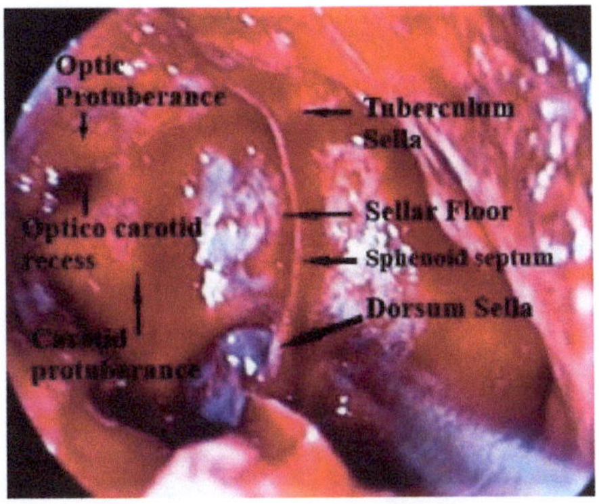

Figure 12. End of the sphenoidal phase with exposure of the sellar floor. Source: Figure by authors.

Hammer and Radberg's initial classification of the sphenoid sinuses into conchal, presellar, and sellar types is still extensively used today (Hammer and Radberg 1962), because it accurately predicts the surgical route utilized in transsphenoidal procedures. Depending on the extension of the pneumatization, Guldner et al. classified the sellar type into incomplete and complete types (Güldner et al. 2012; Hiremath et al. 2018). The modifications and the conventional system concentrate on the posterior limit of pneumatization as well as the ease of accessibility of the sellar floor during transsphenoidal endoscopic surgeries.

8.2.3. Sellar Phase

The endoscope can be fastened to the holder from this point on in the process, freeing both hands of the surgeon. In reality, it is standard procedure for the surgeon to keep using the endoscope while the two instruments are being dynamically moved via one or both nostrils by an aid.

The procedure's sellar phase (Figure 13) adheres to the same guidelines as the microscopic transsphenoidal technique. The sellar floor is opened utilizing a high-speed drill and a Kerrison rongeur, often extending the bone drilling from the tuberculum to the floor of the sellae as well as from one side of the cavernous sinus to the contralateral side. However, its size and shape could be customized depending on the need for lesion removal. The carotid arteries may be more easily identified during such procedures with the aid of an ultrasound Doppler probe, allowing for a safer opening of the dura and subsequent linear, rectangular, or cruciate incisions. The inferior and lateral parts of the lesion are resected before the superior part in cases of macroadenoma. In fact, removing the upper portion first will cause the redundant diaphragm and suprasellar cistern to enter the operating field too early, decreasing the chance to expose and excise the lateral parts of the lesion. The Valsalva maneuver, which causes the suprasellar cistern to protrude into the sellar cavity, can be helpful if the collapse of the suprasellar component of the lesion is not seen.

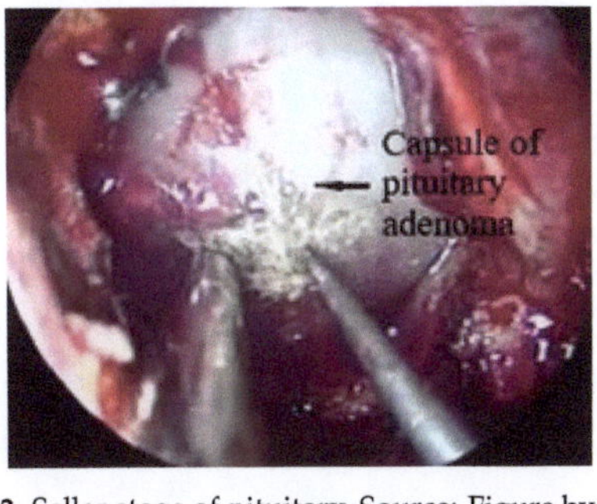

Figure 13. Sellar stage of pituitary. Source: Figure by authors.

Additionally, while performing interior debulking on a microadenoma, it is preferred to detach the tumor pseudocapsule from the pituitary gland to obtain an "enbloc" excision (Oldfield and Vortmeyer 2006).

After the lesion has been removed, an endoscopic examination of the tumor cavity using a 0° and/or an angled telescope is next carried out to see whether any tumor remnants remain.

8.2.4. Sellar Reconstruction

Sellar repair is necessary at the conclusion of the procedure, typically when a peroperative CSF leakage has occurred. Based on the extent of the osteo-dural deficiency and the amount of "dead space" within the sellae, different procedures (intradural and/or extradural repair of the sellae, as well as packing of the sellar tumor cavity with or without packing of the sphenoidal sinus) are used (Cappabianca et al. 2002).

The purpose of this type of repair is to ensure a watertight seal, eliminate dead space, and stop the chiasm from descending into the sellar cavity. To keep the optic system from being compressed, overpacking must be avoided. Except in the event of a small, unanticipated, postoperative CSF leakage, lumbar drainage is no longer used. The middle turbinate is softly repositioned in a medial direction once the endoscope has been gradually removed. There is no use of nasal cavity packing.

8.3. Advantages of Endoscopic Transsphenoidal Surgery

Transsphenoidal endoscopy has a number of benefits for patients (such as less nasal injury, no nasal packing, less perioperative pain, and (typically) rapid recovery) as well as for surgeons (e.g., a wider and closer vision of the surgical area; increased scientific activity, as evidenced by the peer-reviewed literature on the subject in the last ten years; smoother interdisciplinary co-operation, etc.) (Spencer et al. 1999; Snyderman et al. 2007; Cappabianca et al. 2008).

8.4. Complications of Endoscopic Transsphenoidal Surgery

Major morbidity was reported in 1% to 2% of case scenarios and postoperative CSF fistulas in 3.9% of patients in the Ciric et al. study (Ciric et al. 1997), which is taken as the gold standard for transsphenoidal surgery complication questionnaires pertaining to perioperative complications, with further reduced rates among more experienced surgeons (Barker et al. 2003).

The postoperative occurrence of CSF leaks was reported to range from 1.4 to 16.9% by Lobatto et al. in a systematic study (Lobatto et al. 2018). The published frequency of DI varies from 0.3% to 45% and is different, in part, due to inconsistent definitions (Abhinav et al. 2020). Two skilled pituitary groups who utilized accepted definitions for DI or whose surgical experience primarily targeted endoscopic excision of pituitary tumors recently published their postoperative DI frequency with reasonably comparable outcomes (Ajlan et al. 2018; Nayak et al. 2018).

Both investigations indicated a DI occurrence of 26% and 16.6% in 178 and 271 patients, respectively, with only 10% and 4% developing persistent DI (Ajlan et al. 2018; Nayak et al. 2018).

While late hyponatremia is the most frequent reason for unplanned re-hospitalization after pituitary tumor surgery, hypernatremia can also cause substantial morbidity during the perioperative period (Bohl et al. 2016). The majority of delayed hyponatremia (SIADH) cases, which often develop between postoperative days 4 and 7, are a secondary effect of incorrect antidiuretic hormone release. It has a documented incidence of 3.6% to 19.8% (Barber et al. 2014; Hussain et al. 2013; Jahangiri et al. 2014).

Hypothalamic–pituitary axis (HPA) dysfunction is still regarded as a clinical issue. Adrenal insufficiency is the condition that poses the greatest risk to life, with current case studies indicating rates ranging from 3 to 21% (Little et al. 2019).

Nasal structural support can be lost as a result of excessive nasal septum removal, which can lead to external nasal malformation. Extended approaches requiring nasal septal flap repair may increase this risk (Rowan et al. 2016, 2020). When substantial posterior superior segments of the nasal septum and its mucosa as well as the nearby superior and middle turbinate mucosa are removed (structures that form the olfactory cleft), hyposmia or more serious anosmia may result. As a result, while a sufficient surgical corridor is made towards the sellae and a nasoseptal flap is procured, special attention is typically given to maintain these structures (Harvey et al. 2015a, 2015b).

With a reported incidence between 0.2 and 0.4%, injury of the ICA during sellar drilling and exposure or excision of the tumor is uncommon but is linked with considerable morbidity (Perry et al. 2019). Iatrogenic injuries can cause serious stroke, permanent disability, or even death (Chin et al. 2016). Three percent of cases may involve significant epistaxis that requires further treatment (De Los Reyes et al. 2015; Alzhrani et al. 2018).

The self-reported questionnaire study provided by Ciric et al. showed that the mean surgical mortality for each of the three groups was 0.9% (Ciric et al. 1997). Only one (1/1153) perioperative fatality was reported by Agam et al., representing 0.1% of their series (Agam et al. 2019).

Cases with visual impairments and tumors that had invaded any nearby structures were at a higher danger of complication, possibly reflecting a more serious underlying disease, according to a new paper by Agam et al. (2019). Because of scarring and adhesions that make the operative environment more difficult, revision operations for previous transsphenoidal surgery, craniotomies, and radiosurgery were also more likely to result in problems (Esquenazi et al. 2017).

9. Endoscopy in Intracranial Aneurysm Surgery

9.1. General Roles of Endoscope

The utilization of the endoscope in and around aneurysms is made simpler and safer by the benefits of greater illumination; good, close-up views of local anatomic features; and extended visual angles. The endoscope also makes it easier to determine the best clip locations (Yoshioka and Kinouchi 2015).

Endonasal extended transsphenoidal total exposure of the circle of Willis within the brain in situ was shown by Chowdhury et al. to be the best method for observing the circle for variations, including asymmetry in the cadaveric investigation (Figures 14 and 15) (Chowdhury et al. 2012). Taniguchi et al. published that, in their series of fifty-four case scenarios, the endoscope made clear the intricate additional local anatomy in nine cases (16.7%); in five cases (9.3%), the neurosurgeons repositioned the clip based on endoscopic data collected after the initial clip application (Taniguchi et al. 1999).

In a series of research by Kalavakonda et al. (2002), a neuroendoscope was utilized to inspect the applied clip in 75 of 79 cases (95%) and anatomical features in 26 cases (33%). Important details including the perforators, parent artery, their branches, the aneurysm's neck and back wall, the extent of the clipping of the neck, and the incorporation of the parent artery in the clip could all be seen using the endoscope in 15 (19%) aneurysms. In six instances, the clip was moved due to a residual neck or the incorporation of the parent artery, and in one instance, the clip location was altered due to compression of the second nerve (Kalavakonda et al. 2002). In 150 of 180 cases in a recent publication by Fischer et al., a neuroendoscope was utilized to obtain extra topographic data prior to clipping (83%) (Fischer et al. 2012). In four cases, clipping under endoscopic vision was successful. In 130 of the 180 surgeries, endoscopic examination was performed after clipping (Yoshioka and Kinouchi 2015).

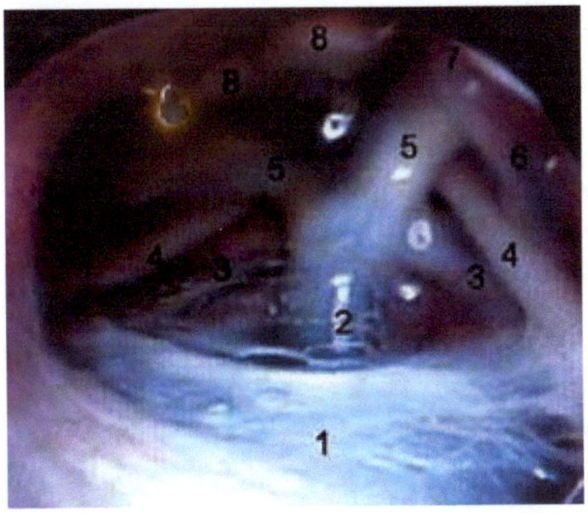

Figure 14. Endoscopic exposure of circle of Willis. 1—Liliequist membrane, 2—basilar artery, 3—superior cerebellar artery, 4—3rd nerve, 5—posterior cerebral artery, 6—posterior communicating artery, 7—P2 segment of posterior communicating artery, and 8—mamillary body. Source: Figure by authors.

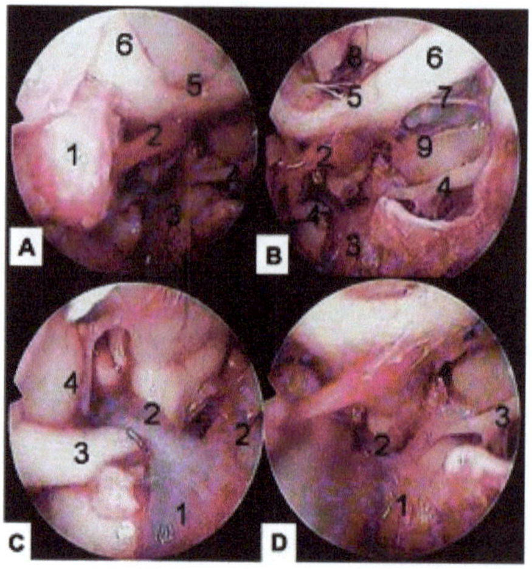

Figure 15. Endoscopic exploration of circle of Willis with pituitary gland mobilization. (**A**,**B**) 1—pituitary gland, 2—pituitary stalk, 3—basilar artery, 4—3rd nerve, 5—optic chiasm, 6—optic nerve, 7—anterior cerebral artery, 8—anterior communicating artery, and 9—medial temporal lobe. (**C**,**D**) 1—basilar artery, 2—posterior cerebral artery, 3—3rd nerve, and 4—medial temporal lobe. Source: Figure by authors.

The mass of the lesion makes it more difficult to insert and fix the endoscope in the operational region, so very large aneurysms typically benefit less from the endoscope than smaller ones in the same place (Galzio et al. 2013). The treatment of brain aneurysms with deep locations particularly benefits from the endoscope. Consequently, the area is another crucial consideration. The usefulness of the endoscope for such aneurysms is restricted when they are superficially placed, such as middle cerebral artery aneurysms, and for distant aneurysms, like pericallosal aneurysms (Yoshioka and Kinouchi 2015). This chapter does not cover the detailed approach to aneurysms.

Additionally, some endoscopic drawbacks have been reported (de Divitiis et al. 2002). During initial examination, the aneurysm may burst due to the endoscope. The endoscope may become worthless if there is blood in the surgical area, so the clot must be cleared before continuing. Instrumentation made especially for endoscopic surgery is still lacking (Kalavakonda et al. 2002). Prior to the development of more recent 3D endoscopes, three dimensional images were not possible.

10. Microvascular Decompression

In general, offending vessels cause hemifacial spasms (HFSs), primary trigeminal neuralgia (TN), and glossopharyngeal neuralgia, which frequently compress the pertinent nerve at the root entry or exit zone (REZ). Microvascular decompression (MVD) is a well-researched and successful treatment (Haines et al. 1980; Antonini et al. 2014; Campos-Benitez and Kaufmann 2008; Pollock and Schoeberl 2010; Apra et al. 2017).

MVD procedures have been performed using endoscopic techniques like endoscopic or endoscope-assisted MVD (E-MVD). Some drawbacks of microscopic MVD (M-MVD) can be addressed in the meantime, as the technique develops and neurosurgeons gain experience in endoscopic surgery. When compared to microscopy, several publications claimed that endoscopy is more effective at locating the zone of neurovascular conflict (Duntze et al. 2011; Chen et al. 2008; Burchiel et al. 1988).

TN is characterized by rostromedial compression of the trigeminal nerve by the lateral pontomesencephalic section of the SCA, which typically runs medial to the trigeminal nerve (Hitotsumatsu et al. 2003; Martin et al. 1980). By using an endoscopic method, the lateral pontomesencephalic section of the SCA can be transferred rostromedially and then anchored at the cerebellar tentorium. While not requiring brain retraction or petrosal vein ligation, a 30° endoscopic vision through the lateral tentorial surface of the cerebellum allows good exposure of the trigeminal nerve from the REZ to the Meckel cave and also reveals the path of the lateral pontomesencephalic portion of the SCA as the culprit artery along the midbrain . The SCA lateral pontomesencephalic segment's perforators can also be seen with a clean endoscopic view. The SCA lateral pontomesencephalic segment's perforators are quite lengthy and do not obstruct transposition to tentorial fixation.

For hemifacial spasm, the flocculus emerges just lateral to the eighth cranial nerve, and the REZ of the facial nerve is placed immediately medial to the eighth cranial nerve in the supraolivary fossette. The root output zone of the seventh nerve is frequently compressed from a caudal direction by the lateral pontomedullary portion of the AICA (Hitotsumatsu et al. 2003; Martin et al. 1980). By using an endoscopic technique, the AICA should be anchored at the petrosal dura and transferred caudally.

The neurovascular structures and relationships surrounding the supraolivary fossette behind the flocculus are clearly visible in a 30° endoscopic view through the petrosal surface of the cerebellum through a retrosigmoid keyhole. After the AICA has been mobilized, the problematic artery can easily be identified as the facial nerve root exit zone. Small perforators may be seen clearly by the endoscope even when they are hidden by obstructions (Ishikawa et al. 2015), and secure identification of perforators helps prevent harm during decompression treatments, particularly for the transposition technique.

It is demonstrated in the meta-analysis by Li et al. (Li et al. 2019) that E-MVD is better when perioperative safety is taken into account, as there are less perioperative problems. Postoperative efficacy, as indicated by the recent cure rate, long-term cure rate, and offending vessel identification rate, was also better with E-MVD. Facial paralysis was much lower in E-MVD, but CSF leakage and dysaudia also exhibited a similar tendency to the prior discussions (Kabil et al. 2005; Badr-El-Dine et al. 2002). The results suggest that EMVD is the best surgical technique for MVD to treat facial spasms and trigeminal or glossopharyngeal neuralgia.

11. Surgery for Craniosynostosis

Craniosynostosis' minimally invasive surgical cure was invented by Jimenez and colleagues (Jimenez and Barone 1998; Jimenez et al. 2004). Before the age of six months, endoscopy-assisted craniosynostosis surgery (EACS) can be used to treat this issue, along with postoperative helmet shaping therapy. Three months old is the ideal age for EACS. With a conventional arsenal and a 0-degree endoscope with a working shaft utilized for endoscopic face lift surgery sans irrigation, the procedure—basically a strip craniectomy—can be carried out. The authors presented a low risk of complications as well as a high percentage of success.

A craniectomy in scaphocephaly is carried out from the anterior to the posterior fontanelle. With powerful scissors, the bone is sliced. The removed strip needs to be 11 cm long and 4–5 cm wide. Wedge-shaped osteotomies or lateral barrel stave osteotomies can be introduced in front of the lambdoid sutures and behind the coronal suture. This endoscopic method has a strong success rate and fewer complications. Furthermore, in their most recent publication, only 9% of the 139 patients needed blood transfusions. Within three weeks following surgery, the children donned a helmet for ten months. Skin problems were infrequent, although probable pressure sores or eczema were given special attention (Jimenez et al. 2004; Sgouros 2013; Shim et al. 2017).

12. Endoscopic and Endoscope-Assisted ICH Evacuation

Endoscope-Assisted Evacuation: It is the term used to describe the formation of a minor craniotomy or craniectomy followed by evacuation using an endoscope and a sucker or combination device beside each other in the lumen of the sheath. In prospective research conducted in 2009 by Kim and Kim, patients with minor ICH (30 cm^3) restricted to the basal ganglia and thalamus were divided into two groups: those who had stereotactically guided active removal (n = 204) and those who underwent conservative care (n = 103); the 1st group had better outcoome (Kim and Kim 2009). At 180 days following initial presentation, patients who received endoscope-assisted evacuation had reduced mean mRS scores (1.2 vs. 3.0 for those who were medically treated) (Hersh et al. 2018).

Endoscopic Evacuation: Pure endoscopic evacuation was employed in one of the early investigations to investigate active MIS ICH evacuation. In this single-center study, accomplished by Auer et al. and published in 1989, the investigators randomly assigned 100 cases (within 48 h of onset) who had supratentorial ICH of more than 10 cm^3 as well as an altered degree of awareness (Auer et al. 1989). When comparing to the medically managed sample, most cases had a 50–70% reduction in hematoma volume following endoscope-assisted surgery and saw considerably lower death and morbidity rates (30 and 60% versus 70 and 75%). The surgery was most beneficial for patients with hemorrhages ≤ 50 cm^3 and who were younger than 60 (Hersh et al. 2018).

13. Spinal Endoscopy

13.1. Introduction

Endoscopic spine surgery is one type of minimally invasive surgery that has evolved from conventional open spine surgery in degenerative disc disease. With the development of and advancements in optics, high-resolution video cameras, endoscopic light sources, high-speed burrs, irrigation pumps, etc., minimally invasive spine procedures are now possible for all sections of the spine using a variety of endoscopic approaches. Less tissue and muscle dissection; less trauma; less blood loss; less disruption of the epidural vascular supply, which prevents epidural fibrosis and scarring; shorter hospital stays; quicker functional recovery; better quality of life; better cosmetic results; and simpler access for recurrent cases are all benefits of endoscopic spine surgery (Choi et al. 2017).

Initially only utilized for lumbar, cervical, and thoracic disc herniations, endoscopic spine surgery is now also employed for spinal canal stenosis, including endoscopic-aided fusion surgeries. In the management of teenage disc herniations, spinal endoscopy can be quite helpful, especially for athletes and those who participate in competitive sports, where minimal tissue stress, cosmetic improvement, and rapid functional recovery are all highly desired outcomes (Choi et al. 2017).

13.2. History of Endoscopic Spine Surgery

Lymen Smith introduced real minimally invasive spine surgery by injecting chymopapain intradiscally, or chemonucleolysis, in 1963 (Hoogland 2003). In order to test the viability of mechanical nuclear debulking, Kambin inserted a Craig cannula using a posterolateral route in 1970. The success rate of the mechanical nucleotomy performed in 1975 (Hijikata et al. 1975) via a posterolateral approach to the disc's nucleus was 64%. Then, using a posterolateral approach, Schreiber and Suezawa created a succession of cannulas, which telescoped one over another, and inserted them into the intervertebral disc's center. Larger forceps could be inserted and nuclear tissue could be evacuated more quickly due to the larger cannulas with an internal diameter (ID) of 7 to 8 mm. For the first time, Friedman and Jacobson used a far lateral procedure for lumbar intervertebral disc herniation, inserting a 40-gauge French thoracostomy tube through an incision above the iliac crest and guiding it to the disc after manually removing disc pieces with forceps (Choi et al. 2017; Friedman 1983). Onik et al. (1985) performed a central nucleotomy in 1985 using a nucleotome, a technology that gained popularity due to its low cost and ease of use. Kambin started using a laser to vaporize disc fragments in 1990, but the laser's large arc of deflection and damage to the neural structure prevented sufficient decompression. The parameters of the safe working area for the posterolateral approach between departing and crossing nerve roots were described by Kambin after an extensive cadaver study. He talked about Kambin's triangle (Figure 16). Adipose tissue and a very small superficial vein loosely surround the triangle (Kambin 1991, 1992; Kambin and Gellman 1983). All prior trials on minimally invasive disc access were blind. Kambin and Sampson published a purely endoscopic visualization method for a non-sequestrated intervertebral disc herniation as an extraforaminal approach; however, this technique eventually developed into a translaminar approach for discectomy (Kambin and Sampson 1986). In 1996, Sofamor Danek began a transforaminal endoscopic discectomy through a foramen (Mathews 1996). Choi et al. made a significant contribution to the reconfiguration of the endoscopic approach by entry to the far lateral intervertebral disc herniation (Choi et al. 2006; Kim et al. 2011).

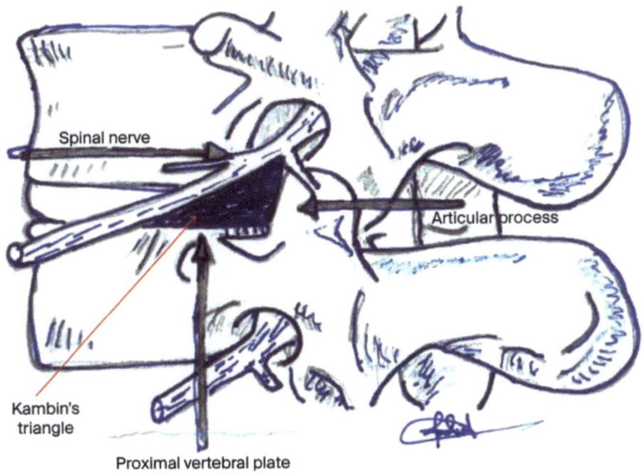

Figure 16. Illustration showing Kambin's triangle. Source: Figure by authors.

13.3. Endoscopic Lumbar Spinal Surgery

13.3.1. Transforaminal Endoscopic Lumbar Discectomy (TELD)

In the TELD, discectomy and decompression are carried out through the foramen between the exiting and traversing roots of the vertebrae. The crucial TELD procedure involves precisely inserting the needle into the disc through the Kambin's safe triangle, which is located between the outgoing and traversing roots. The superior endplate of the inferior vertebra serves as the Kambin's triangle's inferior boundary, while the thecal sac and the crossing nerve root, which is constrained by the facet, serve as its anterior boundary (Figure 16) (Choi et al. 2017).

During percutaneous procedures, the pedicle and associated disc space are utilized as radiographic landmarks. The position of needle insertion in the X-ray view is separated into horizontal lines parallel to the endplates in the anteroposterior view and a posterior vertebral line in the lateral view. For the majority of transforaminal surgeries, the posterior vertebral line and the medial pedicular line are typically used as reference points. To determine the largest and safest working cannula to enter the foramen, the working zone's dimensions are also crucial. Cannulas of 6.5 mm are safer when inserted at the medial pedicular line in the anteroposterior X-ray view, while 7.5 mm cannulas are safer when put at the midpedicular line, according to (Mirkovic et al. 1995) cadaveric study. The majority of functioning cannulas on the market have a diameter of about 7.5 mm.

Standard indications to keep in mind for discectomy.

Contraindications are (Choi et al. 2017):

- Severe disc migration and extensive disc calcification;
- L5-S1 level (special in males; cases with long iliac wings);
- More than single level (relative contraindication);
- Foraminal and spinal canal stenosis (relative contraindication);
- Spondylolisthesis;
- Recurrent intervertebral disc herniation (reoperation);
- Anomalies of the nerve root, like-conjugate root;
- Cauda equine syndrome.

Surgical Approach of TELD

TELD is accomplished in the lateral or prone position while the patient is under local anesthesia (1% lidocaine) as well as sedation with midazolam (0.05 mg/kg, 30 min prior to surgery) and fentanyl (0.8 g/kg, 10 min prior to surgery). Due to superior anatomical alignment, most surgeons choose the prone position. The distance from the midline and the needle trajectory used to target the ruptured fragment, sans entering the peritoneal sac and only grazing the facet, are estimated to determine the skin entry location for the needle depending on preoperative CT scan and MRI. In the C-arm anteroposterior (AP) view, the needle is pointed 10° downwards to form a 10° angle with the upper and lower endplates, sequentially, and advanced further until the first bony hindrance of the facet is felt. A limited adjustment of the trajectory can be made by beveling the needle; doing so allows for more superficial advancement and vice versa, with the needle slightly withdrawn, elevated, and inserted into the foramen while the C-arm is in the side view. The most crucial aspect is a precise and secure entry into the lower third of Kambin's triangle (Figure 16). The lower lumbar spine posterior vertebral line and medial pedicular line are the sites of annular puncture because the lamina is wider and less likely to puncture the dura. Next, puncture the annulus. Conduct a discography by injecting a mixture of 2 to 3 mL radiopaque dye and normal saline mixed in 2:1:2 ratios once the needle has reached the disc's center in AP view. During surgery, dye makes it easier to identify nuclear fragments. Change the needle for a guide wire, and then slide the obturator over the guide wire until it pierces the annulus. With the use of a mallet and tapper, withdraw the guide wire, and then thread the working cannula over the obturator. Insert the endoscope through the working cannula after removing the obturator. When performing a procedure, keep an eye out for any excessive discomfort radiating to the leg that could be caused by compression over the departing root (the traveling root is shielded by a facet), and adjust the needle trajectory as necessary. After the endoscope has been inserted, try to identify the structures, remove the fragment with various forceps, and, if necessary, repair the annular tear using bipolar cold cauterization and a Ho-YAG laser. Thecal sac and transverse root mobility without restriction, recent epidural hemorrhage, and pain relief are indications of sufficient decompression.

Extraforaminal disc herniation, high-grade above or below migrating disc herniations, and a high iliac crest for the L5-S1 level require special modification of the conventional procedure.

For extraforaminal intervertebral disc herniation:

(1) The needle direction needs to be steeper;
(2) The angle of needle insertion should be between 10 and 50%, depending on preoperative images;
(3) The distance from the midline needs to be between 5 and 8 cm;
(4) The midpedicular line should be used in the AP view and the posterior vertebral line should be used in the lateral C-arm view;
(5) The superior endplate of the caudal vertebra should be in the direction of the needle.

For migrated disc herniation:

(1) The entry point of the needle ought to be lower than the disc space, and vice versa for down-migrated disc herniations;
(2) Foraminoplasty (undercutting the non-articular section of the upper facet) or oblique pediculotomy (cutting of medial and upper wall of the lower pedicle) may be necessary for high-grade, down-migrating disc herniation (Choi et al. 2017).

Interlaminar Approach

Due to anatomical restrictions such a high iliac crest or up-migrated intervertebral disc herniation, where the trajectory is not on the plane of herniation, the transforaminal approach can occasionally be challenging at the L5-S1 level. The interlaminar approach can be helpful in certain circumstances. The interlaminar approach is feasible for L5-S1-level intervertebral disc herniation because the interlaminar window is greatest (31 mm) and there is little upper laminar overhang. The use of endoscopic surgery to treat spinal canal stenosis has grown recently (Choi et al. 2017).

13.3.2. Complications

Immediate Complications

- Neural and vascular structure injury;
- Peritoneal sac perforation, including abdominal contents;
- Missed or left fragments;
- Wrong spinal level or side exploration;
- Breakage of instrument.

Early Postoperative Complications

- Psoas muscle hematoma;
- Postoperative development of hematoma;
- CSF cyst formation;
- Infection.

Delayed Complications

- Recurrent intervertebral disc herniation;
- Possible spinal instability (Choi et al. 2017).

13.4. Endoscopic Cervical Spine Surgery

13.4.1. Percutaneous Endoscopic Cervical Discectomy (PECD)

The benefit of performing anterior PECD is that it can be conducted as a day-case procedure under local anesthesia, avoiding the need to fuse that segment and the difficulties associated with it. Additionally, because the patient is awake and conscious, there is ongoing feedback from them throughout the process, making it safer.

Indications: Annular rupture with concordant pain on provocative discography, whether contained or not, and paracentral or central intervertebral disc herniation that does not improve with conservative management for an acceptable period of time with correlating MRI and CT scans.

Contraindications:

- Migrated intervertebral disc herniation;
- Collapse disc space < 5 mm;
- Calcified disc;
- Instability;
- Infection;
- Previous history of anterior cervical spinal surgery (Choi et al. 2017).

13.4.2. Percutaneous Endoscopic Posterior Cervical Foraminotomy

Another endoscopic procedure, posterior cervical foraminotomy, can be used to treat foraminal intervertebral disc herniation, which can sometimes be challenging to treat with PECD. It has the advantages of not damaging the anterior normal disc, allowing for the removal of the herniated foraminal fragment, and avoiding anterior cervical discectomy plus fusion. It is also known as "key hole foraminotomy". It might be used for osteophytic foraminal stenosis.

Indications:

- Foraminal intervertebral disc herniations (mainly one-sided arm pain);
- Single/multilevel foraminal stenosis (one-sided arm pain);
- Persistent symptoms in spite of past anterior cervical discectomy and fusion.

Contraindications:

- Axial neck ache;
- Existence of cervical kyphosis;
- Instability (Choi et al. 2017).

13.5. Thoracic Spinal Endoscopy

13.5.1. Percutaneous Endoscopic Thoracic Discectomy (PETD)

Thoracic disc herniations (TDHs), which make up 0.25 to 0.75% of all disc herniations, are less common than lumbar or cervical disc prolapses. Thus, TDH surgery is extremely uncommon, accounting for approximately 0.15–1.8% of all medically corrected disc herniations. The frequency of TDH is rising today along with the usage of CT scans and MRI. With a posterior or posterolateral approach, PETD has evolved to lessen trauma and improve the postoperative course of TDHs. Jho described the posterolateral procedure for percutaneous endoscopic transpedicular thoracic discectomy in 1997 (Jho 1999). This prevented the need for additional skin cuts in the chest wall, as was necessary with thoracoscopic techniques, for postoperative chest drainage. Later, in 2010, Choi et al. (2010) utilized a 4 mm 0° endoscope and a low-energy, non-ablative laser to demonstrate the safety and effectiveness of PETD from a posterolateral perspective. The current standard of care for thoracic disc herniations has been compared to PETD, which has been described as a safer surgery with superior results.

The indications are the same for conventional thoracic discectomy. The disc has to be soft.

Contraindications:

- Calcified or hard disc;
- Ossified posterior longitudinal ligament;
- Proof of progressive or acute degenerative spinal cord disease;

- Severe disc narrowing;
- Severe spinal cord compression.

Complications:

- Damage to the spinal cord as well as its nerve roots;
- Vascular injury, such as injury to the thoracic aorta or inferior vena cava, can be life threatening;
- Visceral injury to the mediastinal viscera or lung (Choi et al. 2010, 2017; Jho 1999).

14. Endoscopy in Peripheral Nerve Surgery

Since the late 1980s, endoscopic carpal tunnel release (ECTR) procedures have been carried out. Shorter recovery times, reduced postoperative pain, lower postoperative wound sensitivity, and less scarring are benefits of ECTR. Flat learning curves for surgeons; reduced vision, which could lead to incomplete transverse carpal ligament (TCL) sectioning and a higher risk of neurovascular damage; and higher costs are drawbacks. This method produced outstanding outcomes in several published investigations. Using Brown's biportal endoscopic approach, Hankins et al. demonstrated an 82.6% total recovery, while Chen et al. demonstrated a 91% full recovery utilizing Menon's uniportal endoscopic technique (Hankins et al. 2007; Chen et al. 2011). Endoscopy was also used in attempts to cure cubital tunnel syndrome. Among 85 cubital tube releases, Tsai et al. observed a 64% success rate (Tsai et al. 1999). Ahčan and Zorman demonstrated even better outcomes; in their series, 91% of patients experienced a good or outstanding outcome (Ahčan and Zorman 2007). Decompression was accompanied by subcutaneous transposition in the research by Krishnan et al. of eleven treated patients, with outstanding results in 63.7%, good in 27.3%, and satisfactory in 9.1% of cases. While solely "in situ" decompression was conducted in these series (Krishnan et al. 2006).

There have reportedly been endeavors in endoscopic cubital tunnel release. Zlowodzki reported four randomized controlled studies. These investigations utilized the subcutaneous method in two studies and submuscular transposition in the other two. The studies covered 261 patients in all, with a follow-up period of, on average, 21 months. The "in situ" decompression patient group's complication rate was 9%, but the anterior subcutaneous transposition patient group's complication rate was 30% (Mullick and Dellon 2008). Tsai et al. published 85 endoscopic cubital tunnel releases using a 2–3 cm incision along the ulnar nerve (UN) path at the elbow. The authors decompressed the area up to 10 cm proximal as well as 10 cm distal to the medial epicondyle. A total of 64% of the patients in this series demonstrated improvement following surgery, although two of them later underwent transposition surgeries due to reoccurring problems (Tsai et al. 1999). Ahčan and Zorman described endoscopic release of a 20 cm length of UN through a 3.5 cm incision above the cubital tunnel, with good and excellent outcomes obtained in 91% of cases (Ahčan and Zorman 2007).

Brachial plexus endoscopic surgery is still in the research and development phase. Even though technology has advanced greatly over the past few years, there are still situations when the precise location and nature of a lesion cannot be determined, necessitating open surgical examination. In an effort to discover a minimally invasive method for exploring the brachial plexus that would also enable surgical repair of the severed nerve, a few cadaveric studies utilizing surgical robotic systems have been carried out (Mantovani et al. 2011).

Sural nerve harvesting is an intriguing use of endoscopes in peripheral nerve surgery. As is well known, the sural nerve is most likely the most popular donor for nerve transplantation. The typical open method for harvesting sural nerves involves making a succession of very small incisions along this nerve's course. Endoscopic sural nerve harvesting is a new method that has been devised in recent years. The surgery takes about 25 min to complete and only one 12 mm long skin incision is needed, as opposed to three in the traditional open technique (Park et al. 2006).

15. Future Directions

Neuroendoscopic surgery is expected to have a promising future. The sector will gain from additional advancements in camera and optical downsizing, surgical instrument design developments, the development of novel navigation or robotics systems, multiport endoscopy, and improved endoscope-assisted microsurgery using bimanual microdissection techniques. Endoscopic neurosurgery will be extended beyond intraventricular or skull base pathologies to intraparenchymal cranial lesions due to the continued development of endoscopic tools and cutting-edge surgical procedures, such as multiport approaches. These developments are crucial for the development of endoscope-assisted microsurgery in the future.

Other objectives include fully robotic telesurgery, shared control systems, or even remotely operated robotic neurosurgery. To meet future indications for minimally invasive or even ultra-micro-access neurosurgery, nanotechnology breakthroughs are required.

Neuroendoscopy is anticipated to become commonplace in contemporary neurosurgery practices in the future. For aspiring neurosurgeons, institutions should offer training programs (Shim et al. 2017).

Author Contributions: Conceptualization, methodology, validation, formal analysis, investigation, resources, data curation, K.A.K. and A.H.G.; writing—original draft preparation, K.A.K.; writing—review and editing, visualization, supervision, F.H.C. All authors have read and agreed to the published version of the manuscript.

Funding: This research received no external funding.

Conflicts of Interest: The authors declare no conflicts of interest.

References

Abhinav, Kumar, Mathew Tyler, Oliver T. Dale, Ahmed Mohyeldin, Juan C. Fernandez-Miranda, and Laurence Katznelson. 2020. Managing complications of endoscopic transsphenoidal surgery in pituitary adenomas. *Expert Review Endocrinology Metabolism* 15: 311–19. [CrossRef]

Agam, Matthew S., Michelle A. Wedemeyer, Bozena Wrobel, Martin H. Weiss, John D. Carmichael, and Gabriel Zada. 2019. Complications associated with microscopic and endoscopic transsphenoidal pituitary surgery: Experience of 1153 consecutive cases treated at a single tertiary care pituitary center. *Journal of Neurosurgery* 130: 1576–83. [CrossRef]

Ahčan, Uroš, and Peter Zorman. 2007. Endoscopic decompression of the ulnar nerve at the elbow. *The Journal of Hand Surgery* 32: 1171–76. [CrossRef]

Ajlan, Abdulrazag M., Sarah Bin Abdulqader, Achal S. Achrol, Yousef Aljamaan, Abdullah H. Feroze, Laurence Katznelson, and Griffith R. Harsh. 2018. Diabetes Insipidus following Endoscopic Transsphenoidal Surgery for Pituitary Adenoma. *Journal of Neurological Surgery Part B: Skull Base* 79: 117–22. [CrossRef]

Akbari, S. Hassan A., Terrence F. Holekamp, T. Martin Murphy, Deanna Mercer, Jeffrey R. Leonard, Matthew D. Smyth, T. S. Park, and David D. Limbrick, Jr. 2015. Surgical management of complex multiloculated hydrocephalus in infants and children. *Child's Nervous System* 31: 243–49. [CrossRef]

Alberti, O., T. Riegel, D. Hellwig, and H. Bertalanffy. 2001. Frameless navigation and endoscopy. *Journal of Neurosurgery* 95: 541–43. [CrossRef]

Alzhrani, Gmaan, Walavan Sivakumar, Min S. Park, Philipp Taussky, and William T. Couldwell. 2018. Delayed Complications After Transsphenoidal Surgery for Pituitary Adenomas. *World Neurosurgery* 109: 233–41. [CrossRef]

Andresen, Morten, and Marianne Juhler. 2012. Multiloculated hydrocephalus: A review of current problems in classification and treatment. *Child's Nervous System* 28: 357–62. [CrossRef]

Antonini, Giovanni, Antonella Di Pasquale, Giorgio Cruccu, Andrea Truini, Stefania Morino, Giorgia Saltelli, Andrea Romano, Guido Trasimeni, Nicola Vanacore, and Alessandro Bozzao. 2014. Magnetic resonance imaging contribution for diagnosing symptomatic neurovascular contact in classical trigeminal neuralgia: A blinded casecontrol study and meta-analysis. *Pain* 155: 1464–71. [CrossRef]

Apra, Caroline, Jean-Pascal Lefaucheur, and Caroline Le Guérinel. 2017. Microvascular decompression is an effective therapy for trigeminal neuralgia due to dolichoectatic basilar artery compression: Case reports and literature review. *Neurosurgical Review* 40: 577–82. [CrossRef]

Apuzzo, Michael L. J., Milton D. Heifetz, Martin H. Weiss, and Theodore Kurze. 1977. Neurosurgical endoscopy using the side-viewing telescope. Technical note. *Journal of Neurosurgery* 16: 398–400. [CrossRef]

Auer, Ludwig M., Wolfgang Deinsberger, Kurt Niederkorn, Günther Gell, Reinhold Kleinert, Gerhard Schneider, Peter Holzer, Gertraude Bone, Michael Mokry, Eva Körner, and et al. 1989. Endoscopic surgery versus medical treatment for spontaneous intracerebral hematoma: A randomized study. *Journal of Neurosurgery* 70: 530–35. [CrossRef]

Badr-El-Dine, M., H. F. El-Garem, A. M. Talaat, and J. Magnan. 2002. Endoscopically assisted minimally invasive microvascular decompression of hemifacial spasm. *Otology & neurotology* 23: 122–28.

Barber, Sean M., Brandon D. Liebelt, and David S. Baskin. 2014. Incidence, Etiology and Outcomes of Hyponatremia after Transsphenoidal Surgery: Experience with 344 Consecutive Patients at a Single Tertiary Center. *Journal of Clinical Medicine* 3: 1199–219. [CrossRef]

Barker, Fred G., Anne Klibanski, and Brooke Swearingen. 2003. Transsphenoidal surgery for pituitary tumours in the United States, 1996–2000: Mortality, morbidity, and the effects of hospital and surgeon volume. *The Journal of Clinical Endocrinology & Metabolism* 88: 4709–19. [CrossRef]

Barlow, P., and H. S. Ching. 1997. An economic argument in favour of endoscopic third ventriculostomy as a treatment for obstructive hydrocephalus. *Minimally Invasive Neurosurgery* 40: 37–39. [CrossRef]

Bohl, Michael A., Shah Ahmad, Heidi Jahnke, Deborah Shepherd, Laura Knecht, William L. White, and Andrew S. Little. 2016. Delayed Hyponatremia Is the Most Common Cause of 30-Day Unplanned Readmission After Transsphenoidal Surgery for Pituitary Tumours. *Neurosurgery* 78: 84–90. [CrossRef]

Brockmeyer, Douglas, Keyvan Abtin, Lyn Carey, and Marion L. Walker. 1998. Endoscopic third ventriculostomy: An outcome analysis. *Pediatric Neurosurgery* 28: 236–40. [CrossRef]

Burchiel, Kim J., Hadley Clarke, Michael Haglund, and John D. Loeser. 1988. Long-term efficacy of microvascular decompression in trigeminal neuralgia. *Journal of Neurosurgery* 69: 35–38. [CrossRef]

Bushe, K. A., and E. Halves. 1978. Modifizierte Technik bei transnasaler Operation der Hypophysengeschwulste. *Acta Neurochirurgica (Wien)* 41: 163–75. [CrossRef]

Campos-Benitez, Mauricio, and Anthony M. Kaufmann. 2008. Neurovascular compression findings in hemifacial spasm. *Journal of Neurosurgery* 109: 416–20. [CrossRef]

Cappabianca, Paolo, Luigi Maria Cavallo, Felice Esposito, Vinicio Valente, and Enrico De Divitiis. 2002. Sellar repair in endoscopic endonasal transsphenoidal surgery: Results of 170 cases. *Neurosurgery* 51: 1365–71. [CrossRef]

Cappabianca, Paolo, Luigi Maria Cavallo, Oreste de Divitiis, Domenico Solari, Felice Esposito, and Annamaria Colao. 2008. Endoscopic pituitary surgery. *Pituitary* 11: 385–90. [CrossRef]

Carrau, Ricardo L., Hae-Dong Jho, and Yong Ko. 1996. Transnasal-transsphenoidal endoscopic surgery of the pituitary gland. *The Laryngoscope* 106: 914–18. [CrossRef]

Chen, Alvin Chao-Yu, Meng-Huang Wu, Chung-Hsun Chang, Chun-Ying Cheng, and Kuo-Yau Hsu. 2011. Single portal endoscopic carpal tunnel release: Modification of Menon's technique and data from 65 cases. *International Orthopaedics* 35: 61–65. [CrossRef]

Chen, Min Jie, Wei Jie Zhang, Chi Yang, Yi Qun Wu, Zhi Yuan Zhang, and Yong Wang. 2008. Endoscopic neurovascular perspective in microvascular decompression of trigeminal neuralgia. *Journal of Cranio-Maxillofacial Surgery* 36: 456–61. [CrossRef]

Chin, Oliver Y., Ritam Ghosh, Christina H. Fang, Soly Baredes, James K. Liu, and Jean Anderson Eloy. 2016. Internal carotid artery injury in endoscopic endonasal surgery: A systematic review. *The Laryngoscope* 126: 582–90. [CrossRef]

Choi, Gun, Chetan S. Pophale, Bhupesh Patel, and Priyank Uniyal. 2017. Endoscopic Spine Surgery. *Journal of Korean Neurosurgical Society* 60: 485–97. [CrossRef]

Choi, Gun, Sang-Ho Lee, Pradyumna Pai Raiturker, Seungcheol Lee, and Yu-Sik Chae. 2006. Percutaneous endoscopic interlaminar discectomy for intracanalicular disc herniations at L5-S1 using a rigid working channel endoscope. *Operative Neurosurgery* 58: ONS59–ONS68. [CrossRef]

Choi, Joong-Uhn, Kook-Hee Yang, Tae-Gon Kim, Jong Hee Chang, Jin Woo Chang, Byung-In Lee, and Dong-Seok Kim. 2004. Endoscopic disconnection for hypothalamic hamartoma with intractable seizure. Report of four cases. *Journal of Neurosurgery* 100: 506–11. [CrossRef]

Choi, K. Y., S. S. Eun, S. H. Lee, and H. Y. Lee. 2010. Percutaneous endoscopic thoracic discectomy; transforaminal approach. *Minimally Invasive Neurosurgery* 53: 25–28. [CrossRef]

Chowdhury, Forhad H., Mohammod R. Haque, Khandkar A. Kawsar, A. R. A. Shamim, Quazi Deen Mohammod, Mainul H. Sarker, and H. Goel Atul. 2012. Endoscopic endonasal transsphenoidal exposure of circle of Willis (CW); can it be applied in vascular neurosurgery in the near future? A cadaveric study of 26 cases. *Turkish Neurosurgery* 22: 68–76. [CrossRef]

Ciric, Ivan, Ann Ragin, Craig Baumgartner, and Debi Pierce. 1997. Complications of transsphenoidal surgery: Results of a national survey, review of the literature, and personal experience. *Neurosurgery* 40: 225–37. [CrossRef]

de Divitiis, Enrico, Paolo Cappabianca, and Luigi Maria Cavallo. 2002. Endoscopic transsphenoidal approach: Adaptability of the procedure to different sellar lesions. *Neurosurgery* 51: 699–705. [CrossRef]

Delalande, Olivier, and Martine Fohlen. 2003. Disconnecting surgical treatment of hypothalamic hamartoma in children and adults with refractory epilepsy and proposal of a new classification. *Neurologia Medico-Chirurgica* 43: 61–68. [CrossRef]

De Los Reyes, Kenneth M., Bradley A. Gross, Kai U. Frerichs, Ian F. Dunn, Ning Lin, Jordina Rincon-Torroella, Donald J. Annino, and Edward R. Laws. 2015. Incidence, risk factors and management of severe post-transsphenoidal epistaxis. *Journal of Clinical Neuroscience* 22: 116–22. [CrossRef]

Di Rocco, Federico, Masami Yoshino, and Shizuo Oi. 2005. Neuroendoscopic transventricular ventriculocystostomy in treatment for intracranial cysts. *Journal of Neurosurgery* 103: 54–60. [CrossRef]

Duntze, J., C. F. Litre, C. Eap, E. Théret, A. Bazin, A. Chays, and P. Rousseaux. 2011. Adjunctive use of endoscopy during microvascular decompression in the cerebellopontine angle: 27 case reports. *Neuro-Chirurgie* 57: 68–72. [CrossRef]

El-Ghandour, Nasser M. F. 2008. Endoscopic cyst fenestration in the treatment of multiloculated hydrocephalus in children. *Journal of Neurosurgery: Pediatrics* 1: 217–22. [CrossRef]

El-Sayed, Ivan H., Fredrick C. Roediger, Andrew N. Goldberg, Andrew T. Parsa, and Michael W. McDermott. 2008. Endoscopic reconstruction of skull base defects with the nasal septal flap. *Skull Base* 18: 385–94. [CrossRef]

El-Tantawy, Mohammed H. 2018. Endoscopic Fenestration of Multiloculated Post-Infectious Hydrocephalus. *The Medical Journal of Cairo University* 86: 2995–3002. [CrossRef]

Esquenazi, Yoshua, Walid I. Essayed, Harminder Singh, Elizabeth Mauer, Mudassir Ahmed, Paul J. Christos, and Theodore H. Schwartz. 2017. Endoscopic endonasal versus microscopic transsphenoidal surgery for recurrent and/or residual pituitary adenomas. *World Neurosurgery* 101: 186–95. [CrossRef]

Fernández Molina, Guillermo. 2013. Neuroendoscopic management of middle fossa arachnoid cysts. *World Neurosurgery* 79: S19. [CrossRef]

Fischer, Gerrit, Joachim Oertel, and Axel Perneczky. 2012. Endoscopy in aneurysm surgery. *Operative Neurosurgery* 70: ons184–ons191. [CrossRef]

Fortes, Felipe S. G., Ricardo L. Carrau, Carl H. Snyderman, Amin Kassam, Daniel Prevedello, Allan Vescan, Arlan Mintz, and Paul Gardner. 2007. Transpterygoid transposition of a temporoparietal fascia flap: A new method for skull base reconstruction after endoscopic expanded endonasal approaches. *The Laryngoscope* 117: 970–76. [CrossRef]

Friedman, William A. 1983. Percutaneous discectomy: An alternative to chemonucleolysis. *Neurosurgery* 13: 542–47. [CrossRef]

Fries, Georg, and Axel Perneczky. 1998. Endoscope-assisted brain surgery: Part 2—Analysis of 380 procedures. *Neurosurgery* 42: 226–32. [CrossRef]

Fukushima, Takanori, Buichi Ishijima, Kimiyoshi Hirakawa, Norio Nakamura, and Keiji Sano. 1973. Ventriculofiberscope: A new technique for endoscopic diagnosis and operation. Technical note. *Journal of Neurosurgery* 38: 251–56. [CrossRef]

Galzio, Renato J., Francesco Di Cola, Soheila Raysi Dehcordi, Alessandro Ricci, and Danilo De Paulis. 2013. Endoscope-assisted microneurosurgery for intracranial aneurysms. *Frontiers in Neurology* 4: 201. [CrossRef]

Gamea, A., M. Fathi, and A. el-Guindy. 1994. The use of the rigid endoscope in trans-sphenoidal pituitary surgery. *The Journal of Laryngology & Otology* 108: 19–22. [CrossRef]

Gangemi, Michelangelo, Vincenzo Seneca, Giuseppe Colella, Valentina Cioffi, Alessia Imperato, and Francesco Maiuri. 2011. Endoscopy versus microsurgical cyst excision and shunting for treating intracranial arachnoid cysts. *Journal of Neurosurgery: Pediatrics* 8: 158–64. [CrossRef]

Garcia, Delia M., and Keith H. Fulling. 1985. Juvenile pilocytic astrocytomas of the cerebrum in adults. A distinctive neoplasm with favorable prognosis. *Journal of Neurosurgery* 63: 382–86. [CrossRef]

Grotenhuis, André. 2014. Neuroendoscopic Instruments and Surgical Technique. In *Neuroendoscopy: Current Status and Future Trends*. Edited by Spyros Sgouros. Berlin and Heidelberg: Springer, p. 81. [CrossRef]

Guiot, G. 1973. Ventriculo-cisternostomy for stenosis of the aqueduct of Sylvis. *Acta Neurochirurgica* 28: 275–89. [CrossRef]

Guiot, G., J. Rougerie, M. Fourestier, A. Fournier, C. Comoy, J. Vulmiere, and R. Groux. 1963. Explorations endoscopiques intracraniennes. *Presse Medicale* 71: 1225–28.

Güldner, Christian, Sarah M. Pistorius, Isabell Diogo, Siegfried Bien, Andreas Sesterhenn, and Jochen A. Werner. 2012. Analysis of pneumatization and neurovascular structures of the sphenoid sinus using cone-beam tomography (CBT). *Acta Radiologica* 53: 214–19. [CrossRef]

Hadad, Gustavo, Luis Bassagasteguy, Ricardo L. Carrau, Juan C. Mataza, Amin Kassam, Carl H. Snyderman, and Arlan Mintz. 2006. A novel reconstructive technique after endoscopic expanded endonasal approaches: Vascular pedicle nasoseptal flap. *The Laryngoscope* 116: 1882–86. [CrossRef]

Hader, Walter J., James Drake, Douglas Cochrane, Owen Sparrow, Edward S. Johnson, and John Kestle. 2002. Death after late failure of third ventriculostomy in children. Report of three cases. *Journal of Neurosurgery* 97: 211–15. [CrossRef]

Haines, Stephen J., Peter J. Jannetta, and David S. Zorub. 1980. Microvascular relations of the trigeminal nerve. An anatomical study with clinical correlation. *Journal of Neurosurgery* 52: 381–86. [CrossRef]

Halves, E., and K A. Bushe. 1979. Transsphenoidal operation on craniopharyngiomas with extrasellar extensions. The advantage of the operating endoscope [proceedings]. *Acta Neurochirurgica. Supplementum* 28: 362.

Hammer, G., and C. Radberg. 1962. The sphenoidal sinus. An anatomical and roentgenologic study with reference to transsphenoid hypophysectomy. *Acta Radiologica* 56: 401–22. [CrossRef]

Hanieh, A., D. A. Simpson, and J. B. North. 1988. Arachnoid cysts: A critical review of 41 cases. *Child's Nervous System* 4: 92–96. [CrossRef]

Hankins, Christopher L., Michael G. Brown, Randolph A. Lopez, Andrew K. Lee, Joseph Dang, and R. Douglas Harper. 2007. A 12-year experience using the Brown two-portal endoscopic procedure of transverse carpal ligament release in 14,722 patients: Defining a new paradigm in the treatment of carpal tunnel syndrome. *Plastic and Reconstructive Surgery* 120: 1911–21. [CrossRef]

Hardy, J. 1967. La chirurgie de l'hypophyse par voie transspénoïdale. *Union Médicale du Canada* 96: 702–12.

Harvey, Richard J., Joanne Malek, Mark Winder, Andrew Davidson, Tim Steel, Nadine Mrad, Henry Barham, Anna Knisely, and Charles Teo. 2015a. Sinonasal morbidity following tumour resection with and without nasoseptal flap reconstruction. *Rhinology* 53: 122–28. [CrossRef]

Harvey, Richard J., Mark Winder, Andrew Davidson, Tim Steel, Sunny Nalavenkata, Nadine Mrad, Ali Bokhari, Henry Barham, and Anna Knisely. 2015b. The Olfactory Strip and Its Preservation in Endoscopic Pituitary Surgery Maintains Smell and Sinonasal Function. *Journal of Neurological Surgery Part B: Skull Base* 76: 464–70. [CrossRef]

Hersh, Eliza H., Yakov Gologorsky, Alex G. Chartrain, J. Mocco, and Christopher P. Kellner. 2018. Minimally invasive surgery for intracerebral hemorrhage. *Current Neurology and Neuroscience Reports* 18: 34. [CrossRef]

Hijikata, S., M. Yamagishi, T. Nakayama, and K. Oomori. 1975. Percutaneous diskectomy: A new treatment method for lumbar disc herniation. *Journal Toden Hospital* 5: 5–13.

Hiremath, Shivaprakash B., Amol B. Gautam, Keerthy Sheeja, and Geena Benjamin. 2018. Assessment of variations in sphenoid sinus pneumatization in Indian population: A multidetector computed tomography study. *Indian Journal of Radiology and Imaging* 28: 273–79. [CrossRef]

Hitotsumatsu, Tsutomu, Toshio Matsushima, and Tooru Inoue. 2003. Microvascular decompression for treatment of trigeminal neuralgia, hemifacial spasm, and glossopharyngeal neuralgia: Three surgical approach variations: Technical note. *Neurosurgery* 53: 1436–41. [CrossRef]

Hoogland, T. 2003. Transforaminal endoscopic discectomy with foraminoplasty for lumbar disc herniation. *Surgical Techniques in Orthopaedics and Traumatology* 40: 55–120.

Hussain, Namath S., Mackenzie Piper, W. Grant Ludlam, William H. Ludlam, Cindy J. Fuller, and Marc R. Mayberg. 2013. Delayed postoperative hyponatremia after transsphenoidal surgery: Prevalence and associated factors. *Journal of Neurosurgery* 119: 1453–60. [CrossRef]

Ishikawa, Mami, Yuichi Tanaka, and Eiju Watanabe. 2015. Microvascular decompression under neuroendoscopic view in hemifacial spasm: Rostral-type compression and perforator-type compression. *Acta Neurochirurgica* 157: 329–32. [CrossRef]

Jacques, Skip, C. Hunter Shelden, Gilbert D. McCann, Donald B. Freshwater, and Robert Rand. 1980. Computerized three-dimensional stereotaxic removal of small central nervous system lesions in patients. *Journal of Neurosurgery* 53: 816–20. [CrossRef]

Jahangiri, Arman, Jeffrey Wagner, Sung Won Han, Corinna C. Zygourakis, Seunggu J. Han, Mai T. Tran, Liane M. Miller, Maxwell. W. Tom, Sandeep Kunwar, Lewis S. Blevins, Jr., and et al. 2014. Morbidity of repeat transsphenoidal surgery assessed in more than 1000 operations. *Journal of Neurosurgery* 121: 67–74. [CrossRef]

Jankowski, Roger, Jean Auque, Claude Simon, Jean Claude Marchal, Henry Hepner, and Michel Wayoff. 1992. Endoscopic pituitary tumour surgery. *The Laryngoscope* 102: 198–202. [CrossRef]

Jho, Hae-Dong. 1999. Endoscopic transpedicular thoracic discectomy. *Journal of Neurosurgery* 91: 151–56. [CrossRef]

Jimenez, David F., and Constance M. Barone. 1998. Endoscopic craniectomy for early surgical correction of sagittal craniosynostosis. *Journal of Neurosurgery* 88: 77–81. [CrossRef]

Jimenez, David F., Constance M. Barone, Maria E. McGee, Cathy C. Cartwright, and C. Lynette Baker. 2004. Endoscopy-assisted wide-vertex craniectomy, barrel stave osteotomies, and postoperative helmet molding therapy in the management of sagittal suture craniosynostosis. *Journal of Neurosurgery* 100: 407–17. [CrossRef]

Jones, R. F. C., B. C. T. Kwok, W. A. Stening, and M. Vonau. 1994. Neuroendoscopic third ventriculostomy. A practical alternative to extracranial shunts in non-communicating hydrocephalus. *Minimally Invasive Neurosurgery II* 61: 79–83. [CrossRef]

Jones, R. F., W. A. Stening, and M. Brydon. 1990. Endoscopic third ventriculostomy. *Neurosurgery* 26: 86–91. [CrossRef]

Jouanneau, Emmanuel, Emile Simon, Timothée Jacquesson, Marc Sindou, Stéphane Tringali, Mahmoud Messerer, and Moncef Berhouma. 2014. The endoscopic endonasal approach to the Meckel's cave tumours: Surgical technique and indications. *World Neurosurgery* 82: S155–S161. [CrossRef] [PubMed]

Kabil, M. S., J. B. Eby, and H. K. Shahinian. 2005. Endoscopic vascular decompression versus microvascular decompression of the trigeminal nerve. *Minimally Invasive Neurosurgery* 48: 207–12. [CrossRef] [PubMed]

Kalavakonda, Chandrasekar, Laligam N. Sekhar, Pranatartiharan Ramachandran, and Peter Hechl. 2002. Endoscope-assisted microsurgery for intracranial aneurysms. *Neurosurgery* 51: 1119–26. [CrossRef] [PubMed]

Kambin, Parviz. 1991. *Arthroscopic Microdiscectomy: Minimal Intervention in Spinal Surgery*. Baltimore: Urban & Schwarzenberg, pp. 67–1100.

Kambin, Parviz. 1992. Arthroscopic microdiscectomy. *Arthroscopy: The Journal of Arthroscopic & Related Surgery* 8: 287–95. [CrossRef]

Kambin, Parviz, and Harris Gellman. 1983. Percutaneous lateral discectomy of the lumbar spine: A preliminary report. *Clinical Orthopaedics and Related Research (1976–2007)* 174: 127–32. [CrossRef]

Kambin, P., and S. Sampson. 1986. Posterolateral percutaneous suction-excision of herniated lumbar intervertebral discs. Report of interim results. *Clinical Orthopaedics and Related Research (1976–2007)* 207: 37–43.

Kaptain, George J., David A. Vincent, Jason P. Sheehan, and Edward R. Laws, Jr. 2001. Transsphenoidal approaches for the extracapsular resection of midline suprasellar and anterior cranial base lesions. *Neurosurgery* 49: 94–100. [CrossRef]

Karabagli, Hakan, and Volkan Etus. 2012. Success of pure neuroendoscopic technique in the treatment of Sylvian arachnoid cysts in children. *Child's Nervous System* 28: 445–52. [CrossRef]

Kassam, Amin B., Johnathan A. Engh, Arlan H. Mintz, and Daniel M. Prevedello. 2009. Completely endoscopic resection of intraparenchymal brain tumours. *Journal of neurosurgery* 110: 116–23. [CrossRef]

Kawsar, Khandkar A., Mohammod R. Haque, and Forhad H. Chowdhury. 2015. Avoidance and management of perioperative complications of endoscopic third ventriculostomy: The Dhaka experience. *Journal of Neurosurgery* 123: 1414–19. [CrossRef]

Kawsar, Khandkar Ali, Thomas Land, Georgios Tsermoulas, Alessandro Paluzzi, and Shahzada Ahmed. 2020. Novel Surgical Treatment of Recurrent CSF Leak by Temporoparietal Temporalis Myofascial Flap: A Series of 6 Cases. *World Neurosurgery* 147: 1–6. [CrossRef] [PubMed]

Kelly, Patrick J., Bruce A. Kall, Stephan Goerss, and Franklin Earnest. 1986. Computer-assisted stereotaxic laser resection of intra-axial brain neoplasms. *Journal of Neurosurgery* 64: 427–39. [CrossRef] [PubMed]

Kelly, Patrick J., Stephan J. Goerss, and Bruce A. Kall. 1988. The stereotaxic retractor in computer-assisted stereotaxic microsurgery. *Journal of Neurosurgery* 69: 301–6. [CrossRef] [PubMed]

Kim, Daniel H., Gun Choi, and Sang-Ho Lee. 2011. *Endoscopic Spine Proceduresed*. New York: Thieme, pp. 42–58.

Kim, Young Zoon, and Kyu Hong Kim. 2009. Even in patients with a small hemorrhagic volume, stereotactic-guided evacuation of spontaneous intracerebral hemorrhage improves functional outcome. *Journal of Korean Neurosurgical Society* 46: 109–15. [CrossRef]

Krishnan, Kartik G., Thomas Pinzer, and Gabriele Schackert. 2006. A novel endoscopic technique in treating single nerve entrapment syndromes with special attention to ulnar nerve transposition and tarsal tunnel release: Clinical application. *Operative Neurosurgery* 59: ONS89–ONS100. [CrossRef]

Lewis, Adam I., Kerry R. Crone, Jamal Taha, Harry R. van Loveren, Hwa-Shain Yeh, and John M. Tew, Jr. 1994. Surgical resection of third ventricle colloid cyst. Preliminary results comparing transcallosal microsurgery with endoscopy. *Journal of Neurosurgery* 81: 174–78. [CrossRef]

Li, Khan W., Clarke Nelson, Ian Suk, and George I. Jallo. 2005. Neuroendoscopy: Past, present, and future. *Neurosurg Focus* 19: 1–5. [CrossRef]

Li, Youwei, Feng Mao, Fangling Cheng, Chenghao Peng, Dongsheng Guo, and Baofeng Wang. 2019. A meta-analysis of endoscopic microvascular decompression versus microscopic microvascular decompression for the treatment for cranial nerve syndrome caused by vascular compression. *World Neurosurgery* 126: 647–55. [CrossRef]

Little, Andrew S., Daniel F. Kelly, William L. White, Paul A. Gardner, Juan C. Fernandez-Miranda, Michael R. Chicoine, Garni Barkhoudarian, James P. Chandler, Daniel M. Prevedello, Brandon D. Liebelt, and et al. 2019. Results of a prospective multicenter controlled study comparing surgical outcomes of microscopic versus fully endoscopic transsphenoidal surgery for nonfunctioning pituitary adenomas: The Transsphenoidal Extent of Resection (TRANSSPHER) Study. *Journal of Neurosurgery* 22: 1–11. [CrossRef]

Liu, James K., Kaushik Das, Martin H. Weiss, Edward R. Laws, and William T. Couldwell. 2001. The history and evolution of transsphenoidal surgery. *Journal of Neurosurgery* 95: 1083–96. [CrossRef]

Lobatto, Daniel J., Friso de Vries, Amir H. Zamanipoor Najafabadi, Alberto M. Pereira, Wilco C. Peul, Thea PM Vliet Vlieland, Nienke R. Biermasz, and Wouter R. van Furth. 2018. Preoperative risk factors for postoperative complications in endoscopic pituitary surgery: A systematic review. *Pituitary* 21: 84–97. [CrossRef] [PubMed]

Locatelli, Davide, P. Castelnuovo, L. Santi, M. Cerniglia, M. Maghnie, and L. Infuso. 2000. Endoscopic approaches to the cranial base: Perspectives and realities. *Child's Nervous System* 16: 686–91. [CrossRef] [PubMed]

Mantovani, Gustavo, Philippe Liverneaux, Jose Carlos Garcia, Stacey H. Berner, Michael S. Bednar, and Catherine J. Mohr. 2011. Endoscopic exploration and repair of brachial plexus with telerobotic manipulation: A cadaver trial. *Journal of Neurosurgery* 115: 659–64. [CrossRef] [PubMed]

Martin, Richard G., John L. Grant, David Peace, Cynthia Theiss, and Albert L. Rhoton Jr. 1980. Microsurgical relationships of the anterior inferior cerebellar artery and the facialvestibulocochlear nerve complex. *Neurosurgery* 6: 483–507. [CrossRef] [PubMed]

Mathews, Hallett H. 1996. Transforaminal endoscopic microdiscectomy. *Neurosurgery Clinics of North America* 7: 59–64. [CrossRef] [PubMed]

Mirkovic, Srdjan R., David G. Schwartz, and Kenneth D. Glazier. 1995. Anatomic considerations in posterolateral procedures. *Spine* 20: 1965–71. [CrossRef]

Mixter, W. J. 1923. Ventriculoscopy and puncture of the floor of the third ventricle: Preliminary report of a case. *The Boston Medical and Surgical Journal* 188: 277–78. [CrossRef]

Mullick, Tarun, and A. Lee Dellon. 2008. Results of decompression of four medial ankle tunnels in the treatment of tarsal tunnels syndrome. *Journal of Reconstructive Microsurgery* 24: 119–26. [CrossRef]

Nayak, Pratima, Alaa S. Montaser, Jie Hu, Daniel M. Prevedello, Lawrence S. Kirschner, and Luma Ghalib. 2018. Predictors of Postoperative Diabetes Insipidus Following Endoscopic Resection of Pituitary Adenomas. *Journal of the Endocrine Society* 2: 1010–19. [CrossRef]

Nulsen, Frank E., and Eugene B. Spitz. 1951. Treatment of hydrocephalus by direct shunt from ventricle to jugular vein. *Surgical Forum* 1951: 399–403.

Oertel, Joachim, Stefan Linsler, Wolfgang Wagner, Michael Gaab, Henry Schroeder, and Jana Rediker. 2020. Endoscopic Treatment of Intracranial Arachnoid Cysts: A Retrospective Analysis of a 25-Year Experience. *Operative Neurosurgery* 15: 32–44. [CrossRef]

Oi, Shizuo, and Rick Abbott. 2004. Loculated ventricles and isolated compartments in hydrocephalus: Their pathophysiology and the efficacy of neuroendoscopic surgery. *Neurosurgery Clinics of North America* 15: 77–87. [CrossRef] [PubMed]

Oldfield, Edward H., and Alexander O. Vortmeyer. 2006. Development of a histological pseudocapsule and its use as a surgical capsule in the excision of pituitary tumours. *Journal of Neurosurgery* 104: 7–19. [CrossRef] [PubMed]

Onik, Gary, Clyde A. Helms, Leonard Ginsburg, Franklin T. Hoaglund, and James Morris. 1985. Percutaneous lumbar discectomy using new aspiration probe. *American Journal of Roentgenology* 144: 1137–40. [CrossRef] [PubMed]

Otsuki, Taisuke, Hidefumi Jokura, and Takashi Yoshimoto. 1990. Stereotactic guiding tube for open-system endoscopy: A new approach for the stereotactic endoscopic resection of intra-axial brain tumours. *Neurosurgery* 27: 326–30. [CrossRef]

Park, Si-Bog, Samuel Cheshier, Douglas Michaels, Judith A. Murovic, and Daniel H. Kim. 2006. Endoscopic harvesting of the sural nerve graft: Technical note. *Neurosurgery* 58: E180. [CrossRef]

Perneczky, Axel, and Georg Fries. 1998. Endoscope-assisted brain surgery: Part I Evolution, basic concept, and current technique. *Neurosurgery* 42: 219–25. [CrossRef]

Perneczky, Axel, Wibke Muller-Forell, Erik van Lindert, and Georg Fries. 1999. *Keyhole Concept in Neurosurgery: With Endoscope-assisted Microsurgery and Case Studies*. Stuttgart: Thieme, pp. 120–48.

Perry, Avital, Christopher S. Graffeo, Jenna Meyer, Lucas P. Carlstrom, Soliman Oushy, Colin L. W. Driscoll, and Fredric B. Meyer. 2019. Beyond the Learning Curve: Comparison of Microscopic and Endoscopic Incidences of Internal Carotid Injury in a Series of Highly Experienced Operators. *World Neurosurgery* 131: e128–e135. [CrossRef]

Pollock, Bruce E., and Kimberly A. Schoeberl. 2010. Prospective comparison of posterior fossa exploration and stereotactic radiosurgery dorsal root entry zone target as primary surgery for patients with idiopathic trigeminal neuralgia. *Neurosurgery* 67: 633–38. [CrossRef]

Raza, Shaan M., Angela M. Donaldson, Alpesh Mehta, Apostolos J. Tsiouris, Vijay K. Anand, and Theodore H. Schwartz. 2014. Surgical management of trigeminal schwannomas: Defining the role for endoscopic endonasal approaches. *Neurosurgical focus* 37: E17. [CrossRef]

Reinprecht, Andrea, Wolfgang Dietrich, Angelika Berger, Gerhard Bavinzski, Manfred Weninger, and Thomas Czech. 2001. Posthemorrhagic hydrocephalus in preterm infants: Long term follow-up and shunt related complications. *Child's Nervous System* 17: 663–69. [CrossRef] [PubMed]

Rekate, Harold L., Iman Feiz-Erfan, Yu-Tze Ng, L. Fernando Gonzalez, and John F. Kerrigan. 2006. Endoscopic surgery for hypothalamic hamartomas causing medically refractory gelastic epilepsy. *Child's Nervous System* 22: 874–80. [CrossRef] [PubMed]

Robinson, R. G. 1971. Congenital cysts of the brain: Arachnoid malformations. In *Progress in Neurological Surgery*. Edited by H. Krayenbuhl, P. E. Maspes and W. H. Sweet. Basel: Karger Publishers, pp. 133–74. [CrossRef]

Rowan, Nicholas R., Benita Valappil, Jonlin Chen, Eric W. Wang, Paul A. Gardner, and Carl H. Snyderman. 2020. Prospective characterization of postoperative nasal deformities in patients undergoing endoscopic endonasal skull-base surgery. *International Forum of Allergy & Rhinology* 10: 256–64. [CrossRef]

Rowan, Nicholas R., Eric W. Wang, Paul A. Gardner, Juan C. Fernandez-Miranda, and Carl H. Snyderman. 2016. Nasal Deformities Following Nasoseptal Flap Reconstruction of Skull Base Defects. *Journal of Neurological Surgery Part B: Skull Base* 77: 14–18. [CrossRef] [PubMed]

Roxbury, Christopher R., Masaru Ishii, Gary L. Gallia, and Douglas D. Reh. 2016. Endoscopic management of esthesioneuroblastoma. *Otolaryngologic Clinics of North America* 49: 153–65. [CrossRef] [PubMed]

Russell, Stephen M., and Patrick J. Kelly. 2002. Volumetric stereotaxy and the supratentorial occipitosubtemporal approach in the resection of posterior hippocampus and parahippocampal gyrus lesions. *Neurosurgery* 50: 978–88.

Sainte-Rose, Christian, Giuseppe Cinalli, Franck E. Roux, Wirginia Maixner, Paul D. Chumas, Maher Mansour, Alexandre Carpentier, Marie Bourgeois, Michel Zerah, Alain Pierre-Kahn, and et al. 2001. Management of hydrocephalus in paediatric patients with posterior fossa tumours; the role of endoscopic third ventriculostomy. *Journal of Neurosurgery* 95: 791–97. [CrossRef]

Sekhar, L. N., C. Sen, and C. H. Snyderman. 1993. Anterior, anterolateral, and lateral approaches to extradural petroclival tumours. In *Surgery of Cranial Base Tumours*. Edited by L. N. Sekhar and I. P. Janecka. New York: Raven Press.

Sgouros, Spyros. 2013. *Neuroendoscopy: Current Status and Future Trends*. Heidelberg: Springer Science & Business Media.

Shelden, C. Hunter, Gilbert McCann, Skip Jacques, Harold R. Lutes, Robert E. Frazier, Richard Katz, and Rudi Kuki. 1980. Development of a computerized microstereotaxic method for localization and removal of minute CNS lesions under direct 3-D vision: Technical report. *Journal of Neurosurgery* 52: 21–27. [CrossRef]

Shim, Kyu Won, Eun Kyung Park, Dong-Seok Kim, and Joong-Uhn Choi. 2017. Neuroendoscopy: Current and future perspectives. *Journal of Korean Neurosurgical Society* 60: 322–26. [CrossRef]

Siomin, Vit, and Shlomi Constantini. 2004. Basic principles and equipment in neuroendoscopy. *Neurosurgery Clinics of North America* 15: 19–31. [CrossRef]

Snyderman, Carl, Amin Kassam, Ricardo Carrau, Arlan Mintz, Paul Gardner, and Daniel M. Prevedello. 2007. Acquisition of surgical skills for endonasal skull base surgery: A training program. *The Laryngoscope* 117: 699–705. [CrossRef] [PubMed]

Spencer, William R., Kaushik Das, Chedioze Nwagu, Eugene Wenk, Steven D. Schaefer, Augustine Moscatello, and William T. Couldwell. 1999. Approaches to the sellar and parasellar region: Anatomic comparison of the microscope versus endoscope. *The Laryngoscope* 109: 791–74. [CrossRef] [PubMed]

Spennato, P., Giuseppe Cinalli, G. Carannante, C. Ruggiero, and M. L. Del. 2004. Multiloculated hydrocephalus. In *Pediatric Hydrocephalus*. Edited by Giuseppe Cinalli, Wirginia June Maixner and Christian Sainte-Rose. Milan: Springer, pp. 219–44.

Spennato, Pietro, Giuseppe Cinalli, Claudio Ruggiero, Ferdinando Aliberti, Vincenzo Trischitta, Emilio Cianciulli, and Giuseppe Maggi. 2007. Neuroendoscopic treatment of multiloculated hydrocephalus in children. *Journal of Neurosurgery: Pediatrics* 106: 29–35. [CrossRef] [PubMed]

Sufianov, A., G. Sufianova, and I. Iakimov. 2008. Neuroendoscopic procedures in achievement of shunt independence: Outcome analysis of 28 patients with shunt malfunction. *Minimally Invasive Neurosurgery* 51: 158–64. [CrossRef] [PubMed]

Taniguchi, Masaaki, Hiroshi Takimoto, Toshiki Yoshimine, Nobumitsu Shimada, Yasuyoshi Miyao, Masayuki Hirata, Motohiko Maruno, Amami Kato, Eiji Kohmura, and Toru Hayakawa. 1999. Application of a rigid endoscope to the microsurgical management of 54 cerebral aneurysms: Results in 48 patients. *Journal of Neurosurgery* 91: 231–37. [CrossRef] [PubMed]

Teo, Charles. 2000. Endoscopic-assisted tumour and neurovascular procedures. *Clinical Neurosurgery* 46: 515–25.

Teo, Charles, and Peter Nakaji. 2005. Application of endoscopy to the resection of intra-axial tumours. *Operative Techniques in Neurosurgery* 8: 179–85. [CrossRef]

Teo, Charles, and Ralph Mobbs. 2004. Neuroendoscopy. In *Principals of Neurosurgery*. Edited by Setti S. Rengachary and Richard G. Ellenbogen. New York: Elsevier Mosby.

Tisell, Magnus, Odd Almström, Hannes Stephensen, Mats Tullberg, and Carsten Wikkelsö. 2000. How effective is endoscopsic third ventriculostomy in treating adult hydrocephalus caused by primary aqueductal stenosis? *Neurosurgery* 46: 104–9. [CrossRef]

Tsai, Tsu-Min, I-Chen Chen, Mohammed E. Majd, and Beng-Hai Lim. 1999. Cubital tunnel release with endoscopic assistance: Results of a new technique. *The Journal of Hand Surgery* 24: 21–29. [CrossRef]

Unal, Tugrul Cem, and Aydin Aydoseli. 2018. *Endoscopic Third Ventriculostomy*. London: Intechopen, p. 75394.

Vries, J. K. 1978. An endoscopic technique for third ventriculostomy. *Surgical Neurology* 9: 165–68.

Walker, Marion L. 2001. History of ventriculostomy. *Neurosurgery Clinics of North America.* 12: 101–10. [CrossRef] [PubMed]

Wallner, Kent E., Michael Gonzales, and Glenn E. Sheline. 1988. Treatment of oligodendrogliomas with or without post-operative irradiation. *Journal of Neurosurgery* 68: 684–88. [CrossRef] [PubMed]

Wang, Chao, Chuangxi Liu, Yunbiao Xiong, Guoqiang Han, Hen Yang, Hao Yin, Jun Wang, and Chao You. 2013. Surgical treatment of intracranial arachnoid cyst in adult patients. *Neurology India* 61: 60–64. [CrossRef]

Wang, Xuejian, Xiaobiao Zhang, Fan Hu, Yong Yu, Ye Gu, Tao Xie, and Junqi Ge. 2016. Image-guided endoscopic endonasal transmaxillary transpterygoid approach to meckel's cave. *Turkish Neurosurgery* 26: 309–14. [PubMed]

Yamini, Bakhtiar, Daniel Refai, Charles M. Rubin, and David M. Frim. 2004. Initial endoscopic management of pineal region tumours and associated hydrocephalus: Clinical series and literature review. *Journal of Neurosurgery: Pediatrics* 100: 437–41. [CrossRef] [PubMed]

Yoshioka, Hideyuki, and Hiroyuki Kinouchi. 2015. The Roles of Endoscope in Aneurysmal Surgery. *Neurologia Medico-Chirurgica* 55: 469–78. [CrossRef]

Zwagerman, Nathan T., Georgios Zenonos, Stefan Lieber, Wei-Hsin Wang, Eric W. Wang, Juan C. Fernandez-Miranda, Carl H. Snyderman, and Paul A. Gardner. 2016. Endoscopic transnasal skull base surgery: Pushing the boundaries. *Journal of Neuro-Oncology* 130: 319–30. [CrossRef]

Section XII: Functional Neurosurgery

Dementia

Md Moshiur Rahman , Syeda Neyamot-e-Ferdousi and Forhad H. Chowdhury

Abstract: Approximately 47.5 million people are dementia sufferers worldwide. Dementia is a frequent etiology of morbidity and mortality with the growing elderly population. This translates to a vast global economic impact. Risk factors of dementia include oxidative stress, infection, the accumulation of excessive protein deposits in the cerebrum, metal accumulation, and cholinesterase disorders. The bulk of dementias affecting the elderly population are due to Alzheimer's disease, Lewy body dementia, ischemic brain injury, and normal pressure hydrocephalus (NPH). Among the long list of etiologies of dementia, only a few are reversible and treatable. Among the treatable causes, NPH-induced dementia is surgically treatable. In this chapter, avery short discussion and differentiation of common causes of dementia are provided. Surgical management of NPH is discussed in the later part of the chapter.

Abbreviations

AD	Alzheimer's disease	BOLD	blood-oxygen-level-dependent
CSF	cerebrospinal fluid	CT	computerized tomography
BLB	dementia with Lewy bodies	ETV	endoscopic third ventriculostomy
FTD	frontotemporal dementia	fMRI	functional MRI
ICP	intracranial pressure	iNPH	idiopathic normal pressure hydrocephalus
LBs	Lewy bodies	LP	Lumboperitoneal
MRI	magnetic resonance imaging	NFT	neurofibrillary tangle
NPH	normal-pressure hydrocephalus	PD	Parkinson's disease
ROS	reactive oxygen species	VaD	vascular dementia
VP	ventriculoperitoneal	VA	ventriculo-atrial

1. Introduction

The word dementia comes from the Latin demens ("de": private; "mens": intellect, knowledge), referring to the cognitive deterioration of these functions. Dementia is primarily a severe, persistent, and permanent neurological impairment syndrome, a subtype of which is Alzheimer's disease. Acute-onset degenerative dementia has relatively few causes. The word "reversible dementia" is frequently utilized to characterize reversible encephalopathies but is rather inaccurate owing to the connotations correlated with the phrase "dementia". Irreversible, non-progressive cognitive dysfunction describes static encephalopathy, such as that correlated with severe brain damage, stroke, or sensitivity to neurotoxins. Practically, the differentiation between dementia with reversible encephalopathy requires evidence of reversibility via correct therapy of the causative disease. The bulk of dementias affecting the elderly population are due to Alzheimer's disease (approximately 60%), Lewy body dementia (nearly 15%), and ischemic brain injury (nearly 15%), while the other cases of encephalopathy are caused by a vast variety of etiologies.

2. Dementia and Causes

The American Psychiatric Association described dementia as any mental disability or global cognitive loss in an earlier intact individual, marked by the degradation of cognitive, social, emotional, and behavioral capacities, sufficiently extreme to negatively impact on sufferers' everyday lives (American Psychiatric Association 2013). Approximately 47.5 million people are dementia sufferers worldwide (Hügel and Jackson 2015). Hence, dementia has become a frequent etiology of morbidity and mortality with the growing elderly population (Fadil et al. 2009). This translates to a vast global economic impact (Wimo et al. 2013). Risk factors of dementia include oxidative stress, infection, the accumulation of excessive protein deposits in the cerebrum, metal accumulation, and cholinesterase disorders (Choi et al. 2012).

Three primary etiologies of dementia are Alzheimer's disease (AD), vascular dementia (VaD), and dementia with Lewy bodies (DLB). Vascular dementia is due to blockage from a blood clot of one or more cerebral blood vessels. When a large blood artery in the brain is obstructed, it is considered a stroke. However, the most common events that contribute to vascular dementia are a sequence of minor arterial blockages that go undiagnosed for years before manifesting as dementia.

Taking an antiplatelet drug on a daily basis is an effective stroke prevention therapy for those who have acquired atherosclerosis.

About half of the elderly adults with dementia are reported to have neurological signs of more than one etiology of dementia. Mixed dementia, AD, and VaD are frequently encountered together. Depression, thyroid disease, the adverse effects of some drugs, alcohol misuse, vitamin deficiencies, and other factors might induce dementia-like symptoms (not dementia).

Dementia is a syndrome defined as a gradual and irreversible pathological process characterized by a degenerative pathology that causes degeneration and neuronal death in several cerebral regions, causing the brain's function and structure to decline. Furthermore, it is primarily a later-life disorder that is not associated with the natural aging process (Vemuri et al. 2011). DLB, mixed dementia with AD, VaD, Parkinson's disease (PD), Creutzfeldt–Jakob disease, frontotemporal dementia, Huntington's disease, normal hydrocephalus pressure (NPH), and progressive supranuclear palsy are the most common kinds of dementia (de Villemeur 2013; Picascia et al. 2016; Eddy et al. 2016; Reed et al. 2003; Cunningham et al. 2015) (Tables 1 and 2).

Nondegenerative dementia can be due to a variety of causes, including infections, head injuries, brain tumors, subdural hematomas, and clear and spontaneous hydrocephalus strain (Ghosh 2010). Age, sex hormones (Barron and Pike 2012), genetic variables (Chou et al. 2017; Jamal et al. 2017; Kanatsu and Tomita 2017; Loy et al. 2014), and external conditions (chemical exposures and metals) (Uchoa et al. 2016) are all risk factors that might promote dementia. The molecular basis of dementia, neuronal death, and synaptic damage is unknown, and it may differ according to the type of neurodegenerative disorder. However, common characteristics of dementia include the involvement of certain common causes, such as oxidative stress, neuroinflammation, and irregular protein folding (Finkel and Holbrook 2000; Santos et al. 2014; Polidori and Scholtes 2016; Rahal et al. 2014; Chen et al. 2016; Stefaniak and O'Brien 2016; Barrientos et al. 2015; Craig-Schapiro et al. 2010; Shimizu et al. 2011).

Table 1. Chronic degenerative dementias.

Alzheimer's disease
Lewy body dementia
Frontotemporal dementia
Progressive supranuclear palsy
Parkinson's disease
Multiple system atrophy
Corticobasalganglionic degeneration
Huntington's disease
Multiple sclerosis
Mitochondrial disorders
Amyotrophic lateral sclerosis

Source: Authors' compilation based on data from de Villemeur (2013); Picascia et al. (2016); Eddy et al. (2016); Reed et al. (2003); Cunningham et al. (2015).

Table 2. Acute dementias.

Traumatic brain injury
Creutzfeldt–Jakob disease
Neurotoxin exposure
Vascular dementia
Reversible encephalopathies
Infectious disease

Source: Authors' compilation based on data from de Villemeur (2013); Picascia et al. (2016); Eddy et al. (2016); Reed et al. (2003); Cunningham et al. (2015).

3. Diagnosing Dementia

Dementia is diagnosed using mini-mental state examination (MMSE) (Chapter 2; Section 1).

3.1. *Molecular Neuroimaging of the Dementias*

3.1.1. Identification of Abnormal Characters of Cerebral Function Utilizing Molecular Neuroimaging

Irregular trends in dementias can show new insights into how these diseases interrupt brain circuits. They can also be useful when diagnosing differentials. Irregular findings usually include a decreased metabolism or blood supply in different brain areas affected by the disorder and vice versa in some other situations. Molecular neuroimaging was also used to determine abnormal cerebral function patterns in people who are asymptomatic but carry genetic potential factors for dementia.

3.1.2. Physiological Basis of Functional MRI in Dementia

The most widely used fMRI method to classify cortical functions depends on contrast scanning of the interior blood-oxygen-level-dependent (BOLD) signal. The MRI signal during one cognitive state is usually equated to a monitoring task or a responsive standard condition in fMRI investigations. The BOLD fMRI signal, as well as neurovascular coupling, which links cellular functions to hemodynamic alterations, is predicted to vary in healthy aging and during neurodegenerative dementia pathological processes. Changes in cerebral fMRI activation patterns between controls and persons with neurodegenerative dementia could be due to disease-related neuropathological abnormalities as well as variations in fMRI-measured neurovascular coupling. When taken together, BOLD-based fMRI provides a novel and readily accessible method for studying intact human cognition as well as improvements in neural activity associated with stable aging and neurodegenerative-disease-related dysfunctions (Logothetis et al. 2001; Shmuel et al. 2006; Kwong et al. 1992; Ogawa et al. 1992; Buckner et al. 2005; Cavanna and Trimble 2006; D'Esposito et al. 2003; Iadecola 2004).

3.2. Memory Dysfunction in Dementia

3.2.1. Episodic Memory

Episodic memory is a declarative memory device that is utilized to recall a specific event in one's life, such as a date with a friend. Episodic memory is primely characterized by what people with an injured medial temporal lobe cannot recall compared to normal people. The basal forebrain with Broca's medial septum and lateral bands, the presubiculum, the retrosplenial cortex, the fornix, the mammillothalamic tract, and the anterior thalamus nucleus are all important components of the episodic memory network (Mesulam 2000). A lesion in either of these systems may induce the disorder characteristic of episodic memory system dysfunction. Episodic memory loss develops slowly and gradually in degenerative conditions such AD, frontotemporal dementia, and DLB (Solomon and Budson 2003). Episodic memory often deteriorates over time in disorders involving several brain areas, such as vascular dementia and multiple sclerosis. Tumors, medicines, hypoglycemia, traumatic brain injury, and Korsakoff's syndrome are all linked to memory loss. In Azheimer's illness, the hippocampus and amygdala, as well as the parietal, temporal, and frontal lobes, are predisposition sites for pathogenic involvement. Since the hippocampus and other medial temporal lobe anatomical structures are the first and most seriously impacted cerebral areas in AD, episodic memory—particularly, the file cabinet elements of episodic memory—is the first and most severely damaged cognitive function. Telling the same stories, asking the same questions, missing appointments, and leaving the stove on are all common symptoms. Another feature of the disease's episodic memory impairment is that memory is harmed even when many rehearsals maximize information learning or encoding and retrieval demands are reduced with the utilization of a multiple-choice recognition test. "Fast rate of forgetting" is a term used to describe this type of memory loss. Besides fast forgetting, Alzheimer's disease patients often suffer memory disturbances and mistaken memories. Patients with such delusions may believe they have already turned off the burner or taken their medicines, causing them to neglect certain tasks. A hallucination or a delusion can be confused with a false memory. For example, a dementia patient may claim to see and communicate with a long-dead family member. Both AD and moderate cognitive dysfunction are linked to the frontal lobes, but not as much as the medial temporal lobes (Dickerson and Sperling 2009; Schonknecht et al. 2009). Memory distortions and fabricated memories may be caused by frontal lobe impairment in AD. People with AD, on the other hand, have a substantial pathology in the parietal cortex, which can manifest early in the treatment process (McKee et al. 2006).

3.2.2. Semantic Memory

Semantic memory is our storage of factual and conceptual knowledge that is unrelated to any particular memory, for example, the color of a ripe mango or the purpose of a glass. Semantic memory is a declarative and explicit memory system, similar to episodic memory (Schacter et al. 2000). Semiconductor memory is preserved in patients with severe episodic memory loss, such as destruction of the Papez circuit or surgical displacement of the medial temporal lobes (Corkin 1984). In its general sense, semantic memory comprises all of our global information and is unrelated to episodic memory. As a result, it is possible that semantic memory dwells in numerous cortical regions of the brain. Visual pictures are preserved in nearby visual association zones, according to evidence (Vaidya et al. 2002). Semantic memory is located in the inferolateral temporal lobes, primarily on the left, according to a more restricted interpretation supported by the naming and classification tests by which it is normally tested (Damasio et al. 1996; Perani et al. 1999).

The most frequent clinical illness that disrupts semantic memory is Alzheimer's disease (Price and Morris 1999; Greene and Hodges 1996). TBI, stroke, surgical injuries, encephalitis, and tumors are among the conditions that can impact the temporal lobes infero-laterally and induce functional memory (semantic memory) loss. All semantic memory tests, such as single-word interpretation, naming, and visual intelligence, are impaired in patients with semantic dementia. When semantic memory impairment is suspected, the assessment should contain the same elements as an episodic memory disorder work-up.

3.2.3. Procedural Memory

The capacity to learn unconscious cognitive and behavioral abilities and algorithms is referred to as procedural memory. Procedural memory is implicit and non-declarative. Driving a car with a normal transmission or learning to play the violin are two examples. The procedural memory system is clearly separate from the episodic memory system since it is spared in cases with significant episodic memory disorders. Procedural-memory-involving areas are the motor cortex, basal ganglia, and cerebellum (Daselaar et al. 2003; Exner et al. 2002). In Alzheimer's disease, the cerebellum and basal ganglia are relatively excluded. In spite of episodic memory loss, these cases show consistent development and preservation of procedural memory skills (Baird and Samson 2009). Because PD is the most prevalent disorder that disrupts procedural memory, Lewy body dementia is the most common neurodegenerative disorder that disrupts procedural memory. Patients with Huntington's disease with olivopontocerebellar degeneration in the preliminary stages of the disease have reduced procedural memory, while performing relatively normally on episodic memory tests (Heindel et al. 1989; Salmon et al. 1998). Strokes, tumors, and hemorrhages can all affect procedural memory by causing injury to the cerebellum or basal ganglia. Patients with significant depression have trouble with procedural memory tests, which could be due to basal ganglia dysfunction. Analysis of procedural memory disorders is akin to that of episodic memory disorders; management relies on the process of the specific disease. Finally, patients whose episodic memory was harmed by a static disease, such as cerebral encephalitis, were able to rehabilitate successfully by utilizing procedural memory to acquire new skills (Glisky and Schacter 1989).

3.2.4. Working Memory

Concentration, classic fields of attention, short-term memory, and working memory relate to the capability to transiently maintain and utilize necessary data. Working memory is a declarative and explicit form of memory. The working memory has generally been split into three parts: one for processing phonological information, another for processing spatial information, and an executive system for allocating attention resources (Baddeley 1998). Working memory is composed of a network of subcortical and cortical units that alter based on the task (Rowe et al. 2000). The prefrontal cortex is engaged in practically every working memory task (Fletcher and Henson 2001). Subsequent brain regions are commonly linked to prefrontal areas to complete a circuit in the cortical and subcortical area network. More areas on the right cerebral hemisphere are involved in spatial working memory, while more areas on the left side are involved in phonological working memory.

Patients with AD, PD, Huntington's disease, DLB, and less-prevalent illnesses including progressive supranuclear palsy may have problems with working memory (Calderon et al. 2001). Strokes, tumors, multiple sclerosis, head injuries, and other conditions can all affect working memory. Almost every type of aphasia can affect phonological working memory since it entails silent rehearsal of spoken material. Hyperactivity disorder, obsessive compulsive disorder, insomnia, and schizophrenia are among the attention-deficit disorders that can interfere with memory performance (Egeland et al. 2003; Klingberg et al. 2002). Working memory disorders can manifest in a variety of ways, including failure to concentrate or difficulty doing a new job with multiple steps. Working memory impairments are assessed in the same way episodic memory abnormalities are. The treatment is determined by the underlying cause.

3.3. *The Neuropathology of the Dementing Disorders*

3.3.1. Dementia with Lewy Bodies (DLB)

Lewy body dementia is a frequent neurodegenerative etiology of dementia following AD. Okazaki and colleagues (Okazaki et al. 1961) were the first to describe DLB in 1961. Significant quantities of intracytoplasmic inclusions resembling Lewy bodies (LBs) were demonstrated in the cerebral cortex (Kuzuhara et al. 1988; Spillantini et al. 1998). LBs are found in transentorhinal and entorhinal cortex, cingulate gyrus, amygdala, frontotemporal cortex, and insular cortex in DLB, as well as the brainstem, diencephalic regions, and basal forebrain in PD (McKee et al. 1998). The combination of LB pathology and Alzheimer's pathology, as well as neurochemical abnormalities and neuronal loss, in DLB is likely to cause dementia (McKee et al. 1998; Samuel et al. 1996; Apaydin et al. 2002). DLB is frequently associated with AD, and some researchers have classified it as a subset of the disease (Kosaka et al. 1984). DLB, on the other hand, is part of a spectrum of LB diseases, with PD on one end and DLB on the other. Cortical LBs are circumscribed inclusions in the deeper layers of the cortex that are found in medium- to small-sized pyramidal neurons of the cortex. Cortical LBs have a similar ultrastructure to brainstem LBs, but the fibrils are less densely oriented and there is no core to identify (Nussbaum and Polymeropoulos 1997).

3.3.2. Progressive Supranuclear Palsy

Progressive supranuclear palsy macroscopic traits include globus pallidus atrophy, subthalamic hippocampus, and midbrain and pontine tegmentum. Microscopically, tau immune-reactive neurofibrillary tangles, neuropil loops, tufted astrocytes, and inclusions of oligodendroglia occur. Tau abnormalities have been identified in the subcortical parenchyma and neocortex, entorhinal cortex, striatum, globus pallidus, hippocampus, substantia nigra, third nerve nuclei, red nuclei, pontine nuclei, cerebellar dentate nuclei, inferior olives, and spinal cord dorsal horns.

3.3.3. Neurofibrillary Tangle Dementia

The macroscopic pathology of dementia of neurofibrillary tangles frequently demonstrates extensive brain atrophy. The condition is marked by extensive neurofibrillary tangles (NFTs), neuropil threads, and ghost tangles in the hippocampus, entorhinal cortex, transentorhinal, and amygdala, with only infrequent engagement of other neocortical areas.

3.3.4. Vascular Dementia (VaD)

The presence of VaD in autopsy studies differs widely, ranging from 2% to 58% (Barclay et al. 1985; Esiri 2000). Vascular dementia can predominate in older age groups over some other causes of dementia. The heterogeneity of vascular dementia, which frequently coexists with other degenerative pathologies, makes estimating its prevalence difficult (Nolan et al. 1998). When microvascular abnormalities like white matter lesions and amyloid angiopathy are involved, approximately all AD cases have some degree of vascular disease (Kalaria 2000). Much clinical research investigating the relationship between AD and cerebrovascular damage has proved the pathology of large arteries, such as infarctions and hemorrhages, as well as large amounts of small vessel lesions, such as gaps lacunes (Bowling and Beal 1995; Skoog et al. 1993; Snowden et al. 2007). Microvascular disease has been identified as a major cause of dementia in older people (Kalaria et al. 1993; Kövari et al. 2007; Sonnen et al. 2007; White et al. 2002).

Strategic Infarct Dementia

Focal ischemic lesions, which typically consist of small- to medium-sized infarcts in clinically significant brain areas like the anterior cerebral artery area, the dominant angular gyrus, longitudinal hippocampus, unilateral to longitudinal medial thalamus, prevalent caudate nucleus, and basal forebrain, can also occur in dementia syndrome in conjunction with certain influential neurological impairments (Jellinger 2007).

3.3.5. Normal-Pressure Hydrocephalus (NPH)

NPH, also known as hydrocephalus of mal-resorption, is a type of communicating hydrocephalus where the ventricles have an excess of cerebrospinal fluid (CSF) and the cerebrospinal fluid pressure is normal or slightly higher. As the CSF volume builds up in the ventricles, the intracranial pressure inside the skull rises, crushing surrounding brain tissue and causing neurological issues. Dementia, urinary incontinence, and gait abnormalities are the characteristic trinity of symptoms of the condition. Hakim and Adams were the first to demonstrate the condition in 1965 (Adams et al. 1965). NPH is frequently misinterpreted as PD or AD (due to gait and cognitive dysfunction).

Epidemiology

Primary NPH comprises most of the cases. The prevalence of NPH rises with age, and the majority of patients are over 60. It is calculated that it affects less than 1% of people under the age of 65 and up to 3% of those over the age of 65. There is no difference in the occurrence in males and females (Younger 2005; Brean and Eide 2008; Tanaka et al. 2009). The prevalence of NPH is defined to be between 2 and 6% among dementia patients.

Signs and Symptoms

NPH presents a characteristic trilogy of clinical symptoms (called the Hakim's triad or Adam's triad). Gait deviation, dementia, and urinary incontinence make up the trio (usually referred to as "weird walking water" or "wet, wacky, and wobbly").

Approximately all patients have gait abnormalities, which are frequently the first sign. The corticospinal tract motor fibers are impinged on by the swelling of the lateral ventricles. The usual gait impairment in NPH is a wide-based, sluggish, narrow-stepped, "stuck to the floor", or "magnetic" movement. The abnormal gait seen in NPH is similar to those seen in PD. The gait disturbance can be minor, noticeable, or severe: "marked" means the patient has trouble walking due to significant instability; "severe" means the patient is unable to walk without assistance (Krauss et al. 2001; Ropper and Samuels 2009).

Dementia manifests itself as progressive cognitive abnormalities in 60% of cases at the time of treatment. Distortions in the frontal lobe and subcortex are mostly responsible for this (Younger 2005). Planning, organization, focus, and concentration are among the first shortcomings. Taking medications, managing finances, keeping track of appointments, driving, daytime sleeping, short-term memory difficulties, and psychomotor slowness are among the other weaknesses. Late-stage traits include indifference, slowed thinking, less drive, and reduced communication.

Urinary incontinence develops later and affects 50% of cases at the time of management. Urinary dysfunction starts with frequent urination, particularly at night, that escalates to urge incontinence and persistent incontinence (Younger 2005).

In idiopathic NPH (iNPH), apathy is the most frequent behavioral abnormality and it contributes to gait abnormalities. Oropharyngeal dysphagia "falling spells" as well as impulsive, violent conduct, both verbal and physical, are other uncommon signs. Oropharyngeal dysphagia is caused by ventricular dilatation compressing the corticobulbar tract (Allali et al. 2016).

Pathogenesis

Although the exact etiology is uncertain, there is agreement on several processes:

- An imbalance presents between CSF production versus resorption.
- CSF outflow resistance is frequently high.

Over-secretion of CSF or restriction of CSF flow in the ventricles do not cause the condition NPH and should be differentiated from hydrocephalus ex vacuo, which occurs due to brain atrophy (Figure 1).

The primary (sometimes known as idiopathic) and secondary causes of the condition are frequently distinguished. The fundamental cause of main NPH has yet to be discovered (Figure 2). Primary NPH affects adults aged 40 and up, with the elderly being the most commonly affected.

Secondary NPH can afflict people of any age and can be caused by things like subarachnoid hemorrhage, brain surgery (Figure 3), meningitis, traumatic brain injury, or brain radiation.

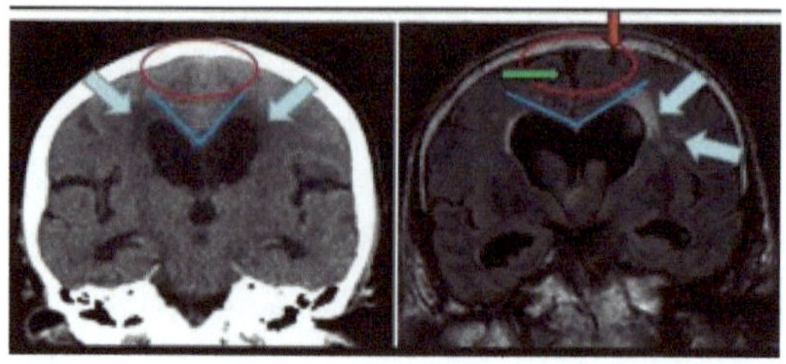

Figure 1. CT scan of head: coronal views. Left image: NPH. Right image: brain atrophy (hydrocephalus ex vacuo). Blue lines are indicating callosal angle. In the red circle, sulci are shown which are prominent in brain atrophy. Source: Figure by authors.

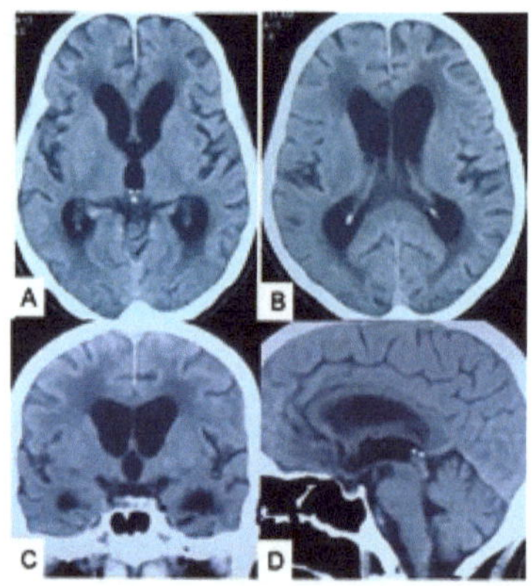

Figure 2. CT scan of head. (**A**,**B**) Axial section, (**C**) coronal, and (**D**) sagittal section showing iNPH. Source: Figure by authors.

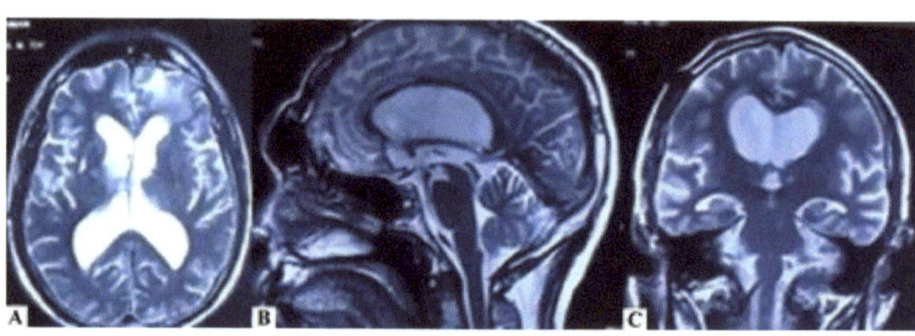

Figure 3. MRI of brain T2W images. (**A**) axial, (**B**) sagittal, and (**C**) coronal showing secondary NPH developed after removal of left frontal meningioma. Source: Figure by authors.

Diagnosis

Along with ventricular enlargement on neuroimaging, cases with suspicion of NPH should have characteristic symptoms. The following are the internationally accepted, evidence-based diagnostic criteria for iNPH:

1: Gradual beginning after 40 years of age, symptoms lasting 03–06 months, clinical evidence of balance or gait impairment, cognitive impairment, or urine incontinence.

2: To show larger ventricles as well as no macroscopic blockage to CSF flow, imaging from MRI or CT scans is required. On imaging, at least one of the temporal horns of the lateral ventricles should be enlarged, with impingement against the falx cerebri at a callosal angle of 90° on the coronal image, indicating changes in brain water content or normal CSF flow (also known as "flow void") at the cerebral aqueduct and fourth ventricle.

MRI scans are the best option. It is difficult to tell the difference between normal and increased ventricular size due to cerebral atrophy. Up to 80% of patients are unidentified and mistreated due to the complexity of diagnosis. Imaging should also demonstrate the lack of any pathology or blockages in the brain. Despite the fact that all NPH cases have enlarged ventricles, not all elderly cases with enlarged ventricles have iNPH.

Hydrocephalus ex vacuo is the medical term for enlarged ventricles caused by cerebral atrophy (Figure 1).

Before deciding on a CSF diversion treatment, the iNPH concordance neuroimaging findings as well as clinical improvement after clinical tests are critical.

Current data of imaging utilized:

1. Evans' index;
2. Magnetic resonance elastography;
3. Callosal angles;
4. Glymphatic MRI;
5. Reversed aqueductal CSF net flow;
6. The SILVER Index: subarachnoid space is enlarged disproportionately;
7. Computerized volumetric assessment of the cranial CSF distribution;
8. Hyperdynamic CSF motion;
9. MRI water apparent diffusion coefficient;
10. Computed tomography perfusion;
11. Arterial spin labeling perfusion MRI;
12. Brain to ventricle ratios at the posterior and anterior commissure levels and three-dimensional (3D) volumetric convexity cistern to ventricle ratios;
13. High-field 3D-MRI study of subarachnoid space (Liew et al. 2019).

The Miller Fisher test is performed with 30–50 mL of CSF removed. To evaluate for symptoms of symptomatic improvement, cognitive function and gait are often examined soon before and within 2–3 h following the LP. The Miller Fisher test is similar to the CSF infusion test or the lumbar test. These tests have a positive predictive value of more than 90% but a negative predictive value of under 50%. CSF pressure should be normal or slightly elevated on the LP. Normal glucose levels, cell contents, and protein levels should all be present in CSF (Marmarou et al. 2005, 2007; Tarnaris et al. 2009).

Treatment

CSF diversion is the first-line treatment for suspected cases of NPH. Shunt surgery has proven to be the only long-lasting and effective treatment for iNPH (Vanneste et al. 1992). The current ideal treatment is the insertion of a ventriculoperitoneal (VP) shunt (Poca et al. 2004).

Kuriyama et al. conducted a statewide, hospital-based study in Japan and found that among patients diagnosed with iNPH the lumboperitoneal (LP) shunt was the top choice (55.1%), followed by the VP shunt (43.2%) (Kuriyama et al. 2017).

In iNPH patients, a modification of the VP shunt that placed the peritoneal end between two epiploic layers of the larger omentum resulted in a satisfactory outcome with no major postoperative problems (Grigorean et al. 2017).

Tudor et al. observed no changes in outcomes (balance, cognitive, function, mobility, and gait) between endoscopic third ventriculostomy (ETV) and normal therapy (VP shunting with a nonprogrammable valve) for iNPH cases in a systematic review (Tudor et al. 2015).

Bayar et al. investigated the efficacy of LP shunt surgery in NPH patients, finding that headache was cured in nearly all cases by the third month, and urinary incontinence, gait disturbance, and cognitive functions were recovered in 72%, 86%, and 65% of cases at the end of the first year, respectively (Bayar et al. 2018).

In a prospective multicenter trial, the efficacy and safety of LP shunts for cases with iNPH were investigated, with the previously completed VP shunt cohort study serving as a historical control group. The authors finally commented that the efficacy and safety of LP shunts with programmable valves for the management of patients with iNPH are comparable to those of VP shunts. Shunt revisions were, however, more common in LP shunt cases than in VP shunt cases (Miyajima et al. 2016). In research, only approximately 40% of iNPH cases improved following shunt operation, and only about 60% indicated their general health state was better than preoperatively using the self-assessed modified Rankin Scale (smRS) (Andrén et al. 2018). Vascular comorbidities, such as hypertension, stroke, diabetes, and cardiac disease, had no effect on the iNPH patients' early outcomes after shunt surgery. Cases with a history of stroke and hypertension, on the other hand, had a less favorable outcome, according to the same study. Surgery for NPH is clearly superior to the natural course or conservative treatment, according to risk–benefit studies (Liew et al. 2019).

Outcome

Eighty-five percent of patients see improvements in their gait. When surgery is performed early in the illness course, approximately 80% of patients' cognitive problems improve. Incontinence recovers in up to 80% of patients, but only in 50–60% of those who had a shunt inserted late in the illness course. Patients with mere gait deviation, mild or no autonomic incontinence, and mild dementia are the most likely to improve. Shunt failure, shunt obstruction, infections such as ventriculitis, under- or over-drainage, and the formation of a subdural hematoma are all risks associated with shunt implantation (Molde et al. 2017; Allali et al. 2017; Jo et al. 2017).

Medication

There are no drugs that can help with iNPH. Acetazolamide and other diuretics are only indicated for use in cases who are not candidates for shunt implantation.

Author Contributions: Conceptualization, methodology, validation, formal analysis, investigation, resources, data curation, writing—original draft preparation, M.M.R. and S.N.-e.-F.; writing—review and editing, visualization, supervision, F.H.C. All authors have read and agreed to the published version of the manuscript.

Funding: This research received no external funding.

Conflicts of Interest: The authors declare no conflicts of interest.

References

Adams, R. D., C. M. Fisher, S. Hakim, R. G. Ojemann, and W. H. Sweet. 1965. Symptomatic Occult Hydrocephalus with Normal Cerebrospinal-Fluid Pressure. *The New England Journal of Medicine* 273: 117–26. [CrossRef] [PubMed]

Allali, Gilles, Magali Laidet, Stéphane Armand, Arnaud Saj, Paul Krack, and Frédéric Assal. 2017. Apathy and higher level of gait control in normal pressure hydrocephalus. *International Journal Psychophysiology* 119: 127–31. [CrossRef] [PubMed]

Allali, Gilles, Valentina Garibotto, and Frèdèric Assal. 2016. Parkinsonism differentiates idiopathic normal pressure hydrocephalus from its mimics. *Journal of Alzheimer's Disease* 54: 123–27. [CrossRef] [PubMed]

American Psychiatric Association. 2013. *Diagnostic and Statistical Manual of Mental Disorders*, 5th ed. Washington, DC: American psychiatric publishing.

Andrén, Kerstin, Carsten Wikkelsö, Nina Sundström, Simon Agerskov, Hanna Israelsson, Katarina Laurell, Per Hellström, and Mats Tullberg. 2018. Long-term effects of complications and vascular comorbidity in idiopathic normal pressure hydrocephalus: A quality registry study. *Journal of Neurology* 265: 178–86. [CrossRef] [PubMed]

Apaydin, Hulya, J. Eric Ahlskog, Joseph E. Parisi, Bradley F. Boeve, and Dennis W. Dickson. 2002. Parkinson disease neuropathology, later-developing dementia and loss of the levodopa response. *Archives of Neurology* 59: 102–12. [CrossRef]

Baddeley, Alan. 1998. Recent developments in working memory. *Current Opinion in Neurobiology* 8: 234–38. [CrossRef]

Baird, Amee, and Séverine Samson. 2009. Memory for music in Alzheimer's disease: Unforgettable? *Neuropsychology Reviews* 19: 85–101. [CrossRef]

Barclay, Laurie L., Alexander Zemcov, John P. Blass, and Fletcher H. McDowell. 1985. Factors associated with duration of survival in Alzheimer's disease. *Biological Psychiatry* 20: 86–93. [CrossRef]

Barrientos, Ruth M., Meagan M. Kitt, Linda R. Watkins, and Steven F. Maier. 2015. Neuroinflammation in the normal aging hippocampus. *Neuroscience* 309: 1–15. [CrossRef]

Barron, Anna M., and Christian J. Pike. 2012. Sex hormones, aging, and Alzheimer's disease. *Frontiers in Bioscience (Elite Edition)* 4: 976–97. [CrossRef]

Bayar, Mehmet Akif, Ayhan Tekiner, Haydar Celik, Ali Yilmaz, Guner Menekse, Timur Yildirim, Fatih Alagoz, Yahya Guvenc, and Yavuz Erdem. 2018. Efficacy of Lumboperitoneal Shunting in Patients with Normal Pressure Hydrocephalus. *Turkish Neurosurgery* 28: 62–66. [CrossRef] [PubMed]

Bowling, Allen C., and M. Flint Beal. 1995. Bioenergetic and oxidative stress in neurodegenerative diseases. *Life Sciences* 56: 1151–71. [CrossRef] [PubMed]

Brean, Are, and Per K. Eide. 2008. Prevalence of probable idiopathic normal pressure hydrocephalus in a Norwegian population. *Acta Neurologica Scandinavica* 118: 48–53. [CrossRef] [PubMed]

Buckner, Randy L., Abraham Z. Snyder, Benjamin J. Shannon, Gina LaRossa, Rimmon Sachs, Anthony F. Fotenos, Yvette I. Sheline, William E. Klunk, Chester A. Mathis, John C. Morris, and et al. 2005. Molecular, structural, and functional characterization of Alzheimer's disease: Evidence for a relationship between default activity, amyloid, and memory. *Journal of Neuroscience* 25: 7709–17. [CrossRef] [PubMed]

Calderon, J., R. J. Perr, S. W. Erzinclioglu, G. E. Berrios, T. R. Dening, and John R. Hodges. 2001. Perception, attention, and working memory are disproportionately impaired in dementia with Lewy bodies compared with Alzheimer's disease. *Journal of Neurology, Neurosurgery & Psychiatry* 70: 157–64. [CrossRef]

Cavanna, Andrea E., and Michael R. Trimble. 2006. The precuneus: A review of its functional anatomy and behavioural correlates. *Brain* 129: 564–83. [CrossRef]

Chen, Wei-Wei, X. I. A. Zhang, and Wen-Juan Huang. 2016. Role of neuroinflammation in neurodegenerative diseases. *Molecular Medicine Reports* 13: 3391–96. [CrossRef]

Choi, Dong-Young, Young-Jung Lee, Jin Tae Hong, and Hwa-Jeong Lee. 2012. Antioxidant properties of natural polyphenols and their therapeutic. Potentials for Alzheimer's disease. *Brain Research Bulletin* 87: 144–53. [CrossRef]

Chou, Ping-Song, Meng-Ni Wu, Mei-Chuan Chou, I. Chien, and Yuan-Han Yang. 2017. Angiotensin-converting enzyme insertion/deletion polymorphism and the longitudinal progression of Alzheimer's disease. *Geriatrics & Gerontology International* 17: 1544–50. [CrossRef]

Corkin, Suzanne. 1984. Lasting consequences of bilateral medial temporal lobectomy: Clinical course and experimental findings in H.M. *Seminars in Neurology* 4: 249–59. [CrossRef]

Craig-Schapiro, Rebecca, Richard J. Perrin, Catherine M. Roe, Chengjie Xiong, Deborah Carter, Nigel J. Cairns, Mark A. Mintun, Elaine R. Peskind, Ge Li, Douglas R. Galasko, and et al. 2010. YKL-40: A novel prognostic fluid biomarker for preclinical Alzheimer's disease. *Biological Psychiatry* 68: 903–12. [CrossRef] [PubMed]

Cunningham, E. L., B. McGuinness, B. Herron, and A. P. Passmore. 2015. Dementia. *Ulster Medical Journal* 84: 79–87. [PubMed]

Damasio, Hanna, Thomas J. Grabowski, Daniel Tranel, Richard D. Hichwa, and Antonio R. Damasio. 1996. A neural basis for lexical retrieval. *Nature* 380: 499–505. [CrossRef] [PubMed]

Daselaar, Sander M., Serge A. R. B. Rombouts, Dick J. Veltman, Jeroen G. W. Raaijmakers, and Cees Jonker. 2003. Similar network activated by young and old adults during the acquisition of a motor sequence. *Neurobiology of Aging* 24: 1013–19. [CrossRef] [PubMed]

D'Esposito, Mark, Leon Y. Deouell, and Adam Gazzaley. 2003. Alterations in the BOLD fMRI signal with aging and disease: A challenge for neuroimaging. *Nature Reviews Neuroscience* 4: 863–72. [CrossRef]

de Villemeur, Thierry Billette. 2013. Creutzfeldt-Jakob disease. *Handbook of Clinical Neurology* 112: 1191–93. [CrossRef]

Dickerson, Bradford C., and Reisa A. Sperling. 2009. Large—Scale functional brain network abnormalities in Alzheimer's disease: Insights from functional neuroimaging. *Behavioral Neurology* 21: 63–75. [CrossRef]

Eddy, Clare M., Ellice G. Parkinson, and Hugh E. Rickards. 2016. Changes in mental state and behaviour in Huntington's disease. *The Lancet Psychiatry* 3: 1079–86. [CrossRef]

Egeland, Jens, Kjetil Sundet, Bjorn Rishovd Rund, Arve Asbjornsen, Kenneth Hugdahl, Nils Inge Landro, Anders Lund, Atle Roness, and Kirsten I. Stordal. 2003. Sensitivity and specificity of memory dysfunction in schizophrenia: A comparison with major depression. *Journal of Clinical and Experimental Neuropsychology* 25: 79–93. [CrossRef]

Esiri, Margaret M. 2000. Which vascular lesions are of importance in vascular dementia? *Annals of the New York Academy of Sciences* 903: 239–43. [CrossRef]

Exner, Cornelia, Janka Koschack, and Eva Irle. 2002. The differential role of premotor frontal cortex and basal ganglia in motor sequence learning: Evidence from focal basal ganglia lesions. *Learning & Memory* 9: 376–86.

Fadil, Halim, Aimee Borazanci, Elhachmia Ait Ben Haddou, Mohamed Yahyaoui, Elena Korniychuk, Stephen L. Jaffe, and Alireza Minagar. 2009. Early onset dementia. *International Review of Neurobiology* 84: 245–62. [CrossRef] [PubMed]

Finkel, Toren, and Nikki J. Holbrook. 2000. Oxidants, oxidative stress, and the biology of aging. *Nature* 408: 239–47. [CrossRef] [PubMed]

Fletcher, Paul C., and R. N. A. Henson. 2001. Frontal lobes and human memory: Insights from functional neuroimaging. *Brain* 124: 849–81. [CrossRef] [PubMed]

Ghosh, Amitabha. 2010. Endocrine, metabolic, nutritional, and toxic disorders leading to dementia. *Annals of Indian Academy of Neurology* 13: S63–S68. [CrossRef]

Glisky, Elizabeth L., and Daniel L. Schacter. 1989. Extending the limits of complex learning in organic amnesia: Computer training in a vocation domain. *Neuropsychologia* 27: 173–78. [CrossRef]

Greene, John D. W., and John R. Hodges. 1996. Identification of famous faces and famous names in early Alzheimer's disease. Relationship to anterograde episodic and general semantic memory. *Brain* 119: 111–28. [CrossRef]

Grigorean, Valentin Titus, Aurelia Mihaela Sandu, Mihai Popescu, Ioan Stefan Florian, Cristian Dumitru Lupascu, and Corina Lupascu Ursulescu. 2017. Our initial experience with ventriculo-epiplooic shunt in treatment of hydrocephalus in two centers. *Neurologia i Neurochirurgia Polska* 51: 290–98. [CrossRef]

Heindel, William C., David P. Salmon, Clifford W. Shults, Patricia A. Walicke, and Nelson Butters. 1989. Neuropsychological evidence for multiple implicit memory systems: A comparison of Alzheimer's, Huntington's, and Parkinson's disease patients. *Journal of Neuroscience* 9: 582–87. [CrossRef]

Hügel, Helmut M., and Neale Jackson. 2015. Polyphenols for the prevention and treatment of dementia diseases. *Neural Regeneration Research* 10: 1756–58. [CrossRef]

Iadecola, Costantino. 2004. Neurovascular regulation in the normal brain and in Alzheimer's disease. *Nature Reviews Neuroscience* 5: 347–60. [CrossRef] [PubMed]

Jamal, Salma, Sukriti Goyal, Asheesh Shanker, and Abhinav Grover. 2017. Computational Screening and Exploration of Disease-Associated Genes in Alzheimer's Disease. *Journal of Cellular Biochemistry* 118: 1471–79. [CrossRef] [PubMed]

Jellinger, Kurt A. 2007. The enigma of vascular cognitive disorder and vascular dementia. *Acta Neuropathologica* 113: 349–88. [CrossRef] [PubMed]

Jo, Kwang Wook, Youngkook Kim, Geun-Young Park, Ik Seong Park, Yongjun Jang, Sohn Dong Gyun, and Sun Im. 2017. Oropharyngeal dysphagia in secondary normal pressure hydrocephalus due to corticobulbar tract compression: Cases series and review of literature. *Acta Neurochirurgica* 159: 1005–11. [CrossRef]

Kalaria, Raj N. 2000. The role of cerebral ischemia in Alzheimer's disease. *Neurobiology of Aging* 21: 321–30. [CrossRef]

Kalaria, R. N., S. U. Bhatti, W. D. Lust, and G. Perry. 1993. The amyloid precursor protein in ischemic brain injury and chronic hypoperfusion. *Annals of the New York Academy of Sciences* 695: 190–93. [CrossRef]

Kanatsu, Kunihiko, and Taisuke Tomita. 2017. Molecular mechanisms of the genetic risk factors in pathogenesis of Alzheimer disease. *Frontiers in Bioscience* 22: 180–92.

Klingberg, Torkel, Hans Forssberg, and Helena Westerberg. 2002. Training of working memory in children with ADHD. *Journal of Clinical and Experimental Neuropsychology* 24: 781–91. [CrossRef]

Kosaka, K., M. Yoshimura, K. Ikeda, and H. Budka. 1984. Diffuse type of Lewy body disease, progressive dementia with abundant cortical Lewy bodies and senile changes of varying degree—A new disease? *Clinical Neuropathology* 3: 185–92.

Kövari, E., Gabriel Gold, F. R. Herrmann, Alessandra Canuto, P. R. Hof, Constantin Bouras, and Panteleimon Giannakopoulos. 2007. Cortical microinfarcts and demyelination affect cognition in cases at high risk for dementia. *Neurology* 68: 927–31. [CrossRef]

Krauss, Joachim K., Michael Faist, Martin Schubert, Jan J. Borremans, Carl H. Lücking, and Wiltrud Berger. 2001. Evaluation of Gait in Normal Pressure Hydrocephalus Before and After Shunting. In *Advances in Neurology, Volume 87: Gait Disorders*. Edited by Evzen Ruzicka, Mark Hallett and Joseph Jankovic. Philadelphia: Lippincott Williams & Wilkins, pp. 301–9.

Kuriyama, Nagato, Masakazu Miyajima, Madoka Nakajima, Michiko Kurosawa, Wakaba Fukushima, Yoshiyuki Watanabe, Etsuko Ozaki, Yoshio Hirota, Akiko Tamakoshi, Etsuro Mori, and et al. 2017. Nationwide hospital-based survey of idiopathic normal pressure hydrocephalus in Japan: Epidemiological and clinical characteristics. *Brain and Behavior* 7: e00635. [CrossRef] [PubMed]

Kuzuhara, S., H. Mori, N. Izumiyama, M. Yoshimura, and Y. Ihara. 1988. Lewy bodies are ubiquitinated. A light and electron microscopic immunocytochemical study. *Acta Neuropathologica* 75: 345–53. [CrossRef] [PubMed]

Kwong, Kenneth K., John W. Belliveau, David A. Chesler, Inna E. Goldberg, Robert M. Weisskoff, Brigitte P. Poncelet, David N. Kennedy, Bernice E. Hoppel, Mark S. Cohen, and Robert Turner. 1992. Dynamic magnetic resonance imaging of human brain activity during primary sensory stimulation. *Proceedings of the National Academy of Sciences* 89: 5675–79. [CrossRef] [PubMed]

Liew, Boon, Kiyoshi Takagi, Yoko Kato, Shyam Duvuru, Sengottuvel Thanapal, and Balamurugan Mangaleswaran. 2019. Current updates on idiopathic normal pressure hydrocephalus. *Asian journal of Neurosurgery* 14: 648–56. [CrossRef] [PubMed]

Logothetis, Nikos K., Jon Pauls, Mark Augath, Torsten Trinath, and Axel Oeltermann. 2001. Neurophysiological investigation of the basis of the fMRI signal. *Nature* 412: 150–57. [CrossRef]

Loy, Clement T., Peter R. Schofield, Anne M. Turner, and John B. J. Kwok. 2014. Genetics of dementia. *The Lancet* 383: 828–40. [CrossRef]

Marmarou, Anthony, Harold F. Young, and Gunes A. Aygok. 2007. Estimated incidence of normal pressure hydrocephalus and shunt outcome in patients residing in assisted-living and extended-care facilities. *Neurosurgical Focus* 22: E1. [CrossRef]

Marmarou, Anthony, Marvin Bergsneider, Petra Klinge, Norman Relkin, and Peter McL Black. 2005. The value of supplemental prognostic tests for the preoperative assessment of idiopathic normal-pressure hydrocephalus. *Neurosurgery* 57: S17–S28. [CrossRef]

McKee, A. C., N. W. Kawall, J. S. Schumacher, and M. Flint Beal. 1998. The neurotoxicity of amyloid beta protein in aged primates. *Amyloid* 5: 1–9. [CrossRef]

McKee, Ann C., Rhoda Au, Howard J. Cabral, Neil W. Kowall, Sudha Seshadri, Caroline A. Kubilus, Jon Drake, and Philip A. Wolf. 2006. Visual association pathology in preclinical Alzheimer disease. *Journal of Neuropathology & Experimental Neurology* 65: 621–30. [CrossRef]

Mesulam, M. Marsel. 2000. *Principles of Behavioral and Cognitive Neurology*. New York: Oxford University Press.

Miyajima, Masakazu, Hiroaki Kazui, Etsuro Mori, and Masatsune Ishikawa. 2016. One-year outcome in patients with idiopathic normal-pressure hydrocephalus: Comparison of lumboperitoneal shunt to ventriculoperitoneal shunt. *Journal of Neurosurgery* 125: 1483–92. [CrossRef] [PubMed]

Molde, Karin, Lars Söderström, and Katarina Laurell. 2017. Parkinsonian symptoms in normal pressure hydrocephalus: A population-based study. *Journal of Neurology* 264: 2141–48. [CrossRef] [PubMed]

Nolan, Karen A., M. Maddelena Lino, Arthur W. Seligmann, and John P. Blass. 1998. Absence of vascular dementia in an autopsy series from a dementia clinic. *Journal of the American Geriatrics Society* 46: 597–604. [CrossRef] [PubMed]

Nussbaum, R., and M. Polymeropoulos. 1997. Genetics of Parkinson's disease. 1997. Genetics of Parkinson's disease. *Human Molecular Genetics* 6: 1687–91. [CrossRef] [PubMed]

Ogawa, Seiji, David W. Tank, Ravi Menon, Jutta M. Ellermann, Seong G. Kim, Helmut Merkle, and Kamil Ugurbil. 1992. Intrinsic signal changes accompanying sensory stimulation: Functional brain mapping with magnetic resonance imaging. *Proceedings of the National Academy of Sciences of the United States of America* 89: 5951–55. [CrossRef] [PubMed]

Okazaki, Haruo, Lewis E. Lipkin, and Stanley M. Aronson. 1961. Diffuse intracytoplasmic ganglionic inclusions (Lewy type) associated with progressive dementia and quadriparesis in flexion. *Journal of Neuropathology and Experimental Neurology* 20: 237–44. [CrossRef]

Perani, Daniela, Stefano F. Cappa, Tatiana Schnur, Marco Tettamanti, Simona Collina, Màrio Miguel Rosa, and Ferruccio Fazio. 1999. The neural correlates of verb and noun processing. A PET study. *Brain* 122: 2337–44. [CrossRef]

Picascia, Marta, Brigida Minafra, Roberta Zangaglia, Luciana Gracardi, Nicolo Gabriele Pozzi, Elena Sinforiani, and Claudio Pacchetti. 2016. Spectrum of cognitive disorders in idiopathic normal pressure hydrocephalus. *Functional Neurology* 31: 143–47. [CrossRef]

Poca, Maria A., Maria Mataró, Maria Del Mar Matarín, Fuat Arikan, Carmen Junqué, and Juan Sahuquillo. 2004. Is the placement of shunts in patients with idiopathic normal-pressure hydrocephalus worth the risk? Results of a study based on continuous monitoring of intracranial pressure. *Journal of Neurosurgery* 100: 855–66. [CrossRef]

Polidori, M. Cristina, and Marlies Scholtes. 2016. Beyond and behind the fingerprints of oxidative stress in age-related diseases: Secrets of successful aging. *Archives of Biochemistry and Biophysics* 595: 50–53. [CrossRef]

Price, Joseph L., and John C. Morris. 1999. Tangles and plaques in nondemented aging and "preclinical" Alzheimer s disease. *Annals of Neurology* 45: 358–68. [CrossRef] [PubMed]

Rahal, Anu, Amit Kumar, Vivek Singh, Brijesh Yadav, Ruchi Tiwari, Sandip Chakraborty, and Kuldeep Dhama. 2014. Oxidative stress, prooxidants, and antioxidants: The interplay. *BioMed Research International* 63: 187–94. [CrossRef] [PubMed]

Reed, Laurence J., Dan Lasserson, Paul Marsden, Nicola Stanhope, Tom Stevens, Fernando Bello, Derek Kingsley, Alan Colchester, and Michael D. Kopelman. 2003. FDG-PET findings in the Wernicke-Korsakoff syndrome. *Cortex* 39: 1027–45. [CrossRef] [PubMed]

Ropper, Allan H., and Martin A. Samuels. 2009. *Adams and Victor's Principles of Neurology*. New York: McGraw-Hill Medical.

Rowe, James B., Ivan Toni, Oliver Josephs, Richard S. J. Frackowiak, and Richard E. Passingham. 2000. The prefrontal cortex: Response selection or maintenance within working memory? *Science* 288: 1656–60. [CrossRef] [PubMed]

Salmon, David P., Tara T. Lineweaver, and William C. Heindel. 1998. Nondeclarative memory in neurodegenerative disease. In *Memory in Neurodegenerative Disease: Biological, Cognitive, and Clinical Perspectives*. Edited by Alexander I. Troster. Cambridge: Cambridge University Press, pp. 210–25.

Samuel, William, Douglas Galasko, Eliezer Masliah, and Lawrence A. Hansen. 1996. Neocortical Lewy body counts correlate with dementia in the Lewy body variant of Alzheimer's disease. *Journal of Neuropathology and Experimental Neurology* 55: 44–52. [CrossRef]

Santos, Jose R., Auderlan M. Gois, Deise M. F. Mendonça, and Marco A. M. Freire. 2014. Nutritional status, oxidative stress, and dementia: The role of selenium in Alzheimer's disease. *Frontiers in Aging Neuroscience* 6: 206. [CrossRef]

Schacter, Daniel L., Anthony D. Wagner, and Randy L. Buckner. 2000. Memory systems of 1999. In *The Oxford Handbook of Memory*. Edited by Endel Tulving and Fergus I. M. Craik. New York: Oxford University Press, pp. 627–43.

Schonknecht, Oskar Dieter Peter, Aoife Hunt, Pablo Toro, Marcus Henze, Uwe Haberkorn, and Johannes Schröder. 2009. Neural correlates of delayed episodic memory in patients with mild cognitive impairment—A FDG PET study. *Neuroscience Letters* 467: 100–4. [CrossRef]

Shimizu, Motohiro, Joji Ishikawa, Yuichirou Yano, Satoshi Hoshide, Kazuyuki Shimada, and Kazuomi Kario. 2011. The relationship between the morning blood pressure surge and low-grade inflammation on silent cerebral infarct and clinical stroke events. *Atherosclerosis* 219: 316–21. [CrossRef]

Shmuel, Amir, Mark Augath, Axel Oeltermann, and Nikos K. Logothetis. 2006. Negative functional MRI response correlates with decreases in neuronal activity in monkey visual area V1. *Nature Neuroscience* 9: 569–77. [CrossRef]

Skoog, Ingmar, Lars Nilsson, Bo Palmertz, Lars-Arne Andreasson, and Alvar Svanborg. 1993. A population-based study of dementia in 85-year-olds. *New England Journal of Medicine* 328: 153–58. [CrossRef]

Snowden, Julie, David Neary, and David Mann. 2007. Frontotemporal lobar degeneration: Clinical and pathological relationships. *Acta Neuropathologica* 114: 31–38. [CrossRef] [PubMed]

Solomon, P. R., and A. E. Budson. 2003. Alzheimer's disease. *Clinical Symposia* 54: 1–44.

Sonnen, Joshua A., Eric B. Larson, Paul K. Crane, Sebastien Haneuse, Ge Li, Gerald D. Schellenberg, Suzanne Craft, James B. Leverenz, and Thomas J. Montine. 2007. Pathological correlates of dementia in a longitudinal, population-based sample of aging. *Annals of Neurology* 62: 406–13. [CrossRef] [PubMed]

Spillantini, Maria Grazia, R. Anthony Crowther, Ross Jakes, Masato Hasegawa, and Michel Goedert. 1998. Alpha-Synuclein in fi lamentous inclusions of Lewy bodies from Parkinson's disease and dementia with Lewy bodies. *Proceedings of the National Academy of Sciences of the United States of America* 95: 6469–73. [CrossRef] [PubMed]

Stefaniak, James, and John O'Brien. 2016. Imaging of neuroinflammation in dementia: A review. *Journal of Neurology, Neurosurgery & Psychiatry* 87: 21–28. [CrossRef]

Tanaka, Naofumi, Satoshi Yamaguchi, Hiroyasu Ishikawa, Hiroshi Ishii, and Kenichi Meguro. 2009. Prevalence of possible idiopathic normal-pressure hydrocephalus in Japan: The Osaki-Tajiri project. *Neuroepidemiology* 32: 171–75. [CrossRef]

Tarnaris, Andrew, Ahmed K. Toma, Neil D. Kitchen, and Laurence D. Watkins. 2009. Ongoing search for diagnostic biomarkers in idiopathic normal pressure hydrocephalus. *Biomarkers in Medicine* 3: 787–805. [CrossRef]

Tudor, Katarina Ivana, Mario Tudor, Jenny McCleery, and Josip Car. 2015. Endoscopic third ventriculostomy (ETV) for idiopathic normal pressure hydrocephalus (iNPH). *Cochrane Database of Systematic Reviews* 7: CD010033. [CrossRef]

Uchoa, Mariana F., V. Alexandra Moser, and Christian J. Pike. 2016. Interactions between inflammation, sex steroids, and Alzheimer's disease risk factors. *Frontiers in Neuroendocrinology* 43: 60–82. [CrossRef]

Vaidya, Chandan J., Margaret Zhao, John E. Desmond, and John D. E. Gabrieli. 2002. Evidence for cortical encoding specificity in episodic memory: Memory—Induced reactivation of picture processing areas. *Neuropsychologia* 40: 2136–43. [CrossRef]

Vanneste, Jeroen, Paul Augustijn, Clemens Dirven, Wee Fu Tan, and Zeger D. Goedhart. 1992. Shunting normal-pressure hydrocephalus: Do the benefits outweigh the risks? A multicenter study and literature review. *Neurology* 42: 54–59. [CrossRef] [PubMed]

Vemuri, Prashanthi, Gyorgy Simon, Kejal Kantarci, Jennifer L. Whitwell, Matthew L. Senjem, Scott A. Przybelski, Jeffrey L. Gunter, Keith A. Josephs, David S. Knopman, Bradley F. Boeve, and et al. 2011. Antemortem differential diagnosis of dementia pathology using structural MRI: Differential-STAND. *Neuroimage* 55: 522–31. [CrossRef] [PubMed]

White, L. O. N., Helen Petrovitch, John Hardman, James Nelson, Daron G. Davis, G. Webster Ross, Kamal Masaki, Lenore Launer, and William R. Markesbery. 2002. Cerebrovascular pathology and dementia in autopsied Honolulu-Asia Aging Study participants. *Annals of the New York Academy of Sciences* 977: 9–23. [CrossRef] [PubMed]

Wimo, Anders, Linus Jönsson, John Bond, Martin Prince, Bengt Winblad, and Alzheimer Disease International. 2013. The worldwide economic impact of dementia 2010. *Alzheimer's & Dementia* 9: 1–11. [CrossRef]

Younger, David S. 2005. Adult Normal Pressure Hydrocephalus. In *Motor Disorders*. Edited by David S. Younger. Philadelphia: Lippincott Williams & Wilkins, pp. 581–84.

Movement Disorders and Other Functional Neurosurgery

Jalal Uddin Mohammod Rumi, Mohammod Selim Sahi and Forhad H. Chowdhury

Abstract: Functional neurosurgery is not usually a life-saving surgery; it is typically used in certain neurological conditions, including intractable or resistant-to-medical-therapy forms. It includes (but is not limited to) surgery for movement disorders (i.e., Parkinson's disease, tremor, and dystonia) in the form of deep brain stimulation (DBS) or lesioning (ablative procedures) in the brain; surgery for spasticity and torticollis; MVD (microvascular decompression for neurovascular compression syndromes, i.e., trigeminal and glossopharyngeal neuralgia, hemifacial spasm, spasmodic torticollis, etc.); surgery for psychiatric disorders; intractable pain surgery; etc. The principles of surgical management of extreme or resistant forms of these conditions will be discussed in abstract form.

Abbreviations

AAD	atlantoaxial dislocation	AICA	anterior inferior cerebellar artery
AVM	arteriovenous malformation	CBD	corticobasal degeneration
CBZ	Carbamazepine	CNS	central nervous system
CRPS	complex regional pain syndrome	CSF	cerebrospinal fluid
CSPTC	cortico-striato-pallido-cortical	CT	computed tomography
CVA	cerebrovascular accident	DRD	dopa-responsive dystonia
DBS	deep brain stimulation	ET	essential tremor
EMG	Electromyography	GKRS	gamma knife radiosurgery
GK	gamma knife	GTS	Gilles de la Tourette's syndrome
GN	glossopharyngeal neuralgia	HIFU	high-frequency focal ultrasound
HFS	hemifacial spasm	MDD	major depressive disease
IPG	implanted pulse generator	MS	multiple sclerosis
MSA	multiple system atrophy	MRgFUS	MR-guided focus ultrasound
MVD	microvascular decompression	NPD	neurosurgery for psychiatric disorders
MRI	magnetic resonance imaging	PD	Parkinson's disease
OCD	obsessive compulsive disorder	PSP	progressive supranuclear palsy
PICA	posterior inferior cerebellar artery	RF	Radiofrequency
REZ	root entry/exit zone	SCM	Sternocleidomastoid
SCA	superior cerebellar artery	TBI	traumatic brain injury
STN	subthalamic nucleus	TENS	transepidermal neurostimulation
TDPD	tremor-dominant Parkinson's disease	TS	Tourette's syndrome
TN	trigeminal neuralgia	VA	vertebral artery
UE	upper extremity		

1. Movement Disorder Surgery

1.1. Introduction

Medication, in conjunction with rehabilitative treatments such as physiotherapy, occupational therapy, and even psychotherapy, is the prime therapy for movement disorders. As the condition advances, these techniques may fail or have unfavorable outcomes, necessitating surgery. In movement disorders such as essential tremor (ET), Parkinson's disease (PD), and dystonia, surgery has become a well-established type of treatment. Other movement disorders, such as tremors linked with multiple sclerosis as well as tics observed in Tourette's syndrome, seem to benefit from surgery (TS). Although surgery cannot cure movement disorders, it does significantly reduce symptoms and, therefore, improve quality of life.

We will give an overview of numerous movement abnormalities in this chapter, with a focus on those that may benefit from neurosurgical intervention. We will also go over the indications, outcomes, and drawbacks of several surgical approaches for movement disorders.

1.2. Definition of Movement Disorders

Movement disorders are defined by impairments in movement planning, control, or execution and are genetically, pathologically, and clinically heterogeneous. Hypokinetic and hyperkinetic disorders are the two most common types. Paucity or slowness of movement (bradykinesia) and an involuntary increase in muscular tone characterize hypokinetic diseases (rigidity). Parkinson's disease and various kinds of parkinsonism are examples of hypokinetic illnesses. Hyperkinetic disorders are characterized by excessive involuntary movement, either spontaneously or in reaction to a voluntary movement or another stimulus. Hyperkinetic disorders can sometimes have a voluntary element. Tremor, tics, dystonia, chorea, myoclonus, and ballismus are all hyperkinetic disorders.

1.3. Parkinson's Disease

PD is an age-linked disease with a progressively growing prevalence beyond the age of 50. It is anticipated that up to 2% of adults over the age of 60 will get the disease (Tanner and Aston 2000). PD is marked by bradykinesia, postural instability, and resting tremor that develops slowly and asymmetrically (Lang and Lang 1998). It progresses slowly and has a long-term response to dopaminergic medicines. The loss of melanin-laden dopaminergic neurons in the substantia nigra zona compacta causes depigmentation of the substantia nigra.

Patients with PD experience a wide range of symptoms of the nonmotor type, including fatigue, depression, cognitive decline, anxiety, visual dysfunction, behavioral disorders, dysautonomia, weight loss, sleep irregularities, aberrant sensations, and pain, in addition to motor dysfunction (Chaudhuri et al. 2006). These nonmotor signs may appear earlier in the disease, but they become increasingly disabling as the disease progresses, contributing mostly to a reduction in quality of life.

Atypical parkinsonism can mirror PD in its early stages, but there are typically "red flags" that point to a different diagnosis. The response to levodopa in atypical parkinsonism is poor from the start, transient, or unsustainable. Progressive supranuclear palsy (PSP), multiple system atrophy (MSA), and corticobasal degeneration are examples of atypical parkinsonisms (CBD).

Medical treatments are effective in the early stages of PD. Patients become less sensitive to treatments as the condition progresses, and medication-related problems occur. These are the patients who have benefited greatly from surgical operations.

1.3.1. Treatment of PD

1. Medical therapy: available medications include levodopa, dopamine agonists (pramipexole and ropinirole), anticholinergics (e.g., trihexyphenidyl), amantadine, MAO-B inhibitors (e.g., rasagiline), COMT inhibitors (e.g., entacapone), and many other. Levodopa is the main medication, in combination with add-on drugs from other groups.
2. Occupational and physiotherapy
3. Surgery
    a. Deep brain stimulation (DBS) to STN, GPi, VIM thalamus, and PPN;
    b. Ablative surgery: radiofrequency thalamotomy, pallidotomy, focus ultrasound thalamotomy, and gamma knife thalamotomy;
    c. Cell therapy;
    d. Gene therapy;
    e. Immunotherapy.

1.4. Tremor

In clinical practice, tremor is one of the most frequent movement disorders. It has been defined as a rhythmic, involuntary, and sinusoidal oscillation of one or more parts of body caused by synchronous or alternating muscle contractions.

Tremors are defined as resting or action tremors, in clinical terms. Postural, kinetic, and intention tremors are the three types of action tremor. When a limb is in a resting position, its weight is completely supported against gravity and it develops a resting tremor. It is common in PD and other parkinsonian disorders, as well as midbrain and rubral tremor. An active contraction of the muscles involved is implied by action tremor. A postural tremor takes place when the body maintains a posture against gravity, such as when the arms are stretched out in front of it. A voluntary movement of the extremity causes a kinetic tremor, such as a tremor in the upper extremity during the finger-to-nose technique. When approaching a target, the amplitude of the intention tremor increases.

Differential diagnosis of tremor includes:

1. Physiologic tremor;
2. Essential tremor;

3. Orthostatic tremor;
4. Task specific tremor;
5. PD and other parkinsonian syndromes;
6. Wilson's disease;
7. Multiple sclerosis;
8. Stroke;
9. Holmes tremor;
10. Neuropathic tremor;
11. Palatal tremor;
12. Dystonic tremor.

Essential tremor (ET) is the most prevalent type of action tremor, which can be postural or kinetic in nature and primarily affects the hands. With a frequency of 4–12 Hz, it is usually bilateral and symmetrical (Louis 2001). In around 95% of patients, the distal arms and hands are afflicted, followed by the head (34%), lower limbs (20%), voice (12%), face, and trunk (5%) (Elble 2000a).

When tremor of the head arises alone or before the beginning of hand tremor, dystonic tremor should be considered a possibility. The frequency of ET tremors diminishes over time, while the magnitude may increase (Elble 2000b).

Because ET frequently has an insidious onset, it is difficult for patients to memorize the exact age of onset. The majority of instances begin after the age of 40. The disease's family manifestations are more likely to manifest at an earlier age.

Although the results differ between studies, the majority suggest a crude prevalence of 4% or greater in those aged 60 and up, with both sexes being equally affected.

The incidence appears to increase exponentially as people become older (Louis 2019).

Apart from physiological tremor, essential tremor is the most prevalent type of tremor. In 50% of patients, a significant reduction in tremor occurs in reaction to a small amount of alcohol, which may aid in diagnosis (Mostile and Jankovic 2010).

Tremor is thought to affect roughly 25–60% of persons with multiple sclerosis. Postural and intention tremors are the most common symptoms of MS. The limbs, head, neck, voice cord, and trunk are all affected by the tremor. The tremor is thought to be cerebellar in origin and to be associated with additional sensory, cerebellar, and corticospinal dysfunction. The symptoms are frequently severe, humiliating, and difficult to manage (Koch et al. 2007).

Holmes' tremor, midbrain tremor, rubral tremor, and Benedikt's syndrome are all terms for a condition that affects the proximal limbs. It is a tremor with a slow frequency (less than 4.5 Hz) with a rest element that becomes worse with postural maintenance and even worse with motion.

The common etiology includes stroke, head injury, demyelinating diseases, infection, and vascular malformation. An MRI study usually discloses structural lesions occurring in the upper brain stem, cerebellum, or thalamus. The most common symptoms/signs associated with HT are hemiparesis, ataxia, hypoesthesia, dystonia, cranial nerve palsy, and dysarthria.

Treatment of Tremor

(i) Medical therapy: propranolol and primidone are two highly effective and widely used drugs for ET. Medical treatment of MS tremor and Holmes' tremor are very unrewarding. Isoniazid, levodopa, ondansetron, clonazepam, and some other drugs are used in these condition, in addition to the drugs used for ET.
(ii) Intramuscular injections of botulinum toxin.
(iii) Surgery:

- Deep brain stimulation (DBS) to the VIM thalamus;
- Ablative surgery: radiofrequency thalamotomy, focus ultrasound thalamotomy, and gamma knife thalamotomy.

1.5. Dystonia

Dystonia is a type of movement disorder that results in abnormal postures, typically repetitive abnormal motions, or both. Dystonic motions are structured, tremulous, and twisting in nature. Dystonia is frequently sparked or exacerbated by deliberate effort and is associated with an overflow of muscular activation (Albanese et al. 2013).

One of the most disabling movement disorders is Parkinson's disease. Its pathogenesis is a network condition engaging the basal ganglia, sensorimotor cortices, and cerebellum that is defined by an abnormal input versus output sensorimotor or plasticity mismatch (Cury et al. 2018).

Dystonia syndromes are classified along three main axes: age at onset, etiology, (childhood onset and adult onset), and body distribution (focal, segmental, multifocal, generalized, and hemidystonia) (Fahn 2011).

Dystonia that starts in childhood has more chance to have a known cause and move from a focal to a widespread form, whereas dystonia that starts beyond the age of 25 commonly affects the craniocervical group of muscles, remains segmental or localized, and is generally non-progressive (Bressman 2004).

Primary dystonia, secondary dystonia, paroxysmal dystonia, and dystonia-plus syndromes are the etiological categories (Fahn et al. 1998).

Primary dystonias are idiopathic, with the exception of genetic alterations in rare cases, and are not accompanied by additional neurologic abnormalities other than tremor and myoclonus. Primary generalized dystonia is uncommon and usually begins in childhood. Primary focal dystonias are more frequent and almost always strike adults in their forties or fifties. These can affect the neck, arm, or face, but leg involvement is uncommon.

Cervical dystonia, the most common kind of focal dystonia, typically manifests itself between the ages of 30 to 50, with restricted head mobility, neck stiffness, and aberrant head postures, as well as irregular tremor of the head. Sensory tactics, such as lightly caressing the chin or face, are widespread and especially effective early in the disease course; this phenomenon is also called the geste antagoniste (Prakash and Lang 2009).

Cranial dystonia: A variety of face, oropharyngeal, and jaw muscles are involved in cranial dystonia. It is frequently linked with cervical muscle involvement (craniocervical dystonia) and occasionally with laryngeal involvement (spasmodic dysphonia). Blepharospasm is a condition in which the orbicularis oculi muscles contract abnormally, causing excessive blinking as well as forced eyelid closure, which can lead to functional blindness (Prakash and Lang 2009).

Oro-mandibular dystonia is characterized by aberrant activity in the lower face, tongue, pharyngeal, and jaw muscles, which can make speaking and swallowing difficult. Spasmodic dysphonia is a vocal cord dystonia; improper adduction, which results in a strangled, strained voice, is more common than abduction, which results in a whispered, breathy voice (Prakash and Lang 2009).

Brachial dystonia: Another type of focal dystonia is brachial dystonia, which is most commonly associated with writing (writer's cramp). Similar issues might arise with pianists and string players. This type of "task specific focal dystonia" can impact a wide range of extremely complicated skills (Prakash and Lang 2009).

Dystonia-plus syndromes are neurological illnesses that include symptoms such as parkinsonism or myoclonus (Prakash and Lang 2009).

Dopa-responsive dystonia (DRD) is a type of generalized dystonia that begins in childhood. As a result of mutations in the gene that codes for GTP cyclohydrolase I, the disorder usually starts in the first decade of life with foot dystonia, gait irregularity, and hyperreflexia. The illness eventually progresses to generalized dystonia with considerable postural instability and gait difficulty. With peak difficulty late in the evening, considerable diurnal variability is a unique trait. A significant, prolonged, and straightforward response to low to moderate dosages of levodopa is the characteristic of this condition (Prakash and Lang 2009).

1.5.1. Treatment Options for Dystonia

1. Medical therapy: available medication includes anticholinergics (e.g., trihexyphenidyl), baclofen, levodopa, benzodiazepines (clonazepam and diazepam), and dopamine depletors (tetrabenazine).
2. Local botulinum toxin injections.
3. Surgery:
    (a) Baclofen pump infusion;
    (b) Deep brain stimulation (DBS) to the GPi and VIM thalamus;
    (c) Ablative surgery: radiofrequency thalamotomy and pallidotomy (Cloud and Jinnah 2010).
4. 'Ruth Chiles Brain spotting technique' for cure of focal dystonia: The author claimed with cases of evidence in her book 'The focal dystonia cure' that most of the focal dystonia can be cured by this technique (Chiles 2022).

1.6. *Stereotactic Neurosurgery*

The *xx*-axis, *yy*-axis, and *zz*-axis are three mutually perpendicular coordinate axes that make up the Cartesian coordinate system. As a result, x, y, and z values can be used to define any point in space. A Cartesian coordinate system is used in stereotactic surgery. By using a computed tomography (CT) scan, magnetic resonance imaging (MRI), and Cartesian-coordinate-based stereotactic frame, anywhere deep in the brain could be reached/approached in a minimally invasive, precise, and reproducible manner. Modern stereotactic planning software helps in MRI and CT scan image fusion and trajectory planning and reduces surgical complication significantly.

Indications for intracranial stereotactic surgery:

1. Biopsy;
2. Radiosurgery;
3. Deep brain stimulation;
4. Radiofrequency ablation;
5. lacement of depth electrode;
6. Aspiration of hematoma or abscess.

1.7. *Surgery for Movement Disorders*

A variety of surgical treatments such as resection, ablation, stimulation, cell therapy, gene therapy, immunotherapy, and others have been utilized to manage cases with movement disorders. Currently, deep brain stimulation (DBS), with its inherent character of adjustability and reversibility as well as strong advocacy and marketing from industry, is the most common surgical procedure for PD, ET, and dystonia. Radiofrequency thalamotomy and other ablative procedures are also performed in selected patients. There have been a number of animal studies and clinical trials of gene therapy, tissue transplantation, and immunotherapy. While these trials have shown the safety of the procedure, clinical benefits have been less encouraging.

1.7.1. Deep Brain Stimulation

Deep brain stimulation (DBS) is basically stereotactic implantation of an electrode leading to a specific part of the brain (Figure 1). An internal pulse generator (IPG) is placed in the chest wall and can deliver the stimulus current pulses. An extension wire passes subcutaneously from the scalp area to the chest wall, thereby connecting the lead to the IPG. DBS applies high-frequency electrical stimulation in the subcortical brain. The selection of an appropriate patient and appropriate target is critical for satisfactory outcomes. The precise placement of a DBS lead in its target of interest is the main challenge of the procedure.

DBS has complicated electrical effects on individual neurons and neuronal networks, affects neurotransmitter concentrations and dynamics, and shapes the microenvironment, which includes astrocytes, microglia, and endothelial cells. DBS also affects neuroplasticity and may cause neurogenesis and neuroprotection (Jakobs et al. 2019).

Targets for DBS

1. Subthalamic nucleus: PD;
2. VIM thalamus: essential tremor, other tremor, and tremor-dominant PD;
3. Globus pallidus interna: dystonia and PD with dyskinesia;
4. Pedunculopontine nucleus: PD with gait instability.

The ideal candidates for DBS among PD patients should fulfill the following criteria (Enslin 2016):

1. Appropriate neuroimaging to exclude possible differential diagnosis;
2. Realistic expectations on the potential result of DBS;
3. No cognitive abnormality and motivated patient and family;
4. Duration of PD more than 5 years;
5. Disabling drug-resistant tremor;
6. Proof of dopamine responsiveness (at least 30% improvement in motor score with dopamine);
7. Problematic dyskinesia and motor fluctuations, in spite of appropriate drug therapy;
8. $\leq$70 years of age;
9. No atypical parkinsonism;
10. Good medical health.

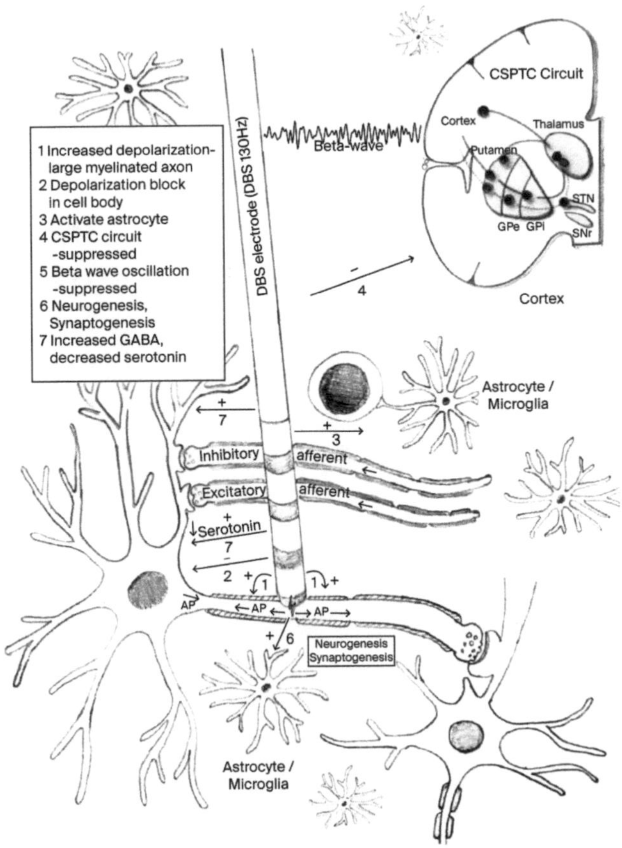

Figure 1. Illustrations showing possible mechanism of action of deep brain stimulation (DBS). CSPTC—cortico-striato-pallido-thalamo-cortical. Source: Figure by authors.

DBS in PD patients has shown long-term improvement in cardinal motor symptoms like tremor, bradykinesia, and rigidity. GPi DBS demonstrated long-term efficacy in the management of generalized and segmental dystonia. Efficacy is more pronounced in primary dystonia than secondary dystonia. Thalamic stimulation seems to be highly effective in TDPD, ET, and dystonic tremor with modest efficacy in Holmes tremor and MS tremor.

Complication of DBS Surgery

1. Intracranial hemorrhage;
2. Infection;
3. Fracture of DBS electrode, lead migration, failure of extension wire, IPG malfunction, and erosion of skin;
4. Dyskinesia, worsening of symptom, speech dysfunction, and dysarthria (Rezai et al. 2008).

1.7.2. Ablative Procedures

Currently, three main ablative procedures that are utilized for movement disorders are RF thermo-ablation, gamma/cyber knife radiosurgery, and high-frequency focused ultrasound (HIFU) thermal ablation. All these surgeries have their foundation in stereotactic principles.

The radiofrequency thermal ablation procedure involves heating a lesion with an intracranial electrode connected to an RF generator to create a lesion. Except at the tip, where the active electrode is placed, this electrode is electrically isolated.

External ablative treatment mode stereotactic radiosurgery offers a large single dose of radiation to a small intracranial target volume while sparing surrounding tissue. Lars Leksell developed gamma knife radiosurgery (GKRS), which takes advantage of gamma rays emitted by excited cobalt nuclei.

Thermal ablation with MR-guided focused ultrasound (MRgFUS) is a promising, noninvasive technology. Using a hemispheric phased array of transducers mounted to the skull, high-frequency focused ultrasound (HIFU) beams are targeted to an intracranial region. This permits ultrasonic waves to flow through a vast area of the skull, preventing overheating and brain injury. Ultrasonic mechanical energy is absorbed and transformed to heat within the focal target volume, causing tissue damage locally at the focus (ter Haar and Coussios 2007).

Radiofrequency for cases with ET and tremor-dominant PD and VIM thalamotomy have been demonstrated to provide considerable tremor control (TDPD). The majority of side effects with RF thalamotomy are temporary due to perilesional edema that goes away with time; nevertheless, persistent ataxia, dysarthria, and motor/sensory deficiency might develop. With bilateral lesions, the chance of dysarthria is much higher. As a result, RF thalamotomy is usually only performed unilaterally (Franzini et al. 2019).

GK thalamotomy and transcranial MRgFUS thalamotomy are noninvasive techniques that eliminate the risk of cerebral hemorrhage and infection associated with open surgery. In patients with TDPD and ET, both of these techniques revealed significant tremor (Witjas et al. 2015; Chang et al. 2018). While GK radiosurgery takes a long time to lesion, MRgFUS allows for rapid lesioning.

RF of the globus pallidus internus pars interna (GPi) was used to treat PD, PD with dyskinesia, and dystonia. In PD, a unilateral pallidotomy is performed on the side that is more symptomatic. Primary dystonic patients, on the other hand, frequently receive bilateral lesioning because they have bilateral extremities and axial symptoms and are more capable of tolerating bilateral lesioning. The cardinal motor symptoms of Parkinson's disease, including tremor, stiffness, and bradykinesia, have been demonstrated to be improved with posteroventral pallidotomy. Pallidotomy may also help with dyskinesias caused by levodopa (Franzini et al. 2019).

2. Surgery for Spasticity

Upper motor neuron pathway lesions cause spasticity in limbs and the trunk. The lack of inhibitory impulse on alpha motor neurons and on gamma motor neurons (intrafusal fibers) results in alpha spasticity and gamma spasticity, respectively. Increased muscle tone, myoclonus, and (sometimes) involuntary movements are the clinical findings in spasticity (Greenberg 2010).

2.1. Etiologies

- Cerebral insult (e.g., stroke, tumor, and vasculitis).
- Spinal cord lesions (cord injury rostral to the conus medullaris, tumor, and vasculitis).
- Multiple sclerosis and congenital abnormalities (e.g., spinal dysraphism and cerebral palsy).

2.2. Clinical Features

- History of etiological event (such as stroke, trauma, etc.).
- Elevated resistance to passive movements.
- Exaggerated deep tendon reflexes.
- Activation of antagonistic muscles simultaneously.
- Characteristic postures (i.e., hyperflexion of thighs or scissoring of legs).
- Pain (sometimes).
- It may confound the patient's ability to sit in a wheelchair, lay in bed, drive modified vehicles, sleep, etc.
- May also foster development of decubitus/contracture ulcers.
- Urge incontinence of bladder.

2.3. Grading Spasticity (The Ashworth Scale)

Assessment should be performed with patient supine and relaxed (Table 1).

Table 1. Ashworth scorer.

Score	Degree of Muscle Tone
1	Normal muscle tone
2	Slight (mild) increase; slight "catch" in flexion and extension
3	More marked (moderate) increase; passive movements easy
4	Considerable increase; difficult passive movements
5	Affected part rigid inflexion and extension

Source: Authors' compilation based on data from Ashworth (1964).

2.4. *Treatment*

2.4.1. Conservative

- Regular physiotherapy.
- Drugs: benzodiazepines, baclofen, and dantrolene.

2.4.2. Surgical

Reserved for spasticity that is refractory to medical management or where side effects of medications are intolerable. Generally, either orthopedic (e.g., tendon release operations (tenotomies) of heel cord or hamstrings, iliopsoas myotomies, etc.) or neurosurgical (e.g., nerve blocks, neurectomies, myelotomy, etc.).

A. Non-lesional procedures

1. Intrathecal baclofen (baclofen pump)—widely used where baclofen is administered intrathecally through a subcutaneously implanted reservoir. Other indications include: CVA (Meythaler et al. 2001), cerebral palsy, TBI, dystonia, and stiff-man syndrome.
2. Intrathecal morphine.
3. Electrical stimulation through epidural electrodes (Richardson et al. 1979).

B. Lesional procedures, with preservation of potential for ambulation

Motor point block (Scott et al. 1985) (intramuscular phenol neurolysis): sensations and remaining voluntary functions are preserved.

Time-consuming phenol nerve block: Akin to motor point block but utilized for more severe spasticity. Here, complete blocking of muscles is desired (Herz et al. 1990).

(i) Selective neurectomies (Scott et al. 1985)

1. Sciatic nerve neurectomy (Herz et al. 1990).
2. Obturator nerve neurectomy: useful for strong hip adductor spasticity that causes scissoring.
3. Pudendal nerve neurectomy: helpful if excessive detrusor dyssynergy interferes with bladder function.

(ii) Percutaneous radiofrequency foraminal rhizotomy
(iii) Midline "T" myelotomy

It intercepts the reflex arc from sensory to motor units without disturbing connections from the corticospinal tract to anterior horn cells (Cury et al. 2018).

(iv) Selective dorsal rhizotomy (Privat et al. 1976)

Intraprocedural EMG and electrophysiological stimulation are used to cut the sensory rootlets engaged in "handicapping spasticity". It may be temporary but seems to work for a minimum of 5 yrs. In cerebral palsy children, it may improve gait in ambulatory cases; in nonambulatory children, their gait is improved, but they may not be able to walk.

(v) Stereotactic thalamotomy or dentatotomy

It may be helpful in cerebral palsy. Usually used for unilateral dystonia, especially shoulders or hips. It should not be utilized if the situation is swiftly progressive.

C. Lesioning procedures, with sacrifice of potential for ambulation (such as in complete cord injuries where Nona lesioning procedures are not indicated as there is no motor function to recover). Utilized in failed percutaneous rhizotomy and "T" myelotomy.

(i) Intrathecal injection of 6 mL of 10% phenol (by weight) in glycerin mixed with 4 ml of iohexol;
(ii) Selective anterior rhizotomy: results in flaccid paralysis and atrophy of muscles;

(iii) Neurectomies plus/minus tenotomies;
(iv) Intramuscular neurolysis by phenol;
(v) Cordectomy (reserved only for patients who do not respond to any other measure; it results in total flaccidity) (Greenberg 2010; Ashworth 1964; Meythaler et al. 2001; Richardson et al. 1979; Scott et al. 1985; Herz et al. 1990; Privat et al. 1976).

3. Torticollis (Wry Neck)

A special type of dystonia due to failure to maintain the head position.

3.1. Etiology

- Congenital torticollis;
- Spasmodic torticollis (Idiopathic)—the sternocleidomastoid (SCM) muscle is shortened in spasm;
- Hemorrhage into the sternocleidomastoid muscle (scaring);
- Extrapyramidal lesions: usually improve by lying down; EMG usually shows abnormal, grouped electrical activities of muscles;
- Psychogenic;
- Torticollis from atlantoaxial rotatory instability—SCM may be in continuous spasm state (unlike that of spasmodic torticollis) (Figure 2);
- Neurovascular compression of the 11th nerve;
- Infection of the cervical spine, i.e., Tuberculosis;
- Cervical adenitis;
- Chari malformation;
- Syringomyelia/syringobulbia;
- Cerebellar tumors in children;
- Bulbar palsies;
- Diplopia from extraocular muscles weakness (Greenberg 2010).

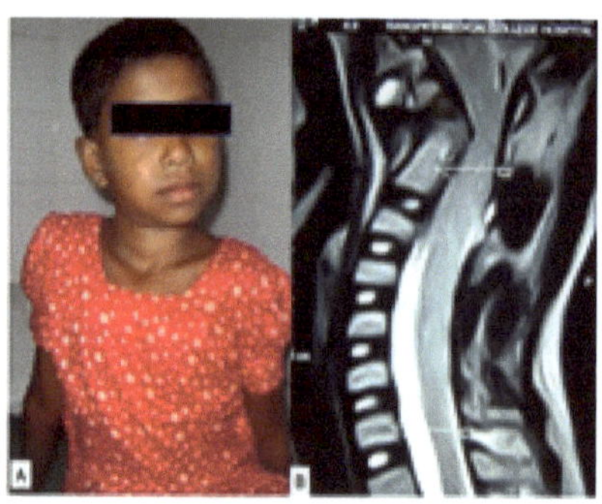

Figure 2. (**A**) Torticollis due to atlantoaxial dislocation (AAD) in a pediatric patient. (**B**) MRI of cervical spine showing AAD. Source: Figure by authors.

3.2. Investigations

1. MRI of brain in accessory and lower cranial nerve protocol and MRI craniovertebral junction;
2. CT scan of cervical spine and craniovertebral junction;
3. EMG of neck muscle.

3.3. Treatment

3.3.1. Conservative

Relaxation training, stretching, physiotherapy, and transepidermal neurostimulation (TENS).

3.3.2. Surgical Procedures

Usually advised for disabling, intractable cases. Options are as follows:

1. Dorsal cord stimulation;
2. Local injection of botulinum toxin—less effective for torticollis;

3. Selective rhizotomy and spinal accessory neurotomy;
4. MVD of accessory nerve root entry zone;
5. Stereotactic lesioning of Forel's H1 field;
6. Sectioning SCM;
7. Treatment of specific etiology, such as Chiari malformation, AAD, etc.;
8. Torticollis of accessory nerve origin.

    - Transection of the anastomotic branches between the 11th nerve and the upper cervical posterior root (C1 anastomotic branch is sensory only);
    - MVD of the 11th nerve (most cases caused by VA, but PICA compression is also described; symptoms relieved a few weeks after operation) (Greenberg 2010; Shima et al. 1988).

4. Trigeminal Neuralgia (TN)

4.1. Introduction

Trigeminal neuralgia (TN) is a condition marked by recurrent, unilateral, short, electric-shock-like pains that are sudden in onset and termination, localized to one or more divisions of the trigeminal nerve, and caused by harmless stimuli. Moreover, there might be simultaneous continuous pain of moderate intensity within the distributions of the involved nerve division/s.

4.2. Diagnostic Criteria

A. Recurrent paroxysms of one-sided face pain in one or more divisions of the fifth nerve, with no radiation beyond, while meeting criteria B and C.

B. Pain manifests itself in all of the following ways:

(1) Lasting anywhere between a fraction of a second and two minutes;
(2) Extreme severity;
(3) The quality is electric-shock-like, sharp, shooting, or stabbing.

C. Triggered by seemingly harmless stimuli in the involved trigeminal distribution;

D. Not adequately explained by another condition (International Headache Society 2018).

4.3. Classification of TN

1. Classical trigeminal neuralgia: vascular compression seen on MRI or during surgery with morphological alterations of the fifth nerve root.
2. Secondary trigeminal neuralgia occurs when a neoplasm in the cerebellopontine angle, multiple sclerosis, or an arteriovenous malformation causes pain (International Headache Society 2018).
3. Idiopathic TN: there are no diagnostic tests that can confirm a lesion or condition that could cause trigeminal neuralgia (International Headache Society 2018).

4.4. Incidence and Pathophysiology

TN is a rare condition, with a yearly incidence of 4.3–27 per 100,000 people. Women are more likely to be affected, and the risk rises with age. In classic TN, the average age of onset is 53 years, while in secondary TN, it is 43 years (Maarbjerg et al. 2017).

The transition from peripheral Schwann cell myelination to central oligodendroglia myelination occurs within the root entry zone (REZ). This area is especially prone to compression by a blood vessel or tumor, which causes demyelination and morphological changes such distortion, indentation, flattening, or atrophy (Maarbjerg et al. 2014). Sensory nerve fibers that have been demyelinated turn hyperexcitable and are capable of producing ectopic impulses, which present as spontaneous pain (Devor et al. 2002). Touch-evoked pain may be caused by ephaptic links between demyelinated A and A fibers (Magerl and Treede 2004).

4.5. Causes

Classical TN caused by microvascular compression by:

- Superior cerebellar artery (SCA—the most frequent);
- Anterior inferior cerebellar artery (AICA);
- Elongated PICA;

- Ectatic vertebrobasilar artery (EVBA) (Figure 3);
- Veins.

Secondary TN caused by:

- Mass lesion epidermoid (Figure 4), schwannoma, meningioma, etc.;
- Multiple sclerosis and white mater plaque.

Idiopathic.

- There is no microvascular compression or other pathology.

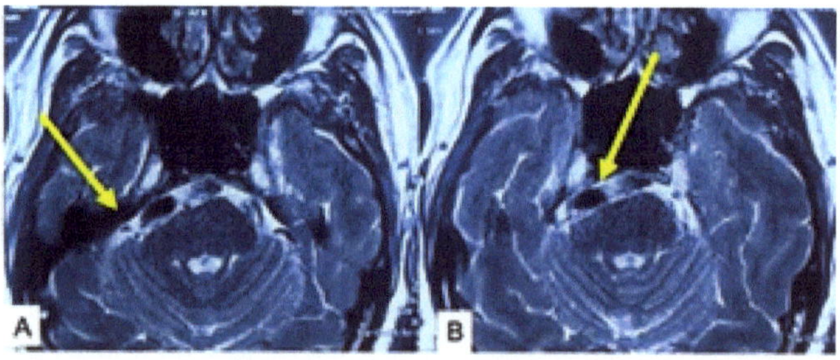

Figure 3. (**A**,**B**) MRI of brain T2W images: axial views showing REZ compression of right 5th nerve (arrow marked) by an ectatic vertebrobasilar artery (EVBA) causing trigeminal neuralgia. Source: Figure by authors.

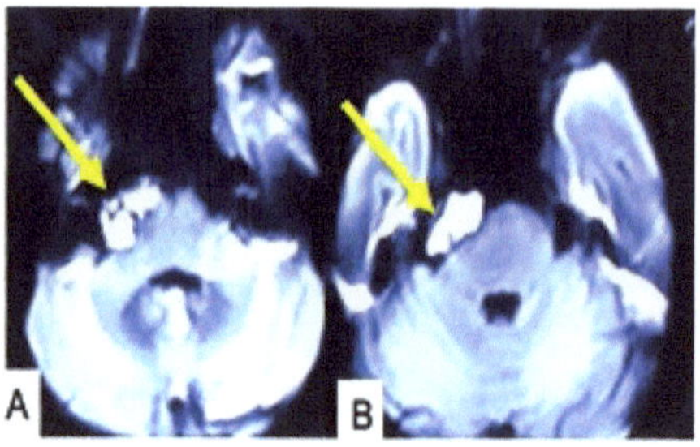

Figure 4. (**A**,**B**) MRI of brain axial DW images showing sided small epidermoid in right cerebellopontine angle (arrow marked) causing TN. Source: Figure by authors.

Intraoperatiive picture of MVD in hemifacial spasm (right side) is shown in Figure 5.

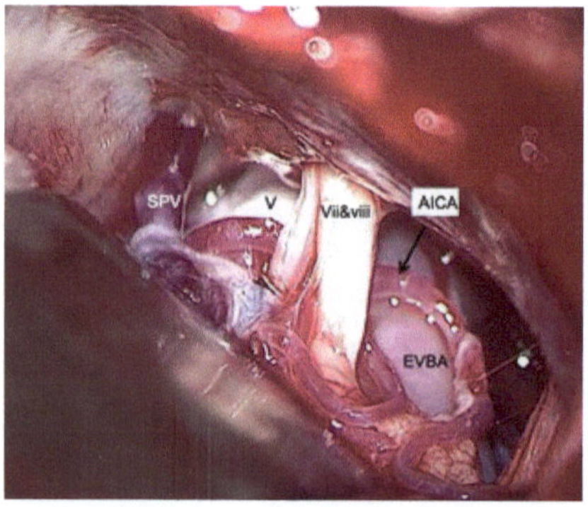

Figure 5. Peroperative picture after right-sided retrosigmoid retromastoid craniotomy showing compression of REZ of 7th (Vii) nerves by ectatic vertebrobasilar artery (EVBA) and anterior inferior cerebellar artery (AICA), causing hemifacial spasm. The patient also had REZ compression of 5th (V) nerves (not in picture) by superior cerebellar artery, causing TN as well. Viii—vestibulo-cochlear nerves. Source: Figure by authors.

4.6. Clinical Features

Short-lasting, paroxysmal, stabbing, shooting, or electric-shock-like pain is characteristic of trigeminal neuralgia. However, 14–50% of cases also have a simultaneous, continuous, dull-aching pain of low intensity (Maarbjerg et al. 2014). Mild autonomic features, such as nasal congestion, lacrimation, rhinorrhea, sweating, and miosis might be present.

The second and/or third trigeminal divisions are most commonly afflicted by TN, and the right side is more involved than the left. Bilateral illness is extremely uncommon and should raise concerns of subsequent TN (Maarbjerg et al. 2017). Innocuous sensory stimulation such as mild contact, chatting, chewing, tooth brushing, and washing the face can all trigger discomfort (Bendtsen et al. 2020).

4.7. Diagnosis

A clinical diagnosis of trigeminal neuralgia exists. Physical and neurological exams are generally normal. Any aberrant neurological results should trigger additional testing to rule out other causes. Three-dimensional (3D) T2-weighted, 3D time-of-flight, and MR angiography, in combination with 3D T1-weighted gadolinium, have proven to be dependable in finding vascular contact and estimating the severity of root compression [MRI of the brain in the TN protocol]. Diffusion tensor imaging and tractography give information about the brain structure that traditional imaging techniques cannot capture (Bendtsen et al. 2020).

Differential diagnosis includes glossopharyngeal neuralgia, painful post-traumatic trigeminal neuropathy, post-herpetic neuralgia, persistent idiopathic facial pain, a cluster headache, a cracked tooth, a primary stabbing headache, and caries or pulpitis.

4.8. Treatment

4.8.1. Medical Treatment

Sodium channel blockers (carbamazepine and oxcarbazepine) are first-choice drugs and were shown to be most effective according to one very-high-quality meta-analysis (McQuay et al. 1995). Zakrzewska and Linskey have demonstrated rates of 100% symptom relief in 70% of patients (Zakrzewska and Linskey 2014). Lamotrigine, baclofen, pregabalin, or gabapentin are used as add-on drugs with CBZ or oxcarbazepine, when the later drugs are ineffective or poorly tolerated.

4.8.2. Surgical Treatment

Microvascular decompression (MVD) is the most effective, albeit most invasive, surgical treatment. It is a nondestructive surgery with a low risk of sensory disturbances, as well as being a good choice for otherwise healthy persons. This procedure results in lasting pain relief in 70% of cases (Tronnier et al. 2001). Here, the offending vessel (usually the superior cerebellar artery) is freed from the REZ by arachnoid dissection and displacement and is kept away from the REZ by Teflon, surgical, cotton, fascia, or muscle. In the case of an ectatic artery, "slinging of artery" may be needed. Common complications are hearing loss, tinnitus, imbalance, facial weakness and facial sensory loss, diplopia (fourth nerve palsy), hemorrhage, infarction, meningitis, seizure, CSF fistula, etc. (Greenberg 2010). MVD cures up to 80% of cases, 10% of cases improve, and 10% fail (mostly due to failure to detect the offending vessel peroperatively, and so re-exploration is needed). Options for failed MVD or recurrent cases are reoperation (MVD), neurectomy, rhizotomy, high cervical spinal tract of trigeminal nerve tractotomy, DBS, thalamotomy, anterior cingulotomy, and motor cortex stimulation (Greenberg 2010; Henderson and Lad 2006).

Percutaneous rhizotomy is a minimally invasive surgical option that involves the selective lesioning of A-delta and C pain nerve fibers with intent to preserve A-alpha as well as beta sensory nerve fibers. Rhizotomy has three types:

(1) Percutaneous balloon compression rhizotomy;
(2) Percutaneous retrogasserian glycerol rhizotomy;
(3) Percutaneous radiofrequency rhizotomy.

The pathway to the trigeminal ganglion for all these techniques is through the foramen ovale. Percutaneous procedures offer variable degrees of pain relief for up to three years (Jones et al. 2019).

4.8.3. Gamma Knife Radiosurgery (GKRS)

It is utilized as a surgical option for patients who are not good surgical candidates or who refuse to undergo more intrusive treatment. This is a stereotactic, outpatient operation that uses high doses (70–80 Gy) of submillimeter radiation beams directed at the trigeminal root entrance zone to promote necrosis, which reduces pain signals over time. A systematic review found a 69% success rate after one year and a 52% success rate after three years (Jones et al. 2019).

5. Hemifacial Spasm (HFS)

5.1. Introduction

Hemifacial spasm (HFS) is a pathological condition of painless, involuntary, intermittent, spasming of facial muscles supplied by the seventh cranial nerve solely in one side. In typical HFS, it commonly starts from the orbicularis oculi and progresses to half of the face (due to compression on the anterio-inferior part of the REZ); the frequency of the spam increases with time, which may impair the vision of the involved side. In atypical forms of HFS, spasms start from the buccal muscle and spread upward over the face (due to compression on the upper or posterior part of the REZ) (Greenberg 2010; Wilkins and Rengachary 1985). Some patients may have hyper-lacrimation of the involved side. HFSs may be restricted to the upper or lower part of the face only.

5.2. Etiopathophysiology

5.2.1. Causes of HFS

1. Neurovascular compression syndrome at the root exit zone (REZ) is the most common cause of HFS (Figures 5–7).

   Culprit vessels may include the following:

- AICA (most common; either pre- or post-meatal);
- An elongated PICA;
- SCA (a tortuous EVBA);
- The cochlear artery;
- A dolichoectatic basilar artery;
- AICA branches;
- Aneurysm or an arterio-venous malformation (AVM);
- Veins (rarely).

2. Idiopathic or unknown cause.
3. Posterior fossa tumor compressing the fascial nerve.

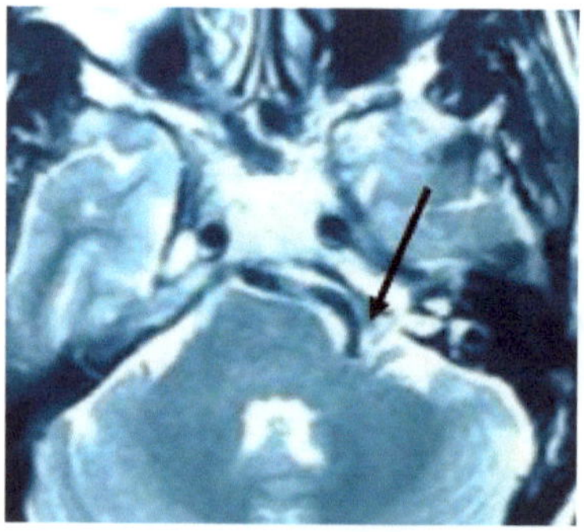

Figure 6. MRI of brain axial view T2W image showing REZ compression of left 7th nerve (arrow marked) by an EVBA, causing intractable HFS. Source: Figure by authors.

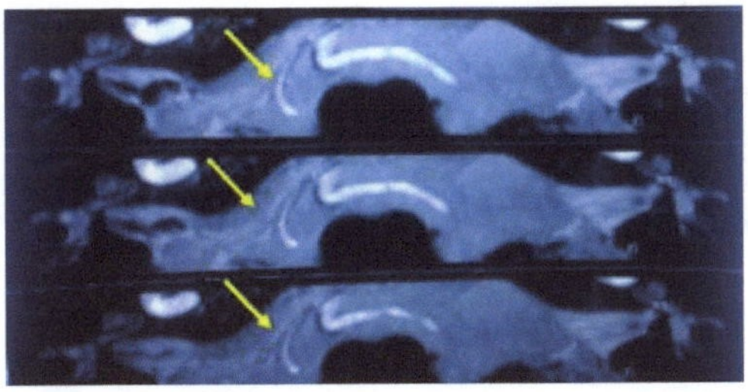

Figure 7. Focused MRA of brain showing compression of REZ of right 7th nerve (arrow marked), causing HFS. Source: Figure by authors.

Here, there is no short-circuit (ephaptic) conduction at the REZ; rather, the facial motor nucleus is engaged secondarily due to compression of the REZ via the kindling phenomenon. HFSs persist during sleep (like palatal myoclonus and unlike all other movement disorders that disappear during sleep). HFS is more common in women than men and the left side is more affected than the right. It may be associated with vestibulo-cochlear nerve dysfunction (hearing loss, vertigo, and tinnitus). Differential diagnoses include blepharospasm and facial myokymia (Greenberg 2010; Wilkins and Rengachary 1985; Yeh et al. 1981; Chowdhury et al. 2018).

5.3. Investigations

HFS is a clinical diagnosis like TN. Any unusual neurological finding(s) requires additional investigations to exclude secondary etiology. Three high-resolution sequences, three-dimensional (3D) T2-weighted, 3D time-of-flight, and MR angiography, as well as 3D T1-weighted gadolinium, may be used to detect vascular contact at the REZ [MRI of the brain in HFS protocol].

5.4. Treatment

5.4.1. Conservative

HFS is usually a neurosurgical condition. Carbamazepine and phenytoin generally do not work. Local injection of botulinum toxin may work temporarily (Greenberg 2010; Moller and Jannetta 1983).

5.4.2. Surgical Management

MVD is the procedure of choice. Techniques include that of TN. Here, the culprit vessel is put away by arachnoid dissection and by placing surgical Teflon, fascia, muscle, etc. (Greenberg 2010). Sometimes, slinging may be needed. Postoperatively, HFS starts to decrease 2–3 days after MVD. Severe spasms that do not improve suggest failure to accomplish satisfactory decompression, and re-exploration should be considered. Complete cure of HFS occurs in about 80% patients. A total of 10% partially improve and 10% provide no response (Moller and Jannetta 1983). Recurrence occurs in 10% of cases within 2 years (Greenberg 2010). Complications include tinnitus, hearing loss, facial weakness, ataxia, etc.

Some ablative techniques are useful for HFS where MVD has failed such as sectioning of divisions of the facial nerve with some paresis.

6. Glossopharyngeal Neuralgia (GN)

GN is often misdiagnosed due to its rarity. The incidence of GN is very low and 70 times lesser than TN (Youmans 1982).

6.1. Pathophysiology

Most GN cases seem to be a manifestation of the compression of a ninth cranial nerve at the REZ by the vessels, usually by PICA or VA. But, GNs can also be due to compression of the nerve by a mass lesion (Chowdhury et al. 2020).

6.2. *Clinical Features*

GN pain is a very severe, lancinating, pricking pain most frequently involved (in the distribution of the ninth and tenth nerves) in the throat and base of the tongue, which usually radiates to the ear. GN can be associated with occasional salivation, coughing, hypotension (Weinstein et al. 1986), syncope (Ferrante et al. 1995), and cardiac arrest. It may be precipitated by swallowing, chewing, and talking. Trigger zones are rarer.

6.3. *Investigations*

MRI of the brain is usually normal. MRI in cranial nerve protocol (GN) may show the culprit vessel at the REZ of the glossopharyngeal ± vagus nerve.

6.4. *Treatment*

6.4.1. Conservative

Pain may be reduced by cocaine application on tonsillar pillars and fossa. Anti-epileptic drugs (carbamazepine and phenytoin) are less responsive.

6.4.2. Microsurgery

Patients with drug intolerance, refractoriness, or both require microsurgery. Presently, MVD is a highly efficacious treatment and should be utilized as the first therapy in drug-resistant GPN with aberrant vessel compression. Surgical therapies for medically intractable GPN that involve the destruction of glossopharyngeal and vagus nerve fibers (neurectomy) are becoming less common. Transection of the preganglionic glossopharyngeal nerve (IX) and upper third of the vagus (X) nerve: IX is easily recognized as it is the dural exit zone in the jugular foramen, where it is separated from the vagus nerve by a dural septum. Early postoperative dysphagia commonly resolves. Cardiovascular events following vagal nerve section are alarming and warrant close monitoring for at least 24 h (Youmans 1982; Chowdhury et al. 2020; Weinstein et al. 1986; Ferrante et al. 1995).

7. Psychosurgery

7.1. *Introduction*

The management of mental diseases has improved, thanks to advances in medication, psychotherapy, and cognitive behavioral intervention. However, a significant number of individuals do not react to treatment, do not maintain their response, or have intolerable side effects. For more than a century, surgery for psychiatric disorders (NPD), also known as psychosurgery, has been used to address these treatment-resistant individuals. Indiscriminate patient selection, initially crude techniques, and a high incidence of complications made psychosurgery one of the most controversial topic in medical science (Neumaier et al. 2017). Over time, a better understanding of pathophysiology has led to more targeted approaches and eventually morbidity and mortality dropped significantly. Contemporary indications for neurosurgery are major depressive disorder (MDD), obsessive compulsive disorder (OCD), and Gilles de la Tourette syndrome (GTS), with level-two evidence of safety and efficacy. Neurosurgical intervention for anorexia nervosa, post-traumatic stress disorder, and addiction are still at the experimental stage (Neumaier et al. 2017).

7.2. *Prerequisites for NPM*

1. Diagnosis should be based on structured interviews.
2. Candidates for surgery should fulfil generally accepted clinical criteria for chronicity, severity, disability, and drug management refractoriness.
3. Patient with OCD should receive at least 20 sessions of cognitive behavior therapy prior to considering surgery.
4. Major depressive disorder should have been found to be nonresponsive to electroconvulsive therapy. Similarly, patients should be administered at least twelve sessions of evidence-based psychotherapy.
5. Informed consent must be obtained from the patient.
6. It is acceptable to take surrogate consent only when the patient is deficient of decision-making capacity. Hospital ethical committee approval for DBS in psychiatric disorders is needed.

7. Patient selection, preoperative evaluation, choice of procedure, and the surgical target should be decided by an expert multidisciplinary team composed of trained functional and stereotactic neurosurgeons working together in a team with neurologists, psychiatrists, and neuropsychologists (Neumaier et al. 2017; Doshi et al. 2019).

7.3. Surgical Procedures

Stereotactic thermal or gamma knife lesioning of various brain targets has been conducted since 1950. In the 21st century, deep brain stimulation has been replacing ablative techniques in developed countries.

Anterior cingulotomy represents radiofrequency or gamma knife lesioning of the anterior cingulate gyrus and the cingulate bundle. In the United States, Scotland, and South Korea, it is the most commonly reported psychosurgical procedure (Ferrante et al. 1995). Cingulotomy has the best results for intractable MADs and, to a lesser extent, OCD and GTS (Nuttin et al. 2014; Leiphart and Valone 2010).

Lesioning of the anterior limb of the internal capsule (Anterior Capsulotomy) is the more favorable ablative technique for OCD. It is the most frequent lesion surgery in Spain, Sweden, Brazil, Canada, China, and Mexico (Ferrante et al. 1995).

Limbic leucotomy represents a summation of bilateral cingulumotomy and subcaudate tractotomy. Use of this procedure is declining.

Bilateral Stereotactic RF ablation of nucleus accumbens has been conducted in China and some other countries for addiction and intractable anorexia nervosa (Li et al. 2013; Wang et al. 2013).

Deep brain stimulation has been popularizing for its inherent reversibility and adjustability. The anterior limb of the internal capsule, the ventral capsule/striatum, the subgenual cingulate, the inferior thalamic peduncle, and the nucleus accumbens are all targets for DBS. The thalamic nuclei anteromedial globus pallidus internus (amGPi) and centromedian–parafascicular (cmPf) complex are two of the most common DBS targets in GTS (Servello et al. 2008; Baldermann et al. 2016).

8. Intractable Pain Surgery

8.1. Introduction

Chronic pain is defined as pain that persists for longer than six months. It can be classified as nociceptive, neuropathic, or cancer-related. Peripheral pain receptors, as well as A-delta and C fibers, are activated in nociceptive pain. Pain signaling or the nervous system's processing of sensory input is distorted in neuropathic pain. Cancer pain is linked to the evolution of the disease, including tissue injury and nervous system impairment, which can cause both nociceptive and neuropathic symptoms. There are two forms of surgical pain treatments: ablative (or, more accurately, destructive) techniques and neuromodulation. Medical therapy must be trialed in maximum dose before consideration for pain surgery.

8.2. Options of Pain Surgeries

8.2.1. Pain Surgeries Particular to Trigeminal Neuralgia and Glossopharyngeal Neuralgia

These includes MVD, rhizotomy, spinal tractotomy of the trigeminal nerve, thalamotomy, cortical stimulation, DBS, and cingulotomy.

8.2.2. Pain Surgeries for Other Intractable Pains

1. Electrical neurostimulation
    (a) Deep brain stimulation: targets include the thalamus and periaqueductal or periventricular gray matter;
    (b) Spinal cord stimulation (Figure 8).

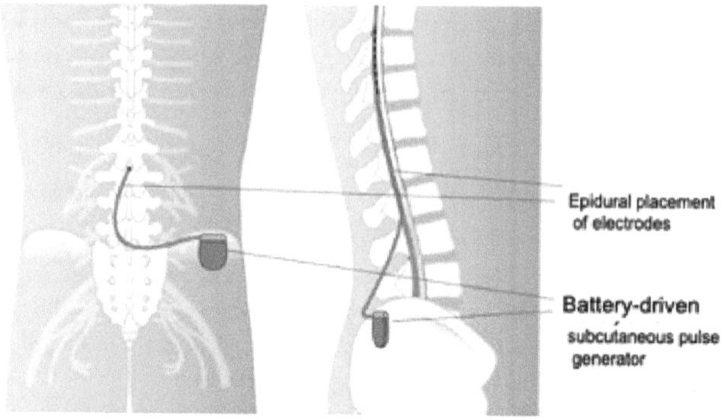

Figure 8. Illustration showing placement of spinal cord stimulator. Source: Figure by authors.

2. Direct administration of drugs into the CNS: epidural, intrathecal, or intraventricular administration of local anesthetics and narcotics.
3. Intracranial ablative/destructive surgeries:
   (a) Bilateral cingulotomy: diminishes the unpleasant effect of pain, sans eliminating the pain (pain persists without bothering the patient).
   (b) Stereotactic medial thalamotomy: controversial—may be useful for some nociceptive malignant pain.
   (c) Stereotactic mesencephalotomy: for one-sided head, face, neck, and/or UE pain. (Radiofrequency is utilized to produce lesion 5 mm lateral to the sylvian aqueduct at the level of the inferior colliculus.)
4. Spinal ablative surgical procedures
   (a) Cordotomy:
      (i) Open;
      (ii) Percutaneous.
   (b) Cordectomy.
   (c) Commissural myelotomy: for bilateral pain.
   (d) Punctate midline myelotomy: for relief of visceral malignant pain.
   (e) Dorsal root entry zone lesion.
   (f) Dorsal rhizotomy: not useful for large areas of involvement.
   (g) Dorsal root ganglionectomy (an extradural/extraspinal procedure).
   (h) Sacral cordotomy: for patients with pelvic pain who have had colostomy and ileostomy. A ligature is tied around the dural sac below the Sl nerve roots.
   (i) Sympathectomy: possibly for causalgia major and complex regional pain syndrome (CRPS).
5. Peripheral nerve procedures
   (a) Nerve block: injection of neurodestructive agents e.g., phenol or absolute.
   (b) Neurectomy: such as intercostal neurectomy in infiltration of the chest wall by malignancy. Types:
      (i) Open;
      (ii) Percutaneously with radiofrequency lesion.
   (c) Peripheral nerve stimulators: very rarely mentioned (Greenberg 2010; Burchiel and Raslan 2019; Young et al. 1985; Marshall 1996; Krieger and Rosomoff 1974).

Because about one-third of patients with advanced cancer suffer from medically refractory and intractable pain, and fear of pain outnumbers fear of death in many of these cases, surgical management of intractable pain should be a top priority. Procedures are available to help these individuals, and the existing data, at least in the case of cordotomy, suggest that neurosurgery should play a bigger role in their care (Burchiel and Raslan 2019).

Author Contributions: Conceptualization, methodology, validation, formal analysis, investigation, resources, data curation, writing—original draft preparation, J.U.M.R. and M.S.S.; writing—review and editing, visualization, supervision, F.H.C. All authors have read and agreed to the published version of the manuscript.

Funding: This research received no external funding.

Acknowledgments: Hafiz Asif Raihan, neurosurgeon, National Institute of Neurosciences and hospital, Dhaka.

Conflicts of Interest: The authors declare no conflicts of interest.

References

Albanese, Alberto, Kailash Bhatia, Susan B. Bressman, Mahlon R. Delong, Stanly Fahn, Victor S. Fung, Mark Hallett, Joseph Jankovic, Hyder A. Jinnah, Christin Klein, and et al. 2013. Phenomenology and classification of dystonia: A consensus update. *Movement Disorder* 28: 863–73. [CrossRef] [PubMed]

Ashworth, Bryan. 1964. Preliminary trial of carisoprodal in multiple sclerosis. *Practitioner* 192: 540–52. [PubMed]

Baldermann, Juan Carlos, Thomas Schueller, Daniel Huys, Ingrid Becker, Lars Timmermann, Frank Jessen, Veerle Visser-Vandewalle, and Jens Kuhn. 2016. Deep Brain Stimulation for Tourette-Syndrome: A Systematic Review and Meta-Analysis. *Brain Stimulation* 9: 296–304. [CrossRef]

Bendtsen, Lars, Joanna Maria Zakrzewska, Tone Bruvik Heinskou, Mojgan Hodaie, Paulo Roberto Lacerda Leal, Turo Nurmikko, Mark Obermann, Giorgio Cruccu, and Stine Maarbjerg. 2020. Advances in diagnosis, classification, pathophysiology, and management of trigeminal neuralgia. *The Lancet Neurology* 19: 784–96. [CrossRef] [PubMed]

Bressman, S. B. 2004. Dystonia genotypes, phenotypes, and classification. *Advances Neurology* 94: 101–7.

Burchiel, Kim J., and Ahmed M. Raslan. 2019. Contemporary concepts of pain surgery. *Journal of Neurosurgery* 130: 1039–49. [CrossRef]

Chang, Jin Woo, Chang Kyu Park, Nir Lipsman, Michael L. Schwartz, Pejman Ghanouni, Jaimie M. Henderson, Ryder Gwinn, Jennifer Witt, Travis S. Tierney, G. Rees Cosgrove, and et al. 2018. A prospective trial of magnetic resonance-guided focused ultrasound thalamotomy for essential tremor: Results at the 2-year follow-up. *Annals of Neurology* 83: 107–14. [CrossRef]

Chaudhuri, Kallol Ray, Pablo Martinez-Martin, Anthony H. V. Schapira, Fabrizio Stocchi, Kapil Sethi, Per Odin, Richard G. Brown, William Koller, Paolo Barone, Graeme MacPhee, and et al. 2006. International multicenter pilot study of the first comprehensive self-completed nonmotor symptoms questionnaire for Parkinson's disease: The NMSQuest study. *Movement Disorder Society* 21: 916–23. [CrossRef]

Chiles, Ruth S. L. 2022. *The Focal Dystonia Cure: Powerful and Definitive Practices to Completely Heal Yourself*. London: Attuned press.

Chowdhury, Forhad H., Jalal U. M. Rumi, Farah Zainab, and Maliha Hakim. 2020. Ganglioneuroma of glossopharyngeal nerve in a patient with glossopharyngeal neuralgia: A case report. *NMC Case Report Journal* 7: 117–20. [CrossRef]

Chowdhury, Forhad Hossain, Mohammod Raziul Haque, Jalal Uddin Mohammod Rumi, and Monir Hossain Reza. 2018. Microvascular Compression caused by Slinging a Tortuous Vertebrobasilar Artery to the Petrous Dura in Hemifacial Spasm: Technical Note. *Arquivos Brasileiros de Neurocirurgia: Brazilian Neurosurgery* 37: 352–61. [CrossRef]

Cloud, Leslie J., and H. A. Jinnah. 2010. Treatment strategies for dystonia. *Expert opinion on Pharmacotherapy* 11: 5–15. [CrossRef] [PubMed]

Cury, Rubens Gisbert, Suneil Kumar Kalia, Binit Bipin Shah, Joohi Jimenez-Shahed, Lingappa Kumar Prashanth, and Elena Moro. 2018. Surgical treatment of dystonia. *Expert Review of Neurotherapeutics* 18: 477–92. [CrossRef]

Devor, Marshall, Ron Amir, and Z. Harry Rappaport. 2002. Pathophysiology of trigeminal neuralgia: The ignition hypothesis. *The Clinical Journal of Pain* 18: 4–13. [CrossRef] [PubMed]

Doshi, Paresh K., Shyam S. Arumugham, Ajit Bhide, Sandeep Vaishya, Amit Desai, Om Prakash Singh, Suresh B. Math, Shiv Gautam, T. S. Satyanarayana Rao, E. Mohandas, and et al. 2019. Indian guidelines on neurosurgical interventions in psychiatric disorders. *Indian Journal of Psychiatry* 61: 13–21. [CrossRef]

Elble, Rodger J. 2000a. Diagnostic criteria for essential tremor and differential diagnosis. *Neurology* 54: S2–S6.

Elble, Rodger J. 2000b. Essential tremor frequency decreases with time. *Neurology* 55: 1547–51. [CrossRef] [PubMed]

Enslin, J. M. Nico. 2016. Surgical management of movement disorders. *South African Medical Journal* 106: 854–57. [CrossRef]

Fahn, Stanley. 2011. Classification of movement disorders. *Movement Disorders* 26: 947–57. [CrossRef]

Fahn, Stanley, S. B. Bressman, and C. D. Marsden. 1998. Classification of dystonia. *Advances Neurology* 78: 1–10.

Ferrante, Luigi, Marco Artico, Barbara Nardacci, Bernardo Fraioli, Fausto Cosentino, and Aldo Fortuna. 1995. Glossopharyngeal neuralgia with cardiac syncope. *Neurosurgery* 36: 58–63. [CrossRef]

Franzini, Andrea, Shayan Moosa, Domenico Servello, Isabella Small, Francesco DiMeco, Zhiyuan Xu, William Jeffrey Elias, Angelo Franzini, and Francesco Prada. 2019. Ablative brain surgery: An overview. *International Journal of Hyperthermia* 36: 64–80. [CrossRef] [PubMed]

Greenberg, Mark S. 2010. *Handbook of Neurosurgery*. New York: Thieme.

Henderson, Jaimie M., and Shivanand P. Lad. 2006. Motor cortex stimulation and neuropathic facial pain. *Neurosurgical Focus* 21: E6. [CrossRef]

Herz, David A., Janice E. Looman, Angela Tiberio, Kevan Ketterling, Robert K. Kreitsch, John C. Colwill, and Oliver D. Grin, Jr. 1990. The management of paralytic spasticity. *Neurosurgery* 26: 300–6. [CrossRef]

International Headache Society. 2018. Headache classification committee of the international headache society (IHS). The international classification of headache disorders, 3rd edition. *Cephalalgia* 38: 1–21. [CrossRef]

Jakobs, Martin, Anton Fomenko, Andres M. Lozano, and Karl L. Kiening. 2019. Cellular, molecular, and clinical mechanisms of action of deep brain stimulation—A systematic review on established indications and outlook on future developments. *EMBO Molecular Medicine* 11: e9575. [CrossRef]

Jones, Mark R., Ivan Urits, Ken P. Ehrhardt, John N. Cefalu, Julia B. Kendrick, Daniel J. Park, Elyse M. Cornett, Alan D. Kaye, and Omar Viswanath. 2019. A Comprehensive Review of Trigeminal Neuralgia. *Current Pain and Headache Reports* 23: 74. [CrossRef] [PubMed]

Koch, Marcus, Jop Mostert, Dorothea Heersema, and Jacques De Keyser. 2007. Tremor in Multiple Sclerosis. *Journal of Neurology* 254: 133–45. [CrossRef] [PubMed]

Krieger, Abbott J., and Hubert L. Rosomoff. 1974. Sleep-induced apnea. Part 1: A respiratory and autonomic dysfunction syndrome following bilateral percutaneous cervical cordotomy. *Journal of Neurosurgery* 39: 168–80. [CrossRef]

Lang, Andres M., and Anthony E. Lang. 1998. Parkinson's disease. *Neurosurgery Clinics of North America* 339: 1044–53. [CrossRef]

Leiphart, James W., and Frank H. Valone. 2010. Stereotactic lesions for the treatment of psychiatric disorders. *Journal of Neurosurgery* 113: 1204–11. [CrossRef]

Li, Nan, Jing Wang, Xue-lian Wang, Chong-wang Chang, Shun-nan Ge, Li Gao, He-ming Wu, Hai-kang Zhao, Ning Geng, and Guo-dong Gao. 2013. Nucleus accumbens surgery for addiction. *World Neurosurgery* 80: S28.e9–S28.e19. [CrossRef] [PubMed]

Louis, Elan D. 2001. Essential tremor. *New England Journal of Medicine* 345: 887–91. [CrossRef] [PubMed]

Louis, Elan D. 2019. The roles of age and aging in essential tremor: An epidemiological perspective. *Neuroepidemiology* 52: 111–18. [CrossRef]

Maarbjerg, Stine, Aydin Gozalov, Jes Olesen, and Lars Bendtsen. 2014. Concomitant persistent pain in classical trigeminal-evidence for different subtypes. *Headache* 54: 173–83. [CrossRef] [PubMed]

Maarbjerg, Stine, Giulia Di Stefano, Lars Bendtsen, and Giorgio Cruccu. 2017. Trigeminal neuralgia—Diagnosis and treatment. *Cephalalgia* 37: 648–57. [CrossRef]

Magerl, Walter, and Rolf-Detlef Treede. 2004. Secondary tactile hypoesthesia: A novel type of pain-induced somatosensory plasticity in human subjects. *Neuroscience Letters* 361: 136–39. [CrossRef]

Marshall, Kenneth A. 1996. Managing cancer pain: Basic principies and invasive treatment. *Mayo Clinic Proceedings* 71: 472–77. [CrossRef]

McQuay, Henry, Dawn Carroll, Alejandro R. Jadad, Philip Wiffen, and Andrew Moore. 1995. Anticonvulsant drugs for management of pain: A systematic review. *BMJ Publishing Group* 311: 1047–52. [CrossRef]

Meythaler, Jay M., Sharon Guin-Renfroe, Robert C. Brunner, and Mark N. Hadley. 2001. Intrathecal baclofen for spastic hypertonia from stroke. *Stroke* 32: 2099–109. [CrossRef]

Moller, Aage R., and Peter J. Jannetta. 1983. Monitoring auditory functions during cranial nerve microvascular decompression operations by direct recording from the eighth nerve. *Journal of Neurosurgery* 59: 493–99. [CrossRef]

Mostile, Giovanni, and Joseph Jankovic. 2010. Alcohol in essential tremor and other movement disorders. *Movement Disorders* 25: 2274–84. [CrossRef] [PubMed]

Neumaier, Felix, Mario Paterno, Serdar Alpdogan, Etienne E. Tevoufouet, Toni Schneider, Jürgen Hescheler, and Walid Albanna. 2017. Surgical Approaches in Psychiatry: A Survey of the World Literature on Psychosurgery. *World Neurosurgery* 97: 603–34. [CrossRef]

Nuttin, Bart, Hemmings Wu, Helen Mayberg, Marwan Hariz, Loes Gabriëls, Thorsten Galert, Reinhard Merkel, Cynthia Kubu, Osvaldo Vilela-Filho, Keith Matthews, and et al. 2014. Consensus on guidelines for stereotactic neurosurgery for psychiatric disorders. *Journal of Neurology, Neurosurgery & Psychiatry* 85: 1003–8. [CrossRef]

Prakash, K. M., and A. E. Lang. 2009. Surgery for Movement Disorder: An overview. In *Textbook of Stereotactic and Functional Neurosurgery*. Edited by Andres M. Lozano, Philip L. Gildenberg and Ronald R. Tasker. Berlin: Springer.

Privat, J. M., J. Benezech, P. Frerebeau, and C. Gros. 1976. Sectorial posterior rhizotomy, a new technique of surgical treatment for spasticity. *Acta Neurochirurgica* 35: 181–95. [CrossRef]

Rezai, Ali R., Andre G. Machado, Milind Deogaonkar, Hooman Azmi, Cynthia Kubu, and Nicholas M. Boulis. 2008. Surgery for Movement Disorders. *Neurosurgery* 62: 809–39. [CrossRef] [PubMed]

Richardson, R. R., L. J. Cerullo, D. G. McLone, F. A. Gutierrez, and V. Lewis. 1979. Percutaneous epidural neurostimulation in modulation of paraplegic spasticity. Six case reports. *Acta Neurochirurgica* 49: 235–43. [CrossRef]

Scott, Brett A., Zelig Weinstein, Robert Chiteman, and Morris W. Pulliam. 1985. Intrathecal phenol and glycerin in metrizamide for treatment of intractable spasms in paraplegia. Case report. *Journal of Neurosurgery* 63: 125–27. [CrossRef]

Servello, Domenico, Mauro Porta, Marco Sassi, Arianna Brambilla, and Mary M. Robertson. 2008. Deep brain stimulation in 18 patients with severe Gilles de la Tourette syndrome refractory to treatment: The surgery and stimulation. *Journal of Neurology, Neurosurgery & Psychiatry* 79: 136–42. [CrossRef]

Shima, Fumio, Masashi Fukui, Katsutoshi Kitamura, Chiharu Kuromatsu, and Tomomi Okamura. 1988. Diagnosis and surgical treatment of spasmodic torticollis of 11th nerve origin. *Neurosurgery* 22: 358–63. [CrossRef]

Tanner, Caroline M., and Diana A. Aston. 2000. Epidemiology of Parkinson's disease and akinetic syndromes. *Current Opinion in Neurology* 13: 427–30. [CrossRef]

ter Haar, Gail, and Constantin Coussios. 2007. High intensity focused ultrasound: Physical principles and devices. *International Journal of Hyperthermia* 23: 89–104. [CrossRef]

Tronnier, Volker M., Dirk Rasche, Jürgen Hamer, Anna-Lena Kienle, and Stefan Kunze. 2001. Treatment of idiopathic trigeminal neuralgia: Comparison of long-term outcome after radiofrequency rhizotomy and microvascular decompression. *Neurosurgery* 48: 1261–68. [CrossRef] [PubMed]

Wang, Jing, Chongwang Chang, Ning Geng, Xuelian Wang, and Guodong Gao. 2013. Treatment of intractable anorexia nervosa with inactivation of the nucleus accumbens using stereotactic surgery. *Stereotactic and Functional Neurosurgery* 91: 364–72. [CrossRef] [PubMed]

Weinstein, Ralph E., David Herec, and Joseph H. Friedman. 1986. Hypotension due to glossopharyngeal neuralgia. *Archives of Neurology* 43: 90–92. [CrossRef] [PubMed]

Wilkins, Robert H., and Setti S. Rengachary. 1985. *Neurosurgery*. New York: McGraw-Hill.

Witjas, Tatiana, Romain Carron, Paul Krack, Alexandre Eusebio, Marianne Vaugoyeau, Marwan Hariz, Jean Philippe Azulay, and Jean Régis. 2015. A prospective single-blind study of Gamma Knife thalamotomy for tremor. *Neurology* 85: 1562–68. [CrossRef] [PubMed]

Yeh, Hwa-Shain, John M. Tew, Jr., and Rafael M. Ramirez. 1981. Microsurgical treatment of intractable hemifacial spasm. *Neurosurgery* 9: 383–86. [CrossRef]

Youmans, Julian R. 1982. *Neurological Surgery*. Philadelphia: W. B. Saunders.

Young, Ronald F., Richard Kroening, Wayne Fulton, Robert A. Feldman, and Israel Chambi. 1985. Electrical stimulation of the brain in treatment of chronic pain. Experience over 5 years. *Journal of Neurosurgery* 62: 389–96. [CrossRef]

Zakrzewska, Joanna M., and Mark E. Linskey. 2014. Trigeminal neuralgia. *BMJ* 348: g474. [CrossRef]

Epilepsy and Epilepsy Surgery

Jalal Uddin Mohammod Rumi and Forhad H. Chowdhury

Abstract: Epilepsy affects approximately 50 million people throughout the world, making it one of the most common neurological disorders. Around 60–70% of epilepsy patients react to treatment, whereas 30–40% become resistant to anti-epileptic drugs. Patients not responding to medical treatment are supposed to undergo evaluation for surgical intervention. Not all cases of drug-resistant epilepsy (DRE) are remediable by surgery. Worldwide, 10.1 million persons with active epilepsy could benefit from surgery every year. Methodical, careful, and skillful presurgical evaluation to select appropriate candidates for surgical intervention and choosing an appropriate procedure are the most critical parts of epilepsy surgery. A short synopsis of epilepsy, including definitions, diagnostic criteria, etiology, classification, and differentials of epilepsy, is given in first part of the chapter. Epilepsy surgery is discussed in the later part of the chapter and includes principles of presurgical evaluation, tools for presurgical evaluation, epileptic conditions remediable by epilepsy surgery, and common surgical procedures for epilepsy.

Abbreviations

AEDs	anti-epileptic drugs	AKA	also known as
AMTL	anteromedial temporal lobectomy	CNS	central nervous system
CT	computed tomography	DNET	dysembryoplastic neuroepithelial tumor
DRE	drug-resistant epilepsy	ECoG	electrocorticogram
ECS	electrical cortical stimulation	EEG	electroencephalogram
EZ	epileptogenic zone	FCD	focal cortical dysplasia
FDA	food and drug administration	FDG-PET	flurodeoxyglucose PET
fMRI	functional MRI	HME	hemimegaencephaly
ILAE	international league against epilepsy	IEEG	intracranial EEG
IVIG	intravenous immunoglobin	LGS	Lennex–Gastaut syndrome
LKS	Landau–Kleffner syndrome	MEG	magnetic encephalography
MTLE	mesial temporal lobe epilepsy	MRI	magnetic resonance imaging
MTS	mesial temporal sclerosis	PET	positron emission tomography
RNS	responsive neurostimulation	SAH	selective amygdalohippocampectomy
SEEG	scalp EEG	SPE CT	single photon emission CT
SRT	stereotactic radiofrequency thermocoagulation	TIA	transient ischemic attack
TLE	temporal lobe epilepsy	VEM	video EEG monitoring
VNS	vagus nerve stimulation		

1. Introduction

Epilepsy affects approximately 51.7 million people worldwide, making it one of the most common neurological disorders. Every year, 4.6 million people are diagnosed with epilepsy for the first time. Epilepsy is more common in LMICs (low- and middle-income countries), with 104 per 100,000 person-years in low-income countries and 78 per 100,000 in middle-income countries, compared to 51 per 100,000 person-years in HICs (High-income income countries). According to various studies, 60–70% of epilepsy patients react to treatment, whereas 30–40% become resistant to anti-epileptic medicines (AEDs) (Kalilani et al. 2018; Kwan and Brodie 2000). Patients not responding to medical treatment are supposed to undergo evaluation for surgical intervention. Not all cases of drug resistance epilepsy (DRE) are suitable for remediation by surgery. Worldwide, 10.1 million persons with active epilepsy could benefit from surgery, and 1.4 million new surgically treatable epilepsy patients are diagnosed each year, potentially increasing the number of surgical candidates (Vaughan et al. 2019). Methodical presurgical evaluation to select appropriate candidates for surgical intervention and choosing an appropriate procedure are the most critical parts of epilepsy surgery.

Definition of epilepsy (ILAE n.d.): Epilepsy is a brain disorder characterized by one or more of the following criteria:

- At least two spontaneous (or reflex) seizures that occur within 24 h.

- One spontaneous (or reflex) seizure, with a danger of subsequent seizures analogous to the overall recurrence risk (at least 60%), following two unprovoked seizures over the next 10 years.
- An epilepsy syndrome is diagnosed.

Individuals who have stayed seizure-free for the last 10 years with no anti-epileptic drug for the last 5 years are regarded as having resolved epilepsy if they had age-based, self-limited epilepsy syndrome but have now past the applicable age.

Definition of Seizure (ILAE n.d.): A seizure is a brief episode of symptoms and/or indications in the brain caused by abnormally high or synchronized neuronal activity. Unless the criteria for epilepsy diagnosis are met, a seizure event does not essentially suggest the presence of epilepsy.

The following are the different forms of epileptic seizures:

- Unknown-onset seizures;
- Focal (localized)-onset seizures;
- Generalized-onset seizures.

1.1. ILAE (International League against Epilepsy) Classification of Seizure Types, Expanded Version

ILAE Classification of Seizure Types is shown in Figure 1.

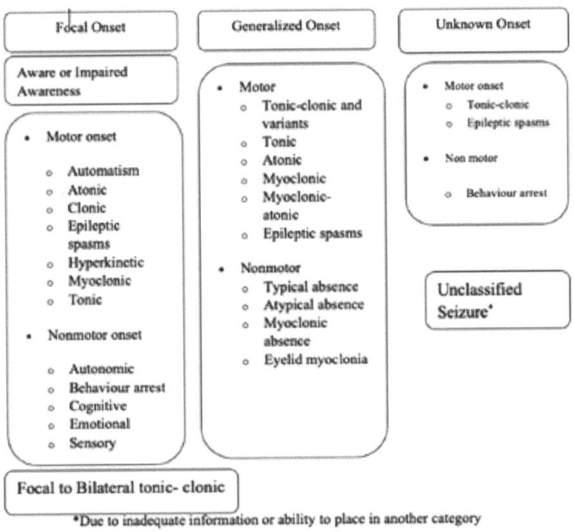

Figure 1. ILAE (International League against Epilepsy) Classification of Seizure Types, Expanded Version. Source: Authors' compilation based on data from Fisher et al. (2017).

1.1.1. Generalized Onset Seizure

A generalized seizure is thought to start somewhere within bilaterally dispersed networks and spread very quickly. Cortical and subcortical structures can be included in bilateral networks, but they do not always contain the entire cerebral cortex. Individual seizure onsets may appear isolated, yet their lateralization and location vary from one seizure to the next.

1.1.2. Focal Onset Seizure

Focal seizures are thought to originate in networks that are restricted to one hemisphere. They could be concentrated in one area or widely spread. Focal seizures could be caused by subcortical structures. Ictal initiation is uniform from one seizure to the next one for each seizure type, with ipsilateral and/or opposite hemispheres showing preferred propagation patterns. During a seizure, semiology (symptoms/signs) can be utilized to determine the specific brain region, lobe, or hemisphere that is engaged in seizure onset and propagation.

1.1.3. Unknown Onset Seizure

Unknown onset seizures are those that cannot be characterized as either generalized or focal in onset seizures. Seizures with uncertain initiation can be characterized as motor (tonic–clonic and epileptic spasm) and nonmotor (behavioral arrest, for example).

1.2. Classification of Epilepsy

Epilepsies are categorized as follows:

- Focal epilepsy;
- Generalized epilepsy;
- Combined generalized and focal epilepsy;
- Unknown epilepsy (ILAE n.d.).

1.2.1. Generalized Epilepsy

Generalized epilepsy patients have a generalized type of seizure, which might involve ictal and/or interictal EEG irregularities (such as generalized spike and wave). A family history of epilepsy or generalized seizures is beneficial.

1.2.2. Focal Epilepsy

Focal epilepsy patients have specific seizure types, which may include ictal and/or interictal EEG abnormalities (for example, focal sharp waves or focal interictal slowing). Patients with hereditary causes and normal imaging can have localized epilepsy; however, imaging that reveals a focal structural brain anomaly may be useful. Unifocal, multifocal, and hemispheric epilepsies are the three types of focal epilepsies.

1.2.3. Combined Generalized and Focal Epilepsy

Patients may have both focal and generalized seizures, as well as interictal and/or ictal EEG irregularities. Patients with Dravet syndrome and Lennox–Gastaut syndrome can experience both generalized and localized seizures.

1.2.4. Unknown Epilepsy

The term "unknown" is utilized when it is impossible to tell whether a patient has focal, generalized, or a combination of focal and generalized epilepsy. This can happen when there is not enough information to define epilepsy, such as when the EEG is normal/uninformative.

1.3. Epilepsy Syndrome

An epileptic syndrome is a collection of signs and symptoms that makes up a distinct epilepsy condition with varied causes (Daroff et al. 2015). A typical age at which seizures begin, distinct seizure types with EEG features, and other criteria, when combined, allow the detection of a specific epileptic conditions. The detection of an epilepsy syndrome is beneficial since it indicates which underlying causes should be explored as well as which antiseizure medication(s) may be most effective (ILAE n.d.). Some epilepsy syndromes are inherently intractable and long trials with medication before considering surgical evaluation seem unwise. Some other syndromes, i.e., Benign Childhood Epilepsy with Centrotemporal Spikes (BECTS), may have poor control of seizures with medication but will ultimately remit and do not need surgery. Surgically remediable epilepsy syndromes will be discussed later.

2. Etiology of Epilepsy

Advances in contemporary neuroimaging (Figure 2) and genetic testing have contributed to a major increase in explaining the underlying causes of epilepsies in recent years (ILAE n.d.). As a result, terms like "idiopathic," "cryptogenic," and "symptomatic" are no longer employed.

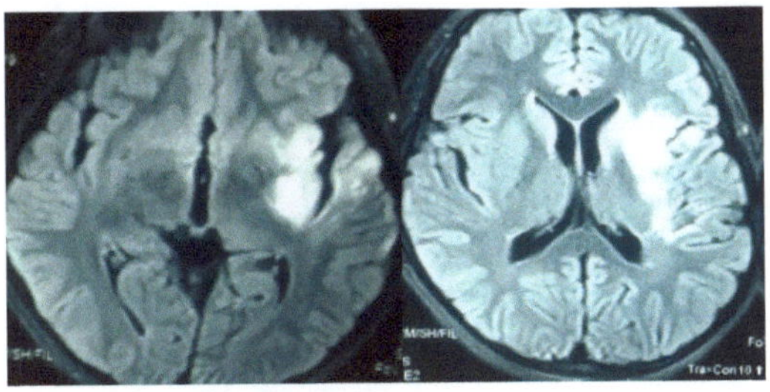

Figure 2. MRI of brain axial views showing insular cortical dysplasia (CD). Source: Figure by authors.

2.1. Etiology Genetic

4p–syndrome, Angelman syndrome, inversion duplication 15 syndrome, Miller–Dieker syndrome, ring chromosomes 14 and 20, terminal deletions of chromosome 1q and 1p, and ring chromosomes 14 and 20 are chromosomal abnormalities with a high association with seizures.

2.2. Structural Etiology

Common structural brain abnormalities associated with epilepsy, including cavernoma-causing, drug-resistant TLE:

- Developmental malformation of the cortex (Figure 2);
- Malformations of blood vessels (Figure 3);
- Sclerosis of hippocampus (Figures 4 and 5);
- Structural abnormalities from hypoxia +/ischemia (Figure 6);
- Head injury (Figure 7);
- Neoplasms (Figures 8 and 9) and porencephalic cysts;
- Cerebral gliosis (Figure 10).

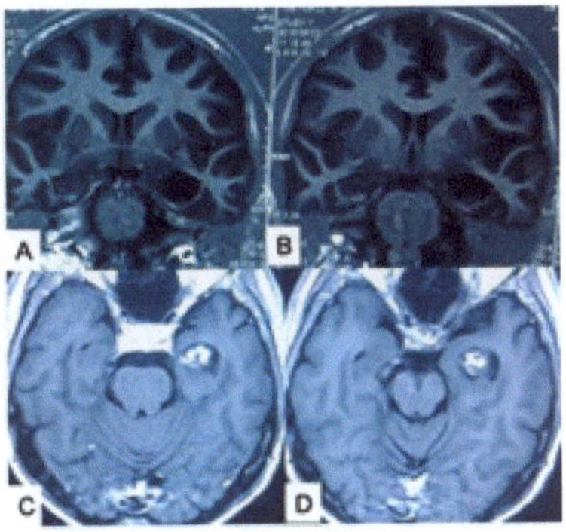

Figure 3. MRI of brain: (**A**,**B**) coronal views and (**C**,**D**) axial views showing hippocampal head. Source: Figure by authors.

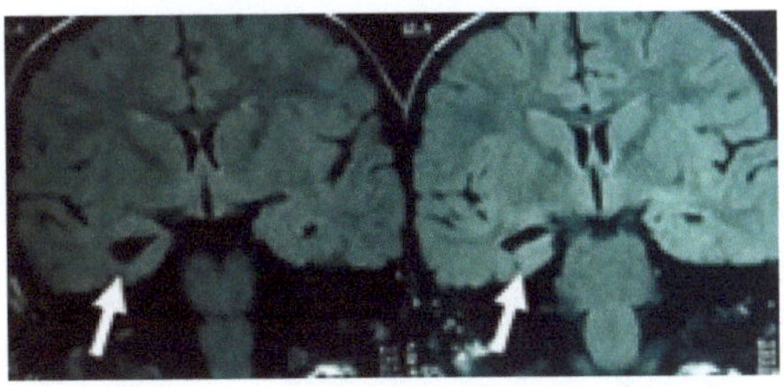

Figure 4. MRI of brain coronal views showing right-sided (arrow indicated) MTS (mesial temporal sclerosis). Source: Figure by authors.

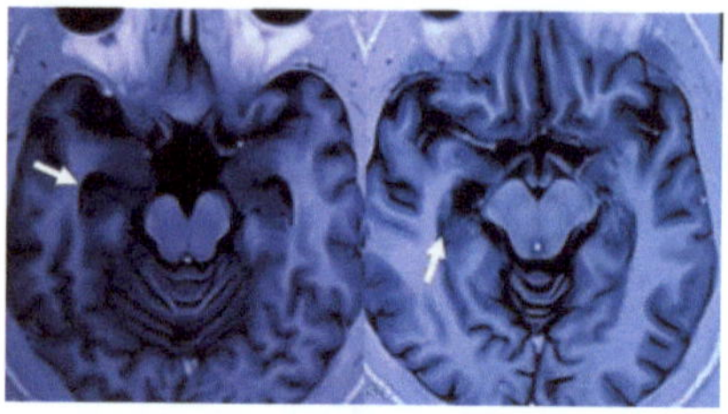

Figure 5. MRI of brain axial views showing right hippocampal head sclerosis (arrow indicated). Source: Figure by authors.

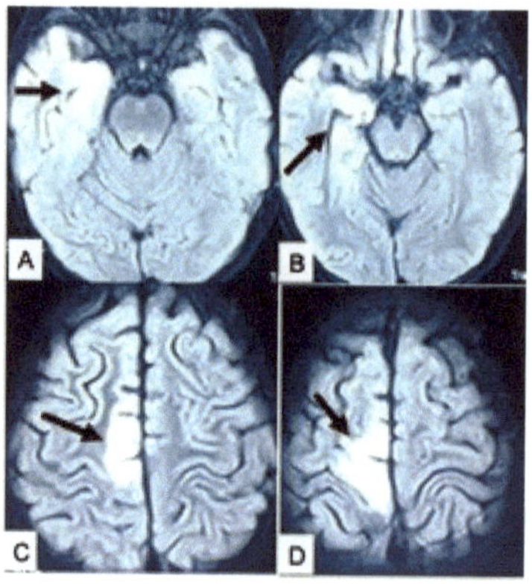

Figure 6. MRI of brain axial views in a 7-year-old girl with a history of birth asphyxia with intractable focal seizures: (**A**,**B**) showing right MTS (arrow indicated) and (**C**,**D**) showing right superior frontal focal CD (arrow indicated). Source: Figure by authors.

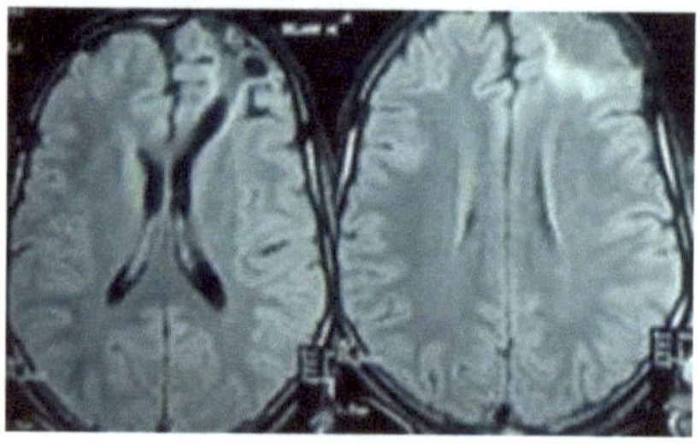

Figure 7. MRI of brain axial views showing post-traumatic left fronto-polar gliosis causing drug-resistant focal seizures. Source: Figure by authors.

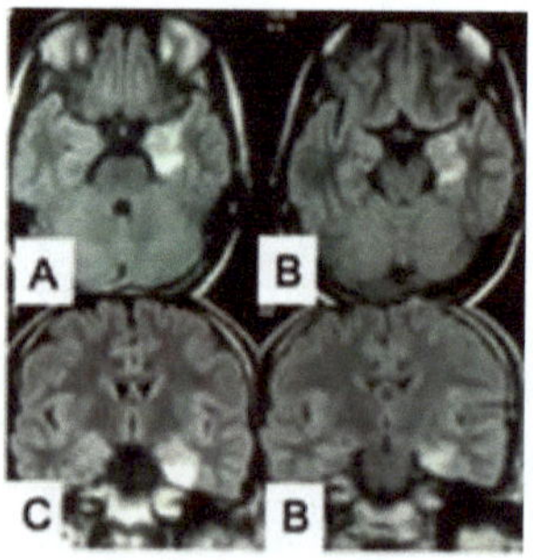

Figure 8. MRI of brain: (**A**,**B**) axial and (**C**,**D**) coronal views showing left amygdalo-hippocampal DNET causing TLE. Source: Figure by authors.

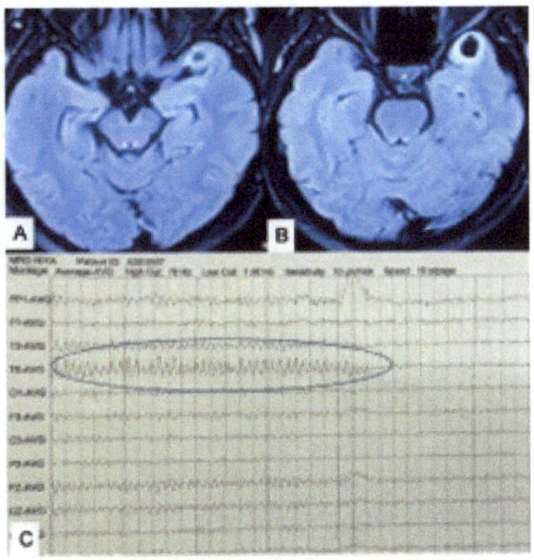

Figure 9. (**A**,**B**) MRI of brain axial views showing left temporal polar cystic lesion causing complex partial seizures. (**C**) Scalp EEG tracing showing left temporal focal discharges. Source: Figure by authors.

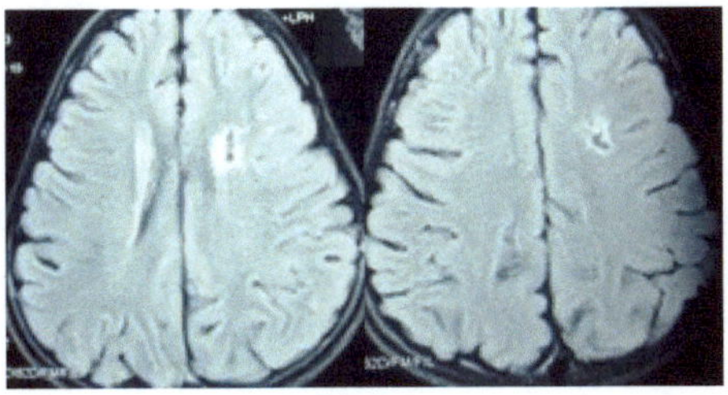

Figure 10. MRI of brain FLAIR axial views showing left frontal subcortical gliosis causing focal seizures. Source: Figure by authors.

2.3. *Metabolic Etiology*

- Creatine problems;
- Deficiency in cerebral folate;
- Deficiency in biotinidase and holocarboxylase synthase;
- Glucose transporter 1 (GLUT1) deficiency;
- Pyridoxine-dependent epilepsy/PNPO deficiency;
- Mitochondrial disorders;
- Folinic acid responsive seizures;
- Peroxisomal disorders.

2.4. *Immune Etiology*

- Antibody mediated etiologies;
- Rasmussen syndrome.

2.5. *Infectious Etiology*

Infectious disease is the most common etiology of epilepsy throughout the world, particularly in developing nations. Infections of the CNS may result in both acute symptomatic epilepsy and seizures (both are linked to the time of the initial infection). HIV, Tuberculosis, cerebral malaria, cerebral toxoplasmosis, subacute sclerosing panencephalitis, and neurocysticercosis are all infectious etiologies.

2.6. *Unknown Etiology*

The term "unknown" is meant to be taken in a neutral manner and used to indicate a type of the underlying etiology of epilepsy which is still unclear; it could be a basic genetic abnormality or a distinct, undiagnosed condition.

3. Epilepsy Imitators

There are a number of disorders linked to recurring paroxysmal occurrences that can mimic epilepsies and lead to misdiagnosis. Epilepsy misdiagnosis rates are high all throughout the world. Video recordings are quite important in determining a precise diagnosis. Epileptic and non-epileptic episodes can coexist under certain circumstances. Common epilepsy imitators are reflex anoxic seizures, syncopal attack, breath-holding attacks, psychogenic non-epileptic seizures, parasomnias, narcolepsy–cataplexy, stereotypies, paroxysmal kinesigenic dyskinesia, paroxysmal nonkinesigenic dyskinesia, hyperekplexia, migraine, shuddering attacks, and TIA (ILAE n.d.).

4. Drug-Resistant Epilepsy

Drug-resistant epilepsy, also called refractory epilepsy or intractable epilepsy, may be defined as "the failure of 02 tolerated and correctly designed and utilized AED regimens (whether as mono or combination therapy) to get persistent seizure independence" (Kwan et al. 2010). Seizure freedom lasting at least three times the longest seizure-free period previous to a new therapeutic intervention is defined as a treatment response in these criteria.

Factors associated with the risk of DRE include early-onset epilepsy, symptomatic generalized epilepsy, the presence of neuropsychiatric disorders, abnormal neuroimaging test results, abnormal EEG, focal EEG slowing, high initial seizure frequency, and a history of febrile seizures (Kalilani et al. 2018; Ko and Holmes 1999).

5. Epilepsy Surgery

5.1. Introduction

Despite much improvement in understanding the pathophysiology of epilepsy, improved imaging facilities, and the availability of newer-generation AEDs, the prevalence of DRE (0.30%) has been somewhat similar over decades. Surgical intervention could assist 10.1 million people with active epilepsy worldwide, and 1.4 million new epilepsy patients per annum could potentially be surgical candidates (Vaughan et al. 2019). Methodical presurgical evaluation to select appropriate candidates for surgical intervention and choosing appropriate procedures are the most important part of epilepsy surgery.

5.2. Principle of Presurgical Evaluation

Presurgical evaluation aims to detect and define the epileptogenic zone, its function, and spatial relation with eloquent brain, as well as to determine the best surgical procedure for that particular case. The following questions should be addressed:

1. Does the person truly have epilepsy? It is quite common that epilepsy imitators are misdiagnosed as epilepsy and treated with AED with ultimate failure and referral to a comprehensive epilepsy management program.
2. Is the epilepsy truly refractory? The selection of an appropriate AED and treatment with the maximum tolerable dose is needed before considering surgery.
3. What is the underlying etiology? Surgery has little effect in a patient with epilepsy secondary to an underlying progressive metabolic or degenerative condition.
4. Is remission still a possibility? Benign rolandic epilepsy patients may have difficult-to-control seizures but ultimately will recover.

5.2.1. Definition of Cortical Zones

The epileptogenic zone (EZ) is an area of the brain that is essential for epileptic seizures to begin. It may contain a "potential epileptogenic zone," which is a region of cerebral cortex that may induce seizures once the presurgical seizure onset zone has been removed, as well as an actual EZ, which is the cortical region producing seizures prior to surgery.

When stimulated by an epileptiform discharge, the symptomatogenic zone of the cortex generates ictal symptoms. It is defined by a thorough examination of seizure semiology, which includes either a detailed history or an examination of ictal video records.

Interictal electrographic spikes are generated in the irritative zone, which is characterized as a region of cortical parenchyma. Interictal spikes trigger EEG (invasive or scalp), functional MRI (fMRI), or magnetoencephalography (MEG) to quantify the irritative zone. This irritative zone, which is frequently greater than the EZ, encompasses all regions where the epileptic focus could potentially be found.

In contrast to the EZ, which is required for the development of epileptic seizures, the seizure start zone is the region of the cerebral cortex from which clinical seizures are (actually) produced. Either calp EEG or invasive EEG techniques are often utilized to locate the seizure onset zone.

A radiographic lesion that causes epileptic episodes is called an epileptogenic lesion. High-resolution MRI is the best way to define this now. However, not all lesions detected in epileptic seizure patients are epileptogenic. It is possible that some radiographic abnormalities have nothing to do with the clinical seizures.

In the interictal stage, the functional deficit zone is mentioned as the area of cortex that is functionally unusual. This dysfunction could be a direct outcome of the lesion's destructive effect, or it could be functionally mediated, i.e., aberrant neuronal transmission affecting cerebral function either locally or far away from the epileptogenic tissue. The functional deficiency zone can be measured using a variety of techniques; some examples include a neurological exam, cognitive testing, EEG evaluation, [^{18}F]fluorodeoxyglucose-PET (FDG-PET) scan, and interictal SPECT.

The eloquent cerebral cortex is the part of the brain that has a specific critical clinical role. The eloquent cortex refers to primary sensory, primary motor, memory, or language skills in the context of epilepsy surgery (Rosenow and Luders 2001).

5.2.2. Modalities/Tools in Presurgical Evaluation

1. History and clinical examination;
2. Neurophysiological assessment;
3. Structural neuroimaging;
4. Functional neuroimaging;
5. Neuropsychological assessment;
6. Intracarotid amobarbital procedure (Wada test);
7. Electrical cortical stimulation.

History and Clinical Examination

Presurgical evaluation starts with detailed clinical history and general and neurological examination. History details include the age of onset of seizures and frequency. The sequence of incidents at the time of a seizure should be obtained from the patient and also from one or more witnesses and compared with videotaped seizures recorded at home and in an epilepsy monitoring unit. The past medical history should include birth history, history of febrile seizures, significant head trauma, and CNS infections. Medication trials and their adverse effects should be noted. Family history of febrile/afebrile seizures and other neurological illness should be taken. Most patient's neurological examinations reveal no findings. In children, the skin should be examined for signs of neurocutaneous disorders. Any focal weaknesses or asymmetric reflexes might have a lateralizing value.

The semiology of seizures is an important aspect of the epilepsy surgery examination. Clinicians can benefit from a thorough examination of seizure semiology. In three-quarters of patients, semiology locates and lateralizes seizures (Elwan et al. 2018).

The following are characteristics that indicate lateralization of the seizure. These characteristics support the idea of lateralization (ILAE n.d.):

- Ictal dystonia or unilateral ictal clonic activity indicate lateralization of the seizure to the opposite hemisphere. The initial forced-head version alludes lateralization to the cerebral hemisphere opposite the head version direction, i.e., if the head rotates to the right side, the seizure initiation is in the left hemisphere.
- Ictal speech does lateralize to the cerebral hemisphere—it is not dominant.
- The dominant hemisphere is affected by ictal aphasia.
- The dominant hemisphere is affected by postictal dysphasia.
- During ictal automatisms, awareness is preserved and lateralized to the non-dominant cerebral hemisphere.
- After ictal nose-wiping, the hemisphere ipsilateral to the nose-wiping hand lateralizes.
- Unilateral eye-blinking does lateralize to the hemisphere on the opposite side.
- The non-dominant hemisphere is affected by ictal vomiting.

However ictal semiology is also an area fraught with pitfalls. Seizures may arise from a "silent" or non-eloquent cortex and then spread to a functional area and express its manifestation. Thus, semiology would indicate the site of seizure propagation instead of the site of seizure onset. Generally, the late features of seizure semiology reflect ictal spread and have less localizing value.

Neurophysiological Assessment

Electroencephalography (EEG): EEGs record the electrical activity of the brain in real time. An interictal scalp EEG (also known as a routine EEG) is used as the initial investigation for seizure disorders. It is a simple, noninvasive procedure where EEG electrodes are put on the scalp according to a standard, international 10/20 system. Recording is conducted for 30 to 60 min. Digital EEG recordings allow reformatting of EEG montages with judicious utilization of filters to improve reporting, hence it is adopted by most epilepsy centers. Routine EEGs very rarely record actual seizures, except generalized absence seizures. The main positive findings of routine EEGs are interictal epileptiform activity, which includes spikes and sharp waves and focal slowing. Both spikes (duration < 70 ms) and sharp waves (duration 70–200 ms) have pointed peaks of negative polarity, in most cases. Epileptiform discharges tend to have aftercoming slow waves. Sharp and spiked waves and focal slowing on the interictal EEG indicate the irritative zone and the functional deficit zone, respectively (Figure 11). Even without an epileptogenic lesion, subtle background asymmetries may be significant for localization and lateralization.

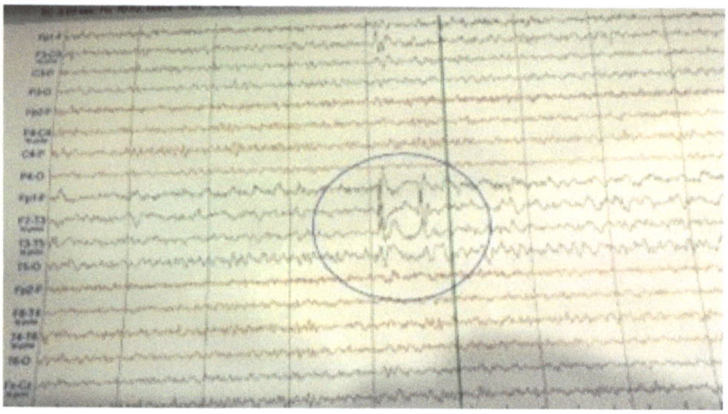

Figure 11. Interictal scalp EEG tracing showing focal electrical discharge from left frontotemporal regions. Source: Figure by authors.

However routine EEGs have important limitations. The electrical activity detected by a scalp EEG is attenuated by the impedance of intervening tissue. Epileptiform discharges are detected only if more than a 6 cm^2 area of cortical surfaces is involved in synchronized activity (Cooper et al. 1965). Interictal activity originating from the midline or deep area do not show up in scalp recordings. Therefore, the yield of the first routine EEG is normal in 50% of patients. With multiple recordings, epileptiform EEGs detected abnormality in more than 90% of epilepsy patients (Salinsky et al. 1987).

Prolonged video EEG monitoring (VEM) is considered a cornerstone of presurgical evaluation. Anti-epileptic drugs are tapered or withdrawn to capture 4–10 habitual seizures. The ictal onset zone is detected by electrographic discharge and clinical manifestations that reflect the symptomatic zone. Placement of additional electrodes increases the precision of localization of the ictal onset zone. Ictal EEG activity should be analyzed in the background of time-locked symptoms and signs. Most video recordings at home miss the initial events, which are more important. VEM provides better opportunities for analysis of seizure semiology. The interpretations are more accurate when ictal events are analyzed in conjunction with simultaneously recorded EEGs. VEM is a sensitive tool to exclude pseudoseizures.

The scalp EEG recorded at the start of the seizure can take at least five different forms (Fisher et al. 2014):

1. Rhythmically evolving frequencies in the theta, delta, or alpha bands;
2. Rhythmic spiking;
3. Spike–wave patterns;
4. Electrodecremental patterns;
5. No change in the scalp EEG.

Similar to routine EEGs, ictal recording of scalp EEGs comes with limitations in detecting deep foci and very focal small partial seizures, which explain the fifth pattern of ictal EEGs mentioned above. Furthermore, signals are obscured by muscle and movement artifacts in tonic–clonic seizures. In the presence of substantial atrophy on the side of the epileptogenic focus, false lateralization of the ictal EEG might occur. The reliability of scalp ictal EEG recordings appears to be contingent on the presence of enough brain in the epileptogenic focus area to provide an amplitude signal that can be distinguished from the surface. Furthermore, the amplitude of the ictal EEG signal from the non-diseased hemisphere surpasses that of the atrophic side during bilateral ictal propagation, resulting in a falsely lateralized image (Chang et al. 2007). Invasive intracranial monitoring is frequently required when MRI and EEG data are inconsistent. Intracranial electroencephalography (IEEG) is an invasive procedure and is utilized only when noninvasive tools fail to define EZ adequately. ILAE-recommended general indications for IEEG are as follows (Jayakar et al. 2016):

1. To properly identify the EZ when noninvasive data are equivocal;
2. To reconcile noninvasive data divergence pointing to two or more areas;
3. To correctly map eloquent cerebral cortical functions;
4. Secondary indications: to confirm the EZ or offer prognostic information by targeted ablation of active areas with thermocoagulation.

There are subdural grid and strip electrodes and depth electrodes of multiple configurations for IEEG. Intracranial EEGs may be recorded intraoperatively or extraoperatively. Craniotomy and placement of subdural and depth electrodes and recording of electrical activity intraoperatively is known as electrocorticography (ECoG) (Figure 12). ECoG records interictal epileptiform discharge and background abnormalities, thus defining the irritative zone. In lesional epilepsy, ECoG-based stepwise resections of tumors and the peritumoral irritative zone improve outcomes significantly (Mikuni et al. 2006). ECoG is unlikely to capture ictal events. Thus, for more complex cases, after the placement of electrodes, IEEGs are recorded extraoperatively.

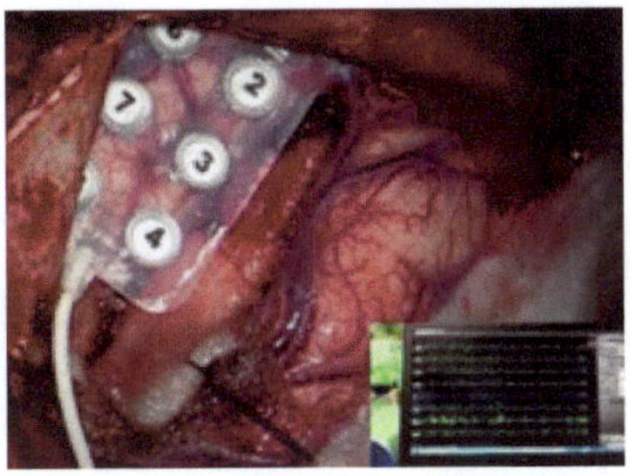

Figure 12. Peroperative electrocorticogram (ECoG). Source: Figure by authors.

Strips can be inserted through burr holes. Craniotomy is needed for grid placement. Depth electrodes could be placed through the burr, via craniotomy, or under neuronavigation guidance but are more commonly placed using the stereotactic method. Some centers practice only stereotactically placed, bilateral multiple electrodes for chronic invasive recording, known as an SEEG. Based on noninvasive evaluations, a hypothesis was to made of a presumptive EZ. Electrodes are placed to cover the EZ and irritative zone and adjacent EC. Cortical stimulation mapping could be conducted through IEEG electrodes after EEG recording is completed. AEDs should be restarted before ECS.

Magnetoencephalography is a promising noninvasive tool for defining the epileptogenic cortex and to delineate the eloquent cortex as well. The MEG signal is generated using the same neurophysiological process as the EEG signal (Barth 1993). Extracranial magnetic fields created by intracellular neuronal currents are detected using an MEG recording device made up of highly sensitive bio-magnetometers. MEG signals, unlike EEG signals, are unaffected by inhomogeneous tissue conductivity. Magnetic source imaging is the co-registration of MEG-determined source localization of epileptic spikes and evoked responses with MRI (MSI). As a result, in extratemporal localization epilepsy, presurgical assessment of MEG spike sources (MEGSS) and evoked responses on MSI is very reliable (Çataltepe and Jallo 2019). MEGSS in temporal lobe epilepsy is not precise enough to locate the source of interictal epileptiform discharges (Ebersole 1997).

Magnetoencephalography is also useful in the localization of the sensory motor cortex, primary auditory cortex, and language area. However, the establishment of an MEG recording system is very expensive and it has a very large running cost. Hence, despite encouraging results in clinical trials, its use in routine clinical set-ups is limited to a few centers. For a minority of patients with intractable localization-related epilepsy, improved clinical application of MEG has the potential to replace invasive subdural and depth electrode recordings.

Structural Neuroimaging

MRI is the mainstay investigation for epilepsy. The ILAE recommends MRI evaluation for all patients who have experienced their first seizure, except patients with genetic generalized epilepsy. Radiologically detected epileptogenic lesions help in syndromic classification and are a predictor of poor seizure freedom with medication and better outcomes following surgery. However, the presence of a lesion does not necessarily mean that it is responsible for seizures. Moreover, multiple lesions do not confirm that the epilepsy is multifocal. The concordance of a radiological lesion with seizure semiology and/or an EEG is to be established. Common pathological indications for DRE include hippocampal sclerosis, malformation of cortical development, epilepsy-associated tumors, Rasmussen encephalitis, hypothalamic hamartoma, arteriovenous malformation, and cavernoma.

The neuroimaging task force of the ILAE recommend the "Harmonized Neuroimaging of Epilepsy Structural Sequences (HARNESS-MRI) protocol" for the evaluation of seizures (Bernasconi et al. 2019). Key features of the HARNESS–MRI protocol are as follows:

1. High-resolution, 3D, T1-weighted MRI in gradient echo sequence with isotropic millimetric voxel resolution; slice thickness of 1.5 mm or less; and no interslice gap.
2. Acquisition of a high-resolution, 3D, fluid-attenuated inversion recovery (FLAIR) sequence in the turbo spin with isotropic millimetric voxel resolution and no interslice gap.
3. High in-plane resolution, 2D, coronal, T2-weighted MRI with sub-millimetric voxel resolution and no interslice gap obtained perpendicular to the long axis of the hippocampus.
4. Available in 1.5 T and 3 T scanners.

In children with FCD, MRI conducted at one year of age is more sensitive as subsequent myelination may hide the features of dysplasia on later scans. MRI should be repeated for patients with DRE if the available scan is not optimized or normal.

Computed tomography (CT) scanning has low sensitivity for identifying small cortical lesions and basal lesions and, therefore, is not a primary imaging modality in epilepsy. However, CT scans should be considered in new-onset seizure patients presenting in the emergency room to rule out intracerebral hemorrhage, subarachnoid hemorrhage, or brain abscess. Furthermore, CT scans may be followed to identify any area of focal calcification, when MRI shows tuberous sclerosis, Sturge–Weber syndrome, or an epilepsy-associated tumor.

Functional Neuroimaging

Blood flow and metabolism in the epileptic zone and eloquent cortex are different from adjacent brain tissue. The epileptic region shows hypometabolism and hypoperfusion in the interictal period and the reverse in the ictal period. During a particular task, blood flow and oxygenation levels increase in the corresponding functional cortex. Functional neuroimaging was developed based on these physiological phenomena (So and Ryvlin 2018).

Functional MRI (fMRI) is a noninvasive and widely available tool for presurgical evaluation of cognitive function and the motor cortex. Functional mapping in fMRI is performed by calculating the blood-oxygen-level-dependent (BOLD) signal change in T2-weighted images while patients engage in functional tasks. fMRI is comparable with IAT for determining hemispheric dominance for language and speech. But, fMRI detects both essential and nonessential language regions. fMRI-based motor cortex mapping is performed when the presumed EZ is adjacent to the motor cortex.

During seizures, blood flow in the epileptic zone (EZ) increases up to three times. For ictal SPECT, patients remain admitted in the video EEG monitoring unit. At the onset of a seizure, ethylene cysteine dimer (ECD) or hexamethyl propylene amine oxime (HMPAO) labeled with 99 mTc is injected. HMPAO/ECD crosses the BBB and is trapped within the neuron in proportion to regional cerebral perfusion during a seizure. Trapped radiotracers emit gamma rays, which are then detected by a rotating camera. The exact timing of the radiotracer is crucial and ictal SPECT is less feasible in very-short-lasting seizures such as myoclonic epilepsy. In SPECT, the EZ displays hyperperfusion. Interictal SPECT depicts normal perfusion or hypoperfusion in the epileptic region and is compared with the ictal image. Interictal SPECT is subtracted from ictal SPECT and the resulting image is co-registered to an MRI (SISCOM). SISCOM improves ictal SPECT's specificity and sensitivity.

In positron emission tomography (PET), various biological substrates leveled with a radioisotope such as ^{18}F, ^{11}C, or ^{15}O are injected intravenously. ^{18}Flurodeoxyglucose (FDG) is the most commonly used radiotracer. FDG is taken up by brain tissue and phosphorylated to FDG-6-phosphate and becomes trapped within the cell. FDG-6-phosphate trapped in the body emits gamma rays, which are identified by a PET camera and used to rebuild quantified tomographic pictures, which are then combined with CT images. As metabolism is low in the epileptic region in the interictal period, FDG PET shows reduced radiotracer uptake in the EZ. The area of hypometabolism detected by PET extends far beyond the EZ; thus, it is less precise for defining EZ. However, PET reliably lateralizes the EZ and, thus, a hypothesis could be made of a presumed EZ for subsequent placement of IEEG electrodes. The FDG-PET findings may guide reviews of MRI images retrospectively and reveal the pathology. Moreover, concordant findings on PET increase confidence in subtle MRI findings (So and Ryvlin 2018).

Neuropsychological Testing

It is standard practice that all epilepsy surgery candidates should receive a presurgical outpatient neuropsychological evaluation. It provides a baseline neurocognitive profile for comparison after surgery. The domains of neuropsychological testing include verbal memory and nonverbal memory, expressive and receptive language skills, verbal fluency, semantic fluency, visuospatial function, general cognitive ability, and higher executive functions. The location of the epileptic focus, the age at which the seizures began, the epilepsy syndrome, and the brain's plasticity all influence the pattern of cognitive deficits. For example, a person with dominant temporal lobe epilepsy would have remarkable language and verbal memory problems.

An identical type of seizure arising on the right (non-language-dominant) side, on the other hand, would usually result in visual memory problems (Bell and Davies 1998). Thus, neuropsychological test findings have lateralizing and localizing value, especially useful in MRI-negative epilepsy to further confirm—or argue against—the assumed epileptogenic zone. Patients with a similar cognitive profile have a better seizure result, while those with a lower baseline intellectual profile have worse postoperative seizure control. Memory and language tests help determine the ipsilateral lobe's functional capacity and the contralateral lobe's functional reserve.

Memory deficit is a common complication of anteromedial temporal lobectomy. Patients with better preoperative memory and language function (i.e., suggesting better functional integrity of the parenchyma to be removed) have a higher risk of postsurgical memory and language deterioration than those with lower scores in this category.

Intracarotid Amobarbital Injection Procedure (IAP, Wada Test)

Dr. John Atsushi Wada developed the procedure in 1949 and it has since been further modified by others. It is the gold standard for determining language and speech hemisphere dominance. The Wada test's more delicate function is to assess memory function in each hemisphere as well as the functional adequacy of the contralateral hippocampus in supporting memory following ipsilateral mesial temporal lobe resection. Additionally, the Wada test aids to predict seizure freedom following surgery.

Anterior circulation feeds the anterior two-thirds of the cerebrum. Short-acting barbiturate introduced into the ICA (internal carotid artery), thus, will induce temporary disruption in the function of the anterior two-thirds the of cerebrum, including the temporal lobe. Prior to the procedure, an angiogram is performed to assess anatomical variation and the extent of cross flow. Then 100–150 mg of sodium amobarbital is injected into one ICA at a time and cognitive ability and language function for each hemisphere are assessed in isolation.

However, the Wada test is an invasive procedure and has potential minor and major complications (Loddenkemper et al. 2008). More importantly, this technique is not standardized and there are reports of false positive and false negative results. At present, in most centers, the Wada test is replaced by noninvasive fMRI (Binder 2011).

Electrical Cortical Stimulation (ECS)

The encroachment of the epileptic zone on the eloquent cortex necessitate precise mapping using cortical stimulation to ensure adequate removal of potential epileptogenic tissue without creating new functional deficits. Extraoperative ECS is performed at the end of IEEG by stimulating subdural and depth electrodes. Intraoperative ECS is performed after ECoG. During stimulation, clinical responses and electrocorticographic changes are monitored. Cortical stimulation at primary and supplementary motor areas produce tonic or clonic movements. Sensory responses are elicited at sensory cortex stimulation. Stimulation of motor or sensory speech areas causes speech arrest (Çataltepe and Jallo 2019). With the availability and increasing accuracy of noninvasive tools such as fMRI, ECS is reserved for MRI-negative epilepsy and complex cases of malformation near eloquent cortex.

5.2.3. Epilepsy Remediable by Epilepsy Surgery

Malformations of Cortical Development

Cortical malformations occur when neuronal proliferation, migration, or cortical structures are disrupted during the development of the cortex (Jamuar and Walsh 2015; Barkovich et al. 2012). The disruption of any of these processes can raise the risk of seizures and neurodevelopmental delays in children (Jamuar and Walsh 2015). Malformations may be focal or multifocal such as focal cortical dysplasia, polymicrogyria, schizencephaly, and hypothalamic hamartomas, which require focal, lobar, or multilobar resection. Malformation may involve most or all of one hemisphere (e.g., hemimegalencephaly), making these patients ideal candidates for some form of hemispherectomy. Less commonly, malformation may be widespread and bilateral, e.g., lissencephaly and subcortical band heterotopia, and not amenable to surgery.

Hemimegalencephaly (HME)

This is a spontaneous congenital brain deformity that is extremely rare. It can be found on its own or in conjunction with a neurocutaneous syndrome. The abnormal growth of a significant piece of one hemisphere, a whole hemisphere, or a hemisphere and part of the opposite side characterizes HME. There may be ipsilateral cerebellar and brainstem hypertrophy, as well as cranial expansion.

Mental retardation, contralateral hemiparesis, intractable epilepsy, macrocephaly, and hemi-anopsia are common clinical characteristics. Motor function and linguistic impairment are typically worse in persons with localized cortical dysplasia. Partial-onset seizures, epilepsia partialis continua, infantile spasms, and drop attacks are all examples of seizures (Terra-Bustamante et al. 2006).

An enlarged cerebrum (proportion or entirety) with a broad gyrus, thicker cortex, neuronal heterotopia, aberrant gray–white matter differentiation, ventricular asymmetry, and internal capsule and basal ganglia abnormalities are all seen on post-natal MRI. The damaged hemisphere may shrink as the disease progresses, and it may not be greater than the contralateral, unaffected hemisphere during imaging. Cortical tubers may or may not exist in the non-HME hemisphere (Terra-Bustamante et al. 2006).

Slow, rhythmic, or rapid activity, as well as multifocal bilateral or unilateral high-amplitude spikes and spike–wave complexes, are all examples of interictal EEG abnormalities. Generalized or independent bilateral discharges are possible. Ictal abnormalities might be made up of a build-up of unilateral or widespread fast rhythmic activity or bilateral independent activity (Terra-Bustamante et al. 2006).

Histopathologic changes include abnormal gyrification, dyslamination, neuronal heterotopia, marked gliosis, and balloon cells (Terra-Bustamante et al. 2006).

For intractable epilepsy, hemispherotomy or functional hemispherectomy is the technique of choice. Following hemispherectomy, patients with HME had a dramatically improved seizure load and quality of life, although less than patients with Rasmussen's encephalitis or congenital vascular anomalies (Ikeda and Mirsattari 2017).

Focal Cortical Dysplasia

Localized patches of cortical lamination disruption characterize focal cortical dysplasias (FCDs), which are frequently linked to epilepsy in both adults and children (Figure 2). In children receiving epilepsy surgery, FCD is the most frequent pathogenic condition (Wyllie et al. 1998). The ILAE Task Force recommends a three-tiered clinicopathological classification system for FCD. Isolated lesions of the neocortex that show as radial (FCD Type Ia) or tangential (FCD Type Ib) dyslamination, microscopically diagnosed in one or more lobes, are referred to as FCD Type I. Cortical dyslamination as well as dysmorphic neurons without (Type IIa) or with balloon cells describe FCD Type II (Type IIb). Cortical dysplasia develops in FCD Type III in conjunction with hippocampal sclerosis (FCD Type IIIa) or epilepsy-related malignancies (FCD Type IIIb) (Blümcke et al. 2011).

MRI characteristics of FCD include cortical thickening, blurring of the gray matter–white matter junction, an enhanced signal on T2-weighted imaging, a radially oriented linear or conical T2 hyperintensity stripe, cortical thinning, and regional brain atrophy. Unfortunately, none of these indicators are dependable or constant (Blümcke et al. 2011).

On MRI, FCD can sometimes go undetected, especially in type I. Furthermore, possible epileptogenic zones are often bigger than lesions shown by MRI, necessitating the use of additional technologies for precise surgical resection planning (Kabat and Król 2012). Extratemporal FCDs are more prevalent, and they have a tendency to encroach on the eloquent cortex. IEEG improves the accuracy of both ictal and interictal data, making it easier to distinguish the EZ. Electrical stimulation using the implanted electrodes can also be used to perform functional mapping.

A discrete epileptogenic focus is removed via focused resection. When the ictal area is big, lobectomy or multilobar resections are considered. When a lesion encroaches into the functional cortex, partial resection combined with multiple subpial resection for the rest of the EZ is the safest surgical strategy.

Rasmussen's Encephalitis

Rasmussen's encephalitis is an uncommon neurological illness marked by inflammation of one cerebral hemisphere, persistent epilepsy, progressive hemiparesis and hemianopia, and cognitive decline. Rasmussen's encephalitis is most likely caused by a T-cell response to one or more antigenic epitopes, with autoantibodies playing a role as well. The inflammatory process in the brain is seen with MRI as T2/FLAIR hyperintensity in the cortical or subcortical region with ipsilateral caudate atrophy. The evolution of signal alteration and atrophy is usually visible on serial MRIs (Chiapparini et al. 2003; Yamazaki et al. 2011). In Rasmussen's encephalitis, seizures are localized and around half of the patients develop epilepsia partialis continuous. Electroencephalography shows continuous high-amplitude delta activity over the injured hemisphere within months of the seizure starting, but epilepsy partialis continua is not always associated with visually evident ictal surface EEG activity (So and Gloor 1991). Interictal aberrations in the non-affected hemisphere can indicate cognitive decline, but they do not appear to be suggestive of bilateral disease (Longaretti et al. 2012).

Choosing the correct time to transition from medical care to surgery is a significant therapeutic challenge for many patients, families, and clinicians, especially when the neurological damage is partial. The sole solution for seizures is anatomical or functional hemispherectomy, which comes at the cost of some functional constraints. Immunomodulatory therapy appears to reduce rather than stop the progression of Rasmussen's encephalitis, with no effect on the final result.

Corticosteroid and intravenous immunoglobulin are used as immunomodulators in Rasmussen's encephalitis, while AED is used to lessen seizure intensity and frequency. However, interventions have thus far merely addressed the symptoms rather than the underlying causes. Total disconnection of the afflicted hemisphere (hemidisconnection), either via hemispherotomy or functional hemispherectomy (Figures 13 and 14), is the only treatment for the convulsions due to Rasmussen's encephalitis (Varadkar et al. 2014).

Temporal Lobe Epilepsy

The commonest epilepsy surgically treated is temporal lobe epilepsy (TLE), which impacts the majority of patients with localization-related epilepsy observed in tertiary epilepsy centers (Téllez-Zenteno and Hernández-Ronquillo 2012).

Based on the anatomical area of seizure onset, TLE can be categorized into two categories. Lateral or neocortical epilepsy occurs when the epileptogenic zone is lateral to the collateral sulcus, while mesial temporal TLE occurs when the epileptogenic zone is medial to the collateral sulcus (MTLE).

The limbic regions that make up the temporal lobe's mesial part are strongly epileptogenic. The fornix connects the anteromesial frontal lobe to the anterior nucleus of the thalamus, and the uncinate fasciculus connects the mesial temporal lobe to the orbitomesial frontal lobe (Duvernoy et al. 2013). The mesial temporal structures are closely linked to the anterolateral neocortical temporal lobe. The two TLE groups frequently share seizure semiology due to the substantial linkages between the mesial temporal structures and the anterior and lateral temporal lobes, as well as other limbic regions (O'Brien et al. 1996; Burgerman et al. 1995).

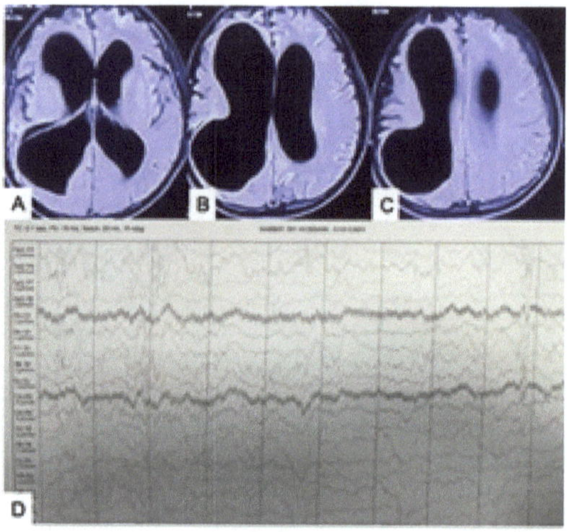

Figure 13. (**A–C**) MRI of brain axial views showing right hemispheric atrophy (with intractable left-sided focal convulsion to generalization). (**D**) Scalp EEG tracing showing multifocal electrical discharges mainly from right-sided leads. (But, left-sided lead spikes and sharps are more pronounced due to more parenchymal tissue-paradoxical affects.) Source: Figure by authors.

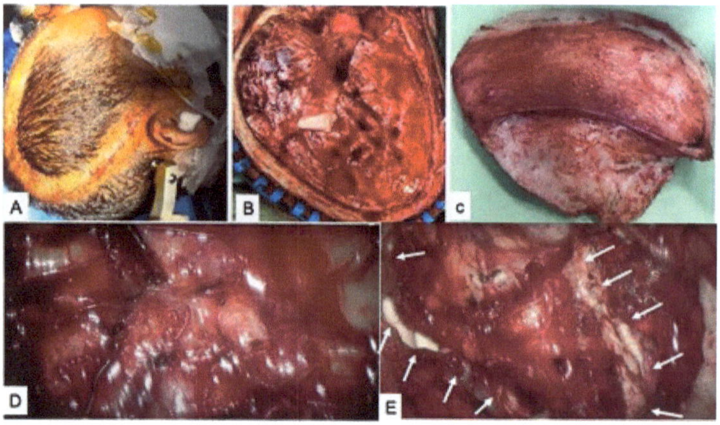

Figure 14. Peroperative pictures of right-sided functional hemispherotomy: (**A**) incision mark, (**B**) after craniotomy, (**C**) craniotomy bone flap, (**D**) right hemisphere before hemispherotomy, and (**E**) right hemisphere after hemispherotomy (arrows marked). Source: Figure by authors.

Behavioral arrest and reduced awareness are common symptoms of temporal lobe seizures. Automatisms, such as oral and/or manual automatisms, are common during seizures. There may be sensory (auditory), cognitive (déjà vu), emotional (terror), or autonomic (tachycardia, epigastric sensation, and color change) characteristics before the onset of diminished consciousness. Postictal confusion is very common.

Ictal speaking, spitting, the urge to urinate, vomiting, drinking, and automatisms with maintained consciousness reflect non-dominant temporal lobe seizure onset. A dominant temporal lobe seizure is indicated by postictal speech difficulties. Upper limb dystonia is a good lateralizing trait since it shifts the seizure to the other hemisphere. On the other hand, manual automatisms frequently occur on the ipsilateral side.

The most prevalent substrate for MTLE is mesial temporal sclerosis, which manifests in MRI as hippocampal atrophy and sclerosis, as well as elevated T2 and FLAIR signal intensity (Berkovic et al. 1991). FCD, cavernoma, epilepsy-associated tumors, and post-traumatic gliosis are some of the other indications for mesial or neocortical TLE.

Despite significant semiological overlap between the two types of TLE, noninvasive testing can usually pinpoint the seizure focus. In a limited number of people, intracranial electrode monitoring may be needed to analyze the lateralization of seizure onset to a temporal lobe (So et al. 1989) or to verify temporal lobar localization in one hemisphere (Olivier et al. 2012).

The standard temporal resection accomplished at most epilepsy facilities is anteromedial temporal lobectomy (AMTL). It mainly entails removing temporal mesial tissues after anterior temporal neocortical resection.

Selective amygdalohippocampectomy (SAH) for MTLE has sparked a lot of attention since Yasargil et al. published their findings (Yasargil et al. 1985). SAH may have the advantage of selectively removing the seizure focus, preserving temporal lobe areas that are not actually epileptogenic.

The outcome on seizure independence is the same as for anteromedial temporal lobectomy at centers with experience in SAH (AMTL) (Little et al. 2009). SAH appears to have better cognitive outcomes than typical temporal resections (Kessels et al. 2004; Gleissner et al. 2004).

Epilepsy Associated Tumors

A neoplasm is the second most prevalent etiology of focal epilepsy (Englot and Chang 2014) among individuals considered for epilepsy surgery, and it is found in roughly 30% of cases intervened in for focal epilepsy (Tassi et al. 2009).

The risk of focal seizures differs based on the tumor's location and histological type. Low-grade neoplasms are, thus, frequently more epileptogenic compared to high-grade tumors (van Breemen et al. 2007).

The biologic activity of epileptogenic tumors is normally benign, yet certain tumors may recur or develop into cancer (Luyken et al. 2003). Gangliogliomas (Figure 15), dysembryoplastic neuroepithelial tumors (DNET), pleomorphic xanthoastrocytoma, diffuse astrocytoma, papillary glioneuronal tumor, oligodendroglioma, pilocytic astrocytoma, and angiocentric gliomas are all examples of epileptogenic tumors.

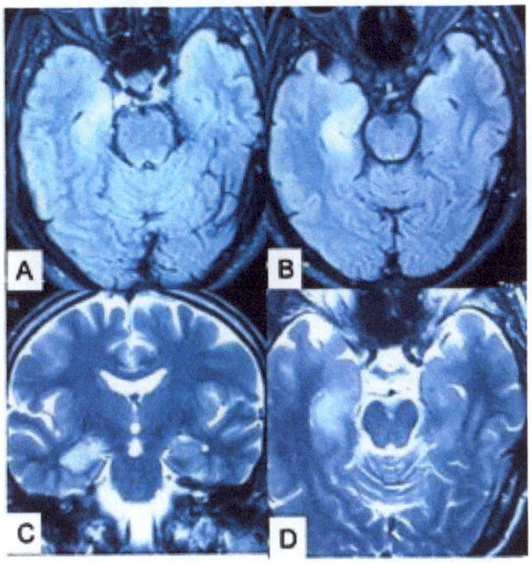

Figure 15. MRI of brain: (**A**,**B**) axial sections and (**C**,**D**) coronal sections showing right-sided medial temporal (hippocampal) ganglioglioma. Source: Figure by authors.

The most common and often only sign of malignant tumors that develops in young adulthood and adolescence is focal seizure.

As a result of the presence of a mixture of solid, calcified, and cystic elements, the MR signal of ganglioglioma is inhomogeneous and variable, with no contrast enhancement; an axial CT scan reveals the calcified element.

DNETs are multinodular, wedge-shaped, "bubbly" intracortical tumors that are usually mistaken for other LGGs. DNETs are more likely than GGs to have a multi-cystic shape and to stay the same size throughout time.

In around 30% of cases, contrast enhancement was discovered. The tumor presents on CT scana as a hypoattenuating cortical–subcortical mass with occasional calcifications. The surrounding inner table of the cranium may also have scalloping. On MRI, DNETs are most commonly seen as multinodular, pseudocystic cerebral cortical lesions that are hypointense on T1W images but hyperintense on T2W images, with or without circumferential vasogenic edema.

Anti-epileptic medicines are frequently ineffective in controlling epilepsy-related tumors, although surgery can provide great benefits (Clusmann et al. 2004). Lesionectomy, extended lesionectomy, and customized resection are among the surgical strategies used. When a tumor is found in the mesial or neocortical temporal lobe, some authors recommend anterior temporal lobectomy.

When the tumor is extratemporal or in the temporal neocortex, most of the authors concur that lesionectomy alone delivers the best seizure reduction result (Cataltepe et al. 2005). However, the effects of temporomesial lesionectomy are debatable (Cataltepe et al. 2005). The involvement of temporomesial areas, according to some writers, may extend and complicate the epileptogenic zone.

Hypothalamic Hamartoma

A hypothalamic hamartoma (HH) is an uncommon, developing, disordered tissue mass that arises from the tuber cinereum and the bottom of the third ventricle and is found in the hypothalamus. Precocious puberty is associated with infraventricular HHs linked to the tuber cinereum. Intraventricular HHs are connected to the third ventricle's floor and cause seizures. Gelastic seizures (GSs) are the commonest type of seizure in pediatric patients; however, patients can also have dacrystic seizures, complicated partial seizures, or other types of seizures. Epilepsy linked to HH is pharmacoresistant and results in severe epileptic encephalopathy and infantile catastrophic epilepsy (Harvey and Freeman 2007).

Scalp electroencephalograms do not exhibit epileptiform discharge in gelastic seizures caused by HH, whereas depth electrodes implanted into the hamartoma clearly indicate epileptiform activity.

The suprasellar cistern and anterior third ventricle are obliterated on non-enhanced CT scans, and the nodule is iso- or hypodense compared to the grey matter. On high-dose, contrast-enhanced CT, HHs do not enhance. On T1WI, signal intensity is frequently isointense to normal gray matter, and on T2/FLAIR, signal intensity is usually isointense to slightly hyperintense. Following contrast injection, HHs do not improve (Saleem et al. 2007).

Surgery appears to be the best technique for acquiring seizure independence and preventing the steady loss of neurocognitive function in HHS patients who were resistant to AED. Surgical options include the transcallosal interhemispheric approach, endoscopic removal, stereotactic radiosurgery (Rosenfeld et al. 2004), and stereotactic radiofrequency thermocoagulation (SRT) (Wang et al. 2009).

The Lennox–Gastaut Syndrome

Lennox–Gastaut syndrome (LGS) is one of the most severe epileptic syndromes. It generally develops between the ages of 3 and 5, but it can also occur later in life, even into adulthood (Camfield 2011; Arzimanoglou et al. 2009). LGS is a clinical diagnosis marked by polymorphous epileptic seizures, primarily axial tonic, atypical absences, and atonic seizures; permanent psychological disturbances; and an electroencephalogram (EEG) that frequently shows either paroxysmal fast activity or slow spike–waves brought on by sleep when superimposed on a slow background (Camfield 2011; Arzimanoglou et al. 2009).

LGS is still difficult to treat and seizures are extremely pharmacoresistant. Patients with LGS who have not responded to pharmacological treatment may be candidates for surgery.

Neuroimaging studies in patients with LGS may have two patterns of findings. MRI may reveal a well-circumscribed lesion, the removal of which will lead to seizure freedom. More usual is that MRI reveals no epileptogenic lesion or lesions that are extensive, bilateral, diffuse, or not well defined and, thus, not removable. In the second situation, it is possible to perform a palliative operation such as corpus callosotomy or vagus nerve stimulation.

The Landau–Kleffner Syndrome

This is an epileptic encephalopathy with the EEG characteristic of continuous spikes and waves during slow sleep (CSWS). During a vital phase of language development, an epileptogenic lesion in the speech area (or that influences the speech cortex) causes the disease.

Neurocysticercosis, subpial gliosis, encephalitis, vasculitis, and neuronal migration disorder have all been recognized as pathologic entities in children with LKS (Cole et al. 1988). In most patients with LKS, however, standard neuroimaging reveals no structural abnormalities.

The onset of language disturbances is temporally linked to the onset of seizures. Seizures are typically low in severity, infrequent, and nocturnal. AEDs, steroids, high-dose benzodiazepines, and IV immunoglobulin have all been used to treat LKS (IVIG). Clinical seizures can be effectively treated with AEDs and other medical treatments; however, cognitive impairments and epileptiform discharge are treated differently.

Surgical options for LKS include lesionectomy, when appropriate, and multiple subpial transection (MST), when there is no identifiable lesion in MRI.

The target of epilepsy surgery for LKS is to obtain seizure freedom and remission of the language problems. AEDs can usually achieve the latter goal in most patients. As a result, the most common reason for considering surgery is to eliminate epileptiform discharge and thereby improve language function. There are reports of excellent outcomes following lesionectomy (Nass et al. 1993).

Morell and colleagues introduced MST for selected children with LKS who failed medical therapy, and the outcome of their series was encouraging (Morrell et al. 1995). A similar outcome was also published by Grote et al. (1999) and Irwin et al. (2001). However, Downes et al. found reason to recommend MST over medical therapy (Downes et al. 2015).

5.2.4. Classification of Epilepsy Surgery

The surgical approach and method in a case with refractory epilepsy is determined by the seizure type, location of epileptic focus, presence or absence of an identifiable pathology on MRI, and its proximity to eloquent brain and the patient's functional baseline. Epilepsy surgery is divided into two types: curative and palliative. Without the use of AEDs, the goal of curative surgery is to fully eliminate seizures and create long-term remission. When "curative" surgery is not an option, palliative surgery is considered. Resection of the epileptic zone, disconnection at the level of white fibers, and neurostimulation are the three basic techniques in epilepsy surgery.

Resective Surgery for Epilepsy

Anteromedial temporal lobectomy (AMTL) and its modifications are the most commonly accomplished surgeries for the management of refractory epilepsy.

In conventional resection (AMTL), the neocortical resection in the non-dominant and dominant temporal lobes is roughly 5 cm and 3.5 cm, respectively. The amygdala and the first 3 cm of the hippocampus are removed (Figure 16). A more extensive hippocampus resection was not linked to a higher risk of seizure freedom after surgery (Schramm et al. 2011). Selective amygdalohippocampectomy (SAH) was created for people with obvious hippocampal sclerosis to prevent the removal of lateral (neocortical) temporal tissue and has been demonstrated to be as effective in controlling seizures (Figure 17) (Tanriverdi et al. 2009). Yasargil advocated for a trans-sylvian route (Siegel et al. 1990), but the same surgery might be performed using an inferior temporal approach or a transcortical method through the middle temporal gyrus.

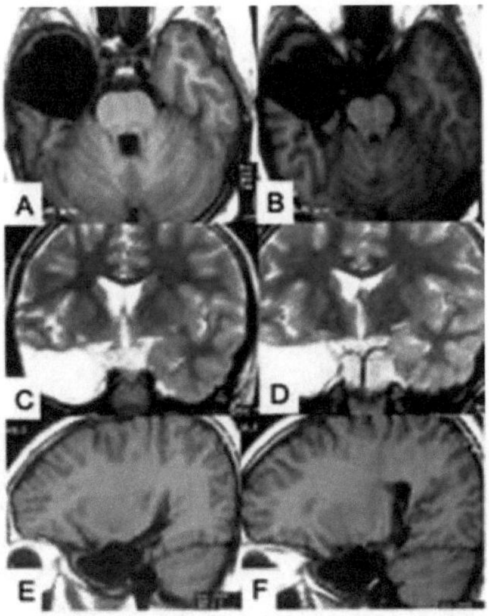

Figure 16. MRI of brain; (**A**,**B**) T1W axial, (**C**,**D**) T2W coronal and (**E**,**F**) T1W sagital postoperative images after right amygdalohippocampectomy plus standard anterior temporal lobectomy in a case of MTS. Source: Figure by authors.

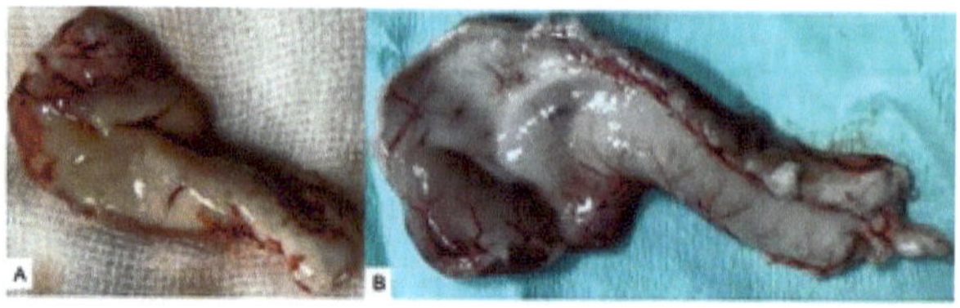

Figure 17. Resected specimens (**A**,**B**) of amygdala and hippocampus after selective amygdalohippocampectomy. Source: Figure by authors.

Approximately 70% of correctly selected patients achieve seizure-free status after ATL, and the majority of those who remain, benefit greatly from seizure reduction and increased quality of life (Engel 1996; Spencer et al. 1984).

When there is a well-demarcated structural lesion, such as a benign tumor, FCD (Figures 18–20), gliosis (Figures 21 and 22), or cavernous malformation, lesionectomy is a viable surgical option if seizure semiology and EEGs are in agreement. In general, removing the epileptogenic brain area completely increases the likelihood of seizure freedom. Overlap with the eloquent cortex makes adequate resection difficult. As a result, the extent of resection should be assessed against these risks and tailored to each individual instance.

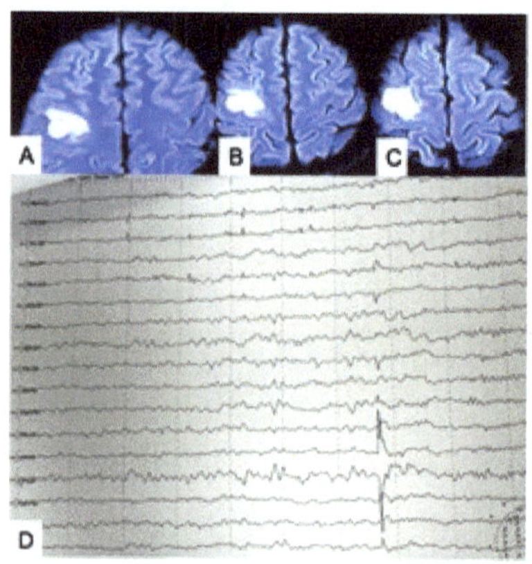

Figure 18. (**A**–**C**) MRI of brain axial sections showing right middle frontal gyrus FCD. (**D**) EEG showing right frontal focal discharge. Source: Figure by authors.

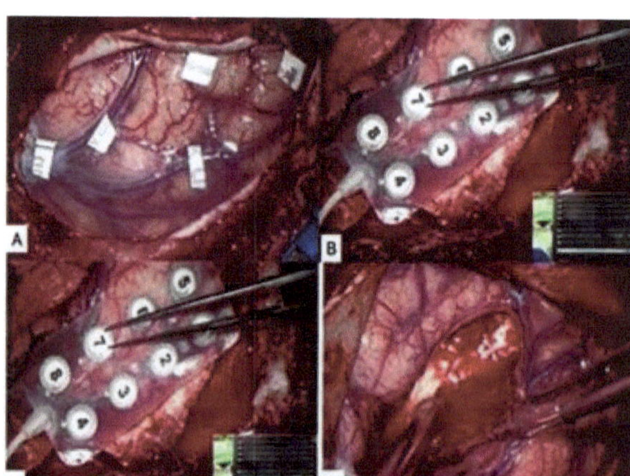

Figure 19. Peroperative (ECoG- and neuronavigation-guided excision) pictures: (**A**) before excision, (**B**,**C**) ECoG-guided excision, and (**D**) after excision. Source: Figure by authors.

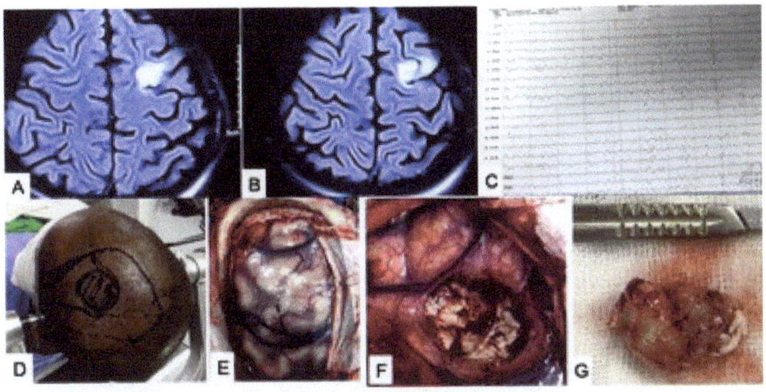

Figure 20. (**A**,**B**) MRI of brain axial sections showing left frontal FCD. (**C**) EEG showing abnormal electrical discharge concordant with lesion. (**D**–**F**) Peroperative pictures of focal excision of lesion. (**G**) Specimen after resection of lesion. Source: Figure by authors.

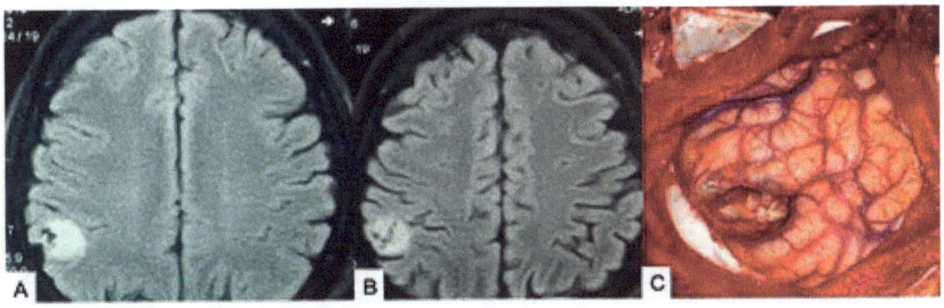

Figure 21. (**A**,**B**) MRI of brain showing right-sided parietal post-neurocysticercosis gliosis. (**C**) Peroperative picture of excision of lesion. Source: Figure by authors.

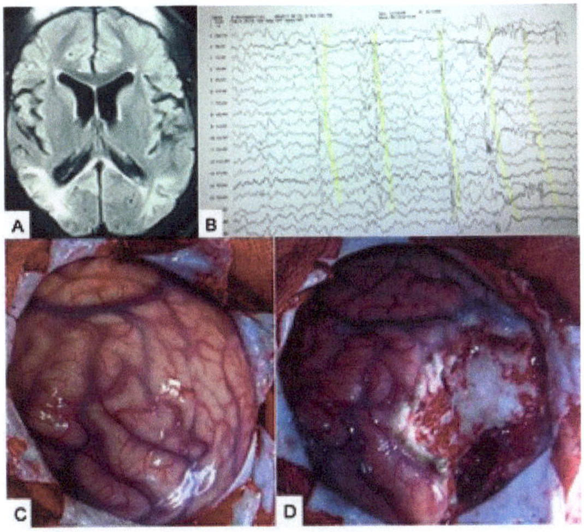

Figure 22. (**A**) MRI of brain axial view showing post-viral-infection occipital gliosis and atrophy (right > left) with resistance epilepsy with a history of repeated severe head injury due to falls. (**B**) EEG showing abnormal electrical discharges predominantly from the right occipital area. (**C**,**D**) Peroperative pictures of right occipital focal excision (patient was hemianopic). Surgical excision eased seizure control with drugs. Source: Figure by authors.

Removal of hemosiderin-stained tissue around the malformation is required in cavernoma. The use of intraoperative cortical mapping and intraoperative electrocorticography (ECoG) (Figure 19) (Van Gompel et al. 2009) and awake craniotomy with neuronavigation-guided (Figure 23) resection improves outcomes and reduces postoperative neurological deficits.

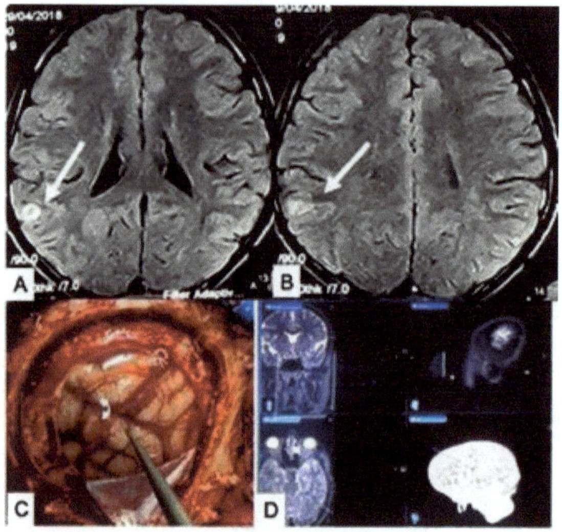

Figure 23. (**A**,**B**) MRI of brain axial sections showing right parietal small FCD. (**C**,**D**) Peroperative identification of lesion with neuronavigation guide. Source: Figure by authors.

After the ictal onset zone and cortical functions have been established using intracranial recordings, most typically utilizing subdural grids or SEEGs, MRI-negative epilepsy usually requires a customized resection.

While open brain resection has traditionally been the basis of surgical treatment, recent advancements have enabled less-invasive ablative treatments such as MRI-guided laser interstitial thermotherapy (LITT). Following is a brief rundown of the many technological approaches and procedures.

Recently, laser ablation under real-time MR thermographic guidance has been shown as an alternative to open resection in patients with hippocampal sclerosis (Willie et al. 2014). Its main advantages are decreased surgical morbidity and better cognitive outcomes (Drane et al. 2015). This approach can also be used for other small, deep epileptogenic lesions.

Laser Ablation Surgery

In both extratemporal and temporal lobe epilepsy, laser ablation surgery has recently been found to be successful in both non-lesional and lesional instances. MTS, FCD, unsuccessful prior open surgery, and deeper lesions relatively inaccessible to open surgery are all examples (Gonzalez-Martinez et al. 2014).

This approach has the advantage of precisely targeting seizure-causing lesions without the need for a craniotomy, leading to less pain as well as a shorter hospital stay. The goal of an MRIgLITT (MRI-guided laser interstitial thermal therapy) system is to use interstitial irradiation or thermal therapy to necrotize soft tissues while employing MRI guidance. This method has been used to treat MTS, cavernous angioma, hypothalamic hamartoma, cortical development abnormalities, and tuberous sclerotic lesions (Gross et al. 2016). MRIgLITT can also be used to treat mesial temporal epilepsy. It has been compared to open surgery in terms of safety, accuracy, and efficacy but provides reduced morbidity (Kang et al. 2016), especially in elderly patients (Waseem et al. 2015).

Corpus Callosotomy

Corpus callosotomy (CC) is a palliative surgical treatment that involves severance of the corpus callosum in the anterior two-thirds or its entirety. The treatment is most commonly utilized for drop attacks, with roughly three-quarters of patients benefiting and more than a third being free of drop attacks (Tanriverdi et al. 2009). Detaching the corpus callosum is thought to stop rapid bilateral seizure spread, which causes loss of consciousness or posture, and so lessens the intensity and frequency of secondary generalized seizures in people who are not surgical candidates. In seizure types that require bi-hemispheric synchrony for seizure expression, CC has the potential to eliminate clinical seizure symptoms. Patients with very refractory, generalized tonic–clonic seizures may benefit from CC in the case of IGE (Cukiert et al. 2009; Jenssen et al. 2006).

Multiple Subpial Transection Procedure

This approach, developed by Morrell in 1989, is largely used to treat refractory epilepsies in which resection is impossible due to the epileptogenic zone being close to, or overlapping, the eloquent cortex (Morrell et al. 1989). Ictal discharges frequently spread along horizontal fibers, whereas cortical activities tend to be organized vertically. Multiple vertical subpial transections are performed in 5 mm intervals of the cortex based on this principle, severing horizontal intracortical fibers but maintaining vertical connections. In an awake patient, MST on the eloquent cortex is frequently combined with the excision of neighboring nonessential cortex. Excision surgery has been found to be more successful than this method (Morrell et al. 1989).

Hemispherectomy

The most favored surgical strategy in the care of children with unilateral hemispheric epilepsy and hemisphere functions that are compromised or projected to become impaired is hemispherectomy (Figures 13 and 14) (Limbrick et al. 2009). Indications for hemispherectomy include Rasmussen syndrome, hemimegalencephaly, Sturge–Weber syndrome, infantile spasms, hemiconvulsion-hemiplegia-epilepsy (HHE) syndrome, multilobar cortical dysplasia, and congenital hemiplegia. In anatomical hemispherectomy, the entire abnormal hemisphere is resected, giving excellent seizure freedom. But, patients develop serious late postoperative complications including superficial cerebral hemosiderosis and hydrocephalus. With subsequent modifications, anatomical hemispherectomy has been almost completely abandoned and replaced by functional hemispherectomy and hemispherotomy. Current functional hemispherectomy surgery removes the temporal and centroparietal portions of the brain, keeping the frontal and occipital poles alive but isolated from the rest of the brain. Around three-quarters of patients have total seizure control after hemispherectomy, with the majority of the remaining patients having better seizure control (Limbrick et al. 2009). Seizure independence generally improves the function of the remaining hemisphere, resulting in enhanced cognitive function and behavior during follow-up.

Non-Resective Surgical Treatments: Neurostimulation

i. Vagus Nerve Stimulation (VNS)—The US Food and Drug Administration (FDA) approved VNS for refractory focal onset epilepsies with or without secondary generalization in cases aged 4 years and up. A battery generator is inserted in the left upper chest wall and tunneled beneath the skin to the vagus nerve in the VNS system. The device is set to send electrical stimulation to the brain via the left vagus nerve. The mean seizure frequency dropped by 26% after one year, 30% after five years, and 52% after 12 years, according to a retrospective assessment assessing the efficacy of VNS in 48 patients with intractable partial epilepsy (Uthman et al. 2004).

ii. Responsive Neurostimulation (RNS)—The FDA authorized RNS in 2013 for medically resistant focal epilepsy. In reaction to ictal discharges recorded by the RNS device, it gives cortical stimuli. This programmable neurostimulator is implanted in the brain and coupled to one or two depth and/or subdural cortical strip electrodes over seizure foci. In the final months of the two-year trial, the randomized investigation of 191 patients found a progressive decrease in the frequency of debilitating seizures in the treatment group (41.5%) compared to the control group (9.4%) (Heck et al. 2014).

iii. Deep Brain Stimulation (DBS)—DBS of the anterior nucleus of the thalamus has been licensed in the European Union as an adjunctive treatment for drug-resistant focal epilepsy in adults since 2010. It is also FDA-approved. In a multicenter trial, the treatment group experienced a 29% reduction in seizures in the first month, analogous to the control group, and at least a 50% seizure decrease in 54% of patients after two years (Fisher et al. 2010).

6. Conclusions

Drug-resistant epilepsy has a remarkable impact on cognitive development and life quality. Many of them can be addressed successfully with surgery. In managing patients with DRE, appropriate utilization of diagnostic tools to identify a patient's suitability for surgical management as well as to determine what type of surgical technique would be safer and most useful to the particular case is critical. Both presurgical examination and surgical approaches will improve as diagnostic and treatment technologies advance.

Author Contributions: Conceptualization, methodology, validation, formal analysis, investigation, resources, data curation, writing—original draft preparation, J.U.M.R. and F.H.C.; writing—review and editing, visualization, supervision, F.H.C. All authors have read and agreed to the published version of the manuscript.

Funding: This research received no external funding.

Conflicts of Interest: The authors declare no conflicts of interest.

References

Arzimanoglou, Alexis, Jacqueline French, Warren. T. Blume, J. Helen Cross, Jan-Peter Ernst, Martha Feucht, Pierre Genton, Renzo Guerrini, Gerhard Kluger, John M. Pellock, and et al. 2009. Lennox-Gastaut syndrome: A consensus approach on diagnosis, assessment, management, and trial methodology. *Lancet Neurology* 8: 82–93. [CrossRef] [PubMed]

Barkovich, A. James, Renzo Guerrini, Ruben I. Kuzniecky, Graeme D. Jackson, and William B. Dobyns. 2012. A developmental and geneticclassification for malformations of cortical development: Update 2012. *Brain* 5: 1348–69. [CrossRef]

Barth, Daniel S. 1993. The neurophysiological basis of epileptiform magnetic fields and localization of neocorticalsources. *Journal of Clinical Neurophysiology* 10: 99–107. [CrossRef] [PubMed]

Bell, Brian D., and Keith G. Davies. 1998. Anterior temporal lobectomy, hippocampal sclerosis, and memory: Recentneuropsychological findings. *Neuropsychology Review* 8: 25–41. [CrossRef]

Berkovic, Samuel F., Frederick Andermann, André Olivier, Roméo Ethier, Denis Melanson, Yvon Robitaille, Ruben Kuzniecky, Terence Peters, and William Feindel. 1991. Hippocampal sclerosis in temporal lobe epilepsy demonstrated by magnetic resonanceimaging. *Annals of Neurology* 29: 175–82. [CrossRef]

Bernasconi, Andrea, Fernando Cendes, William H. Theodore, Ravnoor S. Gill, Matthias J. Koepp, Robert Edward Hogan, Graeme D. Jackson, Paolo Federico, Angelo Labate, Anna Elisabetta Vaudano, and et al. 2019. Recommendations for the use of structural magnetic resonance imaging inthe care of patients with epilepsy: A consensus report from the International League Against Epilepsy Neuroimaging Task Force. *Epilepsia* 60: 1054–68. [CrossRef]

Binder, Jeffrey R. 2011. Functional MRI is a valid noninvasive alternative to Wada testing. *Epilepsy & Behavior* 20: 214–22. [CrossRef]

Blümcke, Ingmar, Maria Thom, Eleonora Aronica, Dawna D. Armstrong, Harry V. Vinters, Andre Palmini, Thomas S. Jacques, Giuliano Avanzini, A. James Barkovich, Giorgio Battaglia, and et al. 2011. The clinicopathologic spectrum of focal cortical dysplasias: A consensus classification proposed by an ad hoc Task Force of the ILAE Diagnostic Methods Commission. *Epilepsia* 52: 158–74. [CrossRef]

Burgerman, Robert S., Michael R. Sperling, Jacqueline A. French, Andrew J. Saykin, and Michael J. O'Connor. 1995. Comparison of mesial versusneocortical onset temporal lobe seizures: Neurodiagnostic findings and surgical outcome. *Epilepsia* 36: 662–70. [CrossRef]

Camfield, Peter R. 2011. Definition and natural history of Lennox-Gastaut syndrome. *Epilepsia* 52: 3–9. [CrossRef]

Çataltepe, Oguz, and George I. Jallo. 2019. *Pediatric Epilepsy Surgery: Preoperative Assessment and Surgical Intervention*. New York: Thieme Medical Publishers.

Cataltepe, Oguz, Güzide Turanli, Dilek Yalnizoglu, Meral Topçu, and Nejat Akalan. 2005. Surgical management of temporal lobetumor-related epilepsy in children. *Journal of Neurosurgery: Pediatrics* 102: 280–87. [CrossRef] [PubMed]

Chang, Victor, Jonathan Edwards, and Oren Sagher. 2007. False Lateralization of Electrographic Onset in the Setting of CerebralAtrophy. *Journal of Clinical Neurophysiology* 24: 438–43. [CrossRef] [PubMed]

Chiapparini, L., T. Granata, L. Farina, E. Ciceri, A. Erbetta, F. Ragona, E. Freri, L. Fusco, G. Gobbi, G. Capovilla, and et al. 2003. Diagnostic imaging in 13 cases of Rasmussen's encephalitis: Can early MRI suggest thediagnosis? *Neuroradiology* 45: 171–83. [CrossRef] [PubMed]

Clusmann, Hans, Thomas Kral, Ulrike Gleissner, Robert Sassen, Horst Urbach, Ingmar Blümcke, Jacek Bogucki, and Johannes Schramm. 2004. Analysis ofdifferent types of resection for pediatric patients with temporal lobe epilepsy. *Neurosurgery* 54: 847–59. [CrossRef]

Cole, A. J., F. Andermann, L. Taylor, A. Olivier, T. Rasmussen, Y. Robitaille, and J. P. Spire. 1988. The Landau-Kleffnersyndrome of acquired epileptic aphasia: Unusual clinical outcome, surgical experience, and absence ofencephalitis. *Neurology* 38: 31–38. [CrossRef]

Cooper, Ray, A. L. Winter, H. J. Crow, and W. Grey Walter. 1965. Comparison of subcortical, cortical, and scalp activityusing chronically indwelling electrodes in man. *Electroencephalography and Clinical Neurophysiology* 18: 217–28. [CrossRef]

Cukiert, Arthur, Jose Augusto Burattini, Pedro Paulo Mariani, Cristine Mella Cukiert, Meire Argentoni-Baldochi, Carla Baise-Zung, Cássio Roberto Forster, and Valeria Antakli Mello. 2009. Outcome after extended callosal section in patients with primary idiopathic generalizedepilepsy. *Epilepsia* 50: 1377–80. [CrossRef]

Daroff, Robert B., Joseph Jankovic, John C. Mazziotta, and Scott L. Pomeroy. 2015. *Bradley's Neurology in Clinical Practice*. Amsterdam: Elsevier, p. 1571.

Downes, Michelle, Rebecca Greenaway, Maria Clark, J. Helen Cross, Nicola Jolleff, William Harkness, Marios Kaliakatsos, Stewart Boyd, Steve White, and Brian G. R. Neville. 2015. Outcome following multiple subpial transection in Landau-Kleffner syndrome andrelated regression. *Epilepsia* 56: 1760–66. [CrossRef]

Drane, Daniel L., David W. Loring, Natalie L. Voets, Michele Price, Jeffrey G. Ojemann, Jon T. Willie, Amit M. Saindane, Vaishali Phatak, Mirjana Ivanisevic, Scott Millis, and et al. 2015. Better object recognition and naming outcome with MRI-guided stereotactic laser Amygdalohippocampotomy for temporal lobe epilepsy. *Epilepsia* 56: 101–13. [CrossRef]

Duvernoy, Henri M., Françoise Cattin, and Pierre-Yves Risold. 2013. *The Human Hippocampus: Functional Anatomy, Vascularization and Serial Sections with MRI*. New York: Springer.

Ebersole, John S. 1997. Defining epileptogenic foci: Past, present, future. *Journal of clinical neurophysiology* 14: 470–83. [CrossRef]

Elwan, Sherif, Andreas Alexopoulos, Diosely C. Silveira, and Prakash Kotagal. 2018. Lateralizing and localizing value of seizure semiology:comparison with Scalp EEG, MRI and PET in patients successfully treated with respective epilepsy surgery. *Seizure* 61: 203–8. [CrossRef] [PubMed]

Engel, Jerome, Jr. 1996. Surgery for seizures. *New England Journal of Medicine* 334: 647–57. [CrossRef] [PubMed]

Englot, Dario J., and Edward F. Chang. 2014. Rates and predictors of seizure freedom in resective epilepsy surgery: Anupdate. *Neurosurgical Review* 37: 389–404. [CrossRef]

Fisher, Robert S., Helen E. Scharfman, and Marco DeCurtis. 2014. How Can We Identify Ictal and Interictal Abnormal Activity? In *Issues in Clinical Epileptology: A View from the Bench*. Edited by Helen E. Scharfman and Paul S. Buckmaster. Dordrecht: Springer, pp. 3–23. [CrossRef]

Fisher, Robert S., J. Helen Cross, Jacqueline A. French, Norimichi Higurashi, Edouard Hirsch, Floor E. Jansen, Lieven Lagae, Solomon L. Moshé, Jukka Peltola, Eliane Roulet Perez, and et al. 2017. Operational classification of seizure types by the International League Against Epilepsy: Position Paper of the ILAE Commission for Classification and Terminology. *Epilepsia* 58: 522–30. [CrossRef]

Fisher, Robert, Vicenta Salanova, Thomas Witt, Robert Worth, Thomas Henry, Robert Gross, Kalarickal Oommen, Ivan Osorio, Jules Nazzaro, Douglas Labar, and et al. 2010. Electrical stimulation of the anterior nucleus of thalamus for treatment of refractory epilepsy. *Epilepsia* 51: 899–908. [CrossRef] [PubMed]

Gleissner, Ulrike, Christoph Helmstaedter, Johannes Schramm, and Christian E. Elger. 2004. Memory outcome after selectiveamygdalohippocampectomy in patients with temporal lobe epilepsy: One-year follow-up. *Epilepsia* 45: 960–62. [CrossRef]

Gonzalez-Martinez, Jorge, Sumeet Vadera, Jeffrey Mullin, Rei Enatsu, Andreas V. Alexopoulos, Ravish Patwardhan, William Bingaman, and Imad Najm. 2014. Robot-Assisted Stereotactic Laser Ablation in Medically Intractable Epilepsy: Operative Technique. *Neurosurgery* 10: 167–72. [CrossRef]

Gross, Robert E., Jon T. Willie, and Daniel L. Drane. 2016. The Role of Stereotactic Laser Amygdalohippocampotomy in Mesial Temporal Lobe Epilepsy. *Neurosurgery Clinics of North America* 27: 37–50. [CrossRef]

Grote, Christopher L., Patricia Van Slyke, and Jo-Ann B. Hoeppner. 1999. Language outcome following multiple subpial transections forLandau-Kleffner syndrome. *Brain* 3: 561–66. [CrossRef]

Harvey, A. Simon, and Jeremy L. Freeman. 2007. Epilepsy in hypothalamic hamartoma: Clinical features. *Seminars in Pediatric Neurology* 14: 60–64. [CrossRef]

Heck, Christianne N., David King-Stephens, Andrew D. Massey, Dileep R. Nair, Barbara C. Jobst, Gregory L. Barkley, Vicenta Salanova, Andrew J. Cole, Michael C. Smith, Ryder P. Gwinn, and et al. 2014. Two-year seizure reduction in adults with medically intractable partialonsetepilepsy treated with responsive neurostimulation: Final results of the RNS System Pivotal trial. *Epilepsia* 55: 432–41. [CrossRef] [PubMed]

Ikeda, Kristin M., and Seyed M. Mirsattari. 2017. Evolution of epilepsy in hemimegalencephaly from infancy to adulthood: Case report and review of the literature. *Epilepsy & Behavior Case Reports* 7: 47–48. [CrossRef]

ILAE. n.d. *EpilepsyDiagnosis.org*. Available online: https://www.epilepsydiagnosis.org/ (accessed on 31 July 2021).

Irwin, Kate, Victoria Birch, Janet Lees, Charles Polkey, Gonzalo Alarcon, Colin Binnie, Martin Smedley, Gillian Baird, and Richard O. Robinson. 2001. Multiplesubpial transection in Landau-Kleffner syndrome. *Developmental Medicine and Child Neurology* 43: 248–52. [CrossRef] [PubMed]

Jamuar, Saumya S., and Christopher A. Walsh. 2015. Genomic variants and variations in malformations of cortical development. *Pediatric Clinics of North America* 13: 571–85. [CrossRef] [PubMed]

Jayakar, Prasanna, Jean Gotman, A. Simon Harvey, André Palmini, Laura Tassi, Donald Schomer, Francois Dubeau, Fabrice Bartolomei, Alice Yu, Pavel Kršek, and et al. 2016. Diagnostic utility of invasive EEG for epilepsy surgery: Indications, modalities, and techniques. *Epilepsia* 57: 1735–47. [CrossRef]

Jenssen, Sigmund, Michael R. Sperling, Joseph I. Tracy, Maromi Nei, Liporace Joyce, Glosser David, and Michael O'Connor. 2006. Corpus callosotomy inrefractory idiopathic generalized epilepsy. *Seizure* 15: 621–29. [CrossRef]

Kabat, Joanna, and Przemysław Król. 2012. Focal Cortical Dysplasia—Review. *Polish journal of radiology* 77: 35–43. [CrossRef]

Kalilani, Linda, Xuezheng Sun, Barbara Pelgrims, Matthias Noack-Rink, and Vicente Villanueva. 2018. The epidemiology of drug-resistant epilepsy: A systematic review and meta-analysis. *Epilepsia* 59: 2179–93. [CrossRef]

Kang, Joon Y., Chengyuan Wu, Joseph Tracy, Matthew Lorenzo, James Evans, Maromi Nei, Christopher Skidmore, Scott Mintzer, Ashwini D. Sharan, and Michael R. Sperling. 2016. Laser interstitial thermal therapy for medically intractable mesial temporal lobe epilepsy. *Epilepsia* 57: 325–34. [CrossRef]

Kessels, Roy PC, Marc PH Hendriks, Jacob Schouten, Marieke Van Asselen, and Albert Postma. 2004. Spatial memory deficits in patientsafter unilateral selective amygdalohippocampectomy. *Journal of the International Neuropsychological Society* 10: 907–12. [CrossRef]

Ko, Tae-Sung, and Gregory L. Holmes. 1999. EEG and clinical predictors of medically intractable childhood epilepsy. *Clinical Neurophysiology* 110: 1245–51. [CrossRef] [PubMed]

Kwan, Patrick, Alexis Arzimanoglou, Anne T. Berg, Martin J. Brodie, W. Allen Hauser, Gary Mathern, Solomon L. Moshé, Emilio Perucca, Samuel Wiebe, and Jacqueline French. 2010. Definition of drug resistant epilepsy: Consensus proposal by the ad hoc Task Force ofthe ILAE Commission on Therapeutic Strategies. *Epilepsia* 51: 1069–77. [CrossRef]

Kwan, Patrick, and Martin J. Brodie. 2000. Early identification of refractory epilepsy. *New England Journal of Medicine* 342: 314–19. [CrossRef] [PubMed]

Limbrick, David D., Prithvi Narayan, Alexander K. Powers, Jeffrey G. Ojemann, Tae Sung Park, Mary Bertrand, and Matthew D. Smyth. 2009. Hemispherot-omy: Efficacy and analysis of seizure recurrence. *Journal of Neurosurgery: Pediatrics* 4: 323–32. [CrossRef] [PubMed]

Little, Andrew S., Kris A. Smith, Kristin Kirlin, Leslie C. Baxter, Steve Chung, Rama Maganti, and David M. Treiman. 2009. Modifications to thesubtemporal selective amygdalohippocampectomy using a minimal-access technique: Seizure and neuropsychological outcomes. *Journal of Neurosurgery* 111: 1263–74. [CrossRef]

Loddenkemper, Tobias, Harold H. Morris, and Gabriel Möddel. 2008. Complications during the Wada test. *Epilepsy & Behavior* 13: 551–53. [CrossRef]

Longaretti, Francesca, Colin Dunkley, Sophia Varadkar, Faraneh Vargha-Khadem, Stewart G. Boyd, and J. Helen Cross. 2012. Evolution of the EEG inchildren with Rasmussen's syndrome. *Epilepsia* 53: 1539–45. [CrossRef]

Luyken, Cordelia, Ingmar Blümcke, Rolf Fimmers, Horst Urbach, Christian E. Elger, Otmar D. Wiestler, and Johannes Schramm. 2003. The spectrum oflong-term epilepsy-associated tumors: Long-term seizure and tumor outcome and neurosurgicalaspects. *Epilepsia* 44: 822–30. [CrossRef] [PubMed]

Mikuni, Nobuhiro, Akio Ikeda, Jun A. Takahashi, Kazuhiko Nozaki, Susumu Miyamoto, Waro Taki, and Nobuo Hashimoto. 2006. A step-by-stepresection guided by electrocorticography for nonmalignant brain tumors associated with long-termintractable epilepsy. *Epilepsy & Behavior* 8: 560–64. [CrossRef]

Morrell, Frank, Walter W. Whisler, and Thomas P. Bleck. 1989. Multiple subpial transection: A new approach to thesurgical treatment of focal epilepsy. *Journal of neurosurgery* 70: 231–39. [CrossRef]

Morrell, Frank, Walter W. Whisler, Michael C. Smith, Thomas J. Hoeppner, Leyla de Toledo-Morrell, Serge J. C. Pierre-Louis, Andres M. Kanner, Janice M. Buclow, Ruzica Ristanovic, Donna Bergen, and et al. 1995. Landau-Kleffner syndrome. Treatment with subpialintracortical transection. *Brain* 118: 1529–46. [CrossRef] [PubMed]

Nass, Ruth, Linda Heier, and Russell Walker. 1993. Landau Kleffner Syndrome: Temporal lobe tumor resection results in goodoutcome. *Pediatric Neurology* 9: 303–5. [CrossRef] [PubMed]

O'Brien, Terence J., Christine Kilpatrick, Vanessa Murrie, Simon Vogrin, Kevin Morris, and Mark J. Cook. 1996. Temporal lobe epilepsy caused bymesial temporal sclerosis and temporal neocortical lesions. A clinical and electroencephalographicstudy of 46 pathologically proven cases. *Brain* 119: 2133–41. [CrossRef]

Olivier, André, Warren W. Boling, and Taner Tanriverdi. 2012. *Techniques in Epilepsy Surgery: The MNI Approach*. New York: Cambridge University Press.

Rosenfeld, Jeffrey V., Jeremy L. Freeman, and A. Simon Harvey. 2004. Operative technique: The anterior transcallosal transseptal inter forniceal approach to the third ventricle andresection of hypothalamic hamartomas. *Journal of Clinical Neuroscience* 11: 738–44. [CrossRef] [PubMed]

Rosenow, Felix, and Hans Luders. 2001. Presurgical evaluation of Epilepsy. *Brain* 124: 1683–700. [CrossRef]

Saleem, Sahar N., Ahmed-Hesham M. Said, and Donald H. Lee. 2007. Lesions of the hypothalamus: MR imaging diagnostic features. *Radiographics* 27: 1087–108. [CrossRef]

Salinsky, Martin, Roy Kanter, and Richard M. Dasheiff. 1987. Effectiveness of multiple EEGs in supporting the diagnosis ofepilepsy: An operational curve. *Epilepsia* 28: 331–34. [CrossRef]

Schramm, Johannes, T. N. Lehmann, J. Zentner, C. A. Mueller, J. Scorzin, R. Fimmers, H. J. Meencke, A. Schulze-Bonhage, and C. E. Elger. 2011. Randomized controlled trial of 2.5-cm versus 3.5-cm mesial temporal resection intemporal lobe epilepsy—Part 1: Intent-to-treat analysis. *Acta Neurochirurgica* 153: 209–19. [CrossRef]

Siegel, Adrian M., Heinz G. Wieser, Werner Wichmann, and Gazi M. Yasargil. 1990. Relationships between MR-imaged total amountof tissue removed, resection scores of specific mediobasal limbic subcompartments and clinicaloutcome following selective amygdalohippocampectomy. *Epilepsy Research* 6: 56–65. [CrossRef]

So, Elson L., and Philippe Ryvlin. 2018. *MRI Negative Epilepsy: Evaluation and Surgical Management*. Cambridge: Cambridge University Press.

So, Norman, and Pierre Gloor. 1991. Electroencephalographic and electrocorticographic findings in chronic encephalitis of the Rasmussen type. In *Chronic Encephalitis and Epilepsy: Rasmussen's Syndrome*. Edited by Frederick Andermann. Boston: Butterworth-Heinemann, pp. 37–45.

So, Norman, Pierre Gloor, L. Felipe Quesney, Marilyn Jones-Gotman, André Olivier, and Frederick Andermann. 1989. Depth electrode investigationsin patients with bitemporal epileptiform abnormalities. *Annals of Neurology* 25: 423–31. [CrossRef]

Spencer, Dennis D., Susan S. Spencer, Richard H. Mattson, Peter D. Williamson, and Robert A. Novelly. 1984. Access to the posterior medialtemporal lobe structure in surgical treatment of temporal lobe epilepsy. *Neurosurgery* 15: 667–71. [CrossRef] [PubMed]

Tanriverdi, Taner, André Olivier, Nicole Poulin, Frederick Andermann, and François Dubeau. 2009. Long-term seizure outcome after corpuscallosotomy: A retrospective analysis of 95 patients. *Journal of Neurosurgery* 110: 332–42. [CrossRef] [PubMed]

Tassi, Laura, Alessandra Meroni, Francesco Deleo, Flavio Villani, Roberto Mai, Giorgio Lo Russo, Nadia Colombo, Giuliano Avanzini, Chiara Falcone, Manuela Bramerio, and et al. 2009. Temporal lobe epilepsy: Neuropathological and clinical correlations in 243 surgicallytreated patients. *Epileptic Disorders* 11: 281–92. [CrossRef] [PubMed]

Téllez-Zenteno, Jose F., and Lizbeth Hernández-Ronquillo. 2012. A Review of the Epidemiology of Temporal Lobe Epilepsy. *Epilepsy Research and Treatment* 2012: 630853. [CrossRef]

Terra-Bustamante, Vera C., Hélio R. Machado, and Américo C. Sakamoto. 2006. Hemimegalencephaly and epilepsy:an overview. *Journal of Epilepsy and Clinical Neurophysiology* 12: 99–105. [CrossRef]

Uthman, B. M., A. M. Reichl, J. C. Dean, S. Eisenschenk, R. Gilmore, S. Reid, S. N. Roper, and B. J. Wilder. 2004. Effectiveness of vagus nerve stimulation in epilepsy patients: A 12-year observation. *Neurology* 63: 1124–26. [CrossRef]

van Breemen, Melanie S. M., Erik B. Wilms, and Charles J. Vecht. 2007. Epilepsy in patients with brain tumours: Epidemiology, mechanisms, and management. *The Lancet Neurology* 6: 421–30. [CrossRef]

Van Gompel, Jamie J., Jesus Rubio, Gregory D. Cascino, Gregory A. Worrell, and Fredric B. Meyer. 2009. Electrocorticography-guided resectionof temporal cavernoma: Is electrocorticography warranted and does it alter the surgical approach? *Journal of Neurosurgery* 110: 1179–85. [CrossRef]

Varadkar, Sophia, Christian G. Bien, Carol A. Kruse, Frances E. Jensen, Jan Bauer, Carlos A. Pardo, Angela Vincent, Gary W. Mathern, and J. Helen Cross. 2014. Rasmussen's encephalitis: Clinical features, pathobiology, and treatment advance. *The Lancet Neurology* 13: 195–205. [CrossRef]

Vaughan, Kerry A., Christian Lopez Ramos, Vivek P. Buch, Rania A. Mekary, Julia R. Amundson, Meghal Shah, Abbas Rattani, Michael C. Dewan, and Kee B. Park. 2019. An estimation of global volume of surgically treatable epilepsy based on a systematic review and meta-analysis of epilepsy. *Journal of Neurosurgery* 130: 1127–41. [CrossRef]

Wang, Wei, Weimin Wang, Xiaofei Guo, Yanjun Zeng, and Xiaodan Jiang. 2009. Hypothalamic hamartoma causing gelastic seizures treated with stereotactic rad iofrequency thermocoagulation. *Epileptic Disorders* 11: 333–38. [CrossRef] [PubMed]

Waseem, Hena, Katie E. Osborn, Mike R. Schoenberg, Valerie Kelley, Ali Bozorg, Daniel Cabello, Selim R. Benbadis, and Fernando L. Vale. 2015. Laser ablation therapy: An alternative treatment for medically resistant mesial temporal lobe epilepsy after age 50. *Epilepsy & Behavior* 51: 152–57. [CrossRef]

Willie, Jon T., Nealen G. Laxpati, Daniel L. Drane, Ashok Gowda, Christina Appin, Chunhai Hao, Daniel J. Brat, Sandra L. Helmers, Amit Saindane, Sherif G. Nour, and et al. 2014. Real-time magnetic resonance-guided stereotactic laser amygdalohippocampotomy for mesial temporal lobe epilepsy. *Neurosurgery* 74: 569–84. [CrossRef] [PubMed]

Wyllie, Elaine, Youssef G. Comair, Prakash Kotagal, Juan Bulacio, William Bingaman, and Paul Ruggieri. 1998. Seizure outcome after epilepsy surgery in children and adolescents. *Annals of Neurology* 44: 740–48. [CrossRef]

Yamazaki, Etsuko, Yukitoshi Takahashi, Noriyuki Akasaka, Tateki Fujiwara, and Yushi Inoue. 2011. Temporal changes in brain MRI findings in Rasmussen syndrome. *Epileptic Disorders* 13: 229–39. [CrossRef]

Yasargil, M. G., P. J. Teddy, and P. Roth. 1985. Selective amygdalo-hippocampectomy: Operative anatomy and surgical technique. In *Advances and Technical Standards in Neurosurgery*. Edited by L. Symon. New York: Springler-Wien.

Section XIII: Peripheral Nerve

Peripheral Nerve Surgery

Forhad H. Chowdhury, Mainul Haque Sarker, Abul Khair, S. M. Monir Hossain and Mohammod Raziul Haque

Abstract: Surgical conditions involving peripheral nerves are nerve injury, nerve tumor, and nerve entrapment. Injury to the nerves is usually caused by a road traffic accident, cut injury, penetrating injury, or blunt injury. Nerve trauma usually occurs in young people and can be devastating. Decision-making regarding surgical repair of the nerves is critical. In properly indicated cases, early surgical repair can provide the best possible outcome. Various types of peripheral nerve tumors can occur; however, schwannoma, neurofibroma, and malignant neurofibroma are the most common. Nerve tumors need proper evaluation and microsurgical management. Entrapment neuropathies are the other type of pathology that may require surgery. Carpal tunnel syndrome is the commonest type of entrapment. This chapter will discuss surgical diseases of the peripheral nerve. Peripheral nerve injury is discussed in the first part of the chapter and peripheral nerve tumors and entrapment neuropathy are discussed subsequently in brief.

Abbreviations

ATLS	advanced life trauma support	BTT	benign triton tumor
CNS	central nervous system	CT	computed tomography
CTR	carpal tunnel release	CTS	carpal tunnel syndrome
EN	entrapment neuropathy	DTF	desmoid-type fibromatosis
DTR	deep tendon transfer	EMG	electromyogram
FEMT	free functioning muscle transfer	FNA	fine-needle aspiration
LHN	lipofibromatous hamartoma of the nerve	HNST	hybrid nerve sheath tumor
IHO	intraneural heterotopic ossification	IPT	inflammatory pseudotumor
MPNST	malignant peripheral nerve sheath tumor	MRI	magnetic resonance imaging
NCS	nerve conduction study	NCT	nerve conduction test
NF	neurofibromatosis	PET	positron emission tomography
PNS	peripheral nervous system	PNI	peripheral nerve injury
VHL	von Hippel–Lindau		

1. Peripheral Nerve Injury (PNI)

1.1. Introduction and History

Peripheral nerve injury (PNI) causes a major disability in working people. The upper limb is the most common site of peripheral nerve injuries of traumatic etiology (Seddighi et al. 2016; Kouyoumdjian 2006). Some serious PNIs have a calamitous effect on a persons' quality of life. Transected nerve fibers regenerate spontaneously with scaring in the traumatic nerve gap, which produces neuroma (Siemionow and Brzezicki 2009). Sensory symptoms, motor function defects, and sometime the development of intractable neuropathic pain are common symptoms (Siemionow and Brzezicki 2009). The principal target of nerve repair is to foster the re-establishment of neural connections of the innervated organs by allowing regrowth of motor, sensory, and autonomic neuronal axons in the distal part of nerve with very minimal loss of axons at the repaired suture line (Seddighi et al. 2016; Brushart 1991).

Aegineta et al. (626–696 AD) were the first surgeons who reported the repair of traumatized peripheral nerves (Aegineta 1528).

In 1873, Huenter was the first surgeon who demonstrated an epineural nerve repair procedure, which exists in use even today (Millesi 1973). In 1892, Cajal proposed that neurotropic growth factors promote regeneration of axons distally to the target organ (Cajal 1892). Sunderland, in 1945, published the principles of microsurgical repair of peripheral nerves. In 1964, Kurze and Smith converted them into a microsurgical technique (Seddighi et al. 2016; Kurze 1964; Smith 1964; Sunderland 1991).

1.2. Peripheral Nerve Anatomy

Understanding of fundamental anatomy for classification and subsequent treatment of a nerve injury is mandatory for a neurosurgeon. The nervous system's cells differ more than those in any other component of the body (Grinsell and Keating 2014; Kandel et al. 2000). The peripheral nervous system (PNS) has three types of cells: neuronal cells, stromal cells, and glial cells. The CNS communicates to the rest of the body through peripheral nerves. Different combinations of motor, sensory, and autonomic neurons make up peripheral nerves. Efferent neurons (motor as well as autonomic) receive information and signals from CNS neurons via dendritic connections, primarily using neurotransmitters. Afferent neurons receive signals from specialized cell types (receptors) via their dendritic connections, such as Pacinian corpuscles for fine sensation (Seddighi et al. 2016; Grinsell and Keating 2014). When a spinal reflex activity is required, these signals are delivered to the CNS to send sensory messages to the brain and to interneurons in the spinal cord (Jobe and Martinez 2013). Fascicules are individual bundles that make up a peripheral nerve. Myelin sheaths cover less than half of peripheral nerve fibers. The remaining unmyelinated fibers run along the surface of Schwann cells in deep gutters. The endoneurium, a network of reticular collagenous fibers, muffles each Schwann cell. The perineurium is a connective tissue layer that wraps around each fascicle. The epineurium, a loose vascular tissue tube, surrounds all of the fascicles (which encloses an individual nerve). Although the endoneurium is longitudinal, the perineurium and epineurium are circular (Sunderland 1990). For irrigation of the axons, micro-vessels (vasa nervosa) divide sequentially across the nerve in line with the structural layers. In the endoneurium, microvascular plexuses travel axially through the epineurium and provide transverse branches into the perineurium, producing a vascular network primarily made up of capillaries. These epineural vessels are more vulnerable to harm than nerve core vessels because of their more peripheral placement (Figure 1) (Seddighi et al. 2016; Grinsell and Keating 2014; Rydevik and Lundborg 1977).

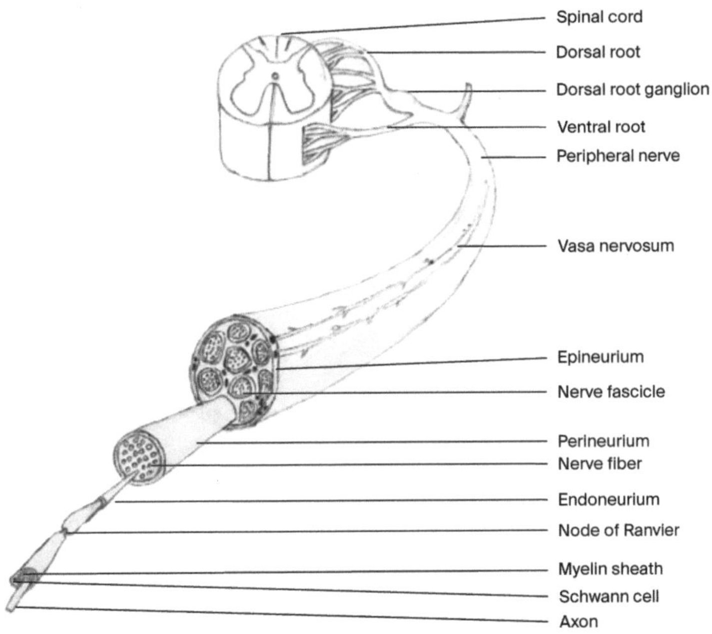

Figure 1. Anatomical organization of a peripheral nerve. Source: Figure by authors.

1.3. Peripheral Nerve Physiology and Trauma Responses

The internal environment of a neuron, like all cells, is diligently controlled. Axoplasmic movement back and forth between the cell body and the axon transports neurotransmitters and structural cell components. Any structural disruption or fault in the axonal or neuronal "lipid bilayer membrane" must be repaired immediately, or an irreversible sequence of apoptosis will begin (Bittner et al. 2000). Axonal degeneration and disintegration occur as a result of a number of events that occur both above and below the traumatic zone. Separated cell bodies and axons (in proximal axon injuries) degenerate through chromatolysis, a type of programmed cell death (apoptosis) (Pfister et al. 2011). From the zone of injury to the sensory or motor receptor, Wallerian degeneration of the distal axonal section of the axon occurs.

Wallerian degeneration takes place 24–48 h following peripheral nerve trauma. Here, both the surrounding myelin and distal axons degenerate (Griffin et al. 2013). The proximal axonal part, likewise, degenerates up to the next neighboring Ranvier node, which is where axonal regeneration occurs. Schwann cells appear as phagocytic cells that phagocytize axonal and myelin debris until there are no more endoneurial tubes. The recruited macrophages release growth factors into the region, stimulating the development of Schwann cells and fibroblasts. Schwann cells form orderly longitudinal columns termed Bungner bands in the empty endoneurial tubes (Pfister et al. 2011). This speed is required for effective axonal regeneration. Axonal regrowth begins at Ranvier's most distal node. A growth cone is formed when 50–100 nodal sprouts mature and elongate distally in response to trophic cues from denervated sensory and motor receptors and local tissue (neurotrophic as well as neurotropic factors) (Lee and Wolfe 2000). In addition, regeneration has motor–axon–motor receptor and sensory–axon–sensory receptor specialization (Grinsell and Keating 2014; Kandel et al. 2000; Brushart 1988). The growth cone also releases protease enzymes to assist axonal regrowth through tissue. Many axonal extensions branch out from the growth cone until they reach a receptor. The surviving neurites are then subjected to axonal pruning. If an endoneurial tube or receptor is not reached, the growth cone branches and grows haphazardly, resulting in a neuroma, which can present as a painful lump (neuroma) (Siemionow and Brzezicki 2009). Studies demonstrate that with severe nerve injury (Pan et al. 2003) axonal regeneration is more disorganized, resulting in fewer axons reaching the distal motor or sensory target due to less optimal axonal regeneration and scarring (Figure 2) (Seddighi et al. 2016; Grinsell and Keating 2014).

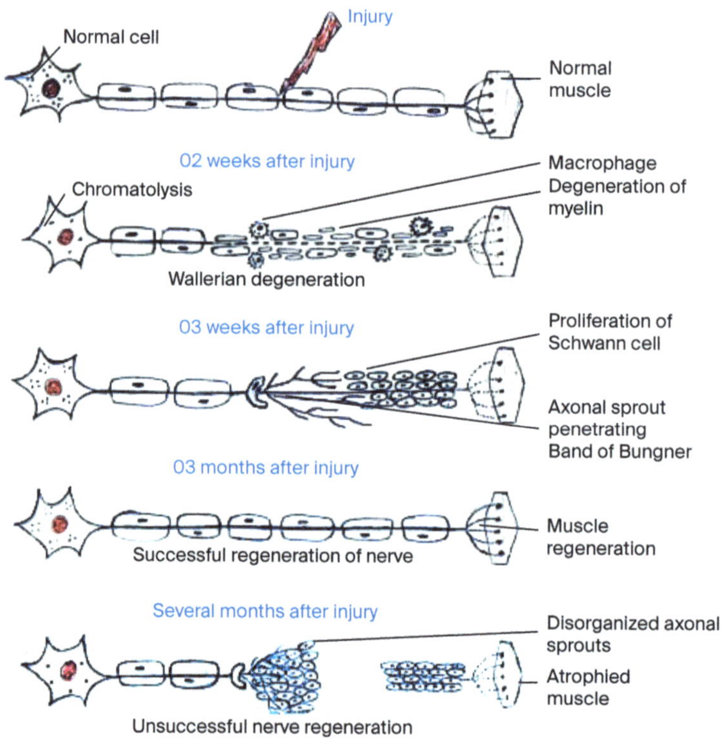

Figure 2. Schematic diagram of degeneration and regeneration of peripheral nerve after injury. Source: Figure by authors.

1.4. Classification of PNI

The Seddon and the Sunderland classifications (Seddighi et al. 2016; Grinsell and Keating 2014; Sunderland 1990; Seddon 1943) are commonly used for PNI, which is shown in Table 1.

Table 1. Classification of PNI.

Seddon Classification		Properties	Sunderland Grade
Neuropraxia		Segmental demyelination	1st degree
Axonotmesis	I	Axon severed but endoneurium intact (ideal condition for regeneration)	2nd degree
	II	Discontinuous axon, discontinuous endoneurial tube, fascicular arrangement, and perineurium preserved	3rd degree
	III	Absence of continuity of endoneurial tubes, axons, perineurium, and fasciculi; intact epineurium (neuroma in continuity)	4th degree
Neurotmesis		Absence of continuity of total nerve trunk	5th degree

Source: Authors' compilation based on data from Seddighi et al. (2016); Grinsell and Keating (2014); Sunderland (1990); Seddon (1943).

1.4.1. Neuropraxia

Neuropraxia (Sunderland grade 1) is the mildest type of PNI, which is a recoverable neuro-conduction interruption that persists for hours to days. Neuropraxia presents with neuro-deficit of the involved nerve. There are minimal or no identifiable histopathologic changes in nerve structure. Early clinical evaluations often demonstrates partial loss of nerve function/s, sparing autonomic function. In patients showing total loss of neuro-function/s, an early single clinical examination cannot differentiate neuropraxia from more serious nerve injuries. PNI grade 1 recovers excellently and spontaneously over days to weeks and seldomly over months (Dumitru et al. 2001; Wilbourn 2002).

1.4.2. Axonotmesis

In axonotmesis-I (Sunderland grade 2) of PNI, the axon is disrupted, but the nerve's connective tissue structures remain relatively unaffected. With low endoneurial edema and fibrosis, the fascicular and endoneurial connective tissue tubes remain intact. Wallerian degeneration takes place in the distal axon following axon division. The proximal axon similarly degenerates for a variable length up to the next Ranvier node. The undamaged endoneurial tube directs the budding terminals of regrowing axons toward the target area. The regrowth rate of a damaged nerve is approximately 1 mm/day or 1 inch/month, which can be utilized for serial clinical assessments of the patient and to estimate the duration to the recovery of function/s. Sunderland grade 2 PNIs normally recover without operation.

Axonotmesis-II (Sunderland grade 3) of PNI occurs when the damage takes place and is confined to endoneurial tubes within the fascicle.

Axonotmesis-III (Sunderland grade 4) of PNI is one where further damage occurs in fascicular tubes and extrafascicular connective tissue. Here, different degrees of interfascicular scaring result in severe obstacles to axonal regeneration, which results in haphazard growth in spite of coarse continuity of the injured nerve. The ultimate traumatic neuroma in injured sites is composed of a connective tissue network entangled with poorly myelinated, fine-caliber axons (Sunderland 1991; Sunderland 1951a; Mackinnon and Dellon 1988).

1.4.3. Neurotmesis (Sunderland Grade 5)

Here, the injured nerve is severed anatomically. It always requires surgical repair, but the timing of surgery is critical. Surgical repair of sharp PNI (e.g., laceration by knife or glass) should be completed within hours to a day or two. A lacerated nerve that has been bluntly wounded should be sutured 3 to 4 weeks following the injury. This time delay permits the longitudinal length of the injury to be completely diagnosed and visible, allowing for nerve clipping to healthy distal and proximal stumps before restoration (Seddighi et al. 2016; Grinsell and Keating 2014; Schmid and Salyapongse 2008; Bittner et al. 2000).

There is no way to tell the differences among the Sunderland grades II and IV without a diagnostic examination. These Sunderland grades are currently solely diagnosed histologically (Pfister et al. 2011).

1.5. Nerve Conduction Studies (NCSs), Electromyograms (EMGs) and MRI

NCSs and EMGs are noninvasive diagnostic procedures that can be used in the case of delayed nerve healing, when muscular fibrillations are present in denervated muscle but not visible right after an injury. As a result, no noninvasive investigative tool can accurately determine the presence or degree (severity) of a PNI in the first few weeks after injury. Clinical examination and/or exploratory surgery are still used to make diagnoses.

NCSs use a voltage stimulator applied to the skin over several locations of the peripheral nerve to be evaluated to examine both sensory and motor function. A surface electrode overlying the muscle bellies supplied by the nerve (motor response) or nerve supply (nervous response) records the evoked response (sensory response).

EMGs are used to assess the electrical activity of resting muscles (the evidence of aberrant spontaneous function such as positive sharp waves and fibrillations) as well as to conduct voluntary motor unit evaluations (Effron and Beasley 2006). Depending on the degree of the injury, fibrillations may not be seen for three to six weeks following PNI (Robinson 2000). NCSs can be performed as a screening test for the absence or presence of conduction blocks, whereas EMGs can provide further data in the form of diminished action potentials (Griffin et al. 2013). So, serial NCSs and EMGs can detect if a PNI is neurapraxic or axonotmetic over time. After three to six months, if there is no spontaneous clinical or NCS/EMG recovery, the nerve must be surgically explored (Grinsell and Keating 2014).

In delayed situations, high-quality MRI imaging (neurograms) in the implicated area/s can reveal the discontinuity of nerves or traumatic neuroma, which can help with surgical decision-making and planning. MRI images are now commonly employed in the treatment of brachial plexus and lumbosacral plexus injuries (Figures 3 and 4).

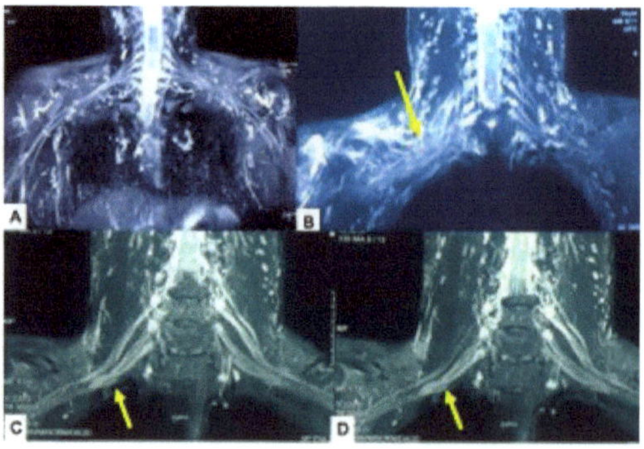

Figure 3. MRI of brachial plexus (BP): (**A**) normal MRI of BP; (**B**) MRI of BP with right-sided pan-brachial plexus injury; and (**C**,**D**) MRI showing right-sided middle and inferior trunks of BP injury. Arrow indicates injury site. Source: Figure by authors.

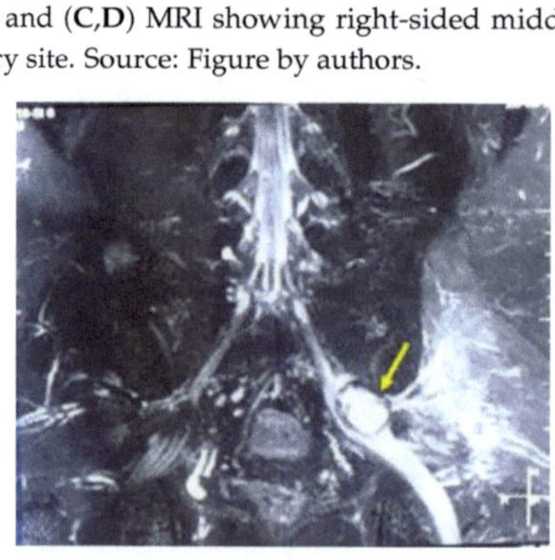

Figure 4. MRI of lumbosacral plexus showing post-stab left lumbosacral trunk injury with neuroma. Arrow indicates injury site. Source: Figure by authors.

1.6. Mechanism of PNI and Neuropathology

PNI increases epineural vascular permeability, which is more sensitive to compression damage than endoneurial arteries, due to its microvascular orientation. Endoneurial arteries are also damaged by sustained and higher pressure levels, as well as more prolonged compression trauma, resulting in intrafascicular edema, which can lead to secondary injury (Hall 2005). PNI can be caused by a variety of traumatic etiologies, including traction, stretch, stab, blow, blunt injury, laceration (transaction), contusion, gunshot wounds, thermal and electrical injuries, compression and ischemia (crush), iatrogenic causes, and injection injuries. Compression damage to nerves is thought to be caused by a variety of causes. Anatomically, restricting a root causes increased tension at that location, compressing blood vessels and causing nerve ischemia, as seen in vasculitis and artherosclorotic disorders (Tapadia et al. 2010; Pham and Gupta 2009).

Crush injuries to the nerve are most commonly caused by compression of the nerve by a blunt item such as a surgical clamp, bat, or another crushing device. Transection injuries (neurotmesis or grade V PNI) are most usually caused by a laceration from a blade, knife, gunshot, or shard of glass (Zochodne and Levy 2005). In actuality, most of these injuries come in a variety of forms (Dellon et al. 1988). Primary exploration and primary microsurgical treatment are the best options for an acute penetrating wound with nerve damage. Most nerve damages from gunshots or high-velocity missile injuries are discovered, contused, or bruised during examination; the contused and divided nerve ends should be sutured to fascial tissue close to each other with a large, non-absorbable suture under moderate distraction (to prevent retraction). Definitive nerve repair should be performed several weeks following the first procedure during secondary exploration (Stanec et al. 1997).

PNI as a result of intramuscular medication injection is a potentially fatal complication. Any nerve can be affected, but the proximal radial nerve and sciatic nerves in the buttocks are the most commonly affected. The needle may cause injury; however, most injuries are due to the toxic effects of the substance delivered into the intraneural region. Traditionally, the needle causes an electric-shock-like sensation down the limb. Severe radiating pain and paresthesia are felt shortly after the medication is injected.

Patients frequently complain afterwards of extreme pain with symptoms such as burning, scalding, and electric-like or numbing discomfort. In a small percentage of instances, delayed onset of neuropathy can develop, with symptoms such as scorching pain, profound discomfort, or annoying paresthesias down the extremity and in the supplying area of the injured nerve. Motor deficiency is generally more common than sensory neuropathic pain when an injury is incomplete (Grinsell and Keating 2014).

1.7. Recovery Time Frame for PNI

Better functional outcomes result from early nerve restoration (Mackinnon 1989). Despite good nerve healing, axonal development is sluggish, averaging only 1–2 mm each day. There is no drug or treatment method for increasing this rate. It takes 12–18 months for muscle reinnervation to achieve functional reinstallation after irreversible motor endplate degeneration (Lee and Wolfe 2000). The sensory renewal process takes longer. For example, ulnar and median nerve lesions at the wrist require axons to regrow over distances of 100 mm (roughly) in order to reach the hand muscles. As a result, functional recovery takes at least one hundred days. More proximal PNIs, such as an upper brachial plexus injury, need nerve regeneration over the gap of up to a meter and take more than 2 to 3 years to reach and reinnervate the arm. Clinically, there may be little or no function restoration in such instances. The target tissue and distal nerve remain denervated during this time because neurons lack target connections (Pfister et al. 2011). Muscle atrophy and fibrosis begin shortly following denervation and reach a halt after 04 months, when 60 to 80% of muscle mass has disappeared (Lee and Wolfe 2000). Although motor endplates develop within the muscle, functional reinnervation is improbable beyond twelve months as a result of fibrosis (Lee and Wolfe 2000). Chronic axotomy of the neurons as well as chronic Schwann cell denervation can cause axon regeneration to fail after PNI (Pfister et al. 2011).

1.8. Treatment Approaches

In the clinical context, the emergency management of a patient with suspected PNI differs dramatically from that of a patient who is in elective or even urgent care. Priority is always given to life-threatening airway, pulmonary, circulatory, and CNS trauma in any acute trauma patient (according to ATLS recommendations) before extremity injuries are handled. Nerve injuries (5%) and brachial plexus injuries (1%) are rather prevalent in polytrauma patients. In more than 60% of cases, this PNI can be detected during the initial clinical phase (trauma encounter).

An asymmetrical neurological finding, with absence of function restricted to one extremity when associated with loss of DTRs, is frequently related to PNI in trauma patients with an altered level of consciousness (Dahlin 2006; Battiston et al. 2009). Nerve function recovery is mostly determined by the nerve's underlying neuropathologic condition; those with a big neurotmetic element seldom recover; however, those with axonotmetic or neuropraxic pathology, or both, may do so over time. The major justification for surgical investigation is a lack of nerve continuity, either clinically or electrophysiologically (Aguayo et al. 1973; Shokrzadeh et al. 2010). The mechanism of injury helps determine the best time to investigate a continuous nerve injury. More focal injuries, such as those caused by gunshot wounds, stab wounds, iatrogenic causes, lacerations, and fracture-related contusions, should be investigated 2 to 3 months following the initial injury (Thomsen and Dahlin 2007). In grade 3 PNI, clinical outcomes range from no recovery to a full restoration of function. In grade 4 PNI, on the other hand, a neuroma in continuity is the most dangerous pathology. Unless surgical excision and repair are considered, functional recovery is rare (Diao and Vannuyen 2000). PNI caused by injection is treated using the same criteria as any other patient with a continuous nerve lesion. The majority of partial and some complete PNIs regenerate without surgery, with early function recovery seeming to be the most important prognostic indicator in these instances. Patients who do not recover spontaneously after 4 months, and those patients with medically refractory neuropathic pain, may be candidates for surgical intervention, including internal and external neurolysis and nerve repair, based on intraoperative results (Seddighi et al. 2016; Grinsell and Keating 2014)

1.8.1. Nerve Repair

For severe axonotmesis and neurotmesis, epineural microsuturing is the mainstay surgical treatment for traumatic peripheral nerve repair (Figures 5–8). This repair should take place in a tension-free, well-vascularized bed. Gross fascicular alignment and matching should be present, as should correct surface epineural vasa nervosum orientation.

Intra-nerve dissection, direct fascicular matching, and fascicular group suturing are all required for group fascicular repair. Intraneural trauma and scarring can obstruct neural regrowth, and this can happen with a major nerve in the distal limb (Lundborg 2000).

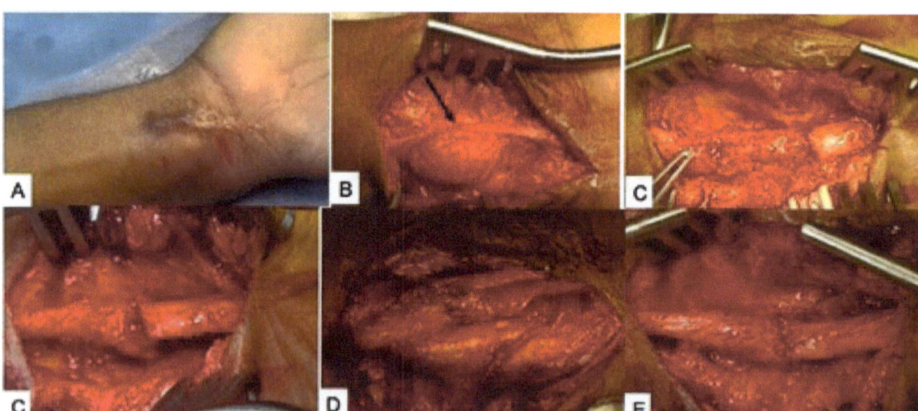

Figure 5. Sequential peroperative images: (**A**) post-traumatic median nerve neuroma at wrist; (**B**) operative exposure of neuroma and nerve; arrow indicating neuroma (**C**) neuroma excision; and (**D–F**) epineural repair of nerve without graft. Source: Figure by authors.

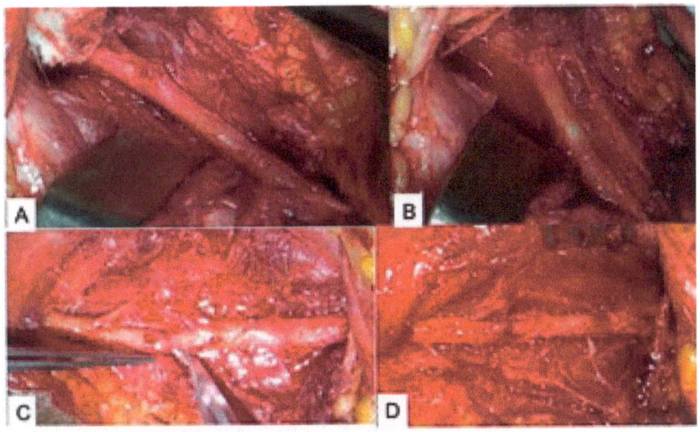

Figure 6. Peroperative sequential images of post-traumatic exposure of radial nerve at midarm (axonotmesis-III). (A–D) Exposure, identification of pathological part, excision and trimming of scar and neuroma, and direct epineural repair. Source: Figure by authors.

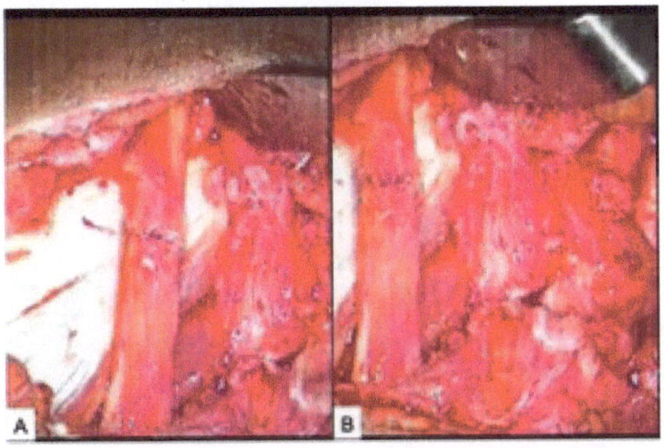

Figure 7. (A,B) Epineural repair of transected common peroneal nerve at popliteal fossa. Source: Figure by authors.

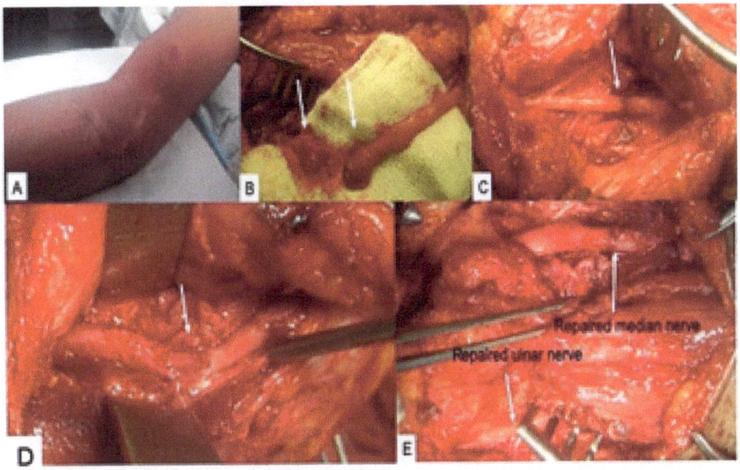

Figure 8. (A) Post-RTA injury of both ulnar and median nerve at and around elbow. (B) Neurotmesis of ulnar nerve; arrows showing both end of ulnar nerve (C) Epineural repair with anterior transposition of ulnar nerve; arrow indicating suture line (D,E) Exposure of median nerve with the same incision (axonotmesis), excision of scar, and epineural repair. Source: Figure by authors.

When there is an interval between the injured nerve ends, and excessive strain is needed for direct epineural healing, nerve grafting is employed; reversed interposition autologous nerve grafts (such as for the sural nerve) are required (Figures 5–13) (Pfister et al. 2011). Single, cable, trunk, interfascicular, and vascularized autologous nerve cable grafts are available. A single graft connects the nerve interval with a donor nerve segment of a similar width. Cable grafts, which use numerous lengths of a lesser-diameter donor nerve, in order to approximate the diameter of the injured peripheral nerve, are used to bridge gaps between large diameter nerves. Expensive sensory nerves, such as the sural and medial antebrachial nerves, are used as donor nerve grafts and are employed in a reversed orientation (Colen et al. 2009). A damaged recipient tissue bed that will not tolerate a non-vascularized nerve transplant will receive a vascularized nerve graft (Terzis and Kostopoulos 2010).

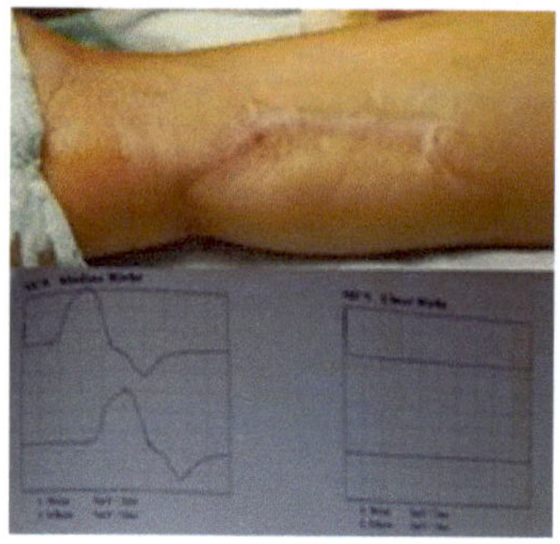

Figure 9. Upper picture showing post-family-violence ulnar nerve injury at wrist and lower forearm. Lower picture showing NCS showing normal activity of median nerve and no activity of ulnar nerve in the same patient of upper picture. Source: Figure by authors.

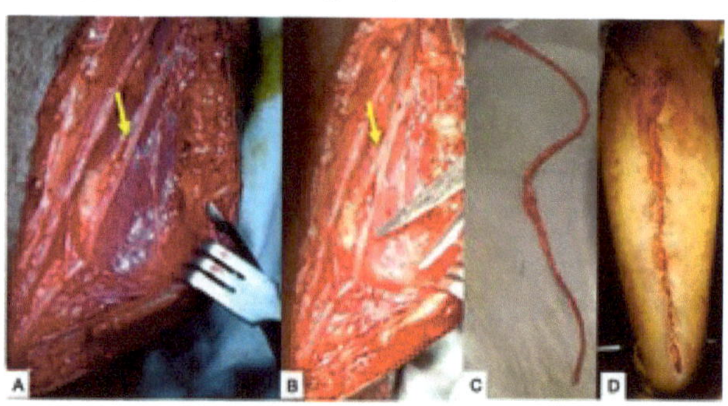

Figure 10. Peroperative pictures of patient of Figure 9: (**A**,**B**) exposure and dissection of sural nerve, arrow indicating sural nerve (**C**) sural nerve after procurement, and (**D**) closure of leg wound after sural nerve procurement. Source: Figure by authors.

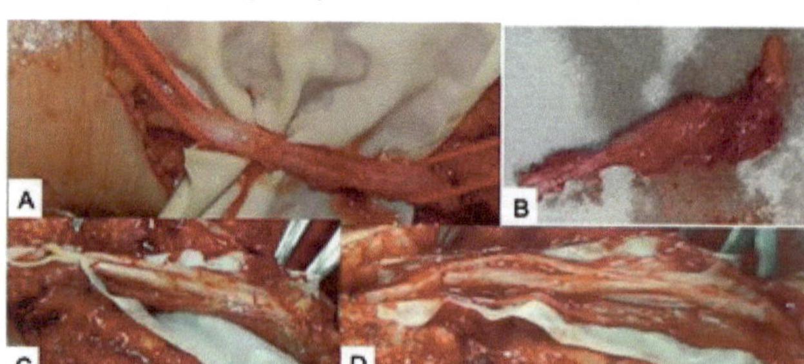

Figure 11. Peroperative pictures of patient of Figure 9. Sequential peroperative images: (**A**) exposure of ulnar nerve, (**B**) excision of neuroma and scar, and (**C**,**D**) "Cables grafting repair" of ulnar nerve by sural nerve graft strands using interfascicular (perineural) sutures. Source: Figure by authors.

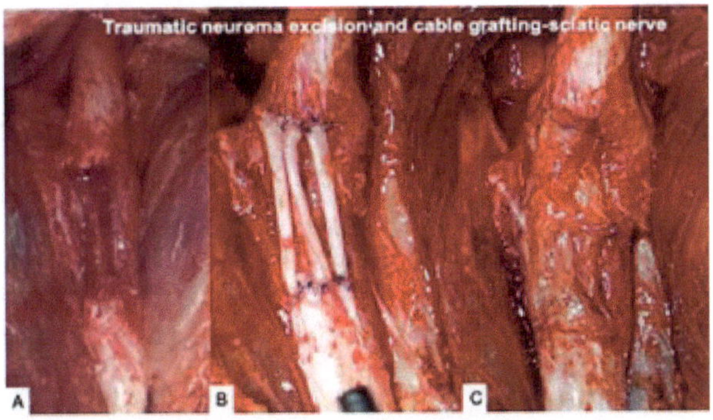

Figure 12. Peroperative pictures of repair of a sciatic nerve (tibial portion injured only) at upper popliteal fossa: (**A**) excision of traumatic neuroma from tibial part of sciatic nerve, (**B**) interfascicular "cable nerve grafting" repair of tibial nerve by sural nerve graft, and (**C**) fascial covering of repaired nerve. Source: Figure by authors.

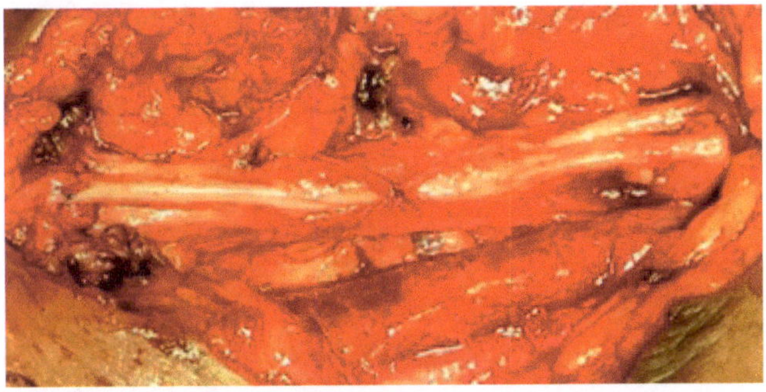

Figure 13. Peroperative picture of interfascicular "cable nerve grafting" repair of sciatic nerve by sural nerve graft at upper thigh. Source: Figure by authors.

The autologous nerve graft passes through Wallerian degeneration, providing only mechanical guidance and a foster structure for axon regeneration (Millesi 1990). Autologous nerve grafts meet the characteristics of an ideal nerve conduit as they elicit a stimulating and permissive environment that includes neurotrophic factors, Schwann cell basal laminae, and adhesion molecules (Siemionow and Brzezicki 2009). Although autografts burn a working nerve (sensory), they are used to replace a more essential wounded nerve (usually motor). At the donor location, there is frequently sensory deficiency and scarring, as well as the possibility of painful neuroma formation (Moore et al. 2009). Fascicle and size mismatch, tissue handling, suture scarring and fibrosis, and the injury itself, as well as any of these factors at the repair site, can all result in poor PNI regeneration. A surgical rule of thumb is that each repair site loses 30–50% of its axons. As a result, roughly 50–70% of the original axons will effectively regrow across the suture line after initial nerve repair. Approximately 25–40% of axons regrow successfully through a nerve transplant with two coaptation sites. Due to persistent axotomy and muscle fibrosis, there will be further axonal loss based on the gap to the sensory/motor target. Numerous conduits and allogenic nerve grafts have been described; however, none of them have proven similar or superior results.

1.8.2. Factors That Dictate the Results of Nerve Repair

Motor axons must be properly attached to motor endplates and axons must land on sensory receptors for functional nerve regeneration. Nerve autografts produce fewer favorable results than original nerve repair. Grafts that extend above the elbow, are longer than 7 cm, are older, and take longer to heal are all bad signs (Lee and Wolfe 2000). The abstract of nerve repair is that early nerve repairs are more result-oriented than late repairs; primary repair is better than the nerve grafts; younger people do better than older people; the distal repair is more effective than the proximal repair; and the short grafts perform better than the long grafts (Sunderland 1990).

1.8.3. Surgical Alternatives to Nerve Repair

Nerve Transfers (Neurotization)

There are alternatives to utilizing healthy donor nerves to treat affected peripheral nerve networks. This is appropriate in injuries to the very proximal nerves and in those who do not have a proximal nerve segment/stump, such as cervical spinal nerve root avulsions. The microsurgical coaptation of a normally functioning nerve donor to an injured nerve is known as nerve transfer/neurotization (Lee and Wolfe 2012). Neurotization is commonly used to regenerate key motor nerves, but it can also be utilized to regenerate critical peripheral sensory nerves. It connects a less-significant limb muscle to a disposable motor donor nerve. The nerve is severed and subsequently attached to the more essential motor nerve's wounded distal end (Seddighi et al. 2016; Grinsell and Keating 2014).

Free Functioning Muscle Transfer

It is a reconstructive treatment for severe and late PNIs, particularly those that have failed after primary surgery, and is a form of free functioning muscle transfer (FFMT) (Siemionow and Brzezicki 2009). A healthy muscle and its neurovascular pedicle are moved to a new site to perform a new function (Carlsen et al. 2009). This could be utilized in a situation when both the nerve and the muscle have been destroyed by a serious acute injury or derangement caused by chronic axotomy as well as muscular fibrosis. Transferring a functioning motor nerve to the FFMT's nerve and restoring the muscle's circulation through microsurgical vascular anastomosis to recipient vessels empowers the muscle. Within a few months, the donor nerve neurotizes the transferred muscle, allowing it to operate independently (Seddighi et al. 2016; Grinsell and Keating 2014).

1.9. Conclusions

In the last half-century, very minor improvements in surgical technique have been made and epineural initial repair remains the gold standard. Microsurgical nerve repair, with end-to-end direct repair or by employing interposition autologous nerve grafts where there is unnecessary strain, is the key to satisfactory results.

2. Peripheral Nerve Tumor Surgery

2.1. Introduction

Peripheral nerve tumors are a diversified group composed of non-neural sheath neoplasms, nerve sheath neoplasms, and sometime non-neoplastic masses (Kokkalis et al. 2019; Seol et al. 2009; Chowdhury et al. 2008b). Nerve tumors of the peripheral nervous system may develop anywhere in the body. Although several cases of malignant peripheral nerve tumors have been reported in the literature (Prudner et al. 2020), the majority of them are benign. Peripheral nerve tumors can take several forms. These tumors could grow within nerves (intraneural tumors) or press against them (extraneural tumors) (Kokkalis et al. 2019; Seol et al. 2009).

2.2. Clinical Presentation and Diagnostic Approach

Swelling or a lump along the course of the peripheral nerve; pain, tingling sensations, or numbness; loss of function in the affected area or weakness; and loss of balance or dizziness are all common clinical symptoms of a peripheral nerve tumor. Depending on the clinical presentation, patients should be thoroughly checked, with particular attention paid to any indicators that may be linked to the presenting symptoms. When a tumor is first noticed, any changes in shape and size, the rate of increasing growth, and any probable B-symptoms that can be attributed to the original diagnosis should be investigated and recorded. It is also worth noting whether there is a family history of tumors. Furthermore, it is important to define whether the symptoms are due to specific events. Following that, a thorough clinical evaluation should be accomplished, beginning with the examination of the tumor and ending with filing of the findings. Regardless of the type of the tumor, regional lymph nodes should be checked on a regular basis. The bulk of clinical symptoms are caused by the tumor mass itself, either through intraneural invasion or involvement of the peripheral nerve, or by the surrounding tissues, primarily due to its size (Kokkalis et al. 2019; Chowdhury et al. 2008b; Mrugala et al. 2005).

2.3. Imaging

The first-choice investigation methods for such tumors are diagnostic ultrasonography (U/S) and MRI. To begin, ultrasound can be utilized to determine the form, integrity, matrix, and size of the mass. More comprehensive observations and features can be obtained by combining MRI imaging of the mass with a neurogram (Figures 14–18). However, tissue biopsy of the tumor is crucial in the end. When a malignant tumor is suspected in peripheral nerve tumors, biopsy is recommended, and tissue biopsy is required to plan the definitive treatment (Sacks et al. 2013; Hsu et al. 2007; Plate et al. 2006; Mavrogenis et al. 2017). The oncological principles of biopsy should be followed during the procedure (Mavrogenis et al. 2014; Webber 2014). It goes without saying that any oncological case is approached as a collaborative effort by dedicated and experienced treating surgeons. Nerve Conduction Tests (NCTs) performed before surgery are not always accurate, but intraoperative electrophysiological monitoring is critical (Kokkalis et al. 2019; Chowdhury et al. 2011).

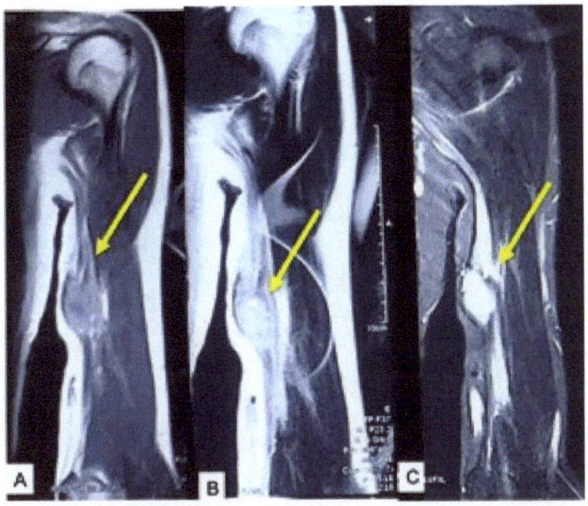

Figure 14. (**A–C**) MRI images of arm showing median nerve schwannoma (arrow-marked). Source: Figure by authors.

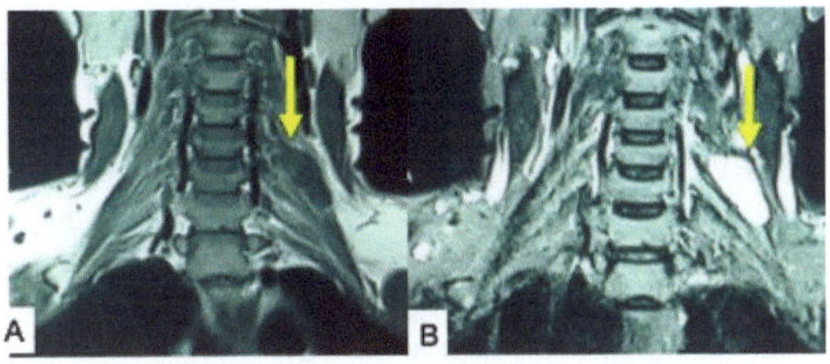

Figure 15. (**A,B**) MRI of brachial plexus showing schwannoma(arrow-marked) of left upper trunk. Source: Figure by authors.

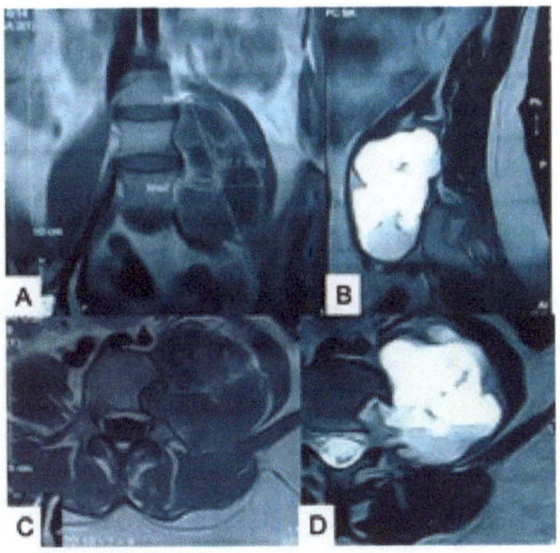

Figure 16. MRI of images: (**A**) coronal, (**B**) sagittal, and (**C,D**) axial images showing left lumbar plexus schwannoma. Source: Figure by authors.

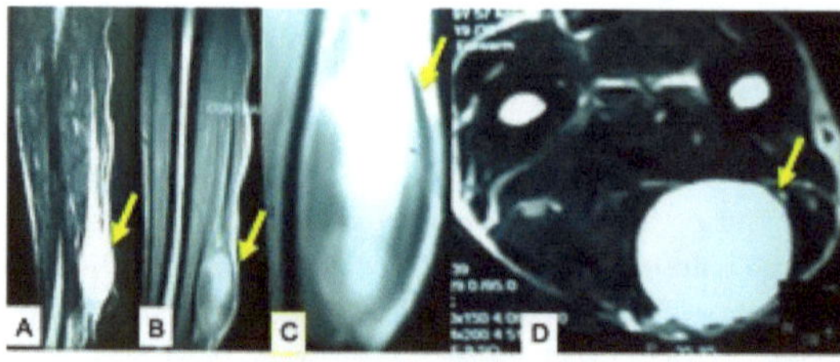

Figure 17. MRI images of thigh: (**A–C**) sagittal and (**D**) axial images showing sciatic nerve schwannoma (arrow-marked) at lower thigh. Source: Figure by authors.

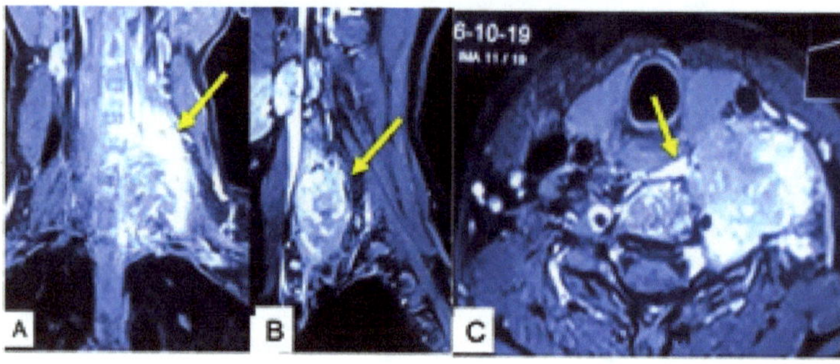

Figure 18. (**A–C**) Contrast MRI of brachial plexus (coronal, sagittal and axial view) showing malignant peripheral nerve sheath tumor (MPNST) (histologically proved) of left brachial plexus (arrow-marked). Source: Figure by authors.

2.4. Benign Neoplasms of Nerve Sheaths or Nerve Sheath Tumors

2.4.1. Schwannoma

Schwannomas are slow-growing nerve sheath neoplasms with no known cause, unless they are associated with neurofibromatosis syndrome (Antonescu et al. 2013). They are Schwann cells that have been encapsulated. Antoni A area of highly organized cellular elements and Antoni B area of loose myxoid elements are biphasic sheath tumors with two components. These two areas' component percentages differ. They can strike at any age, although they are commoner in the 4th to 6th decades (Antonescu et al. 2013). About 90% of schwannomas are sporadic, with 3% in cases with neurofibromatosis-2 (NF-2), 2% in cases with schwannomatosis (of which a very small percentage had familial schwannomatosis), and 5% in patients with or without NF-2 in combination with multiple meningiomas (1% with and 4% without) (Antinheimo et al. 2000). Multiple schwannomas can occur in NF-2 syndrome and in Gorlin–Koutlas syndrome (Antonescu et al. 2013; Goldblum et al. 2014). S-100 protein immunohistochemistry contributes to the differentiation from neurofibromas. Schwannomas are usually benign, yet there have been a few reports of malignant alterations (Chowdhury et al. 2010; Rasbridge et al. 1989; Woodruff et al. 1994; McMenamin and Fletcher 2001). Neurofibromatosis is a group of genetically determined disorders (phakomatoses) that is divided into two types: neurofibromatosis-1 (NF-1) and neurofibromatosis-2 (NF-2) (NF-2). A schwannoma is a slow-growing neoplasm that often goes unnoticed for several years before being diagnosed (frequently in peripheral nerves of the subcutaneous tissues and skin of the neck, head, or the flexor surfaces of the limbs) (Chowdhury et al. 2011; Antonescu et al. 2013). Spinal schwannoma is a less common cancer (Zhang et al. 2018). Large tumors cause neurologic symptoms and pain, which are caused by the mass effect. If the neoplasm begins in the nerve sheath, it is encased in a capsule made up of nerve fibers and epineurium (Goldblum et al. 2014). On T1-weighted imaging, schwannomas have a medium signal intensity, while T2-weighted imaging shows a hyperintense signal (Figures 14–17) (Crist et al. 2017). To avoid or reduce neuro-deficits, it is critical to properly detect the incoming and outgoing fascicles, nerve fibers encountered during microsurgery (Kim et al. 2004) (Figures 19–21). Though rare, the occurrence of a schwannoma in the retroperitoneum has been documented (Figure 16) (Khandakar et al. 2014).

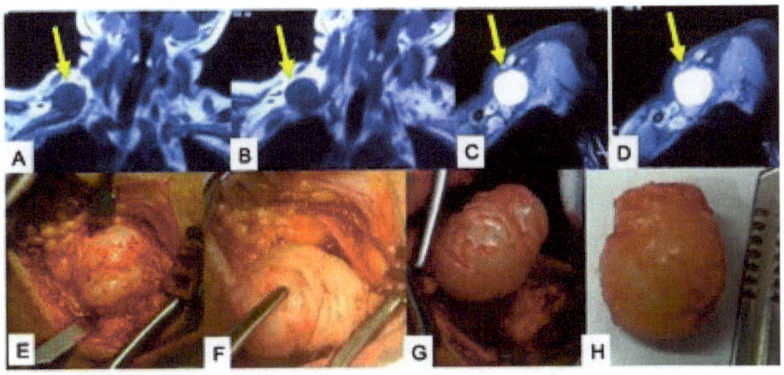

Figure 19. (**A–D**) MRI images showing a right brachial plexus schwannoma (arrow-marked). (**E–H**) Peroperative pictures of the removal of the schwannoma. Source: Figure by authors.

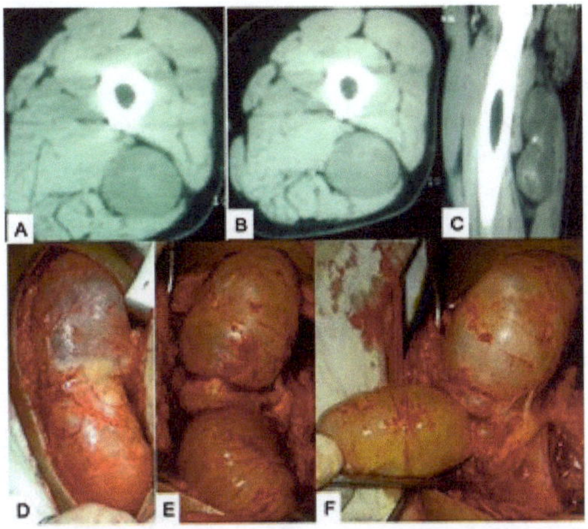

Figure 20. (**A–C**) CT scan of thigh showing a dumbbell-shaped femoral nerve schwannoma. (**D–F**) Sequential images of the removal of the schwannoma. Source: Figure by authors.

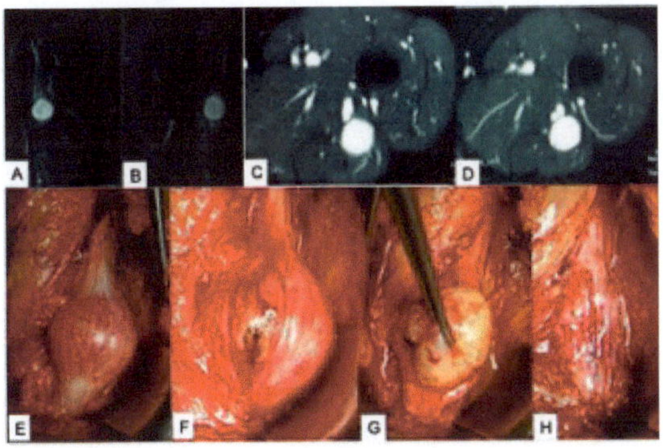

Figure 21. (**A–D**) Contrast MRI of thigh showing a sciatic nerve schwannoma. (**E–G**) Sequential peroperative images of the removal of the schwannoma. (**H**) After removal of the tumor. Source: Figure by authors.

2.4.2. Cellular Schwannoma

Cellular schwannoma is a type of schwannoma that is distinguished by the absence of Verocay structures in Antoni A tissue. They are found in the paravertebral spaces, retroperitoneum, mediastinum, and pelvis, with about 25% in the limbs (Goldblum et al. 2014). Cellular schwannoma was initially misdiagnosed as a low-grade malignant peripheral nerve sheath tumor (MPNST); however, its benign nature has since been confirmed (White et al. 1990; Casadei et al. 1995; Lodding et al. 1990).

2.4.3. Plexiform Schwannoma

Plexiform schwannomas are extremely rare; however, they can cause brachial plexus involvement. They do not change into a cancerous state (unlike plexiform neurofibromas) (Kokkalis et al. 2019; Chowdhury et al. 2008a).

2.4.4. Melanotic Schwannoma

Melanotic schwannomas can become cancerous (unlike other variants of schwannoma). The tumor, which originates from the sympathetic nervous system, is an adult neoplasm characterized by Schwann cells that produce varying amounts of melanin. Psammoma bodies are spherical, laminated bodies that indicate psammomatous melanotic schwannomas (Antonescu et al. 2013; Goldblum et al. 2014; Millar 1932; Fu et al. 1975; Carney 1990; Keskin et al. 2017).

2.4.5. Neurofibroma

Neurofibromas are the most prevalent PNSTs, and they are made up of perineurial-like cells, Schwann cells, fibroblasts, mast cells, and unmyelinated and myelinated axons entangled in a matrix. The World Health Organization (WHO) classifies neurofibromas into five types. The commonest are "localized subcutaneous", which affects the subcutaneous tissues and dermis, with 90% of cases being sporadic and 10% being linked to NF-1; "diffuse cutaneous", which also affects subcutaneous tissues and the dermis; and "localized intraneural", which affects the spinal, cranial, or autonomic nerves sporadically or in association with NF-1. The remaining two types of tissue are only linked to NF-1: "plexiform" and "massive soft" tissue. The "localized cutaneous" has no malignant potential, while the others are prone to cancer (the plexiform neurofibroma to has the highest risk). Certain clinical criteria have been established for the diagnosis of NF-1 and NF-2 (Pilavaki et al. 2004; Longo et al. 2018; Evans et al. 1992). Neuroimaging can aid in the observation and monitoring of the characteristics and appearance of tumors over the course of treatment. The presence of the so-called "target sign" on T2-weighted imaging, which is a central hypointense area attributed to the fibrous and collagen component, is highly indicative but not pathognomonic of the neurofibroma (Patel and Stacy 2012). Moreover, the "reverse target sign" can be seen on T1W images as a central component enhancement (Patel and Stacy 2012). The function of positron emission tomography (PET) in clinical decision-making and evaluation is critical in circumstances where the neurosurgeon must closely monitor all nodular lesions (Meany et al. 2013). The symptoms as well as the clinical and radiological appearances of the malignancies guide treatment. Surgical resection is the primary option if the patient is symptomatic and the diagnosis is unknown. Systematic therapy can help to stabilize plexiform neurofibromas (Packer et al. 2002; Chowdhury et al. 2008b). The final outcome is heavily dependent on factors such as the tumor's location, extent, and involvement, as well as the nerve functional state prior to surgery. The incidence of malignant transformation is a point of contention because the exact incidence is unknown. Individuals with NF-1 face a lifetime risk of malignant transformation (Kokkalis et al. 2019; Hirbe and Gutmann 2014).

2.4.6. Perineurioma

Perineurioma is a rare nerve sheath neoplasm made up totally of perineural cells that develops in middle age. Only a few occurrences have been documented in the literature (Hornick and Fletcher 2005). As sclerosing and reticular tumors, they are either intraneural or extraneural. Localized hypertrophic neuropathy was the name given to intraneural perineuriomas, although they were recognized as real neoplastic lesions based on the presence of perineural cells in the epithelial membrane antigen (EMA) and S-100 protein immunostaining in cross section imaging (Goldblum et al. 2014; Tsang et al. 1992). Perineurioma intraneural is a benign tumor. Muscle weakness or nerve problems are drawing clinical attention to the presence of malignancies. There have been no definitive guidelines established for their management. Even though both are rare, extraneural (soft tissue) perineurioma is more common than intraneural perineurioma (Hornick and Fletcher 2005). Soft-tissue perineuriomas are typically 4 cm in diameter (Goldblum et al. 2014; Hornick and Fletcher 2005). Treatment is similar to that of an intraneural lesion, with the exception that perineuriomas are benign tumors. Sclerosing perineurioma is a rarer kind of perineurioma that solely affects the hand (Goldblum et al. 2014; Fetsch and Miettinen 1997).

2.4.7. Hybrid Nerve Sheath Tumour

The WHO classification of hybrid nerve sheath tumors (HNSTs) was adopted in 2013 and 2016. HNSTs combine the properties of multiple PNST types. The commonest variety is schwannoma/perineurioma, which appears on its own, whereas schwannoma/neurofibroma is linked to neurofibromatosis. Hybrid PNSTs are linked to tumoral syndromes, so neurosurgeons should be cautious (25% of cases with NF-2, whereas the percentage is higher in cases with NF-1, which have tumors with hybrid characteristics) (Antonescu et al. 2013; Antonescu et al. 2016; Ud Din et al. 2019; Harder et al. 2012; Kacerovska et al. 2013).

2.4.8. Nerve Sheath Myxomas (NSMs)/Dermal Nerve Sheath Myxomas

NSM was once referred to as a myxoid variety of neurothekeoma, although it is a benign tumor that is not related to neurothekeoma (Antonescu et al. 2013; Fetsch et al. 2005). It is a type of fibrohistiocytic tumor known as neurothekeoma (Sheth et al. 2011). It is mostly found in the dermis and subdermis layers, with the dorsal paravertebral space being a rare exception (Malkoc et al. 2014). NSM is most common in the limbs, with the digits accounting for roughly 35% of all cases (Fetsch et al. 2005). NSMs are small, slowly developing masses that are usually asymptomatic (except diffuse pain in the involved region). According to Fetsch et al., over half of the patients who received surgical resection experienced one or more recurrences but no proof of malignant change was obtained (Fetsch et al. 2005).

2.4.9. Granular Cell Tumor

Granular Cell Tumors are a type of benign nerve sheath tumor that is modest in size, typically found in the skin, neck, soft tissue of the head, and limbs, as well as the viscera. Surgical excision and nerve grafting are used in treatment (if needed). The recurrence rate is almost 8% (Cheng et al. 2016; Smolle et al. 1985; Adeniran et al. 2004; Wadhwa et al. 2014; Davis 2007).

2.4.10. Benign Triton Tumor

Benign triton tumors (BTTs) are tumors of neural and mature skeletal muscle cells that have only a few reported occurrences. They are also known as hamartomatas. They are more likely to affect big peripheral nerves or plexuses, such as the sacral and brachial plexuses. They are more common in childhood or early childhood (Antonescu et al. 2013; Amita et al. 2013). Symptoms of peripheral neuropathy usually led to a diagnosis (Kokkalis et al. 2019).

2.4.11. Nerve Sheath Ganglions/Intraneural Ganglions

Ganglia are more of a degenerative change than a true tumor. Nerve Sheath Ganglia are cystic forms seen in the epineurium of peripheral nerves that contain transparent, jelly-like fluid. The peroneal nerve is the most typical location of involvement; however, there have been reports of other peripheral nerve involvement as well. The cystic formation is associated with a localized expansion of the nerve. Symptoms arise as a result of the cyst's compression impact. Local surgical excision is one approach, while cyst decompression is an appropriate alternative in cases when nerve integrity is at danger (Goldblum et al. 2014; Gillies and Burrows 1991; Ratanshi et al. 2018).

2.4.12. Benign Neoplasms of Non-Nerve-Sheath Origin or Benign Non-Nerve Sheath Tumors (BNNSTs) of Peripheral Nerves

Lipofibromatous Hamartoma of the Nerves

The median nerve and its digital branches are affected by lipofibromatous hamartoma of the nerves (LHN), also known as neural fibrolipoma (Mavrogenis et al. 2017). It has been linked to macrodactyly or macrodystrophia lipomatosa during birth, according to reports. On T1- and T2-weighted MRI images, LHN exhibits a distinct "cable-like" appearance. Excision is rarely recommended since the tumor is "imbedded" inside the nerve fibers. In symptomatic patients, nerve decompression is advised (Antonescu et al. 2013; Chiang et al. 2010; Uchiyama et al. 2016; Mishra et al. 2017; Tahiri et al. 2013).

Desmoid-Type Fibromatosis

Desmoid-type fibromatosis (DTF) in peripheral nerves is a dangerous neoplasm defined by benign fibroblast infiltration. These tumors appear as a firm mass due to the fibrous tissue. In the literature, sporadic occurrences of DTF have been reported (Ferraresi et al. 2001; Siqueira et al. 2012). These are frequently symptomatic, but there is no consensus on the best therapy; hence, each case should be handled individually based on the symptom(s) (Kokkalis et al. 2019).

Hemangioblastoma

Hemangioblastoma is an uncommon start tumor that affects about 25% of people with von Hippel–Lindau (VHL) syndrome. Even though the majority of cases occur in the CNS, cases from peripheral areas have been documented. Patients with neuro-deficiency symptoms present with increasing neurological symptoms. The standard treatment is surgical removal with clear margins (Doyle and Fletcher 2014; Giannini et al. 1998; Mitchell et al. 2013).

Traumatic Neuromas

Traumatic neuromas are benign tumors that develop after neurotmesis owing to a lack of endoneurium tubes that carry nerve regeneration signals (Figure 5). The important variables in the formation of a traumatic neuroma are axonal regeneration, development, and dissemination. "Traumatic Neuropathic Pain" and dysesthesia are two of the most unpleasant symptoms to deal with. As a mass, a traumatic neuroma appears to be a hard, sometimes painful nodule. Several therapeutic options have been offered, including nerve repair, neuroma excision, neuromodulation, and functional pain surgery, with mixed results (Oliveira et al. 2018; Yao et al. 2017; Kang et al. 2016).

Tumor-like Lesions

Neuritis ossificans or intraneural heterotopic ossification: Intraneural heterotopic ossification has a small number of reports (IHO). A case of neuritis ossificans, or IHO, was reported by Woltman et al. in 1946 and Catalano et al. in 1992 (Woltman and Adson 1946; Catalano et al. 1992). Apposition of fibrovascular tissue along with an intermediate zone of osteoid and a periphery of ossification microscopically characterizes this uncommon lesion. Trauma has been proposed as a risk factor. The clinical evaluation should look for painful mononeuropathy, progressive muscular weakness, focal swelling, and the course of the engaged nerve (Muzaffar et al. 2012; McCarthy and Sundaram 2005; George et al. 2002). When the probability of cancer is doubtful, a biopsy should be performed (as specific varieties of osteoblastic sarcomas exist). IHO is treated symptomatically, and various criteria must be examined in order to avoid iatrogenic nerve injury (Kokkalis et al. 2019).

Inflammatory pseudotumor (IPT) of nerves: IPT is rare and can be mistaken for a variety of malignant and benign neoplasms. IPT was first discovered in the lungs, but it has since been found in practically every anatomic region. It is uncommon in the neck and head, although it most commonly involves the orbit. Pseudotumors of the skull base are uncommon and often act aggressively, resembling a neoplasm (Seol et al. 2009; Chowdhury et al. 2008a).

2.5. Malignant Peripheral Nerve Sheath Tumors (MPNSTs)

2.5.1. Introduction

Sarcomas that arise from peripheral nerves or cells linked to the nerve sheath, such as Schwann cells, fibroblasts, or perineural cells, are known as malignant peripheral nerve sheath tumors (MPNSTs). Because MPNSTs may come from a variety of cell types, the physical appearance can differ greatly from case to case. An MPNST is defined as a sarcoma that originates from a neurofibroma or peripheral nerve. Neurofibrosarcoma, malignant schwannoma, and neurogenic sarcoma are some of the terms that have been used in the past (Prudner et al. 2020; Weiss and Goldblum 2001). When at least one of the following conditions is met, a sarcoma is classified as an MPNST (Prudner et al. 2020):

1. It is caused by a peripheral nerve;
2. It develops from a benign nerve sheath neoplasm that already exists (neurofibroma);
3. On histologic examination, it indicates Schwann cell differentiation.

2.5.2. Epidemiology

MPNSTs are responsible for about 5–10% of all soft-tissue sarcomas. They can exist on their own or in conjunction with NF1. The cause is unknown; however, radiation exposure is a risk factor (Adamson and

Friedman 2004; Amin et al. 2004; Ducatman et al. 1986; Loree et al. 2000). Patients with NF1 account for up to 50% of MPNSTs. NF1 individuals have a 1–2% prevalence of MPNSTs. NF-1 patients have a 10% chance of developing an MPNST in their lifetime. MPNSTs usually strike in adulthood, between the ages of 20 and 50, but they can strike at any age (D'Agostino et al. 1963; King et al. 2000; Huson and Harper 1989; Evans et al. 2002; Ducatman et al. 1984; Ellison et al. 2005).

2.5.3. Clinical Features of MPNSTs

An MPNST usually manifest as a palpable mass that grows in size. The intensity of pain varies. Rapid expansion is more common in the presence of NF1 and should raise concerns about a neurofibroma's malignant change. MPNSTs originating from peripheral nerves can cause radicular discomfort, paresthesias, and motor dysfunction, among other symptoms. The brachial plexus, the sciatic nerve, and the sacral plexus are also examples of major peripheral nerves that grow in tandem with MPNSTs (Prudner et al. 2020).

2.5.4. Imaging

The preferred imaging method is magnetic resonance imaging (MRI). MPNSTs share several imaging features with their benign counterparts. A longitudinal orientation and a fusiform shape in the line of the nerve are two of them. There are, nevertheless, certain distinctions to be made. MPNSTs are more likely to have large tumors (>5 cm), heterogeneity, invasion of fat planes, poorly defined margins, and edema around the lesion (Figure 18) (Friedrich et al. 2005; Pilavaki et al. 2004). The preferred imaging examination for screening for metastases is a chest computed tomography. A bone scan is also recommended to aid in the detection of metastatic bone disease (Prudner et al. 2020). FDG PET assesses the metabolic activity of tumors and metastases (Hruban et al. 1990).

2.5.5. MPNST Staging

Staging identifies the most important aspects of a tumor, allowing for proper planning and therapy. Histologic grade, tumor depth, tumor size, and the absence or presence of metastases all play a role in staging soft-tissue sarcomas (Table 2). The biggest indicators of eventual metastases in the absence of observable metastases are tumor size, histologic grade, and tumor depth (Prudner et al. 2020).

Table 2. The American Joint Committee on Cancer (AJCC) staging system for soft-tissue sarcoma, 6th edition.

Stage	Size	Depth	Grade	Metastases
I	Any	Any	Low	No
II	<5 cm, any depth OR >5 cm	Superficial	High	No
III	>5 cm	Deep	High	No
IV	Any	Any	Any	Yes

Depth is superficial (above the deep fascia) or deep (deep to the deep fascia). Retroperitoneal tumors are regarded as deep. Source: Authors' compilation based on data from Prudner et al. (2020).

A biopsy is an important component of the staging process. It provides a histological tissue diagnosis as well as the ability to detect the lesion's grade. As a result of this data, proper planning of adjuvant therapy, such as chemotherapy or radiation, is possible. It also gives a sense of the prognosis. FNAs, or fine-needle aspirations, are frequently used to determine the existence of malignant cells. However, because it is too small to show the architectural depiction within a neoplasm, it is not commonly used to make an initial diagnosis. FNAs may frequently be successfully utilized to sample tissues of recurrent disease to establish a definitive diagnoses, such as following surgical removal of a neoplasm. True-cut needle biopsy: This sample allows for examination of both individual cells and their architectural layout. This information is frequently needed to make a histopathologic diagnosis. This is frequently performed as a day-case operation in several tertiary care cancer centers under CT guidance. Open biopsy procedure: It is required in some circumstances. An incisional biopsy involves removing a very small piece of tissue from a bigger tumor mass, whereas an excisional biopsy involves removing the tumor mass in its entirety. When a sarcoma is suspected, an incisional biopsy is recommended (Prudner et al. 2020; Mavrogenis et al. 2014; Webber 2014; Ducatman et al. 1986; Ducatman et al. 1984; Hruban et al. 1990).

2.5.6. Surgical Treatment for MPNST

Surgical resection is the principal form of treatment. The purpose of the surgery is to remove the tumor completely and leave tumor-free (broad) margins (Figure 22). This provides the best results in terms of local recurrence as well as distant metastases (Prudner et al. 2020).

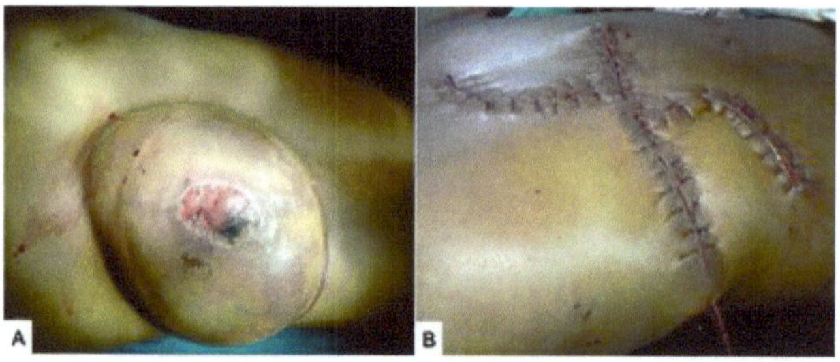

Figure 22. (**A**) Malignant peripheral nerve sheath tumor (MPNST) on back. (**B**) Closure of wound after tumor removal. Source: Figure by authors.

2.5.7. Radiation Therapy

In most soft-tissue sarcomas, radiation treatment is now an integral aspect of local disease control, and it can be used in the preoperative, peroperative, and postoperative periods for MPNST. Radiation therapy, when paired with broad surgical excision, offers local control and overall survival rates comparable to amputation, and the paired-modality treatment typically permits patients to have limb-salvage surgery successfully (Vraa et al. 1998; Yang et al. 1998).

2.5.8. Chemotherapy

Chemotherapy is used to treat systemic diseases that are either too small to detect or too diffuse to be treated locally. Chemotherapy is only used in high-grade cancers where metastatic illness is a possibility. Chemotherapy may be administered both before and after surgery. Chemotherapy's benefits must be evaluated against its side effects, some of which are permanent. As a result, the decision to manage with chemotherapy is influenced by the individual case and their ailment (Prudner et al. 2020).

2.5.9. MPNST Prognosis

MPNST recurrence is described in terms of both local and distant (metastatic) illness. The local recurrence frequency for MPNSTs has been found to be between 40 and 65%, with the distant recurrence frequency being between 40% and 68% (Hruban et al. 1990; Kourea et al. 1998; Wong et al. 1998). The five-year survival rate varies between 16% and 52%. Complete surgical resection, the presence of a low-grade component, and a modest tumor size (less than 5 cm) have all been linked to improved long-term survival (Hruban et al. 1990; Kourea et al. 1998). In recent research, patients managed at a sarcoma facility had an average 84% survival rate (Prudner et al. 2020). This has mostly been ascribed to enhanced imaging, which has resulted in earlier diagnosis, and aggressive therapy with adjuvant and neoadjuvant modalities like chemotherapy and radiation therapy. Patients with metastatic disease at the time of presentation had worse outcomes in this trial (only 33% survival), as one might expect. Patients with NF1 MPNSTs had traditionally been assumed to have a worse prognosis than those with random MPNSTs (Poyhonen et al. 1997). This claim was not supported by a recent report (Kourea et al. 1998; Cashen et al. 2004).

3. Peripheral Nerve Entrapment

3.1. Introduction

"A peripheral nerve lesion occurring without apparent external source and located in one of those anatomical areas where the nerve goes through a limited channel", according to the original definition of entrapment neuropathy (EN) (Wahab et al. 2017; Mumenthaler 1990). These channels are not only very small but they are also often flanked by stiff structures (often a fibro-osseous tunnel or an aperture in fibrous or muscle tissue), which can result in confinement and increased tissue pressures over time (Rempel and Diao 2004). Some ENs are frequent, while others are uncommon, and some are even debatable, as the word has been applied to different compression syndromes caused by external pressure. EN is also known as compression neuropathy or nerve compression syndrome. The joint is a common site for entrapment neuropathy to develop. If left untreated, the strain on the nerve can cause severe discomfort, nerve damage, and eventually muscular weakening and atrophy. Nerve entrapment can also be caused by other disorders such as bone spurs, cysts, joint swelling, and trauma. EN can also be used to describe nerve root compression caused by a prolapsed disc in the spine (Wahab et al. 2017; Chowdhury et al. 2009).

3.2. *Pathological Mechanisms of EN*

A fundamental grasp of the basic nerve damage types is required for the integration of EN mechanisms. Stretch-related, compression, and laceration nerve injuries are the three commonest forms. Stretch-related injuries are caused stretching of the peripheral nerve, as observed in brachial plexus avulsion. Knives and other weapons can cause laceration injuries. The third most common type is compression injury. EN is classified as a compression injury. Seddon (Seddon 1942) divided these injuries into three groups: neurapraxia, axonotmesis, and neurotmesis (Stewart 2000). Sunderland later divided them into five categories based on the severity of the injury (Sunderland 1951b). Most entrapment neuropathies fall into the neurapraxia category. Mechanical compression and ischemia are the two main pathogenic pathways engaged in compression injuries (Burnett and Zager 2004).

Mechanical Compression Mechanism

Wallerian degeneration occurs in acute nerve injuries, although the chronic form of nerve compression injuries was linked to some of the degenerative alterations outlined below. These are thought to be signs of nerve compression caused by mechanical forces.

1. Demyelination and remyelination: This process slows down the nerve conduction in EN (Ludwin and Maitland 1984; Berger and Gupta 2006). Myelin plays an important part in the saltatory conduction of action potentials, and this process is responsible for the slower nerve conduction velocity caused by lighter myelin and a shorter internodal distance (Pham and Gupta 2009).
2. Schwann cell proliferation and apoptosis occur simultaneously: Schwann cells proliferate in the compressed axon segment and distal to the site of compression, yet there is no axonal swelling or degeneration; these changes begin before any discernible drop in nerve conduction velocity (Gupta et al. 2012).
3. Downregulation of myelin-associated protein and axonal sprouting: axonal sprouting occurs in the compressed nerve following a decrease in myelin-associated glycoprotein, which usually restricts axonal growth (Gupta et al. 2006).
4. The dorsal root ganglion response: Growth-Associated Protein 43 is upregulated in chronic nerve compression, which is critical for modulating F-actin behavior in response to extracellular inputs. This increase is restricted to calcitonin gene-related, peptide-positive neurons and part of the small-caliber, isolectin-B4-binding protein. This causes a phenotypic alteration in the dorsal root ganglion, as well as an elevation in glial-derived neurotrophic factor close to the compression site (Chao et al. 2008).

Ischemic Mechanism

The peripheral nerves have a well-developed and structured microvascular system, which is important since action potentials are energy-dependent. The compression of this vascular system in EN will lead the nerves affected to dysfunction. Ischemia is caused by thickening of the microvessel walls that occurs in a compressed nerve. All of these things cause thickening, edema, and fibrosis at the compression site (Mackinnon et al. 1984). Common ENs are listed in Table 3 with involved nerves and sites.

Table 3. Involved peripheral nerves and sites in EN.

Nerve	Site
Suprascapular	Spinoglenoid notch
Medial cord or lower trunk of brachial plexus	Neurogenic thoracic outlet syndrome—cervical band or rib at thoracic outlet
Median	Carpal tunnel (at wrist) Pronator teres syndrome—at elbow, in between heads of pronator teres
Ulnar	i. Guyon's canal / ulnar tunnel—at wrist ii. Bicipital groove/cubital tunnel—at elbow
Posterior interosseous	Radial tunnel—arcade of Frohse: at point of entrance into supinator muscle
Lateral femoral cutaneous nerve—meralgia paraesthetica	Inguinal ligament
Obturator	Obturator canal
Posterior tibial	Medial malleolus and flexor retinaculum: tarsal tunnel
Interdigital plantar—Morton's metatarsalgia	Plantar fascia (heads of 3rd and 4th metatarsals)
Supratrochlear and supraorbital nerves	At supraorbital ridge (intractable migraine)
Greater and lesser occipital nerves	Superior nuchal line (intractable basilar migraine)

Source: Authors' compilation based on data from Ropper and Samuels (2009).

3.3. *Epidemiology of EN*

The most prevalent type of EN is carpal tunnel syndrome (CTS). It is commonest in women over 50. CTS affects women more commonly than men, with a 1.5 per 1000 people yearly incidence compared to 0.5 per 1000 for men (Otoshi et al. 2018).

Cubital tunnel syndrome, on the other hand, is more common in men, with a rate of 24.7 per 100,000 people per annum in the general population. Cubital tunnel syndrome is the second most prevalent EN, with males experiencing it more frequently than women (Otoshi et al. 2018). In the medial elbow overlaying the ulnar coronoid tubercle, men have less fat content than women. In men, the tubercle itself is larger. These anatomical characteristics may explain why men are more likely to develop cubital tunnel syndrome or ulnar neuropathy. Peroneal neuropathy is the most prevalent form of mononeuropathy in the lower limbs and the third most common type of EN. Then, there is tarsal tunnel syndrome, which affects the lower extremities (Dong et al. 2012).

3.4. *Causes and Risk Factors of EN*

EN is often caused by repetitive injuries. These repetitive injuries may take place in the workplace as a result of repeated movements linked to a patient's profession. Accidental trauma such as sprains and fractures can also result in EN. In addition, certain medical conditions can trigger EN. The risk factors are (Wahab et al. 2017; Chowdhury et al. 2009; Otoshi et al. 2018):

- Diabetes mellitus;
- Autoimmune disorders, such as rheumatoid arthritis;
- Endocrine dysfunctions: thyroid dysfunction, acromegaly, and Cushing syndrome;
- Hypertension;
- Local tumors and cysts;
- Pregnancy or menopause;
- Obesity;
- Congenital (birth) defects (e.g., small carpal tunnel);
- Neural disorders;
- Female sex and middle age.

3.5. *Clinical Features of EN*

Symptoms and signs of EN vary based on the type and site of the nerve involved. They usually happen near the compression site, but they can also happen in the surrounding tissues and structures. Aches and pains, tingling or numbness, muscle weakness, diminished flexibility, and trouble with particular activities are all common symptoms (Wahab et al. 2017; Chowdhury et al. 2009; Thomsen et al. 2010; Padua et al. 2016).

3.6. Investigations

Some investigations are used to diagnose EN, especially rarer forms of nerve compression syndrome, and include nerve conduction studies (NCSs), electromyography (EMG), ultrasound, and MRI. Diagnostic testing is not always required for carpal tunnel and cubital tunnel syndrome. They may, however, provide important information indicating the compression's location and intensity (Wahab et al. 2017; Chowdhury et al. 2009; Dong et al. 2012; Thomsen et al. 2010; Padua et al. 2016).

3.7. Treatment Options

Treatment for EN often starts with lifestyle changes and noninvasive therapies. Treating an underlying cause of EN may also relieve symptoms. In severe cases, EN may require surgery.

3.7.1. Lifestyle Changes

Restraining movements that initiate pain, adopting ergonomic strategies at home and at work, or changing job duties may elevate symptoms. When obesity is the etiology, weight reduction can reduce symptoms.

3.7.2. Physiotherapy

Physiotherapy can help to enhance the affected area's flexibility, strength, and range of motion. Physical therapy can also assist with symptoms like numbness and soreness.

3.7.3. Medication

Medication (nonsteroidal anti-inflammatory drugs (NSAIDs) or corticosteroids such as dexamethasone, which are injected directly around the nerve) can aid in relieving symptoms of EN such as inflammation and pain. The type of drug(s) used in EN depends on the severity of symptoms.

3.7.4. Prosthetic Devices

In some cases of EN, a brace or a splint is used to relieve pressure on the nerve.

3.7.5. Surgery

Surgical operations are usually viewed as a last resort in the treatment of these patients. EN does not always necessitate surgery. The type of nerve compression, the degree of compression, and the nerves and structures impacted all influence the surgical treatment. Each technique has its own set of dangers and advantages. Many factors influence the outcome of surgery including the duration and severity of symptoms and underlying general health conditions. Overall, the results of surgery are favorable. If nonsurgical treatment fails to alleviate the pressure on the compressed nerve, surgery may be required. Carpal tunnel release, cubital tunnel release, medial epicondylectomy, ulnar nerve anterior transposition, and tarsal tunnel release are some of the most popular surgical treatments used to treat entrapment neuropathy (Wahab et al. 2017; Chowdhury et al. 2009; Thomsen et al. 2010; Padua et al. 2016).

3.8. Outcomes of EN

The outcomes of EN vary. In very severe, untreated cases, it can result in permanent nerve damage or deficiency of function in the involved area. However, this is relatively rare. When NE is identified and treated early, significant relief can be provided. Many people make a full recovery.

3.9. Carpal Tunnel Syndrome

CTS is caused by compression of the median nerve when it travels through the carpal tunnel (Mumenthaler 1990). It is the most common EN in the world, and it has a substantial effect on the quality of life of those who suffer with it (Thomsen et al. 2010; Padua et al. 2016). However, one of the early signs of CTS is brachialgia paraesthetica nocturna (rising at night due to unpleasant and disturbing sensations in the fingers) (Oyedele et al.

2002). Symptoms of the condition have been found to have a prevalence of 10–20%, whereas definitive CTS has a prevalence of 0.9% to 10% (Al Saleh et al. 2016; de Krom et al. 1992; Ferry et al. 1998; Atroshi et al. 1999; Khedr et al. 2016).

Anatomy and Pathophysiology of CTS

The carpal tunnel (Figures 23 and 24) is an osseo-fibrous tunnel that runs between the carpal bones and the flexor retinaculum.

The nine extrinsic flexor tendons of the thumb and fingers and the median nerve are contained within the tunnel, which is about 2.5 cm distal to its upper limit and densely packed with anatomical components. The pressure within the tunnel varies from 2 to 31 mmHg in healthy people, while it can reach 32–110 mmHg in CTS patients depending on their wrist posture (Werner and Andary 2002). When the wrist is flexed, the pressure within the tunnel is elevated by up to eight times, and if the wrist is extended, by up to ten times (Werner and Andary 2002). The Phalen's test, a clinical test performed in the diagnosis of CTS, has a physiological explanation (Mackinnon 2002). Obesity, diabetes, hypothyroidism/myxedema, acromegaly, ganglion cysts, flexor tenosynovitis, and pregnancy are only a few of the risk factors for CTS. The chance of acquiring CTS increases by 7.4% for every unit increase in body mass index (BMI) (Shiri et al. 2015). It is very common in those who labor with repeated hand movements (England 1999; Violante et al. 2016; van Rijn et al. 2009). It has an idiopathic etiology in up to 50% of cases, mostly in premenopausal women (Dekel et al. 1980).

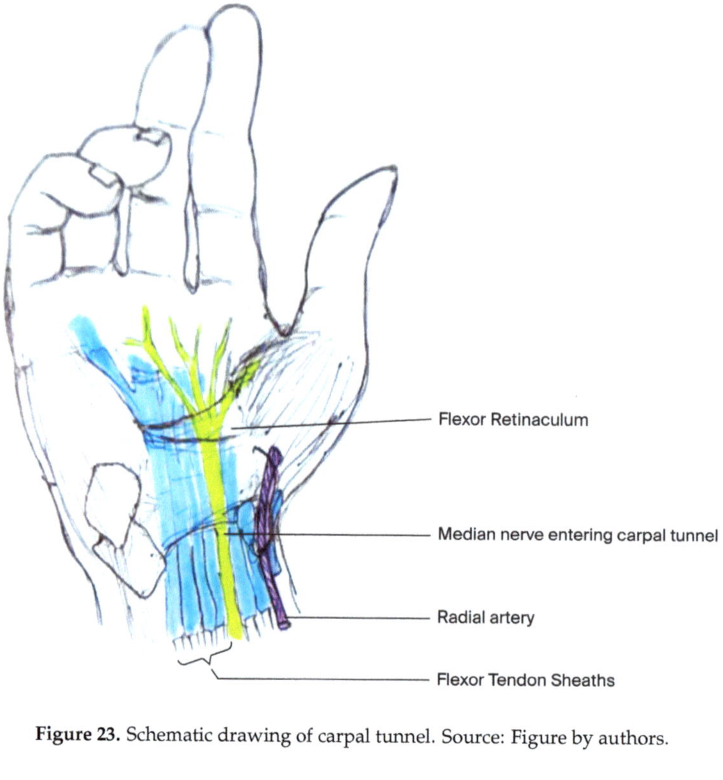

Figure 23. Schematic drawing of carpal tunnel. Source: Figure by authors.

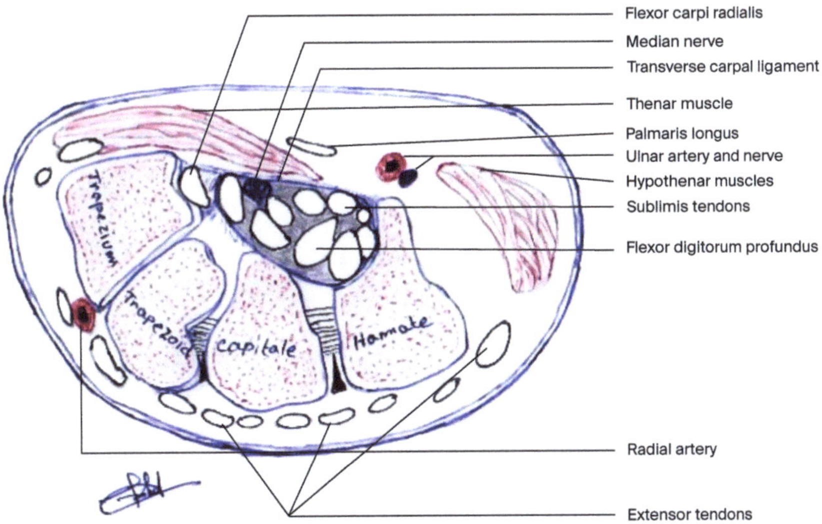

Figure 24. Cross sectional anatomy at wrist showing carpal tunnel and its contents. Source: Figure by authors.

Clinical Presentation of CTS

The thumb and first two and a half fingers are the commonest paresthesias, but some people may experience paresthesias throughout the hand or pain that travels up the arm to the shoulder (Bland 2007). More than 50% of the time, symptoms impact both hands at first, whereas the bulk of the time, symptoms begin on the dominant side. Any one of the symptoms listed below in the median-nerve-supplying zones are highly suggestive of CTS: swelling, dry skin, or color changes in the hand; hand weakness or clumsiness; or hand paresthesias (Bland 2007). Sleep, prolonged arm or hand position, and repetitive wrist/hand movement are the triggers for these symptoms. Changing the hand posture/position or merely shaking the involved hand can bring these sensations to the surface (American Academy of Neurology 1993). Phalen's test, Tinel's signals, and reverse Phalen's test are employed in the clinical examination (Werner et al. 1994). For early CTS diagnosis, a nerve conduction examination is preferred (Fertl et al. 1998).

Confirmation of Diagnosis

Electrophysiological testing in conjunction with clinical testing is a recognized standard method for diagnosis confirmation (Phillips and Juel 1997). The severity of CTS can also be determined via electrophysiology. Although the intensity of nerve conduction studies (NCSs) and symptoms are not strongly correlated, the use of a grading system can aid in the prediction of surgery outcomes. Patients who have moderate-grade NCS abnormalities had a better surgical outcome than those who have very severe or no abnormalities (Stevens 1987; Bland 2001). Other tests include MRI, wrist ultrasonography, and, if necessary, examinations to exclude a systemic disease or underlying cause (Wahab et al. 2017; Dong et al. 2012).

Treatment

Treatment can be conservative or surgical.

Conservative: For situations with milder disease, a conservative approach is used, which includes anti-inflammatory medication (e.g., local steroid injection) and wrist splinting (Wahab et al. 2017; American Academy of Neurology 1993; Peters-Veluthamaningal et al. 2010). A new therapy option is radial extracorporeal shockwaves paired with wrist splinting (Raissi et al. 2017). Another novel therapy option is platelet-rich plasma injection, which has been demonstrated to be effective in the short term (Padua et al. 2016; Uzun et al. 2017; Malahias et al. 2015).

Surgery: For those patients where conservative management failed or those with severe form of disease, carpal tunnel release (CTR) is advised (Wahab et al. 2017; Chowdhury et al. 2009; Bland 2007; Uzun et al. 2017; Shi and MacDermid 2011). The overall result of CTR is very good. Surgical options:

i. Open surgical CTR (Figure 25);
ii. Percutaneous CTR (mini transverse incision at wrist) (Figure 26);
iii. Endoscopic CTR.

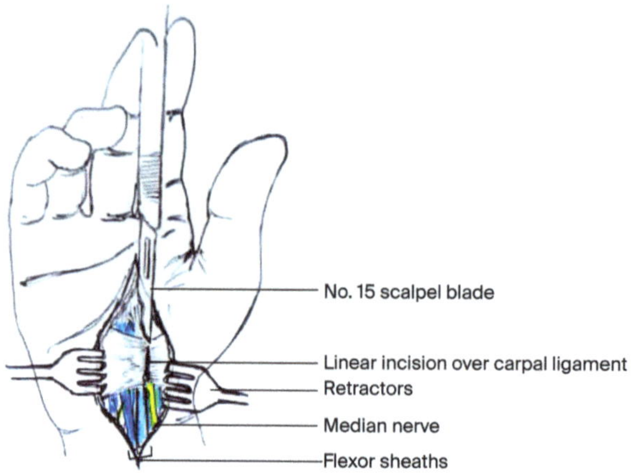

Figure 25. Schematic drawing of open carpal tunnel release. Source: Figure by authors.

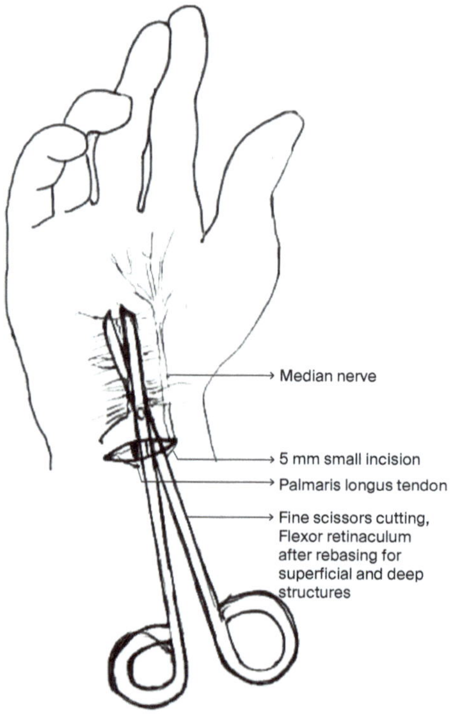

Figure 26. Schematic drawing of percutaneous carpal tunnel release. Source: Figure by authors.

Author Contributions: Conceptualization, methodology, F.H.C. and M.H.S.; validation, formal analysis, investigation, resources, data curation, A.K., S.M.M.H. and F.H.C.; writing—original draft preparation, writing—review and editing, visualization, supervision, F.H.C. and M.R.H. All authors have read and agreed to the published version of the manuscript.

Funding: This research received no external funding.

Conflicts of Interest: The authors declare no conflicts of interest.

References

Adamson, D. C., and A. H. Friedman. 2004. Malignant peripheral nerve sheath tumor of the spine after radiation therapy for Hodgkin's lymphoma. *Clinical Neuropathology* 23: 245–55. [PubMed]

Adeniran, Adebowale, Hikmat Al-Ahmadie, Mary C. Mahoney, and Toni M. Robinson-Smith. 2004. Granular cell tumor of the breast: A series of 17 cases and review of the literature. *The Breast Journal* 10: 528–31. [CrossRef] [PubMed]

Aegineta, P. De re medica. 1528. *Paulou Aiginetou iatrou aristou, biblia hepta. En arche hekastou ton biblion deiknytai ta en ekeino periekomena, Pavli Aeginetae medici optimi, libri septem.* West Ryde: Aldus.

Aguayo, A. J., J. M. Peyronnard, and G. M. Bray. 1973. A quantitative ultrastructural study of regeneration from isolated proximal stumps of transected unmyelinated nerves. *Journal of Neuropathology & Experimental Neurology* 32: 256–70. [CrossRef]

Al Saleh, Jamal, Manal E. L. Sayed, Nahed Monsef, and Ebtihal Darwish. 2016. The prevalence and the determinants of musculoskeletal diseases in emiratis attending primary health care clinics in Dubai. *Oman Medical Journal* 31: 117–23. [CrossRef]

American Academy of Neurology. 1993. Practice parameter for carpal tunnel syndrome (summary statement). Report of the Quality Standards Subcommittee of the American Academy of Neurology. *Neurology* 43: 2406–9. [CrossRef]

Amin, Amit, Asif Saifuddin, Adreienne Flanagan, Daniel Patterson, and Jan Lehovsky. 2004. Radiotherapy-induced malignant peripheral nerve sheath tumor of the cauda equina. *Spine* 29: E506–E509. [CrossRef]

Amita, Krishnappa, S. Vijay Shankar, Kuchangi C. Nischal, and Haleuoor B. Basavaraj. 2013. Benign triton tumor: A rare entity in head and neck region. *Korean Journal of Pathology* 47: 74–76. [CrossRef]

Antinheimo, J., R. Sankila, O. Carpen, E. Pukkala, M. Sainio, and J. Jaaskelainen. 2000. Population-based analysis of sporadic and type 2 neurofibromatosis-associated meningiomas *and schwannomas. *Neurology* 54: 71–76. [CrossRef] [PubMed]

Antonescu, C. R., A. O. Stemmer-Rachamimov, and A. Perry. 2016. Hybrid nerve sheath tumors. In *WHO Classification of Tumors of the Central Nervous System Revised.* Edited by David N. Louis, Hiroko Ohgaki, Otmar D. Wiestler, Webster K. Cavenec, David W. Ellison, Dominique Figarella-Branger, Arie Perry, Guido Reifenberger and Andreas von Deimling. Lyon: IAR, pp. 224–25.

Antonescu, C. R., A. Perry, J. M. Woodruf, C. A. Stratakis, H. Brems, and E. Legius. 2013. Nerve sheath tumors. In *WHO Classification of Tumours of Soft Tissue and Bone.* Edited by Christopher D. M. Fletcher, Julia A. Bridge, Pancras C. W. Hogendoorn and Fredrik Mertens. Lyon: IARC, pp. 170–86.

Atroshi, Isam, Christina Gummesson, Ragnar Johnsson, Ewald Ornstein, Jonas Ranstam, and Ingmar Rosén. 1999. Prevalence of carpal tunnel syndrome in a general population. *JAMA* 282: 153–58. [CrossRef]

Battiston, Bruno, Igor Papalia, Pierluigi Tos, and Stefano Geuna. 2009. Peripheral nerve repair and regeneration research: A historical note. *International Review of Neurobiology* 87: 1–7. [CrossRef]

Berger, Brent L., and Ranjan Gupta. 2006. Demyelination secondary to chronic nerve compression injury alters Schmidt-Lanterman incisures. *Journal of Anatomy* 209: 111–18. [CrossRef] [PubMed]

Bittner, George D., Timothy Schallert, and Jean D. Peduzzi. 2000. Degeneration, trophic interactions, and repair of severed axons: A reconsideration of some common assumptions. *The Neuroscientist* 6: 88–109. [CrossRef]

Bland, Jeremy D. P. 2001. Do nerve conduction studies predict the outcome of carpal tunnel decompression? *Muscle & Nerve* 24: 935–40. [CrossRef]

Bland, Jeremy D. P. 2007. Carpal tunnel syndrome. *BMJ* 335: 343–46. [CrossRef] [PubMed]

Brushart, T. M. 1988. Preferential reinnervation of motor nerves by regeneratingmotor axons. *Journal of Neuroscience* 8: 1026–31. [CrossRef]

Brushart, T. M. E. 1991. The mechanical and humoral control of specificity in nerve repair. In *Operative Nerve Repair.* Edited by Richard H. Gelberman. Philadelphia: JB Lippincott, pp. 215–30.

Burnett, Mark G., and Eric L. Zager. 2004. Pathophysiology of peripheral nerve injury: A brief review. *Neurosurgical Focus* 16: E1. [CrossRef] [PubMed]

Cajal, S. Ramón Y. 1892. La retine des vertebres. *La Cellule* 9: 121–33.

Carlsen, Brian T., Allen T. Bishop, and Alexander Y. Shin. 2009. Late reconstruction for brachial plexus injury. *Neurosurgery Clinics of North America* 20: 51–64. [CrossRef]

Carney, J. Aidan. 1990. Psammomatous melanotic schwannoma. a distinctive, heritable tumor with special associations, including cardiac myxoma and the cushing syndrome. *The American Journal of Surgical Pathology* 14: 206–22. [CrossRef]

Casadei, Gian P., Bernd W. Scheithauer, Takanori Hirose, Marco Manfrini, Cari van Houton, and Michael B. Wood. 1995. Cellular schwannoma—A clinicopathologic, DNA flow cytometric, and proliferation marker study of 70 patients. *Cancer* 75: 1109–19. [CrossRef]

Cashen, David V., Robert C. Parisien, Kevin Raskin, Francis J. Hornicek, Mark C. Gebhardt, and Henry J. Mankin. 2004. Survival data for patients with malignant schwannoma. *Clinical Orthopaedics and Related Research* 426: 69–73. [CrossRef] [PubMed]

Catalano, F., F. Fanfani, A. Pagliei, and G. Taccardo. 1992. A case of primary intraneural ossification of the ulnar nerve. *Annals of Hand and Upper Limb Surgery* 11: 157–62. [CrossRef]

Chao, Tom, Khoa Pham, Oswald Steward, and Ranjan Gupta. 2008. Chronic nerve compression injury induces a phenotypic switch of neurons within the dorsal root ganglia. *Journal of Comparative Neurology* 506: 180–93. [CrossRef]

Cheng, Ron Ron, Jessica A. Forcucci, and Stephen P. Kalhorn. 2016. Intraneural Granular Cell Tumor of a Cervical Dorsal Nerve Root: A Case Report and Review of the Literature. *World Neurosurgery* 86: 511. [CrossRef]

Chiang, Chia-Ling, Meng-Yuan Tsai, and Clement Kuen-Huang Chen. 2010. MRI diagnosis of fibrolipomatous hamartoma of the median nerve and associated macrodystrophia lipomatosa. *Journal of the Chinese Medical Association* 73: 499–502. [CrossRef] [PubMed]

Chowdhury, Forhad H., Md. Raziul Haque, Md. Shafiqul Islam, Khandkar Ali Kawsar, and Mainul Haque Sarkar. 2010. Retoperitoneal Giant Schwann cell Tumors: Report of a Schwannoma and A Malignant Schwannoma. *Journal of Surgical Science* 14: 103–5.

Chowdhury, Forhad H., Md. Raziul Haque, S. M. Noman Khaled Chowdhury, Md. Shafiqul Islam, Syeda Asfiya Ara, and Mainul Haque Sarkar. 2009. Surgical management of carpal tunnel syndrome. A study of 21 cases. *CMSGHJ* 9: 24–29.

Chowdhury, Forhad H., Noman Khaled Chowdhury, Md. Raziul Haque, Md. Shafiqul Islam, Manjural Haque Akhond Chowdhury, and Mainul Haque Sarkar. 2008a. Peripharal nerve tumors: It's Profile and surgical outcome. *CMSGHJ Journal* 8: 11–16.

Chowdhury, Forhad Hossain, Md. Raziul Haque, Md. Shafiqul Islam, and Mainul Haque Sarkar. 2011. Giant schwannoma of median nerve at forearm: A case report. *Journal of Bangladesh College of Physicians and Surgeons* 29: 174–76. [CrossRef]

Chowdhury, Noman Khaled, Md. Raziul Haque, Forhad H. Chowdhury, Md. Shafiqul Islam, Abu Hena Mahboo, and Syeda Asfiya Ara. 2008b. Surgical management of plexiform Neurofibroma: An experience of 11 cases. *CMSGHJ Journal* 8: 32–36.

Colen, Kari L., Mihye Choi, and David T. W. Chiu. 2009. Nerve grafts and conduits. *Plastic and Reconstructive Surgery* 124: e386–e394. [CrossRef] [PubMed]

Crist, Jamie, Jacob R. Hodge, Matthew Frick, Fiona P. Leung, Eugene Hsu, Ming Tye Gi, and Sudhakar K. Venkatesh. 2017. Magnetic resonance imaging appearance of schwannomas from head to toe: A pictorial review. *Journal of Clinical Imaging Science* 7: 38. [CrossRef] [PubMed]

D'Agostino, Anthony N., Edward H. Soule, and Ross H. Miller. 1963. Sarcomas of the peripheral nerves and somatic soft tissues associated with multiple neurofibromatosis (Von Recklinghausen's disease). *Cancer* 16: 1015–27. [CrossRef] [PubMed]

Dahlin, Lars B. 2006. Nerve injury and repair: From molecule to man. In *Peripheral Nerve Surgery: Practical Applications in the Upper Extremity*. Edited by David J. Slutsky and Vincent R. Hentz. Philadelphia: Churchill Livingston, Elsevier, pp. 1–22.

Davis, Gavin A. 2007. Granular cell tumor: A rare tumor of the ulnar nerve. case report. *Neurosurgical Focus* 22: E25. [CrossRef]

de Krom, Marc C. T. F. M., Paul G. Knipschild, Arnold D. M. Kester, Carel T. Thijs, Peter F. Boekkooi, and F. Spaans. 1992. Carpal tunnel syndrome: Prevalence in the general population. *Journal of Clinical Epidemiology* 45: 373–76. [CrossRef]

Dekel, S., T. Papaioannou, G. Rushworth, and R. Coates. 1980. Idiopathic carpal tunnel syndrome caused by carpal stenosis. *British Medical Journal* 280: 1297–299. [CrossRef]

Dellon, A. Lee, Susan E. Mackinnon, and William A. Seiler IV. 1988. Susceptibility of the diabetic nerve to chronic compression. *Annals of Plastic Surgery* 20: 117–19. [CrossRef]

Diao, Edward, and Tammy Vannuyen. 2000. Techniques for primary nerve repair. *Hand Clinics* 16: 53–66. [CrossRef] [PubMed]

Dong, Qian, Jon A. Jacobson, David A. Jamadar, Girish Gandikota, Catherine Brandon, Yoav Morag, David P. Fessell, and Sung-Moon Kim. 2012. Entrapment Neuropathies in the Upper and Lower Limbs: Anatomy and MRI Features. *Radiology Research and Practice* 2012: 230679. [CrossRef]

Doyle, Leona A., and Christopher D. M. Fletcher. 2014. Peripheral hemangioblastoma: Clinicopathologic characterization in a series of 22 cases. *The American Journal of Surgical Pathology* 38: 119–27. [CrossRef]

Ducatman, Barbara S., Bernd W. Scheithauer, David G. Piepgras, and Herbert M. Reiman. 1984. Malignant peripheral nerve sheath tumors in childhood. *Journal of Neuro-Oncology* 2: 241–48. [CrossRef] [PubMed]

Ducatman, Barbara S., Bernd W. Scheithauer, David G. Piepgras, Herbert M. Reiman, and Duane M. Ilstrup. 1986. Malignant peripheral nerve sheath tumors. A clinicopathologic study of 120 cases. *Cancer* 57: 2006–21. [CrossRef] [PubMed]

Dumitru, Daniel, Machiel J. Zwarts, and Anthony A. Amato. 2001. Peripheral nervous system's reaction to injury. In *Electrodiagnostic Medicine*. Edited by Daniel Dumitru, Anthony A. Amato and Machiel Zwarts. Philadelphia: Hanley and Belfus, pp. 115–56.

Effron, Charles R., and Robert W. Beasley. 2006. Compression neuropathies in the upper limb and electrophysiological studies. In *Grabb and Smith's Plastic Surgery*. Edited by Charles H. Thorne, Robert W. Beasley, Sherrell J. Aston, Scott P. Bartlett, Geoffrey C. Gurtner and Scott L. Spear. Philadelphia: Lippincott Williams & Wilkins.

Ellison, Dale A., Julissa Corredor-Buchmann, David M. Parham, and Richard J. Jackson. 2005. Malignant triton tumor presenting as a rectal mass in an 11-month-old. *Pediatric and Developmental Pathology* 8: 235–39. [CrossRef]

England, John D. 1999. Entrapment neuropathies. *Current Opinion in Neurology* 12: 597–602. [CrossRef]

Evans, D. Gareth R., Michael E. Baser, J. McGaughran, Saba Sharif, E. Howard, and Anthony Moran. 2002. Malignant peripheral nerve sheath tumours in neurofibromatosis 1. *Journal of Medical Genetics* 39: 311–14. [CrossRef]

Evans, D. G., S. M. Huson, D. Donnai, W. Neary, V. Blair, D. Teare, V. Newton, T. Strachan, R. Ramsden, and R. Harris. 1992. A genetic study of type 2 neurofibromatosis in the United Kingdom. I. prevalence, mutation rate, fitness, and confirmation of maternal transmission effect on severity. *Journal of Medical Genetics* 29: 841–46. [CrossRef]

Ferraresi, Stefano, Debora Garozzo, and Enzo Bianchini. 2001. Aggressive fibromatosis (desmoid tumor) of the radial nerve: Favorable resolution. Case report. *Journal of Neurosurgery* 95: 332–33. [CrossRef] [PubMed]

Ferry, S., T. Pritchard, J. Keenan, P. Croft, and A. J. Silman. 1998. Estimating the prevalence of delayed median nerve conduction in the general population. *British Journal of Rheumatology* 37: 630–35. [CrossRef]

Fertl, E., C. Wöber, and J. Zeitlhofer. 1998. The serial use of two provocative tests in the clinical diagnosis of carpal tunnel syndrome. *Acta Neurologica Scandinavica* 98: 328–32. [CrossRef]

Fetsch, John F., and Markku Miettinen. 1997. Sclerosing perineurioma: A clinicopathologic study of 19 cases of a distinctive soft tissue lesion with a predilection for the fingers and palms of young adults. *The American Journal of Surgical Pathology* 21: 1433–42. [CrossRef]

Fetsch, John F., William B. Laskin, and Markku Miettinen. 2005. Nerve sheath myxoma: A clinicopathologic and immunohistochemical analysis of 57 morphologically distinctive, S-100 protein- and GFAP-positive, myxoid peripheral nerve sheath tumors with a predilection for the extremities and a high local recurrence rate. *The American Journal of Surgical Pathology* 29: 1615–24. [CrossRef] [PubMed]

Friedrich, Reinhard E., Lan Kluwe, C. Fünsterer, and V. F. Mautner. 2005. Malignant peripheral nerve sheath tumors (MPNST) in neurofibromatosis type 1 (NF1): Diagnostic findings on magnetic resonance images and mutation analysis of the NF1 gene. *Anticancer Research* 25: 1699–702. [PubMed]

Fu, Yao-Shi, Gordon I. Kaye, and Raffaele Lattes. 1975. Primary malignant melanocytic tumors of the sympathetic ganglia, with an ultrastructural study of one. *Cancer* 36: 2029–41. [CrossRef] [PubMed]

George, David H., Bernd W. Scheithauer, Robert J. Spinner, Ueli Buchler, Timothy E. Cronin, Michael T. Reedy, and Byron C. Arndt. 2002. Heterotopic ossification of peripheral nerve ("neuritis ossificans"): Report of two cases. *Neurosurgery* 51: 244–46; discussion 246. [CrossRef] [PubMed]

Giannini, C., B. W. Scheithauer, L. C. Hellbusch, A. G. Rasmussen, M. W. Fox, S. R. McCormick, and D. H. Davis. 1998. Peripheral nerve hemangioblastoma. *Modern Pathology* 11: 999–1004.

Gillies, R. M., and C. Burrows. 1991. Nerve sheath ganglion of the superficial radial nerve. *Journal of Hand Surgery* 16: 94–95. [CrossRef]

Goldblum, John R., Andrew L. Folpe, and Sharon W. Weiss. 2014. Benign tumors of peripheral nerves. In *Enzinger and Weiss's Soft Tissue Tumors*. Edited by John R. Goldblum, Andrew L. Folpe and Sharon W. Weiss. Philadelphia: Saunders, Elsevier, pp. 885–958.

Griffin, Justin W., MaCalus V. Hogan, A. Bobby Chhabra, and D. Nicole Deal. 2013. Peripheral nerve repair and reconstruction. *Journal of Bone and Joint Surgery A* 95: 2144–51. [CrossRef]

Grinsell, D., and C. F. Keating. 2014. Peripheral Nerve Reconstruction after Injury: A Review of Clinical and Experimental Therapies. *BioMed Research International* 2014: 698256. [CrossRef]

Gupta, Ranjan, Laura S. Rummler, Winnie Palispis, Linh Truong, Tom Chao, Kasra Rowshan, Tahseen Mozaffar, and Oswald Steward. 2006. Local down-regulation of myelin-associated glycoprotein permits axonal sprouting with chronic nerve compression injury. *Experimental Neurology* 200: 418–29. [CrossRef]

Gupta, Ranjan, Nima Nassiri, Antony Hazel, Mary Bathen, and Tahseen Mozaffar. 2012. Chronic nerve compression alters Schwann cell myelin architecture in a murine model. *Muscle & Nerve* 45: 231–41. [CrossRef]

Hall, S. 2005. Mechanisms of repair after traumatic injury. In *Peripheral Neuropathy*. Edited by Peter J. Dyck and P. K. Thomas. Philadelphia: Saunders, Elsevier, pp. 1403–33.

Harder, Anja, Martin Wesemann, Christian Hagel, Jens Schittenhelm, Susan Fischer, Marcos Tatagiba, Christoph Nagel, Astrid Jeibmann, Axel Bohring, Victor-Felix Mautner, and et al. 2012. Hybrid neurofibroma/schwannoma is overrepresented among schwan-nomatosis and neurofibromatosis patients. *The American Journal of Surgical Pathology* 36: 702–9. [CrossRef] [PubMed]

Hirbe, Angela C., and David H. Gutmann. 2014. Neurofibromatosis type 1: A multidisciplinary approach to care. *The Lancet Neurology* 13: 834–43. [CrossRef] [PubMed]

Hornick, Jason L., and Christopher D. M. Fletcher. 2005. Soft tissue perineurioma: Clinicopathologic analysis of 81 cases including those with atypical histologic features. *The American Journal of Surgical Pathology* 29: 845–58. [CrossRef] [PubMed]

Hruban, Ralph H., Man H. Shiu, Ruby T. Senie, and James M. Woodruff. 1990. Malignant peripheral nerve sheath tumors of the buttock and lower extremity. A study of 43 cases. *Cancer* 66: 1253–65. [CrossRef]

Hsu, Charles S., Vincent R. Hentz, and Jeffrey Yao. 2007. Tumours of the hand. *The Lancet Oncology* 8: 157–66. [CrossRef]

Huson, S. M., and P. S. Harper. 1989. A genetic study of von Recklinghausen neurofibromatosis in south east Wales. II. Guidelines for genetic counselling. *Journal of Medical Genetics* 26: 712–21. [CrossRef]

Jobe, M. T., and S. F. Martinez. 2013. Canale & Beaty: Campbell's Operative Orthopaedics. In *Peripheral Nerve Injuries*. Philadelphia: Elsevier Mosby, pp. 3063–65.

Kacerovska, Denisa, Michal Michal, Naoto Kuroda, Azusa Tanaka, Radek Sima, Natalja Denisjuk, Boris Kreuzberg, Renata Ricarova, and Dmitry V. Kazakov. 2013. Hybrid peripheral nerve sheath tumors, including a malignant variant in type 1 neurofibromatosis. *The American Journal of Dermatopathology* 35: 641–49. [CrossRef]

Kandel, Eric R., James Harris Schwartz, and Thomas Jessell. 2000. *Principles of Neuroscience*. New York: Mcgraw-Hill, p. 34.

Kang, Jian, Pinglin Yang, Quanjin Zang, and Xijing He. 2016. Traumatic neuroma of the superficial peroneal nerve in a patient: A case report and review of the literature. *World Journal of Surgical Oncology* 14: 242. [CrossRef]

Keskin, Elif, Sumeyye Ekmekci, Ozgur Oztekin, and Gulden Diniz. 2017. Melanotic schwannomas are rarely seen pigmented tumors with unpredictable prognosis and challenging diagnosis. *Case Reports in Pathology* 2017: 1807879. [CrossRef]

Khandakar, Binny, Soumit Dey, Prabir Chandra Paul, Sriparna Medda, Aparna Bhattacharya, and Saikat Datta. 2014. Retroperitoneal giant ancient schwannoma. *Archives of Iranian Medicine* 17: 847–49.

Khedr, Eman M., Gharib Fawi, Mohammed Abd Allah Abbas, Noha Abo El-Fetoh, Ahmed F. Zaki, and Ayman Gamea. 2016. Prevalence of Common Types of Compression Neuropathies in Qena Governorate/Egypt: A Population-Based Survey. *Neuroepidemiology* 46: 253–60. [CrossRef] [PubMed]

Kim, Daniel H., Judith A. Murovic, Robert L. Tiel, and David G. Kline. 2004. Operative outcomes of 546 louisiana state university health sciences center peripheral nerve tumors. *Neurosurgery Clinics of North America* 15: 177. [CrossRef]

King, Allison A., Michael R. Debaun, Vincent M. Riccardi, and David H. Gutmann. 2000. Malignant peripheral nerve sheath tumors in neurofibromatosis 1. *American Journal of Medical Genetics* 93: 388–92. [CrossRef]

Kokkalis, Zinon T., Nikolaos A. Stavropoulos, Andreas F. Mavrogenis, Andreas Panagopoulos, and Panayotis N. Soucacos. 2019. Benign peripheral nerve tumors. *Injury* 50: S77–S83. [CrossRef] [PubMed]

Kourea, Helen P., Mark H. Bilsky, Denis HY Leung, Jonathan J. Lewis, and James M. Woodruff. 1998. Subdiaphragmatic and intrathoracic paraspinal malignant peripheral nerve sheath tumors: A clinicopathologic study of 25 patients and 26 tumors. *Cancer* 82: 2191–203. [CrossRef]

Kouyoumdjian, João Aris. 2006. Peripheral nerve injuries: A retrospectivensurvey of 456 cases. *Muscle and Nerve* 34: 785–88. [CrossRef] [PubMed]

Kurze, Theodore. 1964. Microtechniques in neurological surgery. *Clinical Neurosurgery* 11: 128–37. [CrossRef]

Lee, Steve K., and Scott W. Wolfe. 2000. Peripheral nerve injury and repair. *Journal of the American Academy of Orthopaedic Surgeons* 8: 243–52. [CrossRef] [PubMed]

Lee, Steve K., and Scott W. Wolfe. 2012. Nerve transfers for the upper extremity: New horizons in nerve reconstruction. *Journal of the American Academy of Orthopaedic Surgeons* 20: 506–17. [CrossRef]

Lodding, Pär, Lars-Gunnar Kindblom, Lennart Angervall, and Göran Stenman. 1990. Cellular schwannoma: A clinicopathologic study of 29 cases. *Virchows Archiv A, Pathological Anatomy and Histopathology* 416: 237–48. [CrossRef]

Longo, Jody F., Shannon M. Weber, Brittany P. Turner-Ivey, and Steven L. Carroll. 2018. Recent advances in the diagnosis and pathogenesis of neurofibromatosis type 1 (NF1)-associated peripheral nervous system neoplasms. *Advances in Anatomic Pathology* 25: 353–68. [CrossRef] [PubMed]

Loree, Thom R., James H. North, Jr., Bruce A. Werness, Rina Nangia, Alan P. Mullins, and Wesley L. Hicks, Jr. 2000. Malignant peripheral nerve sheath tumors of the head and neck: Analysis of prognostic factors. *Otolaryngology—Head and Neck Surgery* 122: 667–72. [CrossRef] [PubMed]

Ludwin, Samuel K., and Marion Maitland. 1984. Long-term remyelination fails to reconstitute normal thickness of central myelin sheaths. *Journal of the Neurological Sciences* 64: 193–98. [CrossRef] [PubMed]

Lundborg, Göran. 2000. A 25-year perspective of peripheral nerve surgery: Evolving neuroscientific concepts and clinical significance. *Journal of Hand Surgery* 25: 391–414. [CrossRef] [PubMed]

Mackinnon, Susan E. 1989. New directions in peripheral nerve surgery. *Annals of Plastic Surgery* 22: 257–73. [CrossRef]

Mackinnon, Susan E. 2002. Pathophysiology of nerve compression. *Hand Clinics* 18: 231–41. [CrossRef]

Mackinnon, Susan E., A. Lee Dellon, Alan R. Hudson, and Daniel A. Hunter. 1984. Chronic nerve compression–an experimental model in the rat. *Annals of Plastic Surgery* 13: 112–20. [CrossRef]

Mackinnon, Susan E., and A. Lee Dellon. 1988. *Surgery of the Peripheral Nerve*. New York: Thieme.

Malahias, Michael Alexander, Elizabeth O. Johnson, George C. Babis, and Vasileios S. Nikolaou. 2015. Single injection of platelet-rich plasma as a novel treatment of carpal tunnel syndrome. *Neural Regeneration Research* 10: 1856–59. [CrossRef]

Malkoc, Melih, Tugrul Ormeci, Adem Yılmaz, Ozgur Korkmaz, and Canan Besleyici Tanik. 2014. Nerve sheath myxoma of the dorsal paravertebral space. *International Journal of Surgery Case Reports* 5: 858–60. [CrossRef]

Mavrogenis, Andreas F., Andrea Angelini, Costantino Errani, and Eugenio Rimondi. 2014. Howshould musculoskeletal biopsies be performed? *Orthopedics* 37: 585–88. [CrossRef]

Mavrogenis, Andreas F., Georgios N. Panagopoulos, Andrea Angelini, Jan Lesenský, Christos Vottis, Panayiotis D. Megaloikonomos, Zinon T. Kokkalis, Vasilios Kontogeorgakos, Pietro Ruggieri, and Panayiotis J. Papagelopoulos. 2017. Tumors of the hand. *European Journal of Orthopaedic Surgery & Traumatology* 27: 747–62. [CrossRef]

McCarthy, E. F., and M. Sundaram. 2005. Heterotopic ossification: A review. *Skeletal Radiology* 34: 609–19. [CrossRef] [PubMed]

McMenamin, Máirín E., and Christopher D. M. Fletcher. 2001. Expanding the spectrum of malignant change in schwannomas: Epithelioid malignant change, epithelioid malignant peripheral nerve sheath tumor, and epithelioid angiosarcoma. *The American Journal of Surgical Pathology* 25: 13–25. [CrossRef]

Meany, Holly, Eva Dombi, James Reynolds, Millie Whatley, Ambereen Kurwa, Maria Tsokos, Wanda Salzer, Andrea Gillespie, Andrea Baldwin, Joanne Derdak, and et al. 2013. 18-fluorodeoxyglucose–positron emission tomography (FDGPET) evaluation of nodular lesions in patients with neurofibromatosis type 1 and plexiform neurofibromas (PN) or malignant peripheral nerve sheath tumors (MPNST). *Pediatric Blood & Ccancer* 60: 59–64. [CrossRef]

Millar, W. Gilbert. 1932. A malignant melanotic tumor of ganglion cells arising from thoracic sympathetic ganglion. *The Journal of Pathology and Bacteriology* 35: 351. [CrossRef]

Millesi, Hanno. 1973. Microsurgery of peripheral nerves. *Hand* 5: 157–60. [CrossRef]

Millesi, Hanno. 1990. Progress in peripheral nerve reconstruction. *World Journal of Surgery* 14: 733–47. [CrossRef]

Mishra, Bharat, Jerry R. John, Satyaswarup Tripathy, and Ramesh Kumar Sharma. 2017. Median nerve lipofibrohamartoma: A treatment dilemma. *World Journal of Plastic Surgery* 6: 399–401.

Mitchell, Andrew, Bernd W. Scheithauer, Robert E. Wharen, Joel Franck, and Kris Chan. 2013. Hemangioblastoma of spinal nerve: A report of six cases. *Clinical Neuropathology* 32: 91–99. [CrossRef]

Moore, Amy M., Wilson Z. Ray, Kristofer E. Chenard, Thomas Tung, and Susan E. Mackinnon. 2009. Nerve allotransplantation as it pertains tocomposite tissue transplantation. *Hand* 4: 239–44. [CrossRef]

Mrugala, Maciej M., Tracy T. Batchelor, and Scott R. Plotkin. 2005. Peripheral and cranial nerve sheath tumors. *Current Opinion in Neurology* 18: 604. [CrossRef] [PubMed]

Mumenthaler, M. 1990. Clinical Aspects of Entrapment Neuropathies of Peripheral Nerves. In *Peripheral Nerve Lesions*. Edited by Majid Samii. Berlin/Heidelberg: Springer, pp. 258–69.

Muzaffar, Nasir, Nawaz Ahmad, Aejaz Bhat, and Nissar Shah. 2012. Neuritis ossificans of the radial nerve. *Orthopedics* 35: e589–e591. [CrossRef] [PubMed]

Oliveira, Karla M. C., Lukas Pindur, Zhihua Han, Mit B. Bhavsar, John H. Barker, and Liudmila Leppik. 2018. Time course of traumatic neuroma development. *PLoS ONE* 13: e0200548. [CrossRef] [PubMed]

Otoshi, Kenichi, Shinichi Kikuchi, Nobuyuki Sasaki, Miho Sekiguchi, Koji Otani, Tsukasa Kamitani, Shingo Fukuma, Shunichi Fukuhara, and Shinichi Konno. 2018. The Associated Risk Factors for Entrapment Neuropathy in the Upper Extremity: The Locomotive Syndrome and Health Outcome in Aizu Cohort Study (LOHAS). *Health* 10: 823–37. [CrossRef]

Oyedele, O. O., M. T. Shokunbi, and A. O. Malomo. 2002. The prevalence of hand pain in Ibadan–implications for the carpal tunnel syndrome. *West African Journal of Medicine* 21: 204–7. [CrossRef]

Packer, R. J., D. H. Gutmann, A. Rubenstein, D. Viskochil, R. A. Zimmerman, G. Vezina, J. Small, and B. Korf. 2002. Plexiform neurofibromas in NF1: Toward biologic-based therapy. *Neurology* 58: 1461–70. [CrossRef]

Padua, Luca, Daniele Coraci, Carmen Erra, Costanza Pazzaglia, Ilaria Paolasso, Claudia Loreti, Pietro Caliandro, and Lisa D. Hobson-Webb. 2016. Carpal tunnel syndrome: Clinical features, diagnosis, and management. *The Lancet Neurology* 15: 1273–84. [CrossRef]

Pan, Y. Albert, Thomas Misgeld, Jeff W. Lichtman, and Joshua R. Sanes. 2003. Effects of neurotoxic and neuroprotective agents on peripheral nerve regeneration assayed by time-lapse imaging in vivo. *Journal of Neuroscience* 23: 11479–88. [CrossRef]

Patel, Neel B., and Gregory Scott Stacy. 2012. Musculoskeletal manifestations of neurofibromatosis type 1. *American Journal of Roentgenology* 199: W99–W106. [CrossRef]

Peters-Veluthamaningal, Cyriac, Jan C. Winters, Klaas H. Groenier, and Betty Meyboom-de Jong. 2010. Randomised controlled trial of local corticosteroid injections for carpal tunnel syndrome in general practice. *BMC Family Practice* 11: 54. [CrossRef]

Pfister, Bryan J., Tessa Gordon, Joseph R. Loverde, Arshneel S. Kochar, Susan E. Mackinnon, and D. Kacy Cullen. 2011. Biomedical engineering strategies for peripheral nerve repair: Surgical applications, state of the art, and future challenges. *Critical Reviews in Biomedical Engineering* 39: 81–124. [CrossRef] [PubMed]

Pham, Khoa, and Ranjan Gupta. 2009. Understanding the mechanisms of entrapment neuropathies. *Neurosurgical Focus* 26: E7. [CrossRef] [PubMed]

Phillips, Lawrence H., and Vern C. Juel. 1997. The role of electrodiagnostic testing in carpal tunnel syndrome. *Neurosurgical Focus* 3: e2. [CrossRef]

Pilavaki, Mayia, Danai Chourmouzi, A. Kiziridou, Anna Skordalaki, Thomas Zarampoukas, and Antonios Drevelengas. 2004. Imaging of peripheral nerve sheath tumors with pathologic correlation: Pictorial review. *European Journal of Radiology* 52: 229. [CrossRef]

Plate, Ann-Marie, German Steiner, and Martin A. Posner. 2006. Malignant tumors of the hand and wrist. *Journal of the American Academy of Orthopaedic Surgeons* 14: 680–92. [CrossRef] [PubMed]

Poyhonen, Minna, Solja Niemela, and Riitta Herva. 1997. Risk of malignancy and death in neurofibromatosis. *Archives of Pathology & Laboratory Medicine* 121: 139–43.

Prudner, Bethany C., Tyler Ball, Richa Rathore, and Angela C. Hirbe. 2020. Diagnosis and management of malignant peripheral nerve sheath tumor: Current practice and future perspectives. *Neuro-Oncology Advances* 2: i40–i49. [CrossRef]

Raissi, Gholam Reza, Fatemeh Ghazaei, Bijan Forogh, Seyed Pezhman Madani, Abbas Daghaghzadeh, and Tannaz Ahadi. 2017. The Effectiveness of Radial Extracorporeal Shock Waves for Treatment of Carpal Tunnel Syndrome: A Randomized Clinical Trial. *Ultrasound in Medicine & Biology* 43: 453–60. [CrossRef]

Rasbridge, S. A., N. L. Browse, J. R. Tighe, and C. D. Fletcher. 1989. Malignant nerve sheath tumor arising in a benign ancient schwannoma. *Histopathology* 14: 525–28. [CrossRef]

Ratanshi, Imran, Tod A. Clark, and Jennifer L. Giuffre. 2018. Immediate nerve transfer for treatment of peroneal nerve palsy secondary to an intraneural ganglion: Case report and review. *Plastic Surgery* 26: 80–84. [CrossRef]

Rempel, David M., and Edward Diao. 2004. Entrapment neuropathies: Pathophysiology and pathogenesis. *Journal of Electromyography and Kinesiology* 14: 71–75. [CrossRef] [PubMed]

Robinson, Lawrence R. 2000. Traumatic injury to peripheral nerves. *Muscle Nerve* 23: 863–73. [CrossRef]

Ropper, Allan H., and Martin A. Samuels. 2009. *Adams and Victor's Principles of Neurology*, 9th ed. New York: McGraw-Hill Education.

Rydevik, Björn, and Göran Lundborg. 1977. Permeability of intraneural microvessels and perineurium following acute, graded experimental nerve compression. *Scandinavian Journal of Plastic and Reconstructive Surgery* 11: 179–87. [CrossRef]

Sacks, Justin M., Kodi K. Azari, Scott Oates, and David W. Chang. 2013. Benign and malignant tumors of the hand. In *Plastic Surgery, Volume 6*. Edited by Peter Neligan and James Chang. Philadelphia: Saunders, Elsevier, pp. 311–32.

Schmid, Daniel B., and A. Neil Salyapongse. 2008. Nerve injury and repair. *Current Orthopaedic Practice* 19: 475–80. [CrossRef]

Seddighi, Afsoun, Amir Nikouei, Amir Saied Seddighi, Ali Reza Zali, Seyed Mahmood Tabatabaei, Ali Reza Sheykhi, Fatemeh Yourdkhani, and Shoayb Naeimian. 2016. Peripheral Nerve Injury: A Review Article. *International Clinical Neuroscience Journal* 3: 1–6. [CrossRef]

Seddon, H. J. 1942. A Classification of Nerve Injuries. *British Medical Journal* 2: 237–39. [CrossRef]

Seddon, H. J. 1943. Three types of nerve injury. *Brain* 66: 237–88. [CrossRef]

Seol, J. G., L. A. Loevner, B. W. O'Malley, and M. S. Grady. 2009. Inflammatory Pseudotumor of the Trigeminal Nerve: A Neoplastic Mimic You Do Not Want to Miss. *American Journal of Neuroradiology* 30: 1941–43. [CrossRef]

Sheth, Sachiv, Xinmin Li, Scott Binder, and Sarah M. Dry. 2011. Differential gene expression profiles of neurothekeomas and nerve sheath myxomas by microarray analysis. *Modern Pathology* 24: 343–54. [CrossRef]

Shi, Qiyun, and Joy C. MacDermid. 2011. Is surgical intervention more effective than non-surgical treatment for carpal tunnel syndrome? A systematic review. *Journal of Orthopaedic Surgery and Research* 6: 17. [CrossRef]

Shiri, R., M. H. Pourmemari, K. Falah-Hassani, and E. Viikari-Juntura. 2015. The effect of excess body mass on the risk of carpal tunnel syndrome: A meta-analysis of 58 studies. *Obesity Reviews* 16: 1094–104. [CrossRef] [PubMed]

Shokrzadeh, Ahmad, Afsoun Seddighi, and Amir Saied Seddighi. 2010. Therapeutic Results of Transcutaneous Electrical Nerve Stimulation in Post Laminectomy Syndrome. *Global Journal of Health Science* 2: 137–41. [CrossRef]

Siemionow, Maria, and Grzegorz Brzezicki. 2009. Chapter 8 Current Techniques and Concepts in Peripheral Nerve Repair. *International Review of Neurobiology* 87: 141–72. [CrossRef] [PubMed]

Siqueira, Mario G., Paulo L. Tavares, Roberto S. Martins, Carlos O. Heise, Luciano H. L. Foroni, Marcelo Bordalo, and Roberto Falzoni. 2012. Management of desmoid-type fibromatosis involving peripheral nerves. *Arquivos de Neuro-Psiquiatria* 70: 514–19. [CrossRef]

Smith, James W. 1964. Microsurgery of peripheral nerves. *Plastic and Reconstructive Surgery* 33: 317–29. [CrossRef] [PubMed]

Smolle, J., K. Konrad, and H. Kerl. 1985. Granular cell tumors contain myelinassociated glycoprotein. An immunohistochemical study using leu 7 monoclonal antibody. *Virchows Archiv A, Pathological Anatomy and Histopathology* 406: 1–5. [CrossRef] [PubMed]

Stanec, Sanda, Ivana Tonković, Zdenko Stanec, Dinko Tonković, and Ivo Džepina. 1997. Treatment of upper limb nerve war injuries associated with vascular trauma. *Injury* 28: 463–68. [CrossRef]

Stevens, J. Clarke. 1987. AAEE minimonograph #26: The electrodiagnosis of carpal tunnel syndrome. *Muscle & Nerve* 10: 99–113. [CrossRef]

Stewart, John D. 2000. *Focal Peripheral Neuropathies*, 3rd ed. Philadelphia: Lippincott Williams & Wilkins.

Sunderland, Sydney. 1951a. A classification of peripheral nerve injuries producing loss of function. *Brain* 74: 491–516. [CrossRef]

Sunderland, Sydney. 1951b. The function of nerve fibers whose structure has been disorganized. *Anatomical Record* 109: 503–13. [CrossRef]

Sunderland, Sydney. 1990. The anatomy and physiology of nerve injury. *Muscle & Nerve* 13: 771–84. [CrossRef]

Sunderland, Sydney. 1991. *Nerve Injuries and Their Repair: A Critical Appraisal*. New York: Churchill Livingstone.

Tahiri, Youssef, Liqin Xu, Jonathan Kanevsky, and Mario Luc. 2013. Lipofibromatous hamartoma of the median nerve: A comprehensive review and systematic approach to evaluation, diagnosis, and treatment. *The Journal of Hand Surgery* 38: 2055–67. [CrossRef] [PubMed]

Tapadia, Minal, Tahseen Mozaffar, and Ranjan Gupta. 2010. Compressive neuropathies of the upper extremity: Update on pathophysiology, classification, and electrodiagnostic findings. *The Journal of Hand Surgery* 35: 668–77. [CrossRef]

Terzis, Julia K., and Vasileios K. Kostopoulos. 2010. Vascularized nerve grafts and vascularized fascia for upper extremity nerve reconstruction. *Hand* 5: 19–30. [CrossRef]

Thomsen, Niels O. B., and Lars B. Dahlin. 2007. Injury to the radial nerve caused by fracture of the humeral shaft: Timing and neurobiological aspects related to treatment and diagnosis. *Scandinavian Journal of Plastic and Reconstructive Surgery and Hand Surgery* 41: 153–57. [CrossRef] [PubMed]

Thomsen, N. O. B., Ragnhild Cederlund, Jonas Björk, and L. B. Dahlin. 2010. Health-related quality of life in diabetic patients with carpal tunnel syndrome. *Diabetic Medicine* 27: 466–72. [CrossRef]

Tsang, William Y. W., John K. C. Chan, Louis T. C. Chow, and C. H. Christopher. 1992. Perineurioma: An uncommon soft tissue neoplasm distinct from localized hypertrophic neuropathy and neurofibroma. *The American Journal of Surgical Pathology* 16: 756. [CrossRef]

Uchiyama, Daiji, Toshihisa Oshige, Katsumi Nakamura, and Masamichi Koganemaru. 2016. Carpal tunnel syndrome caused by neural fibrolipoma. *BMJ Case Reports* 2016: bcr2015212819. [CrossRef]

Ud Din, Nasir, Zubair Ahmad, Jamshid Abdul-Ghafar, and Rashida Ahmed. 2019. Hybrid peripheral nerve sheath tumors: Report of five cases and detailed review of literature. *BMC Cancer* 17: 349. [CrossRef]

Uzun, Hakan, Ozan Bitik, Öznur Uzun, Umut Sinan Ersoy, and Erdem Aktaş. 2017. Platelet-rich plasma versus corticosteroid injections for carpal tunnel syndrome. *Journal of Plastic Surgery and Hand Surgery* 51: 301–5. [CrossRef]

van Rijn, Rogier M., Bionka M. A. Huisstede, Bart W. Koes, and Alex Burdorf. 2009. Associations between work-related factors and the carpal tunnel syndrome–A systematic review. *Scandinavian Journal of Work, Environment & Health* 35: 19–36.

Violante, Francesco S., Andrea Farioli, Francesca Graziosi, Francesco Marinelli, Stefania Curti, Thomas J. Armstrong, Stefano Mattioli, and Roberta Bonfiglioli. 2016. Carpal tunnel syndrome and manual work: The OCTOPUS cohort, results of a ten-year longitudinal study. *Scandinavian Journal of Work, Environment & Health* 42: 280–90.

Vraa, S., Johnny Keller, Ole Steen Nielsen, Otto Sneppen, A. G. Jurik, and Olaf M. Jensen. 1998. Prognostic factors in soft tissue sarcomas: The Aarhus experience. *European Journal of Cancer* 34: 1876–82. [CrossRef] [PubMed]

Wadhwa, Vibhor, Safia N. Salaria, and Avneesh Chhabra. 2014. Granular cell tumor of the ulnar nerve: MR neurography characterization. *Journal of Radiology Case Reports* 8: 11–17. [CrossRef]

Wahab, Kolawole Wasiu, Emmanuel O. Sanya, Philip B. Adebayo, Musbaudeen O. Babalola, and Hakeem G. Ibraheem. 2017. Carpal Tunnel Syndrome and Other Entrapment Neuropathies. *Oman Medical Journal* 32: 449–54. [CrossRef]

Webber, N. P. 2014. Biopsy. In *Orthopaedic Knowledge Update: Musculoskeletal Tumors* 3. Edited by J. Sybil Biermann. Rosemont: AAOS, pp. 23–30.

Weiss, Sharon W., and John R. Goldblum. 2001. *Enzinger and Weiss's Soft Tissue Tumors*. St. Louis: Mosby, Inc.

Werner, Robert A., and Michael Andary. 2002. Carpal tunnel syndrome: Pathophysiology and clinical neurophysiology. *Clinical Neurophysiology* 113: 1373–81. [CrossRef]

Werner, Robert A., Cynthia Bir, and Thomas J. Armstrong. 1994. Reverse Phalen's maneuver as an aid in diagnosing carpal tunnel syndrome. *Archives of Physical Medicine and Rehabilitation* 75: 783–86. [CrossRef]

White, Warren, Man H. Shiu, Marc K. Rosenblum, Robert A. Erlandson, and James M. Woodruff. 1990. Cellular schwannoma. A clinicopathologic study of 57 patients and 58 tumors. *Cancer* 66: 1266–75. [CrossRef]

Wilbourn, A. J. 2002. Peripheral neuropathies associated with vascular diseases and the vasculitides. In *Neuromuscular Function and Disease*. Edited by William F. Brown, Charles F. Bolton and Michael J. Aminoff. Philadelphia: Saunders, pp. 1229–62.

Woltman, H. W., and A. W. Adson. 1946. Neuritis ossificans with osteogenic sarcoma in brachial plexus following trauma; report of case. *The Lancet* 66: 372–76.
Wong, William W., Takanori Hirose, Bernd W. Scheithauer, Steven E. Schild, and Leonard L. Gunderson. 1998. Malignant peripheral nerve sheath tumor: Analysis of treatment outcome. *International Journal of Radiation Oncology, Biology, Physics* 42: 351–60. [CrossRef]
Woodruff, James M., Abby M. Selig, Keith Crowley, and Philip W. Allen. 1994. Schwannoma (neurilemoma) with malignant transformation. a rare, distinctive peripheral nerve tumor. *The American Journal of Surgical Pathology* 18: 882–95. [CrossRef] [PubMed]
Yang, James C., Alfred E. Chang, Alan R. Baker, William F. Sindelar, David N. Danforth, Suzanne L. Topalian, Thomas DeLaney, Eli Glatstein, Seth M. Steinberg, Maria J. Merino, and et al. 1998. Randomized prospective study of the benefit of adjuvant radiation therapy in the treatment of soft tissue sarcomas of the extremity. *Journal of Clinical Oncology* 16: 197–203. [CrossRef] [PubMed]
Yao, Chenglun, Xijie Zhou, Bin Zhao, Chao Sun, Keshav Poonit, and Hede Yan. 2017. Treatments of traumatic neuropathic pain: A systematic review. *Oncotarget* 8: 57670–79. [CrossRef] [PubMed]
Zhang, Enlong, Jiahui Zhang, Ning Lang, and Huishu Yuan. 2018. Spinal cellular schwannoma: An analysis of imaging manifestation and clinicopathological findings. *European Journal of Radiology* 105: 81–86. [CrossRef]
Zochodne, D. W., and D. Levy. 2005. Nitirc Oxide in damage, disease and repair of the peripheral nervous system. *Cellular and Molecular Biology (Noisy-le-Grand, France)* 51: 255–67.

Section XIV: Future Directions

Future Directions in Neurosurgery

Bipin Chaurasia and Forhad H. Chowdhury

Abstract: The neurosurgical field is changing swiftly. In the last 100 years, neurosurgery has achieved success and access that was beyond the imagination of a nineteen-century surgeon. What is science-fiction now will be fact tomorrow. Open microsurgery has transformed and is transforming into endoscopic/minimally invasive neurosurgery, which is now, in many cases, aided by robotically assisted surgery. In the near future, neurological and neurosurgical diseases will probably be treated by "biological manipulation". Many researches are defining the future directions of neurosurgery. In this chapter, we will touch on future directions in neurosurgery, i.e., robotics in neurosurgery, neuro stem cell therapy, hydrocephalus research, gene therapy in neurological diseases, and drug addiction surgery.

Abbreviations

ROSA	robotic operating surgical assistant	TBI	traumatic brain injury
MSC	mesenchymal stem cells	NSC	neural stem cells
MAPC	multipotent adult progenitor cells	EPC	endothelial progenitor cells
GBM	glioblastoma multiforme	RNA	ribonucleic acid
GABA	glutamic acid decarboxylase	STN	subthalamic nucleus
ADDC	aromatic amino acid decarboxylase	PD	Parkinson disease
BDNF	brain-derived neurotrophic factor	FGF	fibroblast growth factor
NAc	nucleus accumbens	DBS	deep brain stimulation
CSF	cerebrospinal fluid	NKCC	$Na^+/K^+/2Cl^-$ cotransporter
VP	Ventriculoperitoneal	ETV	endoscopic third ventriculostomy
CPC	choroid plexus cauterization		

1. Introduction

The neurosurgical field and practice are changing very rapidly. In the last 100 years, neurosurgery has achieved success and access that was beyond the imagination of a nineteen-century surgeon. What is science-fiction now will be real tomorrow. Open mechanical microsurgery has converted and is converting to endoscopic/minimally invasive neurosurgery, which is now, in many instances, aided by robotically assisted surgery. In the near future, neurological and neurosurgical diseases will likely to be treated by "biological manipulation". Many researches are defining the future directions of neurosurgery.

2. Robotics in Neurosurgery

2.1. Introduction

Robotic surgery is not as prevalent in neurosurgery compared to other field of surgery like gastroenterology, cardiology, and urology. This is mainly because of anatomical challenges in the complexity of very sensitive brain structures (Gui et al. 2015). "Heartthrob" was the world's first surgical robot, and it was initially utilized in Vancouver, British Columbia, Canada, in 1983. The MKM system, released by Zeiss in 1993, was the first neurosurgery robotic microscope; a robot arm held various instruments, including a microscope head, in the system (Roser et al. 2013; Haegelen et al. 2010).

The first neurosurgical robot commercially available was NeuroMate, which was approved by the FDA. At its most basic level, the neurosurgical robot is made up of the following parts: a robotic arm, controllers that guide the robot (end-effector), feedback sensors, a wireless localization system, and a data processing center (the brain).

Robots can be wholly autonomous, completely reliant, or a hybrid of both autonomous and controlled systems. The most commonly available neuro-robots these days are Neuromate, NeuroArm, SpineAssist, and the Pathfinder (Fomekong et al. 2017; Pak et al. 2015).

2.2. Types of Neuro-Robots

Neurosurgical robots are grossly classified into three categories:

1. Telesurgical robots (master-slave), in which the surgeon remotely controls the activities of the robot.

2. The supervisory surgeon-controlled robot, where the robot assists the surgeon to perform precise tasks.
3. Hand-controlled systems, where the surgeon and the robot both control the instruments utilized to handle and dissect the brain tissue.

2.3. Advantages of Neuro-Robotics

Robotics provides different advantages in surgical tasks (Fomekong et al. 2017; Pak et al. 2015; Kapoor and Rath 2016):

- Helping to improve stereotaxic neurosurgery precision and accuracy;
- In minimally invasive surgery, access to narrow passageways;
- In image-guided surgery, the capability to process enormous amounts of data;
- By stabilizing a surgeon's hand or scaling the surgeon's hand motions;
- The capacity to perform telesurgery, provide a 10-fold reduction in surgeons' physiological tremor, and eliminate surgeons' fatigue.

As compared to modern surgical procedures, robotic surgery provides improved visualization, minimal blood loss, very minimal scarring, a decreased infection rate, less pain, a reduced hospital stay, and early immobilization.

2.3.1. Disadvantages

Despite its many advantages, high costs, the need for high expertise, complicated technical procedure, and time-consuming processes make robotics impractical for many neurosurgeons. At present, robots are utilized primely as stands, freeing up a neurosurgeon's hand and decreasing muscle fatigue (Vougioukas et al. 2003).

2.4. Applications in Neurosurgery

Common robotic procedures in neurosurgery include stereotaxic procedures, endoscopic procedures, applications in robotized microscopes, telepresence, and tumor resection (Chauvet et al. 2017; Tsai et al. 2002).

2.4.1. In Hematoma Evacuation

Robots in neurosurgery assist in stereotactic procedures as well as endoscopic interventions. Hematoma removal with a hand-held endoscope and with robotic endoscopic evacuation has been studied. The findings imply that robotic assistance, at the cost of a somewhat longer procedure time, increases the safety of the target volume excision by increasing the surgeon's solace and dexterity (Kulkarni et al. 2016; Hoshide et al. 2017).

2.4.2. In Functional Neurosurgery

ROSA (robotic operating surgical assistant) Brain, a robotic tool, helps to perform minimally invasive procedures in the brain. The targets can be on the surface or deep within the brain. ROSA can perform many procedures in the brain, including putting an electrode in an epileptic focus for the treatment of epilepsy, which helps in performing biopsies of brain tumors and cortical dysplasia. It also helps in laser ablation in the treatment of hypothalamic hamartoma and in putting electrodes deep inside the brain for movement disorders as a part of deep brain stimulation. Functional procedures are also performed in the spinal cord. ROSA has also proven beneficial in performing stereotaxic biopsies of pontine glioma, with no surgical complications. ETV procedures for pediatric hydrocephalous have been successfully performed, with no complications (Miller et al. 2017; Carai et al. 2017; De Benedictis et al. 2017; Marcus et al. 2015; Hong et al. 2013).

2.4.3. In Spinal Surgery

Spinal robots help not only in the accuracy of the interventions but also by adding the additional benefits of other factors like radiation dosage, minimal invasiveness, and learning curves. Spine surgeries have been successfully performed without complications. In minimally invasive surgeries, robot-assisted transpedicular screw placement in spinal fixation has been performed without any screw misplacements. Roser et al. found that the ideal accuracy with a pure intrapedicular trajectory was 92% in a set of 46 patients with 244 robotic-assisted pedicle screws, with 5.3% of the screws showing a lateral deviation and 2.5% showing a medial deviation. A surgical revision was performed on the patients who had medial screw abnormalities. A total of 65% (30–46) of these patients received intervention using a minimally invasive pure percutaneous technique (Fiani et al. 2017; Ettore et al. 2016).

2.5. Conclusions

Although the utilization of robotics in neurosurgery is still in its early stages, we feel that the few neurosurgical robots now in use in operating rooms have already demonstrated high potential for improving surgical results, particularly when precision and low invasiveness are required.

3. Neuro Stem Cell Therapy

3.1. Introduction

Stem cells are pluripotent cells with the ability to divide into a variety of cell types within the body. The divided stem cells have the capability to remain as stem cells or transform into a different type of cell with a more specialized purpose. They have unique characteristics in that they lack tissue-specific features that would enable them to conduct specialized functional activities. These unspecialized stem cells can differentiate into specialized cells such as blood cells, heart muscle cells, and brain cells. They also have the capability to divide and regenerate for long periods of time, as well as replicate multiple times (Lee 2003; Horita et al. 2006). Stem cells for transplantation can be autologous (person's own cells) or allogenic (from donor). Pre-implantation embryos, aborted fetuses, children, adults, embryos, umbilical cord, amniotic fluid, menstrual blood, and the placenta are all possible sources of stem cells.

Pluripotent stem cells can be used to treat a variety of diseases, pathological conditions, and disabilities, including stroke, Parkinson's and Alzheimer's diseases, cerebral palsy spinal cord injury, Batten's disease (a pediatric lysosomal storage disease that causes neuronal loss), chronic pain, epilepsy, amyotrophic lateral sclerosis, vision restoration, and many other neurodegenerative diseases (Horie et al. 2011; Ourednik et al. 2000).

Embryonic stem cells, e.g., human embryonic cells or mouse-derived cells are derived from the inner cell mass of the embryonic blastula. The main drawback of embryonic cell transplantation is the development of teratomas. Adult stem cells could be a source of autologous cells for transplantation, removing immunological risks. A notable example of this is bone marrow transplantation. When implanted into irradiated recipients, bone-marrow-derived hematopoietic or mesenchymal stem cells can move into the brain and develop into astrocytes, microglia, and possibly neurons.

3.2. Applications in Neurosurgery

3.2.1. Spinal Cord Injury

Stem cells in spinal cord injury not only take part in neuron replacement but also foster functional recovery. They influence the post-traumatic cord milieu by secreting a collection of bioactive chemicals that decrease local immune responses, increase angiogenesis, and inhibit scarring and cell death in a paracrine and autocrine manner. They are also in charge of axon remyelination, sprouting, and directing them to their destinations, as well as the development of functional bridges. Possible mechanisms through which stem cells work and their modes of action have been summarized in Table 1 below.

Direct injection to the wounded location, Subarachnoid Stem Cell Implantation by intra-arterial, Lumber Puncture, and intravenous injections are all options for stem cell delivery. Intranasal (i.n.) administration of stem cells after stem cell implantation using brain stereotactic surgery is another option. The best sort of cells to choose for implantation, their dosage, the best delivery route, and the optimal timing for therapy are all important variables to specify in this discipline. Mesenchymal stem cells from adipose tissue and bone marrow, hematopoietic stem cells, olfactory ensheathing, embryonic cord blood stem cells, and neural precursor cells have all been used to treat spinal cord injuries (Iwanami et al. 2005).

Logistics and ethical issues, the utilization of allogeneic cells demanding immunosuppressive therapy, and the possible tumorigenicity of transplanted cells are some of the disadvantages of using neural stem cells. Autologous cells should be used in cellular treatment if they can be easily obtained, processed in vitro, and reinoculated into the same patient. Stem cells have also found potential in the treatment of spinal and cranial bony defects, as well as intervertebral disc degeneration. Careful selection of patients with spinal cord injuries is necessary for the transplantation of neural stem cells, which have the ability to replace lost tissue after nervous system injury.

Table 1. Mechanism of functional recovery in spinal cord injury.

Events	Consequences	Mechanism
After spinal cord injury	Parenchymal damage	Inflammation-inducted stimulation of host plastic reactions
	Interference	With autologous neural activity
After neuro stem cell therapy	Make up of biochemical deficiency	Missing transmitter discharge ('minipump')
	Growth factor release	Initiation of plastic responses; improvement in survival and activity of host neurons
	Local reinnervation	Re-establishment of synaptic neurotransmitter release
	Reformation of neural circuitries	Reconstruction of functional efferent and afferent connections

Source: Authors' compilation based on data from Iwanami et al. (2005).

3.2.2. In Peripheral Nerve Injury

The peripheral neural system has a stronger capacity for regeneration than the CNS. Embryonic neural stem cells, adipose tissue, bone marrow cells, and the skin and its accompanying structures are all possible sources for peripheral nerve repair. Stem cell therapy's therapeutic potential for damaged peripheral nerves is unclear. According to some evidence, transplanted, neutrally generated embryonic stem cells develop into myelin-forming cells, suggesting that they could be used to treat severely wounded peripheral nerves. The implantation of embryonic stem cells potentiates nerve repair in peripheral nerves (Walsh and Midha 2009).

3.2.3. In Degenerative Intervertebral DISC

Mesenchymal stem cells have been used to try to repair or regenerate the degenerated intervertebral disc. Stem cells have the ability to develop into nucleus-pulposus-like cells capable of producing the physiological, proteoglycan-rich extracellular matrix found in healthy intervertebral discs (Lee 2003).

3.2.4. Traumatic Brain Injury (TBI)

TBIs include concussion, contusions, diffuse axonal injury, and penetrating injury. In all types of TBI, brain cell death occurs when brain tissues are damaged or when blood supply to crucial parts of the brain is disrupted. When neurons die, they are incapable of regenerating or growing, and the sections of the body that they control become disabled. Exogenous stem cells have been found to move to damaged brain tissue and then assist in brain parenchyma repair by further differentiation into substitute damaged cells while producing anti-inflammatory and growth factors, leading to considerable enhancements in neurological function. In recent studies, a variety of stem cells, including neural stem cells (NSCs), mesenchymal stem cells (MSCs), multipotent adult progenitor cells (MAPCs), and endothelial progenitor cells (EPCs), have been discovered to heal neurological damage following a TBI (Boockvar et al. 2005).

The utility of SB623 bone-marrow-derived modified stem cells has showed promise in neuro-regeneration and repair, as well as preserving functional recovery after various forms of injuries. Twenty-eight endothelial progenitor cells are migratory precursor cells that can convert into vascular endothelial cells and contribute to endothelial healing, particularly in the brain following trauma. Mesenchymal cells, the neuroectoderm, the visceral mesoderm, and the endoderm can all be differentiated from multipotent adult progenitor cells. This has the potential to improve information retention, spatial learning, memory retrieval, and dyskinesia following delayed brain injury as well as maintain the blood–brain barrier's integrity during the acute phase of TBI. Neurons, glial cells, and oligodendrocytes can all be formed from neural stem cells. It could be a long-term treatment for neurological recovery following brain damage (Boockvar et al. 2005; Burns et al. 2009).

3.3. Conclusions

Stem cell transplantation appears to be a viable therapeutic option for patients suffering from a variety of neurosurgical illnesses. The expectation that stem-cell-based therapies can restore and sustain function in the spinal cord and brain has been bolstered by recent developments and progress.

4. Gene Therapy in Neurosurgery

4.1. Introduction

Gene therapy is the transfer of nucleic acid as genetic material into somatic cells to provide a therapeutic effect. Gene transfer into the human body can be performed by ex vivo and in vivo approaches. Ex vivo approaches include the process of cell isolation from the patient and genetic modification exterior to the body in a cultivated area and then re-implantation into the patient, while in vivo gene transfer includes transferring a gene by a vector into the subject as a direct target cell transducer. For in vivo gene transfer, issues like the selection of appropriate vectors to carry the genetic load, the efficacy of distribution and targeting, the capacity to regulate gene function or expression in vivo, and safety concerns, especially when viruses are used as vectors, should be addressed (Weihl et al. 1999; Ourednik et al. 2000).

Germ line gene therapy and somatic gene therapy are the two types of gene therapy that can be used. In somatic gene therapy, therapeutic genes are deployed into a patient's somatic cells, or body. Any changes and effects will be limited to one patient only, and it will not be passed along to the patient's children or future generations. In germ line gene therapy, however, sperm or ovum are transformed through the implantation of functional genes into their genomes. This would make the therapy heritable, allowing it to be handed down to future generations (Chiocca 2003; Helm et al. 2000). Most brain tumors are treated with viral gene transfer as viral vectors are increasingly safe and non-immunogenic. While non-viral vectors are less efficient, they are safer, can be produced more easily, and offer reduced pathogenicity. The issue with non-viral vectors is that they link to blood cells or plasma proteins, causing aggregation and capillary blockage. Recombinant herpes simplex virus, retroviruses/lentiviruses, adeno-associated viruses, and adenoviruses are examples of viral vectors. Cationic polymers and cationic lipids are non-viral delivery techniques whose efficacy is determined by saturation, cationic charge, and linker stability.

The main drawback of gene therapy is that the vector cannot cross the blood–brain barrier. Another problem is that it causes immune-mediated vector toxicity. That is why the delivery of a vector into the brain is achieved by stereotactic inoculation of the vector into the wall of the tumor cavity, direct intrathecal or intraventricular administration, and intravascular application by disruption of the blood–brain barrier using an intracarotid infusion of vasoactive compounds and hyperosmolar solutions (Freese et al. 1997; Alden et al. 1999).

4.2. Applications in Neurosurgery

Some of the conditions of the brain treated with gene therapy include Parkinson disease, Alzheimer's disease, ischemic brain diseases, brain tumors, epilepsy, lysosomal storage disease, amyotrophic lateral sclerosis, motor neuron disease, and Huntington's disease.

4.2.1. For Glioblastoma Multiforme

Gene therapy for brain tumors is used especially for glioma. Among gliomas, most studies on gene therapy strategy have been trialed on glioblastoma multiforme, due to its very low survival rate, inaccessibility to respective surgery due to the anatomical site of the tumor, and infiltration from tumor cells into nearby tissues. A combination of thymidine kinase and ganciclovir, called "suicide" gene therapy, has been studied for GBM. The non-toxic prodrug is transformed into a toxic compound that kills tumor cells in transduced cells. The Escherichia coli cytosine deaminase/5-fluorocytosin system, the rat cytochrome P450 2B1/cyclophosphamide system, and the Escherichia coli reductase/CB1954 system have all been employed for gene therapies in experimental animal models for the management of gliomas (Weihl et al. 1999; Ourednik et al. 2000; Helm et al. 2000). Other gene therapy strategies include tumor suppressor genes (such as p53, Fas, ras, TNF-a, and caspases); augmentation of extracellular matrix protein expression; inhibition of angiogenesis; immune system modulation; oncolytic virus eradication; and the utilization of ribozymes, small interfering RNA, and antisense oligonucleotides to induce apoptosis in tumor cells.

4.2.2. For Parkinson's Disease (PD)

Two gene therapy clinical studies for Parkinson's disease are currently underway. One method is to use glutamic acid decarboxylase gene transfer and subsequent GABA synthesis in the subthalamic nucleus (STN). The other employs an ADDC intrastriatal gene transfer strategy (aromatic amino acid decarboxylase) (Chiocca 2003; Freese et al. 1997; Alden et al. 1999) . The newer therapy with gene transfer for the treatment of various brain conditions has gained new popularity after the rapid progress of viral and non-viral vector systems as an alternative to existing pharmacological treatments. Both vector systems, however, have advantages and limitations, thus the search for the optimum one continues. When medicine fails to control PD symptoms, gene therapy is a better option than DBS or subthalamotomy.

4.2.3. For Epilepsy

Gene therapy has been attempted for focal seizures like temporal-lobe-originated seizures, which are medically refractive. It has anti-epileptogenic, antiseizure, and disease-modifying properties. Gene therapy produces a combination therapy based on the replenishment of fibroblast growth factor 2 (FGF-2) and brain-derived neurotrophic factor (BDNF) to counteract epilepsy (Chiocca 2003; Helm et al. 2000).

4.3. Conclusions

The role of gene therapy in many of brain diseases is very promising. However, more preclinical and clinical research is needed in this field to fully understand the potential side effects and develop truly effective treatments for neurological illnesses.

5. Drug Addiction Surgery

5.1. Introduction

Neurosurgery for addiction is not a futuristic concept. On the contrary, neurosurgery to treat addiction to heroine, alcohol, methamphetamine is happening now in many parts of world. In fact, DBS is the preferred method of treatment for this purpose and is well known for its management of Parkinson's symptoms that cannot be treated with medications. It is considered a last-resort therapy if traditional treatment, such as medication to lessen drug cravings, has failed (Li et al. 2013; Lu et al. 2009; Voges et al. 2013).

5.2. Application

When there is substantial relapse frequency after conservative therapy and the negative effects of persistent alcohol consumption on the mental, physical, and social life of these people persist, deep brain stimulation may be considered. Its exact mechanism is unknown, although it is considered to work by modifying the reward circuit, which is dependent on a chemical messenger called dopamine. Dopamine elevations in the nucleus accumbens (NAc) caused by drugs facilitate reward. The medial forebrain bundle, which links the ventral tegmental region and hypothalamus with the olfactory tubercle, and the NAc make up the reward circuit (Gao et al. 2003; Lamphier 1957; Luigjes et al. 2013). The nucleus accumbens, which is often called the "pleasure center" of the brain, is the main nucleus of the brain's reward circuit, where deep brain stimulation electrodes are placed. The neurotransmitter dopamine stimulates cells of the NAc, which elicit pleasurable sensations after taking heroin, etc. An electrical current is transmitted through the electrodes that destroys the cells of the NAc. By destroying the pleasure center, it is easy to get rid of addictions. Surgery is performed in an awake condition where the patient talks during the procedure, so that surgeons know if the electrodes are too close to actual sites that control various functions.

Resetting of the NAc function, according to evidence, can significantly enhance addictive behavior. However, the findings of DBS in clinical trials are still quite preliminary. As a result, the initial priority of future activities should be to confirm the seen improvement in prospective studies employing DBS stimulation procedures that are randomized, double-blind, or crossover. These studies are restricted by small patient numbers, unpredictable long-term follow-up, probable publication bias, and a lack of blinded stimulation, despite their encouraging results (Pelloux and Baunez 2013; Wang et al. 2018).

5.3. Conclusions

Neurosurgeons have worked hard to develop procedures that are both successful and safe for treating addiction. The surgical management of addiction will continue to pursue a safer and more standardized path as technical approaches and the realization of neurophysiology increase, and as the aggregation of high-level clinical trial data occurs.

6. Hydrocephalus Research

6.1. Introduction

Much of the research focuses on finding better ways to prevent, treat, and ultimately cure hydrocephalus. For many, the future is bright if hydrocephalus is detected early and treated appropriately. Recent research has advanced our understanding and brought us closer to a cure. Technological advancements, as well as improved diagnosis and treatment regimens, are allowing an increasing number of persons with hydrocephalus to live full and active lives. There is currently no effective medical treatment for hydrocephalus. Neurosurgical treatment is the primary choice for accurate management at present.

6.2. Medical Research

The choroid plexus produces nearly half of all cerebrospinal fluid (CSF), according to new research. The $Na^+/K^+/2Cl^-$ cotransporter, or NKCC1, is a protein found in the choroid plexus that is responsible for the majority of CSF production. CSF is primarily created by a process known as osmosis, in which water passively accompanies the movement of salts. However, current studies suggests that KCC1 creates cerebrospinal fluid by moving ions across choroid plexus cell membranes while also conveying water via a mechanism built into this unique protein. Because the fluid conveys both salts and water at the same time, this action is known as "cotransport" of water. This finding is particularly significant because, for a long time, people believed that cerebrospinal fluid was produced by a process called osmosis.

Bumetanide, a well-known diuretic medicine that inhibits NKCC1, could eventually lead to novel nonsurgical hydrocephalus treatments, which would be a huge step forward for patients (Steffensen et al. 2018).

TGF-1 (transforming growth factor-1) and VEGF (vascular endothelial growth factor) are two biomarkers found in high concentration in CSF that govern cell differentiation, proliferation, and other important biological activities. TGF-1 has been demonstrated in studies to be released into CSF following an intraventricular hemorrhage and to upregulate genes involved in the formation of extracellular matrix proteins (e.g., fibronectin and collagen). By focusing on pathways that affect the hydrocephalic brain, researchers revealed that certain medical therapies can reduce the rate at which hydrocephalus develops in animal models. Decorin, a growth factor antagonist, has been shown in an animal model to be effective in preventing the development of juvenile communicative hydrocephalus (Merhar 2012; Botfield et al. 2013).

6.3. Surgical Research

The current surgical treatments used are mainly ventriculoperitoneal shunt, endoscopic third ventriculostomy, and combined endoscopic third ventriculostomy (ETV) and choroid plexus cauterization (CPC). Ventriculoperitoneal shunt is the commonly performed procedure for hydrocephalus. The only advances in VP shunt treatment to date include the development of newer types of shunt valves to prevent the complications of over-drainage. Some of the valves available are antisiphon devices, siphon control devices, delta valves, and Orbis-Sigma valves. Hydrocephalus programmable valves are devices that have several differential pressure valves, all of which are differential pressure valves. It is still unclear how much these new advanced technological devices have contributed to patient therapy (Rekate 1997). The use of combination ETV and CPC for hydrocephalus management is also gaining popularity. In research in East Africa, ETV/CPC treatments were shown to be safer, with minimal mortality and morbidity; infection and long-term ETV/CPC failure rates were lower than shunts, along with success rates ranging from 62–82% (Warf et al. 2012).

Researchers have also worked on new protocols to minimize postoperative shunt infections as this is vital in controlling the morbidity and mortality of patients, even though the old protocols to minimize infections are also followed these days. In pediatric neurosurgery, the utilization of standardized protocols to minimize infection is not recent. To prevent infections, a series of steps are taken in the preoperative, peroperative, and postoperative periods, including using a no-touch technique protocol in which the neurosurgeons' hands do not touch the shunt equipment, limiting implant and skin-edge manipulation, and using educated assistants; the operative field has two drapes, neurosurgeons wear double gloves, meticulous surgical techniques are used, antibiotic prophylaxis is initiated, and total shunt revision occurs. Researchers have found that silver or antibiotic-impregnated catheters have the capability to decrease shunt infections and reduce the necessity for shunt replacement. Initial outcomes are promising and a 63% decrease in the relative risk of infections related to shunts for pediatric patients has been demonstrated (Parker et al. 2015; Jenkinson et al. 2014). Even after sticking to a strict protocol to prevent shunt infections, following modern medical and surgical management of hydrocephalus, the results are not promising. Still more research is needed for better results and outcomes.

6.4. Conclusions

Research in the field of the overall management of hydrocephalus patients is promising. More research is needed to better understand the genetics of hydrocephalus, develop models to better understand the condition, employ multidisciplinary opportunities and standardized protocols, emphasize novel bioengineering concepts, improve surgical trials, and produce validated outcome metrics.

7. Culminating Remark

At the conclusion of this chapter, we can say that what we cannot dream of today could become fact in the near future. Investigation and research in neurosurgery and other branches of medicine are growing so fast that it is even possible that the scalpel will no longer be required for treating nervous system diseases in the near future (bad news for neurosurgeons)!

Author Contributions: Conceptualization, methodology, validation, formal analysis, investigation, resources, data curation, writing—original draft preparation, B.C.; writing—review and editing, visualization, supervision, F.H.C. All authors have read and agreed to the published version of the manuscript.

Funding: This research received no external funding.

Conflicts of Interest: The authors declare no conflicts of interest.

References

Alden, Tord D., Debra D. Pittman, Elisa J. Beres, Gerald R. Hankins, David F. Kallmes, Benjamin M. Wisotsky, Kelvin M. Kerns, and Gregory A. Helm. 1999. Percutaneous spinal fusion using bone morphogenetic protein-2 gene therapy. *Journal of Neurosurgery: Spine* 90: 109–14. [CrossRef] [PubMed]

Boockvar, John A., Joost Schouten, Nicolas Royo, Marie Millard, Zak Spangler, Debbie Castelbuono, Evan Snyder, Donald O'Rourke, and Tracy McIntosh. 2005. Experimental traumatic brain injury modulates the survival, migration, and terminal phenotype of transplanted epidermal growth factor receptor-activated neural stem cells. *Neurosurgery* 56: 163–71. [CrossRef] [PubMed]

Botfield, Hannah, Ana Maria Gonzalez, Osama Abdullah, Anders Dæhli Skjolding, Martin Berry, James Pat McAllister, and Ann Logan. 2013. Decorin prevents the development of juvenile communicating hydrocephalus. *Brain* 9: 2842–858. [CrossRef] [PubMed]

Burns, Terry C., Catherine M. Verfaillie, and Walter C. Low. 2009. Stem cells for ischemic brain injury: A critical review. *Journal of Comparative Neurology* 515: 125–44. [CrossRef]

Carai, Andrea, Angela Mastronuzzi, Alessandro De Benedictis, Raffaella Messina, Antonella Cacchione, Evelina Miele, Franco Randi, Giacomo Esposito, Andrea Trezza, Giovanna Stefania Colafati, and et al. 2017. Robot-assisted stereotactic biopsy of diffuse intrinsic pontine glioma: A single-center experience. *World Neurosurgery* 101: 584–88. [CrossRef]

Chauvet, Dorian, Stéphane Hans, Antoine Missistrano, Celeste Rebours, Wissame El Bakkouri, and Guillaume Lot. 2017. Transoral robotic surgery for sellar tumors: First clinical study. *Journal of Neurosurgery* 127: 941–48. [CrossRef]

Chiocca, E. Antonio. 2003. Gene therapy: A primer for neurosurgeons. *Neurosurgery* 53: 364–73. [CrossRef]

De Benedictis, Alessandro, Andrea Trezza, Andrea Carai, Elisabetta Genovese, Emidio Procaccini, Raffaella Messina, Franco Randi, Silvia Cossu, Giacomo Esposito, Paolo Palma, and et al. 2017. Robot assisted procedures in pediatric neurosurgery. *Neurosurgical Focus* 42: E7. [CrossRef]

Ettore, Éric, Emeline Wyckaert, Renaud David, Philippe Robert, Olivier Guérin, and Frédéric Prate. 2016. Robotics and improvement of the quality of geriatric care. *Soins. Gerontologie* 21: 15–17. [CrossRef]

Fiani, Brian, Syed A. Quadri, Vivek Ramakrishnan, Blake Berman, Yasir Khan, and Javed Siddiqi. 2017. Retrospective review on accuracy: A pilot study of robotically guided thoracolumbar/sacral pedicle screws versus fluoroscopy-guided and computerized tomography stealth-guided screws. *Cureus* 9: e1437. [CrossRef]

Fomekong, Edward, Salah Edine Safi, and Christian Raftopoulos. 2017. Spine navigation based on 3-dimensional robotic fluoroscopy for accurate percutaneous pedicle screw placement: A prospective study of 66 consecutive cases. *World Neurosurgery* 108: 76–83. [CrossRef] [PubMed]

Freese, Andrew, Michael G. Kaplitt, William M. O'Connor, Maureen Abbey, David Langer, Paola Leone, Michael J. O'Connor, and Matthew J. During. 1997. Direct Gene Transfer into Human Epileptogenic Hippocampal Tissue with an Adeno-Associated Virus Vector: Implications for a Gene Therapy Approach to Epilepsy. *Epilepsia* 38: 759–66. [CrossRef] [PubMed]

Gao, Guodong, Xuelian Wang, Shiming He, Weixin Li, Qingfeng Wang, Qinchuan Liang, Yaqun Zhao, Fang Hou, Ling Chen, and Aining Li. 2003. Clinical study for alleviating opiate drug psychological dependence by a method of ablating the nucleus accumbens with stereotactic surgery. *Stereotactic and Functional Neurosurgery* 81: 96–104. [CrossRef]

Gui, Haijun, Shilei Zhang, Nan Luan, Yanping Lin, Steve G. F. Shen, and Joy S. Bautista. 2015. Novel system for navigation-and robot-assisted craniofacial surgery: Establishment of the principle prototype. *Journal of Craniofacial Surgery* 26: 746–49. [CrossRef]

Haegelen, Claire, Gustavo Touzet, Nicolas Reyns, Claude-Alain Maurage, Mohamed Ayachi, and Serge Blond. 2010. Stereotactic robot-guided biopsies of brain stem lesions: Experience with 15 cases. *Neurochirurgie* 56: 363–67. [CrossRef]

Helm, Gregory A., Tord D. Alden, Jason P. Sheehan, and David Kallmes. 2000. Bone morphogenetic proteins and bone morphogenetic protein gene therapy in neurological surgery: A review. *Neurosurgery* 46: 1213–22. [CrossRef] [PubMed]

Hong, Wei-Chen, Jui-Chang Tsai, Steven D. Chang, and Jonathan M. Sorger. 2013. Robotic skull base surgery via supraorbital keyhole approach: A cadaveric study. *Neurosurgery* 72: 33–38. [CrossRef]

Horie, Nobutaka, Marta P. Pereira, Kuniyasu Niizuma, Guohua Sun, Hadar Keren-Gill, Angelo Encarnacion, Mehrdad Shamloo, Scott A. Hamilton, Kewen Jiang, Stephen Huhn, and et al. 2011. Transplanted stem cell-secreted vascular endothelial growth factor effects poststroke recovery, inflammation, and vascular repair. *Stem Cells* 29: 274–85. [CrossRef]

Horita, Yoshifumi, Osamu Honmou, Kuniaki Harada, Kiyohiro Houkin, Hirofumi Hamada, and Jeffery D. Kocsis. 2006. Intravenous administration of glial cell line-derived neurotrophic factor gene-modified human mesenchymal stem cells protects against injury in a cerebral ischemia model in the adult rat. *Journal of Neuroscience Research* 84: 1495–504. [CrossRef]

Hoshide, Reid, Mark Calayag, Hal Meltzer, Michael L. Levy, and David Gonda. 2017. Robot-assisted endoscopic third ventriculostomy: Institutional experience in 9 patients. *Journal of Neurosurgery: Pediatrics* 20: 125–33. [CrossRef]

Iwanami, A., S. Kaneko, M. Nakamura, Y. Kanemura, H. Mori, S. Kobayashi, M. Yamasaki, S. Momoshima, H. Ishii, K. Ando, and et al. 2005. Transplantation of human neural stem cells for spinal cord injury in primates. *Journal of Neuroscience Research* 80: 182–90. [CrossRef] [PubMed]

Jenkinson, Michael D., Carrol Gamble, John C. Hartley, Helen Hickey, Dyfrig Hughes, Michaela Blundell, Michael J. Griffiths, Tom Solomon, and Conor L. Mallucci. 2014. The British Antibiotic and Silver-Impregnated Catheters for ventriculoperitoneal shunts multi-centre randomised controlled trial (the BASICS trial): Study protocol. *Trials* 15: 4. [CrossRef] [PubMed]

Kapoor, Indu, and Girija P. Rath. 2016. Robotized surgical assistant in neurosurgery. Anaesthetic implication! *Journal of Neuroanaesthesiology and Critical Care* 3: 151–52. [CrossRef]

Kulkarni, Abhaya V., Jay Riva-Cambrin, Richard Holubkov, Samuel R. Browd, D. Douglas Cochrane, James M. Drake, David D. Limbrick, Curtis J. Rozzelle, Tamara D. Simon, Mandeep S. Tamber, and et al. 2016. Endoscopic third ventriculostomy in children: Prospective TD, multicenter results from the Hydrocephalus Clinical Research Network. *Journal of Neurosurgery: Pediatrics* 18: 423–29. [CrossRef]

Lamphier, Timothy A. 1957. Drug addiction. *Journal of the American Medical Association* 163: 68. [CrossRef]

Lee, Il Woo. 2003. Stem cells and neurosurgery. *Journal of Korean Neurosurgical Society* 33: 1.

Li, Nan, Jing Wang, Xue-lian Wang, Chong-wang Chang, Shun-nan Ge, Li Gao, He-ming Wu, Hai-kang Zhao, Ning Geng, and Guo-dong Gao. 2013. Nucleus accumbens surgery for addiction. *World Neurosurgery* 80: S28.e9–S28.e19. [CrossRef]

Lu, Lin, Xi Wang, and Thomas R. Kosten. 2009. Stereotactic neurosurgical treatment of drug addiction. *The American Journal of Drug and Alcohol Abuse* 35: 391–93. [CrossRef]

Luigjes, Judy, Bart P. de Kwaasteniet, Pelle P. de Koning, Marloes S. Oudijn, Pepijn van den Munckhof, P. Richard Schuurman, and Damiaan Denys. 2013. Surgery for psychiatric disorders. *World Neurosurgery* 80: S31.e17–S31.e28. [CrossRef]

Marcus, Hani J., Archie Hughes-Hallett, Thomas P. Cundy, Guang-Zhong Yang, Ara Darzi, and Dipankar Nandi. 2015. da Vinci robot-assisted keyhole neurosurgery: A cadaver study on feasibility and safety. *Neurosurgical Review* 38: 367–71. [CrossRef]

Merhar, Stephanie. 2012. Biomarkers in neonatal posthemorrhagic hydrocephalus. *Neonatology* 101: 1–7. [CrossRef]

Miller, Brandon A., Afshin Salehi, David D. Limbrick, and Matthew D. Smyth. 2017. Applications of a robotic stereotactic arm for pediatric epilepsy and neurooncology surgery. *Journal of Neurosurgery: Pediatrics* 20: 364–70. [CrossRef] [PubMed]

Ourednik, Vaclav, Jitka Ourednik, Kook I. Park, Y. D. Teng, Karen A. Aboody, Kurtis I. Auguste, Rosanne M. Taylor, Barbara A. Tate, and Evan Y. Snyder. 2000. Neural stem cells are uniquely suited for cell replacement and gene therapy in the CNS. In *Neural Transplantation in Neurodegenerative Disease: Current Status and New Directions: Novartis Foundation Symposium 231*. Edited by Derek J. Chadwick and Jamie A. Goode. Chichester: John Wiley & Sons, Ltd., pp. 242–69. [CrossRef]

Pak, Nikita, Joshua H. Siegle, Justin P. Kinney, Daniel J. Denman, Timothy J. Blanche, and Edward S. Boyden. 2015. Closed-loop, ultraprecise, automated craniotomies. *Journal of Neurophysiology* 113: 3943–53. [CrossRef] [PubMed]

Parker, Scott L., Matthew J. McGirt, Jeffrey A. Murphy, J. Thomas Megerian, Michael Stout, and Luella Engelhart. 2015. Comparative effectiveness of antibiotic-impregnated shunt catheters in the treatment of adult and pediatric hydrocephalus: Analysis of 12,589 consecutive cases from 287 US hospital systems. *Journal of Neurosurgery* 122: 443–48. [CrossRef]

Pelloux, Yann, and Christelle Baunez. 2013. Deep brain stimulation for addiction: Why the subthalamic nucleus should be favored. *Current Opinion in Neurobiology* 23: 713–20. [CrossRef]

Rekate, Harold L. 1997. Recent advances in the understanding and treatment of hydrocephalus. *Seminars in Pediatric Neurology* 4: 167–78. [CrossRef]

Roser, Florian, Marcos Tatagiba, and Gottlieb Maier. 2013. Spinal robotics: Current applications and future perspectives. *Neurosurgery* 72: 12–18. [CrossRef]

Steffensen, Annette B., Eva K. Oernbo, Anca Stoica, Niklas J. Gerkau, Dagne Barbuskaite, Katerina Tritsaris, Christine R. Rose, and Nanna MacAulay. 2018. Cotransporter-mediated water transport underlying cerebrospinal fluid formation. *Nature Communications* 9: 1–3. [CrossRef] [PubMed]

Tsai, Eve C., Stephen Santoreneos, and James T. Rutka. 2002. Tumors of the skull base in children: Review of tumor types and management strategies. *Neurosurgical Focus* 12: e1. [CrossRef]

Voges, Juergen, Ulf Müller, Bernhard Bogerts, Thomas Münte, and Hans-Jochen Heinze. 2013. Deep brain stimulation surgery for alcohol addiction. *World Neurosurgery* 80: S28.e21–S28.e31. [CrossRef]

Vougioukas, Vassilios I., Ulrich Hubbe, Albrecht Hochmuth, Nils C. Gellrich, and Vera van Velthoven. 2003. Perspectives and limitations of image-guided neurosurgery in pediatric patients. *Child's Nervous System* 19: 783–91. [CrossRef] [PubMed]

Walsh, Sarah, and Rajiv Midha. 2009. Use of stem cells to augment nerve injury repair. *Neurosurgery* 65: A80–A86. [CrossRef] [PubMed]

Wang, Tony R., Shayan Moosa, Robert F. Dallapiazza, W. Jeffrey Elias, and Wendy J. Lynch. 2018. Deep brain stimulation for the treatment of drug addiction. *Neurosurgical Focus* 45: E11. [CrossRef] [PubMed]

Warf, Benjamin C., Sarah Tracy, and John Mugamba. 2012. Long-term outcome for endoscopic third ventriculostomy alone or in combination with choroid plexus cauterization for congenital aqueductal stenosis in African infants. *Journal of Neurosurgery: Pediatrics* 10: 108–11. [CrossRef]

Weihl, Chris, R. Loch Macdonald, Marcus Stoodley, Jürgen Lüders, and George Lin. 1999. Gene therapy for cerebrovascular disease. *Neurosurgery* 44: 239–52. [CrossRef]

Section XV: Neurology

Neurological Medical Diseases for Neurosurgeons

Forhad H. Chowdhury, Mohammod Habibur Rahman and Mohammod Bodrul Alam Mondal

Abstract: A deep understanding of neurological medical diseases is very important for a neurosurgeon. It is essential during clinical assessment, radiological evaluation, and surgical decision-making to identify when one should not operate on a multiple sclerosis or motor neuron disease patient. Many of these neurological medical diseases are under trial for neuro stem cell therapy. In this chapter, we will briefly discuss important and frequent neurological medical diseases. We will discuss encephalitis, acute demyelinating encephalomyelitis, multiple sclerosis, transverse myelitis, peripheral neuropathy, Guillain–Barré syndrome, chronic inflammatory demyelinating neuropathy, myasthenia gravis, hereditary muscular disorders, and Wilson's disease.

Abbreviations

AChR	acetylcholine receptor	ADEM	acute demyelinating encephalomyelitis
ADL	adrenoleukodystrophy	AIDP	acute inflammatory demyelinating polyneuropathy
ALS	amyotrophic lateral sclerosis	AMAN	acute motor axonal neuropathy
AMSAN	acute motor sensory axonal neuropathy	ATM	acute transverse myelitis
BAEP	brain stem auditory evoked potential	CIDP	chronic inflammatory demyelinating polyneuropathy
CIS	clinically isolated condition	CK	creatine kinase
CMT	Charcot–Marie–Tooth	CNS	central nervous system
CSF	cerebrospinal fluid	CT	computed tomography
EDSS	extended disability status score	EEG	electroencephalogram
EMG	Electromyography	FSH	Facioscapulohumeral
GBS	Guillain–Barré syndrome	HAART	highly active antiretroviral therapy
INO	internuclear ophthalmoplegia	IVIG	intravenous immunoglobin
LGMD	limb girdle muscular dystrophy	LMN	lower motor neuron
MAC	membrane attack complex	MD	muscular dystrophy
MFS	Miller Fisher syndrome	MG	myasthenia gravis
MND	motor neuron disease	MRI	magnetic resonance imaging
MS	multiple sclerosis	My D	myotonia dystrophica
NCS	nerve conduction study	NMDA	N-methyl D-aspartate
OCN	oligoclonal band	PCR	polymerase chain reaction
PEG	percutaneous endoscopic gastrostomy	PML	progressive myelo leukoencephalopathy
PNS	peripheral nervous system	PPMS	primary progressive multiple sclerosis
RRMS	relapsing and remitting multiple sclerosis	SMA	spinal muscular atrophy
SOD	superoxide dismutase	SSEP	somatosensory evoked potential
UMN	upper motor neuron	VER	visual evoked response
VLCFA	very long chain fatty acid		

1. Encephalitis

1.1. Introduction

Inflammation of the brain is encephalitis. When the meninges and the brain are affected at the same time, the condition is known as meningoencephalitis. In Western nations, there are 7.4 new instances of acute encephalitis for every 100,000 individuals each year. The incidence in tropical nations is 6.34 per 100,000 individuals annually. In 2015, encephalitis is thought to have killed 150,000 people worldwide and afflicted 4.3 million people. Viruses are typically the cause of encephalitis. The incidence of herpes simplex encephalitis is 2–4 per million people per year. Encephalitis is predisposed by immunosuppression or immunodeficiency. The degree of severity may vary and could even result in death (Vos et al. 2016; Meningitis and Encephalitis Information Page 2017; Wikipedia contributors 2022).

1.2. Signs and Symptoms

- In adult patient:

- Fever of acute onset;
- Headache;
- Confusion;
- Seizures (sometimes).

- In infants or children:
  - Irritability;
  - Restlessness;
  - Poor appetite;
  - Fever.
- Neurological examinations
  - Drowsiness, confusion, stupor, or coma;
  - Memory disturbances;
  - Stiff neck, or other signs of meningism (meningoencephalitis) (NHS 2015; Wikipedia contributors 2022).

1.3. Causes

1.3.1. Viral

Viral encephalitis may affect patients as a direct result of an acute infection or as a sequalae of a latent infection. Most cases of viral encephalitis have an unidentified/unknown cause.

- Common viruses:
  - Herpes simplex infection (the commonest identifiable cause);
  - Rabies virus;
  - Measles virus;
  - Poliovirus.
- Rare viral causes:
  - Arboviral flavivirus (West Nile virus and St. Louis encephalitis);
  - Bunyavirus (La Crosse strain);
  - Reovirus (Colorado tick virus);
  - Arenavirus (lymphocytic choriomeningitis virus);
  - HIV infection;
  - Henipavirus infections;
  - Powassan virus.

1.3.2. Bacterial and Other Etiologies

- Bacterial infection (such as bacterial meningoencephalitis);
- Syphilitic encephalitis;
- Lyme disease encephalitis.

Mycoplasma and Rickettsial Encephalitis

- Parasitic:
  - Cysticercosis;
  - Malaria;
  - Toxoplasmosis;
  - Primary amoebic meningoencephalitis.
- Autoimmune:
  - Anti-NMDA receptor encephalitis;
  - Rasmussen encephalitis;
  - Limbic encephalitis.
- Idiopathic:
  - Encephalitis lethargica (Roos and Tyler 2015; Fisher et al. 2015; Kennedy 2004; Wikipedia contributors 2022).

1.4. *Investigations*

Only those who have experienced lethargy, a change in personality, or a lowered or altered level of consciousness for longer than 24 h should be considered to have encephalitis. Several tests are used to determine whether someone has encephalitis:

- MRI of the brain—detect inflammation;
- EEG—abnormal signal;
- CSF study—routine study, culture, PCR test, and antibody detection (anti-NMDA receptor);
- Blood test;
- Urine analysis (Venkatesan et al. 2013).

1.5. *Treatment*

The ideal medication for treating brain infections should have the following characteristics: small size, moderate lipophilicity at pH 7.4, low plasma protein binding level, distribution volume of 1 liter per kilogram, and weak affinity for binding with P-glycoprotein or other efflux pumps on the blood–brain barrier. Certain medications have high blood–brain barrier penetration, including isoniazid, pyrazinamide, linezolid, metronidazole, fluconazole, and some fluoroquinolones.

Here is the course of therapy (based on supportive care):

- Antiviral drugs (if virus is the etiology);
- Antibiotics (if the etiology is bacteria);
- Steroids are utilized to decrease brain edema;
- Sedatives (in restlessness);
- Anticonvulsants;
- Acetaminophen as an antipyretic;
- Decompressive craniotomy (very rare);
- Occupational and physical therapy;
- Pyrimethamine-based continued treatment is frequently utilized to manage toxoplasmic encephalitis;
- HAART (highly active antiretroviral therapy)—in HIV infection;
- Intravenous immunoglobulin (IVIG)—autoimmune encephalitis (Wikipedia contributors 2022).

1.6. *Prognosis*

Status epilepticus, thrombocytopenia, and cerebral edema are indicators of poor prognosis. On the other hand, early diagnosis with a normal encephalogram is connected with good survival rates (Wikipedia contributors 2022).

2. Demyelinating CNS Diseases

2.1. *Acute Disseminated Encephalomyelitis (ADEM)/Post-Infectious Encephalomyelitis*

2.1.1. Introduction

It is an immune-mediated demyelinating disease with an acute onset that is dispersed throughout the central nervous system (CNS) as small demyelinating foci in perivenous locations. Lesions do not exceed multiple sclerosis (MS) size and demyelination is restricted to perivascular regions. Most lesions have a diameter of 0.1 to 1.0 mm. ADEM may develop after viral upper respiratory or gastrointestinal tract infections, viral exanthematous diseases (measles, rubella, chickenpox, etc.), or vaccination (influenza or rabies). The most frequent cause of ADEM is measles, succeeded by varicella zoster (chickenpox) (Lindsay et al. 2011).

2.1.2. Clinical Features

After the viral infection has subsided for a few days or weeks, fever, headache, nausea, and vomiting start to appear. Drowsiness plus multifocal neurological symptoms and signs, including hemispheric, cerebellar, brain stem, spinal cord, and optic nerve involvement, come after meningeal symptoms (neck stiffness and photophobia). Myoclonus is frequent.

The predominant forms are spinal, cerebral, or cerebella; however, the situation is typically mixed. Optic neuritis is a symptom of optic nerve involvement. Rarely are the peripheral nerves involved (Greenberg 2010).

2.1.3. Diagnosis

There is no diagnostic test. Total protein and globulin levels in the CSF are elevated. Diffuse, slow wave activity is visible on an electroencephalogram (EEG). The CT scan is normal. The same level of acuteness of all very small focal white matter alterations seen on an MRI are shown by their simultaneous enhancement with contrast (unlike MS).

When there is a clear-cut prior viral infection or immunization, the diagnosis is simple. It is frequently impossible to distinguish viral infection from acute encephalitis when it quickly precedes it. It could be challenging to distinguish it from acute MS. ADEM is indicated by fever, meningeal symptoms, increased CSF protein > 100 mg per ml, and cell count > 50 per mm^3 (Lindsay et al. 2011; Greenberg 2010).

2.1.4. Treatment

Despite the lack of controlled trials, steroids are used. In the acute phase, large doses are advised. In refractory situations, cyclophosphamide may be utilized (Lindsay et al. 2011).

2.1.5. Outcome

Usually, the sickness manifests in one phase. The death rate is 20%, and 50% of patients fully recover. The severity of the deficiency and a sudden start are linked to a poor prognosis (Lindsay et al. 2011).

2.2. Multiple Sclerosis

2.2.1. Introduction

Multiple sclerosis (MS) is the most common disabling non-traumatic illness to affect young adults (Kobelt et al. 2017). It is a white-matter-only, idiopathic, demyelinating illness involving the spinal cord, optic nerves, and brain (particularly corticospinal tracts and the posterior columns). The peripheral nerve myelin is not affected (Greenberg 2010). Its basic reason is yet unknown. MS is a complicated disease; numerous genes as well as a number of known environmental factors, including vitamin D or ultraviolet B light exposure, Epstein–Barr virus infection, obesity, and cigarette smoking, all modestly increase disease risk (Ascherio 2013; Dobson and Giovannoni 2018). Most cases begin between the ages of 10 and 59, peaking between 20 and 40. The female and male sex ratio is 2:1. Near the equator, prevalence is less than 1 per 100,000 people and varies with latitude (Lindsay et al. 2011).

2.2.2. Pathology

Plaques are small, dispersed lesions with a greyish color that range in size from 1 millimeter to several centimeters and are found in the white matter of the CNS. The lesions have a perivenous distribution and are in close proximity to veins (particularly, postcapillary venules) (Lindsay et al. 2011).

2.2.3. Pathogenesis

Immune deficiency: There has been talk of immune insufficiency. Deviations in normal immune status may be the cause of "relapses and remissions", and this may explain the possibility of a latent virus persisting. Plaques' T lymphocytes and macrophages may become sensitive to myelin antigens.

Genetic and hereditary factors seem to be important. Multiple sclerosis seems to run in families. As a result, histocompatibility antigens have been studied (HL-A). MS has been linked to A3, B7, B18, and DW2/DRW2, according to research. A total of 30% of monozygotic and 5% of dizygotic twins have concordance. More often than affected males, affected women pass MS to their children, indicating that mitochondrial genes play a role in inheritance.

Viruses: The establishment of MS may be influenced by viruses; infection may take place in a genetically or immunologically predisposed host. Varicella zoster, rubella, measles, and herpes simplex have all been linked to elevated serum as well as CSF antibody titers after recurrence.

Biochemical: A biochemical effect has not been observed. Myelin looks normal prior to disintegration, and the suggested excess of lipids in the diet or malabsorption of polyunsaturated fatty acids remain untested.

In conclusion, the cause is likely complicated and multifactorial (Lindsay et al. 2011; Dobson and Giovannoni 2018).

2.2.4. Clinical Categories

1. Relapsing and remitting: This stage is experienced by 70% of MS patients. With every assault, recovery is almost complete. This stage of the sickness could last for years. There is no established reason why relapses occur.

2. Secondary progressive and relapsing/remitting secondary progressive: Relapsing and remitting MS (RRMS) events are eventually succeeded by an additive loss of function with disability as well as an incomplete recovery. A total of 20% of all patients are currently in the chronic progressive stage. Six to ten years after the onset of symptoms, the condition typically switches from relapsing and remitting to secondary progressive.

3. Primary progressive MS (PPMS): This kind, which affects 15% of all patients, is typical in late-onset MS (>45 years). Relapses are typically absent in the context of gradual progression, and symptoms and signs are typically spinal.

4. Benign: 10 years after commencement, this condition is defined as low-disability (extended disability status score—EDSS 3). The real frequency of these situations is impossible to estimate, and individuals could eventually become severely disabled. The sporadic, unintentional discovery of MS in autopsies lends credence to a benign variety.

It is crucial to recognize the various MS phases when choosing patients to receive novel disease-modifying therapies. Specific scales, like the Kurtzke score/EDSS, can be used to quantify the degree of disability.

[EDSS is a ten-point, non-linear score scale where 1 = no symptoms/signs, 6 = requires a walking aid to achieve a short distance, 8 = restricted to bed or wheelchair, and 10 = death due to MS (Lindsay et al. 2011; Dobson and Giovannoni 2018; Greenberg 2010)].

2.2.5. Clinical Features

An exploration of the symptomless, prodromal, and symptomatic phases of MS is required to understand the condition. When a patient manifests with a clinically isolated condition (CIS), MS is often assumed. Depending on where the eloquent lesion is, this may be mono- or polysymptomatic. Optic neuritis, spinal cord, and brainstem syndromes are the most often observed presentations; nevertheless, a wide range of less-frequent presentations occur, encompassing cortical presentations like dominant parietal lobe syndromes.

Relapses of MS classically start off slowly over the course of a few hours to a few days, hit a plateau after a few weeks, and then slowly recover. In the early stages of MS, the gross clinical recovery after relapses frequently seems complete; yet, most relapses leave some injury behind. For instance, after acute optic neuritis, gross visual acuity may improve, but defects in contrast sensitivity, color vision, and depth perception are still present. As the neuronal reserve is gone, relapse recovery becomes imprecise, neurological abnormalities mount, and a chronic handicap results.

Approximately 10 "asymptomatic" lesions are observed on MRI for every clinical incident. Location and size play a role in symptomatology; a very small lesion in an eloquent area is more likely to result in symptoms. Lesions that are seen on an MRI are solely the tip of the iceberg; there are a lot more lesions that are microscopic in size and many more in deep or cortical grey matter.

After the onset of RRMS, secondary progressive MS often appears 10 to 15 years later and gradually progresses from sporadic relapses to a progressively worsening condition. Instead of a clear transition between disease categories, relapses take place against a background of slow progression until progression becomes dominant. Early MS symptoms like cognitive decline and MRI atrophy suggest that neurodegeneration has been present since the disease's clinical beginning.

Primary progressive onset (PPMS), which often involves one dominant neural system and gradual accumulation of progressive impairment, occurs in 5%–15% of cases. The most typical PPMS manifestation is a progressive spastic paraparesis, but other well-known PPMS subtypes include cerebellar ataxia, sensory ataxia, cognitive loss, and progressive visual loss.

There are fewer people who have PPMS now than there were previously. This raises ethical concerns regarding the classification of MS into different subtypes and is likely linked to the fact that there are no approved therapies for PPMS. Cases may be classified as experiencing relapsing MS after receiving treatment. The pharmaceutical industry used this fictitious categorization of MS into distinct disorders to obtain interferon beta approval under the Orphan Drug Act in the USA.

With a maximum recorded incidence of 2.9/100,000 people, pediatric MS is much less common than adult-onset MS. Treatment is decided based on recurrent demyelination events that are spatially and temporally isolated. As pediatric MS may be multicentric at onset, it might be challenging to differentiate it from acute disseminated encephalomyelitis. Although relapse rates may be higher, physical recovery is frequently more thorough. In cases where the diagnosis is suspected, referral to a pediatric neurologist with experience in demyelinating illnesses is advised because only a few therapies are approved for use in children.

According to the 2013 changes to the clinical course of MS, MS can be conceived of as a single disease living within a continuum ranging from relapsing ('inflammatory dominant') to progressive ('neurodegeneration dominant'). Currently, false distinctions among the cases with progressive and the cases with relapsing disease are made in MS definitions. Instead, it is preferable to think of these categories as locations along a disease continuum that also includes prodromal (or radiologically isolated) disease.

Symptoms at Onset

1. General symptoms, such as fatigue, headaches, sadness, and aches in the limbs, may indicate psychoneurosis.
2. In a young patient, trigeminal neuralgia may be the first sign of multiple sclerosis.

Motor Symptoms

Among motor symptoms, monoparesis and paraparesis are more prevalent. Quadriparesis and hemiparesis are less frequent. Increased muscle tone, hyperactive deep tendon reflexes, an extensor plantar reflex, and a lack of abdominal reflexes are all warning signs.

Sensory Symptoms

Due to demyelination of the posterior column, numbness and paresthesia can be frequent, frequently mild, and temporary. Lesions to the posterior column affect the ability to feel joint position and vibration. When the cervical posterior column is involved, Lhermitte's sign occurs, and sudden neck flexion causes the limbs to feel "shock-like." Dysesthesia is a disagreeable sensation of burning, coldness, or warmth caused by spinothalamic tract lesions.

Loss of Vision

Acute optic neuritis (Retrobulbar neuritis): Loss of vision typically accompanied by a central scotoma, followed by weeks of recovery. This frequently happens to young adults. The loss of vision happens gradually over several days and is frequently accompanied by pain while moving the eyes (irritation of the dura around the optic nerve). Only color vision is compromised in milder instances. Usually, only one eye is damaged, but sometimes both eyes may be affected at the same time.

Visual impairment can range from a modest central scotoma to total blindness. In up to 50% of patients, a fundoscopy reveals swelling caused by papillitis. The difference between papilledema and papillitis is reduced visual acuity.

Investigation: VERs (visual evoked responses) show delayed conduction. High-resolution MRI confirms the presence of plaque.

Treatment: IV or oral steroid.

The incidence of repeated optic neuritis is greater when oral steroids are used. Within the following two years, it becomes apparent that intravenous steroids decrease the likelihood of later developing MS. Most patients (90%) regain their vision. The ocular neuritis study group observed that, within 2 years, clinically confirmed MS had manifested in 12% of individuals. After then, the annual risk was 5–6%.

Acute, double-sided optic neuritis is less frequent than one-sided illness and the likelihood of developing MS is lower. A transverse myelitis may occasionally follow (neuromyelitis optica). Leber's hereditary optic neuropathy can be distinguished from other conditions by testing mitochondrial DNA.

Disturbance of Ocular Movement

Demyelination that affects the third, fourth, or sixth cranial nerves' brain stem pathways can cause diplopia. When supranuclear or internuclear connections are implicated, abnormal eye movements can occur with or without diplopia. Internuclear ophthalmoplegia (INO), which originates from a lesion in the medial longitudinal fasciculus, is pathognomonic of MS in young people. Other symptoms include nystagmus (rare), pupillary abnormalities, involvement of the III nerve, or involvement of the II nerve due to sympathetic engagement in the brain stem (Horner's syndrome).

Other Clinical Features

Ataxia of gait and limb incoordination (cerebellar or sensory type), intention tremor and dysarthria (cerebellar involvement), sphincter disruption, and impotence are some other conditions that can cause vertigo of the central type, as can emotional instability, paresthesia, dysarthria, pain, ataxia, photopsia (visual scintillations), depression or euphoria, dysarthria, dysarthria, ataxia, and epilepsy (Lindsay et al. 2011; Dobson and Giovannoni 2018; Greenberg 2010).

2.2.6. Investigations

Neurophysiological Testing

May detect a second asymptomatic lesion.

1. Visual evoked potential (VEP) detects visual pathway defects;
2. SSEP (somatosensory evoked response) may identify central sensory pathway pathologies;
3. BAEP (brain stem auditory evoked potential) may find brain stem pathologies.

Cerebrospinal Fluid (CSF) Study

On rare occasions, a moderate pleocytosis, primarily lymphocytes, is discovered. The total protein level can be higher. In 50–60% of instances, gamma globulin levels rise.

Agar or acrylamide electrophoresis of CSF reveals distinct bands that are absent from serum. Up to 95% of individuals with a diagnosed condition and 50–60% of patients following the initial incident have these bands. In contrast to other inflammatory neurological illnesses, OCBs (oligoclonal bands) are not unique to MS and do persist forever (Lindsay et al. 2011).

MRI of Brain and Spine

Longer relaxation times and a stronger signal on T2W are results of myelin degradation. Gliosis causes alterations that are comparable. The presence of periventricularly distributed white matter abnormalities is suggestive but not definitive of MS. Gadolinium's paramagnetism will reveal any active inflammation. If both the MRI and CSF (oligoclonal band) results are negative, MS will be ruled out. Following a single bout of demyelination, MR may be able to predict the long-term consequences (e.g., transverse myelitis or optic neuritis). People who have abnormalities in their cranial MR will relapse earlier than people who do not. MRI findings do not correlate enough with disability; however, newer methods may be more accurate indicators of illness development.

Diagnosis demands the absence of alternative illnesses and the occurrence of two or more events of symptoms attributed to demyelination, at least thirty days apart at separate sites in the CNS. For clinical investigations that integrate clinical elements with research findings, research criteria have been devised. According to the McDonald criteria (McDonald et al. 2001), a diagnosis can be made following a single clinical episode based on MRI evidence of the occurrence of new lesions.

After a year of increasing deficit, primary progressive MS can be identified by the presence of CNS plaques, oligoclonal bands in CSF that are not matched, and the elimination of other diagnoses (Lindsay et al. 2011; Greenberg 2010).

2.2.7. Differential Diagnosis

Due to MS's wide range of potential signs and symptoms, practically all other illnesses that might produce localized or diffuse CNS dysfunction are included in the differential diagnosis. Conditions that, both clinically as well as on diagnostic tests, may appear to closely resemble MS include the following (Greenberg 2010):

1. ADEM: Usually a single time event. May also have a CSF-Oligoclonal band. Corpus callosum engagement is rare;
2. CNS lymphoma;
3. Other closely linked demyelinating diseases, like Devic's syndrome;
4. Vasculitis;

5. Encephalitis: individuals are generally very ill;
6. Chronic white matter alteration: found in elder patients.

2.2.8. Treatment

Symptom management will frequently require an integrated multi-specialty approach, especially when the disease advances.

Acute Relapse

Methylprednisolone 3 gm i.v. over 3 days. It can also be administered orally.

Modification of Natural Course

Relapsing and remitting MS: Beta interferon and glatiramer acetate decrease the relapse frequency by approximately 30%.

A monoclonal antibody called natalizumab lowers the relapse rate by more than 60% and lessens disability, but it also increases the danger of getting PML-progressive multifocal leucoencephalopathy (01 in 1000). It is, therefore, only offered to people with severe illness.

Mitoxantrone is a chemotherapeutic drug that can be utilized in cases of aggressively severe disease but carries a risk of leukemia and cardiotoxicity.

Trials for a variety of other agents are ongoing.

Primary and secondary progressive MS: Currently, no efficacious disease-modifying agents are available (Lindsay et al. 2011; Dobson and Giovannoni 2018; Greenberg 2010).

2.3. Acute Transverse Myelitis

2.3.1. Introduction

Acute transverse myelitis (ATM) indicates inflammation of the spinal cord, and the etiologies encompass infectious/post-infectious, idiopathic, and autoimmune.

2.3.2. Etiology

Many so-called "causes" remain unproven. Generally agreed etiologies include the following (Greenberg 2010):

1. Infectious and post-infectious
    (a) Primary infectious transverse myelitis
        (i) Viral ATM: myelitis with viral encephalomyelitis, poliomyelitis, herpes zoster, and rabies;
        (ii) Bacterial ATM: encompassing tuberculoma of the cord;
        (iii) Spirochetal ATM: syphilitic myelitis;
        (iv) Fungal (blastomycosis, cryptococcosis, and aspergillosis);
        (v) Parasitic (echinococcus, paragonimiasis, schistosomiasis, and cysticercosis).
    (b) Post-infectious ATM: includes post-exanthematous and influenza
2. Post-traumatic
3. Physical agents
    (a) Decompression sickness;
    (b) Electrocaution;
    (c) Radiation.
4. Paraneoplastic syndrome: the commonest primary is lung; however, ovary, prostate, and rectum malignancy may cause ATM.
5. Metabolic
    (a) Pernicious anemia;
    (b) Diabetes mellitus;
    (c) Chronic liver disease.
6. Toxins

(a) Cresyl phosphates;
(b) Spinal anesthetics;
(c) Intra-arterial contrast materials;
(d) Myelographic contrast dye;
(e) After chemonucleolysis.

7. Arachnoiditis
8. Autoimmune

(a) MS (particularly Devic's syndrome);
(b) Post vaccination (rabies and smallpox).

9. Collagen vascular disease

(a) Mixed connective tissue disease;
(b) Systemic lupus erythematosus.

2.3.3. Clinical Presentation

ATM affects just 1–8 people per million each year. Age of onset range: 15–55 years. Patients may have a viral-like prodrome. Clinical features may include the following (Sherrell 2022):

- Backpain or radicular pain;
- Progressive muscle weakness;
- Paralysis, often starting in the legs;
- Diminished touch and temperature sensations;
- Numbness, tingling, and burning;
- Sexual malfunction;
- Raised urinary incontinence or urgency;
- Fatigue;
- Constipation.

The thoracic level is the most common sensory and presenting level. ATM is rarely the initial symptom of MS.

2.3.4. Progression

Progression is generally fast, with most attaining maximal neuro-deficit by 24 h, but the interval between the first symptom and highest deficit varies from 2 h to 14 days (Berman et al. 1981).

2.3.5. Evaluation

CSF Study

Normal during acute phase, but there may be elevated protein or pleocytosis levels or both.

MRI of Spine

In an individual developing acute paraplegia/myelopathy, particularly when ATM is considered a possibility, the initial investigation should be an urgent MRI. It excludes hemorrhage and other compressive myelopathy. MRI may be normal, however, there may be fusiform-shaped cord swelling with T2W signal changes at the involved level.

2.3.6. Treatment

High-dose steroid therapy (methylprednisolone). In nonresponsive cases, plasma exchange or intravenous immunoglobin (IVIG) can be tried (Absoud et al. 2017).

2.3.7. Prognosis

Good recovery takes place in 30% of patients. Death due to respiratory failure is rare (5%) (Lindsay et al. 2011).

2.4. *Leukodystrophies*

The normal development of myelin may be hampered by inborn metabolic abnormalities. Although certain genetic illnesses occasionally show their initial symptoms in adulthood, they typically first appear in infancy or youth.

The varieties have been identified:

- Metachromatic leukodystrophy;
- Adrenomyeloneuropathy or adrenoleukodystrophy (ADL);
- Globoid cell leukodystrophy.

Sex-related ADL is marked by adrenal hypofunctions and abnormal myelin in the CNS and peripheral nerves. A failure in the beta oxidation of very long chain fatty acids (VLCFA), which accumulate in the blood as well as skin fibroblasts, is the cause of the clinical presentation, which is quite varied. Lorenzo's oils, a dietary supplement, decrease them and may halt the advancement of this fatal disease. Female heterozygote carriers may have symptoms of a progressive myelopathy with late onset (Lindsay et al. 2011; Greenberg 2010).

3. Motor Neuron Disease (Amyotrophic Lateral Sclerosis)

3.1. *Introduction*

Motor neuron disease (MND)/amyotrophic lateral sclerosis (ALS) is a progressive neurodegeneration condition involving of upper and lower motor neurons. A total of 2 per 100,000 people are affected per year, with a prevalence of 6 per 100,000. Familial ALS is responsible for 5% of cases of MND and is generally inherited as a dominant trait. The male/female ratio is 1.5:1. The average age of onset is 55 years. Average survival after diagnosis is 03 years. Pathologically, various levels of the CNS and peripheral nerves may be affected:

1. Atrophy of the primary motor cortex;
2. The corticobulbar tract;
3. Nuclei of the cranial nerve;
4. The corticospinal pathway;
5. Neurons of the anterior horn.

Microscopically, there is a loss of neurons in the primary motor cortex, anterior horns, and cranial nerve nuclei. There is evidence of downsizing of corticospinal and corticobulbar fibers. There is no inflammatory response in the involved areas (Lindsay et al. 2011; Gaudette et al. 2000).

3.2. *Etiology*

The cause of MND is unknown. It seems that cell bodies of motor neurons (upper and lower) die spontaneously. Mutations in the SOD1 gene (superoxide dismutase enzyme producer) may be the cause in some familial ALSs (20%). These are responsible for about 2% of cases with ALS. However, other possible causes include viral infection, toxins, or mineral deficiencies (Lindsay et al. 2011).

3.3. *Clinical Presentation*

3.3.1. At Onset

A total of 75% of people have asymmetrical limb weakness and atrophy.

Clinical characteristics that are bulbar or pseudobulbar: dysphagia or dysarthria (25%).

The crucial element in both bulbar-onset as well as limb-onset diseases is the involvement of both lower and upper motor neurons together with normal sensation. Approximately 3–5% of instances of dementia include frontal dementia. Emotional instability can happen (Lindsay et al. 2011; Greenberg 2010; Arora and Khan 2022).

3.3.2. Limb-Onset ALS

Corticospinal pathways and anterior horn cells are affected in ALS with limb-onset. Increased muscle tone, exaggerated tendon jerks, extensor plantar reflex, and an asymmetrical occurrence of weakness are all symptoms of corticospinal tract degeneration. A slowly progressing type of MND that only affects the cortical spinal tract is primary lateral sclerosis. Involvement of the anterior horn cells causes muscular atrophy, weakness, and fasciculations. Muscle cramping could occur. The degree of weakness does not indicate that weakness is as bad as bulbar-onset disease. Possible hand wasting can occur (Lindsay et al. 2011; Greenberg 2010; Arora and Khan 2022).

3.3.3. Bulbar-Onset Disease (Progressive Bulbar Palsy)

Bulbar-onset disease has a mixer of corticobulbar plus lower cranial nerve motor nuclei degeneration, which results in difficulty chewing, an expressionless face, nasal regurgitation, and an exaggerated jaw jerk.

As the pathology advances, the motor system is affected at all levels. Individuals with limb-onset get bulbar features, and vice versa. Weakness of respiratory muscles finally happens and is the frequent etiology of death.

Rare clinical scenarios are dyspnea from respiratory muscles dysfunction, recurrent chest infections from cryptic aspiration, or significant weight loss (Lindsay et al. 2011; Greenberg 2010; Arora and Khan 2022).

3.3.4. Rare Clinical Types and Differentials

1. Primary lateral sclerosis is an asymmetrical upper motor neuron condition that progresses relatively slowly.
2. The "flail arm" variety refers to severe weakening and atrophy of the arms with solely mild weakening of the legs. Typically, this progresses more slowly.
3. Progressive muscular atrophy (may mimic multifocal motor neuropathy along with conduction block, spinal muscular atrophy, limb girdle dystrophy, lead neuropathy, or diabetic amyotrophy).
4. ALS like syndrome:
    - Hexosaminidase deficiency;
    - Paraproteinemias;
    - Lymphoproliferative disease;
    - HIV infection;
    - Lead poisoning;
    - Hyperparathyroidism and hyperthyroidism (produce hyperreflexia and muscle wasting);
    - Pseudobulbar palsy in cerebrovascular disease or multiple sclerosis.

3.3.5. Never in MND

- Bladder is never involved;
- Sensory deficits do not occur;
- Ocular muscles are never involved (Lindsay et al. 2011; Greenberg 2010; Arora and Khan 2022).

3.4. Investigations

Common investigations:

- Nerve conduction studies show normal results;
- EMG shows fibrillation;
- MRI (to excludes compression of spinal cord or foramen magnum);
- Thyroid hormones and calcium studies rule out metabolic or endocrine disease;
- In certain cases, screening for paraproteinemia, lymphoreticular disorders, and hexosaminidase deficiency.

Investigation of suspected MND:

- Mixed upper and lower motor neuron (ALS) syndrome:
    - Electromyography and nerve conduction studies (NCSs).
    - MRI of the brain and spinal cord.
    - Routine blood tests, serum electrophoresis, and thyroid function.
    - HIV test, if there are risk factors.
- Pure lower motor neuron syndrome:
    - Genetic investigations (if slowly progressive, indicating spinal muscular atrophy).
    - Electromyography/NCSs for conduction block.
    - Routine blood tests, serum electrophoresis, and thyroid function.
- Pure upper motor neuron syndrome:
    - MRI of the spinal cord and brain.
    - Folate/B12.
    - Central motor conduction time (utilizing transcranial magnetic stimulation techniques, rarely available).

- Lumbar puncture (Lindsay et al. 2011; Greenberg 2010; Arora and Khan 2022).

3.5. El Escorial Criteria for Diagnosis of MND/ALS

Existence of the following:

- LMN signs in at least two extremities;
- UMN signs in at least one area (cervical/bulbar/ lumbosacral);
- Advancement of disease.

Absence of the following:

- Neurogenic sphincter disturbance;
- Sensory signs;
- Other clinically present PNS/CNS disease;
- Rule out ALS-like syndromes (Brooks 1994; Lindsay et al. 2011).

3.6. Treatment

The main goal of treatment is to control symptoms while providing the patient, and their family, with support as they worsen and their requirements change.

To fully comprehend the ailment and its natural history, counseling is necessary. Meeting the difficulties of each stage of sickness with the help of a nurse professional is essential, and it is ideal to discuss feeding concerns and ventilatory support options in advance so that informed decisions can be made. With medical, legal, and ethical constraints, providing patients with complete care can be difficult.

3.6.1. Symptomatic Treatment

Dysarthria and anarthria—speech evaluation and communication assistance when required.

Dysphagia and aspiration—PEG (percutaneous endoscopic gastrostomy).

Nutrition—calculate calorific components and supplement nutrition with vitamins.

Muscular weakness—walking aids, physiotherapy, splints, etc.

Respiratory failure—Respiratory failure is unavoidable when critical capacity declines. When this goes under 75% or orthopnea begins in patients who do not have extensive bulbar involvement, noninvasive ventilatory support should be taken into account. Recent studies show that this can enhance quality of life. It is less clear what function invasive mechanical ventilation will serve. Rarely, ALS can begin with initial respiratory failure prior to talking about therapy options. This poses a serious managerial conundrum.

3.6.2. Disease-Modifying Agent Treatment

Riluzole is an energy-buffering and anti-glutamate agent. A 100 mg/day dose is safe with a minimal effect, prolonging life by 02 months (Lindsay et al. 2011; Greenberg 2010; Arora and Khan 2022).

4. Inherited Motor Neuron Disorders

4.1. Spinal Muscular Atrophies (SMAs)

The second commonest fatal autosomal recessive illness in Caucasians is spinal muscular atrophy (after cystic fibrosis). The anterior horn cells' deterioration defines the disease. There is symmetrical muscular atrophy and weakening here.

Three forms of recessive SMA are distinguished based on the age of onset, the extent of muscular damage, and the duration of survival (all varieties mapped to the 5q12.2-q13.3 gene locus).

The odds of a parent passing SMA on to their children are 1/10,000, or just under 1%.

4.1.1. Type I—Werdnig–Hoffmann Disease (Acute Infantile SMA)

The incidence of this autosomal recessive condition is 01:25,000 live births.

Clinical characteristics include decreased fetal movements in the final stages of pregnancy along with newborn hypotonia and weakness.

Every motor developmental milestones is postponed, and 95% of cases pass away by 18 months.

4.1.2. Type II—Kugelberg–Welander Disease (Late Infantile or Juvenile SMA)

Pathology is akin to Werdnig–Hoffmann disease.
Clinical pictures includes:

- The involved muscles are limb girdle muscles.
- It progresses slowly. Median age of death: 12 years. The dominant form is the one that progresses through childhood.

4.1.3. Type III—Adult-Onset SMA

Occurs between second and fifth decade where progressive weakness of limb girdle muscles is seen.

Differentiation from progressive muscular atrophy form of ALS is difficult. A benign clinical course suggests the former.

4.1.4. Scapuloperoneal and Distal Forms

Distinction from Charcot–Marie–Tooth (CMT) disease types I and II as well as scapuloperoneal dystrophy is clinically challenging and differentiation may solely be attained on neurophysiological and histological grounds.

4.1.5. Spinal and Bulbar Muscular Atrophy/Kennedy's Syndrome

It is an X-linked, adult-onset neurogenic muscle atrophy with late distal and bulbar involvement (Gene Locus: Xq11-q12). At over 40 years old, fasciculations begin, followed by muscular atrophy and weakening. Both facial fasciculations and bulbar symptoms are typical. The Babinski sign is unfavorable. A long lifespan is possible.

4.1.6. Management of SMAs

There is nothing specific. Supportive care and genetic counselling are needed (Lindsay et al. 2011; Greenberg 2010; Arora and Khan 2022; Teoh et al. 2017).

5. Peripheral Neuropathies

5.1. Introduction

Diffuse peripheral nerve lesions that cause weakness, sensory disturbance, and/or altered reflexes are referred to as peripheral neuropathy. A single nerve condition known as mononeuropathy is frequently caused by entrapment or trauma. The involvement of two or more nerves, typically as a result of a systemic disorder, is referred to as mononeuropathy multiplex (like vasculitis, arteritis, or diabetes mellitus) (Greenberg 2010).

5.2. Etiology

Diabetes mellitus, alcoholism, and Guillain–Barré are responsible for 90% of cases. Other causes encompass vasculitis/arteritis, monoclonal gammopathy, acute idiopathic polyneuritis, hepatitis-C-virus-linked cryoglobulinemia, Sjogren's syndrome, etc. (Table 1) (Greenberg 2010).

Table 1. Mnemonic for etiologies of peripheral neuropathy—"GRAND THERAPIST".

Guillain–Barré syndrome	**T**raumatic
	Hereditary (e.g., Charcot–Marie–Tooth)
Renal (uremic neuropathy)	**E**ndocrine or **E**ntrapment **R**adiation
	Alcoholism
Amyloid or **A**IDS	**P**orphyria or **P**sychiatric or **P**araneoplastic or **P**seudoneuropathy or **P**MR
Nutritional (B6 and B12 deficiency)	**I**nfectious/post-infectious (like Hansen's disease)
Diabetes or **D**rugs	**S**arcoidosis or "**S**ystemic" **T**oxins [such as heavy-metal toxicity (plumbism)]

Source: Authors' compilation based on data from Greenberg (2010).

5.3. Clinical Features

Peripheral neuropathies may present as a deficiency of sensation, pain, incoordination, weakness, and as difficulty in ambulating.

5.4. Evaluation

Work-up for peripheral neuropathies of unknown cause:

1. Blood work: Hb-AIC, ESR, TSH, and vitamin B_{12};
2. EMG and NCS;
3. MR nervogram.

5.5. Treatment

Treatment is provided according to etiology.

6. Guillain–Barré Syndrome (GBS)

6.1. Introduction

Acute demyelinating polyneuropathy Guillain–Barré syndrome (GBS) was initially reported in 1859. It has ascending motor weakness, sensory dysfunction, and autonomic dysfunction, all of which are commonly followed by prodromal disease (generally a gastrointestinal or respiratory infection). It is believed that it has an autoimmune foundation. GBS was once regarded as a singular clinical entity. Acute inflammatory demyelinating polyneuropathy (AIDP), acute motor axonal neuropathy (AMAN), acute motor–sensory axonal neuropathy (AMSAN), and Miller Fisher syndrome (MFS) are the four primary clinical and electrophysiological subgroups of GBS. AMAN is restricted to pure motor involvement, AMSAN is a more serious disease with motor–sensory involvement, and AIDP is characterized by demyelination.

6.2. Incidence and Etiopathogenesis

About two incidents occur for every 100,000 people annually. It typically happens 1 to 3 weeks following a viral illness or other infection, or following immunization. GBS can develop following viral infections, such as varicella zoster, mumps, and cytomegalovirus (CMV). Additionally, Mycoplasma, Campylobacter infections, vaccinations with vaccines and antitoxins, surgery, trauma, and sometimes malignancy and immunodeficiency are associated with it. Responses to peripheral nerve myelin are cell- and antibody-mediated. In some patients, a T-cell-mediated attack on the myelin basic protein is developed; others develop antibodies to myelin gangliosides or glycoproteins. If segmental demyelination is severe, it might cause subsequent axonal damage. Peripheral nerves and nerve roots experience lymphocyte infiltration within the perivascular space. Cytokines, which are released by lymphocytes and macrophages, harm Schwann cells and myelin. Regeneration is not possible after nerve cell loss and axonal damage (Lindsay et al. 2011).

6.3. Clinical Features

6.3.1. Symptoms

GBS has a variety of clinical characteristics. The most frequently presenting symptoms are weakness and sensory disruption. Typically, a progressive ascending motor weakness, ranging from difficulty walking to paralysis, begins in the lower limbs. Respiratory failure could result from the weakening progressing to the respiratory muscles. There may also be ophthalmoplegia and concomitant bulbar paralysis in cases of facial nerve palsies.

The sensory sensations of paresthesia, numbness, and discomfort are possible. Lower-back pain is frequently felt and can be very severe. In 80% of patients, paresthesia and numbness begin distantly and progress in a manner comparable to motor weakness (Pascuzzi and Fleck 1997; Tandel et al. 2016; Lindsay et al. 2011; Greenberg 2010).

6.3.2. Signs

The results of a clinical examination reveal a flaccid areflexic paralysis. Within 2 weeks after the initiation of symptoms, muscle atrophy can start and can be severe. Arrhythmias, blood pressure swings, urine retention, paralytic ileus, and hyperhidrosis are all symptoms of autonomic dysfunction, which is a prevalent condition. If severe, this might be related to unexpected death (Pascuzzi and Fleck 1997; Tandel et al. 2016; Lindsay et al. 2011; Greenberg 2010).

6.4. Clinical Types of GBS

6.4.1. AIDP

The most prevalent type, known as acute inflammatory demyelinating polyneuropathy (AIDP), affects 85 to 90% of patients and is identified pathologically by demyelination, lymphocytic infiltration, and macrophage-mediated removal of myelin. Clinical signs include hypo- or areflexia together with symmetrical, ascending motor weakening. Myelin sheaths wrapping peripheral nerve axons are inflamed and destroyed by activated macrophages as part of the underlying pathogenic process. This causes the conduction of peripheral nerves to slow down and become blocked, which weakens muscles. In severe cases, axonal damage could develop later. Antibody binding occurs after nerve terminal axon damage in AIDP, and this route typically results in membrane attack complex (MAC) development with the breakdown of the terminal axonal cytoskeleton as well as mitochondrial injury.

6.4.2. Acute Motor Axonal Neuropathy (AMAN)

AMAN is more prevalent in young people and during the summer in China and Japan. There is a connection to previous Campylobacter jejuni infection.

6.4.3. MFS

Miller Fisher syndrome (MFS) includes ataxia, areflexia, and ophthalmoplegia but usually not weak limbs. Characteristics are serum IgG antibodies against a particular ganglioside (anti-GQ1B antibodies).

6.4.4. AMSAN

It is a GBS variety that can be proven through electrophysiological investigations that involves both motor and sensory fibers. It is more severe and is accompanied by a protracted or even limited recovery. AMAN-like clinical traits are present; however, there are additional sensory symptoms. The fundamental pathogenic mechanism is identical to that of AMAN (i.e., antibody mediated axonal injury).

Chronic inflammatory demyelinating polyneuropathy, a chronic variant of GBS, has been identified. The clinical characteristics resemble those of AIDP; however, they proceed more slowly or recur more frequently (Hughes and Cornblath 2005; Greenberg 2010; Lindsay et al. 2011).

6.5. Investigations

Most patients have high CSF protein levels, although this does not happen until the second/third week of sickness. Normally, cells are missing; however, in 20% of cases, up to 50 cells per mm^3 can be observed (Lindsay et al. 2011).

6.5.1. Nerve Conduction Studies

These can be typical if they are conducted early on in the illness. Multifocal demyelination findings are quickly followed by decreased motor conduction, conduction block, and extended distal motor latencies.

6.5.2. Ancillary Tests

These are carried out to find any triggering infections and can include bacterial and viral tests. Electrolytes are examined for immune complex glomerulonephritis and improper antidiuretic hormone secretion.

Clinical history, CSF analysis, neurophysiological testing, and the elimination of acute spinal cord illness, myasthenia gravis, and porphyria all contribute to the diagnosis.

A number of subtypes of antibodies have been linked to them:

- AMAN: anti-GD1a and GM1;
- Acute sensory neuropathy: anti-GD1b.

6.6. Treatment

The best probability of a successful result is supportive care in an HDU or ICU with the exclusion of respiratory and autonomic problems. Impending respiratory failure symptoms call for voluntary intubation for ventilation. Tracheotomy should be performed when the need for breathing support is likely to last longer than two weeks.

Where the degree of immobility renders thrombosis a potential risk, low-molecular-weight heparin (subcutaneous) must be administered with supporting stockings.

In order to hasten recovery and enhance results, both plasma exchange (PE) and intravenous immunoglobulin (IVIG), 0.4 g/kg/day for 05 days, are equally beneficial. Blood is circulated via an extracorporeal cell separator during plasma exchange. Human albumin solution or fresh frozen plasma (FFP) is used to replenish the blood's plasma fraction. During the procedure, anticoagulants are given.

Plasma exchange is used to get rid of antibodies linked to the underlying autoimmune response. Due to its simplicity of administration, IVIG is the favored treatment; however, there are several drawbacks, vasomotor instability, including flu-like symptoms, congestive heart failure, thrombotic events (including myocardial ischemia and strokes), temporary renal failure, and allergy. There is a very slight chance of infection. Treatment is typically delayed in milder instances and provided to patients who are unable to walk. There is no need for steroids (Tandel et al. 2016; Hughes and Cornblath 2005; Pascuzzi and Fleck 1997; Lindsay et al. 2011; Greenberg 2010).

6.6.1. Intravenous Immunoglobulin

GBS can be effectively treated with intravenous immunoglobulin (IVIG), which has been shown to hasten recovery in a manner analogous to plasma exchange. When given within 02 weeks of the start of symptoms, it is most helpful. IVIG is superior to plasma exchange in a number of ways. It has fewer adverse effects, is more readily accessible, and requires less labor. IVIG indications include respiratory depression and muscular weakness.

By inhibiting Fc receptors, IVIG, which is made up of pooled donor IgG antibodies, may lessen the degree of autoimmune inflammation in GBS. This stops the Fc component of antibodies from binding, hence stopping antibody-mediated cell death. Additionally, complement activation is changed. IgA deficiency and prior allergic reactions to IVIG are examples of contraindications (linked to anaphylactic reactions to blood products). IVIG side effects can range from mild to severe and include nausea, headaches, fluid overload, abnormal liver function tests, acute renal failure, venous thromboembolism, and anaphylaxis. Dermatological diseases like erythroderma and fluid overload are also possible side effects. There is no proof that additional rounds of therapy are helpful (Tandel et al. 2016; Hughes and Cornblath 2005; Pascuzzi and Fleck 1997; Lindsay et al. 2011; Greenberg 2010).

6.7. Outcome

The death rates is 2%. A total of 10% of those who advance to respiratory failure are moderately impaired and 20% are severely disabled. In milder diseases, the result is fantastic. The recurrence rate is 3% (Lindsay et al. 2011).

7. Chronic Inflammatory Demyelinating Polyneuropathy (CIDP)

Unlike Guillain–Barré, it rarely affects the respiratory function or cranial nerves and has a gradual or variable course from weeks to months. Segmental demyelination followed by remyelination (onion bulb development) and sparse mononuclear inflammatory change are pathological features. All neuropathies have a 3% prevalence and a five per million incidences.

The age of onset is 35 years on average (fluctuating course in younger patients; progressive course in older patients).

In about two-thirds of patients, IVIG, plasma exchange, or steroids are effective. Steroids should be administered first in moderate/severe cases (cost and convenience of usage), followed by IVIG, and then PE if the response is insufficient. Immunosuppressive medications (such as azathioprine, cyclosporin, or cyclophosphamide) are used in resistant instances despite minimal evidence (Lehmann et al. 2019; Lindsay et al. 2011).

Outcome with Therapy

Thirty percent are symptom-free, 45% are mildly disabled, and 25% are severely disable (Lehmann et al. 2019; Lindsay et al. 2011).

8. Neuromuscular Junction Disorder: Myasthenia Gravis (MG)

8.1. Introduction

MG is a neuromuscular transmission disease characterized by weakness and fatigability of some or all muscle units, as well as weakness that worsens with prolonged or frequent effort or that is eased by rest toward the end of the day. The nicotinic postsynaptic receptors for acetylcholine are destroyed by an autoimmune process, which causes this disease.

A total of 5 cases out of 100,000 are myasthenia gravis, making it a rare disease. An immunological basis for the disease is suggested by the rise in autoimmune diseases in both patients and first-degree relatives, as well as by the relationship of the condition with particular histocompatibility antigens (HLA-B7, B8, and DR2) in the body.

8.2. Etiology

Antibodies attach to the receptor sites, destroying them (complement mediated). Ninety percent of patients have acetylcholine receptor antibodies (AChR antibodies), which can be detected by radioimmunoassay in their serum.

The thymus's function: In 80% of cases, thymic abnormalities are present. The thymus' primary job is to influence the development of T-cell lymphocytes, which take part in immunological responses. Numerous conditions, such as systemic lupus erythematosus, that may be related to myasthenia gravis have thymus dysfunction.

8.3. Pathology

Alterations are seen in the thymus as well as in muscles.

Muscle biopsies may demonstrate abnormalities:

- Lymphocytic infiltration linked to very small necrotic foci of muscle fiber injury.
- Muscle fiber atrophy.
- Diffuse muscle necrosis plus inflammatory infiltration (when linked to thymoma).

A biopsy of a motor point may reveal aberrant motor endplates. Terminal nerve branching that is excessively lengthy and crooked is visible after supravital methylene blue staining. ACh receptors are destroyed by light and electron microscopy, and the secondary folds of the postsynaptic surface are simplified.

8.4. Clinical Features

Up to 90% of cases present in early adult life (less than 40 years of age). The female–male ratio is 2:1. The disease may be selective, involving particular groups of muscles.

Several clinical varieties are identified:

- CLASS I—solely ocular muscle (20%);
- CLASS II—mild generalized weakness;
- CLASS III—moderate generalized and mild to moderate ocular-bulbar weakness;
- CLASS IV—severe generalized and oculo-bulbar weakness;
- CLASS V—myasthenic crisis.

CLASSES II–V comprise 80% of cases. Nearly 40% of CLASS I will ultimately become widespread. The rest exist purely in an ocular manner throughout the course of the disease. Respiratory muscle engagement is associated with serious illness.

8.4.1. Cranial Nerve Symptoms and Signs

- Ptosis and muscular paresis are brought on by ocular involvement.
- A weak jaw might cause the mouth to hang open.
- Face muscles that lack strength appear expressionless.

- When patient smiles, a characteristic smile is produced by buccinator weakness (myasthenic snarl).

Bulbar engagement may lead to dysphagia, dysphonic dysarthric speech, nasal regurgitation, and nasal intonation to speech.

The presence of fatiguing is valuable in attaining a diagnosis as well as in following up the response to therapy.

Fatiguing of other bulbar muscles can be shown by:

- Blowing out cheeks against pressure.
- Counting as far as possible in one breath, etc.

The tongue occasionally demonstrates the characteristic triple grooved appearance with a two lateral plus one central furrow.

8.4.2. Limb and Trunk Symptoms and Signs

The head may droop if the muscles in the neck are weak. Muscles in the proximal limbs are most frequently impacted. Moving against a persistent opposition can reveal fatigue. On repeated testing, limb reflexes frequently become overactive and wear out. A total of 15% of instances result in muscle wasting. The weakness is made worse by anxiety, illness, pregnancy, medicines that affect neuromuscular transmission, and stress.

8.5. Differential Diagnosis

Distinguish from the following:

- General debility/weakness (like chronic fatigue syndrome) as well as functional weakness.
- Progressive ophthalmoplegia (like oculopharyngeal dystrophy and mitochondrial myopathy).
- MS—dysarthria, fatigue, and diplopia with a remitting and relapsing course.
- Lambert–Eaton myasthenic syndrome.

8.6. Natural History

10%—long period remission;

20%—short period remission (1 to few months);

30%—progress to death;

40%—varying degree of disability worsen by exercise.

8.7. Investigation

8.7.1. Pharmacological Testing

Anticholinesterase drugs are utilized to finalize a diagnosis.

Tensilon (edrophonium)—To combat the side effects of muscarinics, a short-action, 2–4 min injection of 2–10 mg was slowly combined with atropine pretreatment (nausea and bradycardia—resuscitation facilities should be available). When objective testing reveals a definite improvement in a deficiency, this is encouraging. A saline injection control with a blinded monitoring person can be helpful. The Tensilon test can result in a false positive in Lambert–Eaton syndrome and a negative result in ocular myasthenia.

8.7.2. Serological

A total of 90% of patients have anti-AchR antibodies, which are almost exclusively specific to this illness. Only 60% of cases of ocular myasthenia display antibodies. The severity of the disease is correlated with titer magnitude. A percentage of patients who do not have anti-AchR antibodies have anti-Muscle-Specific Kinase (anti-MUSK) antibodies.

There is overlap with other autoimmune illnesses, as evidenced by the occurrence of other antibodies, such as microsomal, colloid, rheumatoid factor, and gastric parietal cell antibodies. A total of 90% of patients with thymoma and 30% of all patients have anti-striated muscle antibodies.

8.7.3. Electrophysiological

The decrementing response is a reduction in the amplitude of the compound muscle action potential produced by repeated supramaximal nerve stimulation. Different stimulation rates—even those as low as 3/second—can result in a decrementing response.

Single-fiber electromyography is a more accurate indicator of neuromuscular function and is typically increased (95% of mild instances are abnormal). It measures "Jitter", which is the time interval variability of action potentials from two single muscle fibers of the same motor unit.

8.7.4. Additional

A significant mediastinal mass will be shown on a chest X-ray, although a minor thymoma cannot be ruled out. All recently diagnosed cases should have a chest CT scan.

8.7.5. Treatment

Protecting respiration with intubation and, if required, ventilation is the top priority in critically ill patients.

Anticholinesterase Drugs

This is a well-established form of therapy. Anticholinesterase medications prevent the enzyme cholinesterase from degrading acetylcholine, which enhances receptor activation. More acetylcholine is, hence, accessible to influence neuromuscular transmission.

To combat side effects (vomiting, nausea, muscle fasciculations, diarrhea, and increasing weakness), atropine, a muscarinic inhibitor, may be needed. Anticholinesterases seldom completely relieve symptoms, and high doses can cause cholinergic crisis.

Cholinergic crisis:

- Deteriorating weakness;
- Increased salivation, sweating, and bronchial secretions;
- Miosis;
- Ultimate respiratory failure.

Atropine can veil initial warning symptoms of this potentially life-threatening condition.

Steroids

Steroids are a sensible choice in generalized and profound ocular disease (rare) since this disorder is immune-mediated. The first dose of prednisone is 60 mg/day. Before improvement, there may be a brief period of decline. As a result, low-dose regimens are frequently favored, starting cautiously with prednisone 25 mg every other day. When a reaction happens, the dose is decreased.

Immunosuppressants (Other than Steroids)

These drugs (cyclosporine and azathioprine) are applied in individuals who do not respond to steroids or who need an unacceptably large dose of a steroid for maintenance.

Thymectomy

There are two indications for thymectomy:

1. Presence of a thymoma;
2. When MG is widespread and the utility of surgery outweigh the dangers.

A trans-sternal approach is preferred over a supra-sternal approach as it provides more chance of total removal.

Within 5 years of surgery, 70% of cases stay in remission.

Plasmapheresis

Plasma filtration has a short-term benefit by removing antibodies and other circulating components (4–6 weeks). Over a period of 6–8 days, 1.5–2 liters of plasma are swapped 3–5 times. The method is costly and fraught with risks (metabolic disturbance, hypotension, and thrombo-embolism). It is employed to stabilize refractory cases and, in severe illness, to prevent thymectomy.

Immunoglobulin (IVIG)

Administered intravenously daily for 5 days at a dose of 400 mg/kg in place of plasmapheresis. Acetylcholine receptors may be blocked by the mechanism. A favorable reaction lasts for two to three months in 75% of individuals. The cost of treatment is high, and complications and long-term implications are unknown. Anticholinesterases should not be necessary for the full duration of the sickness. These medications may be stopped after the disease is under immunological control.

8.7.6. Emergency Treatment—Myasthenic/Cholinergic Crises

- Find and manage the precipitating etiology, e.g., drug interaction, infection, or overdose;
- Position the patient at 45°, clean airway, give O_2, and, if in obvious respiratory failure, intubate plus ventilate for the duration, as needed.

Myasthenic Crisis

- Neostigmine IV, 08–12 mg/day;
- Inj. atropine 0.5 mg 8 hourly;
- Prednisolone 100 mg/day;
- Consideration for IVIG or plasmapheresis;
- Switch to oral anticholinesterases when patient is able to swallow.

Cholinergic Crisis

- Discontinue all anticholinesterases;
- Regularly check for respiratory function (especially vital capacity);
- Wean from ventilation at the right time;
- Restart oral anticholinesterases at a low dose followed by a gradual increase (Trouth et al. 2012; Gilhus et al. 2019; Lindsay et al. 2011; Greenberg 2010).

8.7.7. Neonatal Form of MG

This happens in a group of infants or mothers with MG.

- Indicated by poor sucking /crying as well as floppy extremities.
- Become symptomatic within 48 h of birth and may exist until the end of the third month.
- Occurs due to passive transplacental transfer of IgG (acetylcholine receptor antibodies).
- Therapy with anticholinesterases is needed until spontaneous resolution occurs. Remission takes place after exchange transfusion. This can occur even when the infant's mother has been in remission for many years (Trouth et al. 2012; Gilhus et al. 2019; Lindsay et al. 2011; Greenberg 2010).

8.7.8. Congenital Myasthenias

Pre-, post-, and mixed synaptic abnormalities are the cause of these non-immunologic illnesses. Although onset might be postponed until adulthood; they typically manifest in infancy. Muscle groups in the extremity (with concomitant skeletal anomalies when early age of onset), bulbar, ocular, and respiratory systems are particularly susceptible to fatigue. Electrophysiological evaluation is complicated, there are no AChR antibodies, and some patients respond to anticholinesterases or 3,4-diaminopyridine as supportive therapies (Trouth et al. 2012; Gilhus et al. 2019; Lindsay et al. 2011; Greenberg 2010).

9. Inherited Myopathies

9.1. Inherited Muscle Disorders

The muscular dystrophies (MD) are gradually deteriorating muscle illnesses that are genetically determined and characterized by cycles of fatty tissue replacement and muscle regeneration. Defects in the dystrophin-related glycoprotein complex are linked to a variety of diseases. Congenital myopathies have a more favorable prognosis and are characterized by morphological muscular defects without necrosis. The metabolic myopathies exhibit aches and weariness.

9.1.1. Xp2.1 Dystrophies (Duchenne and Becker Muscular Dystrophy)

Xp2.1 is where the dystrophin gene is found. While deletions inside the middle rod domain are linked to the milder Becker Dystrophy, point mutations and deletions involving the terminal domains are more frequently linked to the serious clinical phenotype of Duchenne.

Duchenne Muscular Dystrophy

Clinical Features: The prevalence of Duchenne muscular dystrophy is 01:3500 male births. It is characterized by delayed motor development in the early years, which is often seen between 1 and 3 years of age. Contractures, scoliosis, and eventually loss of ambulation occur around the age of 12. Although it occurs in 80% of cases, pseudohypertrophy of muscles, especially the calf, is not a pathognomonic sign.

The child is unable to climb steps or get out of a low chair, and when they try to get up from the ground, Gower's placard warns that he will "climb up him" (not diagnostic; however, implicative of pelvic muscle weakness).

Investigations: A diagnosis may be made through gene testing of serum. Due to the size of the dystrophin gene, many procedures only screen a small portion of it. Therefore, a "negative test" does not exclude it, necessitating a muscle biopsy and immunological investigations. This shows that dystrophin is not present. By using PCR, female carriers may be found.

Creatine kinase (CK): Markedly increased (several thousand times). At birth, the enzyme is increased, and female carriers have higher levels.

Electrocardiogram: In 80% of electrocardiograms, conduction problems are visible together with tall precordial R waves with deep left precordial Q waves. To identify developing cardiomyopathy, repeat echocardiography should be performed occasionally.

Electromyography—demonstrates serious myopathic change.

With the utilization of scoliosis surgery, active treatment of contractures, and noninvasive ventilation, the expected lifespan has increased from late teens to late 20s or early 30s. Although the ideal regimen is still unknown, corticosteroids decrease development and delay the onset of impairment. Death occurs due to a lack of oxygen in the lungs, an infection, or "suddenly" (possibly due to a heart condition). Coordinating long-term care for afflicted people should be performed in advance rather than in response to the progression of the illness.

Becker Dystrophy

From Duchenne dystrophy to the milder illness Becker dystrophy, abnormalities in the dystrophin gene may be linked to a range of manifestations. The incidence of Becker muscular dystrophy is lower than that of Duchenne muscular dystrophy (1:35 000), and it typically manifests later in life with limb girdle involvement and pseudohypertrophy. Some female bearers of the mutation may also experience these later, lesser manifestations. Cardiac involvement, which is unrelated to the mutation or the degree of limb muscle dysfunction, may cause symptoms in up to 10% of affected people and female carriers.

With serum DNA analysis, a diagnosis is made in up to 80% of instances. A diagnosis is made in the remaining cases using a combination of immunohistochemistry evidence of a relatively absent dystrophin, high CK, the clinical type, and pedigree analysis.

9.2. Muscular Dystrophies

9.2.1. Dystrophies with Particular Patterns of Weakness

Facioscapulohumeral (FSH)

A contraction of 3.3 kB repeats at locus 4q35, which is linked to an autosomal dominant disease of varied severity. The prevalence is 1–2:100,000. The exact mechanism through which this mutation results in illness in unknown.

The clinical pictures are:

- Facial muscle weakness (may be asymmetrical or mild);

- Periscapular weakness resulting in winging of the scapula as well as rising up of the scapulae on abduction;
- Humeral muscles weakness;
- A primely proximal lower-limb type of weakness leading to a dromedary or camel-backed gait. Pseudohypertrophy is not a characteristic feature.

The degree can range from severe childhood types to later-onset, potentially asymptomatic diseases. Only the highest limit of 1.5–2 or normal CK levels may be increased. Although secondary inflammatory change on a biopsy may result in an incorrect diagnosis of polymyositis, muscle biopsy and EMG will demonstrate myopathic abnormalities but lack specific characteristics. Heart involvement is not a characteristic. Some early onset cases (Coat's syndrome) are complicated by high-rate sensorineural deafness as well as exudative retinal telangiectases. The magnitude of respiratory muscle involvement affects the prognosis. Some patients might benefit from ventilator support.

Scapuloperoneal

It is a condition affecting the proximal muscles of the upper and lower limbs that is dominant or recessive. Beginning in maturity, foot drop is succeeded by scapular deltoid, bicep, and tricep weakness. It is challenging to distinguish from inflammatory muscle disease and spinal muscular atrophy.

Distal

Apart from myotonic dystrophy, distal weakness brought on by primary dystrophies is uncommon. It is described that both autosomal dominant and recessive patterns can initially affect the muscles of the upper or lower limbs. Some have been linked to muscle fiber vacuolation.

Emery–Dreifuss

Although uncommon, its cardiac consequences make it significant. There are reports on dominant and X-linked forms. Spinal contractures provide the impression of hyperextension. Early ankle and elbow contractures occur. Scapuloperoneal dispersion may be weak. Virtually all heart abnormalities are life-threatening, yet ventricular tachyarrhythmias do occur sometimes. Patients will need to be paced and may have defibrillators implanted. Having weak respiratory muscles is possible.

Oculopharyngeal

The PABP2 gene on chromosome 14 has a modest GCG trinucleotide expansion, which is responsible for this extremely uncommon pattern of weakness. It is autosomal-dominant in inheritance. It occurs with an average onset age of 50 years and features dysphagia, ptosis, and ophthalmoparesis. Limb weakening could occur. Rimmed vacuoles and filamentous intranuclear inclusions are visible in muscle biopsies.

Limb Girdle Syndromes and Limb Girdle Muscular Dystrophy (LGMD)

Both secondary and primary myopathies frequently appear with slowly worsening proximal weakness. A wide variety of proteins with various activities contribute to the LGMD phenotype. Recessive forms occur more often than dominant types. A variety of conditions, such as non-dystrophic Desmin myopathy; metabolic, toxic, and endocrine myopathies; inflammatory polymyositis, etc., can cause weakness in the limb girdle distribution.

9.2.2. Myotonic Dystrophy (MyD)

A non-coding region at location 19q13.3 has an unstable trinucleotide repeat expansion that leads to myotonic dystrophy, an autosomal dominant multisystem condition. Because of its indirect effects on nearby genes, this expansion is thought to be harmful. It has a 5 per 100,000 incidence and can manifest at any age. While neuromuscular characteristics may not be obvious, the disorder is typically distinguished by the presence of MYOTONIA, which is the inability of muscles to immediately relax once a contraction has ended.

Clinical Presentations

- Cataracts.
- Smooth muscle disorder, constipation, gut motility dysfunction, and bladder emptying malfunction.
- Cardiac muscle disease, dilated cardiomyopathy, and atrio-ventricular block.

- Respiratory failure because of diaphragmatic and intercostals weakness, swallowing impairment, and central sleep apnea.
- Diabetes because of insulin resistance.
- Testicular atrophy and subfertility.

Diagnosis

Clinical diagnosis is simple in situations of classic adult onset when myotonia, frontal baldness, cataracts, and progressive distal plus bulbar dystrophy are present. In mild situations, where cataracts could be the only symptom, clinical diagnosis may be more challenging. DNA diagnosis is made possible through direct measurement of the CTG repeat size using Southern blotting on peripheral leucocytes. Patients contain 50 to several thousand CTG repeats, compared to normal people who have 5 to 37.

The management of problems and genetic counseling place a premium on disorder recognition. The extensive clinical diversity (phenotype) of MyD is caused by the genetic defect instability (number of repeats) between generations. Females run the risk of giving birth to a baby who is critically ill and may not make it through the neonatal period due to respiratory failure. Occasionally, people first present with respiratory failure or sudden death, either spontaneously or after anesthesia.

Two rare, alternative illnesses are taken into consideration when molecular studies are negative while clinical symptoms are suggestive:

1. Dystrophia myotonica type 2;
2. Proximal myotonic myopathy.

9.3. Dystrophies: General Principles and Investigation

9.3.1. General Principles

Despite the fact that some types of dystrophy may be impossible to diagnose or rule out, the following practical concerns are universal:

1. Genetics: It is obvious how different inheritance styles affect the patient's family. Even if molecular diagnosis has not been made but an inherited muscle illness is suspected, assistance from a clinical geneticist should be sought to discuss this. The phenotype of LGMD varies greatly, and isolated occurrences may indicate a novel dominant mutation. Patients should be informed of these issues, as well as those of their spouses.

2. Cardiac disease: Emery–Dreifuss syndrome, in which life-threatening conduction deficits are unavoidable, as well as Xp2.1-related dystrophies and polymyositis exhibit this, which is of utmost importance. ECGs should be performed every 12 months in the absence of a confirmed diagnosis, and echocardiography should be conducted as well if signs of heart failure start to appear.

3. Respiratory failure: Diaphragmatic weakness is associated with respiratory failure, a common symptom of Xp2.1, MD, LGMD; other types of MD; and inflammatory muscular disease. Sleep-disturbed breathing may also result from some congenital myopathies' late degeneration. It is crucial to be aware of this because such patients typically benefit from noninvasive nocturnal ventilatory support.

9.3.2. Investigations

Creatine kinase (CK): The injured muscle membrane releases this sarcoplasmic enzyme. Rhabdomyolysis and muscular dystrophies are associated with high levels, although normal readings do not rule out lesser muscle illness.

Neurophysiology: Normal investigations do not rule out muscle disease, but they may be able to distinguish between neurogenic and myopathic weakness and show indications of muscular membrane damage (such as in inflammatory myopathies).

Muscle biopsy: Some illnesses can be diagnosed with routine staining of frozen material, but others require immunohistochemical analysis and appropriate mutation research (e.g., muscular dystrophies). Deciding between a needle biopsy and an open biopsy is challenging; the former is less unpleasant but simpler, while the latter may be preferred to reduce sample mistakes (González-Jamett et al. 2018; Lindsay et al. 2011; Greenberg 2010).

10. Neurometabolic Diseases: Wilson Disease

10.1. Introduction

It is also known as hepatolenticular degeneration. It is an autosomal recessive disease identified by the storage of intracellular copper with hepatic and neurological dysfunctions.

10.2. Pathology

The putamen and the globus pallidus experience cavitation and neuronal death. The liver displays the symptoms of severe cirrhosis. All organs acquire copper, but the kidney, nail beds, and Descemet's membrane in the eye are particularly susceptible. Ceruloplasmin, a type-2 globulin that typically binds 98% of the copper in plasma and delivers copper to enzymes, is insufficient (cytochrome oxidase). All organs experience deposition due to a rise in loosely bound copper/albumin. Urinary copper levels are higher.

10.3. Clinical Presentations

There are two clinical types:

- Acute:
    - Bradykinesia, behavioral change, involuntary movements, and severe liver dysfunction (common);
    - If not treated, death in 02 years from liver failure.
- Chronic
    - Significant proximal wing-beating tremor;
    - Dysarthria, rigidity, and dystonia;
    - Choreoathetosis;
    - Psychosis, behavioral disorder, and dementia;
    - Liver dysfunction is less severe;
    - If not treated, death within 10 years.

The storage of copper in Descemet's membrane produces a golden brown "Kayser-Fleischer ring" that can be observed by the naked eye or using a slit lamp and is pathognomonic.

10.4. Diagnosis

Biochemical evidence of an aberrant copper metabolism supporting the following, any patient with atypical hepatic and/or neurological characteristics should be evaluated for:

- Decreased ceruloplasmin (<20 mg/dL);
- Increased unbound serum copper;
- Raised urinary copper clearance;
- Liver biopsy and copper metabolism tests with radioactive ^{64}Cu;
- MRI (T2W) demonstrates putaminal and thalamic hyperintensity.

Biochemical studies will find decreased ceruloplasmin in carriers and in patients without symptoms in their families. In copper-transporting ATPase, more than 20 mutations have been found. There is no diagnostic genetic testing available.

10.5. Treatment

Provide a low-copper diet as well as chelating medication, such as penicillamine—1.5–1 g per day. Trientine is a good substitute if patients experience side effects including allergy, skin rash, bone marrow suppression, or glomerulonephritis, which are frequent.

The patient will require therapy for the rest of their lives. Normal life expectancy is compatible with adequate treatment. With time, Kayser–Fleischer rings will vanish (Członkowska et al. 2018; Rodriguez-Castro et al. 2015; Lindsay et al. 2011; Greenberg 2010).

Author Contributions: Conceptualization, methodology, validation, formal analysis, investigation, resources, data curation, F.H.C. and M.H.R.; writing—original draft preparation, writing—review and editing, F.H.C.; visualization, supervision, M.B.A.M. All authors have read and agreed to the published version of the manuscript.

Funding: This research received no external funding.

Conflicts of Interest: The authors declare no conflicts of interest.

References

Absoud, Michael, Peter Brex, Olga Ciccarelli, Onyinye Diribe, Gavin Giovannoni, Jennifer Hellier, Rosemary Howe, Rachel Holland, Joanna Kelly, Paul McCrone, and et al. 2017. A multicentre randomiSed controlled TRial of IntraVEnous immunoglobulin compared with standard therapy for the treatment of transverse myelitis in adults and children (STRIVE). *Health Technology Assessment Volume* 21: 1–50. [CrossRef] [PubMed]

Arora, R. D., and Y. S. Khan. 2022. Motor Neuron Disease. In *StatPearls [Internet]*; Treasure Island: StatPearls Publishing. Available online: https://www.ncbi.nlm.nih.gov/books/NBK560774/ (accessed on 3 May 2022).

Ascherio, Alberto. 2013. Environmental factors in multiple sclerosis. *Expert Review of Neurotherapeutics* 13: 3–9. [CrossRef] [PubMed]

Berman, Miriam, Shad Feldman, Milton Alter, Nelly Zilber, and Esther Kahana. 1981. Acute transverse myelitis: Incidence and etiologic considerations. *Neurology* 31: 966–71. [CrossRef] [PubMed]

Brooks, B. Rix. 1994. El Escorial World Federation of Neurology criteria for the diagnosis of amyotrophic lateral sclerosis. Subcommittee on Motor Neuron Diseases/Amyotrophic Lateral Sclerosis of the World Federation of Neurology Research Group on Neuromuscular Diseases and the El Escorial "Clinical limits of amyotrophic lateral sclerosis" workshop contributors. *Journal of the Neurological Sciences* 124: 96–107. [CrossRef] [PubMed]

Członkowska, Anna, Tomasz Litwin, Petr Dusek, Peter Ferenci, Svetlana Lutsenko, Valentina Medici, Janusz K. Rybakowski, Karl Heinz Weiss, and Michael L. Schilsky. 2018. Wilson disease. *Nature Reviews Disease Primers* 4: 21. [CrossRef] [PubMed]

Dobson, Ruth, and Gavin Giovannoni. 2018. Multiple sclerosis—A review. *European Journal of Neurology* 26: 27–40. [CrossRef] [PubMed]

Fisher, D. L., S. Defres, and T. Solomon. 2015. Measles-induced encephalitis. *QJM* 108: 177–82. [CrossRef] [PubMed]

Gaudette, Mara, Makito Hirano, and Teepu Siddique. 2000. Current status of SOD1 mutations in familial amyotrophic lateral sclerosis. *Amyotrophic Lateral Sclerosis and Other Motor Neuron Disorders* 1: 83–89. [CrossRef]

Gilhus, Nils Erik, Socrates Tzartos, Amelia Evoli, Jacqueline Palace, Ted M. Burns, and Jan J. G. M. Verschuuren. 2019. Myasthenia gravis. *Nature Reviews Disease Primers* 5: 30. [CrossRef]

González-Jamett, Arlek Marion, Jorge Alfredo Bevilacqua, and Ana María Cárdenas Díaz. 2018. Hereditary Myopathies. In *Muscle Cell and Tissue—Current Status of Research Field*. Edited by Kunihiro Sakuma. London: IntechOpen. [CrossRef]

Greenberg, Mark S. 2010. *Handbook of Neurosurgery*. New York: Thieme.

Hughes, Richard A. C., and David R. Cornblath. 2005. Guillain-barre syndrome. *The Lancet* 366: 1653–66. [CrossRef]

Kennedy, P. G. 2004. Viral encephalitis: Causes, differential diagnosis, and management. *Journal of Neurology, Neurosurgery, and Psychiatry* 75: i10–i15. [CrossRef] [PubMed]

Kobelt, Gisela, Alan Thompson, Jenny Berg, Mia Gannedahl, Jennifer Eriksson, MSCOI Study Group, and European Multiple Sclerosis Platform. 2017. European Multiple Sclerosis Platform. New insights into the burden and costs of multiple sclerosis in Europe. *Multiple Sclerosis Journal* 23: 1123–36. [CrossRef] [PubMed]

Lehmann, Helmar Christoph, David Burke, and Satoshi Kuwabara. 2019. Chronic inflammatory demyelinating polyneuropathy: Update on diagnosis, immunopathogenesis and treatment. *Journal of Neurology, Neurosurgery & Psychiatry* 90: 981–87. [CrossRef]

Lindsay, Kenneth W., Ian Bone, and Geraint Fuller. 2011. *Neurology and Neurosurgery Illustrated*. London: C L Elsevier, pp. 1–31.

McDonald, W. Ian, Alistair Compston, Gilles Edan, Donald Goodkin, Hans-Peter Hartung, Fred D. Lublin, Henry F. McFarland, Donald W. Paty, Chris H. Polman, Stephen C. Reingold, and et al. 2001. Recommended diagnostic criteria for multiple sclerosis: Guidelines from the International Panel on the diagnosis of multiple sclerosis. *Annals of Neurology* 50: 121–27. [CrossRef]

Meningitis and Encephalitis Information Page. 2017. Available online: https://catalog.ninds.nih.gov/sites/default/files/publications/meningitis-encephalitis.pdf (accessed on 29 October 2017).

NHS. 2015. Symptoms of Encephalitis. Available online: https://www.nhs.uk/conditions/encephalitis/ (accessed on 5 January 2015).

Pascuzzi, Robert M., and James D. Fleck. 1997. Acute peripheral neuropathy in adults: Guillain-Barré Syndrome and Related Disorders. *Neurologic Clinics* 15: 529–47. [CrossRef] [PubMed]

Rodriguez-Castro, Kryssia Isabel, Francisco Javier Hevia-Urrutia, and Giacomo Carlo Sturniolo. 2015. Wilson's disease: A review of what we have learned. *World Journal of Hepatology* 18: 2859–70. [CrossRef]

Roos, K. L., and K. L. Tyler. 2015. Meningitis, Encephalitis, Brain Abscess, and Empyema. In *Harrison's Principles of Internal Medicine*, 19th ed. Edited by Dennis L. Kasper; Anthony S. Fauci and Stephen L. Hauser. New York: McGraw-Hill Education.

Sherrell, Zia. 2022. What is Transverse Myelitis? Available online: https://www.medicalnewstoday.com/articles/transverse-myelitis (accessed on 31 July 2022).

Tandel, Hemal, Jigar Vanza, Nilima Pandya, and P. Jani. 2016. Guillain-barré syndrome (GBS): A review. *European journal of pharmaceutical and medical research* 3: 366–71.

Teoh, Hooi Ling, Kate Carey, Hugo Sampaio, David Mowat, Tony Roscioli, and Michelle Farrar. 2017. Inherited Paediatric Motor Neuron Disorders: Beyond Spinal Muscular Atrophy. *Neural Plasticity* 2017: 6509493. [CrossRef]

Trouth, Annapurni Jayam, Alok Dabi, Noha Solieman, Mohankumar Kurukumbi, and Janaki Kalyanam. 2012. Myasthenia gravis: A review. *Autoimmune Diseases* 2012: 874680. [CrossRef]

Venkatesan, Arun, Allan R. Tunkel, Karen C. Bloch, A. S. Lauring, J. Sejvar, A. Bitnun, J. P. Stahl, A. Mailles, M. Drebot, C. E. Rupprecht, and et al. 2013. Case definitions, diagnostic algorithms, and priorities in encephalitis: Consensus statement of the international encephalitis consortium. *Clinical Infectious Diseases* 57: 1114–28. [CrossRef]

Vos, Theo, Christine Allen, Megha Arora, Ryan M. Barber, Zulfiqar A. Bhutta, Alexandria Brown, Austin Carter, Daniel C. Casey, Fiona J. Charlson, Alan Z. Chen, and et al. 2016. Global, regional, and national incidence, prevalence, and years lived with disability for 310 diseases and injuries, 1990–2015: A systematic analysis for the Global Burden of Disease Study 2015. *Lancet* 388: 1545–602. [CrossRef] [PubMed]

Wikipedia contributors. 2022. Encephalitis. Available online: https://en.wikipedia.org/w/index.php?title=Encephalitis&oldid=1103898820 (accessed on 15 August 2022).

Section XVI: Rehabilitation

Neurorehabilitation in Neurosurgery

Taslim Uddin and Forhad H. Chowdhury

Abstract: Neurorehabilitation is an important pillar in the management of neurosurgical patients. Neurorehabilitation is an integrated interdisciplinary care program including a set of interventions to help people with disabilities to acquire and maintain optimal functioning in their environment, permitting them to attain maximum independence and social reintegration. This chapter is an abstract of the rehabilitation approach to neurosurgical conditions, including trauma (to the brain, spine, and nerves), stroke, and tumor, and post-surgical care.

Abbreviations

ADLs	activities of daily living	ASIA	American Spinal Injury Association
CIMT	constraint-induced movement therapy	EMG	Electromyography
FES	functional electric stimulation	ICH	intracranial hematoma
ICF	International Classification of Functioning, Disability, And Health	ICU	intensive care unit
MS	multiple sclerosis	MRI	magnetic resonance imaging
NMES	neuromuscular electric stimulation	OT	occupational therapy
OPD	outpatient department	PET	positron emitting tomography
PMR	physical medicine and rehabilitation	PT	Physiotherapist
SAH	subarachnoid hemorrhage	SCI	spinal cord injury
SDH	subdural hematoma	SLT	speech and language therapist
tPA	tissue plasminogen activator	TBI	traumatic brain injury
WHO	World Health Organization		

1. Introduction and Concepts

Neurorehabilitation is the provision of an integrated interdisciplinary care program that includes a set of interventions to help people with disabilities to acquire and maintain optimal functioning in their environment, allowing them to attain maximum independence and social reintegration (Australian Rehabilitation Alliance 2011). This chapter is dedicated to the rehabilitation approach to neurosurgical conditions, include trauma (to the brain, spine, and nerves), stroke, and tumor, and post-surgical care.

The International Classification of Functioning, Disability, and Health (ICF) is a framework for categorizing and organizing data on functioning and disability developed by the World Health Organization (WHO). It set up a common vocabulary and conceptual structure for defining and measuring disability and health. The purpose of a neurosurgical rehabilitation program is to assist each patient in regaining the best level of independence, function, and quality of life possible. Body structures, body function, activities, and participation are all referred to as "functioning". It refers to the positive or negative features of the relationship between a person's health condition(s) and their surrounding circumstances (environmental and personal factors). Activity limits, impairments, and participation restrictions all fall under the umbrella term "disability". It refers to the unpleasant features of the interaction between a person's health condition(s) and their surrounding circumstances (environmental and personal factors) (www.wcpt.org).

Modern rehabilitation exercises are founded on the concepts of disability, impairment, and handicap, as mentioned by the WHO, which have recently been redefined as "impairment", "activity" and "participation". Rehabilitation is a functional method that consists of four fundamental components: (1) lowering disability; (2) learning new abilities and applying them to reduce the impact of impairment; (3) acquiring new skills and applying them to reduce the impact of disability; and (4) changing the environment surrounding physical and socioeconomic circumstances so that people with disabilities can participate as much as possible.

Symptoms such as muscular weakness, paralysis, poor coordination, and lack of feeling, as well as seizures, disorientation, pain, and altered degrees of consciousness (Sandberg et al. 2009), can be caused by biochemical, structural, or electrical irregularities in the spinal cord, brain, or nerves leading to or from them. Stroke, intracranial hemorrhage (ICH), subdural hematoma (SDH), brain tumor, aneurysm, Parkinson's disease, multiple sclerosis

(MS), spinal cord injury (SCI), traumatic brain injury (TBI), and other neurological conditions such as spinal disc herniation and peripheral nerve injuries can all benefit from neurorehabilitation (Kaldis and Desai 2015).

Many of the neurological and neurosurgical patients may have short-term or long-term functional disability in relation to activities of daily living (ADLs). Rehabilitation interventions proved beneficial in a number of studies including low-income resource settings and patients with stroke, SCI, TBI, brain tumor, spinal disc prolapse, or peripheral nerve injuries (Uddin et al. 2019b; Al Hasan et al. 2009; Lee et al. 2019; Uddin et al. 2019a).

The usual approach involves a multidisciplinary rehabilitation team guided by a physical medicine rehabilitation physician (also commonly known as physiatrist), a neurosurgeon, and a number of rehab professionals. Box 1 explains the rehabilitation team for neurosurgical conditions; however, this number is not limited and other members—like a pressure ulcer dressing specialist, recreation therapist, or vocational therapist— may need to be included as per requirements in special cases, depending on the nature and length of the rehabilitation process.

Box 1. Rehabilitation Modalities. Source: Box by authors.

Rehabilitation modalities include the following:

(a) Pathological basis of diagnosis and evaluation of disability for rehabilitation;
(b) Mobility, pain, spasticity, cognitive function improving medications, and physical modalities;
(c) Nutrition;
(d) Proper positioning at bed and at mobility;
(e) Heat and cold modalities;
(f) Neuromuscular electric stimulation (NMES);
(g) Assistive technology (AT);
(h) Mobility aids and assistive devices;
(i) Functional electric stimulation (FES), e.g., breathing pacemaker;
(j) EMG biofeedback;
(k) Behavioral, cognitive, and communication therapy.

In a recent review paper on emerging therapies, the following principles were used to produce an enhanced functional state: redistribution of leftover control, augmentation using artificial control, and regeneration. Peripheral nervous system "rewiring"; neuromodulation via spinal epidural excitation and brain stimulation (DBS); external robotics to substitute for a deficiency in motor control; brain–computer interfaces to promote control, when very little remaining control persists; and biological therapies involving stem cells, aiding in the recovery of previously unrecoverable injuries, are examples of such interventions (Iaccarino et al. 2015; Wilson et al. 2013). Patients with spinal cord damage, stroke, cerebral palsy, traumatic brain injury (TBI), brachial plexus injury, severe dystonia, spina bifida, and a variety of other disorders and injuries may benefit from such therapies. This chapter emphasizes several operations, processes, and therapies that represent major modalities of restorative functional and reconstructive neurosurgery, as well as contemporary technology breakthroughs, discoveries, and implementations. Rehabilitation techniques vary and are provided depending on a case-by-case disability assessment, as determined during a patient-centered rehabilitation team meeting.

Providing a detailed description and case-based analysis of disability assessment and rehabilitation protocols is beyond the scope of this current topic; however, an attempt will be made to briefly describe the rehabilitation perspectives of some common neurosurgery-related problems. Readers may refer to physical medicine rehabilitation (PMR) text books for further knowledge (Frontera et al. 2019).

2. Spinal Cord Injury (SCI)

Trauma, malignancies, vascular abnormalities, viral diseases, and developmental disorders are all causes of SCI. SCI is linked to a wide range of functional impairments, with motor deficits being a typical and persistent presenting feature that has an impact on a variety of health-related difficulties, as well as other functional issues and ADLs. Tetraparesis (47.2%) is the commonest neurologic condition, followed by paraparesis (20.4%), total paraplegia (20.2%), and total tetraplegia (11.5%) (Frontera et al. 2019).

The International Standards for Neurological and Functional Classification of Spinal Cord Injury is a widely recognized system for describing the extent and level of injury based on a thorough sensory and motor examination of neurological function (Hakkinen et al. 2005; Johansson et al. 2009; American Spinal Injury Association 1992). The word "tetraplegia" has replaced "quadriplegia" to describe spinal cord injury to the cervical area. The American Spinal Injury Association (ASIA) Impairment Scale in Table 1 describes the severity of an injury. It is a variation of the Frankel Classification that does not utilize the phrases "paraparesis" or "quadraparesis". This scale assigns a letter grade to individuals ranging from "A" for complete recovery to "E" for full recovery (Frontera et al. 2019).

Table 1. American Spinal Injury Association (ASIA) Impairment Scale.

ASIA Scale	Description
A	Complete: no motor or sensory function is preserved in the sacral segments S4–S5.
B	Incomplete: sensory but not motor function is preserved below the neurologic level and extends through the sacral segments S4–S5.
C	Incomplete: motor function is intact below the neurologic level, and most of the key muscles below the neurologic level have a muscle power grade less than 3.
D	Incomplete: motor function is intact below the neurologic level, and the majority of key muscles below the neurologic level have a muscle power grade greater than or equal to 3.
E	Normal: motor and sensory function is normal.

Source: Authors' compilation based on data from American Spinal Injury American Spinal Injury Association (1992).

The definition of incomplete and complete SCI is now dependent on the sacral-sparing definition.

Muscles are graded on a scale of 0–5. A grade 3/5 muscle is considered to have intact innervation if the next most rostral muscle has 4/5 strength. Key muscles are considered for C5 through T1, as well as L2 through S1, in Box 2.

Box 2. Key muscles for SCI patients. Source: Box by authors.

C5: Flexors of elbow (brachialis and biceps)
C6: Extensors of wrist (extensor carpi radialis brevis and longus)
C7: Extensors of elbow (triceps)
C8: Flexors of finger (flexor digitorum profundus) to the middle finger
T1: Abductors of small finger (abductor digiti minimi)
L2: Flexors of hip (iliopsoas)
L3: Extensors of knee (quadriceps)
L4: Dorsi flexors of ankle (tibialis anterior)
L5: Long toe extensors (extensor hallucis longus)
S1: Ankle plantar flexors (gastrocnemius, soleus)

The objectives of care for a patient with SCI include a comprehensive continuum of care from the point of injury to the acute care hospital, resuscitation and specialist rehabilitation medical and surgical care (depending on the case), multidisciplinary inpatient rehabilitation care, and step-down and pre-home care to community and vocational care services.

'Time is Spine,' as shown in Figure 1, is a crucial idea that emphasizes the relationship between the time period of damage and pathophysiological changes, as well as the significance of targeted therapies during the acute injury phase to improve long-term results. While there is no cure for the neurological sequelae of SCI, numerous novel therapies are now being tried in clinical trials and have shown promise in improving long-term functional recovery.

Model rehabilitation care has been shown to be effective, and people with SCI typically demonstrate considerable spontaneous motor and sensory improvement in the first 3–6 months after injury, although substantial spontaneous improvement beyond the first year is uncommon, and only about 1% of people with SCI have full neurologic healing at discharge from the hospital.

Concerns over sexual and bowel–bladder functions are also prevalent in SCI patients requiring continuous monitoring by the caring rehabilitation team either during the hospital stay or when back in the community.

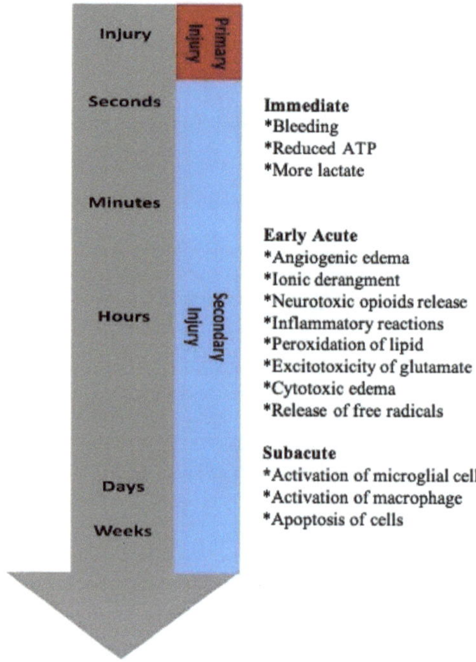

Figure 1. Time is Spine. There are two types of spinal cord injuries: primary and secondary. The first physical injury sets off a chain reaction of subsequent biochemical damage that lasts during the immediate, early acute, and subacute stage. Source: Authors' compilation based on data from Wilson et al. (2013).

3. Spinal Canal Stenosis and Disc Surgery

Low back pain has a high lifetime incidence, and it limits functional activities, resulting in increased health-care consumption and leading to disability and job loss. With the surge in surgical procedures for these disorders, diagnoses of spinal stenosis and disc prolapse are on the rise. Discectomy for intervertebral disc prolapse has greater success rates, ranging from 65–90%, but residual back and leg discomfort, as well as recurrent herniation, remain the most common postoperative problems in lumbar disc surgery, necessitating the attention of a rehabilitation physician. Only 35% of operating surgeons gave written postoperative instructions; referral to rehabilitation therapy was minimal, and 18% of operating surgeons recommended the utilization of a lumbar corset after surgery, with others prohibiting sitting or promoting bed rest. According to research, an intensive postoperative exercise program consisting of stretching and stabilizing exercises, graded behavioral activities, and neuromuscular training with thermotherapy modalities resulted in a faster return to work (Hakkinen et al. 2005).

There are differences in the intensity and type of rehabilitation prescribed for disc surgery patients, including in difficult cases such as failed back surgery syndrome. A graded exercise regime with supporting education given to patients in the postoperative period has proven effective (Johansson et al. 2009).

4. Traumatic Brain Injury (TBI)

TBI is a prominent cause of seizure disorders, disability, and mortality around the world; however, rehabilitation facilities are in short supply. TBI has a wide range of severities, ranging from concussion to a permanent vegetative states, with mild, moderate, and severe classifications. Acute care rehabilitation concentrates on coma emergence and recovery prognosis, with rehabilitation therapy beginning from the first day after trauma and ranging from the ICU through community care. A description of the comprehensive multidisciplinary rehabilitation team involved in a TBI patient's care for assessment of post-traumatic amnesia and pain management is provided in Box 3.

Box 3. Comprehensive multidisciplinary rehabilitation team involved in TBI patient's care. Source: Authors' compilation based on data from Lee et al. (2019).

1. The patient and family members/care giver;
2. Physical medicine rehabilitation physician;
3. Other medical specialties: neurosurgery, orthopedic surgery, and urology;
4. Allied health care professionals and skilled personals: rehabilitation nurse (RN), physiotherapist (PT), occupational therapists (OT), prosthetics and orthotics (P&O), medical social worker, nutritionist, clinical psychologist, speech and language therapist (SLT), and rehab case manager.

Therapeutic modalities are described in Box 1. Exercise, including pharmacologic therapy, can target long-term cognitive and motor effects. Individualized specific rehabilitation protocols prescribed by the physical medicine rehabilitation physician for these patients are discussed in Box 4. They are instituted at three levels of treatment: (a) inpatient, (b) OPD, and (c) home- and community-based facilities. Heterotopic ossification, dystonia, agitation, and spasticity are some of the functionally limiting and therapy-impeding complications of severe TBI.

Box 4. Prescription of rehabilitation protocols in TBI patients. Source: Authors' compilation based on data from Lee et al. (2019).

- Health education and training of the caregiver for pressure ulcer prevention, understanding of the complications, and time-demanding rehabilitation protocols;
- Prescription of neuropharmacological medications and agents;
- Nutritional attainment;
- Cognitive rehabilitation therapy;
- Pain management;
- Management of contractures: serial casting, splinting, and orthotic prescription;
- Cognitive rehabilitation therapy;
- Bowel and bladder management;
- Spasticity management: phenol blocks, botulinum toxin, baclofen pump, and use of pharmacological and non-pharmacological agents;
- Comprehensive dysphagia and communication management;
- Brain stimulation therapy;
- Rehabilitation robotic therapy.

Most patients recover swiftly from mild TBI; however, education about recurrent exposure is crucial, as the sequelae of many injuries can be devastating. Moreover, sleep disturbances, migraines, visuospatial impairments, and cognitive dysfunction are all dealt with throughout therapy (Lee et al. 2019).

5. Rehabilitation of Stroke Patients

Stroke is the absence of neurological function due to an abrupt interruption of relatively constant blood supply to the brain. It is the world's second major cause of death. Ischemic and hemorrhagic strokes are the two main types of strokes. Ischemic strokes are produced by a disruption in the brain's blood flow, whereas hemorrhagic strokes are caused by a blood vessel rupture or an aberrant vascular structure. Acute ischemic strokes constitute 87% of strokes and subarachnoid hemorrhages (SAHs) account for 3%, which is important information in neurosurgery (Kicielinski and Ogilvy 2019). The need for integrated stroke care grows as the load of stroke pathology grows and treatment choices develop.

In medically neglected, lower-income areas around the world, the rates of mortality and disability from stroke are at least 10 times higher than in the most industrialized nations. When compared to Primary Stroke Centers, Comprehensive Stroke Centers showed faster tPA administration and a higher rate of mechanical thrombectomy.

Acute stroke care is quickly changing, and rehabilitation physicians and neurosurgeons are still vital members of the care team.

The rehabilitation team, led by the rehabilitation medicine physician, assess the functional disability status, socioeconomic backgrounds, and comorbidities (usually in association with the neurophysician or neurosurgeon) from the first day of hospital care. A large team, comprising the patient and their family and friends, rehabilitation physicians, other caregivers, occupational and physical therapists, speech–language pathologists, nurses, psychologists, recreation therapists, nutritionists, social workers, and others, is required for stroke rehabilitation. The team set the goal of care either as an intensive phase of inpatient care or OPD/day care. The traditional model of rehabilitation still remains the gold standard of care and includes proper bed positioning, nutritional aspects including dysphagia management, bowel–bladder care, chest–limbs physiotherapy, spasticity, speech therapy, and mobility. Constraint-induced movement therapy (CIMT) and robotics are two potentially useful therapeutic approaches for arm motor rehabilitation. High-intensity therapy, fitness training, and repetitive-task training are all promising strategies for improving the components of gait. The prescription of proper assistive devices for mobility, transcranial magnetic stimulation, programs for cognitive therapy, and functional electrical stimulation are the other rehabilitation programs offered to stroke patients (Dionísio et al. 2018).

The Lokomat robotic assistive device offers novel gait training options in stroke therapy while removing the physical therapist's need to perform long, repetitive movements in an unnatural position. Repeated assessments of the stroke patient, as well as communication and coordination among team members, are critical to improve the efficiency and effectiveness of stroke rehabilitation.

6. Rehabilitation of Patients with Brain Tumor

Brain tumors can be classified into two general groups: primary and secondary. The most common primary brain tumors are gliomas, which include astrocytoma, oligodendroglioma, and ependymoma. Some other mostly benign types are also described, e.g., meningiomas, schwannomas, craniopharyngiomas, etc. Secondary brain tumors are usually metastatic. Magnetic resonance imaging (MRI), intraoperative MRI, computed tomography (CT), magnetic resonance spectroscopy, and positron emission tomography (PET) are some of the advanced imaging techniques used in diagnosis. Surgery, radiation, and/or chemotherapy are commonly used to treat brain tumors, whether they are metastatic or primary, benign or malignant (AANS 2024).

The goal of the operating neurosurgeon is to remove as much tumor as feasible while avoiding damaging brain tissue that is critical to the patient's neurological function (such as the capability to walk and speak; cognitive function; etc.). Common surgical complications include prolong hospital stays, pneumonia, and venous thrombosis, giving rise to deconditioning of the musculoskeletal and cardiorespiratory system, requiring attention from the physical medicine rehabilitation physician and rehabilitation team assessment as a long-term patient (De la Garza-Ramos et al. 2016). The rehabilitation approach is focused on the identification of a specific problem and the prescription of an individualized institute- or home-based rehabilitation protocol. The basic guidelines are discussed above in **??** 2–4. Interested readers may consult physical medicine rehabilitation text books and advanced webpages for further information (Frontera et al. 2019; John Hopkins Medicine n.d.).

7. Conclusions

Ultimately, the outcome of a neurosurgical patient depends on many factors and neurorehabilitation is one of the most important factors. Any patient with neurosurgical intervention needs proper postoperative neurorehabilitative care, otherwise it may not produce any benefit to the patient.

Author Contributions: Conceptualization, methodology, validation, formal analysis, investigation, resources, data curation, writing—original draft preparation, T.U.; writing—review and editing, visualization, supervision, F.H.C. All authors have read and agreed to the published version of the manuscript.

Funding: This research received no external funding.

Conflicts of Interest: The authors declare no conflicts of interest.

References

AANS. 2024. Brain Tumors. Available online: https://www.aans.org/Patients/Neurosurgical-Conditions-and-Treatments/Brain-Tumors (accessed on 9 November 2024).

Al Hasan, Suzon, Zahagir Alam, Maliha Hakim, Md Abdus Shakoor, A. K. M. Salek, Md Moniruzzaman Khan, Syed Mozaffar Ahmed, Md Abdur Rashid, Monirul Islam, Md Taslim Uddin, and et al. 2009. Rehabilitation of Patients with Paraplegia from Spinal Cord Injury: A Review. *Journal of Chittagong Medical College Teachers' Association* 20: 53–57. [CrossRef]

American Spinal Injury Association. 1992. *International Standards for Neurological Classification of Spinal Cord Injury*. Chicago: American Spinal Injury Association, pp. 1–23.

Australian Rehabilitation Alliance. 2011. *The Need for a National Rehabilitation Strategy: Working towards a Clear and United Rehabilitation Strategy for Australia (Position Statement)*. Canberra: ARA.

De la Garza-Ramos, Rafael, Panagiotis Kerezoudis, Rafael J. Tamargo, Henry Brem, Judy Huang, and Mohamad Bydon. 2016. Neurosurgical complications following malignant brain tumor surgery: An analysis of 2002–2011 data. *Clinical Neurology and Neurosurgery* 140: 6–10. [CrossRef] [PubMed]
Dionísio, Ana, Isabel Catarina Duarte, Miguel Patricio, and Miguel Castelo-Branco. 2018. The Use of Repetitive Transcranial Magnetic Stimulation for Stroke Rehabilitation: A Systematic Review. *Journal of Stroke and Cerebrovascular Diseases* 7: 1–31. [CrossRef] [PubMed]
Frontera, Walter R., Joel A. DeLisa, Bruce M. Gans, Lawrence R. Robinson, William Bockenek, and John Chae. 2019. DeLisa's Physical Medicine and Rehabilitation: Principles and Practice. Available online: https://www.wolterskluwer.com/en/solutions/ovid/delisas-physical-medicine-and-rehabilitation-principles-and-practice-2540 (accessed on 8 May 2020).
Hakkinen, Arja, Hannu Kautiainen, Harri Sintonen, and Jan Ylinen. 2005. Health related quality of life after lumbar disc surgery: A prospective study of patients. *Disability and Rehabilitation* 27: 94–100. [CrossRef] [PubMed]
Iaccarino, Mary Alexis, Saurabha Bhatnagar, and Ross Zafonte. 2015. Rehabilitation after traumatic brain injury. *Handbook of Clinical Neurology* 127: 411–22. [CrossRef] [PubMed]
Johansson, Ann-Christin, Steven J. Linton, Leif Bergkvist, Olle Nilsson, and Michael Cornefjord. 2009. Clinic-based training in comparison to home-based training after first-time lumbar disc surgery: A randomised controlled trial. *European Spine Journal* 18: 398–409. [CrossRef] [PubMed]
John Hopkins Medicine. n.d. Physical Medicine and Rehabilitation. Available online: https://www.hopkinsmedicine.org/physical_medicine_rehabilitation/services/programs/tbi-stroke-rehab.html (accessed on 4 June 2020).
Kaldis, Teresa, and Purvi Desai. 2015. Rehabilitation of Neurosurgical Conditions. In *Comprehensive Guide to Neurosurgical Conditions*. Edited by Abhishek Agrawal and Gavin Britz. Berlin: Springer. [CrossRef]
Kicielinski, Kimberly P., and Christopher S. Ogilvy. 2019. Role of the Neurosurgeon in Acute Ischemic Stroke Treatment From Triage to Intensive Care Unit. *Neurosurgery* 85: S47–S51. [CrossRef] [PubMed]
Lee, Su Yi, Bhasker Amatya, Rodney Judson, Melinda Truesdale, Jan D. Reinhardt, Taslim Uddin, Xiang-Hu Xiong, and Fary Khan. 2019. Clinical practice guidelines for rehabilitation in traumatic brain injury: A critical appraisal. *Brain Injury* 33: 1263–71. [CrossRef] [PubMed]
Sandberg, Mark A., Shane S. Bush, and Thomas Martin. 2009. Beyond diagnosis: Understanding the healthcare challenges of injured veterans through the application of the International Classification of Functioning, Disability and Health (ICF). *The Clinical Neuropsychologist* 23: 1416–32. [CrossRef] [PubMed]
Uddin, Taslim, Moshiur Rahman Khasru, Mohammad Tariqul Islam, Mohammad Ali Emran, Mohammad Shahidur Rahman, Mohammad Abdus Shakoor, Abul Khair Mohammad Salek, Syed Mozaffar Ahmed, Mohammad Moniruzzaman Khan, Mohammad Ahsan Ullah, and et al. 2019a. Rehabilitation in Bangladesh. *Physical Medicine and Rehabilitation Clinics of North America* 30: 795–805. [CrossRef] [PubMed]
Uddin, T., Mohammad T. Islam, Farooq A. Rathore, and Colleen O'Connell. 2019b. Disability and rehabilitation medicine in Bangladesh: Current scenario and future perspectives. *The Journal of the International Society of Physical and Rehabilitation Medicine* 2: 168–77. [CrossRef]
Wilson, Jefferson R., Nicole Forgione, and Michael G. Fehlings. 2013. Emerging therapies for acute traumatic spinal cord injury. *CMAJ* 185: 485–92. [CrossRef]

MDPI AG
Grosspeteranlage 5
4052 Basel
Switzerland
Tel.: +41 61 683 77 34

MDPI Books Editorial Office
E-mail: books@mdpi.com
www.mdpi.com/books

www.ingramcontent.com/pod-product-compliance
Lightning Source LLC
Chambersburg PA
CBHW040852230926
51850CB00012BA/2929
* 9 7 8 3 0 3 6 5 6 9 2 3 9 *